Pocket Guide to
Cultural Health Assessment

Pocket Guide to
Cultural Health Assessment

Third Edition

CAROLYN ERICKSON D'AVANZO, RN, DNSc
Associate Professor
School of Nursing
University of Connecticut
Storrs, Connecticut

ELAINE M. GEISSLER, RN, CTN, PhD
Tolland, Connecticut

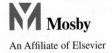
Mosby
An Affiliate of Elsevier

Mosby

An Affiliate of Elsevier

11830 Westline Industrial Drive
St. Louis, Missouri 63146

NOTICE

Nursing is an ever-changing field. Standard safety precautions must
be followed, but as new research and clinical experience broaden
our knowledge, changes in treatment and drug therapy may become
necessary or appropriate. Readers are advised to check the most current
product information provided by the manufacturer of each drug to be
administered to verify the recommended dose, the method and duration
of administration, and contraindications. It is the responsibility of the
treating physician, relying on experience and knowledge of the patient,
to determine dosages and the best treatment for each individual patient.
Neither the publisher nor the author assumes any liability for any injury
and/or damage to persons or property arising from this publication.

Previous edition copyrighted 1998, 1994 by Mosby, Inc.

ISBN-13:   978-0-323-01858-6
ISBN-10:   0-323-01858-0

Vice-President, Nursing Editorial Director: Sally Schrefer
Executive Editor: Michael S. Ledbetter
Senior Developmental Editor: Lisa P. Newton
Project Manager: Joy Moore
Design Manager: Gail Morey Hudson
Cover Design: Carol O'Leary

Printed in China

Last digit is the print number: 9   8   7   6   5   4   3

◆ CONTRIBUTORS

Suher M. Aburawi, PhD, MPhil, MSc, B Pharm
Assistant Professor
College of Pharmacy
Al-Fateh University
Tripoli, Libya

Adebowale A. Adeyemo, MD
Senior Lecturer
College of Medicine
University of Ibadan;
Consultant Pediatrician
University College Hospital
Ibadan, Nigeria

Salim M. Adib, MD, DrPH
Assistant Professor of Community
    Medicine
Health Sciences Center
Kuwait University
Jabriyah, Kuwait

Tjandra Yoga Aditama, SpP(C), MHA, DTM&H
President
Indonesian Association of
    Pulmonologists;
Persahabatan Hospital
Jakarta, Indonesia

Fernando Alarçon, MD
Chief
Department of Neurology
Eugenio Espejo Hospital;
Professor of Neurology
Central University of Ecuador
Quito, Ecuador

Fawwaz Shakir Mahmoud Al-Joudi, BVMS, MSc, PhD
Associate Professor
Department of Chemical
    Pathology
School of Medical Sciences
Universiti Sains Malaysia
Malaysia

Lynn L. Amowitz MD, MSPH, MSc
Instructor in Medicine
Brigham and Women's Hospital,
    Harvard Medical School;
Fireman and Health and Human
    Rights Fellow
Physicians for Human Rights
Boston, Massachusetts

Mary Arevian, MPH, RN
Assistant Professor
School of Nursing
Faculty of Medicine
American University of Beirut
Beirut, Lebanon

Haider Al Attia, MBChB, DTCD, FRCPI, FRCP (G)
Consultant Physician in Internal
    Medicine
Mafraq Hospital
Abu Dhabi, United Arab Emirates

Edoh Azankpé, M Mgt
Primary School Teacher
Ministry of National Education
Lomé, Togo

Jorge Azofeifa, B Biol, MSc, DrScHum
Profesor Asociado
Escuela de Biologia
Instituto de Investigaciones en
    Salud (INISA)
Universidad de Costa Rica
San José, Costa Rica

Virginia C.F. Ballance, BA (Hons), MA, MLS
Nursing and Health Sciences
    Librarian
Hilda Bowen Library
College of the Bahamas
Freeport, Bahamas

Gunay Balta, PhD
Faculty of Medicine
Hacettepe University
Institute of Child Health &
    Pediatric Hematology
Ankara, Turkey

Chiwoza R. Bandawe, PhD, MA
Senior Lecturer in Social
    Psychology;
Head of Department of Community
    Health
College of Medicine
University of Malawi
Blantyre, Malawi

Slavka Barlakova, MSc
Parasitological Institute of the
    Slovak Academy of Sciences
Slovak Republic

Deborah E. Bender, PhD, MPH
Professor
Department of Health Policy and
    Administration
School of Public Health;
Fellow
Carolina Population Center at The
    University of North Carolina
Chapel Hill, North Carolina

Griffin Benjamin, MD, MPH, DM
Consultant, Mental Health
Ministry of Health
Roseau, Dominica;
Psychiatrist and Public Health
    Specialist
Family Medical Clinic
Pottersville, Dominica

Liris Benjamin, MB, BS, PhD
Physician
Family Medical Clinic
Pottersville, Dominica

Henrietta Bernal, RN, PhD
Professor
University of Connecticut School
    of Nursing
Storrs, Connecticut

Dawn Bichel, BSc
Technical Consultant
Pan American Health
    Organization,
Regional Office of the World
    Health Organization
Washington, DC

Alexandre R. Bisdorff, MD
Neurologist
Hôpital de la Ville
Esch-sur-Alzette, Luxembourg

Marija Bohinc, RN, BCS, MA
Senior Lecturer
University of Ljubljana
University College for Health
    Studies
Ljubljana, Slovenia

Snezana Bosnjak, MD, PhD
Senior Scientific Associate
Institute for Oncology and
    Radiology of Serbia
Department Clinical
    Pharmacology/Oncologic
    Intensive Care Unit
Belgrade, Yugoslavia

Richard G. Bribiescas, PhD
Assistant Professor
Department of Anthropology;
Director
Reproductive Ecology
    Laboratory
Department of Anthropology
Yale University
New Haven, Connecticut

**Major Franklin H.G. Bridgewater,
    MB, BS, FRACS, FRCS (Eng)**
3rd Health Support Battalion
Royal Australian Army Medical
    Corps
Australia

Boris Brkljačić, MD, PhD
University Hospital Dubrava
Zagreb, Croatia

Bonnie J. Brownlee, PhD
Associate Dean for Undergraduate
    Studies;
Associate Professor
School of Journalism
Indiana University
Bloomington, Indiana

Catherine Bungener, PhD
Professor of Psychology
University of Burgundy
Dijon, France

**Gemma Burford, MBiochem,
    MSc**
Project Officer
Global Initiative for Traditional
    Systems (GIFTS) of Health
Green College, University of
    Oxford
Oxford, United Kingdom;
Co-Director, Aang Serian
Monduli, Tanzania

Michel Carael, MD
Professor
Faculty of Social Economical and
    Political Sciences
Free University of Brussels
Brussels, Belgium

**Angel Arturo Escobedo Carbonell,
    MD, MS Epid, MS Soc Comm**
Clinical Parasitologist
Primary Healthcare Clinic
Vedado, Cuba

Hugo Cardenas, PhD
Professor
Faculty of Chemistry and Biology
Universidad de Santiago de Chile
Santiago, Chile

Barbara Carpio, RN, MScN, MScT
Associate Professor
School of Nursing
Faculty of Health Sciences
McMaster University
Hamilton, Ontario, Canada

Sung Ok Chang, PhD, RN
Assistant Professor
College of Nursing
Korea University
Seoul, South Korea

**Santanu Chatterjee, MBBS,
    DTM&H**
Consultant Physician
Travel and Tropical Medicine;
Physician,
Wellesley Medicentre
Calcutta, India

Maria Adriana Felix Coler, MS
Substance Abuse Counselor
Willimantic Center
Willimantic, Connecticut

**Marga Simon Coler, EdD, RN,
    CS, CTN, FAAN**
Professor Emeritus
University of Connecticut
Storrs, Connecticut;
Collaborating Professor
Universidade Federal da Parai'ba
Parai'ba, Brasil

Shirley Cooke
Surgical Technologist
University of Connecticut Health
    Center
Farmington, Connecticut

Rosa Ribeiro Costa, RN
Unidade de Cuidados Intensivos
    Polivalente
Hospital de Santo António dos
    Capuchos
Lisbon, Portugal

**Ould El Joud Dahada, PhD,
    MPH**
Epidemiologist
Ministère de la Santé et des
    Affaires Sociales;
Direction de la Planification
Coopération et Statistiques
Nouakchott, Mauritania

Georges Dahourou, Dr Pharm
Directeur
EXALAB
Burkina Faso

Lorraine Antolin D'Avanzo, BS,
    OTR/L
Occupational Therapist
Orlando, Florida

William D'Hoore, MD, PhD
Professor
Ecole de Santé Publique
Université Catholique de Louvain
Brussels, Belgium

John Dixon, BEc, MEc (ANU),
    PhD (UWS)
Professor
Department of Social Policy and
    Social Work
University of Plymouth
Plymouth, United Kingdom

Tinh Do Hoang, BA
Clayton B. Wire Elementary
    School
Sacramento, California

Josef Dolejs, PhD
National Radiation Protection
    Institute
Prague, Czech Republic

Emma Dube, Dipl Nurs
Nursing Assistant and Counselor
    on HIV/AIDS and STIs
The Salvation Army
Mbabane, Swaziland

Eric Dumonteil, PhD
Laboratorio de Parasitología
Centro de Investigaciones
    Regionales "Dr. Hideyo Noguchi"
Universidad Autónoma de
    Yucatán
Mérida, Yucatán, Mexico

Ahmed M. EL Hassan
Emeritus Professor of Pathology
'nstitute of Endemic Diseases

University of Khartoum
Khartoum, Sudan

Laurie Elit, MD, FRCS(c), MSc
Assistant Professor
McMaster University;
Gynecologic Oncologist
Hamilton Regional Cancer Centre
Hamilton, Ontario, Canada

Bodil Ellefsen, RN, Dr Polit
Associate Professor
Institute for Nursing Science
University of Oslo
Oslo, Norway

Angela Ellis, MA
Doctoral Candidate
University of Wisconsin
Madison, Wisconsin

Maria Ellul, BPpharm (Hons),
    MSc(Aber), RPHN
Health Promotion Department
Malta

Arthur Engler, DNSc, RNC,
    APRN
Assistant Professor
School of Nursing
University of Connecticut
Storrs, Connecticut

Ana Veríssimo Ferreira, MS
Assistant
Escola Superior de Educação de
    Santarém
Santarém, Portugal

Malene Kongsmark Flanding, BA
Masters Candidate
Institute of Anthropology
The University of Copenhagen
Copenhagen, Denmark

Igor Y. Galaychuk, MD, PhD
Surgical Oncologist;
Associate Professor
Ternopil State Medical Academy
Ternopil, Ukraine

Adama Dodji Gbadoé, MD
Infectiology and Onco-Hematology
    Division
Department of Pediatrics
Tokoin University Hospital
Lomé, Togo

Bette Gebrian, RN, MPH, PhD
Director of Public Health
Haitian Health Foundation
Jeremie, Haiti

Lynne S. Giddings, BA (Hons),
    MN, PhD
Associate Professor
School of Nursing and Midwifery
Auckland University of Technology
Auckland, Aotearoa, New Zealand

Eglantina Gjermeni, MSW
Lecturer
Social Work Department
University of Tirana
Tirana, Albania

Nel Glass, RN, Dipl Neurosci
    Nurs, BA, MHPEd, FNC
    (NSW), FRNCA
Associate Professor
School of Nursing and Health
    Care Practices
Southern Cross University
New South Wales, Australia

Marshall Godwin, B Med Sc,
    MSc, MD
Associate Professor;
Director
Centre for Studies in Primary Care
Department of Family Medicine
Queen's University
Kingston, Ontario, Canada

Marino J. González, MD, MSc,
    PhD
Associate Professor of Public
    Policy and Health Policy
Department of Economics and
    Administrative Sciences
Universidad Simón Bolívar
Caracas, Venezuela

Miro Gradisar, PhD
Associate Professor
Faculty of Economics
University of Ljubljana
Ljubljana, Slovenia

Devon Graham, PhD
President/Scientific Director
Project Amazonas, Inc,
Florida, USA/Loreto, Peru;
Adjunct Professor
Florida International University
Miami, Florida

Nomsa Mary Gule, Dipl Nurs
Nursing Assistant and Counselor
    on HIV/AIDS and STIs
The Salvation Army
Mbabane, Swaziland

Gabriel Hakizimana, MSc,
    PhD(c)
Département de Médecine Sociale
    et Préventive
Groupe de recherché
    Interdisciplinaire en Santé
Université de Montréal
Montréal, Quebec, Canada

Elín M Hallgrímsdóttir, MN, BSc,
    ICN, RN
Head of Continuing Education
Research Institute
University of Akureyri
Akureyri, Iceland

Abdul Manaf Hamid, MD,
    MPH&TM
Department of Community
    Medicine
Universiti Sains
Penang, Malaysia

Patricia Jane Harry
Diabetes Projects Trust
Auckland, New Zealand

Edlira Haxhiyemeri, PhD
Chief, Social Work
Department of the Faculty of
    Social Sciences

University of Tirana
Tirana, Albania

Anselm Hennis, MB, BS, MSc, MRCP (UK), PhD
Lecturer
Chronic Disease Research Centre
School of Clinical Medicine and Research
University of the West Indies
Bridgetown, Barbados

Eleanor K. Herrmann, EdD, RN, FAAN
Professor Emerita
University of Connecticut
Storrs, Connecticut

Mary Ruth Horner, PhD
Program Operations Advisor
JHPIEGO
Baltimore, Maryland

Muntaser Eltayeb Ibrahim, MSc, PhD
Department of Molecular Biology
Institute of Endemic Diseases
University of Khartoum
Khartoum, Sudan

Klaus Jaffe, PhD
Professor
Universidad Simón Bolívar;
Researcher
IVIC
Caracas, Venezuela

Theano Kalavana, MSc H Psych
PhD Candidate
University of Cyprus
Nicosia, Cyprus

Sam Kariuki, PhD, MSc, DVM
Senior Research Scientist
Kenya Medical Research Institute
Kenya, Africa

Laima M. Karosas, MSN, APRN
Family Nurse Practitioner
The Connecticut Hospice
Branford, Connecticut

Tafadzwa Steven Kasambira, MD, MPH
Pediatric Resident
Children's Hospital Boston/Boston Medical Center
Boston, Massachusetts

Moses N. Katabarwa, BSc, MPH, MA, PhD
Country Representative
Carter Center
Global 2000
Kampala, Uganda

Vered Kater, RN, BA, MSN, CNS
Henriette Szold Hadassah-Hebrew University
School of Nursing
Jerusalem, Israel

Marja Kaunonen, PhD, RN
Senior Lecturer
Department of Nursing Science
University of Tampere
Tampere, Finland

Munir Ahmed Khan, PhD, MA, BA (Hons), MSc
Research Fellow
Department of Rural Health
University of Melbourne
Melbourne, Australia

Hassina Khelladi, MS
University of Sciences and the Technology of Houari Boumedienne
Algeria

Jörg Klewer, MD, PhD, FRIPH
Public Health
Dresden Medical School
Dresden, Germany

Hester Klopper, RN, BA CUR, M CUR, PhD, MBA
Professor and Head
Department of Nursing Education
University of the Witwatersrand
Republic of South Africa

Gennadij G. Knyazev, PhD, Dr Sci
Principal Research Scientist
State Research Institute of Physiology
Siberian Branch of the Russian Academy of Medical Sciences
Novosibirsk, Russia

Robert Kohn, MD, MPhil
Associate Professor of Psychiatry and Human Behavior
Brown University
Butler Hospital
Providence, Rhode Island

Kenneth Y.Y. Kok, MBChB, FRCS, FRCSEd, FAMS
Acting Head
Department of General Surgery
Ripas Hospital
Bandar Seri Begawan, Brunei Darussalam

K.A.L.A. Kuruppuarachchi, MBBS, MD, MRCPsych (UK)
Senior Lecturer
Department of Psychiatry
Faculty of Medicine
University of Kelaniya
Ragama, Sri Lanka

Andrea Cvitković Kuzmić, MD, PhD
Children's Hospital Zagreb
Zagreb, Croatia

Ulrike Kylberg, BScN, MPH
Lecturer
Halmstad University
Halmstad, Sweden

Eric Ledru, MD, PhD
Département de Médecine Moléculaire
Institut Pasteur
Paris, France

Wai-man Lee, BSc, MA, PhD
Assistant Professor
Department of Nursing and Health Sciences
Hong Kong Polytechnic University
Hong Kong, China

M. Rubí Gamboa Léon, BSc
Laboratorio de Parasitología
Centro de Investigaciones Regionales "Dr. Hideyo Noguchi"
Universidad Autónoma de Yucatán,
Mérida, Yucatán, Mexico

Lori Leonard, ScD
Assistant Professor
Bloomberg School of Public Health
Department of International Health
The Johns Hopkins University
Baltimore, Maryland

Durodami Radcliffe Lisk, MB, BS, FRCP, FWACP
Associate Professor
Department of Medicine
College of Medicine and Allied Health Sciences
University of Sierra Leone
Sierra Leone

Joseph D. Lynch, MD, FACC
Associate Professor of Medicine
Creighton University School of Medicine
Omaha, Nebraska;
Medical Director and Interim Executive Director
Institute for Latin American Concerns (ILAC)
Santiago, Dominican Republic

Teresa L. Lynch, RN, C, MA
Director
Institute for Latin American Concern (ILAC);
Adjunct Professor
School of Nursing
Creighton University
Omaha, Nebraska

Cheryl Cox Macpherson, PhD
Professor
St. George's University
School of Medicine
St. George's, Grenada

Elizabeth N. Mataka, BSW
Executive Director
Family Health Trust
Lusaka, Zambia

Ricardo Matos, MD
Unidade de Cuidados Intensivos
   Polivalente
Hospital de Santo António dos
   Capuchos
Lisbon, Portugal

Stephen McGarvey, PhD, MPH
Director
International Health Institute
Brown University
Providence, Rhode Island

Maggi McLeod, BA, CAE
Executive Director
Canadian Relief Fund for
   Chernobyl Victims in Belarus
Canada

Ismat Fayez Mikky, BSN, MSN,
   PhDc, RN
Doctoral Candidate
University of Connecticut
Storrs, Connecticut;
Lecturer and Instructor
IUG, Gaza
Palestinian National Authority
Palestine

Erin O'Donnell Miller, BA
Graduate Student
University of Wisconsin
Madison, Wisconsin

Amal K. Mitra, MD, MPH, DrPH
Associate Professor
Center for Community Health
University of Southern Mississippi
Hattiesburg, Mississippi

Claudia Montilla, PhD
Associate Professor
School of Arts and Humanities
Universidad de los Andes
Bogotá, Columbia

Tomas Morcinek, MD
Psychiatric Hospital Bohnice
Prague, Czech Republic

Rui Moreno, MD, PhD
Unidade de Cuidados Intensivos
   Polivalente
Hospital de Santo António dos
   Capuchos
Lisbon, Portugal

Slavianka Moyanova, PhD
Associate Professor
Institute of Physiology
Bulgarian Academy of Sciences
Bulgaria

Myint Aye Mu, MB, BS, M Med Sc
Research Scientist
Department of Medical Research
   (Physiology)
Myanmar

Sachiyo Murashima, PhD, RN,
   PHN
Professor
Department of Community Health
   Nursing
University of Tokyo
Tokyo, Japan

Brenda Murphy, BA, MA
Department of Communication
   Studies
University of Malta
Msida, Malta

Abdulrahman Obaid Musaiger,
   BSc, MPH, DrPH
Director
Environmental and Biological
   Programme
Bahrain Center for Studies and
   Research
Manama, Bahrain

Mark Muscat, MD, MTropMed, MSc
Department of Public Health
Msida, Malta

Jean-Claude Mwanza, MD
Senior Lecturer
Department of Ophthalmology
Kinshasa University Hospital
Kinshasa, Congo;
PhD Fellow
Centre for International Health
University of Bergen
Bergen, Norway

Khaled Ahmed Nagaty, PhD, MSc, BSc
Assistant Professor
Faculty of Computers and Information Sciences
Ain-Shams University
Cairo, Egypt

Lisa Natoli, RN, MPH
Critical Care Nurse
Victoria, Australia

Haq Nawaz, MD, MPH
Program Director
Preventive Medicine Residency Program
Griffin Hospital
Derby, Connecticut;
Clinical Instructor in School of Medicine;
Lecturer in School of Epidemiology
Yale University
New Haven, Connecticut

Abraham N. Ndiwane, MSc, RN, EdD
Assistant Professor
School of Nursing
Northeastern University
Boston, Massachusetts

Félix Neto, PhD
Professor Catedrático
Faculdade de Psicologia e de Ciências da Educação
Universidade do Porto
Portugal

Kizito Bishikwabo Nsarhaza, PhD
Technical Officer
Division for Africa
Regional Support Department
United Nations Joint Program on HIV/AIDS
Geneva, Switzerland

Francine Ntoumi, PhD
Research Unit Albert Schweitzer Hospital
Lambaréné, Gabon

Nodira Ochilova
Bachelor Degree Candidate
Karshi State University
Karshi, Uzbekistan

Robert O'Donovan, Jr, BA, MS
Associate Country Director
The Eurasia Foundation—Georgia Office
Tbilisi, Georgia

Geeta Oodit, MA
International Planned Parenthood Federation
London, United Kingdom

Shehzad Parviz, MD
Fellow
Department of Infectious Disease
West Virginia University
Morgantown, West Virginia

Elisabeth Patiraki-Kourbani, RN, BSc, PhD
Assistant Professor
Nursing Faculty
University of Athens
Athens, Greece

Bettina F. Piko, MD, PhD
Senior Lecturer in Behavioral Sciences
University of Szeged
Szeged, Hungary

Nurgün Platin, RN, BS, MS, PhD
Professor of Nursing
Director of School of Health
  Sciences
Koc University
Istanbul, Turkey

Draga Plecas, MD, PhD
Professor
Institute of Environmental Health
  and Nutrition
School of Medicine
University of Belgrade
Belgrade, Yugoslavia

Anja Poulsen, MD
Department of Epidemiology
  Research
Statens Serum Institut
Copenhagen, Denmark

Ndola Prata, MD, MSc
Project Coordinator for the Bay
  Area International Group
Institute of Human Development
  and School of Public Health
University of California
Berkeley, California

Katharine Quanbeck, RN
Medical Missionary
Evangelical Lutheran Church in
  America
Madagascar

Stanley D. Quanbeck, MD, FAAFP
Medical Missionary
Evangelical Lutheran Church in
  America
Madagascar

Yahia Ahmed Raja'a, PhD
Assistant Professor of Community
  Medicine
Sana'a University
Sana'a, Yemen

Katja Rask, MNSc, RN
Doctoral Candidate
Department of Nursing Science
University of Tampere
Tampere, Finland

Mary-Elizabeth Reeve, PhD, MPH
Manager
Global Programs
March of Dimes Birth Defects
  Foundation
White Plains, New York

Helen D. Rodd, BDS (Hons), FDS (Paed), PhD
Department of Child Dental Health
University of Sheffield
Sheffield, United Kingdom

Markus Roselieb, MD, DTM&H
Medical Director
Science Development and
  Management Ltd
Bangkok, Thailand

Lori Rosenstein, BA
Former Peace Corps Volunteer
Gold Canyon, Arizona

Majid Sadeghi, MD
Assistant Professor of Psychiatry
Tehran University of Medical
  Sciences
Tehran, Iran

Mohamed Sakho, MD
Research Project on Hemorrhagic
  Fever in Guinea;
Doctoral Candidate
Marshall University
Huntington, West Virginia

Afif Ben Salah, MD, MSc, PhD
Associate Professor of
  Epidemiology
School of Medicine
Tunis, Tunisia

Hilkka Sand, MNSc, RN
Doctoral Candidate
Department of Nursing Science
University of Tampere
Tampere, Finland

Mary G. Schaal, RN, EdD
Acting Chair
Department of Nursing
Thomas Jefferson University
Philadelphia, Pennsylvania

Euan M. Scrimgeour, MD,
    FRACP, DTM & H
Associate Professor of Infectious
    and Tropical Diseases
College of Medicine
Sultan Qaboos University
Muscat, Sultanate of Oman

Conrad Shamlaye, MBChB, MSc
    (Epid), MSc (Health Econ)
Special Advisor to the Minister of
    Health
Victoria, Mahe, Seychelles

Nigel J. Shanks, MD, PhD, MBA
Chief Medical Officer
Ras Gas Co, Ltd
Qatar

David Simmons, MA, MBBS,
    MRCP, FRACP, MD, FRGS
Professor
University of Melbourne
Victoria, Australia

Kathleen Slobin, PhD
Associate Professor of Sociology
North Dakota State University
Fargo, North Dakota

Helena Slobodskaya, MD, PhD,
    Dr Sci
Leading Research Scientist
State Research Institute of
    Physiology

Siberian Branch of the Russian
    Academy of Medical Sciences
Novosibirsk, Russia

Jason B. Smith, PhD, MPH
Senior Scientist
Health Services Research
Family Health International
Research Triangle Park, North
    Carolina

Soe Soe, MB, BS, M.Med.Sc,
    PhD
Deputy Director
Department of Medical Research
Myanmar

Manana Sopromadze, MS
English Teacher
The School of Tomorrow
Tbilisi, Georgia

Şabine Stordeur, RN, MsN, PhD
École de Santé Publique
Université Catholique de Louvain
Brussels, Belgium

Hamlet Suarez, MD
Director
Laboratory of Audiology and
    Vestibular Pathophysiology
School of Medicine
British Hospital
Montevideo, Uruguay

Jean Claude Tabuteau, MD
Senior Physician
Palm Beach County Department
Palm Beach, Florida

Giorgio Tamburlini MD, PhD
Head
Unit for Health Services Research
    and International Health
Department of Pediatrics
Institute for Child Health
IRCCS Burlo Garofolo
Trieste, Italy

Velibor B. Tasic, MD, PhD
Consultant Pediatric Nephrologist
University Children's Hospital
Skopje, Macedonia

Tesfaldet Tecle, MSc, PhD
Karolinska Institutet
Department of Clinical Virology
Huddinge University Hospital
Stockholm, Sweden

Valentina Teosa, PhD
Associate Professor
International Relations
    Department
Moldova State University;
Scientific Director of Labor
    Institute
Chisinau, Republic of Moldova

Narbada Thapa, PhD, MSc, BSN
Lieutenant Colonel
Shree Birendra Hospital, Chhauni;
Visiting Associate Professor
Maharajgunj IOM
Trivuban University
Kathmandu, Nepal

Helle Ussing Timm, MSc, PhD
Senior Researcher
The University Hospitals Centre
    for Nursing and Care Research
Copenhagen, Denmark

Sheila Tlou, PhD
Professor of Nursing;
Director
HIV/AIDS Coordinating Center
University of Botswana
Gaborone, Botswana

Thomas Tolfvenstam, MD, PhD
Karolinska Institutet
Department of Clinical Virology
Huddinge University Hospital
Stockholm, Sweden

Chhan D. Touch, MSN, RN,
    CS-FNP
Family Nurse Practitioner

Lowell Community Health Center/
    Metta Health Center
Lowell, Massachusetts

Mary P. Van Hook, PhD
Director
School of Social Work
University of Central Florida
Orlando, Florida

Frits van Merode, BSc, MSc,
    BPhil, MPhil, PhD
Professor
Department of Health,
    Organization, Policy and
    Economics
University Maastricht
Maastricht, Netherlands

Charles Savona Ventura, MD,
    DScMed, FRCOG, ACertOG,
    MRCPI
Institute of Health Care
University of Malta
Gnardamagia, Malta

Claude Vergès de López, EdD
Clinical Professor of Ethics;
Assistant Professor of Pneumology
Panama University;
Pediatric Pulmonologist
Hospital of the Child
Panama

Adriana Vilan, Dipl Nurs, BA
Health Risk Analyst
Risk Management Department
Nike EHQ
Hilversum, The Netherlands

Carol Vlassoff, PhD
Representative
Pan American Health Organization/
    World Health Organization
Paramaribo, Suriname

Isileli Fakakovi Vunileva
Diabetes Liaison Officer
Diabetes Projects Trust
Otara, Auckland, New Zealand

Steve R. Weaver, RN, BScN (Hons), MPH
Lecturer
Department of Nursing Education
University of the West Indies
Mona, West Indies

Inga Wegener, Dipl Nurs
Bachelor Degree Candidate
The University for Applied Science
Hamburg, Germany

Henry Wilde, MD, FACP
Professor of Medicine
Chulalongkorn University
Bangkok, Thailand

Frances Kam Yuet Wong RN, PhD
Associate Professor;
Associate Head
Department of Nursing and Health Sciences
Hong Kong Polytechnic University
Hong Kong, China

Irena Wrońska, PhD
Professor
Faculty of Nursing and Health Care Sciences
Medical University
Lublin, Poland

Patricia Laure Yepassis-Zembrou, MD, MPH
Doctoral Candidate
Health Services/International Health Program
University of Washington
Seattle, Washington

Zhao Yue, MS
Associate Professor
Department of Nursing
Tianjin Medical University
Hong Kong, China

Danuta Zarzycka, RN, MN, PhD
Assistant Professor

Medical University
Lublin, Poland

Michael Zimmermann, MD
Senior Scientist
The Laboratory for Human Nutrition
Swiss Federal Institute of Technology
Zürich, Switzerland

CONSULTANTS
Nelly P. Alamo, BSN
Charge Nurse
Certified Medical-Surgical Nursing
Medical Telemetry Unit
Paradise Valley Hospital
National City, California

Abdulbari Bener, PhD, MFPHM, ITMA, FRSS
Professor
Department of Community Medicine
United Arab Emirates University
Abu Dhabi, United Arab Emirates;
Advisor
World Health Organization
Geneva, Switzerland

Noriah Khamid Caron
Nurse Recruiter
Singapore

Kathleen R. Clerie, BSN, RN
Charge Nurse
Post-Partum Center
West Boca Medical Center
Boca Raton, Florida

Erin Conrad, BA, MA
Co-Coordinator
U.S.–El Salvador Sister Cities
El Salvador

Leon Fay, MD
Staff Physician and Faculty
Greater Lawrence Family Health Center
Lawrence, Massachusetts;

Assistant Clinical Professor
Family Medicine and Community
  Health
Tufts University School of Medicine
Boston, Massachusetts

Hartwig Huemer, MD
Associate Professor;
Lecturer
University of Innsbruck Medical
  School
Innsbruck, Austria

Lesikar Ole Ngila
Chairman
Aang Serian Traditional Health
  Care Project
Arusha, Tanzania

Narinee Persaud
Certified Nursing Assistant

Church Homes, Inc.
Hartford, Connecticut

Mohammed Yunus Rafiki
Co-Director
Aang Serian Traditional Health
  Care Project
Arusha, Tanzania

Nana Thrane, MD, PhD
Department of Pediatrics
Herning Central Hospital
Herning, Denmark

**Paul Zakowich, MD, FACP,
  FAMS**
American International Clinic;
Medical Advisor for the U.S.
  Embassy
Singapore

Each day the population of the world grows more diverse. This diversity is evident in the varieties of cultural groups that exist today, their differing worldviews and concepts of reality, their changing sociodemographic composition, their amazing variety of social, economic, political, and religious institutions, and their many concepts of health and illness. This diversity exists both within and between groups. It may lead to intergroup and intragroup conflict as one way of life comes into contact with another, and people with different belief systems fail to understand each other's point of view about daily life, social relations, political and economic organizations, and health-seeking behaviors. Diversity may also result in greater understanding and tolerance of different ways of life and different ways of thinking, feeling, and behaving. It is the latter that we hope will persevere as the world becomes more diverse in all spheres of human life, including health and illness.

Health care providers tend to focus on the aspects of diversity that directly affect health and illness, such as patterns of disease in ethnic/racial groups, and the distribution and determinants of biological, behavioral, and environmental risk factors. They tend to draw conclusions about the overall health of cultural groups by assessing health status indicators such as morbidity and mortality rates across age, gender, socioeconomic, and ethnic/racial groups; life expectancy at birth; and level of literacy. In reality, it is false and misleading to separate the health of population groups from the cultural dimension and the social, political, economic, religious, biological, chemical, and physical environments in which population groups live. Culture, health status, and environment, in all of its dimensions, form an intricate web that can both promote or inhibit the attainment of health and wellness.

Health care providers need to go beyond sensitivity to diversity if they are to effectively assess the health of culturally diverse groups and the individuals that comprise them. They must become competent in the use of culture for resolution of problems that impact the health of individuals, their families, and the groups or communities in which they reside. They also must become proficient in assessing the environmental context, which directly and indirectly affects health status. In this new edition of the *Pocket Guide to Cultural Health Assessment*, Drs. D'Avanzo and Geissler provide a ready resource of cultural, epidemiological, and ecological information. The information provided in this *Pocket Guide* is the first step on the path to culture competence by health care providers. Culture is like a double-edged sword. On one hand, it allows individuals in social groups to live together in relative harmony through shared values, beliefs, and practices. On the other hand, it creates social disharmony through ethnocentrism: the tendency to judge others based on one's own values, beliefs, and practices, which are considered to bᵉ true and just. Plus, the variety of social groups in the world and the diversity of environmental contexts in which they exist lead to great intergroup variation in the values, beliefs, and practices that arise in an attempt to meet the basic needs of existence. Likewise, individuals within the same social group have many different life experiences that contribute to intragroup variation in the degree to which they adhere to the norms commonly attributed to their culture. Members of a society often have different perspectives and interpretations of the same situation because of factors such as age, marital status, family structure, gender, income, education level, religious views, and degree of involvement in the situation.

Such intergroup and intragroup variation makes the task Drs. D'Avanzo and Geissler have undertaken in this *Pocket Guide* a vital necessity and a daunting challenge. The challenge here is that health care providers, as well as persons from all walks of life, need quick access to a variety of information to interact effectively with individuals from different cultural groups. However, it is unlikely that anyone, not even experts in trans-cultural health care, can describe all of the permutations of culture and varieties of human experiences that exist in the world. To accommodate these cultural variations, the authors have compiled basic cultural, epidemiological, environmental, and geographical information about cultural groups throughout the world. This *Pocket Guide* is not intended as the definitive word on any one cultural group or nation; however, it does provide us with a snapshot of the cultural diversity that exists and that we must understand to fulfill our dual roles as citizens and providers of culture-competent health care.

Readers need to heed the caution that information in the *Pocket Guide* must not be used to stereotype individuals or groups. This information can be a basis for exploring the degree to which people we encounter from the groups and nations represented may or may not adhere to the cultural norms commonly attributed to them. Another crucial step is to realize that a group's world view gives rise not only to culture but also health culture—the values, beliefs, and practices they hold about health promotion and illness prevention; the causation, detection, and treatment of illness; the care of ill and well individuals; who to go to for assistance; and the social roles, relationships, and expectations that guide the person-provider encounter. As a result, concepts of health, illness, and care cannot readily be separated from general cultural values, beliefs, and practices.

Another important point for the reader is the realization that health behavior is influenced by the situation at hand. As individuals have different experiences with life and health care and are exposed to other health-culture orientations, what they do and believe to be true today about health and illness may be quite different when we next see them. The fluidity of cultural values, beliefs, and practices should again caution against stereotyping, analyzing behavior out of context, or interpreting situations from solely our point of view or health-culture orientation.

A fifth crucial tenet of culture competence is learning about the diverse cultural groups that surround us is through participant-observation. Although most of us cannot go to each place the authors take us in the *Pocket Guide*, we can use a variation of participant-observation to gain a greater depth and breadth of knowledge about the cultural groups in our own region. We can learn about cultural groups through the media, such as documentaries, novels, newspaper articles, ethnographies, and research studies. We can go to markets and restaurants in ethnic neighborhoods and learn about ethnic foods and the role they play in health and illness. We can attend religious ceremonies at places of worship and learn the role of rituals and religion in health promotion and treatment of illness. Additionally, we can share the joy of life-celebrations such as marriages, births, and graduations, as well as the sorrow of their losses and misfortunes. We can take time to go back and talk with patients and families about their health concerns and beliefs about care. We can explore ethnic neighborhoods and learn about the cultural symbolism embodied in arts and crafts found there. We can learn ethnic games and begin to understand about competitiveness and cooperation. In short, we can be investigative reporters learning and experiencing the who, what, when, where, and why of the human diversity that surrounds us. When we do that, we will be able to understand the factors that affect our patients' health behavior and decision-making. We will also come to learn more about ourselves and how our behavior affects others.

Lydia DeSantis, PhD, RN, FAAN, CTN
Professor
University of Miami School of Nursing
Coral Gables, Florida

The present trend in transcultural theory (and we agree with it) is that individuals within any given culture vary markedly. The earth is populated with a vast mosaic of cultures representing every imaginable variety of learned and environmentally generated beliefs and practices. For each person, his or her own culture is deeply ingrained and comfortable, guiding both the conscious and covert activities and behaviors of daily life, including health and illness. Yet culture is also a dynamic influence, meeting changing needs of groups, as well as individuals within those groups.

In his book *Pandaemonium*, Senator Daniel Patrick Moynihan speculates that in the next 50 years there may be 150 or so new nations on the world map that have been "created for the purpose of giving one or another ethnic group a realm of its own." Reflective of Moynihan's prognostication, twenty-three independent nations have already emerged, with the largest number having evolved from the dissolution of the Soviet Union. They are as follows:

Armenia	Latvia
Azerbaijan	Lithuania
Belarus	Moldova
Bosnia and Herzegovina	Tajikistan
Estonia	Turkmenistan
Georgia	Ukraine
Kazakhstan	Uzbekistan
Kyrgyzstan	

The following nations emerged from the former Yugoslavia and Czechoslovakia:

Croatia
Czech Republic
Macedonia
Serbia and Montenegro (new Yugoslavia)
Slovakia
Slovenia

Two other nations, Eritrea and Palau, have gained independence. Zaire has been renamed "The Democratic Republic of Congo" and must not be confused with its neighbor "The Republic of Congo." Many of these newly independent nations have not yet published professional health literature in the English language that is appropriate to this guide. This is frustrating for readers who desire equality in the categories and the amount of information among countries. This edition's immunization schedules from the World Health Organization (WHO) are more complete; only a handful of nations have not provided these data. AIDS rates for most of the countries of the planet are included in this edition, and in some cases when this was not available contributors accessed in-country data. These figures, however, should be considered only as a trend because statistical data change in sometimes-unanticipated ways.

The theory about the "melting pot" phenomenon in the United States that expects immigrants to become Americanized linguistically and culturally is passé. Even the theory about the "salad bowl" phenomenon, in which different cultures are expected to live together in peaceful coexistence, is being rejected. At this critical juncture in history the move toward cultural homogeneity is strengthening. Many of the "new" countries on the previous page came into existence because of the intense—and for some, deadly—struggle for cultural homogeneity. For many of these nations, little or no information on their health care beliefs and practices exists in the literature to date. This dearth of information will improve over time, and the reader is encouraged to keep abreast of the health care literature for guidance in the delivery of culturally competent health care. One of the greatest weaknesses of a guide such as this is *stereotyping*. The reader is **strongly cautioned against** the false assumption that people from one country or geographic area are clones, holding the same beliefs held by their neighbors. The borders of countries are politically determined and often bear no relationship to cultural values. The differences *within* one culture may be as great as variations between two different cultures. Stewart and Bennett (1991) remind us that the tendency to stereotype can be overcome "… by approaching every cross-cultural situation as a kind of experiment. They should assume that some kind of cultural difference exists but that the nature of the difference is unclear. Using available generalizations about the other culture, they can formulate a hypothesis and then test it for accuracy…. The hypothesis should be tested by acting tentatively as if it were accurate and by watching carefully to see what happens …."

Galanti (1997) makes an effective distinction between stereotyping and generalizing with the story of Rosa, a Mexican woman: "[If] I say to myself, Rosa is Mexican, so she must have a large family, I am stereotyping her. Stereotyping closes the mind to potential differences. But if I think Mexicans often have large families and wonder whether Rosa does, I am generalizing and using information I have learned about Mexican culture as a starting point to gain further understanding. By not stereotyping Rosa, I remain receptive to further questioning and assessment of her as a unique individual."

We proceeded with this project because of the reality of the work-a-day world. When you have a patient from an unfamiliar culture you can rarely say, "Excuse me. I'll be back in a few hours (or a few days) after I learn about your culture." The information you need to access is scattered throughout a multitude of journals and books, and most information is not readily accessible.

This guide places at your fingertips some very basic information about peoples of the countries of our world, *when and where you need it*. People from various countries and health care professionals who have worked extensively abroad provide important in-depth knowledge of respective cultures. Although some intra-ethnic differences in cultures are noted, usually only the dominant culture, or aspects common to many groups, are included. That limitation was difficult to make because most countries consist of numerous ethnic and/or racial groups. To include them all would result in a multivolume encyclopedia that is beyond the scope of this guide. The United States and Canada are made up of a myriad of cultural groups from all over the world and therefore were not included in this guide.

The purpose of this edition is to help focus your attention on the potential variations a culturally diverse client may, **or may not**, exhibit. It is based on generalizations that must not be mentally converted into stereotypes by the user. Pull out this guide when you are faced with someone from a culture that is unfamiliar to you. Use this guide to start quickly and efficiently increasing your awareness and understanding of *potential* similarities and differences—the generalizations. Unless you are conscious of the cultural patterns of behavior a patient might exhibit, you will not think to address them in your assessment. To be culturally competent with a few cultures that you routinely encounter in your practice is a *must*. To be culturally competent with the many cultures with which you may on occasion be faced is unrealistic. To not use a guide such as this for fear of stereotyping only impedes movement toward delivery of culturally relevant health care. We are willing to risk criticism for stereotyping; but in return, we ask you to thoughtfully build on the information inside these pages with an individualized cultural assessment. Several good assessment guides are available, such as the following:

Andrews MM, Boyle JS: Andrews/Boyle transcultural nursing assessment guide. In Andrews MM, Boyle JS: *Transcultural concepts in nursing care,* ed 2, Philadelphia, 1995, Lippincott.

Giger and Davidhizar's transcultural assessment model. In Giger JN, Davidhizar RE: *Transcultural nursing: assessment and intervention,* ed 2, St. Louis, 1995, Mosby.

Leininger MM: Leininger's acculturation health care assessment tool for cultural patterns in traditional and non-traditional lifeways, *J Transcultural Nurs* 2(2):40, 1991.

Orque MS, Block B, Monrroy KSA: Block's ethnic-cultural assessment guide. In *Ethnic nursing care: a multicultural approach,* St. Louis, 1983, CV Mosby.

Spector RE: *Guide to heritage assessment and health traditions,* Stamford, Conn, 1996, Appleton & Lange.

Tripp-Reimer T: Cultural assessment. In Bellack JP, Bamford PA: *Nursing assessment: a multidimensional approach,* Monterey, 1984, Wadsworth.

CITED REFERENCES

Galanti GA: *Caring for patients from different cultures,* ed 2, Philadelphia, 1997, University of Pennsylvania Press.

Moynihan DP: *Pandaemonium: ethnicity in international politics,* Oxford, England, 1993, Oxford University Press.

Stewart EC, Bennett MJ: *American cultural patterns: a cross-cultural perspective,* Yarmouth, Me, 1991, Intercultural Press.

SPECIAL RECOGNITION
The following sources were especially helpful in the preparation of this manuscript and deserve special recognition for their contributions:

Brunner B editor in chief: Time Almanac 2001, Boston, 2000, Information Please. This source is cited for demographic and geographic data.

Wright JW editor: 2001 The New York Times Almanac, New York 2000, Penguin Reference Books. This source is cited for demographic and geographic data.

Publications of the STD/AIDS Program of the Pan American Health Organization and World Health Organization.

World Health Organization for immunization schedules.

◆ ACKNOWLEDGMENTS

We deeply appreciate the many contributors worldwide who updated and expanded the cultural content of this edition. Their in-depth knowledge of the countries they represent has been invaluable. We also warmly thank the editors and individuals at Mosby/Elsevier who assisted and guided this edition, with special thanks to Michael Ledbetter, Lisa Newton, Lisa Neumann, and Mary Parker.

Carolyn Erickson D'Avanzo
Elaine M. Geissler

◆ CONTENTS

Pocket Guide to
Cultural Health Assessment

◆ AFGHANISTAN (ISLAMIC EMIRATE OF)

MAP PAGE (866)

Lynn L. Amowitz

Location: Afghanistan is a landlocked country surrounded by mostly rugged mountains. Covering approximately 655,200 km² (252,907 square miles), Afghanistan (which is roughly the size of Texas) is split east to west by the Hindu Kush mountain range (the foothills of the Himalaya mountains) and wedged between Turkmenistan to the northwest, Tajikistan to the north, China to the northeast, Pakistan to the east and south, and Iran to the west. With the exception of the southwest, which is primarily desert, most of the country is covered by high, snowcapped mountains and until the recent drought, was characterized by deep valleys and lush agricultural land. Although Afghanistan has never had a census, it is estimated that it has approximately 25 million people, including refugees.

Major Languages	Ethnic Groups	Major Religions (Islam 99%)
Dari (Afghan Persian)	Patten 38%	Sunni Muslim 80%
Pashto	Tajik 25%	Shi'a Muslim 20%
Hazara	Other (Chahar Aimaks,	Other (Hindus, Sikhs,
Turkik (Uzbek and	Turkmen, Baloch,	and Jews) 0.1
Turkmen)	Kuchi nomads, and	
Uzbek	others) 37%	
Other (Balochi		
and Pashai)		

Health Care Beliefs: Acute sick care; traditional. Acute sick care is the only option because of the destruction of the health care system. In fact, many areas have no facilities for either chronic or acute care. Illness is sometimes believed to be punishment for sins. Expression of illness, especially depressive symptoms, is regarded as a spiritual weakness; otherwise, health is controlled by "God's will." The appearance of good health in males is important, therefore they seek care less than women and sometimes delay care to preserve their dignity. Health is rarely discussed outside of the family and is considered private.

Predominant Sick Care Practices: Magical-religious. People wear charms and amulets to ward off evil spirits. They believe that evil spirits manifest themselves in numerous central nervous system diseases. A medicine man known as a *hakim* uses various methods for helping those with either physical or psychological illnesses. Herbal medications, holy water, or visits to holy sites and shrines may be used to help those with ailments.

Ethnic/Race Specific or Endemic Diseases: About 5% of people in rural areas have access to safe drinking water; in urban areas, 39% have access. Approximately 42% of all deaths are a result of diarrheal diseases; about

1

85,000 children younger than 5 years of age die annually from diarrheal diseases. Measles, a vaccine-preventable disease, infects 35,000 children each year. Among women of reproductive age, tuberculosis is rampant. Tuberculosis causes 15,000 deaths per year, and women account for 12,000 to 13,000 of these deaths. Other prevalent diseases include chloroquine-resistant malaria (which is rare in Kabul—Afghanistan's capital—and is limited to a belt in the east), cholera, and cutaneous leishmaniasis. Because of land mine injuries, 3% to 4% of the population has physical disabilities. Extreme rates of depression, suicide attempts, and suicidal ideation were rampant among women during the Taliban regime. There are no reported estimated prevalence rates (World Health Organization [WHO]) for HIV/AIDS.

Health Team Relationships: The last 23 years of conflict in Afghanistan have left the health care system in shambles. Of its 31 provinces, 23 have no regional hospital, and 50% of the regional hospitals serve the population of Kabul (25% of Afghanistan's total population). Of the 31 provinces, 10 have 1 or no regional, provincial, or district hospital. The provinces of Parwan and Kapisa have no hospitals at all. Although these provinces are not far from Kabul, travel into Kabul for most people requires walking on secondary roads that are difficult to follow and contain land mines. There are approximately 4 hospital beds per 10,000 people, and 6 million people either have insufficient health care services or have no services of any kind. Although hospitals, health posts, and clinics are listed as health care "structures," they are not all staffed, supplied, or used as health care facilities. Many of the structures serve as interim housing for internally displaced (refugees within their own country) families, function as stables, or are in ruins. The vast majority of hospitals lack windows, doors, heat, sanitary conditions, water, or electricity. Hospitals commonly have rodents, other small animals, and insects. Because of a lack of medical school graduates, an exodus of qualified health care providers to other countries, and the lack of a government certification system, many doctors, nurses, and midlevel health care workers are calling themselves "qualified" although they have no official training. During the Taliban regime there were no female health care provider graduates. Subsequently, female health care providers are few, leaving many women without care because they prefer that their providers be women. Corruption has become a method of survival in the medical system. Private doctors own most pharmacies, and private fees are unaffordable for most.

Families' Role in Hospital Care: The severe shortage of health care providers (1.8 doctors per 10,000 people) means that family members must provide food, medications, comfort, and care to patients admitted to any hospital.

Dominance Patterns: In 1996 the Afghan government was displaced by members of the fundamentalist Islamic Taliban movement, which placed severe restrictions on women. In November 2001, the Taliban was removed from power and an interim government put in place. Although women's rights were more severely restricted by the Taliban, during the past 23 years the freedoms to which women were entitled had sharply declined. The literacy rate for females is only 16%; however, this is long-standing issue with a multifactorial origin. In traditional Afghan society, schools are coeducational during the younger years, separate in the high school years, and again coeducational in institutes of higher learning. Because of a severe lack of female teachers, ongoing war, the need for women and girls to help support families, traditional norms and cultural beliefs, many girls and women during the last 20 or more years have not had the opportunity to pursue an education. During the 1970s and 1980s, however, women outnumbered men as students at Kabul University. Eighty-five percent of the country is sustained by agriculture and in the rural areas is farmed by women as well as men; this was even the case during the Taliban. Carpet weaving, needle arts, and tailoring are common skills among Afghan women. Before the Taliban regime 40% of doctors, 70% of teachers, and 50% of civil servants were women. Family interdependence with strict obedience to elders, particularly to the father, is the norm. Dating is prohibited, arranged marriages by family members are the norm, and dowries are still a common part of marriage proposals. Marriages to first cousins are extremely common, as are the genetic consequences of this family pairing. Households headed by widows now make up 20% to 22% of the homes in Afghanistan.

Eye Contact Practices: Direct eye contact is considered rude and immodest between those of the opposite sex.

Touch Practices: Physical affection among family members is common, especially between parents and children. Affection among couples or adults is unlikely to be observed except by family members. Children are consoled by a rhythmic, coarse, patting on the back or an extremity. Public displays of affection occur among same-sex friends but never among couples. Men greet each other with a fast hug in which both chests meet, somewhat off center, or they extend a hand (or both hands if they know each other well), which is held throughout the greeting. This hand gesture is not a handshake; the extended open hand is held between the other person's hands. It is also not uncommon to see friends of the same sex (men or women) holding hands as they walk. When a man greets a woman, he places one or both open hands (with the fingers together) gently on his heart as sign of respect, accompanied by a subtle nod or lowering of the eyes.

Perceptions of Time: Years of war have distorted time perceptions. The people of Afghanistan long for the future, but the immediacy of present needs usually eclipse futuristic thoughts or goal planning. Time is expressed as days or months before or after Ramadan, the holy month of fasting. Questions relating to dates should be asked in relation to the last

Ramadan. Most people express their ages relative to the number of Ramadans that have passed in their lives.

Pain Reactions: Expressions of pain are considered signs of weakness, therefore many are stoic and seem to have an enormous tolerance to pain. Children have not developed this ability and are uninhibited when crying because of pain. Women may describe depression (as do women in many other societies) as an all-over body pain. The desire for dignity inhibits many men from mentioning pain.

Birth Rites: Afghanistan has one of the highest infant mortality rates (165 per 1000 live births) and child mortality rates (257 per 1000) in the world; tetanus neonatorum is a major cause of infant deaths. One in four children dies before the fifth birthday (which translates to 270,000 deaths annually). Women have no or very little control over reproduction and are still blamed by their families if they do not give birth to a boy. Divorce is very uncommon and not done as the women and their children will suffer if they are divorced. Because having up to four wives is permitted, a man will marry another wife if one is deemed infertile. Maternal mortality is the highest in the world, with 1700 women dying per 100,000 live births; compared to 8 women per 100,000 in the United States. In other words, approximately 45 women each day—one woman every 30 minutes— die from pregnancy-related problems. Marriages at young ages and stunted growth caused by chronic malnutrition have led to smaller pelvic outlets and resulted in high rates of obstructed births, which have dire consequences for mothers and infants. Hemorrhages are believed to be the most common cause of death. Because no health care providers are available to attend births (with 0.2 traditional birth attendants per 1000 births and only 0.5 midwives per 1000 births), women who begin to bleed die. Even minor bleeding is deadly because the women are usually anemic as a result of folate and iron insufficiencies, malnutrition, and tuberculosis.

Death Rites: Relatives and friends come to the home of the family to express sympathy and contribute money if it is needed. The body remains in the home with a *mullah* (a religious authority) or close relatives who read from the Koran throughout the night. The body is washed by relatives or specialists, wrapped in new, white clothing, and placed in a simple wood coffin. The body must be buried within 24 hours (and is never cremated). Two days after the burial, a ceremony is held in the mosque or house of the deceased and is followed by a meal. Headstones are usually pieces of slate. The direction of the surface or edge on the grave identifies the sex of the person in the grave.

Food Practices and Intolerances: Because food is not inspected for contaminants, water and milk products must be boiled for safety. Using the hands to eat is the norm. The diet consists primarily of nan (flat bread), rice, and meat (usually lamb). Very few vegetables and fruits are available

Infant Feeding Practices: Exact breast-feeding practices are largely unknown, but it is thought that only 25% of women exclusively breast-feed their infants from birth to 3 months. There is some evidence that women may be feeding their infants tea and tea-soaked nan (flat bread) as early as 3 months, which may be contributing to the high rates of death and malnutrition so prevalent among Afghan children. In regions where they are available, tea and zoof (fried linseeds and cooking oil) provide energy and fat-soluble vitamins. Children in the central Hazarajat area of Afghanistan have the highest rates of malnutrition and during the past few years have begun eating grasses and roots to avoid starvation. Ongoing war, land mines, and lack of access to mountainous areas have presented challenges for the United Nations World Food Program attempting to deliver sustainable food products to the country. Diarrheal diseases (which account for 42% of all deaths), primarily from unsafe drinking water, are the major cause of death among children. Approximately 85,000 children per year die from treatable or preventable diarrheal diseases. Chronic malnutrition affects as many as 50% of children younger than 5 years. Two thirds of the children show signs of protein-energy malnutrition; 10% have acute malnutrition. More than half of all children in Afghanistan have growth stunting from chronic malnutrition.

Child Rearing Practices: Children are an economic asset; they work to supplement the household income. Child labor (such as in carpet weaving and agricultural work) is common in rural areas, and approximately 50,000 children are working on the streets of Kabul. During the Taliban regime, schools were either underground or above ground, depending on which Taliban group was in power in that particular area of the country. Only 3% of girls and 39% of boys had been enrolled in school, but those figures are changing as Afghanistan rebuilds. Although access is still an issue for some, in the summer of 2002 it was estimated that about 600,000 girls had been enrolled in school. Among boys, physical punishment as a form of discipline is customary. Boys are valued more than girls, although there are no reported consequences for having girls (such as abandonment or drowning of female infants). For the most part, children are the center of the family and are attended to by both parents, although parents assume different roles.

National Childhood Immunizations: BCG at birth; OPV at 6, 10, and 14 weeks; DPT at 6, 10, and 14 weeks; and measles at 9 months. However, fewer than 20% of children are completely immunized against childhood illnesses. It is estimated that 40% of all childhood deaths are from measles, a vaccine-preventable disease. Rates for fully immunized 1-year-old children are as follows: BCG, 48%; DPT, 35%; polio, 35%; measles, 40%; and tetanus, 19%.

Other Characteristics: The term "Afghan" refers to a person in Afghanistan; "Afghani" is the monetary unit. Afghans have been designated by the

United Nations High Commission on Refugees as the largest group of refugees in the world for the seventeenth year in a row. As of September 2001, more than 3.7 million refugees lived in neighboring countries, with the vast majority living in Pakistan (2 million) and Iran (1.5 million). Women and children comprise 75% of those who are refugees outside of the country or displaced within the country. One of the most heavily mined countries in the world, Afghanistan is scattered with about 8 million land mines or unexploded artillery. Approximately 100 land mine injuries occur each week, with children younger than 18 years old accounting for half of these injuries. Since September 2001, Afghanistan has been the world's largest opium producer.

BIBLIOGRAPHY

Amowitz LL et al: *Women's health and human rights in Afghanistan: a population-based assessment*, Boston, 2001, Physicians for Human Rights.

Amowitz LL, Iacopino V: Women's health and human rights needs, *Lancet Persp* 356(suppl 65), December 2000.

Carlisle D: Lifting the veil, *Nurs Times* 91(37):22, 1995.

Lipson JG, Omidian PA: Afghan refugee issues in the U.S. social environment, *West J Nurs Res* 19(1):110, 1997.

Lipson JG, Omidian PA, Paul SM: Afghan health education project, *Public Health Nurs* 12(3):143, 1995.

Rasekh Z et al: Women's health and human rights in Afghanistan, *JAMA* 280(5):449, 1998.

Save the Children (January 11, 2002): *Afghanistan: children in crisis*. Retrieved February 9, 2002, from http://www.reliefweb.org

United Nations Children's Fund: *UNICEF/CIET Multiple indicator cluster survey*, 1997, New York.

United Nations Children's Fund (February 2002): *Information statistics by country: Afghanistan*. Retrieved February 14, 2002, from http://www.unicef.org/statis/Country_1.html

United Nations High Commission for Refugees (February 13, 2002): *Afghanistan humanitarian update No. 52*. Retrieved February 14, 2002, from http://www.reliefweb.int/w/rwb.nsf

World Health Organization (January 21, 2002): *Health in Afghanistan situation analysis*. Retrieved February 9, 2002, from http://www.reliefweb.org

World Health Organization-Afghanistan: *Country health profile*, unpublished report, December 2001.

◆ ALBANIA (THE REPUBLIC OF)

MAP PAGE (860)

Eglantina Gjermeni, Edlira Haxhiymeri, and Mary P. Van Hook

Location: Albania is located in the southwestern part of the Balkan Peninsula. It has a total land area of 28,748 km² (11,096 square miles), 34.8% of which is forests, 15% is pastures, 24.3% is arable land, and 4% is lakes. Its land area is mainly mountainous, with an average altitude of

714 m above sea level, which is double that of other areas of Europe. Albania borders the former Republic of Yugoslavia to the north, Greece to the south and southeast, and the Adriatic and Ionian Seas to the west.

Major Languages	**Ethnic Groups**	**Major Religions**
Albanian (official dialect: Tosk)	Albanian 95% Greek 3% Vlach, Gypsy, Serb, Bulgarian 2%	Muslim 70% Albanian Orthodox 20% Roman Catholic 10%

The total population of Albania is 3,354,300; 51% are women. With an average age of 28.6 years, Albania has a younger population than the rest of Europe, and the majority (64%) are younger than 34 years. The Albanian population was growing at about 1% a year until 1999; since that time, population growth has been declining. The majority of people are employed in agriculture (53.2% of men and 66.1% of women). Others work for the public sector (20.4% of men and 21.7% of women) or the nonagricultural private sector (26.4% of men and 12.2% of women). Albanian is an Indo-European language. Religion does not have a strong influence on the life of the residents because religious practices were not allowed during the Communist regime from 1967 to 1990. Since 1990 the country has undergone significant social and political changes and is currently going through a delicate transition toward a market economy and democratic governance.

Health Care Beliefs: Acute sick care; magical-religious. Although medical treatment dominates in the country, people believe some illnesses are caused by the supernatural power of God, therefore they pray that God's power will heal them. Some people pretend to possess special powers that can influence the course of diseases and cure people. Although it is illegal, these individuals purport that they can cure a malady caused by the "evil eye," an illness caused when one person looks at another with malice. Younger people are beginning to undergo regular examinations for prevention purposes. Health education has improved significantly in the last century. During the Communist regime, people were given lectures in health care and medical treatment, and courses were organized to teach older people and women about symptoms of usual diseases and ways of curing them. These efforts have improved the health care knowledge of the general population, so people no longer try to diagnose themselves and instead seek the advice of the doctor. Generally, Albanians do not go to a doctor before they have a problem to prevent problems from developing.

Predominant Sick Care Practices: Biomedical; traditional. Medical care is preferred for the treatment of disease, even in rural and remote areas of the country. Generally Albanians respect the advice of doctors, who are highly respected and trusted by the people. Although medical technology is not updated, people can go hospitals and centers to be examined for health problems, especially in the major cities. Albanians have no cultural preference for injections or oral treatment. Doctors are seen for crisis care only. Herbalists also practice in the country; the majority have inherited their knowledge for preparing different medicines to cure certain diseases. Some herbalists practice in arrangements with medical institutions. Herbal treatment is used for diarrhea, gastrointestinal complaints, sore throats, urinary disorders, and kidney problems. Teas of oregano, parsley, or rosemary are the most frequently used herbal treatment. Abortion used to be taboo, but as a result of a law legalizing abortion, it is now carried out in safe hospital-like conditions under the supervision of a doctor. (The 1999 abortion rate was 344 per 1000 births.) Abortions also take place in the private clinics of well-known doctors and are accompanied by family planning information. Two types of women receive service at these clinics: rich women and unmarried women.

Ethnic/Race Specific or Endemic Diseases: The major causes of death among adult Albanians are of cardiovascular origin, followed by cancer, accidents and violence, and respiratory system diseases. Acute respiratory tract infections, particularly pneumonia, are a leading cause of death in children. The majority of ill children (about 83%) are taken to an appropriate health care provider. In 1999 the life expectancy was 76.4 years for women and 71.7 years for men. The World Health Organization's (WHO) estimated prevalence rate for HIV/AIDS in adults ages 15 to 49 is 0.01%. WHO has no estimates for children from birth to 15 years. HIV/AIDS is not currently a major health problem in Albania. Based on several government reports, between 1993 and 1998 there were 38 cases of HIV infection and four cases of AIDS. In addition, 14 cases of syphilis and 22 cases of gonorrhea were documented. Based on research from the Institute of Public Health, the majority of people who tested positive for HIV were between 20 and 30 years of age. Men (31) were more likely than women (7) to report being infected with HIV. Many Albanian women do not have accurate information about the transmission of the virus or where to seek testing. For example, a recent survey found that only 25% of women ages 15 to 49 know all three of the major ways to prevent HIV transmission. Another 55% believe that having one uninfected sex partner can prevent HIV transmission. Less than 2% of women correctly stated that AIDS could not be transmitted by supernatural means, and 12.6% stated that AIDS could not be spread by mosquito bites. Of all Albanian women of reproductive age, 23% know where to go to get tested for HIV infection, but only 0.7% has been tested. Younger people tend to talk freely about homosexuality and disease preventive sexual practices. Older people consider sex and homosexuality to be private issues and generally do not discuss them openly. Albania has a young population, with more than 64% of its people younger than 34 years.

Health Team Relationships: The doctor is the primary authority in hospital settings, and nurses are subordinate. Nurses are afforded more respect if they are the only health care professionals in a particular setting. Doctors and nurses practice primarily in hospitals, all of which are public. Some new and well-equipped private clinics are also being set up in Albania, and the best doctors practice in them after finishing their work in the public hospitals. Doctors are licensed for practice and guided by a professional code with strict guidelines for professional and patient relationships. Recently some attempts have been made to include social workers and psychologists on hospital medical teams.

Families' Role in Hospital Care: Families rally around people who are sick and continue to play an important role in their care. Family members are expected to stay with the patients while they are in the hospital, providing food and basic hygiene, although the nurses and cleaning staff members offer some service. It is expected that friends will visit people who are ill. The pensions of older adults are very important sources of support for many multigenerational migrant families. Older adults without families can be especially vulnerable because of lack of status and support, although the number of abandoned older adults is relatively small as compared with other Eastern European countries.

Dominance Patterns: Until recently, a patriarchal type of family was dominant, with two to three generations living together under the same roof and males having a higher status. When Albania opened up to the international community in 1990, migration from rural to urban areas contributed to the breakdown of this patriarchal family structure. The principle of gender equality is new in Albanian society and has not yet been embraced by a significant percentage of the population. Women do not play an important role in the decision-making process, although many women are well educated and professionally trained. Women's nongovernmental organizations play an important role in increasing public awareness about the role of women in political and social life. As a result of this long-term pattern of oppression, women have been identified as particularly vulnerable to abuse because of the tensions associated with this transition period. Some young women have been forced into prostitution, whereas other women experience physical violence from family members. Women's nongovernmental organizations are active in helping such women.

Eye Contact Practices: It is customary to hold eye contact with other people while talking. Women (especially women in rural areas) do not look at their husbands or other males and are expected to look down. In conversation with friends, not looking into their eyes signifies a lack of respect or sincerity.

Touch Practices: Touch is common, especially among individuals of the same sex. It is quite normal for Albanian men to shake hands, hug, and kiss when greeting each other. The same is true for women, who may repeat the kisses on the cheeks several times, depending on how much they have missed the person. Members of the opposite sex are more restrained unless they have a very close relationship, such as brother and sister, mother and son, or husband and wife or other close relatives. Albanians hug and kiss children, even when they are babies, and only in rare cases will young mothers ask people not to kiss their babies. When children are sick, touching their foreheads, and holding and hugging them are ways they are comforted. Albanians believe their patterns of touch are based on their Mediterranean origins, and they are generally warm and expressive. Although welcomed among fellow countrymen, the physical closeness that is usual for Albanians is not always welcomed by people from other cultures who are more accustomed to boundaries and privacy.

Perceptions of Time: Punctuality has not traditionally been a very important value. Regardless, views have been changing, especially in the last 10 years, with punctuality becoming more important and appreciated. Albanians hope for a better future, although it is hard for them to ignore the difficulties of the present, or to forget the sacrifices of the past. They are a people who live mainly between the past and the present as they try to establish a future-oriented view.

Pain Reaction Patterns: Albanians typically have a high tolerance for pain and discomfort. Women are not expected to cry out in pain during labor. Loud verbal expressions in response to pain are considered shameful.

Birth Rites: Pregnancy is considered as a very delicate and sacred period, and the family takes great care to offer her the best quality and quantity of food they can. Male babies are often preferred over females. Sexual intercourse continues during pregnancy; it is enjoyed as a "safe period" when no pregnancy precautions need to be taken. Tetanus toxoid injections are given during pregnancy to protect infants from neonatal tetanus, a major cause of infant death caused primarily by unsanitary conditions during childbirth. Professionals typically care for women during and following their delivery, and about 99% of deliveries occur under the supervision of skilled personnel. Such care is more common in urban areas (100%) than rural areas (98.6%). Doctors assist in nearly 57% of births, nurses in about 37%, and professionally trained midwives in 10%. Women are frequently treated for infections that develop because of imperfect sanitation conditions at maternity hospitals. Women usually go home after the first or the second day after delivery, unless they have problems requiring special treatment. At home, new mothers have an older woman—often their mothers or mothers-in-law, who care for them during the first 2 weeks after birth. The first 40 days after birth are considered dangerous for the newborn baby and mother, and they are protected from the "evil eye" by not being allowed to go out or have contact with people considered by the family to be unfriendly. Mothers are warned not to become emotionally upset or to see visitors outside the door of the house because of the belief that her breast milk will stop. Mothers are encouraged to breast-feed and eat food that increases milk production. Babies must be named and legally registered within the first

40 days, but if an infant dies within 40 days after birth, no ceremony accompanies the burial. Visitors, friends, and family are expected to come and visit the family of the newborn and bring gifts, clothes, or money to help the family, but the mother's family of origin customarily buys most of the clothes and the crib. Parents usually decide on the name of the baby, but in rural areas where traditional family structures predominate, grandparents may name it using their names or others. Mothers who work during their pregnancy are allowed a 1-year leave, after which they may return to work. Many women prefer not to stay at home for a full year, however, especially those who work in the private sector, because they do not want to lose their full salary. The infant mortality rate is 28 deaths per 1000 live births; the rate for children younger than 5 years is 33 per 1000.

Death Rites: Death is believed to be a result of natural and supernatural causes. Relatives and friends expend considerable effort to be present when death nears, and the family begins expressing their grief through crying and wailing at the moment the person dies. Family members and close friends of the deceased dress in black and official suits, and visits are expected from all relatives, friends, and neighbors. The body is buried 24 hours after death. If the deceased is a young woman, she is dressed in a white bridal dress, and if a young man dies, he is dressed in a bride-groom's suit. Autopsies are not routinely performed. The whole family is in mourning for at least 40 days, and visitors are usually given a strong Turkish coffee or *raki*, a strong Albanian liquor. In turn, they are supposed to bring coffee, cigarettes, or money to help the family of the deceased. The family offers meals out of respect for the dead person, and they continue to be provided during the first week after the burial ceremony, on the fortieth day, and at the 6-month and 1-year anniversaries, at which time these activities of respect are considered finished. Family members continue to visit the cemetery and bring flowers to the tomb, especially on sacred days, special anniversaries or birthdays, or to mark special family events.

Food Practices and Intolerances: Most people eat three times a day. The largest meal is generally lunch, consisting of meat and vegetables that are well cooked and rice, pasta, or beans. Supper in the evening is lighter, with leftovers from lunch or some light food. As the economy has undergone a transition over the past 10 years, there is an increasing tendency for people to work during the day and thus many now prefer the largest meal in the evening.

Infant Feeding Practices: Approximately 9% of children younger than 4 months are exclusively breast-fed, a level considerably less than recommended. At ages 6 to 9 nine months, 24% of children are being fed breast milk and solid or semisolid foods. By 12 to 32 months, only 6% are still being breast-fed. Four percent of children younger than age

5 are underweight for their age, 17% have stunted growth, and 4% are severely emaciated. Children whose mothers have a secondary education or more are least likely to be underweight and stunted compared with children of mothers with less education.

Child Rearing Practices: The family has a very important role in Albanian society. Unfortunately, children who do not live with their families for various reasons (e.g., physical or mental handicaps, death of the parents, the inability of single parents or emigrating parents to care for them) may not be integrated into society and are at increased risk for abuse. The Albanian culture underscores the necessity for disciplining children, even through corporal punishment. Traditionally, it is expected that when adults speak, children will remain quiet and listen to them. Many children have several caretakers. Maternal and paternal grandparents are usually considered to be the most appropriate and trustworthy caretakers, and they frequently assume this responsibility when the parents are working. Parents pay significant attention to the education of their children, and often sacrifice for their children's education. The education of girls is considered much more important for the family in order to save them from family slavery, although worries about girls' safety have hindered the education of some young women. Social disruption during the transition period has made education more difficult, in that some village schools were destroyed, and many teachers left for more profitable occupations. Children most likely to receive an inadequate education include Gypsies, children of illegal migrants to the cities, and children without families. Drug abuse is a growing problem facing the youth in Albania because of easy access to drugs and doubts about the future.

National Childhood Immunizations: BCG at birth and 6 to 7 years; DPT at 2, 4, 6, and 24 months; OPV at 2, 4, 6, and 24 months and 6 to 7 years; hep B at birth and 2 and 6 months; MR at 12 months and 5 years; DT at 6 years; and Td 14 years. Of children ages 12 to 23 months, 80% have received a BCG vaccination; 71% have received the first dose of DPT by 12 months. Subsequent DPT coverage declines to 61% for the second dose and 52% for the third dose. Similarly, 57.3 % of children receive their first dose of polio vaccine by 12 months, but only 28.7% receive the third dose. By 12 months, 61% receive the measles vaccine. Girls and boys are vaccinated at roughly the same rate, but vaccination compliance is highest among children whose mothers have secondary education or more. Rural children are more likely to be vaccinated than urban children.

BIBLIOGRAPHY

Ekonomi M: *Albania in figures*, September 2000, Tirana, Albania, Institute of Statistics.
Ministry of Health: *Household living condition survey*, Albania, Tirana, October 1988.

recommended by the holy texts of the Koran for a child's first 2 years of life. Weaning usually occurs at about 2 years of age. The decline in fertility (3.8 children per woman at the beginning of 1990s compared with 7.4 in 1970) is partially attributed to women marrying at older ages and the educational improvement of girls. Infant mortality is a sensitive indicator of health, socioeconomic, and nutritional adequacy, and although still high, the rate is decreasing. In 2000 the infant mortality rate was 51.1 deaths per 1000 live births.

Child Rearing Practices: Muslims consider children to be blessings from the Creator because children immortalize the human race. A childless couple is doomed to failure because the Algerian man remarries to procreate. Children are treated affectionately, and warm kisses by all family members are common. Grandmothers play an active role in caregiving, especially when mothers are employed outside of the home. Disciplining of children is carried out by the mother, and the father intervenes only at the request of the mother. The father is authoritarian. Although his role becomes more prominent later in the child's life, children almost always retain a very close relationship with their mothers. Young children are enrolled in nursery school. The educational system has the mission of ensuring the development of children's personalities and their preparation for meaningful life by the acquisition of general scientific and technological knowledge. All Algerians have the right to education and training, and school is compulsory for all children 6 to 16 years. The educational system has three teaching levels—fundamental, secondary, and university—and is free at all levels. Classes are taught in Arabic, with the exception of university classes, in which students can choose the French language.

National Childhood Immunizations: BCG at birth; DPT at 3, 4, 5, and 18 months; OPV at birth, 3, 4, 5, and 18 months, and at 6, 11 to 13, and 16 to 18 years; measles at 9 months and 6 years; and DT at 6, 11 to 13, and 16 to 18 years, and then every 10 years. Because hepatitis B is becoming a more significant health problem, all children born after 2001 began receiving the vaccine for hepatitis. Three doses are administered: one at birth, at 1 month, and at 5 months. The incidence of measles has significantly declined and is believed to be a consequence of a second dose of measles vaccine given at 6 years. Since the introduction of these vaccines, diseases such as poliomyelitis, measles, diphtheria, and whooping cough have decreased 95%. Diphtheria deaths have decreased from 50 in 1994 to 4 in 1999; measles deaths from 61 in 1995 to none since 1998; and poliomyelitis has been eradicated, with no registered cases since 1997. Vaccines are free in at all public health sites. Levels of immunization attained are as follows: BCG, 97%; first dose of DTCP, 92%; second dose of DTCP, 89%; third dose of DTCP, 85%; and measles, 79%.

BIBLIOGRAPHY

Activité, emploi et chomage, No 330, 2ième Trimestre 2000, Office National des Statistiques.

Bencharif A, Baba B: *A Propos de 1000 Cas Enfants Présentant des Angines, Rhinopharingites et Bronchites à Répétition*, Congrès International de Mésothérapie, Sao Paolo, Brasil, 1998.

Compact disc, *Encarta Encyclopedia 1999*, Microsoft.

Démographie Algérienne, No 326, 2000, Office National des Statistiques.

Enquête National sur les Objectifs de la Fin Décennie Santé Mère et Enfant EDG Algérie 2000 MICS2, Rapport de Synthèse, Alger 2001, République Algérienne Démocratique et Populaire, Ministère de la Santé et de la Population, Institut National de Santé Publique. Available as PDF format file on http://www.ands. dz/insp/edg.html

Hachid M: *Les premiers Berbères entre Méditérranée*, Tassili et Nil, Edisud.

Hachid M, Le Tassili des Ajjer: *Aux sources de l'Afrique 50 siècles avant les Pyramides*, Edif2000, Alger.

Oizon R: *Encyclopédie Générale Larousse*, volume 1, ISBN 2-03-009810-8.

Situation Epidémiologique de l'Année 2000 sur la Base des Cas Déclarés à l'INSP, Relevé Epidémiologique Mensuel, Algérie, Vol XI, No V, Annuel 2000. Available as PDF format file on http://www.ands.dz/insp/rem.htmlwww.ons.dz

World Health Organization (June 2000): *Epidemiological fact sheets by country, Geneva*. Retrieved March 1, 2002, from http://www.unaids.org/hivaidsinfo/statistics/june00/fact_sheets/index.html

World Health Organization (2001): *WHO vaccine-preventable diseases: Monitoring system*, Geneva, Retrieved March 1, 2002, from http://www.who.int/vaccines/

◆ ANDORRA (PRINCIPALITY OF)

MAP PAGE (860)

Location: Andorra is an autonomous, semiindependent coprincipality under the suzerainty of France and the Spanish bishops of Urgel (Spain). It is a landlocked country in southwestern Europe between France and Spain in the eastern Pyrenees Mountains. The total land area is 468 km^2 (181 square miles); about 2.5 times the size of Washington, DC. About 35% is forest and woodland. The climate is temperate, with cold, snowy winters and warm, dry summers. The total population is 67,627, with about 72% between the ages of 15 and 64.

Major Languages	Ethnic Groups	Major Religions
Catalan (official)	Spanish 43%	Roman Catholic 90%
French	Andorran 33%	Other 10%
Castilian Spanish	Portuguese 11%	
	French 7%	
	Other 3%	

About 20% are native-born inhabitants of Catalan ancestry and language. The rest of the population consists primarily of immigrants (both legal and illegal) from Spain, France, and Portugal who were attracted by the excellent economy and lack of income taxes. It is estimated that about half of the Roman Catholics are active church attendees. Other religions include Islam (in the roughly 2000 North African immigrants), New Apostolic Church, Church of Jesus Christ of Latter Day Saints, Protestant denominations including Anglican and Reunification churches, and Jehovah's Witnesses.

Ethnic/Race Specific or Endemic Diseases: The World Health Organization (WHO) has no reported prevalence statistics on the human immunodeficiency virus (HIV) or the acquired immunodeficiency syndrome (AIDS) for Andorra. Rabies is a risk. Life expectancy at birth is 80.57 years for males and 86.57 years for females.

Touch Practices: Handshaking is the accepted form of greeting.

Birth Rites: The birth rate is 10.29 births per 1000 people, and the fertility rate is 1.25 children born per woman. Medical care is excellent in Andorra.

Food Practices and Intolerances: The cuisine is primarily Catalan. Local dishes include *coques* (flat flavored cakes), *trinxat* (potatoes and cabbage), *truites de carreroles* (mushroom omelets), and local sausages, cheese, and pork.

National Childhood Immunizations: DPT at 2, 3, 4, and 15 months; OPV at 15 months and 5 years; hep B at birth and 2 and 6 months; HIB at 2, 3, 4, and 15 months; MM at 5 and 6 months; IPV at 2, 3, and 4 months; MMR at 15 months and 5 years; DT at 5 years; and Td at 15 years. Vaccinations reported in 1997 were as follows: third dose of DTP, 90%; third dose of hep B, 75%; MCV, 90%; third dose of OPV, 90%; and second dose of TT, 90%.

Other Characteristics: Andorra is a stable, highly developed democracy. Previously impoverished and isolated, since World War II it has developed a successful tourist industry.

BIBLIOGRAPHY

Portella E, Goicoechea J, Penella J. A cross-sectional study on vaccine coverage and seroprevalence in schoolchildren in Andorra. *Soz-Praventivmed* 38(4):245–248, 1993.
http://encarta.msn.com/find/Concise.asp?ti=00C6F000
http://www.odci.gov/cia/publications/factbook/geos/an.html
http://www.wtg-online.com/data/and/and460.asp

◆ ANGOLA (REPUBLIC OF)

MAP PAGE (863)

Ndola Prata

Location: Angola is a former Portuguese colony on the southwest coast of Africa. The total land area is 1,246,700 km^2 (481,352 square miles).

For the past 40 years, the country has been at war, first against the Portuguese colonial regime, and after gaining independence in 1975, against itself in a civil conflict. After 16 years of continuous hostilities mainly confined to the countryside, a cease-fire accord was reached in May 1991. Aided by the United Nations (UN) military presence, Angola held its first multiparty general elections in September 1992. However, election results sparked a new bout of violence as the opposition party contested the victory of the ruling party. This major round of hostilities lasted through 1993 and continued, although at a much lower scale, until the signing of the Lusaka Peace Protocol in November 1994. Subsequent attempts by the two sides to put the peace process back on track were ineffective, and in December 1998 the war resumed. At the time of this writing the civil war in Angola is still raging.

Major Languages	**Ethnic Groups**	**Major Religions**
Portuguese (national)	Ovimbundu 37%	Indigenous beliefs 47%
Bantu and other	Kimbundu 25%	Roman Catholic 38%
local languages	Bakongo 13%	Protestant 15%
	Mestico 2%	
	European 1%	
	Other 22%	

The country has many local languages spoken by the different ethnic groups. The major ethnolinguistic groups are Kimbundu, Kikongo, Umbundu, Tchokwe, Ngangela, and Kuanhama. Nevertheless, not all the people of each ethnic group use their language for communication; the most widely used is Portuguese, a colonial language.

Health Care Beliefs: Magical-religious. Disease is generally perceived as something that is induced by somebody else and therefore needs special attention. Even those who regularly use conventional health care services consider this as an important component of the treatment process. When the first signs of disease are noticed in a child (the first health problem after birth), mothers and grandmothers immediately seek protection for the child, fearing a series of health problems that in many cases may end up in death or disability. This protection usually requires a visit to a spiritual healer who gives the child a small, red bag to be worn on a string wrapped around the waist. The red bag contains dried plants, roots, small parts of animal bones or teeth, and animal skin. All these combined elements supposedly protect against curses. In addition, when a child is sick, parents are supposed to practice sexual abstinence.

Predominant Sick Care Practices: Biomedical; traditional. Both conventional and traditional medicine practices are prevalent in Angola. Conventional medical care is offered through the national health system, which includes public health facilities, private for-profit facilities, and private not-for-profit organizations (nongovernmental organizations and church services). Traditional medicine is offered by two types of traditional doctors (*curandeiros*). Some focus on spiritual treatment involving rituals and ceremonies calling on dead people's spirits to help determine who is responsible for causing the disease. In this way, punishments may be prescribed or payments to the offended person may be made. Other treatments focus on treating the disease with herbs, local plants, and oils. Some healers practice both types. People of all classes of the population frequent both types of healers. Although herbal healers cover a vast range of diseases, spiritual healers are very popular for mental health, skin diseases, infertility, and chronic diseases. The decision to seek care is based on specific ethnic groups' norms, family values, and traditions; access to care; affordability of care; and beliefs in the type of health service available. Treatments for very common and often-fatal diseases such as malaria, acute respiratory tract infections, diarrhea, and measles are known to be better and faster when they involve conventional health care services. For other diseases that are more difficult to self-diagnose, traditional healers are used first, and conventional medicine is used as a last resource. Lack of access to health care and money can be deterrents to care. Public health services are free but often lack medicines, supplies, and treatments, and the person may have to wait a long time to be seen by a health professional. Traditional healers are not free, but prices are set based on the client's ability to pay, and payments can be made in kind or in installments.

Ethnic/Race Specific or Endemic Diseases: The infant mortality rate is 124 per 1000 live births, and the child mortality rate is 209 per 1000 live births. The most prevalent diseases are the infectious communicable diseases, which include childhood vaccine-preventable diseases (i.e., measles, polio, tetanus), diarrhea, acute respiratory tract infections, and malaria. Tuberculosis has an estimated annual incidence rate of 225 per 100,000 people. Malnutrition is a major problem, especially for children younger than 5 years. Results from the 1996 national Multiple Indicator Cluster Survey (MICS) show that approximately 49% of children younger than 5 years have stunted growth, and 38% are underweight. According to the same survey, 28% of children younger than 5 years reported having had diarrhea in the 2 weeks preceding the survey, and 48% had experienced an acute respiratory tract infection. Other endemic diseases that affect the morbidity of the population but are not major killers are trypanosomiasis, schistosomiasis, leishmaniasis, lymphatic filariasis, onchocerciasis, and other tropical diseases. The World Health Organization's (WHO) estimated prevalence rate for HIV/AIDS in adults ages 15 to 49 is 2.78%. The estimated number of children from birth to 15 years who are living with HIV/AIDS is 7900. The most commonly affected people are women ages 20 to 39 years and men ages 20 to 49 years. An estimated 200,000 Angolans are living with HIV; 26,200 of them have AIDS. More than 35% of all reported cases are young people ages 15 to 29. Since the beginning of the epidemic in Angola, more than 31,000 have died of AIDS-related diseases—8000 in 1998. In 1987 the Ministry of Health created a National Program to Fight AIDS to coordinate national prevention efforts and donor support activities. Although Angola seems to have much lower HIV prevalence rates than its neighboring countries, two factors must be taken into account: (1) underreporting resulting from limited clinical and laboratory capacities for diagnosis and (2) the isolation of populations and difficulties traveling around the country because of the civil war.

Health Team Relationships: The delivery of health care services is driven by doctors; however, it is estimated that there is only one doctor for every 20,000 people. Most of the health centers are entirely run by nurses and even in major urban areas, health centers do not have permanent doctors. Therefore nurses are responsible for the delivery of primary health care services in the country. The relationships between doctors and nurses are usually good. In general, public servants are not well paid, and the nurses working in the public sector are in this category. Nonetheless, the work they do is so important and appreciated by their community that even though they are paid low salaries, they are committed and dedicated to their patients. Patients' attitudes toward health professionals are generally respectful because the community considers health care workers to be authorities.

Families' Role in Hospital Care: Angolan families—extended as well as nuclear—come together during times of sickness. When a person is hospitalized, at least one member of the family stays with the person at the hospital 24 hours a day. Family members to accompany the ill are chosen based on closeness to the sick person, the history of the illness, and time availability, and they usually take turns in the hospital. Some hospitals (including pediatric hospitals) do not allow family members to stay overnight, but even then family members stay within the vicinity of the hospital. It is not unusual to see what could be described as a "camping ground" of family members in the hospital yard in the evening. This support is very important for those who are sick. Even though they cannot see their family for most of the day, they are reassured that somebody is always nearby. Food for those who are hospitalized in public facilities is usually prepared at home. Angolans believe that hospital food is of poor quality (and in reality, most of it is) and does not meet the specific needs of each patient. Depending on the disease, people tend to prepare specific meals according to family norms. For example, it is common practice to feed sick people with very high-protein meals that are also high in sodium and cholesterol. Depending on the disease, this practice may not be detrimental (e.g., for patients who are very weak from a prolonged and debilitating infectious disease or because they have had surgery and massive loss of blood). It may be, however, if a specific diet needs to be followed (e.g., for those with high blood pressure or diabetes). Lack of knowledge on the part of the family, coupled with lack of communication with health providers, and hospitals' insufficient response to patient needs can slow down recovery time. Besides food preparation and keeping the individual company, family members also help with changing linens, bathing, and other activities.

Dominance Patterns: The common perception that sub-Saharan African countries are male-dominated societies applies to Angola. However, economic power dovetails with gender relations and plays a tremendous role in the balance of power or dominance by either reinforcing or offsetting traditional gender roles. Although gender is as an individual (and less mutable) attribute, economic power derives from the familial situations of the individual and is relative to that of the partner. Most often, when a couple marries and forms a new family, the man comes from the wealthier family and thereby has decision-making and economic power over his wife. Such a man usually defers to the judgment of his own mother or another maternal figure to the extent that his decisions in family matters tend to reflect her will. These important family concerns vary and can include factors such as type of food consumed, place of residence, health-seeking behavior, family size, and child-rearing practices. In the less common scenario, in which the wife comes from a wealthier family, the situation is reversed. Because the couple tends to be financially dependent on the wife's family, the wife dominates the relationship, and her family has more of a voice in the decision-making. Beyond the family circle and related dynamics, Angolan women face a landscape of vastly different opportunities and possibilities that depend largely on class and education. The majority of Angolan women assume a broad spectrum of domestic responsibilities, including food preparation, household chores, and child rearing duties. At the same time, many women serve in positions of importance in society (e.g., ministers, vice ministers, CEOs, army and police officers). Angola, like many other societies, continues to wrestle with the tensions and contradictions that often accompany the changing roles of women. In general, women are respected in their roles, and their contributions to society are accepted. In addition to gender relationship and economic disparities, intergenerational dynamics continue to play a significant role in social interactions. As a general rule, respect comes with age. Because older adults usually live with their children, they are positioned to be involved in the family's organization and, therefore, wield considerable influence in shaping decisions.

Eye Contact Practices: Eye contact practices vary depending on the age and profession of the people involved and whether they come from a rural or an urban background. Most ethnic groups consider eye contact with the speaker a sign of defiance if an older adult or someone with higher status in the family or social hierarchy is speaking. Common practice dictates that children do not make eye contact with adults regardless of the setting. In other relationships, nonverbal communication differs depending on the setting. Although rural people do not tend to make eye contact, it is more acceptable in urban settings.

Touch Practices: Angolans consider themselves to be especially affectionate and they place a high premium on communicating warmth, friendliness, and welcoming greetings. Social touching is used to communicate platonic affection within and between genders. Demonstrative behavior usually involves hugging, embracing, and social kissing on the cheek not only when greeting friends and acquaintances but also when making first introductions. Moreover, all social groups engage in tactile behavior to express camaraderie and affection. Parents and the entire society instill such demonstrative behavior early on by teaching children to exchange social kisses during introductions and salutations with other children and all adults.

Perceptions of Time: In general, perception of time varies between urban and rural people. In general, rural people are more punctual, and those from urban areas have a less strict perception of time. With respect to health care (in the public sector only), it is unheard of for patients to be late for appointments, because waiting to be seen is the norm.

Pain Reactions: Reactions to pain differs according to the type of pain and the health condition involved. For example, it is quite normal to emit loud sounds or even scream during the birth of a child. Screaming during deliveries or other health procedures not involving anesthetics (such as suturing, tooth removal, cleaning of wounds, and injections) does not necessarily reflect the amount of pain being experienced but rather helps relieve stress and fear. In all other health circumstances, pain (including pain in children) is usually experienced in silence. The amount of a patient's pain is usually recognized by health professionals through the person's facial expressions, lack of responsiveness to basic questions, and the use of pain-relieving body positions. When asked if they are in pain, it is not uncommon for patients to respond, "just a little." This does not mean that the pain should be disregarded; it should be investigated further.

Birth Rites: Traditionally, women have their babies at home. A 1996 national survey indicates that even in urban areas, 78% of births take place at home (and 90% of births in rural areas are at home). In addition, only 64% of women have access to antenatal care; 49% have had tetanus vaccine, and 39% have had a trained health professional at their birth. Part of the strategy to decrease maternal mortality is to shift births from homes to health centers, but this effort has not been successful, even in urban areas. Factors affecting lack of success are inadequate access to high-quality maternity services and the inability to carry out certain customs during and after delivery. For example, women prefer to have their babies at home because of the warm support provided by family and friends during the delivery. No family members are allowed in the maternity ward, which is contrary to Angolan customs that place a high value on family support. Thus hospital delivery means that women will experience the birth among strangers (i.e., health professionals). During delivery, it is customary for attendants to sit on, or to put pressure on the women's abdomen when it is believed that the woman is not pushing strongly enough. In other situations a birth attendant sweeps a broom (not necessarily a clean one) down the abdomen of the woman. When the expulsion of the placenta is delayed, husbands blow into an empty bottle just outside the delivery room until the placenta is completely expelled. After delivery, mothers are given coconut milk to drink and dried salted fish to eat, which are believed to help increase their milk production. Postpartum baths are also part of the norm in Angola and are very hot (almost like a sauna). The water for the bath is boiled with special plants and roots, and during the bath an older woman (such as the mother or mother-in-law) massages the woman with a piece of cloth (such as a towel). This practice is observed at home even when the delivery occurs in a health facility. The arrival of a son is highly celebrated, but daughters are also celebrated. While growing up, girls do most of the housework, including taking care of the younger siblings. After marriage, daughters usually live and work close to their husband's family. Sons are expected to stay with their family of origin and provide for their parents in their old age by providing shelter when they can no longer take care of themselves. In summary, to the average Angolan family, a good mix of boys and girls is considered a blessed fertility outcome. The national family planning program was started in the mid-1980s as part of the maternal and child health service. Its main objective was to improve the well-being of mothers through child spacing. Since the program's inception, free family planning services have been offered in public health facilities. However, the program has been plagued by shortages of properly trained health workers, limited choices of contraceptive methods, and frequent interruptions in supply. Being clinic-based, family planning information only reaches those who seek services, leaving the majority of the population, especially adolescents and young adults, uninformed. Angola has one of the lowest rates of contraceptive use in sub-Saharan Africa. In 1996, contraceptive use was estimated to be 8.2% (for all methods)—13% in urban areas and 4.2% in rural areas. The maternal mortality rate is one of the highest in the world (1500 women per 100,000 live births) and reflects health care in general, and the state of reproductive health care in particular. So-called indirect causes of maternal deaths contribute to the high maternal mortality statistics. In Angola, 25% of the total maternal deaths are a result of malaria, and another 25% are caused by complications from abortions. Abortions are illegal but permitted for medical or social reasons. The personnel who do most of the illegal abortions are not properly trained, so the procedures are often complicated by infections and bleeding, which usually require assistance at a health facility.

Death Rites: Death at a young age is perceived to be caused by a curse, whereas older people die upon a call from a higher power. Therefore the rituals and ceremonies vary according to the age of the deceased. In both cases, corpses are washed and nicely dressed before burial (a practice that is not observed during cholera epidemics). Family members usually kiss the deceased, and only adults (men and women) can participate in the ceremonies. Children and close family members of the deceased are allowed in the room only for the farewell kiss. The ceremonies are attended by extended family and friends and last for a minimum of 7 days, when mourners dress in black, and any kind of entertainment (e.g., listening to the radio) is prohibited. The mourning house stays open all day and night, and groups of people take turns singing and dancing the death rites dance. After the burial, people are given food and large amounts of alcoholic beverages. After the seventh day of the celebration of mourning the family starts to disperse, and life is supposed to resume as it was before.

Food Practices and Intolerances: The most important meal of the day is lunch. In the northern part of the country the most important source of carbohydrates is the cassava root, whereas in the central and the southern regions corn is the staple. Depending on availability, people eat local vegetables and meat or fish (dried or fresh) with their cassava or corn. Both are usually eaten with a sauce that has a peanut or palm oil base. In rural areas, it is acceptable and usual practice to eat with the hands, whereas the urban population tends to eat with a fork, knife, and spoon.

Infant Feeding Practices: Angola has a very high prevalence of breast-feeding. About 98% of children are breast-fed for a mean duration of 25 months. However, exclusive breast-feeding does not last very long, and only 12% of children younger than 4 months are solely breast-fed. Mothers tend to start food supplementation between the ages of 2 and 3 months. Colostrum is perceived as weak milk, so to compensate, some mothers (in urban areas) feed their children formula in bottles, while mothers in rural areas may use fresh goat milk. Solid food is introduced fairly early—at 3 or 4 months—and consists of porridge made out of corn or cassava flour. Even though children at that age are still being breast-fed, at least one meal a day is solid food. These feeding practices are often associated with diarrheal diseases because of contamination, inability to digest the food, or that infants may not have had a chance to fully benefit from the immunological attributes of breast milk. A child is usually nursed at will, and it is not unusual to see breast-feeding in public places.

Child Rearing Practices: Except for some urban, more westernized families, disciplining children (or other child rearing duties) is mainly a mother's task. Fathers are usually considered to be authoritarian figures and discipline the children when mothers ask. Otherwise, the role of the father starts later in the child's life. Even though fathers participate in parental decisions, mothers usually announce these decisions. Until the age of 1 or 2 years, children have a very close relationship with their mothers. Very frequently, children sleep with their mothers (or another adult female), and they are carried on their mother's back wherever they go (except for urban women employed in the formal sector of the economy). Frequently, women get pregnant while still breast-feeding, which alters these practices.

National Childhood Immunizations: BCG at birth; DPT at 2, 4, and 6 months; OPV at birth and 2, 4, and 6 months; measles at 9 months; yellow fever at 9 months; CBAW × 5. DTP boosters are also recommended. The reported percent of the target population fully vaccinated by antigen is BCG, 59.5%; OPV, 27.5%; DTP, 23.9%; measles, 45.5%; and yellow fever, 21.1%.

Other Characteristics: In 2000, Angola had an estimated population of 13 million, with an average annual population growth rate of 2.9%. The total fertility rate in 1996 was estimated to be 6.9 pregnancies per woman (6.8 in urban areas and 7 in rural areas), but Angola is a very sparsely populated country, with only 9 people per square kilometer. The majority of the population resides in rural areas, and the per capita income was $380 (U.S. dollars) in 1998. Although seen as a country with unique economic potential, Angola is among the poorest countries in sub-Saharan Africa, with 61% of its population living below the poverty line. Only 16% of the population has access to basic sanitation, 32% has access to safe water, and 24% has access to formal health care. Since civil war resumed in December 1998, more than 3 million people have been displaced, primarily in the provinces of Bie, Huila, Huambo, and Malanje. Because of these factors, life expectancy at birth is estimated to be only 45 years for men and 48 for women.

BIBLIOGRAPHY

Agadjanian V, Prata N: *2000: Trends in Angola's fertility*. Paper presented at the Workshop on Prospects for Fertility Decline in High Fertility Countries. Population Division, Department of Economic and Social Affairs, United Nations Secretariat. New York, July 2001.

Agadjanian V, Prata N: War and reproduction: Angola's fertility in comparative perspective. *J South African Studies* 27(2):329–347, June 2001.

Carvalho A et al 1996. Characteristics of contraceptive acceptors in Luanda, Angola, *African J Fertil Sexual Reprod Health* 1(2):109–114.

Instituto Nacional de Estatistica: *Inquerito de indicadores multiplos* (MICS), INE (GMCVP), UNICEF—Angola, 1998.

United Nations Security Council: *Report of the Secretary General on the United Nations Office in Angola*, October 10, 2001.

World Bank: *World development indicators database*, Washington, DC, 2000, The Bank.

◆ ANTIGUA AND BARBUDA

MAP PAGE (858)

Location: Antigua and Barbuda are eastern Caribbean islands. Antigua, the larger of the two, is low lying, deforested, and subject to droughts, with an average rainfall of only 45 inches a year. Barbuda is a wooded, coral island. The islands are about 300 miles southeast of Puerto Rico. Their total land area is 442 km^2 (171 square miles), which is about 2.5 times the size of Washington, DC. (Antigua has 281 km^2, and Barbuda has 161 km^2 total land area.) Their capital is St. John's. Temperatures are in the mid-70s in the winter and mid-80s in the summer with northeast trade winds. The total population is 66,970, and the gross domestic product (GDP) per capita is $8,200.

Major Languages	Ethnic Groups	Major Religions
English (official)	African (almost entirely)	Anglican (predominant)
Local dialects	People of British,	Other Protestant, some
	Portuguese, Lebanese,	Roman Catholic
	and Syrian origins	

Health Care Beliefs: Active involvement; health promotion. Because the major health risks are now lifestyle related, significant efforts have been made to increase health promotion programs to address these risks. *Project Lifestyle* is a program designed to be introduced in grades 1 to 2 and progress throughout the school curriculum. The major focus of the program is on "weighing right, eating right, doing daily physical exercises, and having a positive self-concept." It is hoped that program will stem the present trend of noncommunicable disease incidence.

Predominant Sick Care Practices: Limited biomedical. Medical care is very limited on Antigua and Barbuda, and few resources are available for the treatment of serious illnesses or emergencies. In 1995, Hurricane Luis severely disrupted health facilities, including a much-needed cardiac care center. Poor maintenance and unsound structural designs led to severe damage in the main hospitals and six other health facilities. Efforts are being made to increase the ability of these facilities to endure severe weather.

Ethnic/Race Specific or Endemic Diseases: Chronic diseases and obesity have almost entirely replaced the previous risks of infectious diseases and malnutrition. Cardiovascular diseases are prevalent, and congestive cardiac failure is emerging as a significant problem. A recent study reported the following causes for congestive failure: hypertension (41%), ischemia (44%), valvular-related (12%) and alcohol-related (2%) causes, idiopathic (5%) causes, and mixed (7%) causes. Diabetes is prevalent, and dengue fever remains a risk. Risk for childhood-onset insulin-dependent diabetes mellitus (IDDM) is a major concern for adolescents. The most prevalent types of cancer in males have been reported as skin (26.3%), prostate (22.8%), and upper respiratory and alimentary tract (10.5%) cancers. In women, the major cancers have been breast (23.1%), cervix uteri (22.3%), and skin (15.3%) cancers. Medical conditions are also emerging that are associated with toxicity from the ingestion of cocaine that has been packaged for transportation to other regions. The World Health Organization (WHO) has no published estimated prevalence rates for HIV and AIDS. However, the following statistics (the most recent available) are available locally and illustrate the effectiveness of education and prevention efforts in the islands: two deaths and a rate of 3.1% in 1990, eight deaths and a rate of 12.1% in 1996, seven deaths and a rate of 10.4% in 1997, and four deaths and a rate of 6% in 1998.

Birth Rites: The islands reached replacement-level fertility in the 1980s, a trend believed to reflect changes in the national economy that created greater job opportunities for women. The birth rate is 19.5 births per 1000 population, and the infant mortality rate is 22.33 deaths per 1000 live births. The total fertility rate is 2.31 children born per woman. Life expectancy at birth is 68.45 years for males and 73.14 for females.

National Childhood Immunizations: DPT at 2, 4, and 6 months; OPV at 2, 4, and 6 months; hep B at 2, 4, and 6 months; HIB at 2, 4, and 6 months; MMR at 1 and 5 years; DT at 5 years; and Td at 15 years. The following immunization coverage in the target population has been reported (1999): DTP3, 99%; MCV, 99%; and Pol3, 99%.

Other Characteristics: Water management is a major concern because fresh water sources are very limited. The islands are considered to be a minor transshipment point for narcotics bound for the United States and Europe but are more significant as a center for laundering drug money. During discussions, several people may engage in simultaneous conversations, making frequent interruptions and having loud verbal battles. Such discourse is valued as a normal part of interpersonal relationships.

BIBLIOGRAPHY

Gibbs T, van-Alphen D: Impact of Hurricane Luis on the health services of Antigua and Barbuda, *World Health Stat Quart* 49(3-4):200, 1996.

Handwerker WP: West Indian gender relations, family planning programs and fertility decline, *Soc Sci Med* 35(10):1245, 1992.

McSwain M, Martin TC, Amaraswamy R: The prevalence, aetiology and treatment of congestive cardiac failure in Antigua and Barbuda, *West Ind Med J* 48(3):137, 1999.

Menyuk P, Menyuk D: Communicative competence: a historical and cultural perspective. In Wurzel JS: *Toward multiculturalism*, Yarmouth, Me, 1988, Intercultural Press.

Simon LC: Cancer incidence and mortality in Antigua/Barbuda, *West Ind Med J* 40(2):74, 1991.

Simon LC: The cocaine body packer syndrome, *West Ind Med J* 39(4):250, 1990.

Sinha DP: Project Lifestyle: Developing positive health lifestyles for schoolchildren in Antigua, *J School Health* 62(10):449, 1992.

Tull ES et al: Incidence of childhood-onset IDDM in Black African-heritage populations in the Caribbean, *Diabetes Care* 30(3):309, 1997.

http://www.odci.gov/cia/publications/factbook/geos/ac.html

http://www.carec.org/data/aids/index.htm

http://travel.state.gov/antigua_barbuda.html

◆ ARGENTINA (ARGENTINE REPUBLIC)

MAP PAGE (859)

Location: Argentina, the eighth largest country in the world, is a land of plains from the Atlantic Ocean to the Chilean border and contains the high peaks of the Andes. Its bordering countries are Bolivia, Brazil, Chile, Paraguay, and Uruguay. The north is swampy, and the central populated area has fertile land used for agriculture or grazing. The south boasts Patagonia, with its cool, arid steppes. The climate is primarily temperate—arid in the southeast and sub-Antarctic in the southwest. The total land area is 2,736,690 km^2 (1,056,362 square miles) Argentina is considered to be a medium-income nation with a developing economy and has a gross domestic product (GDP) per capita of $10,000. The total population is 37,384,816, and 63% of the population is between 15 and 64 years. Literacy rates are high: 96% for males and females alike.

Major Languages	Ethnic Groups	Major Religions
Spanish (official)	White 97%	Roman Catholic 92%
English	Mestizo, Amerindian,	Protestant 2%
Italian	other non-White	Jewish 2%
German	groups 3%	Other 4%
Amerindian languages		

Less than 20% of Roman Catholics are reported to be practicing Catholics. The majority of the White Argentinians are of European origin, of primarily Spanish and Italian descent. Argentina has 17 Amerindian languages, including Quechua, Mapuche, Guarani, Tobas, and Matacos.

Health Care Beliefs: Active involvement: health promotion important. Since the 1990s, several bills have passed that mandate the creation of various health promotion and disease prevention programs, such as family planning, sex education, and sexual health services. Numerous difficulties have been encountered, particularly involving the provision of contraceptives, which seems to be primarily a result of the alliance of the country with the Roman Catholic Church. Therefore poor women who depend on public health services for assistance with family planning are particularly vulnerable and unable to control their reproductive destiny.

Predominant Sick Care Practices: Biomedical: curative and preventive. Reforms that took place in the 1990s opened up to competition—internally and from private insurers—the union-administered social insurance system for workers. The current system is a combination of government-sponsored social health insurance and individual private insurance. The movement toward a managed care approach is affecting distribution of health care resources, with the poor receiving the least, although some free hospital clinics exist. Medical standards are highest in urban areas, and rural areas have less adequate services.

Ethnic/Race Specific or Endemic Diseases: Endemic diseases and conditions include malaria (which is regional), tuberculosis, Chagas' disease, animal-borne helminthiases, intestinal parasites, histoplasmosis, paracoccidioidomycosis (northwest), leishmaniasis, trichinosis, typhoid fever and rotavirus, and severe diarrhea in children. People are at risk for Argentine hemorrhagic fever, dengue fever (which is endemic in neighboring countries), *Escherichia coli* infection, measles, yellow fever, cholera, hepatitis A and B, hantavirus, botulism, and *Helicobacter pylori* infection. Argentina has one of the highest automobile accident rates in the world. Cigarette smoking rates (which are high) contribute to respiratory diseases. The World Health Organization's (WHO) estimated prevalence rate for HIV/AIDS in adults ages 15 to 49 is 0.69%. The estimated number of children from birth to 15 years living with HIV/AIDS is 4400. The estimated number of adults and children who died of AIDS in 1999 is 1800, and since the beginning of the epidemic the estimated number of children who have either lost their mother or both parents to AIDS while they were younger than 15 years of age is 8900. Life expectancy at birth is 71.67 years for males, and 78.61 years for females.

Health Team Relationships: Population studies indicate that families are very likely to protect patients from knowing their diagnosis, prognosis, and treatment. Health professionals themselves seem to want to truthfully discuss patients' health situations.

Dominance Patterns: The society is generally patriarchal, with deference given to the father; however, he considers the opinions of the rest of the family. Traditional gender roles are strong, particularly in rural areas and among less educated individuals.

Eye Contact Practices: Direct eye contact is commonly maintained.

Touch Practices: Touching during conversations is quite usual, and males may touch each other without any sexual connotation.

Perceptions of Time: Argentinians have a relaxed attitude toward punctuality.

Birth Rites: The maternal mortality rate is 100 per 100,000 live births. The birth rate is 18.59 births per 1000 population, and the infant mortality rate is 18.31 deaths per 1000 live births. The total fertility rate is 2.47 children born per woman.

Food Practices and Intolerances: Argentinians consume large amounts of beef. Mixed grilles (*parrillada*), which contain almost every part of the animal, are popular, as are Italian foods such as gnocchi (*noquis*). Argentinean ice cream is famous for its quality. Drinking *mate* (Paraguayan tea) from a shared gourd is a ritual of acceptance between individuals.

National Childhood Immunizations: BCG at birth and 6 years; OPV at 2, 4, 6, and 18 months and 6 years; hep B at birth and 2 and 6 months; DTPHH at 2, 4, 6, and 18 months; MMR at 12 months; and Td at

16 years, then every 10 years. The following immunization coverage in the target population has been reported: BCG, 99%; first dose of DTP, 88%; third dose of DTP, 66%; third dose of HIB, 66%; MCV, 56%; and Pol3, 85%.

Other Characteristics: Argentina is being used more and more as a transshipment country for cocaine headed for Europe and the United States and as a money-laundering center. Domestic consumption of drugs has increased dramatically.

BIBLIOGRAPHY

Grimberg M: Knowing about AIDS and sexual precautions among low-income women from the Southern area of Buenos Aires (notes for defining prevention policies), *Cad Saude Publica* 17(3):481, 2001.

Johnson GA: Palliative care in Argentina: a gringo's perspective, *Am J Hospice Palliat Care* 10(4):11, 1993.

Mercer R et al: The need for youth-oriented policies and programmes on responsible sexuality in Argentina, *Reprod Health Matters* 9(17):184, 2001.

U.S. Agency of International Development: Agency program fights Argentine virus, *Front Lines* 31(10):4, 1991.

http://www.odci.gov/cia/publications/factbook/geos/ar.html

http://travel.state.gov/argentina.html

◆ ARMENIA

MAP PAGE (861)

Mary Arevian

Location: The smallest of the former Soviet republics, Armenia achieved independence in 1991. It is a landlocked country in the southern Caucasus. The terrain includes rugged mountains and excellent pastures. The total land area is 29,800 km² (11,506 square miles). On December 7, 1988, a devastating earthquake destroyed Armenia's infrastructure and resulted in approximately 500,000 adults and children who were homeless, who had disabilities, or whose parents had both been killed. Furthermore, about 250,000 Armenian refugees from Azerbaijan took refuge in Armenia as a consequence of problems in Nagorni Karabagh. According to a recent census, the total population of the country is 2,970,000.

Major Languages	Ethnic Groups	Major Religions
Armenian	Armenian 93%	Armenian Orthodox 44%
	Yezidi 3%	Other 6%
	Other 4%	

Health Care Beliefs: Acute sick care; biomedical; traditional. The previous emphasis on the importance of health promotion and disease prevention has decreased, partly because of the lack of infrastructure needed to provide public health services. Health care is primarily treatment of disease. Disease is not viewed as a punishment from God for sinning but as fate. Alternative treatments are not used for illness; people go to clinics or hospitals for biomedical treatment. Medication use is highly predominant among the people, and doctors who do not prescribe drugs are not considered to be good doctors. People are used to taking medications even without prescriptions. Armenia is rich in many kinds of herbs, so herbal treatments are also popular. Many kinds of teas are used to treat respiratory, urinary, digestive, and other ailments. Another common practice is the utilization of locally prepared ointments and creams. Although some of these herbs are beneficial in treating certain ailments, others can be harmful. It is essential that researchers study their herbs and accordingly encourage or discourage their use. Alcohol consumption and smoking are viewed as part of the typical social and cultural behavior of males. Recently broadcasted televised programs have been relating health hazards to lifestyle choices, but the lack of public policy is a significant obstacle. Vigorous advertising campaigns promoting cigarettes and alcoholic drinks pose great challenges to the fairly insignificant health promotion programs.

Predominant Sick Care Practices: Biomedical. Most of the hospitals were built during the 1960s and 1970s, except for the few constructed by European countries in the area of the 1988 earthquake. Because of a persistent lack of funds, most of the hospitals have not been renovated. Diagnostic and therapeutic equipment is very old, very basic, and poorly maintained. The unequal distribution of health care facilities between urban and rural populations has created a large gap in health care between the two.

Ethnic/Race Specific or Endemic Diseases: According to the Ministry of Health, the major health problems in order of importance include coronary artery disease, cancer, gastrointestinal disorders, infectious diseases, diabetes, and perinatal complications. The World Health Organization's (WHO) estimated prevalence rate for HIV/AIDS in adults ages 15 to 49 is 0.01%. The estimated number of children from birth to 15 years living with HIV/AIDS is less than 100. Although the rate seems low compared with other countries, young women are especially vulnerable. Because of high unemployment, many have become sex workers to support their families. Some progress has been made in promoting HIV awareness and prevention programs, especially those involving the youth. Many factors contribute to the difficulties with establishing effective prevention programs including social attitudes, such as the "not in our country" attitude. In addition to the false belief that HIV and AIDS are not a potentially serious problem in Armenia, sex and sexual issues are taboo subjects, hindering frank and open discussions about HIV and other sexually transmitted diseases. Changing these deep-seated social attitudes will take much effort and time. Despite the existing attitudes, positive steps are being taken. Armenia has adopted a national program for HIV/AIDS prevention.

With the help and collaboration of governmental, nongovernmental, and international organizations, a positive outcome may be attained in the near future.

Health Team Relationships: The health care system is centralized, bureaucratic, medically oriented, and male dominated despite the numerous female physicians who occupy positions with less power. Communication among health care personnel is generally unidirectional, moving from doctors to therapists and nurses, and takes the form of instructions and orders. Health care service workers are paid by the government; however, if families do not pay bribes, their family members may not be admitted to a hospital or even when admitted may not receive basic services such as, bathing, turning, and feeding. Because hospitals are paid by the government based on the amount of time a bed is occupied, the length of stay may be somewhat extended.

Families' Role in Hospital Care: Families are the sole supporters of their sick family members. They are responsible for provision of food, medications, syringes, needles, intravenous equipment, and all other necessities. It is common to see visitors carrying bags of food to the hospital for their relatives, and doctors and nurses are invited to eat from the food brought in for patients.

Dominance Patterns: Males are dominant. The family has very important meaning as a support system, so family members generally stay close. Older members are taken care of by their families, and it is a disgrace if a family has institutionalized an older family member. Women in general are the torchbearers and preservers of life values, religious beliefs, and motherhood customs. Throughout history the Armenian woman has had an important role in maintaining the family—and through family maintenance in preserving the nation. During a recent visit to Armenia (March 2002) Marlin Haas, the general secretary of the International Socialist Women's Organization, mentioned that Armenia has established good traditions with regard to women's roles in political and community areas. Haas noted the equal voting privileges of men and women during the First Republic of Armenia in 1918 and the presence of women in parliament. However, in spite of the fact that 60% of those who have received a higher education are women, women constitute only 3% of parliament. To really understand the status of women in Armenia, it is important to refer to historical events that had a significant impact on their role and status. For 600 years during the Turkish occupation, Armenian men saw women as inferior slaves and servants. When Armenia became part of the United Soviet Socialist Republic (which lasted from 1920 to 1991), if they were to survive, women had to learn to be rough and manage hard labor; and it was assumed that men and women were equal in the society. However, during this period of history, while women did the hard work, men turned to the pleasures of smoking, drinking, and having extramarital sex. For a man to have an extramarital lover became a sign of prosperity and a symbol of manhood. For the sake of maintaining family peace, women silently adapted to the situation. It is now usual to see men enjoying themselves with other men and women while their wives are busy with household responsibilities, as well as their work outside the home. The current status of the Armenian woman is a paradox. On one hand, she is highly educated and has entered highly esteemed professions such as medicine, law, and engineering. On the other hand, she is still a subordinate "slave" or "servant." Only a very small proportion of women are active in the political arena or other significant societal or community activities.

Eye Contact Practices: Direct eye contact is usually unacceptable.

Touch Practices: Men usually greet each other and women by shaking hands. Friendly kissing between men and women is not acceptable.

Perceptions of Time: Punctuality was not important in the past. If an appointment does not take place 9 AM, it could very easily be at 9 PM; if it was not today, it could very easily be tomorrow. More recently, Armenians, particularly younger people, seem to be more concerned about the value of time and the importance of being punctual.

Pain Reactions: Men are known for their stoicism, and they are not expected to openly express their feelings of pain. It is acceptable for women to scream during painful experiences, or to cry in a loud voice during sad occasions. Armenian men also are not supposed to express love openly.

Birth Rites: Doctors typically deliver babies in hospitals. Abortion is the primary birth control method, with an average of 15 abortions for a 35-year-old woman. Vasectomy is not generally a culturally acceptable option for the Armenian man. As many as one in three women are infertile as the result of sexually transmitted disease and unsafe abortions.

Death Rites: Relatives, friends and neighbors are required to attend at the time of death. Funeral services are held both at the church and at the place of burial. Fortunes may be spent on decorating the cemeteries. Cemeteries are visited after every family and religious occasion, such as Christmas and Easter.

Food Practices and Intolerances: Births, baptisms, marriages, and deaths have special significance for Armenians. They usually celebrate happy and sad occasions with food and drink. Armenian people are very generous, and during any visit to their homes food and drink is offered. They usually offer all that they have, even if it means that they may have nothing for the next day. Men usually get seated at the table, and women serve the meal.

Infant Feeding Practices: Breast-feeding declined after the 1988 earthquake. Many mothers complained their milk was not sufficient for the baby or that they were under too much stress. At that time, formula preparations were available because many charitable organizations were donating infant formula. However, currently it is very difficult for an average family to afford formula.

Child Rearing Practices: Mothers are the primary caregivers for their children, but if they have to return to work grandmothers and even great grandmothers supervise the children. This shift in caregiving is not a problem because the family is usually traditional and extended. The age of marriage is generally young (about 20) for men and women. Many couples get married while still at the university studying. Because it is difficult to find housing, living with parents or even grandparents has become the norm rather then the exception. The literature typifies the Armenian mother as being kind, virtuous, and sacrificial.

National Childhood Immunizations: BCG at birth and 7 and 12 years; DPT at 3, 4 1/2 , 6, and 18 months; DT/Td at 6, 16, 26, 36, and 46 years; OPV at 3, 4 1/2 , 6, 18, and 20 months and 6 years; measles at 12 months; and mumps at 15 months.

BIBLIOGRAPHY

António B et al: *A situação social em Portugal*, 1960–1999, Instituto de Ciências Sociais da Universidade de Lisboa, Lisboa, 1999.

Aztak Daily, Beirut, March, 21, 2002.

Aztak Daily, Beirut, March 27, 2002.

Bernal H et al: Community health nursing in a former Soviet Union republic: a case study of change in Armenia, *Nurs Outlook* 43(2):78, 1995.

Hertzberg DL: The interdisciplinary team: the experience in the Armenian pediatric rehabilitation program: Project HOPE pediatric rehabilitation education program, *Holistic Nurs Practice* 7(4):42, 1993.

Jinbashian, S.: The woman of Armenia. *Hai Sird* 154:32–38, 2002.

Kalayjian AS: Mental health outreach program following the earthquake in Armenia, *Issues Ment Health Nurs* 15(6):533, 1994.

Ministry of Health of Armenia: *The present health status of the Republic of Armenia: its analysis and the rationales for its improvements and development.* Report presented in a conference in Yerevan, Armenia, May 1991.

Ugularian A: HIV/AIDS in the Transcaucasus, *Hai Sird* 155:10–12, 2001.

www.min-saude.pt

◆ AUSTRALIA (COMMONWEALTH OF)

MAP PAGE (856)

Nel Glass

Location: Australia consists of two land masses: the larger one is known as *mainland Australia* and the smaller is known as *Tasmania*. It has an area of 7,682,300 km² (2,965,368 square miles) and is situated in the Southern Hemisphere. Australia is surrounded by the Pacific Ocean on its east, the Southern Ocean on its south, the Indian Ocean on its west, and the Timor and Arafura Seas on the north. The closest neighboring country is Papua-New Guinea.

Major Languages	Ethnic Groups	Major Religions
English	White 95%	Anglican 26%
Aborigine	Asian 4%	Roman Catholic 26%
	Aborigine, other 1%	Other Christian 24%
		Other 24%

Australia is a multicultural country with many immigrants from non–English-speaking countries. Consequently, several other languages as well as English are spoken, predominantly by immigrants. Children can elect to learn languages such as Japanese, Italian, German, and French in schools. In aboriginal cultures, children and adults can choose to learn some of the major indigenous languages such as Ngaanyatjarra and Kariol. In the last 2 decades, although the trend toward cultural and racial diversity has increased, it is now feared that current world instability and associated terrorism may negatively affect current and future refugee status and immigration. It is clearly evident that a stronger sense of unified nationalism predominates in troubled times, and as a result many Australians tend to revert to and uphold Anglocentric and Eurocentric ways of living.

Health Care Beliefs: Active involvement; health promotion. Australians are the recipients of good health care services, and the adopted underlying national health trends are consistent with health developments and improvements occurring in other developed countries. Australians' life expectancy has increased since 1960; in 1990 it was ranked ninth and seventh out of 24 countries for females and males, respectively, which is better than the United States and United Kingdom and is almost equivalent to Canada. Ongoing health promotion campaigns aim to improve physical and emotional health through the media, community health centers, hospitals, the Australian government, and schools. As mentioned, Australia is becoming more holistic in its approach to health care. Therefore Australians now consider alternative health care treatments as valid in their overall approach to health care, and it is expected that individuals will take some level of responsibility for their own health care maintenance and improvement. In general, Australians are responding to this challenge well and are becoming more informed about their health status.

Predominant Sick Care Practices: Biomedical; alternative. When people are ill, most seek out traditional health care services, such as medical doctors and nurses in community health centers or hospitals. However, during the last 2 decades, trends toward using alternative health care are increasing. This may be partly the result of an increasing dissatisfaction with conventional medicine, specifically regarding medical outcomes and medical encounters. It may also be associated with a strong desire to view health holistically. Consequently, Australians are now choosing health care practitioners such as chiropractors, osteopathic doctors, masseurs, naturopathic doctors, and acupuncturists more regularly. Some choose medical doctors who combine alternative and conventional medicine in their health care approaches. For those with mental illness, most utilize counselors, crisis workers, and psychotherapists rather than the more traditional health workers such as social workers and medical doctors. Most patients are becoming more interested in understanding their physical and emotional health status and being part of decision-making regarding their own health care. Therefore health promotion is considered to be a significant component of health care for providers and consumers. Although less is known about mental illnesses in the general population, these illnesses are not usually feared—with the exception of suicide by young men, which is the leading cause of death in adolescents ages 15 to 24 years in Australia.

Ethnic/Race Specific or Endemic Diseases: The group of people with the most major health issues relative to specific diseases are the indigenous people, and their health status is generally considerably poorer than that of other Australians. The major indicators for this situation are attributed to their broader social and economic disadvantages, but the exact magnitude of their ill health is not known by precise statistical information. High-quality survey data are lacking because of uncertainties about the size and composition of the indigenous population, as well as incomplete death registrations, hospital records, cancer registries, and communicable disease notifications. However, it is known that life expectancy at birth for indigenous Australians from 1991 to 1996 was estimated to be 56.9 years for males and 61.7 years for females, which is considerably lower than the overall Australian estimates in 1996 of 75.6 years for males and 81.3 years for females in the general population. The figures for the Australian indigenous population are similar to those for Australians born at the beginning of the twentieth century, when life expectancy was 55 years for Australian males and 59 years for Australian females. In terms of overall mortality from 1995 to 1997, in the combined states of Western Australia, the Northern Territory, and South Australia, approximately three times more indigenous people died than did members of the total Australian population. The death rates for indigenous people have exceeded those for all Australians in every age group. The major causes of deaths among indigenous people are cardiovascular diseases, injuries, respiratory diseases, cancer, and diabetes, which combined accounted for approximately 75% of all deaths. Australia has not reached the epidemic proportions that were predicted for HIV/AIDS almost 2 decades ago. The World Health Organization's (WHO) estimated prevalence rate for HIV/AIDS in adults ages 15 to 49 is 0.15% (approximately 14,000 people). The estimated number of children from birth to 15 years living with HIV/AIDS is 140. Epidemiological data have revealed that although the HIV incidence peaked in 1984, it then decreased markedly. This trend continued in the 1990s, with a decrease in new AIDS cases from 954 in 1994 to 273 in 1998. As indicated, researchers predict that this proportion of decline will be sustained. At the end of 1998, approximately 10,800 people living in Australia were infected with HIV. It is also predicted that although the number of people living with HIV/AIDS may increase slightly, it is a good thing because it is a result of the introduction of antiretroviral therapy and its associated longer survival.

Health Team Relationships: In traditional health care settings such as hospitals, predominantly all health care team members are respected for their knowledge and decision-making skills. Although in some settings, health care workers may defer more to medical doctors' decision making, currently there is a greater level of equity than in previous years. Since the advent of the basic bachelor's degree qualification for all registered nurses (RNs) and the fact that many RNs have either clinical nurse specialist or clinical nurse consultant status (in New South Wales in particular, independent nurse practitioner status), nurses are significantly more recognized for their contributions to health care. Although older patients may defer more to medical doctors, most younger patients expect to have nurses either interdependently or solely involved in their health care decisions.

Families' Role in Hospital Care: During the last decade, it has become more acceptable to have significant others involved in health care decisions, regardless of whether these people are family members. It is not unusual for patients who are terminally or acutely ill to have a family member or significant other staying with them overnight in the hospital for support. This has been a common practice for the care of hospitalized children for more than 2 or 3 decades. It is acceptable for family members and significant others to bring food and drinks into health care settings, and visiting hours have extended to all day in many health care institutions.

Dominance Patterns: Although Australia is a patriarchal society, since the women's liberation movement of the late 1960s, women have become increasingly aware of their rights and are more assertive. As a result, a strong women's health movement developed in the country, and women have responded proactively to improve their health status. For example, in the past decade the media has paid significant attention to the nature, effects, and interventions related to domestic violence and sexual abuse for women and children.

Eye Contact Practices: Eye contact is considered an indicator of trust and effective interpersonal communication between individuals. Females tend to demonstrate and sustain eye contact more than males. However, in many indigenous cultures, it is considered rude for indigenous and non-indigenous people to make direct eye contact, so averting the gaze is recommended.

Touch Practices: The extent of touching generally indicates degrees of comfort between people, and it tends to vary according to gender. For women, regardless of sexual orientation, touching other women during interpersonal interactions is more frequent than with men. Women touch men less often because men are likely to perceive such behaviors as having sexual connotations. In contrast, heterosexual men touch other men less frequently than they touch women, because they may be perceived as gay.

Perceptions of Time: It is considered respectful to be punctual for formal professional appointments; however, people are much more relaxed about punctuality in social engagements. In general, people do not expect others to arrive at an exact time for such engagements—often, within 30 minutes of the set time is considered acceptable. Australians generally focus on living in the present, but future planning for holidays and travel are common in Australian culture.

Pain Reactions: Pain reactions vary by gender, and it is more socially acceptable for women to speak about their feelings. Therefore women disclose more openly the characteristics and levels of their pain than men. Australian culture is presently more accepting of men's discussing their feelings, rather than expressions of pain. In an effort not to appear "weak" many men appear more stoic than women.

Birth Rites: Birth is celebrated and valued enormously within Australian culture, and after a birth people focus more on the health of the newborn than its gender. Discussions concerning gender preference tend to be more implicit than explicit; nevertheless, fathers often have a desire to have a boy. Consequently, women in traditional families may keep having children until a boy is born. In an emerging trend, more women are having children outside of traditional families. For example, lesbians are having children more than ever before, and their partner is often both a support and co-parent. Many single heterosexual women also are choosing to have children regardless of whether they have a partner to help with the pregnancy and child rearing. It is also evident that fewer women are choosing abortion as an option for an unplanned pregnancy, and fewer single women are choosing adoption. In 1995, it was reported that 95.1% of births in New South Wales took place in hospitals. Notwithstanding, more women are having their babies at home and in birthing centers. Home births tends to occur in certain geographical areas such as the Far North Coast region of New South Wales, where there is a concentration of home birth midwives and a focus on sustaining greater degrees of autonomy in health and healing. During home births in particular, the mother is directly involved in major decisions regarding her antenatal and postnatal care, more so than during any other birthing practice. During hospital births, the focus is on doctor-directed care antenatally and post-natally. Although no specific diet is usually followed by pregnant women, it is common practice for women to strictly avoid alcohol and other drugs for the duration of the pregnancy.

Death Rites: Women tend to speak more openly about their feelings regarding death and dying, and men tend to remain more reserved about their feelings. In health care, family and significant others are considered important parts of the dying process if the person who is dying wants them to participate. Children are often encouraged to express their feelings through art. Although more people tend to die in hospitals, more people are choosing to die in their own homes. In acute care facility and hospital deaths, organ donation is becoming more common, but people tend to resist autopsies more because they are perceived as unnecessary. After a person's death, family members and significant others are encouraged to view the body as part of their own healing process. More people are cremated because of the ever-increasing space problem created by burying people. At funerals, more family members and significant others are participate in the actual ceremony—for example, by speaking about the person who has died or playing their favorite music. After the funeral service, which may or may not be held in a church, it is becoming more common for a wake to be held to celebrate the person's life.

Food Practices and Intolerances: During the last decade, Australians have focused more on healthy eating and are consuming less processed foods, saturated fats, and red meat. Although chicken, seafood, and potatoes are still very popular foods, most people tend to consume diets with a high fiber concentration and with a greater amount of fresh fruit and vegetables than in the past. However, children and adolescents tend to adopt a very stable meat-eating diet, with boys ages 14 to 16 eating more meat than girls in the same age group. During the summer months, with the increased temperatures, many Australians eat meals outdoors at home and in cafes and restaurants. In general, dining in Australia is very social and relaxed, and cafes and restaurants usually have outdoor eating areas, which are very popular with most diners. Alcohol is readily available and consumed regularly. More cafes and restaurants have adopted either a "bring you own" (BYO) alcohol policy or are licensed to serve alcohol. Beer and white wines are the most popular drinks.

Infant Feeding Practices: Consistent with an increasing public health focus, between 50% and 60% of mothers breast-feed their babies in the first 6 months. Moreover, a recent health policy, Health Throughout Life, indicated that the target for 2000 was to have 80% of women breast-feeding. Therefore health care organizations and associated professionals such as midwives, nurse lactation consultants, and medical doctors are strong advocates for breast-feeding. In some instances, health care professionals are even unsupportive of mothers who choose bottle-feeding. Nevertheless, the more common health care practice is to educate mothers on the benefits of breast-feeding and ultimately support her informed decision. Breast-feeding mothers are strongly encouraged to visit family and child health centers and nursing mothers' groups for support. However, social barriers often prevent breast-feeding from continuing for the appropriate duration. For example, it is socially unacceptable to breast-feed in public, and mothers who are paid employees find it difficult to accomplish, especially for those in lower socioeconomic groups. Breast-feeding practices have decreased in indigenous cultures where it was common for children to be breast-fed for 2 years. It is more prevalent for non-urban rather than urban Aboriginal mothers to breast-feed. In a research study with urban Aborigines in Melbourne, 98% of indigenous mothers began breast-feeding, but only 50% were still breast-feeding after 3 months and only 32% were breast-feeding after 6 months. More recently, another study with urban Aborigines in Brisbane found that although breast-feeding had been initiated by 59% of the mothers, after 4 months only 24.6% of the mothers were still breast-feeding.

Child Rearing Practices: Child rearing practices have been changing over the last 2 decades because of several interwoven social factors. First, the overall birth rate in Australia has declined in the last 2 decades from 1.97 in 1976 to 1980 to 1.76 in 1998. Women are giving birth later in life, and fertility is greatest in the 30- to 34-year group. Second, women's workforce participation is not decreasing—specifically, the married women's labor force participation has increased, and women are more involved in part-time work than full-time work. Third, many Australians have moved away from their parents and the geographical area where they lived as children, so the notion of the extended family being widely available for support with child rearing is diminishing. Consequently, child rearing in the immediate family, particularly of children younger than 5 years, rests with mothers rather than fathers. Because many mothers are now working several days per week, some of the child rearing is the responsibility of child-care workers. Child rearing in Australian families has become less strict, in that although discipline is still the norm, parents are more likely to reward positive behavior in children rather than punish them for negative behaviors. The old adage of "children should be seen and not heard" is not followed extensively, and parents concentrate more on improving family communication. Therefore the ways children are responding, thinking, and feeling are critical to family stability and growth.

National Childhood Immunizations: DTP at 2, 4, 6, and 18 months and 4 years; OPV at 2, 4, and 6 months and at 4 and 15 to 19 years; hep B at birth and at 2 and 6 months or three doses from 10 to 13 years; HIB at 2, 4, and 12 months; MMR at 12 months and 4 years, also women who have just given birth or are of child-bearing age; Td at 15 to 19 years, then 50 years. A major primary health program encourages parents and caregivers to immunize their babies. Currently, children have to be immunized or participate in an alternative program before they are able to enroll in school at age 5 years. In 2000, 249,600 live births were recorded in Australia, and of these births, 249,000 babies were immunized, resulting in a prevalence of 99.75%.

BIBLIOGRAPHY

Australia. In *Macquarie world atlas*, Macquarie University, Sidney, Macquarie Library Pty Ltd, 1994.

Australian Bureau of Statistics: *Australia now: health—suicide*, Canberra, Australia, 1999, Australian Bureau of Statistics.

Australian Bureau of Statistics and Australian Institute of Health and Welfare: *The health and welfare of Australia's Aboriginal and Torres Strait Islander peoples*, Canberra, Australia, 1999, Australian Bureau of Statistics.

Australian Institute of Health and Welfare: *Australia's Health 2000: the seventh biennial report of the Australian Institute of Health and Welfare*, Canberra, Australia, 2000, Australian Institute of Health and Welfare.

Baylor J: Conception through adolescence. In Crisp J, Taylor C, eds: *Potter and Perry's fundamentals of nursing* St Louis, Mosby, 2001.

Bottomley G: Identification: ethnicity, gender and culture, *J Intercult Stud* 18(1):41–49,1997.

De Looper M, Bhatia K: *International health: how Australia compares*, Canberra, Australia, 1998, Australian Institute of Health and Welfare.

Davis K, Glass N: Safe sex and student nurses in rural Australia: nurses' knowledge and practices: part 1, *Cont Nurs* 12(1), 2002 (in press).

Eastwood H: Why are Australian GPs using alternative medicine? Postmodernism, consumerism and the shift towards holistic health, *J Soc* 36(12):133–156, 2000.

Galligan B: Reconstructing Australian citizenship, *Quad* November (1):11–18, 1998.

Glass N: The contested work place: reactions to RNs doing degrees, *Coll* 5(1):24–31, 1998.

Glass N: *Interpersonal relating study guide*, Lismore, Australia, 1999, Southern Cross University.

Glass N: Speaking feminisms and nursing. In Greenwood J, ed: *Nursing theory in Australia: development and application*, Melbourne, 2000, Pearson Education.

Gracey M: Infant feeding and weaning practices in an urbanizing traditional, hunter-gatherer society, *Pediatrics* 5(2):1276–1277, 2000.

Gray E: Household work for men and women: implications for future childrearing decisions, *J Aust Stud* March, pp. 85–97, 2000.

Hayman N et al: Breastfeeding and weaning practices of an urban community of indigenous Australians, *Asia Pac J Clin Nutr* 9(3):232–234, 2000.

Holmes W et al: Initiation rate and duration of breastfeeding in the Melbourne Aboriginal community, *Aust NZ J Pub Health* 21:500–503, 1997.

Laing D et al: The development of meat-eating habits during childhood in Australia, *Int J Food Sc Nut* 50(1):29–38, 1999.

Mathers C et al: *The burden of disease and injury in Australia*, Canberra, Australia, 1999, Australian Institute of Health and Welfare.

McIntryre E et al: Determinants of infant feeding practices in a low socio-economic area: identifying environmental barriers to breastfeeding, *Aust NZ J Pub Health* 23(2):207–209, 1999.

Rissel C, Rowling L: Intersectoral collaboration for the development of a national framework for health promoting schools in Australia, *J Sch Health* 70(6):248–250, 2000.

Sargent M et al: *The new sociology for Australians*, ed 4, Sydney, 1997, Longman.

Scott JA: Attitudes toward breastfeeding in Perth, Australia—qualitative analysis, *J Nut Edu* 29(5):244–49, 1997.

Semenza N: Nutrition. In Crisp J, Taylor C, eds: *Potter and Perry's fundamentals of nursing*, St Louis, 2001, Mosby.

Siahpush M: Why do people favour alternative medicine? *Aust NZ J Pub Health* 23(3):266–271,1999.

Taylor L, Pym M: New South Wales midwives data collection 1995. *NSW Public Health Bulletin* December (7; suppl 2):1–39, 1996.

Taylor R, Salkeld G: Health care expenditure and life expectancy in Australia—how well do we perform? *New Doct* 66:13–20, 1996–1997.

United Nations AIDS and World Health Organization: *Epidemiological fact sheet on HIV/AIDS and sexually transmitted infection 2000 update*, Geneva, 2000.

United Nations: *World population prospects: the 2000 revision*, New York, 2000.

World Health Organization: *Vaccines, immunizations and biologicals: immunization profile Australia*, Geneva, 2001.

http://www.abs.gov.au/ausstats

◆ AUSTRIA (REPUBLIC OF)

MAP PAGE (860)

Consultant: Hartwig Huemer

Location: Austria is a landlocked nation in central Europe and includes much of the mountainous territory of the eastern Alps, with many snow fields, glaciers, and snowcapped peaks. Its boundaries are Germany and the Czech Republic to the north, Hungary and the Slovak Republic to the east, Slovenia and Italy to the south, and Switzerland and Liechtenstein to the west. The total land area is 83,858 km^2 (32,377 square miles). The climate is temperate—cool summers and cold winters with frequent rain in the low land and snow in the mountains. The Alps are to the west and south, and the land is flat or sloping to the north and east. The population of 8,131,111 is concentrated in the eastern lowlands, and 68% of the population is between 15 and 64 years. The gross domestic product (GDP) per capita is high at $23,400, and the literacy rate is 98%.

Major Languages	Ethnic Groups	Major Religions
German	German 98%	Roman Catholic 78%
	Croatian and Slovene 1%	Protestant 5%
	Other (Hungarian,	None, 17%
	Czech, Slovak, Roma) 1%	

More than 40,000 gypsies (Roma and Sinti) lived in Austria in the early 1990s. They do not tend to assimilate into Austrian life, living among themselves, often on the outskirts of cities.

Health Care Beliefs: Active involvement; health promotion important. Austrians take an active role in preventing disease. Since the mid 1980s, the Austrian health authority has introduced a program of preventive check-ups under the auspices of various health insurance plans.

Predominant Sick Care Practices: Biomedical. In 1993, Austria adopted a social welfare system of health care guaranteeing social security for all its citizens; 99% are covered by state-required health insurance. Austrians pay into compulsory health insurance plans funded by employers. The self-employed and retired Austrians qualify for less comprehensive plans. With the exception of a flat rate charged for filling prescriptions and 10% of the overall charge for hospitalization of dependents, inpatient and outpatient treatments are free for all individuals covered by the insurance plans. Austrian medicine is not "socialized" in the sense that physicians are not employees of the state. However, fees are regulated, allowing an exceptionally high degree of coverage for the population at large.

Ethnic/Race Specific or Endemic Diseases: Cardiovascular diseases, cancer, and respiratory and liver conditions are major causes of morbidity. The incidence of insulin-dependent and non-insulin-dependent diabetes is increasing. About 20% of women and 45% of men smoke more than 20 cigarettes a day. Most adults consume alcohol (mostly wine and beer) regularly, and the incidences of cirrhosis of the liver and cardiovascular disease are among the highest in Europe. Approximately 250,000 Austrians are alcoholics (twice as many of whom are men). After Hungary and Finland, Austria has one of the highest suicide rates (and men are three times more likely to commit suicide than women). Despite this statistic, the average life expectancy is high: 74.52 for males and 80.99 for women. Endemic diseases include goiter (particularly in the Alpine regions), Lyme borreliosis, Austrian tick-borne encephalitis (TBE), and echinococcosis (multilocularis). Austrians are also at risk for tularemia, visceral leishmaniasis (which is imported from Mediterranean regions), and hepatitis A, B, and C (which are largely imported by immigrants from areas of high endemicity). The World Health Organization's (WHO) estimated prevalence rate for HIV/AIDS in adults ages 15 to 49 is 0.23%. The estimated number of children from birth to age 15 years living with HIV/AIDS is less than 100. The estimated number of adults and children who have died since the beginning of the epidemic is 1200.

Health Team Relationships: Most physicians are in private practice but rely on contracts with specific insurance agencies, which regulate fees for services rendered. Nursing education is in the process of being reformed and is gradually moving from hospital-based training to university-based education. Dependence on the doctor is typical, initiative is not rewarded, and nurses are expected to follow orders for everything except basic nursing care.

Dominance Patterns: Austria had a patriarchal family structure based on gender-specific divisions of labor until the early 1990s, when marriage as a partnership became more common. In 1976 the law established the principle of equal rights and duties for married men and women that extended to child care. Discrimination against women is illegal, and the concept of equal rights extends to unpaid work by women in households and single parents. However, women still bear the major responsibility of child rearing and housework, and the income differential between the sexes is still significant. Highly educated women are more likely to be employed; 84% of women ages 30 to 55 with university degrees are employed.

Perceptions of Time: The past is valued. Traditional approaches to healing are still considered important, although Austrians emphasize biomedical approaches. Punctuality in business and social situations is valued.

Birth Rites: Families have an extensive support system. It is illegal for pregnant women to work 8 weeks before and after the birth, and they receive full net pay. Natural childbirth and the father's presence in the delivery room are becoming more popular. Parents of newborns can take 2 years of maternity or paternity leave, or it can be split between the parents. The parents receive monthly support during these 2 years, and they must be rehired at equal pay and status after this time. By 1991 the rate of first-born children born to single mothers was higher than 33%. This may reflect more tolerant attitudes and the fact that the social welfare system provides more benefits to single mothers than married ones. Infant mortality rates are 4.5 deaths per 1000 live births, and the fertility rate is 1.39 children born per woman.

Food Practices and Intolerances: The main meal is at midday; a light meal is eaten in the early evening, and another is consumed at the end of the day. The Austrian diet is high in fat, carbohydrates, and sugar, which contributes to the high incidence of cardiovascular disease and the steadily increasing incidence of diabetes.

Child Rearing Practices: Parents receive special payments from the government when their children are between 1 and 4 years. Child maintenance allowances are provided until children are 10 years, and then the allowances continue until the age of 21 years if the child is living at home, in school, or unemployed. Payments are also increased until age 27 years if the person is enrolled in vocational training or the university.

National Childhood Immunizations: DTP at 3, 4, 5, and 15 to 18 months; MMR at 14 months and 7 and 13 years for girls only; HIB at 3, 4, 5, and 15 to 18 months; hep B at 3, 4, and 15 to 18 months and 13 years; IPV at 3, 4, 5, and 15 to 18 months; OPV at 7 at 15 years; DT at 7 and 15 years; and, as recommended, middle European tick-borne encephalitis vaccine.

Other Characteristics: Austria is a transshipment point for Southwest Asian heroin and South American cocaine destined for Western Europe. It is reported that anti-Semitism still remains in as much as 25% of the population. Prejudice also extends towards the Roma (gypsies), Serbs, Turks, Poles, and Romanians.

ACKNOWLEDGMENT: Hartwig Huemer is a consultant on immunizations for Austria.

BIBLIOGRAPHY

Boerckel K: Childbirth education in Austria, *Int J Childbirth Educ* 6(1):39, 1991.

Clift JM: Nursing and health services in Austria, *Nurs Adm Q* 16(2):60, 1992.

Clift JM: Nursing education in Austria, Germany, and Switzerland, *IMAGE: J Nurs Sch* 29(1):89, 1997.

Haidinger G, Waldhoer T, Vutue C: The prevalence of smoking in Austria, *Prevent Med* 27(1):50, 1998.

http://lcweb2.loc.gov/cgi-bin/query/r?frd/cstudy:@field(DOCID+at0082)

http://www.impf.at/home/home.html?allg_impfungen.html

http://www.odci.gov/cia/publications/factbook/geos/au.html

◆ AZERBAIJAN (REPUBLIC OF)

MAP PAGE (861)

Lisa Natoli

Location: Azerbaijan (formerly the Azerbaijan Soviet Socialist Republic) is in Transcaucasia. It is bordered to the west by Armenia, to the south by Iran, to the north by Georgia and Daghestan, and to the east by the Caspian Sea. It is 87,000 km^2 (33,582 square miles), a total area that includes the autonomous republic of Nakhchivan and the disputed area of Nagorno-Karabakh. Despite being relatively small, cultural practices in Azerbaijan can be radically different in the various cities and regions. Differences also exist within regions, where people's attitudes toward issues may vary depending on geographical location and religious trends. (Two major orientations of Islam exist: Shiites and Sunnites.)

Major Languages	Ethnic Groups	Major Religions
Azeri (official)	Azeri 90%	Muslim 93%
Russian	Dagestani 3%	Russian Orthodox 3%
Armenian	Russian 3%	Armenian Orthodox 2%
Other	Other 4%	Other 2%

Azeri is very similar (about 80%) to Turkish. In recent years, its written nature has changed to Latin script, although most people other than primary school children prefer and better understand the Cyrillic script. This is an important consideration when developing health education materials for which the target and facilitator groups need to be considered. Russian is widely spoken, especially among professionals, although some people find this offensive because of the nature of the historical links with Russia.

Health Care Beliefs: Acute sick care; traditional. Azerbaijan is far from a health-promoting society. A man living in Baku (known for its mix of nationalities, religions, and idiosyncrasies between ethnic groups) once shared the following scenarios with this author to illustrate the perception of how these different groups might handle a potential health problem.

Abraham (i.e., a Jewish person) visits a hospital: "Please doctor, help! I'm afraid my heart's going to give me a pain in a few days."

Ivan (i.e., a Russian or Christian person) visits a hospital: "Please doctor, help! I have an awful heartache."

Mamed (i.e., an Azeri or a Muslim) is brought to a hospital on a stretcher, and his relatives say to the hospital personnel: "We're afraid he has already died!"

The health promotion activities that exist are largely driven by external agencies working in the country. Many local nongovernmental organizations have emerged since the fall of the Soviet Union, and are also becoming more involved in health promotion programs and campaigns, although they depend heavily on foreign financial support to do so. Mental illness, although poorly understood, is not feared. It is believed that the "source of mental illness is God's will." Heated cups are commonly placed on the skin in the home to treat less serious illnesses such as common colds and the flu.

Predominant Sick Care Practices: Biomedical; traditional; magical-religious. Azeris are very focused on seeking intervention (whether medical or traditional) for even the slightest complaint. Treatment is often quite invasive (i.e., multiple, self-administered, injectable drugs), lacking in a research base, tinged with mythology, and sometimes outright dangerous. Health-care–seeking behavior varies enormously between urban and rural areas. In Baku (the capital), people visit a doctor and then seek out traditional healers if they do not improve. In the rural regions, this situation is likely to be the opposite, and women in particular wear amulets to keep illness away. As a whole, Azeris are quite religious, and they usually pray that God will cure their ill health.

Ethnic/Race Specific or Endemic Diseases: Poverty, as it does in any country, has a dramatic impact on health. The transitional economy coupled with the effects of conflict has resulted in many more vulnerable groups with special needs. Azerbaijan has more than 600,000 internally displaced people (refugees within their own country) and approximately 7000 isolated older adults and socially vulnerable people. The World Bank estimates that more than 1 million people live below the poverty level, and about 20% of these families are in crisis. The unemployment level is conservatively estimated to be about 65%. Chronic and lifestyle-related diseases such as diabetes, heart disease, cancer, and smoking- and alcohol-related illnesses prevail. Domestic violence has become more of an issue and may be linked to the social consequences of unemployment, such as increased alcohol consumption. Tuberculosis (multiple resistant forms) affects all groups but especially those who are more vulnerable because of poor or cramped living conditions and malnutrition. Prisoners and internally displaced people who are living in camps are examples of such groups. The tuberculosis situation also worsened because an effective management strategy was not adopted in Azerbaijan until 2000. Sexually transmitted diseases are extremely prevalent, as are reproductive-health–related problems in women. Abortion is viewed as a common and acceptable form of contraception and is often performed using dangerous and unhygienic methods. In addition to the problems already mentioned, internally displaced and poor rural people have numerous more common and seasonally linked complaints. As might be expected, these people have illnesses related to hygiene and living conditions such as head lice and scabies, diarrhea, respiratory tract infections, and toxoplasmosis. Malaria was a significant problem in the mid-to late 1990s but has been well controlled by the Roll Back Malaria campaign. The International Federation of Red Cross and Red Crescent Societies cited 1400 cases among approximately 32,000 internally displaced people and the local surrounding community in 1996; in 2000, only 50 people in this same group (which had marginally reduced in size) had malaria. A malaria rate cannot be reported because of uncertainties about the total population. Vaccine-preventable diseases including measles, pertussis, diphtheria, and tetanus continue to affect children. As in other Central Asian, former Soviet countries, and Russia, the potential for human immunodeficiency virus (HIV) infection to become an explosive epidemic exists in Azerbaijan. Lack of awareness is a major risk factor for HIV transmission, particularly among teenagers, who in other countries are among the most frequently infected. Other important risk factors relate to the level of prostitution (which has increased since the transition), population movement driven by the economic situation in and out of the country (movement to areas of high HIV prevalence), the increasing prevalence of injected drug use, and the inadequate supply of disposable injecting equipment. The World Health Organization's (WHO) estimated prevalence rate for HIV/AIDS in adults ages 15 to 49 is 0.01%. The estimated number of children from birth to 15 years living with HIV/AIDS is less than 100. According to the National AIDS Control and Prevention Center, as of April 1, 2001, 287 cases of HIV were reported in Azerbaijan. However, because of the lack of general population surveillance, this is certainly a gross underestimate of the true situation.

Health Team Relationships: The health team is definitely doctor driven, and nurses are the subordinate group. This situation is reflected in the attitudes of patient groups toward these health professionals.

Families' Role in Hospital Care: Families have a very important role in the support and care of hospitalized relatives, a practice that is commonplace throughout the country, regardless of city or region. Close relatives (family members) visit two to three times a day. They always bring food and feel the responsibility to do so, even if food is provided by the hospital.

Dominance Patterns: Azerbaijan is clearly a male-dominated culture, with women being the submissive group. This dominance is exemplified by practices such as the woman walking a step behind her husband, or sitting in the back of the car, or in the case of younger women, being chaperoned by a male sibling when socializing. Men are the decision makers of the household, and generally this structure is accepted and unchallenged. However, in and around the capital of Baku women are becoming more liberated.

Eye Contact Practices: Eye contact practices do not seem to have cultural significance and are very individual.

Touch Practices: Azeris are warm people. In public, it is more acceptable for touching between the same sex rather than between males and females (although holding hands between men and women is common in the capital but very unlikely in rural areas). It is not uncommon to see female friends walking together arm in arm or males greeting each other with a kiss and embrace. This is not to say that homosexuality is culturally acceptable. In fact, it is poorly understood—kept "in the closet" and despised and even considered a disease that can be cured with injections and therapy.

Perceptions of Time: Although it varies among individuals, punctuality is generally not considered very important, although people are more likely to be on time for business appointments. If people are invited to a wedding party, only a few guests will arrive at the precise time detailed on the invitation. Traditions are respected and maintained, more so in the rural regions. Older people complain that the younger generation is losing their traditions. However, many traditional practices, such as arranged marriages (often to cousins), still occur, even though the young people involved may not approve of them. They often have little choice because of family and cultural pressures.

Pain Reactions: Pain tolerance is an individual issue, although women joke that men are the weaker sex and less tolerant of pain.

Birth Rites: A male first child is more celebrated than a daughter because if a female child is born next, she will have an older brother to watch over her. After birth, the mother does not take a bath, although showering is acceptable. For 40 days after the delivery, mothers do not wash clothes or participate in heavy work. They are cautious about cold water and cold in general and avoid certain foods believed to affect breast-feeding. In extremely religious, superstitious, or traditional families, women remain indoors for the first 40 days, and guests are not welcome during this time because they may bring an infection into the house.

Death Rites: On the one hand, death is a very painful experience for those who are grieving, but it is also accepted as a part of everyday life. Family members are present, but children are usually prevented from witnessing the dying process. After death, tents are erected in the yard or street outside the home of the family of the deceased for 7 days. During this time, men come and pay their respects, and women sit in the side rooms and serve food. Muslim corpses are buried with their heads facing Mecca, and if possible on the same day of the death. Only men visit the burial site, whereas women stay and mourn outside the home of the deceased. This is meant to protect women from the pain of grief. This writer was saddened to hear a story about a mother who had a stillborn child and was not allowed to see or hold her baby. (Obviously, these feelings are tinged with Western, personal, and cultural biases.) On the third, seventh, and fortieth day after death and at each anniversary, relatives give gifts (usually meat) to friends and neighbors on behalf of the deceased. Men in mourning do not shave for 40 days after the death of a loved one. Organ donation and autopsies are strictly forbidden. Autopsies are occasionally performed in criminal cases, but even under these circumstances they are not acceptable for the majority of the population.

Food Practices and Intolerances: People generally eat with a spoon or fork but rarely with a knife, and it is acceptable to eat with the hands. The cuisine has strong Iranian, Turkish, and Russian influences. Typical Azeri fare usually consists of a lot of meat—mainly lamb, beef, or mutton but not pork (although it is available in Western dining establishments). Bread is very important to the Azeris, and *tandir bread* and wafer-thin *lavash* is served with almost every dish. In Islamic cultures the respect for bread is real and heartfelt. Tradition says that to share bread with others opens your soul to one another, creating a bond not easily broken. A typical meal might begin with yogurt (*qatic*); Russian *stalichni* salad (potato with diced vegetables and mayonnaise); a plate of garnishes such as tomatoes, cucumbers, radishes, coriander, spring onions, basil, or whatever is in season; cheese (*pendir*); and perhaps some sausage. Fresh produce is very seasonal, so in winter months the selection changes considerably, and the cucumbers or other vegetables may be pickled. This is often followed by soup—some variation of meat, vegetables, and potatoes (or *dolvga* in summer, which is made with yogurt, spring onions, and cucumbers). *Dolma*, leaves stuffed with lamb and herbs, are common and *plov*, meat and rice pilaf, may also be served. *Shaslyk*, or kebabs (lamb, chicken, or *lule*—a minced kebab) follow and may include sturgeon (which is typically served with a delicious tart pomegranate sauce). Fruit juice, sweet carbonated drinks, beer, and vodka (essential for the endless toasts) are the typical drinks. Tea (*chai*) usually brings an end to the meal but is also the predominant social drink and is consumed in vast quantities throughout the day. Tea is the Azeri symbol of hospitality; it is drunk from pinch-waist glasses and sweetened with jam or sugar. It is customary to drink tea through sugar cubes placed between the teeth. On the street, newspaper cones of black seeds (*tum*), boiled chick peas, sunflower seeds, or nuts are often sold. Also popular are *pirozshki*—Russian-style cold donuts filled with spiced potato—and Azeri *kutab*—thin pancakes with spinach or meat—as are the Georgian *khajapyuri*, which are cheese pastries. Seasonal fresh fruit and dried fruits and nuts are common and cheap. Street vendors also sell cakes and pastries, fruit buns, spiced cookies, nut rolls, baklava, and halva.

Infant Feeding Practices: People in urban areas seem to have a good understanding of the importance of breast-feeding, and many agencies have worked doggedly during recent years to reinforce this idea. The United Nations Children's Fund (UNICEF) guidelines promote exclusive breast-feeding for the first 4 to 6 months and encourage weaning foods in addition until 2 years of age. However, in rural settings numerous misconceptions about infant feeding exist. For example, mothers often delay initiation of breast-feeding (i.e., do not give the baby colostrum) and introduce early supplementary fluids. Some mothers believe that giving sweet tea in the first month of life will protect the infant against hepatitis.

Child Rearing Practices: The level of discipline used with children is an individual family matter, although it is considered to be strict. Children may sleep with their parents, but this practice is often determined by living conditions. Mothers and grandmothers are responsible for disciplining children, although grandmothers are renowned, as they are in many cultures, for spoiling their grandchildren.

National Childhood Immunizations: BCG at birth; DTP at 2, 3, 4, and 18 months; OPV at birth ad 2, 3, 4, and 18 months; measles at 12 months; and DT at 6 years. Unfortunately, because of issues such as a lack of vaccines in rural regions, poor compliance with cold-chain practices, poor tracking of disease, and inaccurate childhood records, coverage is probably far less than official documents indicate. In recent years, Azeris have tended to react to outbreaks of diseases, such as diphtheria and measles, rather than work proactively to vaccinate the population adequately.

BIBLIOGRAPHY

Claeys P et al: Sexually transmitted infections and reproductive health in Azerbaijan, *Sex Trans Dis* 28(7):372, 2001.

Kasumov VK, Guseinov FZ: Current malaria situation in Azerbaijan, Meditsinskaia Parazitologiia January-March (1):18, 2001.

Miraldi E, Ferri S, Mostaghimi V: Botanical drugs and preparations in the traditional medicine of West Azerbaijan (Iran), *J Ethnopharmacol* 75(2–3): 77, 2001.

Vitek CR, Velibekov AS: Epidemic diphtheria in the 1990s, *J Infect Dis* 181(suppl 1):73, 2000.

◆ BAHAMAS (COMMONWEALTH OF)

MAP PAGE (858)

Virginia C.F. Ballance

Location: The Bahamas is an independent Commonwealth country composed of more 700 islands, of which approximately 22 are inhabited.

The Bahamas is between Florida's east coast, Cuba, and Haiti. Though small, the country is spread over a large region, and it has a total land area of 13,940 km^2 (5,382 square miles). The population is more than 300,000, of which more than 200,000 live on the urbanized New Providence Island, location of the capital and largest city, Nassau. Much of the rest of the population lives on Grand Bahama Island, the site of the country's second-largest city, Freeport. The balance of the people live on the sparsely populated outlying islands of the archipelago, islands called the *Family Islands*, or the *Out Islands*. The majority of inhabitants (about 85%) are of West African ancestry—descendants of slaves and freemen who were brought either directly from Africa to the Caribbean or from the United States during the American Revolution. The remainder of the people has European ancestry. Other significant immigrant groups to the Bahamas, in addition to those from Great Britain and the United States, have been Greeks, Lebanese, and Chinese.

Major Languages	Ethnic Groups	Major Religions
English (official)	Black 85%	Baptist 35%
Creole (among Haitian immigrants)	White 12%	Anglican 20%
	Other 3%	Roman Catholic 20%
		Other (Protestant, Greek Orthodox, Jewish) 25%

Health Care Beliefs: Active involvement; health promotion. Diet-related, noncommunicable diseases (e.g., obesity, cardiovascular diseases, type II diabetes, hypertension, stroke) are leading causes of mortality and morbidity among Bahamians. As a result of the country's shift from communicable to preventable noncommunicable diseases, the government has implemented health promotion and health education campaigns that have become a vital component of the health care system. The government has launched major initiatives to educate the public about HIV and AIDS and other sexually transmitted diseases, breast-feeding, family planning, drug abuse, and child abuse. Also promoted is attaining a healthy lifestyle through diet and exercise. Alcoholism and substance abuse (especially cocaine addiction) are the major behavioral disorders, followed by depression, psychotic, and psychosocial disorders. Mental illness is discussed openly, although some stigma is still attached to having been treated for a psychiatric illness. Some groups in society are fatalistic—ill health is "just one of those things." Others may believe that they have been "fixed" with a spell by someone who practices *obeah*, a form of witchcraft.

Predominant Sick Care Practices: Biomedical; traditional; magical-religious. Bahamians enjoy universal access to health care through government hospitals and clinics or from private hospitals and private doctors. Approximately 450 doctors are practicing in the public and private sectors. Nassau has much more adequate health services than the Family Islands. When ill, older Bahamians are inclined to self-medicate using "bush medicine"—homemade remedies of locally grown herbs and bark from trees. The plants used are determined by the ailment. These remedies may be bush tea infusions, poultices, and salves or simply bathing in water with herbs. Younger Bahamians tend to go to the pharmacy to purchase over-the-counter drugs to self-medicate before seeking medical attention. Therefore the pharmacist is frequently the first point of contact in the health care system. In the Family Islands, where there are no pharmacies, patients are first seen at the government clinic or by the local nurse.

Ethnic/Race Specific or Endemic Diseases: Sickle cell anemia is common in people of African origin. Although malaria and dengue hemorrhagic fever are not endemic to the Bahamas, given the large number of immigrants and frequent travel of Bahamians to areas where malaria and dengue are a problem (primarily Haiti and Cuba), Bahamians are at risk for these diseases. The main health problems among adult Bahamians are HIV and AIDS, accidental injuries, substance abuse, hypertension, diabetes, heart attacks, and cancer. High rates of hypertension and diabetes in the general population result from poor eating habits, a lack of exercise, and excessive alcohol consumption. However, Bahamians have a low rate of smoking—the Bahamas is the most smoke-free nation in the world. Obesity is emerging as a serious health issue; 48.6% of the population is classified as obese, and females (53%) are more likely to be obese than males (43%). Food-borne illnesses continue to plague the general population, a problem that is generally the result of eating contaminated conch (a mollusk) and poorly prepared foods sold at fairs and by street vendors. The World Health Organization's (WHO) estimated prevalence rate for HIV/AIDS in adults ages 15 to 49 is 4.13%. The estimated number of children from birth to 15 years living with HIV/AIDS is 150. AIDS is the leading cause of death among Bahamian men and women ages 15 to 44. From 1983 to 2000 a total of 3810 AIDS cases were reported, and an additional 4537 individuals were infected with HIV. The disease is primarily found in heterosexuals, with a male/female ratio of 1.2:1. The Bahamas has stringent HIV/AIDS reporting procedures and vigilantly follows up new cases. All women reporting to government clinics for antenatal care are tested for HIV infection.

Health Team Relationships: In the government-run hospitals and private sector, the doctor dominates the health team. In the government community health clinics and some of the private walk-in clinics, nurse practitioners primarily provide the services. Overall, nurse-doctor relationships are good. Nurses tend to dominate the wards in the hospital. Patients' attitudes toward doctors and nurses vary. In a small country such as the Bahamas, people tend to be very familiar with one another because of family ties.

Families' Role in Hospital Care: Families do not stay with patients in the hospital. However, in the public hospital it is quite common for families to bring patients food from home or outside restaurants, fruit baskets, flowers, or bottled water and other drinks. In the public hospital, male nurses and male family members are not allowed in the labor and delivery rooms. Visiting hours are observed; however, mothers are permitted to stay longer in the pediatric wards.

Dominance Patterns: Although Bahamian society is matriarchal and the preponderance of homes are headed by single mothers, men still dominate the professional and political arenas.

Eye Contact Practices: Direct eye contact is not an issue in Bahamian society. Bahamians are very friendly and are always willing to chat and talk or greet friends and family.

Touch Practices: Bahamians have no particular rules about touching. They shake hands, embrace, or kiss when greeting others.

Perceptions of Time: In the normal daily life, arriving on "Bahamian time," or later than scheduled, is quite acceptable. Bahamians often pine for days gone by and the loss of their traditions and culture. The Bahamas of the twenty-first century is heavily influenced by its closest neighbor, the United States, through television, cable, the Internet, newspapers, and increasingly by family links. Many Bahamians seek higher education in the United States and return with the social mores of American culture.

Pain Reactions: Reaction to pain is very individual. Some people are naturally rather dramatic and may exaggerate their pain, whereas older men may be much more stoic. Overall, Bahamians are not shy about showing their emotions.

Birth Rites: As do people of many other cultures, Bahamians have many superstitions about pregnancy and birth, predictions of the sex of the infant, and protection of an unborn child from harm. All children are now born in hospitals or clinics and unless complications occur during the delivery, mothers are discharged within a day or two. All new mothers are visited at home by a community health nurse and attend community health clinics for follow-up education. Bahamians have no particular preference for gender, although boys carry on the family name.

Death Rites: Death is accepted as part of life and when possible, family members are present for the funeral and offer prayers for the soul of the family member. Organ donation is not widely practiced in the Bahamas, and no stigma is attached to performing autopsies.

Food Practices and Tolerances: The Bahamian diet is high in sodium, simple sugars, and fat. More than half the population is overweight. The full figure, which Bahamians call a "Gussy-mae" or "solid" figure, is the norm. The diet is dominated by rice cooked with peas, bread, and fried chicken, followed by pork and beef. Consumption of seafood and fish is relatively low in comparison; they are primarily eaten at Christmas or on special occasions. Overall, consumption of fruits and vegetables is relatively low. A typical meal might consist of fried or baked chicken (or pork spare ribs), peas and rice, macaroni and cheese, cole slaw, and baked potatoes or boiled corn. Breakfast might consist of sardines or corned beef hash and grits. Another favorite is pea soup with ham and dumplings. Fast food restaurants, such as McDonald's, Wendy's, Kentucky Fried Chicken, and Burger King, are heavily patronized. Utensils are used for eating.

Infant Feeding Practices: Breast-feeding is not the norm among Bahamian women. Although many mothers (approximately 60%) attempt breast-feeding, more than 90% introduce bottle-feeding by the end of the first week of the infant's life, and often before leaving the hospital or clinic.

Child Rearing Practices: Generally, Bahamian children are raised under the edict, "spare the rod, spoil the child." In single-parent families, the mother, grandmother, or legal guardian is responsible for discipline. Children tend to be very quiet and polite around adults in authority such as school teachers or police officers.

National Childhood Immunizations: DTP at 2, 4, 6, and 15 months; OPV at 2, 4, and 6 months and 4 years; MMR at 1 and 4 years; HIB at 2, 4, and 6 months and 4 years; and DT at 4 years. The community health clinic system provides free childhood vaccinations.

BIBLIOGRAPHY

Bahamas handbook and businessman's annual, Nassau, Bahamas, 2002, Etienne Dupuch Jr Publications.

Craton M, Saunders G: Islanders in the stream: a history of the Bahamian people, Athens, Ga, 1992–1998, University of Georgia Press.

Pan American Health Organization: *Bahamas: basic country health profiles, summaries 1999*. http://www.paho.org/english/SHA/prflbah.htm (January 22, 2002).

World Health Organization (June 2000): *Epidemiological fact sheets by country-Geneva*. Retrieved March 1, 2002, from http://www.unaids.org/hivaidsinfo/statistics/june00/fact_sheets/index.html

World Health Organization (2001): *WHO vaccine-preventable diseases: monitoring system, Geneva*. Retrieved March 1, 2002, from http://www.who.int/vaccines/

◆ BAHRAIN (KINGDOM OF)

MAP PAGE (864)

Abdulrahman Obaid Musaiger

Location: In 2002 the state of Bahrain became the Kingdom of Bahrain, which consists of an archipelago of about 36 small islands and is situated halfway down the Arabian Gulf about 24 km from the eastern coast of Saudi Arabia. The total land area is 710 km^2 (274 square miles). Based on the latest census, the population of Bahrain is 650,604; 62.4% are Bahraini, and 37.6% are non-Bahrainis who are mainly from the Indian subcontinent, Iran, the Far East, and Western countries.

Major Languages	Ethnic Groups	Major Religions
Arabic (official)	Bahraini 62%	Islam (Sunni and Shia) 98%
English	Asian 32%	
Farsi	Other Arab groups 4%	
Urdu	Other 2%	

English is widely used in business and banking, and Farsi (Persian) is used by families with origins in Iran.

Health Care Beliefs: Active involvement; traditional. Most Muslim nationals believe in the concept of envy as a cause of illness. For example, if someone casts an "evil eye" toward another because of jealousy, the recipient may develop an illness, a serious disease, or some misfortune as a result. If the affected person strongly believes that the cause of the disease or misfortune is a result of another's envy rather than of physiological factors, the person is likely to go to a healer, or *shaikh*, who will use the words of the holy Koran for treatment.

Predominant Sick Care Practices: Biomedical; magical-religious. Bahrain has two systems for health care delivery: primary and secondary. The government of Bahrain manages and finances 75% of the national health care system provided by public hospitals and health centers. The other 25% of the funding is obtained through various sources provided by the Ministry of Health. Health care services are available for everyone, even those in rural areas. The government of Bahrain provides free primary, secondary, and tertiary health care for all nationals. Non-nationals are also eligible for care at significantly subsidized rates. The private system is administered through private hospitals, clinics, and polyclinics, and generates its own income through services provided to the public. Traditional medicine is rarely practiced for severe illnesses, but when a minor disease develops, some people prefer traditional healing.

Ethnic/Race Specific or Endemic Diseases: More recently, noncommunicable diseases such as heart disease, diabetes, obesity, dental carries, and some types of cancer have become the major public health problems. Diseases of the circulatory system are the major cause of death (30% of deaths), followed by neoplasms (13%), conditions originating in the perinatal period (8%), diseases of the respiratory system (6%), and injury and poisoning (6%). Changes in dietary habits and in lifestyle have also had a significant impact on the nutritional and health status of the community. Whereas infectious disease and lack of proper nutrition were previously considered the main health problems, no cases of diphtheria, pertussis, neonatal tetanus, or poliomyelitis have been reported since

1990. Although gonococcal infections dropped markedly (from 65.6 per 100,000 in 1990 to 34 per 100,000 in 2000), syphilis incidence increased to 220 cases (31.8 per 100,000) in 2000 from 37 cases (7.4 per 100,000) in 1990. Pulmonary tuberculosis incidence also substantially increased to 160 cases (23.2 per 100,000) in 2000 as compared with 91 cases (18.1 per 100,000) in 1990. The World Health Organization's (WHO) estimated prevalence rate for HIV/AIDS in adults ages 15 to 49 is 0.15%. WHO has no estimates for children from birth to 15 years. Life expectancy increased by 14.3 years for males and 15 years for females between 1965 and 1998 and was reported to be 71.1 and 75.3 years, respectively, in 1998.

Health Team Relationships: Nurses and doctor work together compatibly in heath services. The doctor is responsible for diagnosis and surgery, whereas the nurse provides support for most other needs. Doctors usually have at least a bachelor's degree in medicine and more. Nurses can either have a diploma from high school or a bachelor of science in nursing.

Families' Role in Hospital Care: Family members are usually not allowed to stay with patients in hospitals. However, most hospitals have some private rooms where one or two members of the family can stay with patients and take care of them (under certain circumstances). In pediatric wards, many hospitals allow mothers to stay with their children, especially if the children are quite young. Food from outside of the hospital is not permitted for patients on special diets (e.g., those with diabetes, cancer, or heart disease) but is allowed for other patients. Many families bring comforting traditional foods for their family members.

Dominance Patterns: The participation of women in social and economic life is increasing dramatically. Employed Bahraini women now account for 23.5% of the total working population. Women have recently been given the right to vote, a privilege formerly given only to men. Women play an active role in the lifestyle of the family, especially in feeding and taking care of children. Housemaids, particularly from India, Sri Lanka, and the Philippines also play an important role in taking care of children and house management in most middle- and upper-class families. A considerable discrepancy in illiteracy rates still exists—7.5% of males versus 17% of females are illiterate.

Eye Contact Patterns: Direct eye contact from nonrelated males to women, especially when they are with their husbands, is not acceptable. This avoidance of eye contact is seen as a sign of respect. Women are also not expected to make direct eye contact with men other than their husbands or close relatives.

Touch Practices: Physical touching conveys a type of congenial, in-depth feeling among friends, but people only touch members of the same sex. It is not acceptable for men to touch women or vice versa.

Perceptions of Time: Because of high levels of education and awareness, time perception in Bahrain is much more similar to Western standards. Being punctual is more important than it is in many other Arab countries.

Pain Reactions: When men or women have pain, they usually first seek help from other family members. Further decisions about seeking treatment are then made based on the severity and cause of the pain.

Birth Rites: Bahrainis have no taboos associated with pregnancy. After birth, special foods (*hesso* and *gellab*) are usually given to mothers with the belief that they will help them regain good health and strength. Hesso consists of eggs, watercress seeds, and fat, whereas gellab consists of wheat flour, watercress seeds, fat, and spices. However, many women no longer believe in the efficacy of these traditional foods. Bahrainis have no preference for the gender of newborns. When women get married, their children have the family name of the husband. As a result of improvements in socioeconomic conditions and health services, infant mortality decreased from 20.2 in 1990 to 8.6 in 2000. Fertility rates were consistent at 2.5 children per woman in 2000 (3.3 for Bahrainis and 2 for non-Bahrainis) compared with 3.4 in 1990 (3.9 for Bahrainis and 2.7 for non-Bahrainis).

Death Rites: When a family member dies, the family usually receives condolences and consolation from others for 3 days either in the home of a family member or in a hall linked to the mosque. Women have a separate place to receive condolences from other women. Organ donation has become extremely acceptable because Islamic leaders have increased public awareness about this topic.

Food Practices and Intolerances: Food habits have become more diversified. Breakfast usually consists of eggs, cheese, legumes, bread, jam, fermented fish (*mehiawa*) and many other foods. At lunch, rice with lamb or beef, chicken, or fish, is common. On the weekend (Thursday and Friday), many families prefer to have lunch somewhere other than the home. Supper is usually diversified, and it is common for families to purchase food from outside vendors such as from local and Western fast food establishments. Food habits have changed dramatically during the past 40 years as a result of the increase in the country's income from oil revenue. The consumption of traditional foods such as fish, rice, dates, and vegetables has gradually decreased, and Bahrainis are consuming more beef, chicken, eggs, milk, fat, sugar, and canned and fast foods.

Infant Feeding Practices: Prolonged breast-feeding lasting 2 years, which is promoted by Islamic culture, is no longer practiced. Most women breast-feed their infants for 3 to 9 months and begin to introduce solid foods at 3 to 4 months. The majority of women practice mixed feeding (breast-feeding and bottle-feeding).

Child Rearing Practices: Child rearing practices are very permissive today, but still remain within the cultural context and customs of Bahrain. For example, most families do not allow their children, especially their girls, to be outside of the home unattended in the evening. Physical punishment of children has decreased but is still practiced in some families of lower social class.

National Childhood Immunizations: BCG at birth for Bahrainis, and 5 to 6 years (school entry) for non-Bahrainis; DTP at 2, 4, 6, and 18 months and 5 to 6 years; OPV at 2, 4, 6, and 18 months and 5 to 6 years; hep B at 2, 4, 6, and 18 months; HIB at 2, 4, 6, and 18 months; MMR at 12 months, 5 to 6 years, and 12 years; Td at 13 years, also for Haj pilgrims and after injury; and TT for pregnant women. Overall, immunization coverage is increasing in Bahrain. In 2000 the immunization coverage reached 95% for BCG, 97% for the third dose of DTP, third dose of oral polio, and third dose of hepatitis B because about 85% of all registered live births are immunized free of charge by the public health centers. The coverage of the first dose of MMR reached 98.4%, with 87.4% provided by public health centers. Coverage of the second dose of MMR reached 92.4%, with 87.4% provided by public health centers. In addition, 71.8% of pregnant women received two doses or more of TT (65.5% provided by the public health centers).

BIBLIOGRAPHY

Ministry of Health: *Health statistics*, 2000, Bahrain, 2001.
Central Statistics Organization: *Results of 2001 census*, Bahrain, 2002.
Musaiger AO: *The state of food and nutrition in Bahrain*, Riyadh, Saudi Arabia, 1993, United Nations Children's Fund—Gulf Area Office.
Musaiger AO: The state of nutrition in Bahrain, *Nutrition Health* 14:63–74, 2000.

◆ BANGLADESH (PEOPLE'S REPUBLIC OF)

MAP PAGE (866)

Amal K. Mitra

Location: Bangladesh (formerly East Pakistan) was liberated from Pakistan in December 1971 after a 9-month war. It is bordered by India on the north, east, and west and by the Bay of Bengal and Myanmar (formerly Burma) on the south. The area is 144,000 km^2 (51,264 square miles), with a total estimated population of more than 131 million (approximately half of the U.S. population). The capital is Dhaka. Bangladesh, a country of rivers, has seven major rivers: Padma, Meghna, Jamuna, Brahmaputra, Madhumati, Surma, and Kushiara. Bangladesh is low lying (less than 183 m [600 feet]) and subject to tropical monsoons, frequent floods, and famine. The average rainfall is between 47 and 136 inches. Bangladesh is one of the poorest countries in the world, with 36% of its population living below the national poverty line and a gross national per capita income of $370 (U.S. dollars).

Major Languages	Ethnic Groups	Major Religions
Bangla (Bengali; official)	Bengali 98%	Muslim 83%
English (widely spoken by literate)	Bilhari and tribal 2%	Hindu 16%
		Christian and

Health Care Beliefs: Passive role; acute sick care. Illness is considered to be caused by a curse. Rural Bangladeshis seek an explanation at several levels for unexpected life events: factors such as fate, inherited qualities, the environment, and individual behavior. For example, people usually consider miscarriages or stillbirths to be a result of "bad eye" (*ku najar*) of evil spirits (*jeen, bhut*). This is the same phenomenon as the "evil eye" spoken of in other cultures where a person with bad intent looks at a potential victim and causes illness. However, modern medicine is growing in popularity among literate and urban people, especially for acute illnesses.

Predominant Sick Care Practices: Biomedical; magical-religious. Muslims and Hindus in poor communities and in villages still believe in wearing amulets (*tabij*) as a complementary or an alternative method to cure diseases or protect themselves from illnesses. Most people believe in the efficacy of allopathic medicine, although they also use complementary and alternative treatments including homeopathy, ayurvedic medicine, and spiritual treatments. Those who are illiterate continue to believe that evil spirits and God's will can cause illness, and they prefer injections and intravenous fluid infusions to cure illnesses. Total withdrawal of foods or use of easily digested cereals (*sagu*) or barley water are common practices during fever. Faith healers, such as magic healers (*ojha*) and mystical mendicants (*fakirs*), exorcise the evil air and offer consecrated water (*pani para*) for the relief of symptoms. Poor people may prefer fakirs, herbalists (*kobiraj*), and ojhas because these healers spend time with patients and do not always charge a fee. In villages, where the majority of the people live, untrained rural practitioners outnumber qualified allopathic doctors. However, government health facilities offer modern treatments in every town and city. No provisions have been made for health insurance for the people, and those visiting government health centers and hospitals pay a nominal fee per visit. On the other hand, those who can afford to do so pay a high cost for health care services in private clinics. People can also obtain medicines at pharmacies without having a prescription.

Ethnic/Race Specific or Endemic Diseases: Food- and water-borne diseases such as diarrhea, dysentery, parasitic diseases, typhoid fever, and hepatitis are common among all age groups. Acute respiratory tract infections and diarrhea are the major causes of death in children younger than 5 years. Among the insect-borne diseases, malaria is highly prevalent, especially in Chittagong Hill Tracts, Sylhet, and Mymensingh. Chloroquine-resistant malaria is a growing problem in the country, and a recent upsurge of dengue fever caused many deaths. Another emerging disease that has become a disaster in the country is arsenic poisoning. Arsenic concentrations in tube-well water have been found to be higher than the maximum permissible limit of 0.05 mg/L, affecting almost half of the total population. Malnutrition is a significant health problem, affecting at least 56% of children younger than 5 years. Deficiency disorders, including vitamin A, iodine, and iron deficiencies, are serious public health problems. About 30,000 children younger than 6 years become blind each year because of vitamin A deficiencies alone, and poor nutritional status and severe infections are important predictors. In 1973 the government of Bangladesh instituted a plan for distributing large doses of vitamin A capsules to all children between 1 and 6 years at 6-month intervals. More than 60% of the Bangladeshi population has biochemical iodine deficiencies, prompting health authorities to encourage the use of iodized salt. The problem of goiter caused by iodine deficiencies is primarily clustered in the northern districts and flood-prone areas of the country. The World Health Organization's (WHO) estimated prevalence rate for HIV/AIDS in adults ages 15 to 49 is 0.02%. The estimated number of children from birth to 15 years living with HIV/AIDS is 130. National surveillance from 1989 through 1996 reported 1.13 people with HIV per 1000 people in Bangladesh, which makes it one of the lower prevalence countries in the world. According to 1999 estimates, a total of 13,000 people were living with HIV/AIDS, and 1000 people had died of the disease. The rate among male heterosexuals was significantly higher than that for females (3.4 per 1000 versus 0.29 per 1000, respectively), and infected people were concentrated in two districts, Sylhet and Chittagong, which border India and Myanmar, respectively.

Dominance Patterns: In this patriarchal society, women's activities may be severely restricted, and they are often physically secluded as a result. Both years of schooling received and socioeconomic status are poorer among women than among men. According to the World Bank report of 2000, illiteracy rates are considerably higher among women than men (70.1% versus 47.7%). Unlike most countries in the world, life expectancy is slightly shorter among women than men in Bangladesh (60.33 for women versus 60.74 in men). An indicator of poor women's health is their high maternal mortality rate. About 60,000 women of reproductive age (ages 15 to 44 years) die each year, 25% of whom die from pregnancy complications. The use of contraceptives, however, has increased in recent years, providing women with greater control over reproduction.

Birth Rites: The umbilical cord may be cut with the clean inner strip of a bamboo stalk. Rural, traditional custom requires the mother to reach a water source unaided to wash herself and her clothing immediately after birth. After delivery, numerous rituals are performed. Plum branches are placed on the door of the home to protect against evil spirits, and the Muslim holy Iman chants the birth announcement. The mother chants prayers and stays indoors, and only the husband may visit. Traditionally, this rest period of 7, 21, or even 40 days for the mother after birth is practiced, but depends on the economic status and traditional values of the family.

Death Rites: A holy Iman does not have to be present at death; however, a Muslim may recite the declaration of the faith: "There is no God but God, and Muhammad is his messenger." Family members wash the body according to Islamic tradition. Autopsy is uncommon because the deceased must be buried intact. For Muslim burial the body is wrapped in special pieces of cloth and buried in the ground without a coffin. Muslim tradition forbids organ donations or transplants. Hindus cremate the bodies of everyone except for children ages 10 or younger, whom they bury.

Food Practices and Intolerances: Rice is the staple food. Most people eat two big meals of rice, vegetable curry, and lentil (*daal*) soup. Muslims eat beef but do not eat pork or turtle meat. Hindus do not eat beef, and certain castes of Hindus eat pork. Some food items, such as eggs and meats, are considered harmful during illness. Cow's milk is the most common cause of food intolerance in infants and young children.

Infant Feeding Practices: Breast-feeding is almost universal and usually continues to some degree until the child is 1 year of age. For the first 3 days, the infant also is spoon-fed sugar water. Families who are economically deprived breast-feed infants until introducing supplementary foods, and then the male infants may receive higher quality supplementary nutrition. Sixty percent of mothers bottle-feed using commercial milk and starchy food by the time the infant is 3 months, and 80% do so by 5 months. This additional food usually is provided in a diluted form. Family food such as rice and vegetables are introduced between 6 months and 1 year.

Child Rearing Practices: Because of economic and cultural influences, boys receive preferential treatment in terms of family food allocation and health care practices, resulting in an increased mortality rate in girls after the neonatal period ends. Recent studies show that two times more girls than boys die as a result of delayed initiation of care at home, and prolonged illnesses before hospital admission.

National Childhood Immunizations: BCG at birth; DPT at 6, 10, and 14 weeks; OPV at 6, 10, and 14 weeks and 9 months; measles at 9 months; TT at 15 to 49 years, + 1 month + 6 months + 1 year + 1 year. Bangladesh adopted the Universal Program on Immunization recommended by WHO and the United Nations Children's Fund (UNICEF). Women of child-bearing age and pregnant women should be given two doses of TT during the second or third trimester of pregnancy to protect infants from tetanus. The last dose of TT should be 1 month before delivery. Bangladesh is also one of the participating countries in Southeast Asia for the Global Polio Eradication Initiative of WHO. According to WHO, the total number of confirmed polio cases in Bangladesh dropped from 393 in 1999 to 198 in 2000 to 0 in 2001.

BIBLIOGRAPHY

Ahmed SM et al: Gender, socioeconomic development and health-seeking behaviour in Bangladesh, *Soc Sci Med* 51(3):361–371, 2000.

Bhuiya A, Streatfield K: Feeding, home-remedy practices, and consultation with health care providers during childhood illness in rural Bangladeshk, *J Diarrhoeal Dis Res* 13(2):106–112, 1995.

Bloem MW et al: The role of universal distribution of vitamin A capsules in combating vitamin A deficiency in Bangladesh, *Am J Epidemiol* 142:843–855, 1995.

Fauveau V, Chakraborty J: Women's health and maternity care in Matlab. In Fauveau V, ed: *Matlab: women, children and health, ICDDRB*, pp. 109–132, 1994.

Islam M et al: HIV/AIDS in Bangladesh: a national surveillance, *Int J STD AIDS* 10:471–474, 1999.

Koenig MA, D'Souza S: Sex differences in childhood mortality in rural Bangladesh, *Soc Sci Med* 22(1):15–22, 1986.

Mitra AK et al: Predictors of serum retinol in children with shigellosis, *Am J Clin Nutr* 68(5):1088–1094, 1998.

Mitra AK, Kabir I, Khan MR: Severe urticarial eruption in an infant, *Indian Pediatr* 28:787–789, 1991.

Mitra AK, Rahman MM, Fuchs GJ: Risk factors and gender differentials for death among children hospitalized with diarrhea in Bangladesh, *J Health Popul Nutr* 18(3):151–156, 2000.

Smith AH, Lingas EO, Rahman M: Contamination of drinking water by arsenic in Bangladesh: a public health emergency. *Bull WHO* 78:1093–1103, 2000.

Yusuf HK et al: Iodine deficiency disorders in Bangladesh, *Indian J Pediatr* 63(1):105–110, 1996.

World Health Organization (June 2000): *Epidemiological fact sheets by country, Geneva*. Retrieved March 1, 2002, from http://www.unaids.org/hivaidsinfo/statistics/june00/fact_sheets/index.html

World Health Organization (2001): *WHO vaccine-preventable diseases: monitoring system, Geneva*. Retrieved March 1, 2002, from http://www.who.int/vaccines/

◆ BARBADOS

MAP PAGE (858)

Anselm Hennis

Location: Barbados is the most easterly island in the Caribbean archipelago, has a total land area of approximately 430 km^2 (166 square miles), and is 483 km north of Venezuela. Based on the census conducted in 2000, preliminary reports estimate the total population at 268,792; 52% is female. Barbados was ranked 31 in the Human Development Index for 2001, which is the highest ranking for a developing country. Current life expectancy at birth is 76.6 years (compared with 76.8 years in the United States), and the gross domestic produce (GDP) per capita is $14,353 (U.S. dollars). The adult literacy rate exceeds 97%, and more than 75% of households have telephones.

Major Languages	Ethnic Groups	Major Religions
English	Black African 93%	Protestant 67%
	Mixed (White and Black) 4%	Roman Catholic 4%
	White, other 3%	None or other 29%

Health Care Beliefs: Active involvement; health promotion important. Given the fact that the majority of illnesses in the population are related to lifestyle, the Ministry of Health, the Pan American Health Organization, the Barbados Association of Medical Practitioners, the University of the West Indies, the Heart Foundation of Barbados, and the Diabetes Association of Barbados, among others, are making significant efforts to promote changes in health behaviors. Although the people have widespread knowledge about the benefits of dietary modifications and increased physical activity to prevent chronic, noncommunicable disease, much more needs to be done before public health benefits will become apparent in the population. Indigenous practices such as using herbs for the treatment of illness are more likely to be practiced by the older members of society, although they are frequently used in conjunction with prescribed therapies. Generally, the people fear mental illness. Anxiety neuroses are quite common, accounting for the majority of psychiatric disorders causing people to seek help. Data about schizophrenia indicate an incidence rate of about 2.8 per 10,000, which is consistent with other Caribbean countries and somewhat higher than European rates.

Predominant Sick Care Practices: Biomedical; traditional. The island's easily accessible health care system includes a tertiary care hospital and an island-wide ring of nine primary care polyclinics, all managed by the government and providers of free care to the public. In addition, drugs listed on the national formulary are free for individuals in the public sector, whereas formulary drugs are also free privately to all nationals for chronic diseases, including diabetes, hypertension, asthma, cancer, and epilepsy. Approximately 400 doctors live on the island, and the people seek medical care from this group.

Ethnic/Race Specific or Endemic Diseases: Certain diseases are more likely in particular ethnic groups. For example, sickle cell disease occurs almost exclusively in individuals of African origin, but the overall number of cases is relatively low. The principal illnesses are the chronic, noncommunicable diseases, including cardiovascular diseases and diabetes. In 1999, diseases of the pulmonary circulation and other forms of heart disease, cerebrovascular disease, diabetes mellitus, and ischemic heart disease were ranked (in descending order) as the principal causes of death in Barbados. Malignancies were ranked as the fifth leading cause of death. The World Health Organization's (WHO) estimated prevalence rate for HIV/AIDS in adults ages 15–49 is 1.17%. The estimated number of children from birth to 15 years living with HIV/AIDS is less than 100. From the beginning of the epidemic until December 2000, a total of 2379 individuals have been infected with HIV. Among those whose gender was known, almost two thirds (64.2%) were male. The cumulative number of AIDS cases recorded during this period was 1354, and 1071 people died. During 2000, 178 new cases of AIDS were reported; 136 were male and 42 were female. The impact of HIV infection is significant—it now accounts for almost 80% of deaths among males ages 15 to 45 years. Between 1997 and 1999, HIV/AIDS was one of the five principal causes of death among children younger than 5 years (although it accounted for only three deaths).

Health Team Relationships: Health teams are doctor driven, with relationships being influenced by factors such as the clinical setting and the personalities of those involved. In other words, the doctors tend to dominate, whereas nurses play a greater role in the provision of care in public health settings.

Families' Role in Hospital Care: Families do not stay with hospitalized relatives, and it is considered inappropriate to bring outside food to patients.

Dominance Patterns: Although males dominate this culture, women play a principal role in the household. They are often role models and major breadwinners in families in which men "visit, " the term used for single female-headed households.

Eye Contact Practices: People do not avoid eye contact, and they are likely to assert themselves regardless of their gender or status.

Touch Practices: Excessive touching is unacceptable. Touching usually occurs only when individuals greet others, and generally only involves the hands.

Perception of Time: Consistent with the easygoing Caribbean ethos, the people do not emphasize punctuality in contemporary life. "Arriving on Caribbean time" means arriving later than planned. However, people in the formal business world pay more attention to timeliness. Unfortunately, the importance of past traditions is being lost rapidly. The culture is heavily influenced because of easy access to cable and satellite television and the Internet, and because of the island's proximity to the United States.

Pain Reactions: Pain reactions vary significantly and are uniquely individual.

Birth Rites: The vast majority of births take place in a hospital. Women who have had no complications go home with their infants within a day or two and come back for a routine medical follow-up. Because of the progressively acculturating society, practices followed after birth that were used a generation ago have now essentially disappeared. However, infant boys tend to be celebrated more than infant girls.

Death Rites: Perceptions of death are largely colored by religious beliefs, and in this predominantly Christian society, concepts of death and the afterlife are based on biblical perspectives. Family members usually attend the passing of a loved one in clinical and community settings when feasible. However, a considerable anathema to autopsy exists in the Barbadian society, and not surprisingly, the concept of organ donation has not been embraced. Therefore the island has no established transplantation programs based on cadaveric organ donation.

Food Practices and Intolerances: The principal grain eaten is rice, which is often cooked with a variety of peas, and meals based on macaroni and potatoes are also popular. Chicken is probably the most frequently consumed meat product. Popular local dishes include rice and peas and beef stew with servings of vegetable salads, and the national dish is flying fish and *cou cou*. Cou cou is a dish prepared from cornmeal cooked with okra, and flying fish is a highly regarded local delicacy. Knives and forks are required implements for eating.

Infant Feeding Practices: Breast-feeding is considered highly desirable and is actively promoted in the antenatal clinics.

Child Rearing Practices: Child rearing practices are based on the model that requires children to be disciplined. Social class influences patterns of discipline; for example, smacking (hitting) may be more prevalent among the working-class groups.

National Childhood Immunizations: BCG at 5 years; DPT at 3, $4\frac{1}{2}$, 6, and 18 months and $4\frac{1}{2}$ years; OPV at 3, $4\frac{1}{2}$, 6, and 18 months and $4\frac{1}{2}$ years; and measles at 15 months. More than 90% of children in the general population have been immunized.

BIBLIOGRAPHY

Annual report of the chief medical officer for the years 1997-1999, September 2000, Barbados Ministry of Health.

Health conditions in the Caribbean, Scientific Pub. No. 561, 1997, Pan American Health Organization.

Health in the Americas, vol II, Scientific Pub. No. 569, 1998, Pan American Health Organization.

Leske MC et al: The Barbados eye study: prevalence of open angle glaucoma, *Arch Ophthalmol* 112:821–829, 1994.

United Nations Development Program: *Human development report 2001*, 2001, Oxford University Press.

World Health Organization (June 2000): *Epidemiological fact sheets by country, Geneva*. Retrieved March 1, 2002, from http://www.unaids.org/hivaidsinfo/statistics/june00/fact_sheets/index.html

World Health Organization (2001): *WHO vaccine-preventable diseases: monitoring system, Geneva*. Retrieved March 1, 2002, from http://www.who.int/vaccines/

◆ BELARUS (REPUBLIC OF)

MAP PAGE (861)

Maggi McLeod

Location: Located in Eastern Europe, with Poland on the west and Russia on the east, Belarus is one of the cofounders of the Commonwealth of Independent States. Belarus contains hilly lowlands with forests, swamps, peat marshes, rivers, and lakes. The population in Belarus was 9,972,900 in 2001.

Major Languages	Ethnic Groups	Major Religions
Byelorusian (official)	Byelorusian 81%	Eastern Orthodox 80%
Russian	Russian 12%	Other or none 20%
	Polish 4%	
	Ukrainian 2%	
	Other 1%	

Health Care Beliefs: Acute sick care; passive role. Health care is primarily crisis care. Currently people have little interest in prevention, although awareness is developing. Illness and disease are not viewed as a punishment from God but are thought of fatalistically—as a part of life. People do not use alternative treatments for illness; they go to a clinic for biomedical treatment.

Predominant Sick Care Practices: Biomedical. Ill people seek medical care in local clinics. In cities the clinics are located throughout residential neighborhoods. In smaller towns, these clinics reside within the local hospital. Villages often have no clinic, and people are expected to go to the nearest town for assistance, usually by infrequent bus service. Once treated at a clinic, a patient may be referred to a specialist for testing, provided with a prescription for the ailment, or referred to hospitals if more serious treatments are needed. Hospitals are located throughout the major cities and within the principal towns of the regions or counties. Although regional hospitals provide all hospital services, those in the major centers such as Minsk often specialize in certain surgical procedures or treatments. Prescriptions for medications can be filled at numerous pharmacies, and patients attempt to find the best price because they pay for all medications. Services other than medications are provided by the state.

Ethnic/Race Specific or Endemic Diseases: Since the 1986 nuclear power station disaster in Chernobyl, the incidences of thyroid cancer, common oral health diseases, gastroduodenal pathological conditions, hematological diseases, cancerous tumors, and disturbances of the immune system have increased. Of these increases, only the significant increase in the rate of thyroid cancer has been directly linked by the world scientific community to this accident because many of the other diseases can also be attributed to other factors such as diet. The World Health Organization's (WHO) estimated prevalence rate for HIV/AIDS in adults ages 15 to 49 is 0.28%. The estimated number of children from birth to 15 living with HIV/AIDS is less than 100.

Health Team Relationships: Like most Western countries, doctors are the principal authorities on health issues, and nurses play a supporting role.

Families' Role in Hospital Care: Families find and pay for all medications for their hospitalized family members. It can be difficult to find certain prescribed medications because many of the most popular drugs are not readily available. All other services are free.

Dominance Patterns: Belarus has a matriarchal society. The family is a mutual support system, so siblings remain close even after marriage. Families are expected to look after their aging parents, and often the parents move in with one of their children as they become less able to live on their own.

Eye Contact Practices: Direct eye contact is acceptable.

Touch Practices: Similar to people in most Western countries, men usually greet each other by shaking hands, and women are frequently seen walking arm in arm.

Perceptions of Time: Punctuality is not particularly important in Belarus. Although those who are involved in business with people from other countries are becoming more concerned with punctuality on a professional level, within their personal lives punctuality remains unimportant.

Pain Reactions: People in Belarus are known for their stoicism in physically and emotionally painful situations, so their reactions are largely invisible.

Birth Rites: Birth rites and death rites in Belarus are determined by religion rather than culture. People in Belarus are primarily Eastern Orthodox; the other primary religion is Roman Catholic. The birth and death rites practiced here are more affected by these religions than anything specific to Belarus.

Death Rites: Relatives are not required to be present at the time of death, and few specific death rites exist. Individuals who are Eastern Orthodox follow the rites of their church, which are more specific to Orthodox rituals than to the culture of Belarus. Traditional funerals involve church services, and mourners say prayers at the place of burial. Having the bones of a dead person in a grave is a source of consolation and connection. Cremation is strongly discouraged, and some believe that this practice was introduced by the godless and enemies of the church. It is believed that alms in memory of the dead can bring special benefits to the deceased. Sometimes special burial funds are available to pay for burials of poor parishioners.

Food Practices and Intolerances: People primarily believe that the noon meal should be the largest meal of the day. However, in a society in which most families are not home for the noon meal, this custom can only be practiced on weekends and holidays. Belarusians, like people of many other cultures, enjoy entertaining and are extremely generous in sharing what they have with friends and family. They love to celebrate any occasion and will have a large celebratory meal—usually late in the evening—whenever possible. The staples in a Belarusian diet include potatoes, bread, and smoked sausages that come in many varieties. Tea is the most popular beverage by far, as is compote (a homemade fruit juice) served at room temperature. Ice is not used in cold drinks.

Infant Feeding Practices: Breast-feeding is considered the best source of nutrition for newborns so if possible, new mothers choose to breast-feed. However, no stigma is attached to formula diets if a mother is unable to produce milk. The mother introduces mashed fruit and vegetables, creamed cereals, rice, and potatoes at about 6 months of age.

Child Rearing Practices: Mothers are the primary caregivers for children and are allowed, by law, to take up to 3 years for maternity leave. However, they can return to work as soon as several weeks after the birth of their child. The mother's return to work depends almost solely on the family's financial situation because mothers are not paid for maternity leave. In a country in which two incomes are almost essential, it is becoming much more common for mothers to take much shorter leaves after the birth of a child. Parents frequently ask grandparents to look after children whose mothers have returned to work.

National Childhood Immunizations: BCG: at birth and at 6 to 7 and 14 to 15 years; DTP at 3, 4 to 5, 6, and 18 months; OPV at 3 to 4, 5 to 6, 18, and 24 months, and at 6 to 7 and 14 to 15 years; measles at 5 to 6 years; MMR at 12 months; DT at 5 to 6 years; and Td at 11 to 12 and 15 to 16 years.

BIBLIOGRAPHY

Belarus: a story of change: 1999, Press agency of the Commonwealth of Independent States Secretariat (CIS).

Darmoyan V: Director, Language Training Centre, Services for Open Learning (SOL) Minsk (affiliated with SOL UK).

McLeod M: Executive Director, Canadian Relief Fund for Chernobyl Victims in Belarus.

Ministry of Statistics and Analysis of the Government of Belarus: *Statistical review of Belarus*, Minsk, 2001.

◆ BELGIUM (KINGDOM OF)

MAP PAGE (860)

Sabine Stordeur and William D'Hoore

Location: Historically, Belgium was a shield state created by England, Prussia, and The Netherlands in 1830 against the French Empire. Belgium, a neighbor of France, Germany, The Netherlands, and Luxembourg, has an opening onto the North Sea. Belgium has a total land area of 30,000 km^2 (11,580 square miles) and is a small, highly developed, and densely populated country (10 million inhabitants) at the crossroads of Western Europe. It is a federal state with three relatively autonomous regions: Flanders in the north, where the language is Dutch (Flemish), Wallonia in the south, where the language is French, and the centrally located Brussels, the capital of Belgium and Europe, an area that is officially bilingual but mostly French speaking. A small region in the east of Wallonia cites German as the official language.

Major Languages	Ethnic Groups	Major Religions
Flemish (Dutch)	Fleming 58%	Roman Catholic 75%
French	Walloon 31%	Protestant, other 25%
German	Mixed, other 11%	

The governing of the country is complicated by its particular structure, with three language communities and the multilingual, multicultural, and multinational status of Brussels. Flanders has about 55% of the 10 million Belgian inhabitants, Brussels 10%, and Wallonia the remaining 35%. If unemployment is calculated according to international norms (i.e., people are counted based on whether they are actually looking for a job rather than whether they are entitled to benefits), the calculated unemployment rate becomes almost half of the official rate and comparable to the relatively low U.S. rate. One recurrent problem is the integration of the many Islamic immigrants (mostly Moroccans and Turks). It is often difficult for these people, many of whom have low-level skills and a poor knowledge of the language and culture, to find good jobs. Although economic immigration has basically been stopped, Belgium, like other European countries, has problems with the growing numbers of people from Third World and Eastern European countries, people who are either demanding asylum or entering the country illegally. The Flemish and Walloon cultures differ in several respects. As expected, the Flemish are more similar to the more disciplined Northern European Germanic culture, and the Walloon culture is more similar to the more life-embracing Mediterranean Latin culture. Regardless, they have more things in common than most are willing to admit publicly. Another character trait is the democratic attitude about rights and duties or access to public goods. However, Belgians make distinctions among classes or social strata.

Health Care Beliefs: Active involvement; health promotion and alternative medicine important. In Belgium, medicine and medical care are based on the Western scientific model. Because science is recycled by common sense, traditional folk beliefs are replaced by pseudoscience. The "common sense model" is similar to the French model (*anthropologie de la maladie*), best described by François Laplantine, in which disease is seen as exogenous and evil. The model of health and disease is relatively rational and includes factors relating to religion and nature. Belgians believe that good food brings good health. For example, Belgians think that garlic purifies blood and know that spinach contains iron, which is good for growth. The use of food supplements, vitamins, and biofood is spreading among well-educated people. No intimidating health programs are in place, but healthy behaviors such as exercise, practicing safe sex, being temperate, staying lean, and refraining from smoking are promoted. Many Catholics believe that praying and going on a pilgrimage can help heal, especially severe diseases such as cancer. Other communities have their own rituals. According to the 1997 National Health Survey, 8% of the population sought help from alternative medical professionals in the year before the survey, mainly from homeopathic doctors, chiropractors and osteopathic doctors, and acupuncturists. Alternative medicine is practiced primarily but not solely by qualified doctors and physiotherapists, although most qualified doctors are skeptical about alternative medicine. Until recently, alternative medicine was a privilege only enjoyed by people of high socioeconomic status because the services were not reimbursed. However, insurances now tend to cover osteopathic care.

Predominant Sick Care Practices: Biomedical; use of alternative medical practices increasing. Health care responsibilities are shared by the national Ministry of Public Health and the Dutch-, French-, and German-speaking Community Ministries of Health. In theory, all Belgians must be covered by one of the branches of social insurance, which is based on the principle of "solidarity" (i.e., with the employed paying for the unemployed and the healthy paying for the ill). A special social security scheme exists for vulnerable groups (e.g., widows, people with disabilities, retired people, orphans). The municipalities within each province play a part in the organization of social assistance for people with low incomes. The country now has a mean of 5.5 hospital beds per 1000 people because of a gradual decrease in the number of hospital beds during the last decade as there was increased emphasis on ambulatory care. There are 35.5 physicians per 10,000 inhabitants, half of which are general practitioners. The health system focuses on cures rather than prevention. Access to health care is virtually free, and people may choose their own doctors. Most people (93%) have a family doctor, and women have more contact (seven contacts per year) with health care practitioners than men (4.8 per year). Frequency of contact is influenced by subjective health, not by socioeconomic status. Patients may seek help from several providers— general practitioners and specialists—simultaneously for the same health problem. In other words, there are no "gate keepers." Generally, the doctors make the decision to refer their patients to hospitals, although many direct emergency admissions occur. Dental care is more costly than medical care, consequently, the mean number of contacts is 1.9 per person per year. In addition, 6.3% of Belgians never go to the dentist, and dental health is associated with socioeconomic status.

Ethnic/Race Specific or Endemic Diseases: Morbidity and mortality rates are typically similar to those in other developed countries. The most frequent causes of death are (from highest to lowest) cardiovascular diseases (33% of all deaths), including ischemic heart disease and cerebrovascular events; digestive tract cancer, respiratory tract cancer (7%); chronic obstructive bronchopneumopathy; genitourinary tract cancer; bone cancer; breast cancer; pneumonia; influenza; suicide (2%); lymphoma and leukemia; and motor vehicle accidents (1.5%). In men, 37% of deaths could be prevented through primary prevention measures (e.g., diseases such as lung cancer, prostate cancer, and ischemic heart disease); in women, 41% could be prevented by primary prevention measure (e.g., diseases such as lung cancer and breast cancer). In Brussels in 1999 the incidence of tuberculosis was 15 cases per 100,000 native Belgians and 75 cases per 100,000 immigrants, whereas in Wallonia the incidence was 10 cases per 100,000 and in Flanders was 7 cases per 100,000. In 1999 and 2000, Brussels had 23 and 47 cases of meningitis, respectively (which is an incidence of 2.4 and 4.8 per 100,000 respectively). The World Health Organization's (WHO) estimated prevalence rate for HIV/AIDS in adults ages 15 to 49 was 0.15%. The estimated number of children from birth to 15 years living with HIV/AIDS was 300. The number of people living with HIV/AIDS was estimated to be 7700, and deaths from HIV/AIDS were estimated to be less than 100.

Health Team Relationships: Medicine, dentistry, and pharmacological medicine, which are all classified as "healing arts," can only be practiced by those who have a doctor of medicine, surgery, or obstetrics diploma, a dentistry diploma, or a pharmacy diploma, respectively. Limited and clearly defined services can be provided by midwives and by certain people with a master's degree in sciences (e.g., clinical biology). Three types of nursing services exist: basic nursing, technical nursing, and nursing that is supervised by a doctor. In Belgium, two nursing diploma levels exist. The curriculum of the first diploma is a 3-year practical training program in vocational schools, which is taken after graduation from the secondary modern school, although it is in fact complementary secondary teaching. The first diploma represents the minimum level required for nurses who want to practice in Belgium or in any other European country. The second diploma curriculum is also a 3-year training program and results in a bachelor's degree. The bachelor's degree is more theoretical and is generally completed with a specialization (e.g., pediatric nurse, psychiatric nurse). Several paramedical professions (e.g., physiotherapy) are classified in a third category of health care providers. In hospitals, doctors have a dominant position because of the social recognition of their clinical expertise. Signs and symbols of doctor's prominence include the length of their university studies (7 to 13 years), their salaries (which are 2 to 10 times the average nurse's salary), and their hierarchical position (a medical director is one of the top managers of hospitals). The nursing director is generally subordinate to medical and general directors. This situation is generally accepted. It is possible that current health team hierarchies arise from the varying relationships among doctors and between doctors and other health care workers. More professional relationships exist among doctors (involving accountability to peers and significant commitment to patients), whereas doctors and other health care workers have more bureaucratic relationships.

Families' Role in Hospital Care: In Belgium, relatives participate very little in patient care. Strict visitor schedules are followed by all hospital units to limit the access of the family to the facility. The visits of close relatives are primarily courtesy visits, however, husbands and wives visit more frequently to help manage laundry, assist with personal hygiene, and provide companionship. In pediatric units, mothers frequently visit with young children, sometimes all day and all night, principally to support them emotionally.

Dominance Patterns: Belgians are materialistic and epicurean. Belgians love the "good life," which is reflected in their excellent food and drink, comfortable housing, reliable medical and social services, and highly developed traffic and communications infrastructure. Belgians do not want to impress other people with their achievements or convince others of their righteousness. They tend to be rather reserved and introverted during their first introductions to other people but are sincerely warm and friendly after people get to know them better. They are happy when they can enjoy a safe and comfortable life with their family and friends, and they highly value privacy. They do not like moralizing or telling other people how they should behave (an attitude for which they criticize their neighbors in Holland), and they choose "live and let live" (*chacun chez soi*) as the basis for their philosophy of life. The expression "a Belgian compromise" was created to characterize the typical—and usually less than optimal—solutions used by Belgians to solve their conflicts. Complex issues are settled by conceding something to all parties concerned, using an agreement so complicated that nobody completely understands all its implications. In spite of the apparent inefficiency of these settlements, the compromises do seem to work in practice because they tend to stop existing conflicts and allow life to proceed with few fights or obstructions. In Belgium, established formal rules and fixed patterns of life (e.g., career structures, laws) are used to enhance security, and broad differences in wealth and power exist among individuals. Theoretically, women are as likely as men to hold important positions. Practically, more men are in higher positions, and more women are in lower positions. Nevertheless, two people who have the same job have the same power, regardless of their gender.

Eye Contact Practices: When people talk, they look others directly in the eyes but do not sustain the gaze, because a persistent look can seem inappropriate or even threatening. Conversely, an elusive look is irritating and could be perceived as a lack of attention or frankness. A handshake is accompanied by direct eye-to-eye contact.

Touch Practices: A handshake or up to three kisses on the cheek during greetings and farewells is common.

Perceptions of Time: Belgians are generally punctual, but they expect to wait about 15 minutes for medical appointments. When doctors who are not on time explain why they are late (e.g., too many patients, an emergency case), patients are generally tolerant and accept longer waiting times.

Pain Reactions: Belgians are not extremists in the expression of pain. They are neither extremely stoic nor excessively emphatic. They try to explain their pain, identify its origin, and ask for a remedy, although many individual differences exist. They are particularly grateful if someone (such as a doctor, nurse, or physiotherapist) helps relieve their pain. Pain is not considered a result of fate, although it is considered redemptive by some Catholics. In hospital or outpatient care settings, professional initiatives to control pain are highly individual. No "analgesic" culture yet exists, although many recent changes relative to relief of pain have occurred. Certain patients, such as children and those who are terminally ill, receive better pain management services.

Birth Rites: Medical professionals are extremely involved in pregnancy and delivery. From the announcement of the pregnancy, the mother undergoes blood sampling for various factors (e.g., HIV, cytomegalovirus [CMV], toxoplasmosis, German measles, hepatitis B, blood type) and urine analysis (e.g., for glucose and albumin). During the 9 months of pregnancy, the pregnant woman often has three ultrasounds, but she frequently has more to establish the well-being of the baby. Most parents want to know the sex of the baby by about the sixth month. In the 15th week of pregnancy, various tests are done to detect possible malformations and problems (e.g., spina bifida, Down syndrome). If such a malformation is detected, the future parents, the doctor, and possibly a psychologist discuss different possibilities (e.g., termination of pregnancy), considering the parents' preferences and the child's expected future quality of life. Parents often meet with other parents in the same situations to help them make a decision. Cigarette smoking and the subsequent risk of sudden infant death is the focus of numerous advertising campaigns. Doctors prescribe sessions of antenatal physiotherapy intended to teach breathing and self-control techniques for the delivery and more importantly to strengthen the urinary sphincter and firm the perineum. With the onset of contractions, gynecologists perform the initial examination, and then the woman is supervised by a midwife and assessed by fetal monitoring equipment. Mothers or the medical team frequently request epidural anesthesia, and the father often attends the delivery. Episiotomies are common, and 9.7% of deliveries are done by cesarean section. The mean hospital stay is 4 days. The first name is chosen by the parents before birth, as are the godfathers and godmothers (in Christian families). After birth, a sequence of visits begins. First come grandparents, then the godfather and godmother, followed by the siblings and friends. All bring presents such as baby clothes, toys, and nursery items. Infants are usually christened several months after birth. Beginning in July 2002, fathers began receiving 12, rather than 3, days off after the birth of a child. Maternity leave is 14 weeks, and women are paid 90% of their salaries. Today, prospective parents are equally happy with the birth of a girl or boy, and even the Belgian royal family adopted the principle of primogeniture to show equality between the sexes. Abortion is "illegal" in Belgium except under three circumstances: a threat to the mother's health exists, psychological or social distress exists, or the fetus has an incurable disease. In other words, abortion is discouraged but not forbidden. In 2001 the total fertility rate was 1.61 children born per woman, the birth rate was 10.74 births per 1000 people, and the infant mortality rate was 4.7 deaths per 1000 live births. The life expectancy at birth for the total population is 77.96 years (74.63 for males and 81.46 for females).

Death Rites: Half of Belgian deaths occur in hospitals, and the other 50% occur at home or elsewhere. Death is perceived differently according to the age of the person who died. A child's death is always considered unacceptable and unjust, and people feel that it simply should have been prevented. More and more frequently, if a child dies in a hospital, parents try to incriminate medical staff members and find medical errors. Deaths of older adults are less shocking and need less explanation and justification. If death occurs after an illness, it usually occurs in the hospital. Nevertheless, outpatient care organizations help people with chronic illnesses such as cancer or AIDS stay at home to die. Bereaved people inform others of the death of loved ones by sending a death notice to them personally or to the local papers. The body is often sent to a funeral home, where it is dressed and put on view for 2 to 3 days. On the day of the funeral, people wear black, and the family receives condolences. Some women wear black dresses for a year, but this practice is not standard anymore. In Christian families, a church service is part of the funeral. Most deceased people are buried, but some are cremated. Many advertising campaigns have been organized to inform people about organ donation. People are assumed to be amenable to organ donation unless they have filled out a specific document of disagreement that has been recorded in the federal database.

Food Practices and Intolerances: The main meal is the evening meal. Staples include cheese, bread, fruit, and vegetables, and beer or wine are the usual beverages. The country is famous for its mussels and fries (French-fried potatoes), waffles, and endive. Belgians have a passion for fine chocolates, and exceptional chocolatiers fill the marketplaces of every city. More beer is consumed than wine, and many of the beers are crafted by small breweries whose family recipes and techniques are generations old. Beer laces the national dish, *carbonnades flamandes*, a Flemish beef stew. Belgians love potatoes and are fond of game and meat. Charcuterie, a basket of bread, and beer often comprise the meals, but fish and seafood are important as well. Hearty soups play a big role in the cuisine, and the so-called *waterzooies* are the most typical soups. Medieval cookery still influences the cuisine through condiments, mustards, vinegars, and dried fruits that lend a sweet-sour and sweet-salty flavor to dishes. Almonds and spices are used in abundance, and fresh herbs lace appetizers, salads, meats, and even desserts. Belgians do not practice any particular food restrictions (although they do not eat insects or animals that are kept as pets, such as cats, dogs, or pet birds), and they enjoy frogs, snails, and any kind of seafood. Seasonal foods include Christmas turkey, spring asparagus, Easter lamb, June strawberries, apples and pears, nuts, shrimps, mussels (the best of which are available in September, October, November, and December), and black and white pudding for the New Year. The usual food and drinks include coffee, *rollmops* (herring rolled in vinegar), sandwiches called *pistolet fourré*, and tomato meatballs. Foreign restaurants such as Italian, Chinese, Vietnamese, French, and Arabian restaurants are also common and appreciated. Belgians like to meet and have a beer in cafes (the popular local bars), and regular customers are known as *habitués*.

Infant Feeding Practices: Breast-feeding is emphasized more and more, although parents are not pressured about their choice. In 2000, 68% of mothers chose breast-feeding, compared to 64% in 1996. Numerous associations have been created to support mothers who breast-feed. Breast-feeding mothers can prolong their postnatal maternity leave by an additional 16 weeks.

Child Rearing Practices: Belgian child rearing practices are not excessively strict nor are they too permissive. Children receive a traditional Western education, a happy medium between rigorous English rules and Italian permissiveness. Discipline is fundamentally the same for boys and girls; however, gender roles are acquired early during the educational process. Because of the European single market, European authorities are playing a greater part in education policy. This trend is quite evident in their role in important issues such as teaching new technologies at school, issues involving the children of immigrants, equal opportunities for boys and girls, equivalence rating of diplomas, and exchange programs such as those involving Erasmus, Comenius, Lingua, and Leonardo.

National Childhood Immunizations: Only vaccines against poliomyelitis are compulsory in Belgium. The first three doses should be administered before the age of 18 months (at 2, 4, and 13 to 14 months), and the last dose is administered at 6 years. Other inoculations are recommended, particularly for children who are frequently in community environments (such as day care): DPT at 2, 3, 4, and 13 months; DT/Td at 6 and 16 years; *Haemophilus influenzae* B at 2, 3, 4, and 13 to 14 months; hep B at 3, 4, and 13 to 14 months; and MMR at 15 months and 11 to 12 years.

Other Characteristics: Belgians appreciate compliance and good manners. For example, it is generally considered impolite for men to carry on a conversation while their hands are in their pockets or while they are wearing a hat. In more formal situations (meeting one's boss or applying for a job), it would be unacceptable. In the same way it would be impolite for a man not to take his hat off when speaking to a woman and unacceptable to wear a hat into a church. Women would not be expected to remove their hats in the same situations. These rules are similar to those common in France. Pointing at someone with a finger is also impolite. Social rules are based on social status, age, and hierarchy. In public, people tolerate minor expressions of love between heterosexuals (e.g., holding hands, kissing). Acceptable public behaviors are the same as those in most Western European countries. Belgians like moderate physical exercise, and football, bicycling, and tennis are all considered national sports. A marked difference between the Flemish and Walloon people is the prevalence of short-distance bicycling. In Flanders, many people ride bicycles, whereas only schoolchildren ride them in Wallonia.

BIBLIOGRAPHY

Axtell RE, ed: *Do's and taboos around the world*, ed 2, New York, 1990, John Wiley & Sons.

Bietlot M et al: *La santé en Belgique, ses communautés et ses regions—résultat de l'enquête de santé par interview*, 1997, Belgium, 2000.

Glen S: A family affair: the health of children and their families: paediatric nurses in Denmark, France, Belgium, and Holland, *Nurs Mirror* 155(24):24, 1982.

Heylingen F: *Belgium, society, character and culture—an essay on the Belgian identity*, 2001, http://pespmc1.vub.ac.be/BelgCul2.html.

Hospital Committee of the European Community, ed: *Hospital services in the E.C. organisation and terminology*, Leuven, Belgium, 1993, Hospital Committee of the European Community.

Institut Belge de l'Economie de la Santé, ed: *Aspects socio-économiques des soins de santé en Belgique*, Bruxelles, Belgique, 1998.

Institut Belge de l'Economie de la Santé, ed: *Compendium de statistiques de la santé 2001*, Bruxelles, Belgium, 2001.

Institut Scientifique de la Santé Publique, ed: *Statistique de décès en Communauté Française 1992–1994*, Bruxelles, Belgium, 1999.

Nonneman W, van Doorslaer E: The role of the sickness funds in the Belgian health care market, *Soc Sci Med* 39(10):1483, 1994.

Observatoire de la Santé de Bruxelles-Capitale, ed: *Tableau de bord de la santé— région de Bruxelles capitale 2001*, Bruxelles, Belgium, 2001, Observatoire de la Santé de Bruxelles-Capitale.

Office de la Naissance et de l'Enfance, ed: *Analyse de données de la banque de données médico-sociales et d'études associées de l'ONE*, Bruxelles, Belgium, 2002.

Szpalski M et al: Health care utilization for low back pain in Belgium: influence of sociocultural factors and health beliefs, *Spine* 20(4):431, 1995.

Wilson H: Community nursing in Belgium, *Nurs Times* 86(29):56, 1990.

◆ BELIZE

MAP PAGE (857)

Eleanor K. Herrmann

Location: Belize is a Central American nation (which was formerly British Honduras) that faces the Caribbean Sea to the east and is bounded on the north by Mexico and on the south and west by Guatemala. The coastline, just a few feet above sea level, is flat and swampy and fringed with islets (called *cayes*) and a 212 km (132-miles) coral barrier reef—the longest coral reef in the Western Hemisphere. The entire northern and southern coastal areas are lowland plains. In the south the terrain rises gradually inland to the Maya Mountains; the highest peak is 1,259 m (3,699 feet). Approximately 93% of the country is still classified as forest. The climate is subtropical, and the country lies in the path of the Atlantic hurricane belt.

Major Languages	Ethnic Groups	Major Religions
English(official)	Mestizo 44%	Roman Catholic 62%
Spanish	Creole 30%	Protestant 30%
Garifuna	Maya 11%	Other or none 8%
Maya	Garifuna 7%	
Ketchi	Other 8%	
Creole		

Health Care Beliefs: Passive role; acute sick care. Regular physical examinations are usually not practiced. However, emphasis on preventive care is increasing. Before seeking medical aid, people use home remedies or over-the-counter medications. People believe dark rum relieves headaches; hot Coca Cola or pure lime juice relieves diarrhea; and that they should avoid consuming hot foods, cold drinks, and heavy foods at night to ward off colic and nightmares. They make soup of the bones of spoiled fish to cure illness caused by eating the spoiled fish.

Predominant Sick Care Practices: Biomedical; herbal; magical-religious. Sick care practices vary according to ethnic groups and geographical location. Women with Obeah beliefs read cards. Dream books may be consulted to interpret the significance of dreams. They believe in the power of the "evil eye" (*mal ojo*), and among women the expression "cut your eye at someone" means to cast the evil eye. Family herb recipes are often used before or with biomedical treatment. People seek nurses and doctors for advice and care. Each of the six districts of Belize has a government hospital. In addition, Belize has health centers and rural health posts, and most centers have a mobile clinic that periodically visits small, remote villages. Belize does not have a national health insurance system.

Ethnic/Race Specific or Endemic Diseases: Chloroquine-sensitive malaria (no risk in urban areas) and dengue fever are major health threats. Schistosomiasis, sickle cell anemia, diabetes, and hypertension are present in the population.

Children are especially susceptible to acute respiratory tract infections or diarrhea from unsafe food handling, inadequate personal hygiene, untreated water, and poor sanitation facilities. The World Health Organization's (WHO) estimated prevalence rate for HIV/AIDS in adults ages 15 to 49 is 2.01%. The estimated number of children from birth to 15 years living with HIV/AIDS is less than 100. HIV/AIDS is a growing problem in Belize. This country is reported to have the highest rate of HIV infection per person in Central America.

Health Team Relationships: Patients do not usually question doctors. Doctor-nurse relationships are superior-subordinate relationships, with nurses assuming the subordinate role. Female chaperones are usually present when male doctors perform physical examinations for females. Male nurses usually do not provide intimate physical care for patients. Belize has no medical school, although it does have a school of nursing, which in 2000 became a department within the new University of Belize.

Families' Role in Hospital Care: Families are encouraged to assist with patients' care and act as their advocates. Some families bring food daily. Chronically ill older adults are often cared for at home but are hospitalized for acute illnesses. Currently, mentally ill adults are hospitalized in Belize's only mental hospital, but the country has plans to decentralize psychiatric care to the districts and include acute care facilities, halfway houses, and day care centers.

Dominance Patterns: Households are headed by men in name only. In reality the society is matriarchal.

Eye Contact Practices: Many people do not maintain direct eye contact, especially with authority figures.

Touch Practices: Greetings are usually formal.

Perceptions of Time: People adhere to schedules and are conscious of being on time.

Pain Reactions: Expressive reactions predominate. Cancer is commonly suspected if a reason for pain is not apparent or identified. It is often believed that if the presence of pain is denied, it will go away.

Birth Rites: The average number of births per woman is 4.6; 19% are born to mothers younger than 20 years. Half of the children are born to single mothers and are referred to as *outside children*. In addition to having nurse midwives, Belize has a program to train traditional birth attendants, who are recognized as primary health care workers by the Ministry of Health.

Death Rites: People are demonstrative in their expressions of grief. Religious services are generally held for the deceased. Funeral processions include many cars and people. Burial in above-ground vaults is customary in coastal areas. Life expectancy is 68.2 years for men and 71.8 years for women.

Food Practices and Intolerances: Rice, red beans, and fish are food staples and are highly seasoned with pepper. Corn is a staple among Indian groups. The diet is high in carbohydrates.

Infant Feeding Practices: Breast-feeding is encouraged, but only 24% of infants are exclusively breast-fed for their first 3 months. Ethnicity influences the decision to breast-feed. To discourage bottle-feeding, no Belizean hospitals accept free or low-cost supplies of infant formulas.

Child Rearing Practices: Disposable diapers are used except in rural areas, where cloth or no diapers is the custom. Toilet training begins as soon as the child can sit up. In school, sex education is presented coeducationally to 10- to 12-year-old boys and girls. Knowledge of contraception is excellent in Belize; 95% of women of child-bearing age (15 to 44 years) know of at least one modern method. Children are raised with strict discipline until the boys are 13 and the girls are 16 years. Grandmothers are frequently involved in child care. Child abuse is a taboo subject.

National Childhood Immunizations: BCG at birth; DTP at 2, 4, and 6 months; OPV at 2, 4, and 6 months and 4 to 5 years; hep B at birth and 2 and 4 months; HIB at 2, 4, and 6 months; MMR at 1 year and 4 to 5 years; DT at 4 to 5 years; and Td at 10 to 11 years, during the fourth month of pregnancy, and +1 month. High levels of immunization against diphtheria, pertussis, whooping cough, tetanus, tuberculosis, polio, measles, mumps, and rubella have been achieved. Full immunization before a child's first birthday is more likely among those living in towns, Creole children, and children of mothers who have nine or more years of schooling.

Other Characteristics: In 1995 the population was approximately 215,500. Forty-one percent of the population is younger than 14 years. Skin color and physical features can influence status and opportunity.

BIBLIOGRAPHY

Belize Information Service and Central Statistics Office: *Belize in figures, 1991*. Belize City, 1991, Government Printery.

Esquivel K: *The right to a future: A situation analysis of children in Belize*, Belize, 1997 National Committee for Families and Children and UNICEF Belize.

Johnson S: Personal communications, 1969–2000.

McClaurin I: *Women of Belize: gender and change in Central America*, New Brunswick, NJ, 1996, Rutgers.

UNAIDS/World Health Organization: *Belize: Epidemiological fact sheet on HIV/AIDS and sexually transmitted infections*, 2000, www.unaids/hivaidsinfo/statistics/june00/fact_sheets/index.html

◆ BENIN (REPUBLIC OF)

MAP PAGE (862)

Inga Wegener

Location: Benin is a small country (115,000 km² or 44,390 square miles) on the western coast of Africa, with the Atlantic Ocean to the south (121 km² of coastline), Togo to the west, Burkina Faso and Niger to the north, and Nigeria to the east. Benin has three climate zones: in the south it is humid (subtropical), in the middle it is semidry (semiarid), and in the north it is hot and dry (sub-Saharan).

Major Languages	Ethnic Groups	Major Religions
French (official)	African 99%	Indigenous beliefs 70%
Tribal languages	European 1%	Muslim 15%
		Christian 15%

Benin has five major trading languages and about 50 overall dialects or languages. The five major languages are Fon in the south, Yorouba in the southeast, Dendi in the central region, and Barriba and Haussa in the north.

Health Care Beliefs: Passive role; traditional. Public health service workers and social workers participate in health promotion and disease prevention programs that are based on United Nations Children's Fund (UNICEF) suggestions, such as vaccination programs (*programme elargie de vaccination* [PEV]), weight control for babies, and nutritional education for mothers. During the last 10 years, health promotion activities for the general public have increased greatly. People in Benin fear mental illness, especially people in areas where voodoo is practiced (in the south and middle of Benin). The people believe in the "evil eye" (the belief that a person can make others ill by looking at them), and they protect themselves with fetish-related items (cris-cris).

Predominant Sick Care Practices: Biomedical; magical-religious. The people seek help from traditional healers or doctors depending on the health problem. They frequently visit traditional healers for help with psychological problems and conditions such as epilepsy, fever, or cramps. Amulets are worn around the neck or limbs and believed to ward off a variety of illnesses. Scarification, the process of cutting the skin so as to produce a pattern of scars, is sometimes believed to be a protection against tetanus. Whether to use a doctor depends primarily on finances because patients have to pay for everything in advance. If it is really necessary, most individuals attempt to visit either a doctor, nurse, or midwife. Dispensaries are disseminated throughout the country.

Ethnic/Race Specific or Endemic Diseases: Sickle cell disease is race specific, affecting only black people. The most prevalent disease in Benin is malaria, followed by diarrheal diseases, which are the major reason children between birth and 4 years die. Respiratory tract infections are also very common. Malnutrition is generally widespread, and certain illnesses, such as measles, are accompanied by nutritional taboos that put children at an even greater risk of death. For example, in the south of Benin, children infected with measles are not allowed to have protein, therefore they usually develop kwashiorkor or marasmus and frequently die. The prevalence of various diseases is somewhat unclear due to the lack of accurate reporting. It is known that the number of people with HIV/AIDS is increasing. The World Health Organization's (WHO) estimated prevalence rate for HIV/AIDS in adults ages 15 to 49 is 2.45%. The estimated number of children from birth to 15 years living with HIV/AIDS is 3000. Prostitutes have an infection rate of about 70%, and it is estimated that about 3% of the entire population is infected. However, it is likely that the rates are much higher because people in the country tend to deny the existence of the disease. When someone dies of AIDS, people say that the person died of something else such as diarrhea or a cough. The people of Benin tend to believe HIV/AIDS is something fabricated by white people who are attempting to force Africans to use condoms so that they will have fewer children.

Health Team Relationships: An established hierarchy exists among doctors, nurses, and midwives. If doctors are present, they are the unquestioned leaders of the health team and it is very difficult to criticize them. In dispensaries without doctors, a "main" nurse (which may be a man) is in charge. Health care workers tend to be very strict and dominating in their treatment of patients, and they generally do not exhibit much sympathy or pity.

Families' Role in Hospital Care: Normally, family members stay with patients while they are in the hospital. The families take care of everything, such as providing food and clothing, changing sheets, and bathing the patient. The nurses are responsible for giving medications, cleansing wounds, and other ordered treatments. Compared with the role of the nurse in Western countries, the helping role of the nurse in Benin is very limited.

Dominance Patterns: Men are dominant, and the roles of men and women are strictly defined. Regardless, men and women attempt to have independent incomes. Men are responsible for paying the fees associated with health care and education and are also responsible for the care of the family's cattle. Women are expected to raise the children, work in the fields, prepare the food, and care for the other domestic animals. However, often men are unwilling to pay medical fees. It can be very difficult to convince a father to spend money on a sick child. Women have few rights regarding family planning, and they cannot use birth control unless their husband agrees. The husband decides how many children his wife will have because having numerous children is considered a sign of strength or power. Having large families is also considered beneficial for women because the more children she has, the greater her social status.

Eye Contact Practices: Eye contact varies in the different regions of Benin and among the various ethnicities. For example, the Bariba believe it is impolite to make direct eye contact with another person. In southern Benin, however, avoiding direct eye contact is a sign of respect. Someone in a lower social class may avoid direct eye contact with a person of higher social status, although this is not always the case.

Touch Practices: Physical touching is acceptable and usually quite frequent. People tend to "look more with their hands than with their eyes."

Perceptions of Time: An African proverb says, "There is nothing more than time." Punctuality is not considered particularly important, so it varies significantly from person to person. Traditions also play an important role in cultural and daily life in that the future is far less important than the present.

Pain Reactions: Normally, most individuals avoid expressing their pain, and women are relatively quiet during labor. In certain social situations, such as being beaten at a police station, it is considered important to scream as much as possible.

Birth Rites: In certain villages the mother takes a hot seated bath if her baby is delivered at home. The placenta is buried next to the family's house. A son is often more celebrated than a daughter. Regardless, a family who already has four or five sons would be anxious to have a daughter because daughters stay with the family, and sons leave.

Death Rites: The people of Benin have large death ceremonies, especially for older and important people. When children or young people die, the ceremonies are small. Funerals are important ceremonies, and the deceased person is frequently celebrated on the yearly anniversary of the death. Ceremonies last at least 3 days. All family members bring money and often buy new cloth (*pagne*) for the whole family so that they can be dressed in the same material. More than 2 months' salary may be spent on the funeral, or cattle may be sold to pay for it. Organ donations and autopsies are uncommon.

Food Practices and Intolerances: The basic foods are corn, millet, cassava, sweet potatoes, small fish, gumbo, tomatoes, onions, and meat if it is available. The food is usually eaten with the right hand, but forks are also used. Their favorite foods are corn puree (pâte) and meat (i.e., chicken, fish, beef). People in Benin have food taboos, such as not eating certain foods when ill.

Infant Feeding Practices: Infants are breast-fed as long as possible. Breast-feeding is one way a woman can practice birth control because it often delays future pregnancies. Some people in the southern region of Benin participate in a practice called gavage. When children are no longer being breast-fed, their mothers may force-feed them liquid food, which can lead to aspiration pneumonia.

Child Rearing Practices: Children are raised in a family group in which not only parents but also aunts and older sisters assume responsibilities. In rural areas the whole family sleeps in one room because the huts are too small to separate children from parents; infants are always with their mothers. Young children are not educated until they are about 3 years because it is more likely that they will survive if they can reach this age. At this point, they are expected to behave and follow the orders given by the family. Fathers and other men of the family are the most respected members of society.

National Childhood Immunizations: BCG at birth; DTP at 6, 10, and 14 weeks; OPV at birth and 6, 10, and 14 weeks; measles at 9 months; and TT CBAW. Benin has a national immunization program, which is well accepted by the population. Medical staff members regularly travel to the villages to provide immunizations. Social workers also monitor immunization rates during weight control sessions. In endemic areas, people also receive the meningococcal meningitis vaccine.

BIBLIOGRAPHY

Alihonou E et al: Contraception continuation and its determinants in Benin, *Contraception* 55(2): 97, 1997.

Cleland JG, Ali MM, Capo-Chichi V: Postpartum sexual abstinence in West Africa: implications for AIDS control and family planning programmes, *AIDS* 13(1):125, 1999.

Hounsa AM et al: An application of Ajzen's theory of planned behaviour to predict mothers' intention to use oral rehydration therapy in a rural area of Benin, *Soc Sci Med* 37(2):253, 1993.

Murphy JE: Bush nursing in Benin, *JCN* 10(4):15, 1993.

Sargent C: The implications of role expectations for birth assistance among Bariba women, *Soc Sci Med* 16:1483, 1982.

Wright J: Female genital mutilation: an overview, *J Adv Nurs* 24:251, 1996.

World Health Organization (June 2000): *Epidemiological fact sheets by country, Geneva*. Retrieved March 1, 2002, from http://www.unaids.org/hivaidsinfo/statistics/june00/fact_sheets/index.html

World Health Organization (2001): *WHO vaccine-preventable diseases: Monitoring system, Geneva*. Retrieved March 1, 2002, from http://www.who.int/vaccines/

◆ BHUTAN (KINGDOM OF)

MAP PAGE (866)

Location: Bhutan is a small, mostly mountainous country on the southeast slope of the Himalayas, with China to the north and west and India to the south and east. A succession of lofty and rugged mountains reaches 7315 m (24,000 feet), separated by deep and sometimes high fertile valleys and savannas. The climate is tropical in the southern plains and has thick forests. Most people live in the intermediate areas between the plains and the high mountains. The capital is Thimpu, and the total land area is 47,000 km² (18,100 square miles), about the size of Switzerland. The climate in the central valleys is characterized by cool winters and hot summers, whereas the Himalayas region has severe winters and cool summers. The country's name means "land of the thunder dragon," a reference to the violent storms that originate in the Himalayas. The total population (as reported by nongovernmental sources) is 2,005,222; however, the Bhutanese government states that the country's population is about 600,000. The discrepancy is a result of the official census, which did not count people of Nepali origin. About 40% of the population comprises infants and children from birth to 14 years of age. Bhutan is one of the smallest and least developed economies and is based on agriculture and forestry. The per capita gross domestic product (GDP) is $1060.

Major Languages	Ethnic Groups	Major Religions
Dzongkha (official)	Ngalop, Sharchop,	Lamaistic Buddhism 70%
Nepalese dialects	ethnic Nepalese	Indian- and Nepalese-
Tibetan dialects	75%	influenced Hinduism 25%
	Indigenous and	Other 5%
	migrant tribes 25%	

Lamaistic Buddhism is the state religion, but Hindus have de facto religious freedom. Bhutan has four major ethnic groups: the Ngalop, of Tibetan origin; the Sharchop, of Indo-Mongoloid origin; indigenous tribal people; and Nepalese.

Health Care Beliefs: Acute sick care; passive role. Bhutan has a stable, traditional social structure. Most individuals take a passive role when ill. Rather than preventing disease, people in Bhutan tend to seek care only when they are acutely ill. Some believe that events are determined by "the fates," or the deities, and cannot be changed. Using treatments and foods that are considered "hot" versus "cold" (according to Hindu ayurvedic classification), for illness is common in order to bring the body back into equilibrium. For example, herbal medicine is considered "cold," while Western medicine is considered "hot." As more Westernized medical care becomes available, beliefs about health care have begun to include both traditional and modern viewpoints. For example, researchers in a recent study attempted to evaluate traditional treatments and factors that people believed caused diarrhea. Natural causes were reported more frequently than supernatural causes, with the most important being teething (76%), followed by "cold" food; 57.5%), stale food (52.5%), hot food (41%), and dirty water (38%). However, the terminology individuals used to describe dehydration indicated strong links to supernatural causes, and people had insufficient information relative to diarrhea management. For example, about 83% of mothers said they continue breast-feeding when their infants have diarrhea, but 75% said that they occasionally or always withhold fluids and 58% said that they withhold food as well.

Predominant Sick Care Practices: Biomedical; traditional; magical-religious. People believe that sickness comes to those who have been evil. Indian ayurvedic medicine and Tibetan herbal medicine are practiced.

People have faith in the local healers. Bhutan's medical system improved in the 1960s with the establishment of the Department of Public Health and openings of new hospitals and dispensaries throughout the country. Western medical care has gradually begun to be introduced since the 1980s. As of the early 1990s, Bhutan had 29 general hospitals (including 5 leprosy hospitals, 3 army hospitals, and 1 mobile hospital), 46 dispensaries, and 15 malaria eradication centers. In 1988, the country had 932 hospital beds and a severe shortage of personnel, with only 142 doctors and 678 paramedics. Training has been provided for health care assistants, nurses' aides, midwives, primary health care workers, and village volunteers. Medical facilities are still limited, and some medications are in short supply. Individuals (primarily visitors) with serious medical problems are often sent to other countries for treatment.

Ethnic/Race Specific or Endemic Diseases: Diseases that are endemic are dengue fever, malaria in rural areas, respiratory diseases including tuberculosis, iodine-deficiency goiter, leprosy, cholera, parasitic diseases, typhoid fever (including antibiotic-resistant strains), hepatitis A and B, and vitamin A deficiency in certain areas. People are at risk for various gastrointestinal diseases caused by parasites, altitude sickness, rabies, leprosy, and injuries from motor vehicle accidents. Hand washing and sanitary waste disposal are not practiced in some areas, which contaminates drinking water. Young women may self-inflict burns in response to family quarrels. The World Health Organization's (WHO) estimated prevalence rate for HIV/AIDS is less than 0.01%. WHO has no estimates for children from birth to 15 years. No AIDS cases and no evidence of HIV infection have yet been found in Bhutan. Tests of army recruits, patients at antenatal clinics, and other various groups have all revealed negative results.

Dominance Patterns: Developmental programs have led to additional opportunities for women. The National Women's Association of Bhutan is working to improve the economic status of women, and opportunities have opened up in the fields of nursing, administration, and teaching. Women occupy a secondary position in business and civil service, although the Bhutanese constitution guarantees equality. Nepalese tribal and communal customs dictate women's roles, but they differ by ethnic group and are usually determined by caste. Status is measured by land ownership, occupation, and perceived religious authority. In some sense, women have a dominant social position in that land is often passed on to daughters instead of sons. Traditional society is matriarchal and patriarchal; the head of the family is often the one held in highest esteem. Women's social status is indicated by the color of their *kira*, or ankle-length dress. Men and women wear scarves and shawls, and the specific ways of folding the scarves, as well as their designs and colors, designate status. The laws in the 1990s still allowed a man to have as many as three wives if he had the first wife's permission. The first wife also had the power to sue for divorce and alimony if her husband married additional wives without her consent.

Infant Feeding Practices: The median duration of breast-feeding is 28 months, and infants are fed on demand day and night. Semisolid food is introduced at the median age of 3 months. Studies show that on average the median duration of postpartum amenorrhea is about 12 months. In general, the only reason women stop breast-feeding within 2 years is because of a new pregnancy. One particular study shed light on the relationship of breast-feeding to infant health. In a study of mothers who had given birth 30 to 36 months previously in a traditional community, infants who were weaned during a subsequent pregnancy did not gain as much weight and had more infections than infants weaned at a later date less abruptly. People believed that the breast milk of a pregnant woman could "rot" and make a child ill. They also believed that if the mother became pregnant and the child developed diarrhea, she should immediately stop breast-feeding, a practice that deprived the child of important nutrients needed to combat the diarrhea. The birth rate in Bhutan is 36.22 births per 1000 people, and the total fertility rate is 5.13 infants born per woman. The infant mortality rate is 110.99 deaths per 1000 live births. Life expectancy at birth is 52.79 for males and 51.99 for females. Literacy rates are 56.2% for males and 28.1% for females.

Food Practices and Intolerances: Rice and corn are staples, and yak cheese is a staple for people who live in the mountains. Meat soups, spiced chilies, beef, pork, goat, and poultry are also eaten. Beverages include beer made from cereal grains and tea with butter. People have limited access to potable water.

National Childhood Immunizations: BCG at birth; DTP at 6, 10, and 14 weeks and 18 months; OPV at birth, at 6, 10, and 14 weeks, and at 18 months; hep B at 6, 10, and 14 weeks; measles at 9 months; Vitamin A at 6 months × 3, also school children every 6 months; and TT after first contact and at 4 weeks, 6 months, and next pregnancy. Because good health results from past virtue, people do not always believe that immunizations can affect their future health. However, the country has achieved high percentage rates of immunizations: BCG, 97%; DTP1, 99%; DPT3, 92%; Pol3, 98%; and TT2 plus, 76%.

Other Characteristics: Except for members of the royal family and a few other noble families, Bhutanese do not have surnames. They may be given two names, but neither is considered to be a family name. Some people adopt their village name, wives keep their own names, and children may have names that are not connected to either parent. In addition, approximately 96,500 Bhutanese refugees live in refugee camps in southeast Nepal. Because of ethnic persecution, these ethnic Nepalese were forced to leave after new citizenship policies were enacted by the Bhutanese government. Some of them were tortured, causing anxiety, depression, posttraumatic stress disorder, persistent somatoform pain disorder, and dissociative (amnesia and conversion) disorders.

BIBLIOGRAPHY

Bibbings J: VSO nursing in Bhutan, *Nurs J Clin Pract Educ Manage* 3(47):9, 1989.

Bibbings J: Wound care in a developing country, *Nurs J Clin Pract Educ Manage* 4(41):29, 1991.

Bohler E, Bergstrom S: Premature weaning in east Bhutan: Only if the mother is pregnant again, *J Biosoc Sci* 27(3): 253, 1995.

Bohler E, Ingstad B: The struggle of weaning: Factors determining breastfeeding duration in east Bhutan, *Soc Sci Med* 43(12):1805, 1996.

Morrow RC: A paediatric report on Bhutan, *J Trop Med Hygiene* 90(40):155, 1987.

Nutritional assessment of adolescent refugees—Nepal, 1999, *Morb Mort Wkly Rep* 49(38):864, 2000.

Stapleton MC: Diarrhoeal diseases: Perceptions and practices in Nepal, *Soc Sci Med* 28(6):593, 1989.

Van-Ommeren M et al: Psychiatric disorders among tortured Bhutanese refugees in Nepal, *Arch Gen Psych* 58(5):475, 2001.

http://encarta.msn.com/find/print.asp?&pg=8&ti==0411C000&sc=0&pt=1

http://lcweb2.loc.gov/cgi-bin/query/r?frd/cstdy:@field(DOCID+bt0042)

http://www.odci.gov/cia/publications/factbook/geos/bt.html

http://travel.state.gov/bhutan.html

◆ BOLIVIA (REPUBLIC OF)

MAP PAGE (XXX)

Deborah E. Bender

Location: Bolivia is a small land-locked country in the central part of South America. It is bordered on the west by Peru and Chile, on the south by Argentina, and on the east by Brazil and Paraguay. The total land area is 1,098,580 km² (424,162 square miles). Lake Titicaca, the highest navigable lake in the world, is on its western border with Peru. Three distinct cultural regions divide the country. The mountainous area of western Bolivia is the most traditional, the high valley area in the central portion of the country is home to many recent immigrants because of its moderate climate, and the eastern plains area is modernizing rapidly—culturally and economically. Bolivia has slightly more than 8 million people. By some estimates, 80% to 90% of the population is Amerindian. About 30% of the people are Quechua Indians, descendents of the Inca. Recent estimates indicate that 63% of the population resides in urban areas. Since a period of hyperinflation in the mid-1980s, rapid immigration from rural to urban areas has exacerbated already strained economic and residential conditions in periurban areas.

Major Languages	Ethnic Groups	Major Religions
Spanish	Quechua 30%	Roman Catholic 95%
Amerindian languages	Aymara 25%	Protestant 5%
	Mixed 30%	
	White 15%	

Spanish is the official language. Quechua, Aymara, and Guarani are the three most commonly spoken Amerindian languages. The country is experiencing a resurgence of interest in preserving its native tongues, even among urban, educated people. It is not uncommon to find families who speak Spanish and another language in the home.

Health Care Beliefs: Active involvement; traditional. Traditional medicine is practiced in several forms. The *kallawayas*, traditional itinerant healers (mostly older adults) who travel from market to market, are among the most well known of Bolivian indigenous healers. Many of their amulets, including charms, plants, and llama fetuses, can be found in open markets if a person knows where to look. Herbs and other locally grown plants are widely used for their medicinal qualities. Leaves or flowers may be boiled in water to produce a *mate*, or tea. The coca leaf is widely used in mate to relieve stomachaches and headache distress caused from high altitudes. Other plants are useful in relieving the swelling caused by mumps, to induce abortion, to aid in circulation, and to assist in clotting of cuts and wounds. Many rural residents still rely heavily on traditional practices; however, more and more individuals are selecting traditional or modern treatments based on their perceived effectiveness.

Predominant Sick Care Practices: Biomedical; magical-religious. Western and indigenous health care practices are prevalent in Bolivia. Western health care is offered through (1) the national public health system, (2) one of several employment-linked prepaid health plans called *seguros sociales*, (3) health nongovernmental organizations or church-affiliated services, or (4) a small, fee-for-service private sector. In the public health sector, great strides have been made in reducing infant and maternal mortality rates through immunization campaigns and a broad-based maternal reproductive health program.

Ethnic/Race Specific or Endemic Diseases: The most prevalent illnesses are the communicable and infectious diseases typical of childhood. These include vaccine-preventable diseases and acute respiratory illnesses such as pneumonia. Disease rates are improving as a result of periodic national immunization campaigns and promotion of improved health practices through census-based community efforts for improved child survival and growth. Diarrhea is prevalent in Bolivian children, and it has been reported in research studies that about 25% of children younger than 3 years experienced diarrhea within the 2 weeks before data gathering. Twice as many of these cases of diarrhea occurred in infants 6 to 23 months rather than infants younger than 6 months. Nationally, 84% of mothers interviewed in the same survey reported knowing about oral rehydration therapy (ORT), a public health treatment for diarrhea. Still, only 67% of mothers without education, compared with 97% of those who completed middle school or more, reported knowing about ORT. Endemic diseases include goiter, which is most prevalent near the vast salt lakes of Uyuni, where few leafy green vegetables grow and diets have insufficient iodine. (In other areas of the country, salt is iodized.) Chagas' disease, resulting from the bite of an insect that often lives in housing roof straw, is also endemic in the highland valleys of Bolivia. The disease causes death at middle age, often from cardiac complications. Community-based eradication programs are slowly changing the incidence of the disease. According to information made available by the Pan American Health Organization (PAHO), the first case of AIDS was reported in 1985. The World Health Organization's (WHO) estimated prevalence rate for HIV/AIDS in adults ages 15 to 49 is 0.10%. The estimated number of children from birth to 15 years living with HIV/AIDS is less than 100. By 1996 a total of 123 cases had been reported in addition to 111 cases of asymptomatic infection with HIV. Ninety-two percent of the cases were in the 15- to 49-year-old age group, and 75% of the patients were male. The transmission routes were sexual contact (92%), blood transfusions (6%), and perinatal transmission (2%). Cases of HIV/AIDS infection were reported in eight out of the country's nine regions.

Health Team Relationships: Health care is driven by doctors. More doctors graduate each year than can be absorbed into the economy. Nursing is a low-paid, low-status profession. Graduate training in public health is offered at the University of San Andres in La Paz, at the University of San Simon in Cochabamba, and more recently at several private colleges and universities. Because of the sizeable disparities in education and socio-economic status between doctors and many of their patients, patients commonly cite lack of trust and poor communication as barriers to quality care. Language is another barrier and is particularly a problem for rural residents and recent migrants to urban areas who have settled in heavily populated periurban areas.

Families' Role in Hospital Care: In rural areas, it is not unusual for family members stay with a hospitalized patient, preparing their food and changing their linens. In more urban areas, where there are more health resources, family members may supplement services offered by the hospital, although it is not required.

Dominance Patterns: Stereotypically, Latino cultures promote male dominance. At the same time, men are as concerned as women about the health and well being of their families. Occasionally, the perspectives of outsiders perpetuate traditional cultural patterns. For example, in the 1990s, when Bolivia agreed to institute an innovative family planning and reproductive health program, many health care consultants were afraid that the campaign efforts would be thwarted by men through their labor organizations, the *sindicatos*. The anticipated conflicts were never an issue. In fact, when men were invited to family planning sessions in a reproductive health project in Cochabamba, they came and listened and were just as shy and uncomfortable—and eager to learn—as the women. One man said, "We need to know these things; today things are different. We cannot afford to have as many children as we had in the past." Whether he wanted the knowledge to enforce his dominance or help rear his family is largely in the eyes of the beholder. The literacy rate is 83% overall, 90% for males and 70% for females.

Eye Contact Practices: It is typical in Latino cultures to lower the eyes as a sign of respect. Because of the tremendous differences in social class and education between health care providers and patients, communication barriers can be troublesome if the providers have not been educated about how to overcome the problem.

Perceptions of Time: Punctuality varies from urban to rural areas. However, perceptions of time everywhere in Bolivia are more relaxed than they are in the United States. Most Bolivians are on time for appointments in general, but this is somewhat flexible. However, most interesting is the expectation that Americans ought to be precisely on time for meetings and appointments. For Americans working in Bolivia, this cultural juxtaposition creates some interesting situations. Patients often complain of long wait times for scheduled appointments at clinics or hospitals.

Pain Reactions: Bolivians, especially Amerindians, tend to be somewhat stoic. Regardless, as in much of the world, children cry when stuck with an immunization needle, and adults cringe when in pain.

Birth Rites: Recent program initiatives of the National Ministry of Health encourage all women to give birth in hospital settings. During the past decade, rates of hospital deliveries have doubled to approximately 50% to 55% of deliveries. Still, many families are too far from a hospital or lack trust in Western medicine. Certain common beliefs surround pregnancy and childbirth. During pregnancy women are advised to avoid sun and heat and refrain from lifting heavy things. Pregnant women do not eat spicy foods because they think it can cause bleeding. The first signal of pregnancy is the cessation of menstrual bleeding, and women believe that the blood is accumulating for the birth. Swelling of the feet and hands during pregnancy is regarded as a good sign; it suggests that the blood is accumulating as it should. Bolivian women like a warm, intimate setting for birth. They believe that cold and wind should be avoided because they think that they may cause fever and chills during the postpartum period. During the delivery, women drink warm teas, or mates, to stimulate the flow of blood, facilitate the birth, and aid in delivery of the placenta. After delivery the husband or another close family member washes the placenta and buries it in a protected place, often beneath the foundation of the house. The burial of the placenta ensures that the mother and infant will live a contented life. Many women, particularly those with rural origins, are reluctant to give birth in hospitals because of their lack of respect for this practice. To encourage women to deliver in hospitals, some are giving women the placenta for traditional burial.

Some hospitals are also encouraging women to allow their infants to remain in the hospital room with them at all times. Many women prefer to give birth standing because they are assisted by the forces of gravity. Regardless, hospitals usually place women in horizontal positions, which helps the doctors and nurses. Again, with the establishment of the national reproductive health movement in Bolivia in the early 1990s, accommodations for various delivery preferences have been made in many facilities. Maternal mortality rates are still high (390 per 100,000 live births) because of the low percentage of births (52.9%) that are attended by trained personnel. The infant mortality rate is 59 per 1000 live births. A late 1980s study of illegal abortions in a hospital in La Paz set in motion a series of changes resulting in the previously mentioned reproductive health and family planning program. The 1980 to 1988 maternal mortality rate for Bolivia was 480 deaths per 100,000 live births. Estimates from various sources suggest that as many as 30% of these deaths were associated with induced abortions. A 1998 survey found that 89% of women of reproductive age and men between 15 and 64 had heard of at least one family planning method. The number of people who actually use birth control is considerably smaller. Among all women who knew of at least one method, only 30.5% had used a modern method. (Birth control pills and intrauterine devices are the most commonly used methods.) Some 36.6% report using a traditional method (such as the rhythm method or withdrawal before ejaculation). Of married women, 43.3% reported using a modern method and 51.7% reported using a traditional method. Fears about contraceptive use are still common, but widespread recognition of the increasing costs of raising a child is propelling many young couples to space births and plan their family size. Life expectancy at birth is 60 for males and 63.4 for women.

Death Rites: In some rural areas, newborn infants are not named until 7 days after birth because of fears that the infant may die. Also, many infants born in rural areas are not registered at birth, so that if the infant dies during the first few months of life, the family would not have spent related fees in vain. During the cholera epidemic of the early 1990s, the traditional practice of washing the body of the deceased in community waters became particularly alarming to public health officials and dangerous to residents downstream. These ritual washings were temporarily prohibited, and the public media aired educational messages alerting Bolivians to the dangers of this practice.

Food Practices and Intolerances: The potato is the staple of the Bolivian diet, and more than 300 varieties have been identified. Bolivians freeze-dry potatoes by soaking them in water and exposing them to the sun or the freezing nights of the June winter, making potatoes available year round. The freeze-dried potato, or *chuñyo*, is considered a national delicacy. Rich soups that provide necessary liquids are a part of every dinner, which is served at midday.

Infant Feeding Practices: Breast-feeding is prevalent in Bolivia. According to a recent survey, 97% of infants born in the past 3 years were breast-fed at some time. About 61% of infants younger than 2 months were breast-fed exclusively, and 30% of children were still receiving some breast milk at 24 months. Mate (herbal tea) is often the first food given to a newborn, a practice that may be related to the Incan practice of giving newborns broth made from tender corn boiled for 3 days. At high altitudes (such as in La Paz, where water boils at 88° C), the boiling temperature may not be high enough to kill water-borne bacteria, thus making the infant vulnerable to diarrhea. Although most women do give colostrum, which is secreted the first few days after birth and offers immunological benefits, to their infants, in some areas women think colostrum is damaging and discard this yellowish liquid until the preferred breast milk comes in.

Child Rearing Practices: People who live in rural areas or who have recently migrated from a rural to an urban area swaddle their infants, and the mothers carry them on their back in brightly woven blankets. Mothers can then easily nurse their infants by simply slipping them forward under their arms.

National Childhood Immunizations: BCG at birth; DTPHH at 2, 4, and 6 months; OPV at birth and 2, 4, and 6 months; MMR at 1 year; yellow fever for those in high-risk areas; and Td at 15 to 45 years × 3. The Pan American Health Organization reports the following immunization percentages for children younger than 1 year: DPT, 82%; OPV3, 82%; BCG, 93%; and measles, 98%.

BIBLIOGRAPHY

Bailey PE et al: A hospital study of illegal abortion in Bolivia, *Bull Pan Am Health Org* 22(1):27–41, 1988.

Bastien JW: *Healers of the Andes: Kallawaya herbalists and their medicinal plants*, Salt Lake City, 1987, University of Utah Press.

Bastien JW: *The kiss of death: Chagas' disease in the Americas*, Salt Lake City, 1998, University of Utah Press.

Bender DE, Rivera T, Madonna D: Rural origin as a risk factor for maternal and child health in peri-urban Bolivia, *Soc Sci Med* 37(11):1345–1349, 1993.

The Bolivian Times, http://www.latinwide.com/boltimes/

Bryan RT et al: Community participation in vector control: lessons from Chagas' disease, *Am J Tropical Med Hygiene* 50(suppl 6):61–71, 1994.

McCann MF et al: Neonatal feeding practices in periurban Bolivia, *Ecology Food Nutr* 38:427–450, 1999.

Ministerio de Previsión Social y Salud Publica: *Normas nacionales para atención integral al niño, al escolar, al adolescente y a la mujer*, La Paz, Bolivia, June 1992.

Pan American Health Organization (November 4, 2001): *Bolivia: country profile*, http://www.paho.org/English/SHA/prflbol.htm.

Perry H et al: The census-based, impact-oriented approach: its effectiveness in promoting child health in Bolivia, *Health Pol Planning*, 13(2):140–51, 1998.

Sardan MG, Ochoa LH, Vargas AG: *Encuesta nacional de demografía y salud*, Calverton, MD, 1998, INE/ENDSA and Macro International/DHS+ Program.

United Nations Children's Fund: *The state of the world's children*.
United Nation's Children's Fund: *Statistical data by country*, *Bolivia*, http://www.unicef.org/statis/Country_1Page21.html

---

◆ BOSNIA-HERZEGOVINA (REPUBLIC OF BOSNIA AND HERZEGOVINIA)

MAP PAGE (860)

Marshall Godwin

Location: Formerly part of Yugoslavia, Bosnia-Herzegovina is located on the Balkan Peninsula in southeastern Europe. It borders on the Adriatic Sea (20 km), Croatia (930 km), and Yugoslavia (530 km), with a total land area of approximately 51,000 km^2 (19,686 square miles) The terrain consists primarily of mountains, valleys, and an area of flat, arable land in the south formed by the River Neretva, which flows south to the Adriatic. Two other rivers, the Vrbas and the Bosna, flow northeast into the Sava River. The Sava River flows eventually into the Danube River, which empties into the Black Sea. Within Bosnia and Herzegovina's recognized borders, the country is divided into the joint Bosniak/Croat Federation (about 51% of the country) and the Bosnian Serb-led Republika Srpska (RS; about 49% of the country). Bosnia-Herzegovina generally has hot summers and cold winters. However, the southern parts near the Adriatic Sea tend to have milder, wetter winters and longer summers, not unlike the climate in Italy or other northern Mediterranean countries.

Major Languages	Ethnic Groups	Major Religions
Serbo-Croatian (also known as Serbian, Croatian, or Bosnian)	Bosniak 44% Serb 31% Croat 17%	Slavic Muslim 40% Orthodox 31% Roman Catholic 15% Protestant 4% Other 10%

The previous percentages are based on 1991 census data that calculate the total population of Bosnia-Herzegovina at 4 million. The 1992 to 1995 war has since then caused major shifts in the population. Approximately 250,000 people were killed, 1.5 million were internally displaced (refugees within their own country), and many thousands left the country as refugees and have not returned. The exact composition of the country by religion and ethnic groups is currently unknown. Some estimate that the current total population is between 2 and 3.8 million. The Serbo-Croatian, Croatian, Bosnian, and Serbian languages are all essentially the same language with some very minor word and phrase differences. The language has a Slavic origin and is related to the languages spoken in Poland and the Czech Republic. However, it also has a major Latin influence, and many medical terms of Latin origin are readily recognizable. Although they all speak the same language, Bosnia-Herzegovina has three very distinct ethnic and religious groups. The Bosnian Serbs, who are Orthodox Christians, live primarily in the northeastern and southeastern parts of the country bordering on Yugoslavia. The Bosnian Croats live primarily in the southwestern part of the country bordering on Croatia and are Catholic. The Bosnian Muslims, or Bosniaks, live in the central and south central part of the country.

Health Care Beliefs: Active involvement; holistic. The people of Bosnia-Herzegovina seek help for medical conditions primarily from doctors. However, there is a major emphasis on vitamins, traditional teas, and other remedies, which is common in Eastern Europe. Doctors themselves often suggest these remedies, if anything because of the lack of affordable medications.

Predominant Sick Care Practices: Biomedical; traditional. The medical system is based on the eastern European polyclinic model. The major cities have hospitals; the cities and larger towns have large, outpatient, multi-specialist clinics; and spread throughout the cities, towns, and rural villages are smaller clinics, or *ambulantas*, run by general practitioners. The primary care system is very rudimentary, with the general practitioners referring most patients to specialists for the simplest conditions. This situation is changing as international aid organizations—governmental and non-governmental—work to upgrade the skills and knowledge of local practitioners, introduce modern approaches in the medical schools, and establish effective postgraduate training programs. Administrators manage clinics and hospitals, but doctors are in the dominant position. Nurses only have a high school education and lack many of the skills possessed by nurses in Western health care systems.

Ethnic/Race Specific or Endemic Diseases: Smoking is extremely prevalent, and the diet includes large amounts of red meat. Not surprisingly, heart disease is very common. Programs aimed at decreasing lifestyle risk factors for cardiovascular disease are just beginning and so far have been minimally effective. Posttraumatic stress disorder (PTSD) and depression are common because of the mental trauma experienced by so many people in the 1990s war. Poverty also affects the mental and physical health of many displaced people, who live as refugees within their own country. Many are still unable to return to the part of the country in which they were born and raised because of remaining ethnic hatred. HIV and AIDS are not yet common, and the blood supply is not being screened for HIV/AIDS. The World Health Organization's (WHO) estimated prevalence rate for HIV/AIDS in adults ages 15 to 49 is 0.04% but is definitely rising. WHO has no estimates for children from birth to 15 years. Tuberculosis is fairly common because of poverty and a lack of readily available treatments. The birth rate is 13 per 1000 people, the infant mortality rate is 24 per 100 live births, and the death rate is 8 per 1000 people. The life expectancy is 69 years for men and 75 for women.

Health Team Relationships: Doctors are the dominant health care providers, and nurses serve in assistant roles. Health care is rarely based on a team approach and tends to be dictated by the responsible doctor. Specialists make most of the important decisions about patient care, with the general practitioners following their recommendations with little question.

Families' Role in Hospital Care: The role taken on by the family is largely determined by the economic situation. For the most part, hospitals have limited resources, including a shortage of supplies and medications and too few nurses, so families help with care-taking tasks and bring in food for the patient.

Dominance Patterns: As in most European societies, white men are nominally dominant in society. There are large numbers of women in the workforce, and they also run most aspects of home life. Women still take on the traditional role of homekeeper and childraiser but at the same time often work in business or government offices (if they live in the city) or on the farm (if they live in rural areas). Many roles of authority, such as heads of important governmental and nongovernmental departments and deans of colleges, tend to be male. At the primary care level, many doctors are women.

Eye Contact Practices: Direct eye contact is acceptable.

Touch Practices: Bosnians greet each other as people do in many European societies. Regardless of gender, two people who do not know each other well greet with a handshake. A man and woman meeting for the first time usually shake hands but on subsequent meetings will greet each other with a kiss on both cheeks. *Dobar dan*, meaning "good day," is the standard verbal greeting.

Perceptions of Time: Whether because of a relaxed or lackadaisical attitude or just because of poor organizational skills, people often forget or miss meetings. They tend to focus on the present and future rather than on past traditions.

Pain Reactions: Like Westerners, women typically express their pain more than men.

Birth Rites: Infants are usually born in hospitals. A 1995 report found that only 2% to 11% of mothers with children younger than 4 months were breast-feeding.

Death Rites: The treatment of the dead follows standard Christian and Muslim traditions. In the large cities, some graves are marked by crosses and some by Islamic symbols—all in the same cemetery. Since the war, the newer cemeteries have tended to be either Christian or Muslim but not both.

Food Practices and Intolerances: In the Muslim areas of the country, people do not eat pork. Lamb is a favorite meat throughout the country, and restaurants selling only lamb dishes often line the roads between cities. Outside these restaurants, whole lambs cook outdoors over large rotisserie barbecues. The diet overall is high in meat. *Civap cici* (pronounced "chevap-chee-chee"), a dish consisting of ground meat (lamb and beef) served in a bread pocket, is a favorite fast food at lunchtime, as are meat pies. They tend to be very greasy, similar to a Western hamburger. Cafes and cafe-bars are common, as are dessert and ice cream shops. The people eat plenty of vegetables as well. Yellow and red peppers are a favorite and are often stuffed with minced meat, as are onions and tomatoes. Fruits are readily available from the Dalmatian coast of Croatia. Vegetables, fruits, meat, and fish with very reasonable prices are all readily available in large quantities in the open markets. Unfortunately, many poor people still cannot afford them. Throughout Bosnia-Herzegovina but especially in Herzegovina, fish is a popular dish and is readily available from the Croatian fishermen on the Adriatic (Dalmatian) coast. Squid (*ligne*) is also popular, as are trout from fish farms along the various rivers.

Child Rearing Practices: Child rearing in Bosnia-Herzegovina varies greatly. As in many eastern European and Western countries, child care ranges from loving, caring methods where children are guided (firmly if necessary), to a strict authoritarian approach in which corporal punishment is the norm.

National Childhood Immunizations: BCG at 1 and 7 years; DTP at 1, 2, and 4 years; OPV at 1, 2, 4, 7, and 14 years; measles at 7 years; DT at 7 and 14 years; and TT at 18 years. The country has a fairly strong public health system that encourages vaccination.

Other Characteristics: In the cities, adolescents and young adults who can afford to do so dress well in the latest Western styles (although they do have a tendency to dress in black pants, skirts, shirts, and jackets). Hundreds of very well-groomed people can be seen walking around or sitting in cafes smoking and drinking in downtown Sarajevo in the evening. Going out for the evening is the social event of the day because people have very little else to do. However, outside the cities in the small towns and countryside, a person is more likely to see a woman dressed in old but colorful clothes—looking like something out of the last century—walking behind a herd of sheep and driving them along with a stick. Another common sight would be a man and his son in a horse-drawn cart full of hay, moving slowly along the narrow road as cars edge their way past. As the country rebuilds from the war and 50 years of communist rule, the contrast between those who are becoming wealthy and those who are remaining poor or are refugees is becoming more and more striking.

BIBLIOGRAPHY

http://www.bosnet.org/bosnia/
http://www.cia.gov/cia/publications/factbook/geos/bk.html
http://www.ohr.int/

◆ BOTSWANA (REPUBLIC OF)

MAP PAGE (863)

Sheila Tlou

Location: Botswana is a semiarid, land-locked country in sub-Saharan Africa with an area of almost 582,000 km^2 (224,652 square miles). The country has long borders with South Africa, Namibia, and Zimbabwe and a 700-m border with the Republic of Zambia, the world's shortest international border. Most of the country's land mass is taken up by the Kalahari Desert, but the political and economic capital, Gaborone, is located in the southeast, close to the border with South Africa. The northern regions of the country have a wide variety of wildlife. Since its independence, Botswana has become renowned for its good governance, intolerance for corruption, and respect for legal processes. Botswana was one of the world's poorest countries when it achieved independence in 1966. Fortuitously, the nation discovered large diamond reserves shortly after independence, which have driven its economy ever since. The government began channeling resources into development, including improving the nation's road network, schools, and health facilities with new hospitals, clinics, health centers, and mobile clinics. Village life is extremely important for Batswana; most residents identify with the village from which they came and maintain a second residence in their natal village for weekends or vacations.

Major Languages	**Ethnic Groups**	**Major Religions**
English (official)	Batswana 95%	Christian 50%
Setswana	Bakalanga, Bakgalagadi,	Indigenous beliefs 50%
	Basawara, Baherero 4%	
	White 1%	

The population of Botswana, which is small relative to the size of the country, is growing very rapidly and was estimated at about 1.6 million in 1999. In 1996 the life expectancy was 69 for women and 63 for men. Most of Botswana's people belong to the Setswana-speaking group, or *merafe*, but the country also includes small numbers of people of Asian and European origin. In the past, each of these *merafe* occupied a separate area, acknowledged the supremacy of the chief (*kgosi*) as the ruler in the community, and constituted a single political unit under the ruler's leadership and authority. In 1963, during constitutional talks concerning the new nation of Botswana, it was decided that to ensure national unity, the people's allegiance should be to the nation of Botswana rather than to individual *merafe*. The chiefs (*dikgosi*) thus lost some of their powers, and a new government was elected for the whole country. *Dikgosi* were recognized by the creation of a House of Chiefs, whose major role is to advise the government on *merafe* and customary matters. The concept of *kgotla* is as old as Tswana culture and a foundation for Botswana's modern democracy. *Kgotla* is a village meeting place where all matters pertaining to village policies, developments, and even disputes are discussed and agreed on. *Kgotla's* are usually situated next to the chief's home so that s/he can consult any time as the need arises. Population migration in the villages is characterized by traditional seasonal movements between tribal villages, agricultural lands (*masimo*), and cattle posts (*meraka*). Therefore it is very difficult to determine the true size of any village population. The population distribution of Botswana is skewed, with 48.3% being younger than age of 15 and 8% older than the age of 60. The majority (78%) of the population resides in the rural areas and depends on subsistence agriculture and other informal activities for their livelihood. Health services delivery has improved tremendously since independence, and the country has universal free education.

Health Care Beliefs: Acute sick care; traditional. The people believe that only traditional healers are competent to treat certain diseases, one of which is mental illness. The whole family rather than the individual receives treatment and is encouraged to take the medicines or perform the prescribed rituals in a cohesive manner so that the sick person is cured. One such cure is *go phasa*, or cleansing of the family by the sacrifice of a goat or sheep to the ancestors. The animal is slaughtered, and all the meat is cooked. The traditional healer then prays over the meat and asks the ancestors to heal or reconcile with the family. The meat is eaten by all the clan members and any villagers who choose to participate. All the meat has to be eaten at one meal. Not even the dogs are allowed to have the bones because they are considered meat for the ancestors. The bones are later buried within the family yard or compound by the traditional doctor. Older people in Botswana are important for their knowledge of traditions, including traditional practices relating to illness and its cause. Ethnographical material gathered from folk healers and rural families with members who have disabilities has provided a picture of the people's conceptions of their bodies and how possible illnesses emerge. No concepts of disease transmission through bacterial or viral infections are involved in Tswana folk medicine. The heart is considered the central organ of the body and the primary origin of feelings, thoughts, and emotions. Episodes of illness invariably lead to questions such as "Why has this happened to me" and "Why is this happening now?" Tswana healers may decide that a disease is caused by witchcraft, an ancestor's anger, breaking a taboo related to pollution, or God's will. Although the first three causes involve specific rituals or behavioral measures, "God's will" is often the diagnosis people resort to when treatment attempts have failed. Such a diagnosis calls for acceptance and stoic resignation.

Predominant Sick Care Practices: Biomedical; magical-religious. After achieving independence, Botswana inherited a largely curative, hospital-based health care delivery system; however, the majority of the population had no access to any services at all. In 1975 a separate Ministry of Health was established to improve the health of the nation. The government of Botswana is committed to the idea that primary health care is the best way of improving people's health and promoting development. Primary health care services tackle the health problems of the community by providing health promotion, preventive, curative, and rehabilitative services. The primary health care approach also focuses on the community and encourages it and its individuals to take responsibility for improving their health. This approach encourages the community to help identify health problems; set priorities for action; and plan, organize, and manage health care programs. Women, especially those in middle age, are traditionally the custodians of health care in the community and are a key resource in health care planning and implementation of programs. As mothers-in-law and grandmothers, they are the major decision makers in matters pertaining to the health of the family.

Ethnic/Race Specific or Endemic Diseases: The major causes of inpatient mortality and morbidity include pneumonia, pulmonary tuberculosis, cardiopulmonary diseases, malaria, intestinal infections, and obstetrical complications, none of which are specific to a particular race or ethnic group. Despite the improvement in infant mortality rate and overall health since the late 1960s, the HIV/AIDS pandemic of the late 1990s began a reversal of the gains. The World Health Organization's (WHO) estimated prevalence rate for HIV/AIDS in adults ages 15 to 49 is 35.80%. The estimated number of children from birth to 15 years living with HIV/AIDS is 10,000. Botswana is currently experiencing one of the fastest growing rates of HIV infection in the world. About 300,000 of Botswana's 1.7 million people have been infected with HIV. It is currently estimated that 14% of the total population and 25% of sexually active and economically productive adults have been infected. According to estimations and projections by the U.S. Bureau of the Census, the life expectancy in Botswana in 1996 was down from an initial 61 years to 45 years as a result of the HIV/AIDS epidemic. By 2010, it is estimated that the life expectancy in Botswana will decrease to 33 years. In 1996, as a result of lowered fertility and the premature death of children and adults, the population growth rate in Botswana decreased from an estimated 2.55 per 100 to 1.6 per 100 as a result of AIDS; a negative population growth rate (0.4%) is projected for the year 2010. The HIV epidemic is expected to have large macroeconomic repercussions because of the death of many individuals in their productive years. Heterosexual intercourse has been the predominant mode of HIV transmission. In addition, transmission from mother to child has contributed to the rapidly growing epidemic. Women have been hit hardest by HIV infection. Recent data indicate that 56% of people ages 15 to 49 who are infected are women. In addition, women have the physical and emotional burden of giving birth to infants with HIV, and they are expected to assume much of the care-giving responsibilities for people with AIDS. Poverty, unemployment, legal and sociocultural disadvantages, dependence on partners for financial support, and lack of empowerment in negotiating sexual and reproductive matters all contribute to HIV infection rates among women. If women refuse to have unprotected sex with their partners, they may put themselves at risk for physical and sexual abuse. Although the mortality rate of children younger than 5 is increasing, Botswana's situation is still significantly better than those of other southern African countries primarily because of the significant money the country has invested in basic social services, notably health and education.

Health Team Relationships: In the formal sector, nurses are the backbone of the country's health care system. They are usually the only ones in health care facilities, thus they are responsible for providing preventive, curative, and rehabilitative health care services to the whole population. Their duties include supervising primary health care workers and mobilizing communities, especially women, to become responsible for self-care health tasks. Health facilities, especially ones in the rural areas, have very few doctors. Most of the doctors rely on nurses and have developed very good working relationships with them. Client care is considered a team effort, with the doctor or the nurse practitioner as the team leader.

Families' Role in Hospital Care: Once admitted into a hospital, the patient becomes the responsibility of that hospital. Hospital personnel care for adults, and family members do not stay with them. If a child younger than 5 years is hospitalized, a relative can stay with the child in the children's ward. Hospital food is usually good and nutritionally balanced, so relatives do not have to bring patients any food from home (although they may bring delicacies such a *jugo beans [ditloo]* and *phane [phane/caterpillar]*, which are not served in hospitals).

Dominance Patterns: Girls have always dominated the elementary and high schools because they start formal schooling around age 6, whereas boys, who are cattle herders, have to wait until around age 12. Literacy has thus been a source of empowerment for women, and at the university levels women comprise about 49% of the student body. Inequities in career education are reflected in employment opportunities. Women constitute about 35% of the total formal employment sector, and most of them are in the low-paying service sectors such as education, nursing, and social and community work. Botswana has one of the highest percentages of women in government positions in Africa, and the position of women compared with men in Botswana society is continually improving. Regardless, numerous women still live in poverty. Botswana has a cultural practice of unequal distribution of inheritance. Sons are given the bulk of the property after their father's death, and daughters receive little or nothing. The basic assumption is that the sons will become responsible for all dependent family members. Although this practice worked well in the past, it is not currently effective because the concept of the extended family is quickly disintegrating. Older adults, who are mostly women, often live in social isolation and poverty and receive very little support from their children. Certain legal acts and customary laws still cause women to be in a subordinate position, thereby affecting their ability to act independently without a husband or legal guardian's consent. Marriage decreases a woman's ability to acquire and control property; in most marriages the husband is the sole administrator of their joint estate. The rising rate of divorce and single parents has created another group of women who are seriously affected by the inheritance custom: female heads of households. In 1996, 48% of rural households and 33% of urban households were headed by women. Male-headed households have three times the earning power of female-headed households because women usually have no cattle and tend to pass their poverty on from generation to generation. Botswana has definite customs regarding interactions in intergenerational relationships. Young people are taught to be both well-mannered and productive citizens. They are expected to obey anyone who is older and although they can express themselves when they disagree, they must do so constructively and in a way that is respectful of age and experience. Older people are also expected to behave responsibly and not use their age to exploit others. Under the constitution of Botswana, every person is entitled to certain rights and liberties regardless of race, place of origin, political opinion, color, creed, or sex. In reality, certain traditional values and attitudes still dictate that women should be subordinate to their husbands and male relatives. Women are responsible for rearing children and performing household tasks. Some of the tasks connected with the production and preparation of food, such as tilling small pieces of land, sowing, weeding, and harvesting, are traditionally assigned to women. The tasks of hunting, herding cattle, participation in public life, and other leadership roles are generally men's responsibilities. Although marriage under the traditional Setswana system is potentially polygamous because it permits a man to have more than one wife, polygamous families are actually rare. Marriage is usually consummated by the transfer of *bogadi* ("bride wealth") from the man's family to the woman's family except in tribes that have abolished the practice. The marriage is considered an arrangement not only between husband and wife but also between families. Thus after marriage, the wife moves to her husband's family home or his own home if he has already built one. When she lives with her parents-in-law, she becomes *ngwetsi*, or daughter-in-law, and is expected to behave decently, bear children, and perform all the tasks that go with motherhood. Her situation in the new home depends on the relationship she has with her in-laws, which varies from family to family. The woman is expected to have a child during the first year of marriage, after which her social status goes up significantly, especially if the first child is a boy.

Eye Contact Practices: Eye contact during a normal conversation is a sign of honesty, but it can also be perceived as a sign of insolence and stubbornness during an emotionally charged conversation. For example, when an adult is scolding a young person, the child is expected to be attentive and bow the head to show remorse. These behaviors are not gender specific.

Touch Practices: The most appropriate and almost compulsory form of touch is the handshake, which symbolizes recognition of a person's worth as a human being, even if the person is not welcome. People are considered cold and unwelcoming when they do not offer their hand while greeting others, even if the people see one another every day.

Perceptions of Time: Before the advent of the clock, time was measured by describing the position of the sun (e.g., break of dawn, midday, before or after sunset). In the new era, modern timekeeping is the norm, and even *kgotla* meetings in the rural areas are scheduled based on the clock. Punctuality has always been the norm, so people are usually punctual and try to finish their business on time.

Pain Reactions: From the onset of menstruation, girls are encouraged to be stoical and bear the pain of menstrual cramps "like proper women" in preparation for the even greater pain of childbirth. Thus women are expected to be quiet during childbirth and only make a few grunts. A woman who screams during childbirth becomes the butt of jokes for quite a few months. This kind of pain tolerance is somewhat expected even by some nurses, who have been known to readily ask a screaming woman whether the elders of her household gave her proper instructions on birth. Men are also expected to be stoical and withstand pain, although unlike women, men have no biological tests of their manhood such as childbirth.

Birth Rites: No special customs surround the birth of an infant. Circumcision of girls has never been practiced. Some ethnic groups circumcised boys during initiation in schools, but the practice halted when the schools were taken over by modern educational systems. Although infant boys are preferred, girls are also welcomed, loved, nurtured, and even educated, mostly because of their potential to bring in wealth through *bogadi* at marriage. About 98% of pregnant women go to antenatal clinics, and 92% of births are supervised by health personnel. However, only 38% of women use modern methods of family planning. Infant mortality rates are 45 per 1000 live births, and fertility rates are 4.2 children per woman. Most Batswana believe that children's personalities and emotional dispositions are determined by the mother's physical and mental health during pregnancy. Thus pregnant women, even pregnant teenagers, receive as much love and care as possible. They are encouraged to eat well but not "eat for two." Traditional Batswana beliefs focused on certain foods and their affect on pregnancy and birth. For example, they believed that eating eggs would block the birth canal and prolong labor, whereas eating intestines would give a boy infant a very long penis. Today such food restrictions are extremely rare because of health education about the importance of nutrition in pregnancy and the prevention of anemia among women. Trends in child mortality, which is an important human development indicator, show that the steady expansion of health services throughout the country has been associated with an impressive reduction in the mortality rate of children younger than 5 years.

Death Rites: Botswana's current success in home-based care programs for people with AIDS and other terminal illnesses stems from the fact that most people prefer to die in the presence of supportive family members. It is believed that after death, people join the ancestors, hence it is acceptable for older people to die but not for young people because they have not experienced life on earth. Many families are being traumatized by deaths of young people with AIDS. Autopsies are usually acceptable as the modern way of determining cause of death. Organ donation is not acceptable because of the belief that the person who had organs harvested would either be resurrected without limbs and organs or not be resurrected at all. Certain taboos and rituals surround death and family bereavement. For example, children of the bereaved are usually moved to a relative's home not only to spare them emotional turmoil but also to protect them from bad luck and contact with any evil spirits that may be lurking. A bereaved widow or widower undergoes cleansing rituals by a traditional doctor and is expected to abstain from sex for a year. Women are also expected to wear black mourning clothes for at least 6 months but usually not more than a year. Because of increased urbanization and cross-cultural marriages, some of the rituals are no longer observed.

Food Practices and Intolerances: The Setswana diet has changed a lot, and people eat varieties of foods from other cultures. However, corn, millet, and sorghum are the staples for most families. Numerous varieties of beans are also eaten, usually with a relish of green leafy vegetables (in season or preserved) and meat such as beef, venison, chicken, or mutton or other meat from wild animals. Watermelons and sweet reed are particularly well liked because they are seasonal. The most popular dish is *seswaa*, meat that is cooked until it comes off the bone and is then pounded. *Seswaa* is eaten at funerals, weddings, and other festive or solemn occasions. It is acceptable to eat with the hands as well as with knives and forks.

Infant Feeding Practices: Breast-feeding is the norm for most Batswana women, and the median duration is 16 months for urban and 18 months for rural women. Weaning foods in the form of mashed bananas, cereals, and a special vitamin-enriched soft porridge that is supplied free at clinics are introduced at 4 months. Women who cannot breast-feed because they are infected with HIV are provided with free infant formula from the clinics for 12 months. All employed mothers whose infants are younger than 12 months are entitled to an extra hour off during the day to feed their infant.

Child Rearing Practices: Traditionally, children were reared by the extended family and socialized by all the clan members. They were taught to be well mannered, courteous, disciplined, respectful, and part of the community. This form of socialization has been taken over by the nuclear family. Although the same values are stressed, the process is not as comprehensive as it was in the past.

National Childhood Immunizations: BCG at birth; DPI at 2, 3, and 4 months; D1 at 6 years; measles at 9 months; OPV at 2, 3, and 4 months; and hep B at birth and at 2 and 9 months. No cases of polio have been reported since 1989, and HIV vaccine trials began in August 2002. An important indicator of the health status of a country's children is the proportion of children immunized against potential life-threatening diseases. The Botswana Family Health Survey (BFHS) III report of 1996 revealed good immunization coverage of children younger than 5 years: measles, 74.2%, and BCG, 98.7%

Other Characteristics: Since its independence in 1966, Botswana has rapidly evolved from a poor country into a middle-income, politically stable, and multiracial country. It has a relatively good infrastructure, and most people have access to safe water and education, health, and other public services. This transformation has resulted in a good standard of living and health indicators that are some of the best in Africa. However, these improvements are threatened by HIV/AIDS because most of the funds that could be used for development projects are being channeled toward HIV/AIDS prevention, care, and support activities.

BIBLIOGRAPHY

Botswana Government: *Country profile 1995*, Gaborone, Botswana, 1996, The Government Printer.

Ingstad B, Bruun F, Tlou S: AIDS and the elderly Tswana: the concept of pollution and consequences for AIDS prevention, *J Cross-Cultural Gerontol* 12:357–372, 1997.

Mathebula U: *Needs and experiences of caregivers of PLWA in Francistown*, master's thesis, Gaborone, Botswana, 2000, University of Botswana.

Ministry of Health: *Safe motherhood in Botswana: a situational analysis*, Gaborone, Botswana, 1996.

Ministry of Health, AIDS/STD Unit: *Eighth sentinel surveillance in Botswana, 1999*, Gaborone, Botswana, 2000.

Ministry of Health, AIDS/STD Unit: *Botswana HIV and AIDS second medium term plan (MTP II) 1997-2002*, NACP 38, Gaborone, Botswana, 1997.

Ministry of Health, AIDS/STD Unit: *Community home based care for people with AIDS in Botswana. Operational guidelines*, NACP 30, Gaborone, Botswana, 1996.

Ministry of Health, AIDS/STD Unit: *Programme to prevent mother-to-child transmission (MTCT) of HIV in Botswana*, Gaborone, Botswana, 2000.

Ministry of Health, Family Health Division: *Botswana MTCT pilot project January 2000 review*, Gaborone, Botswana, 2000.

Molokomme A: *A woman's guide to the law*, Gaborone, Botswana, 1984, Women's Affairs Unit, Ministry of Home Affairs.

Molokomme A: A summary of women's legal status under Botswana family law. In Matlakala D, ed: *Women and the law in Botswana*, pp. 2–6, Gaborone, Botswana, 1987, Ministry of Home Affairs.

Mugabe M, Kgosidintsi N: *Botswana males and family planning*, Gaborone, Botswana, 1996, National Institute of Research.

Schapera I: *Married life in an African tribe*, London, 1941, Crown Books.

Schapera I: *A handbook of Tswana law and custom*, London, 1970, Frank Cass and Company.

Staugard F: *Traditional medicine*, Gaborone, Botswana, 1985, Ipelegeng.

Tlou SD: *The experience of the menopause among Botswana women*, doctoral dissertation, 1990, Chicago 1990, University of Illinois at Chicago.

Tlou SD et al: *Community responses to initiatives to prevent mother-to-child transmission of HIV in Botswana*, Washington, DC, 2000, ICRW.

Tlou T, Campbell A: *A history of Botswana*, Gaborone, Botswana, 1984, McMillan Publishers.

UNAIDS: *Report on the global HIV/AIDS epidemic*, Geneva, 2000.

UNAIDS and the World Health Organization: *HIV in pregnancy: a review*, Geneva, 1999.

UNAIDS and the World Health Organization: *AIDS epidemic update*, Geneva, 1999.

United Nations Children's Fund: *The state of the world's children*, New York, 1997, The Fund.

World Health Organization: *Primary health care*, Geneva, 1978, WHO.

◆ BRAZIL (FEDERATIVE REPUBLIC OF)

MAP PAGE (859)

Marga Simon Coler and Maria Adriana Felix Coler

Location: Comprising nearly half of South America, Brazil is the fifth largest and the sixth most populous country in the world. It is divided into five geographical regions and 26 states, and the centrally located capital (*distrito federal*) is Brasilia. The total land area is 8,511,965 km^2 (3,286,475 square miles). Forests cover 60% of the country, and Brazil is the home of the Amazon River (6296 km [3912 miles]) and the world's largest tropical rain forest.

Major Languages	Ethnic Groups	Major Religions
Portuguese	White 55%	Roman Catholic
English	Mixed white and black 38%	(official) 80%
Spanish	Black 6%	Other or none 20%
French	Other (Japanese, Arab, Amerindian) 1%	

The white population comprises Portuguese, German, Italian, Spanish, and Polish people. The overall population is estimated to be 172,860,370. In 1994 the per capita income (in U.S. dollars) was $1980 per year. In 1991, 75.47% of the inhabitants lived in urban areas. Brazil reflects African, Indian, Portuguese, and Dutch cultures in the north and northeast regions and German and Italian influences in the south. São Paulo has one of the largest Japanese communities in the world. A developed country, Brazil has two distinct classes (rich and poor) and a small but growing middle class.

Health Care Beliefs: Both active and passive involvement; selective health promotion. The recently inaugurated Unified Health System (SUS) places emphasis on primary health care and focuses on health promotion and illness prevention. Health agents and public health monitors are very involved in community intervention. The people in the middle class are actively involved, whereas people who are poor are more passive.

Predominant Sick Care Practices: Biomedical; holistic; magical-religious (especially in interior Brazil). Pharmacies run by homeopathic doctors are common, and acupuncture is being used more frequently. Pharmacists and even pharmacy owners prescribe medications and treat illnesses, especially for people in the lower socioeconomic class. Use of medicines made at home using teas made of plants, leaves, and roots is common and reflects the heritage and beliefs of Indians and ancestors. In addition, some people seek assistance from *rezadeiras*, women with the power to cure through prayer. The government pays about 80% of hospital costs for health problems listed in the Diagnosis-Related Group (DRG) classification system. Private health plans are common among people of the middle class. It is also common for people to self-medicate using over-the-counter medications including antibiotics. Narcotics require a prescription.

Ethnic/Race Specific or Endemic Diseases: The endemic diseases in Brazil are dengue fever, hemorrhagic dengue fever, AIDS, cholera, tuberculosis, and schistosomiasis. Brazil's compulsory reportable diseases are cholera, whooping cough, dengue, diphtheria, acute cases of Chagas' disease, diseases of meningicocci or meningitis, yellow fever, typhoid fever, hantavirus, hepatitis B and C, visceral leishmaniasis, Hansen's disease, leptospirosis, malaria (in areas where it is not endemic), *Haemophilus influenzae* infection, poliomyelitis, acute flaccid paralysis, peste, human rabies, rubeola, syndrome of congenital rubeola, sarampo, congenital syphilis, AIDS, tetanus, tuberculosis, and chloroquine-resistant malaria. Diseases preventable through immunization are sarampo, diphtheria, pertussis, neonatal tetanus, tetanus, yellow fever, human rabies, hepatitis B, and typhoid. Brazilians are at risk for work-related, iatrogenic, maternal and neonatal, and asthmatic and respiratory conditions, as well as malnutrition and dysentery. The World Health Organization's (WHO) estimated prevalence rate for HIV and AIDS is 0.57%. The estimated number of children from birth to 15 years living with HIV/AIDS is 9900. From 2000 to 2001 the HIV/AIDS infection rate was 13,932 cases per 100,000 people.

Health Team Relationships: The term *doutor* is used indiscriminately to express respect and affection. Nurses are addressed by their title (*enfermeira*) followed by their first name. Within the patriarchal and capitalist health care system, nurses tend to internalize their oppressed role. Concepts of class and social status are strong.

Families' Role in Hospital Care: The family assumes some responsibility for direct care. Family members may bring food or take turns staying with the patient 24 hours per day. It is common for family members to take part in decision making about referrals and procedures such as surgeries. In some situations, such as the chronic stage of terminal diseases, one member represents the family. That member is chosen based on aspects such as level of education, social status, and leadership skills.

Dominance Patterns: The extended family may include godparents and godchildren who may have been chosen because of their prestigious social status in the community. Godparents are chosen by the parents as a sign of recognition and respect for important members of the community. Godparents are expected to help provide quality medical care to godchildren as needed, although it is common for godparents and godchildren never to see each other after the baptism. Sons and daughters address their parents in the third person (i.e., *"o senhor"* or *"a senhora"*). One tradition of Brazilian children is asking for their parents' blessing and then kissing the parents' right hand. This custom is not as common among younger Brazilians but remains popular in northeastern Brazil. When a person has more than one last name, the mother's name precedes the father's. Even if it is no longer used, having the same last name, or family name, can give family members a sense of belonging.

Eye Contact Practices: Direct eye contact, like other body language, is common between sexes and among social classes.

Touch Practices: Use of the body and touch to make personal and social contact is generally the "tropical" way of relating. Women and men greet each other by shaking hands or kissing on both cheeks. An *abraço*, or embrace, indicates a very close relationship or feelings of affection. Greetings among those in professional relationships are limited to a handshake. Touching while talking is common.

Perceptions of Time: Brazilians are casual about punctuality and focused on the present. The future is measured in decades or generations, and definitions of "early" and "late" are flexible. Arriving late can reflect a successful social standing. Immediate rewards are preferred to delayed gratification.

Pain Reactions: Pain is expressed vocally, through moans and groans, although stoicism is not unheard of. People from the interior of the country tend to somaticize their physical problems.

Birth Rites: Fathers are not usually present during labor and delivery, although the presence of some family members during natural births or cesarean sections is common. Circumcision of male infants is not routine. Girls may have their ears pierced soon after birth, often while they are still in the hospital. Mothers are expected to rest for 60 days after birth, and fathers usually take a week off from work. Working parents continue to collect their salaries, and working mothers usually have flexible hours including extra time during the day to breast-feed. Other family members may assume the role of primary caregiver, while parents return to activities such as work or school. Tubal ligation in women after the birth of two children (of one boy and one girl) is a common practice in the middle and upper classes. This procedure is difficult to obtain for mothers in the lower class. Infants are usually delivered by cesarean section. In 2000 the estimated birth rate was 18.84 per 1000 people, and the infant mortality rate was 38.04 deaths per 1000 live births. The life expectancy at birth was 58.54 years for men and 67.56 years for women.

Death Rites: Death rites are class dependent. People who are poor carry their dead to a cemetery, often in a cardboard casket or hammock. In small towns the ritual may involve the entire community, and towns-people may join the family procession. Small businesses are closed, and activities are suspended as a sign of sympathy and respect. Children dressed in long white robes (so that they represent angels) often lead the procession by carrying a large crown made of natural or artificial flowers. Male relatives such as brothers, sons, or grandsons are the pallbearers and are followed by close relatives and friends. Brazilians sing religious or popular songs and pray during the ceremony. Individuals from the middle and upper classes are buried in wooden caskets, and hearses are often used. People who are poor can rent a plot for 2 years, after which time another body is buried on top of the one already interred. In some family graves, one body may be buried on top of another as well. Embalming and cremation are very expensive and only practiced in some regions (such as the south) .The body is surrounded by flowers, and only the head shows during the service. The body is usually buried the day after death. In the middle and upper classes, the funeral procession is done in cars rather than walking and is limited to the cemetery grounds. A cemetery worker is paid by the month to maintain the gravesite for the family.

Food Practices and Intolerance: Yams, bread, and couscous are common for breakfast, although cereals are becoming more popular. The main meal is eaten at noon and consists of rice, beans, mashed potatoes, pasta, and meat or fish. The consumption of vegetable and salads is increasing. The trend in middle-class families in which both parents work outside the home is to eat the noon meal at a self-service restaurant or a luncheonette, although going back home is still a popular choice because most jobs include a 2-hour lunch break. If eating out, a *coxinha*, *pastel*, or a sandwich is not uncommon. Supper, a light meal (or soup or leftovers from lunch), is eaten in the evening.

Infant Feeding Practices: Breast-feeding is generally short term. The attitude of the father can be the most significant factor in duration of breast-feeding. *Mingau*, a filling formula made of a thickening agent (e.g., flour of manioc, corn, or rice) and water is used, especially by poor families, to fill the stomach of a hungry infant or toddler. Slight obesity in infants or children is considered a sign of health.

Child Rearing Practices: Children are treated affectionately. Parents inhale the scent of a child before kissing the child. Warm embraces from all family members are common. Pacifiers are tied to the diaper or kept on a cord around the infant's neck to keep them from becoming lost or contaminated; safety issues with this procedure are generally ignored. Grandmothers play an active role in caregiving, especially when the mother works outside the home. Children from middle and upper classes are enrolled in private or parochial schools. Students in lower classes receive a public education. Young children are enrolled in a *crèche* (day care) or kindergarten. The normal school day is half a day (in the morning, afternoon, or evening). Children in the lowest socioeconomic bracket often work rather than going to school, and homeless children are numerous in large cities. Research on education has focused on the cognitive abilities of these homeless children and their capacity to use "street knowledge" to learn math and geography. Some of them find jobs as tour guides, demonstrating their ability to memorize historical facts (such as events, places, and famous people) even though they have poor reading skills.

National Childhood Immunizations: BCG at birth and 6 years; DPT at 2, 4, 6, and 15 months; OPV at 2, 4, 6, and 15 months; hep B at birth and at 1 and 6 months; HIB at 2, 4, and 6 months; measles at 9 months; MMR at 15 months; rubella at 12 to 49 years; yellow fever at 9 months; TT CBAW × 3; antisarampo at 9 months; trivalent immunization (sarampo, rubeola, and pertussis) at 12 months; and DT at 7 years.

BIBLIOGRAPHY

Brasil, Ministério da Saúde: *Datasus. Indicadores básicos de morbidade e fator de risco*, 20001. File://A:\morbididade Br.htm

Brasil, Ministério da Saúde: *Indicadores básicos de morbidade e fator de risco*, 2001, File://A:\AIDS Br.htm

Brasil, Ministério da Saúde, Fundação Nacional de Saúde, Centro Nacional de Epidemiologia: *Portaria no. 1.461/GM/MS Informe Epidemiológico do SUS* 9(1), 2000.

Dias J: Problemas e possibilidades de participação comunitária no controle das grandes endemias no Brasil, *Cardernos de Saúde Publica* 14 (suppl 2): 29–37, 1998.

Dias J et al: Espoco geral e perspectivas da doença de Chagas no nordeste do Brasil, *Cadernos de Saúde Pública* 16 (suppl 2), 2000.

Rachid M, Schechter M: *Manual de HIV/AIDS*, Rio de Janeiro, Brazil, 2001, Revinter, Ltda.

Scheper-Hughes N: *Death without weeping*, Berkeley, CA, 1992, University of California Press.

U.S. Government, Central Intelligence Agency: Washington, DC, New York, 2000, Bartleby.com File://A:\education.yahoo.com/reference/factbook/br/popula.html

◆ BRUNEI DARUSSALAM (STATE OF)

MAP PAGE (867)

Kenneth Y.Y. Kok

Location: Brunei Darussalam ("abode of peace") has an area of 5,765 km² and is situated on the northern coast of the island of Borneo. It is a sovereign, independent, democratic, Muslim monarchy, according to Sunni beliefs. About 66.2% of the population lives in the Brunei/Muara District, where the capital, Bandar Seri Begawan, is situated.

Major Languages	Ethnic Groups	Major Religions
Malay (official)	Malay 68%	Muslim (official) 67%
English	Chinese 15%	Buddhist 13%
Chinese	Indigenous 6%	Christian 10%
	Other 11%	Indigenous, other 10%

Malay is the official language, but English is widely used in business and commerce. The estimated population was 338,400 in 2000. The discovery of oil in the western part of the country in the 1920s ushered in a new economic era, and the development of offshore exploration in the 1960s set Brunei Darussalam on the path to economic prosperity. Since the beginning of 1984, when Brunei Darussalam became independent, a ministerial system of government has been in place; His Majesty the Sultan and Yang Di-Pertuan serve as the prime minister and head of state.

Health Care Beliefs: Active involvement; increasing emphasis on health promotion. With noncommunicable diseases high on the list of causes of mortality and morbidity in the country, Brunei Darussalam has identified health promotion as one of the main initiatives as stipulated in the National Health Care Plan 2000–2010. Although health promotion activities have long been in place, it is only recently that concentrated and concerted efforts have been made. The National Committee on Health Promotion has identified seven priority areas that need attention within 5 years: nutrition, food safety, tobacco control, mental health, physical activity, healthy environment and settings, and women's health. The population is young, with 51.2% younger than 25 years. Therefore all prevention and promotion health services are programmed to give priority to health problems of the young. Patients with mental illness are still being stigmatized. However, with the introduction of an open-door policy of hospital psychiatric departments and improvement in the quality of care, the number of patients seeking psychiatric consultation has steadily increased, with patients being more open and less worried about stigma and shame.

Predominant Sick Care Practices: Biomedical; traditional; magical-religious. All services provided to citizens and permanent residents are primarily funded through the general treasury. The health care budget is allocated by the Ministry of Finance and administered by the Ministry of Health. The Ministry of Health budget in 1999 was approximately B$208 million (USD$122 million), about 7.2% of the total national government budget. Health care is free for all citizens, permanent residents, and expatriate government employees, and for others it is heavily subsidized. Services are also created to be accessible to all the population. Citizens are sent overseas at the government's expense for medical care not available in Brunei Darussalam. Remote areas are reached by a flying doctor service that makes regular visits three times a week by helicopter. Traditional medicine, or *ubat kampong*, administered by local healers, or *bomoh*, is quite popular. Frequently patients are not forthcoming about the fact that they have consulted the *bomoh*, therefore asking about traditional medicine when taking a history from a patient is essential. Traditional medicine is part of the people's traditional belief system and has been practiced for centuries. It is believed, especially among older adults, that disease is the work of evil entities in another realm that have been disturbed in some way. In addition, unrealistic expectations patients have regarding hospital care often leads to dissatisfaction. If they do not have instantaneous improvement in their conditions, they resort to options such as alternative and traditional medicines. Fear of the hospital and its unfamiliar surroundings also cause patients to seek out traditional methods; *bomohs* are usually well-known members of the community who reside in the same or nearby villages. *Bomohs* primarily use herbal concoctions, and few scientific evaluations of these herbal plants have been done. Additional studies are needed not only to assess the treatments' effectiveness but also to investigate possible drug reactions and interactions. Alternative medicine such as homeopathy and reflexology are also used.

Ethnic/Race Specific or Endemic Disease: Because of the steady rise in the standard of living, mortality rates have declined in all segments of the population. An analysis of the major causes of death in the past 30 years indicates that the causes are no longer infectious diseases such as tuberculosis and pneumonia. The predominant diseases are now chronic degenerative diseases, such as cancer and cardiovascular disease, related to modern lifestyles. The five leading causes of inpatient morbidity in 1999 were acute upper respiratory tract infections, asthma, pregnancy with abortive outcomes, and acute lower respiratory tract infections. The leading causes of death were (in order of magnitude) malignant neoplasms, heart disease, diabetes mellitus, cerebrovascular disease, bronchitis and asthma, automobile accidents, hypertensive diseases, and pneumonia. The average life expectancy has increased and is among the highest in the Asian region, a change that reflects the enhanced health, social, and economic environments. Other global health indicators such as infant and maternal mortality have decreased and are among the best in Asia. A list of 39 communicable diseases based on international and local priorities are notifiable: out of these, 24 were reported in 1999. Chicken pox continues to be the most prominent of the communicable diseases, comprising 73.5% of reported cases. The remaining 26.5% of diseases cases consist of tuberculosis, gonococcal infections, food poisoning, cholera, and other diseases. No indigenous cases of malaria have been reported since 1969 and no poliomyelitis cases since 1978. In August 1987, Brunei Darussalam was entered in the World Health Organization's (WHO) official register of areas where malaria has been eradicated. The unabated global spread of HIV/AIDS is a matter of grave concern. The World Health Organization's (WHO) estimated prevalence rate for HIV/AIDS in adults ages 15 to 49 is 0.2%. WHO has no estimates for children from birth to 15 years. As of December 2001 the number of people infected with HIV was 564. Vigilance regarding AIDS is being maintained through a national control program. Life expectancy at birth is 74.9 and 78.2 years for men and women, respectively.

Health Team Relationships: The lowest level of doctor is the medical officer; the next is the senior medical officer, and at the top of the hierarchy is the specialist. Major decisions about patient management are solely the responsibility of the specialist. The medical staff works closely and constantly consults with the nursing staff regarding patient care, but the overall care of the patient is carried out by the specialist. A college in Brunei Darussalam offers a 3-year nursing course. The country is experiencing a trend toward subspecialty nursing, so the college offers diploma courses in operating theater, intensive care, and accident and emergency nursing. Nurses play an active role in general patient management and more specialized care such as infection control, diabetes management, and oncology. The doctor and patient usually have a good rapport. A patients' charter was launched 3 years ago, so patients are now more aware of their rights. Health care professionals are respected, trusted, and highly esteemed by patients and the general public. In 1999, 309 medical doctors and 50 dentists were registered to practice, with a ratio of doctors to the population of 1:1070. To overcome the shortage of local doctors in various disciplines, the government continues to employ expatriates on contract.

Families' Role in Hospital Care: Family ties are strong. Grown children are expected to care for their aging parents, so putting parents in a facility for older adults is not well regarded. The family usually has a dominant figure, either the head of the household or the grandfather. Consultation with this person regarding health matters is advisable, and written consent should be obtained from the dominant family member before any investigative or therapeutic procedure is carried out on the patient. Visiting and bringing food to hospitalized relatives are common practices. Occasionally, all extended family members visit the relative at the same time, making visiting hours on the ward a noisy affair, especially during joyous occasions such as childbirth. It is common for a family member to spend the night with a sick relative in the hospital ward.

Dominance Patterns: The pattern of male dominance is slowly changing, a transition that is evident in the recent appointment of women to top government positions: the attorney general and the permanent secretary to two government ministries. However, men are still dominant in families, and major family decisions are made by the head of the household, who is either the father or grandfather.

Eye Contact Practices: Direct eye contact between opposite sexes is allowed and expected during conversation.

Touch Practices: Public displays of affection such as kissing are unacceptable. When shaking hands with a member of the opposite sex, a man generally refrains from extending his hand unless the woman offers it first.

Perceptions of Time: Punctuality is not a major issue during festive occasions such as wedding receptions and gatherings; being 30 minutes late is acceptable. Almost all patients are on time for health clinic appointments, and most arrive at the clinic at least 30 minutes to an hour before scheduled appointments.

Pain Reactions: Pain reactions seem to be related to age. Young people seek medical advice as soon as they experience pain or discomfort. Older individuals tend to keep any discomfort to themselves and do not inform their relatives, probably because they do not want to burden a relative or disrupt routine activities. Patients tend to be fairly reserved in expressions of pain, a practice that is evident after surgeries because it is usually a caring relative who requests analgesics for the patient.

Birth Rites: Certain traditional beliefs, such as avoiding certain foods, surround pregnancy and birth. For example, it is believed that consumption of papaya and pineapples may lead to miscarriages, and consumption of squid may lead to placental deformities. The expectant mother is not allowed to wrap a towel around her neck because people believe this causes the umbilical cord to loop around the neck of the fetus. People also believe that hammering or nailing a wall could lead to a miscarriage. The pregnant woman is not allowed to sit in the doorway because it is believed to lead to difficult labor. Nearly all births are in hospitals; childbirth at home is rare today because hospitals are easily accessible. After birth a black thread is tied at the base of both of the mother's big toes. She is advised to keep warm and avoid "cold" foods, so she is not allowed to drink cold water or eat "cold" foods such as cucumber, spinach, or pineapple. She is not allowed to bathe until 3 days after birth. Some women sleep near burning charcoal to keep warm. The woman's abdomen is wrapped with herbs, and she receives traditional massages to improve her muscle tone and aid uterine involution. These activities are practiced for 40 days, during which sexual activities are prohibited. The country has experienced a significant reduction in its fertility rate, giving rise to a change in the age structure of its population. The total fertility rate decreased from 3.78 children per woman in 1981 to 2.7 in 1999, with a sharp decrease in pregnancies in women younger than 25 (largely because of later first marriages) and older than 40 (caused by fertility curtailment by women who have attained their desired family size). This change in population structure will cause significant growth in the proportion of the population age 15 and older. The infant mortality rate is 5.9 per 1000 live births, and the maternal mortality rate is 0 per 1000 live births.

Death Rites: Death is thought of as the path into the next world. Muslim burial is carried out within 1 day, and the body is wrapped in special white cloth and buried without a coffin. Cremation is not allowed. Relatives and close friends offer ritual prayers either at the home of the deceased person or at the mosque. Prayers are recited on three consecutive nights; 7, 14, 40, and 100 days after death; and yearly thereafter. Autopsies are uncommon and organ donations (from cadavers) are not allowed because the body must be buried intact. In hospitals, it is common for a dying person to request to die at home surrounded by close relatives.

Food Practices and Intolerances: Islamic law forbids the consumption of pork and alcohol, and only *halal* meat may be consumed—meat slaughtered according to Muslim rites. Most western, Southeast Asian, Middle Eastern, international, Chinese, and traditional Malay foods are easily available in major hotels, in family-owned restaurants, at hawker stalls, and at fast-food chain restaurants. After surgery, patients avoid certain foods such as prawns and shellfish because they are believed to inflame wounds and delay healing. The consumption of supplementary foods or natural tonics is common after illness, surgery, or childbirth. Among the popular tonics are fish essence with wild ginseng and cordyceps, chicken essence, and ostrich tonic with cordyceps. These tonics are believed to stimulate blood circulation, improve the complexion, reinforce the body's energy, regenerate muscles, relieve edema, and enhance the body's resistance to disease.

Infant Feeding Practices: All mothers are encouraged to breast-feed their babies; however, because of the change in social structure, working women are finding it increasingly difficult to continue breast-feeding after the first month. To reeducate women and encourage breast-feeding, the Baby-Friendly Hospital Initiative, in collaboration with WHO, has been introduced at major hospitals.

Child Rearing Practices: Parents are quite permissive, although it is the responsibility of both parents to discipline the children. Corporal punishment has been abolished in schools but is still acceptable in the home. Children usually sleep with parents until they are 4 or 5 years old, and they are sent to nursery schools at the age of 3. Formal religious education begins at the age of 8 or at school (grade primary 3). The *istiadat berkhatan* (circumcision ceremony) marks a boy's coming of age and is usually performed between ages 10 and 12. The operation is performed at designated health clinic or hospitals. Female circumcisions are not performed.

National Childhood Immunizations: BCG at birth and 6 years; DTP at 6, 12 to 14, and 18 to 22 weeks and at 5 years; OPV at 6, 12 to 14, and 18 to 22 weeks and at 5 years; hep B at birth and at 1 and 6 months; MMR at 12 months and 10 to 13 years; and TT at weeks 28 and 32 of pregnancy, and during the next pregnancy.

Other Characteristics: The culture is predominantly influenced by Islam. To indicate refusal of offered food, it is polite to touch the plate lightly with the right hand. The right hand is always used to give or receive, because the left is considered unclean. When sitting on the floor, a person should sit cross-legged rather than with the legs stretched out in front. The polite way to summon someone is to use all four fingers of the right hand with the palm facing down while motioning them towards you; the index finger is never used. It is customary to leave footwear at the door when entering a Muslim house.

BIBLIOGRAPHY

Ministry of Health, Brunei Darussalam: *The millennium report* 2000, Brunei Darussalam, 2000.
Ministry of Health, Brunei Darussalam: *National health care plan (2000–2010): a strategic framework for Action*, June 2000.
Ministry of Industry and Primary Resources, Department of Agriculture: *Medicinal plants of Brunei Darussalam, part two*, Brunei Darussalam, 1994.

◆ BULGARIA (REPUBLIC OF)

MAP PAGE (860)

Slavianka Moyanova

Location: Bulgaria is situated in the Balkan Peninsula in southeastern Europe and is bordered on the north by Romania, east by the Black Sea, south by Turkey and Greece, and west by Serbia and the Republic of Macedonia. Bulgaria is now called the *Republic of Bulgaria* but was known as the "People's Republic of Bulgaria" from 1947 to 1990. The capital and largest city is Sofia. More than half of Bulgaria is hilly or mountainous. The Balkan Mountains cross the country from its north-western corner to the Black Sea. The northern side of the Balkan Mountains slopes gradually to form the northern Bulgarian plateau, which ends at the River Danube. In the southern and southwestern parts of the country are the Rhodope and Rila mountains. The population of Bulgaria is about 8 million, and the total land area is 110,910 km^2 (42,822 square miles).

Major Languages	Ethnic Groups	Major Religions
Bulgarian	Bulgarian 84%	Christian (Bulgarian
	Turkish 9%	Orthodox) 84%
	Roma-Gypsy 5%	Muslim 12%
	Other 2%	Other 4%

The first Bulgarian kingdom was created from Bulgarians and Slavs in the seventh century. In the Middle Ages, Bulgaria competed with the Byzantine Empire and greatly influenced the cultural life of the region. Ethnic Turks are the descendants of Osmani Turks who settled in Bulgaria during the 500 years when it was a province of the Ottoman Empire. Ethnic Bulgarians who converted to Islam are recognized as a separate group called *Pomaks*. The Bulgarian Orthodox Church is an autonomous branch of the Eastern Orthodox Church. Most ethnic Turks and Pomaks are Muslims; some groups of Gregorian-Armenians, Protestants, Jews, and Roman Catholics also exist.

Health Care Beliefs: Acute sick care; some magical beliefs. Health prevention practices are ignored by the population and the health care system; no resources in the National Insurance Fund are targeted for prevention purposes. According to a health survey carried out in the last national census of the Bulgarian population, only 16% of the population had ever been offered any type of illness prevention program; those who had been offered services were primarily offered vaccinations. A very small percentage of the population believes that illness may be eradicated by magical intervention. Psychotherapy is not valued in the culture.

Predominant Sick Care Practices: Biomedical; traditional and alternative medicine. Matters of health and medicine in Bulgaria are under the overall control of the Ministry of Health. Before the democratic political reforms in 1989, the health care system guaranteed each resident free access to medical care. A reform in the public health system is currently underway in Bulgaria and should result in the financial responsibility for provision of medical services being assumed by the National Insurance Fund but financed by employers and workers. Doctors and other health care practitioners in the diagnostic and consulting centers (DCCs) or medical centers contract with the fund to provide care. Patients pay a nominal sum for each visit to a general practitioner, who may refer them to a specialist if necessary. Free care is provided for all children, and unemployed people may make arrangements with their general practitioner for medical care and to apply for free hospitalization. The hospitals are government controlled. The government covers the greater part of the costs, and medical services are provided by salaried doctors and other health care personnel. The numbers of private doctors working outside the government hospital system (who are primarily dentists) or in private health centers are increasing. In hospitals and DCCs, only traditional medical treatment is offered. Before going to a doctor, Bulgarians rely primarily on the family and seek help from doctors only as a last resort. Although the majority of Bulgarians trust the care received from doctors, they usually self-medicate and buy their drugs without a doctor's prescription. Deeply religious individuals believe that going to a priest for confession and prayer will relieve their suffering. Indigenous and alternative health care practices are also used, particularly massage therapy, meditation, herbal medicine, therapeutic touch, biofeedback, and homeopathy. Such practices are usually used to treat phobias, arthritis, anxiety, back problems, and headaches. Several newspapers and many books in Bulgaria are devoted to alternative medicine; the use of medicinal herbs, especially in the form of tea, is common. Medicinal herb treatments are based on centuries-old healing traditions, and recipes for the preparation of herb tea are passed down from mothers to family, friends, and colleagues. Although Bulgaria has many medicinal herb shops, many people prefer to gather herbs themselves. Very few people go to doctors because of colds, sore throats, or coughs. Some doctors combine alternative and traditional medicine, prescribing synthetic drugs along with herbs, plant extracts, and natural nutrients. Other doctors practice homeopathy as well. Nutrient supplements such as antioxidants are available in Bulgaria, but they are very expensive and few people can afford to buy them.

Ethnic/Race Specific or Endemic Diseases: The morbidity rates of certain diseases (e.g., sexually transmitted diseases such as syphilis, gastrointestinal diseases, hepatitis B, tuberculosis) are much higher in the Roma ethnic group than in the rest of the population. Diseases related to iodine deficiencies are endemic in southeastern Bulgaria in spite of national preventive actions for use of salt with iodine added. Nephritis, nephrolithiasis, and other kidney diseases are endemic in northwestern Bulgaria. The illnesses that affect Bulgarians most are circulatory system diseases, primarily hypertension and stroke (which affect 21.3% of the population). The most widespread diseases among children are asthma and bronchitis, and the percentage of children and young people affected with these conditions has doubled in the past 4 years. Overall, subjective opinions of health status, obtained in a recent survey, point to deteriorating health in Bulgaria. In a survey conducted in March 2001, 45% of the rural population and 38% of the urban population reported that their health had deteriorated during the 4 previous years. According to data of the same survey, more people began seeking health care, especially older adults. The survey also demonstrated that people's estimates regarding their "expected duration of life in good health" had substantially decreased. The World Health Organization's (WHO) estimated prevalence rate for HIV/AIDS in adults ages 15 to 49 is 0.01%. WHO has no estimates for children from birth to 15 years. The official number of Bulgarians who are infected with HIV is 153.

Health Team Relationships: Despite the relatively high doctor/patient ratio (1:296), Bulgarian doctors are overwhelmed with work, partly because of the enormous number of sick people. Nurses play a subordinate role in the health care system. Since 2000, all Bulgarians have been allowed to choose and change their general practitioner every 6 months if desired. Everyone is at liberty to determine the qualifications of doctors and dentists, which creates a market perspective and natural competition among doctors. Health reforms are occurring, but Bulgaria still has many problems involving the balance between the rights and obligations of patients and doctors. Doctors and nurses work as a team, especially in preclinical centers, and the relationships are usually good because the doctors select and hire the nurses. Nurses working with general practitioners do a great deal of the administrative work and are low-paid health workers. In hospitals the health care teams consist of several doctors and nurses, and roles and responsibilities are strictly defined. Nurses are university educated.

Families' Role in Hospital Care: Because resources in hospitals are less than optimal, family members usually stay with the patient, particularly when the illness is serious. Family members supplement services offered by the hospital by bringing additional food, changing linens, and buying drugs when necessary.

Dominance Patterns: In today's younger families, men and women carry equal weight in certain decision-making processes, but they do not have equal obligations at home. Women do the cooking, the cleaning, the washing, and most other household chores. In older families the father is the head of the household and the main decision maker. Typically, the man reads a newspaper or watches television after work and then moves to the table and waits for dinner to be served.

Eye Contact Practices: Direct eye contact is very important in social and business situations. Not maintaining a direct gaze is considered impolite or a sign of disinterest. Children are taught to make direct eye contact with teachers, with friends of their parents, and during all conversations.

Touch Practices: A brief, light handshake is the usual form of greeting when a person, including a child, is introduced to another person. The handshake often occurs when greeting and parting and in all social situations. If a man is seated, he stands to shake hands with another person. A woman offers her hand first, but a seated woman is not obliged to stand when a man enters the room. When good male friends greet one another, a warm and long handshake may be accompanied by a light touch on the forearm or elbow or by a light embrace. Patting on the back is not very acceptable. Close female friends who are greeting after not seeing each other for a long time may hug lightly, kiss one or both cheeks, or brush the cheeks as if kissing. When conversing, people stand about half a meter from one another. Casual body contact among strangers (e.g., while waiting in line) is avoided.

Perceptions of Time: Punctuality is not an inherent national value. The majority of people are punctual in work situations, but few get to private appointments on time. Because of long lines, patients in the DCCs usually wait for long periods for previously arranged appointments with general practitioners. Patients consider long waiting times for diagnostic tests and other procedures to be a hindrance to good health care.

Pain Reactions: Bulgarians differ in their degree of response to pain according to gender, age, and culture, although patients seek complete explanations of the meaning of their pain and its relief. Some dramatize their pain, reacting expressively, whereas others deny pain and display stoicism. The dramatic reaction is more common among Bulgarians. Men react more expressively and women more emotionally. Older patients, who are more vulnerable to chronic pain, tend to feel increasingly discouraged, helpless, and hypochondriacal in a system that does not adequately respond to their needs.

Birth Rites: All births in Bulgaria occur in hospitals, and women who are at high risk for pregnancy complications are under the care of doctors. Women with high-risk pregnancies may stay at home for the entire pregnancy. Childbirth preparation classes do not exist, and family members (including the husband) are not allowed to be present during the delivery. Women and their infants remain in the hospital for 4 to 5 days, and the infants are brought to them from the nursery four or five times daily for feedings. About 10 to 15 years ago, infants were wrapped tightly around the hips, but this practice has stopped because the practice was causing joint articulation problems.

Death Rites: Details of death rites in urban and rural areas differ. The usual practice in urban areas is to hire a private funeral home to organize all burial rites. The body is dressed in nice clothing and placed inside a coffin that will be sent to a cemetery. Depending on the preference of the relatives, the coffin stays either in a church or a ritual home, where either a priest conducts a funeral service or an official civil person reads a eulogy. Family members, friends, and colleagues of the deceased person pay their last respects. One by one they walk by the coffin, putting many flowers on and around the body, after which condolences are offered to family members. At the cemetery by the grave, family and friends have one more chance to say goodbye to the deceased person, and then all are invited for a plate of biscuits, boiled wheat, and bread. In rural areas, family and friends say goodbye to the deceased in the person's home, where the body stays 1 or 2 days after death. The body is then transported from the home to the cemetery in a procession and is followed by a gathering. Eastern Orthodox Christian practice discourages cremation, but it is practiced because of a lack of cemetery space in larger cities. Autopsies are not well accepted by Bulgarians but are performed for forensic reasons in cases of violent death; for other purposes, close relatives generally consult one another about the decision. Organ donation is valued, and people consider the receipt of a donated organ to be a second chance at life and a greatly valued gift. A system of registration for organ donation is in process. Those who object to donation of their organs record their objections so that the information can be retrieved in the event of their death. The majority of people believe that family wishes should override those of a patient after a patient has died. Even when patients consent to be organ donors, doctors respect families' wishes if the families object. Parents of young children seldom allow donations of the children's organs after their death.

Food Practices and Intolerances: Large meals are eaten at midday and in the evening, and foods with ginger-flavored sauces are preferred. Popular foods include stuffed peppers, green beans, white brined cheese, meat and vegetable hash (*musaka*), hotchpotch (*guvetch*), stuffed cabbage or vine leaves, yogurt, salad with sauerkraut, mixed vegetable salad (tomatoes, roasted and peeled peppers, and cucumber) topped with grated white cheese (*Shops' salad*), and cold chopped cucumber soup (*tarator*). Because vegetables are the preferred food, most people preserve them in cans in the summer for use in winter, when they are very expensive to purchase.

Infant Feeding Practices: All new mothers understand the importance of breast-feeding, not only for infant health but also for infant-mother attachment. They know that colostrum and breast-feeding help their infants resist the bacteria and viruses that cause illness. The majority of Bulgarian women do their best to breast-feed as long as possible, and doctors and nurses in the hospital assist with breast-feeding techniques.

Child Rearing Practices: Child rearing depends on the family's culture and parental views of proper behavior. Younger families tend to be more permissive than older families. Children usually sleep with parents, but after about 10 years of age they move to a separate room if possible. All parents expect their children to be quiet and obedient, but because it is financially necessary for both parents to work, not enough time may be spent with children, and they can become defiant and delinquent. Severe physical punishment or abuse is not accepted, and most parents bring their children up with loving discipline involving suggestions, explanations, and advice. According to the law, children in Bulgaria reach adulthood at age 18. A large-scale discussion involving all levels of Bulgarian society is now taking place regarding what should be permitted and prohibited for children younger than age 18. Just before Christmas Eve in 2001, seven children between 10 and 17 years were trampled and suffocated in a disco club as crowds of young people were trying to make their way through a narrow passage to the club's door. Now children younger than 16 are prohibited to consume liquor or go to disco or computer clubs without an identification card and an accompanying parent or older person. It is thought that although the teaching of moral values should primarily come from parents and school, the government has a role to play and should restrict certain activities.

National Childhood Immunizations: BCG at birth and at 7 and 11 years; OPV at 2, 3, 4, 14, and 24 months and 7 years; DTP at 2, 3, 4, and 24 months; MMR at 13 months and 12 years; hep B at birth and at 1 and 6 months; Td at 7, 12, 17, 25, and 35 years; and TT at 45, 55, 65, 75, and 85 years.

Other Characteristics: The head motions indicating "yes" and "no" are the opposite of those used in the United States, which can cause considerable confusion during conversations among Bulgarians and certain foreigners.

BIBLIOGRAPHY

Axtell RE, ed: *Do's and taboos around the world*, ed 2, New York, 1990, John Wiley & Sons.

Balabanova D, McKee M: Patterns of alcohol consumption in Bulgaria, *Alcohol Alcoholism* 34(4):622, 1999.

Bulgaria, *Microsoft encarta 98 encyclopedia*, 1993–1997, Microsoft Corporation.

Cukuranovic R et al: Balkan epidemic neuropathy: a decreasing incidence of the disease, *Pathol Biol* 48(6):558, 2000.

Joint United Nations Program on HIV/AIDS, World Health Organization: *AIDS epidemic update, December 2001*, http://www.unaids.org/epidemic_update/report/dec01/

Kaneva R et al: A linkage study of affective disorders in two Bulgarian gypsy families: results for candidate regions on chromosomes 18 and 21, *Psychiatr Genet* 8(4):245, 1998.

National Statistical Institute, Bulgaria: *Census 2001 and main results from the survey into health status of Bulgarian population in March 2001 and some comparisons with data of previous surveys*. Retrieved March 1, 2002, from http://www.nsi.bg/Census/Census-i.htm

World Health Organization (June 2000): *Epidemiological fact sheets by country*, Geneva. Retrieved March 1, 2002, from http://www.unaids.org/hivaidsinfo/statistics/june00/fact_sheets/index.html

World Health Organization (2001): *WHO vaccine-preventable diseases: monitoring system: 2001 global summary*, Geneva. Retrieved March 1, 2002, from http://whqlibdoc.who.int/ - hq/2001/WHO_V & B_01.34.pdf

◆ BURKINA FASO

MAP PAGE (862)

Eric Ledru and Georges Dahourou

Location: Burkina Faso (formerly Upper Volta) is landlocked in West Africa and consists of plains, low hills, and high savannas, with desert in the north. The total land area is 274,200 km^2 (105,869 square miles). Burkina Faso is a Sahelian West African country with poor water resources. Distribution of precipitation varies during the year, with a long dry season from November to May. Harmattan, a hot and dry wind, sweeps the country and carries dust clouds from March to May. Because the country has no access to the ocean, important migratory flows of people occur between the harbors of Abidjan (Côte d'Ivoire) and Lomé (Togo). A high contingent of Burkinabe people (about 1 million) is working outside Burkina Faso in more developed countries (primarily Côte d'Ivoire and Ghana), which also contributes to high regional migratory flows.

Major Languages	Ethnic Groups	Major Religions
French (official)	Mossi, Gurunsi, Senufo,	Muslim 50%
Tribal languages	Lobi, Bobo, Mande,	Indigenous beliefs 40%
	Funlani 40%	Christian (Roman
	Other 60 %	Catholic) 10%

Tribal languages are spoken by 90% of the population. Burkina Faso has one of the higher population densities among West African countries (approximately 12 million inhabitants). The majority (84%) of the population lives in rural villages. Burkina Faso is one of the poorest nations in the world. Its economy is primarily based on agriculture, which relies on rudimentary methods. Most of the land area is arid and suitable only for nomadic herders. Although still mainly a rural country, urbanization is rapidly occurring, promoted by the high mobility of active populations in search of economic opportunities; the suburbs of the main cities (Ouagadougou and Bobo-Dioulasso) are growing rapidly as well.

Health Care Beliefs: Acute sick care; traditional. Health promotion and disease prevention are challenges in Burkina Faso. The country is poorer and less developed than the average sub-Saharan African country and has a younger population, fewer medical facilities, low vaccination coverage, and lower quality of housing and water supply and storage. Diseases may be blamed on supernatural forces. Animism is widespread, but there is official disapproval of animist practices. The first line of health care is often assured by *tradipraticians*, or traditional indigenous healers. The cost of seeking care from traditional healers is about half the cost of modern medical care and may be paid with an in-kind payment, such as a chicken, for services rendered. Although modern medicine is well accepted and perhaps preferable for most health needs, access to biomedical medicine is scarce and expensive.

Predominant Sick Care Practices: Magical-religious; traditional; biomedical where available. Burkina Faso has adopted a primary care strategy and has a five-tier national health system. The *Poste de Santé Primaire (PSP)* is village based and staffed by paramedical staff members. The *Centre de Santé et de Promotion Sociale (CSPS)* provides first-level care with certified personnel such as nurses and midwives. Family planning methods are available at this level. According to surveys, most family planning providers are midwives, and much of the training is on-the-job rather than formal. The *Centre Medical (CM)* is for first-level referrals and provides all services including surgery; theoretically, a doctor is available. The *Centre Hospitalier Regional (CHR)* provides family planning services including sterilization for medical reasons. Burkina Faso has two national hospitals, one in Ouagadougou and one in Bobo-Dioulasso. In addition, it has 104 foreign and 61 national nongovernmental health organizations that address particular health issues such as water supply and education of women. Unfortunately, many Burkinabe people consider the hospital a place to die, which results in delayed referrals to health services and high in-hospital mortality rates. As in many African countries, the additional disease burden caused by late-stage complications of infection with HIV (wasting, opportunistic diseases, tuberculosis) has been overwhelming health care facilities. The health system has two types of traditional medical practitioners: the previously mentioned tradipraticians, who use herbal medicine, and witches or wizards. Tradipraticians primarily alleviate symptoms such as abdominal and head pain but occasionally purport to cure diseases such as malaria. They use leaves, barks, and roots that are harvested according to a ritual, one that is often in harmony with the cycle of the plant. The tradipraticians usually provide their services for small gifts such as a few cola nuts or a little money. Some of them even refer their patients to the CSPS. Other less reputable tradipraticians claim to cure such problems as AIDS, gonorrhea, and infertility. These types of practitioners only work for money. All have public offices, but the more reputable practitioners are discreet and their reputation increases based on their works. Witches and wizards are practitioners who use spells. They are renowned, and people are in awe of them. They are consulted only by people with strong beliefs in animistic traditional practices.

Ethnic/Race Specific or Endemic Diseases: Endemic diseases are chloroquine-resistant malaria, meningitis, intestinal nematode infections, tuberculosis, hepatitis, cardiovascular diseases, rabies, and HIV/AIDS. Malaria is associated with high morbidity in adults, creating disabilities that preclude working in this class of age. Burkina Faso has an agropastoral population, and the natural pasture of livestock has great importance in the economical and social structure of the country. The main zoonotic diseases, which can be acquired by contact with livestock, are bacterial (tuberculosis, brucellosis, and anthrax). Rabies is endemic and mainly transmitted to humans through dogs. The World Health Organization's

(WHO) estimated prevalence rate for HIV/AIDS in adults ages 15 to 49 is 6.4 %. More than 200,000 orphans live in the country as a result of their parents dying of AIDS. The estimated number of children from birth to 15 years living with HIV/AIDS is 20,000. It is estimated that AIDS-related mortality will be equal to malaria-related mortality by 2020. Heterosexual transmission is the main method of HIV infection. Although an effort has been made to reduce risk of HIV transmission through transfusions, contamination still occurs. The risk of transmission through ritual scarification or circumcision is also a factor. Pregnant women infected with HIV transmit the virus to one out of three of their children. AIDS cases in adults are clustered in those from 25 to 45 years (i.e., the economically active individuals in the society). Migration, roads, and prostitution combined with infrequent use of condoms (even by those with multiple sexual partners) allow the HIV epidemic to spread rapidly. Helminthiasis may increase the susceptibility to the infection. The high rate of HIV-related mortality in Africa is primarily related to low access to health care in the early phases of the disease. Wasting is the most common AIDS-defining illness in West Africa. AIDS is called *kpéréki* (meaning "losing weight/dying") among those in the Lobi ethnic group. One of the main determinants of this wasting is reduced food intake, not only because of the economic problems of people infected with HIV, who are often marginalized, but also because of anorexia, which is part of the disease. Treatment of opportunistic diseases, which could be accomplished using low-cost generic drugs, is nonexistent in most rural settings, partly because of social rejection of the disease. Although *Mycobacterium tuberculosis* infection can be spontaneously controlled in most healthy people, it cannot be controlled in immunodeficient people with HIV infection. Therefore when individuals with HIV/AIDS are exposed to other factors, such as high population density, poor hygiene, and zoonotic transmission of *M. tuberculosis* infection, their disease progresses more rapidly. The HIV/tuberculosis complex is a new paradigm of the synergistic interactions among poverty, hygiene, and disease. Compliance to antituberculosus treatment is difficult to obtain because of economic problems and the mobility of the population. African trypanosomiasis, or "sleeping sickness," is a reemerging disease, and its control has been neglected during the last decades. Adenopathies in the first stages of the disease and wasting in the more advanced stages can be misdiagnosed as HIV infection or AIDS if biological facilities are not available (which is the typical situation in most of health facilities in the country). Hemorrhagic fever outbreaks such as Rift Valley fever outbreaks are clearly linked to the proliferation of mosquitoes caused by dam and irrigation projects. Schistosomiasis (contracted by swimming in stagnant water) is another example of vector-borne disease boosted by irrigation projects. Malaria, schistosomiasis, and arboviruses are also associated with rice production. Introducing rice cultivation in areas in which malaria is not under control can speed the transmission of the disease. Pesticides (such as pyrethroids) that are used currently against mosquitoes are predicted to cause resistant strains of malaria. Activation of most of the health efforts in the struggle against the emerging HIV epidemics may contribute to the reemergence of previously controlled, or "hidden," diseases in Burkina Faso. In addition, cerebrovascular diseases, ischemic heart diseases, and diabetes, which are linked to an occidental way of life that includes use of tobacco, nutritional imbalances, and a critical lack of education and information about their associated health risks, are emerging problems primarily in the urban centers (but also in the entire country with regard to tobacco consumption).

Health Team Relationships: In rural areas, health workers are always respected. People are in awe of them, and they belong to the local worthies. When people distinguish among different kinds of health care workers, the doctor is always at the top of the hierarchy. In rural areas without doctors, the nurses, who are entitled to prescribe and to perform some surgeries, are in charge of the PSPs. In hospitals, nurses are the primary link in the health care chain and are usually very knowledgeable and efficient. Doctors do not always recognize nurses' abilities.

Families' Role in Hospital Care: Frequently hospitals do not have enough of certain health workers (e.g., doctors, nurses, nursing auxiliaries, stretcher bearers). For example, when a patient needs an x-ray, family members have to carry the patient to the x-ray room. The family also provides personal care, washes bedding, and brings food to augment what is served in the hospital. Most importantly, the family has to observe the patient and alert staff members to potential problems. If surgery is required, the family joins together to pay for the various materials (e.g., compresses, antibiotics) that are needed. Therefore the family's contribution is vital. Some districts such as Bobo-Dioulasso have only one doctor for 20,000 inhabitants. Traditional medicine is not practiced in hospitals because people are in awe of hospital medical staff members.

Dominance Patterns: The rationale for determining who is worthy of receiving health care resources is based on productivity in Burkinabe society rather than on gender. Although children are not productive, women are believed to be as productive as men in the household, so their health is valued equally. The status of women is low in marriage and in society. It is estimated that they work about 16 hours daily, with their time divided between agriculture and domestic work, including food processing and preparation. Adding to this burden is limited access to fuel and water. Men and older adults make the decisions, social and economic. Public life continues to be dominated by men, and few women participate in the government. About 95% of women work in subsistence agriculture or in jobs using low levels of technology. Various nongovernmental organizations have been attempting to change their status by teaching them job skills. In addition, a commission for strengthening the roles and positions of women in the development process has existed since 1993 but has had little effect on participation of women in the decision-making process. The 1991 constitution also prohibits sexual discrimination and gives men and women equal rights in marriage, inheritance, and land access. Most women are not aware of their rights because of lack of information and education, illiteracy (90%), and traditions. About 70% of women have been subjected to genital cutting.

Eye Contact Practices: Eye contact can be related to religion. For some Muslim people the house is divided into two areas to prevent contact between males and females. When a woman talks to a man (e.g., husband, brother-in-law, friend of husband) and looks at him directly, she is considered a woman of little virtue. In the presence of a hierarchical chief or someone in a clan who has higher social status, direct eye contact is avoided as a mark of respect.

Touch Practices: People walk arm-in-arm only in cities. Women do not shake men's hands—a constant in all Burkina Faso ethnical groups.

Perceptions of Time: The saying "time is money" does not apply in Burkina Faso because time in West Africa involves natural references such as sunrise or sunset. It is also disrespectful to shorten a discussion to go to an appointment. The significance of current actions is determined in reference to "ancestor's time." According to tradition, the present is a repetition and a recapitulation of previous acts, not a race against time.

Pain Reactions: The various ethnic groups differ in their pain reactions. For example, the behavioral code for the Fulani ethnic group is self-discipline and stoicism regarding expressions of emotional or physical pain. Regardless of his ethnic group a man does not show his feelings in public because to do so is a mark of weakness. During childbirth, it is acceptable for women of the Bobo group to express pain, whereas among the Mossi and Lobi it is not.

Birth Rites: Women generally want to have girls, and men want to have boys. Most families prefer a boy first to carry on the lineage. High fertility rates result in high infant mortality rates (97 per 1000 live births) and maternal mortality rates (about 930 per 100,000 live births, one of the highest in the world). Because of the lack of treatment for most pregnant women infected with HIV, transmission of the virus from mother to infant takes a high toll in infants. Life expectancy at birth is low (45 years), worse than most West African countries. Acute respiratory diseases, diarrhea, and malaria are the primary killers of children younger than 5 in rural areas. Large families are the norm, and women are likely to have seven children during their lifetime. Therefore the government's present emphasis on family planning is significant because reducing family size could greatly reduce the number of deaths. Infant mortality rates are estimated to be 60% lower in families in which the mother has had secondary education. Young women are also highly sensitive to diseases because of iterative pregnancies and late weaning, which leads to micronutrient deficiencies and anemia. Using non-sterile instruments used to cut umbilical cords and applying karite nut butter to the cord results in numerous cases of neonatal tetanus. Trained birth attendants (whose knowledge varies greatly), professional midwives, or traditional "old women" assist women with most births. Some sick infants are treated only by the family, depending on which type of health care services are nearby, the family's ethnic group, and the parent's educational level. Fulanis often keep their pregnancies secret, and the mother gives birth alone or with her mother's help. Gurmace mothers often give birth with assistance from the husband's family, and an "old woman" or birth attendant usually attends Rimaibe births.

Death Rites: Cremations do not take place in Burkina Faso, and burial rituals differ according to religion, social status, and ethnic group. Muslims are usually buried quickly, whereas burial of some Mossi or Bobo chiefs is delayed for several days. Some ethnic groups (e.g., Dagari) bring the body back to the village. Children are buried immediately with little ritual, whereas burials of older adults are often festive occasions.

Food Practices and Intolerances: Millet or maize (corn) pastry is the usual food of most rural Burkinabe. In Mossi country, bean and pea pastries are also eaten. Meat is only consumed when available and may be from bush game or farm animals. Protein malnutrition is linked not only to the economic situation, the long dry season, and the susceptibility of cattle to sleeping sickness (in areas where glossina flies transmit the disease, which impairs stock breeding) but also to the lack of community health education on healthy childhood feeding practices (e.g., adequate use of available local foods). This lack of health education is associated with the low level of schooling received by many mothers. The combination of numerous parasitical infections and malnutrition increase the children's susceptibility to malaria and bacterial and viral diseases.

Infant Feeding Practices: Maternal breast-feeding increases the vertical (mother-to-infant) transmission of AIDS, and no clear consensus exists regarding a strategy to prevent this method of transmission. Early initiation of bottle-feeding can create nutritional problems because of issues such as a lack of access to clean water. Vitamin A deficiencies are also common in children and can promote the development of ocular diseases.

Child Rearing Practices: Education is necessary for the society's advancement. Increasing the level of schooling (of girls especially) is a key strategy for improving economic and health development. For example, vaccine coverage often parallels rates of schooling. Girls rarely go to a formal school. Adult women teach them about traditions and sex, and many taboos are involved. Boys are subjected to initiation rituals that follow very strict rules and ensure perpetuation of the culture. Nearly

50% of the Burkinabe is younger than 15 years, and the overall schooling rate is low; only about 29% of primary-school-age children receive a basic education. Lack of information about hygiene and disease influences high mortality rates in children; 75% of deaths of children younger than 5 years are linked to infectious diseases. Survey data indicate that households allocate significantly fewer resources to the care of sick children than they do to sick adults because children are not considered productive in terms of family survival.

National Childhood Immunizations: BCG at birth; DPT at 2, 3, and 4 months; yellow fever at 9 months; OPV at birth and at 2, 3, and 4 months; and measles at 9 months. According to a study done in 1994, the coverage immunization rate in the city of Bobo-Dioulasso was more than 90% for BCG in newborns and the second injection of DTCP in infants. Nevertheless, this percentage fell to 77% for the third injection of DTCP and for the administration of the vaccines against measles and yellow fever. These insufficient coverage rates are even worse in most poorly accessible rural areas. Despite governmental efforts, this low rate of immunization coverage explains the failure of the country to eradicate poliomyelitis before 2000, a goal that has been achieved in South America. Epidemic outbreaks of yellow fever are also associated with insufficient immunization coverage. Cholera cases are frequently reported and linked to common factors such as low accessibility to water, poor hygiene practices, and poor-quality drinking water. The harmattan winds carry meningitis germs each year; immunization against meningitis is achieved through mass campaigns, but the vaccine composition now has to be adapted to new types of the germ.

BIBLIOGRAPHY

Abidoye RO: A study of prevalence of protein energy malnutrition among 0–5 years in rural Benue State, Nigeria, *Nutr Health* 13:235–247, 2000.

Carnevale P et al: Diversity of malaria in rice growing areas of the Afrotropical region, *Parassitologia* 41:273–276, 1999.

Coulibaly ND, Yameogo KR: Prevalence and control of zoonotic diseases: collaboration between public health workers and veterinarians in Burkina Faso, *Acta Tropica* 76:53–57, 2000.

Diagbouga S et al: Lack of direct correlation between CD4 T-lymphocyte counts and induration sizes of the tuberculin skin test in human immunodeficiency virus type seropositive patients, *Int J Tuberculosis Lung Dis* 2:317–323, 1998.

Gidel R et al: Epidemiology of human and animal brucellosis in western Africa. The results of six studies in the Ivory Coast, Upper Volta, and Nigeria, *Dev Biol Standard* 31:187–200, 1976.

Gidel R et al: Mycobacteria of animal origin isolated by the Muraz Center from 1965 to 1968: technics of isolation and identification; results, *Revue d'Elevage et de Médecine Vétérinaire des Pays Tropicaux* 22:495–508, 1969.

Jouan A et al: Epidemic of Rift Valley fever in the Islamic republic of Mauritania. Geographic and ecological data, *Bulletin de la Société de Pathologie Exotique et de ses Filiales* 83:611–20, 1990.

Kotler DP: Management of nutritional alterations and issues concerning quality of life, *J AIDS Hum Retrovirol* 16:S30–S35, 1997.

Ledru E et al: Prevention of wasting and opportunistic infections in HIV-infected patients in West Africa: a realistic and necessary strategy before antiretroviral treatment, *Cahiers Santé* 9:293–300.

Ledru S et al: Impact of short-course therapy on tuberculosis drug resistance in South-West Burkina Faso, *Tuberculosis Lung Dis* 77:429–436, 1996.

Lopez AD, Murray CCJL: The global burden of disease, 1990-2020, *Nature Med* 4:1241–1243, 1998.

Molyneux DH: Vector-borne infections in the tropics and health policy issues in the twenty-first century, *Trans Roy Soc Trop Med Hyg* 95:233–238, 2001.

Moreno S et al: Brucellosis in patients infected with the human immunodeficiency virus, *Eur J Clin Microbiol Inf Dis* 17:319–326, 1998.

Morgan D, Whitworth J: The natural history of HIV-1 infection in Africa, *Nature Med* 7:143–145, 2001.

Morten Rostrup, MSF International Council: *Drugs for neglected diseases working group* http://www.neglecteddiseases.org/>www.unaids.org

Taverne B: How to manage HIV seropositive or AIDS patients in rural Burkina Faso. *Cahiers Santé* 7:177–186, 1997.

UNAIDS/World Health Organization: *Epidemiological fact sheet 2000 update*, http://www.unaids.org/>www.unaids.org

World Health Organization: Weekly *Epidemiol Rec* 70:261–268, 1995.

Würthwein R et al: Measuring the local burden of disease. A study of years of life lost in sub-Saharan Africa, *Int J Epidemiol* 30:501–508.

◆ BURUNDI (REPUBLIC OF)

MAP PAGE (XXX)

Gabriel Hakizimana

Location: Burundi is an enclaved country of 28,784 km^2 (11, 111 square miles) in the African Great Lakes region and is surrounded by Zaire to the west, Tanzania to the south and east, and Rwanda in the north. The population is 6.3 million, with a density of 243 people per km^2, the largest in Africa after Rwanda. Low-altitude areas are composed of plains and peripheral depressions. The weather is tropical with moderate temperatures, and the rainy season lasts 4 to 5 months. The central highlands make up most of the country. The most rainy and cold region is above an altitude of 2000 m, and the dry season lasts from June to August.

Major Languages	Ethnic Groups	Major Religions
Kirundi (official)	Hutu (Bantu) 85%	Roman Catholic 75%
French (official)	Tutsi (Hamitic) 14%	Protestant 15%
Swahili	Twa (Pygmy) 1%	Animist 5%
		Muslim 5%

The Hutu and Tutsi are best known for their recent bloody clashes. The Twas are considered pariahs of the society and live completely outside of the dominant political, social, and economical networks of the country.

The Ganwa are aristocratic princes falsely assimilated into the Tutsi by Belgian colonialists and oppressed by successive Tutsi power since the fall of the monarchy in 1966. The available population ratios probably reflect unpublished Belgian surveys from before 1960. No ethnic survey has been documented. All these ethnic groups share the same language and culture, worship the same God, Imana, and have lived since the seventeenth century under the rule of the same monarchy. Kirundi is the only language spoken without regional and ethnical variants by 100% of the Burundese. French is the first foreign language learned in school. It is used primarily among public servants and intellectuals such as university-educated people. English begins during secondary school and could become the leading foreign language in the next 25 years because of its growing influence in the Great Lakes region. Swahili is spoken mainly in urban neighborhoods, markets, and commercial settings. Religious information for the country comes from national demographic surveys, but religious practice is often marked by syncretism. Numerous Christians still practice ancestral rituals despite relatively successful campaigns by the churches to suppress these traditional beliefs.

Health Care Beliefs: Traditional; increasing emphasis on health promotion. The great majority of the population acknowledges the importance of preventive and health promotion services such as immunization, prenatal care, and infant and child care even if the services are not optimal. Because of the current context, individuals define *health* and *illness* specifically, mentioning causes of each. Being *healthy* is having housing, being able to conduct daily activities, and feeling well. Being *ill* is having insufficient or poor-quality food and poor hygiene. People believe that eating well and having access to good hygiene are necessary to maintain good health. In rural areas, people would add that it is necessary to have good crop production to have good health, a response that results from the consequences of crop destruction during ethnic upheaval. Approximately 90% of the population often does not use modern health care services because they consider them too expensive and inadequate (e.g., lacking in quality drugs, staffed by poorly prepared caregivers). Nurses tend to refer patients to traditional healers for diseases beyond their abilities to treat such as liver diseases, mental conditions, and diseases believed to be caused by sorcery.

Predominant Sick Care Practices: Biomedical; traditional; magical-religious. One century of Christianity and many decades of colonialism have not eliminated ancestral heath practices. Despite the impact of modern public health programs to improve hygiene and sanitation, introduce immunization, and control transmissible diseases, the Burundese traditional healer is still a powerful figure in health care. Baerts and Lehmann (1999) explained the place of traditional medicine in the society:

Schematically, the modern health professional can and wants to deal only with the specific organic health problems of his African patient, which does not satisfy the care seeker because when the disease lasts, it becomes for him the sign of a perturbation or a conflict between himself, his family, his clan, or an angry ancestor … It is then necessary to seek the hidden reasons of the disease, to manage them and sometimes, if God, Imana, agrees, to heal it.

Thus the population of Burundi alternates between imported occidental medicine characterized by the administration of pharmaceutical drugs and traditional medicine marked by the personality of the healer and the healer's symbolic rituals and connections with the invisible world. Healers and masters of divination sometimes play the same role. The healer is an herbalist but also a psychologist who cures traditional "poisoning" and chases away evil aggressors. The herbs are expected to heal a person psychologically and physiologically. The master of divination acts in the domain of traditional religious beliefs. He imitates the healer in the sense that he guesses the origins of the evil or sickness and exorcises it by various plants and sacred rituals. He may produce talismans of wood or antelope horns filled with various elements used as protection against evil and to ensure the good health and fecundity of the users. The master of divination has no relationship with God but is connected to the spirits. Because of the socioeconomic crisis in the country, religious sects are emerging that recommend their believers seek healing by prayer. These two health systems have always coexisted. The current difficulties come from the unprecedented collapse of the public health system because of the political and economic crisis in 1993. According to the Ministry of Health, this crisis has broken a weak national health system, suppressed supervision structures, and made ineffective the planning and coordination process. The system lacks essential drugs, vaccines, medical instruments, and qualified personnel. Most health professionals were killed or work in urban areas for security reasons. Burundi's network of 365 health centers, which offered a package of preventive, curative, and promotional services to the community and about 30 referral hospitals for medicine and surgery, were entirely destroyed. The health insurance system implemented by the government in 1984 to allow equitable low-price access to care for families in public health facilities is ineffective.

Ethnic/Race Specific or Endemic Diseases: Burundi has a predominance of infectious and parasitic diseases. Malaria is the major public health problem, with an annual incidence of about 2500 cases per 10,000. Since 1990, malaria has been prevalent in the highlands at altitudes of more than 1400 m, locations where the disease was previously nonexistent. This outbreak is related to environmental factors, population movements, decreases in population immunity, and drug resistance. Respiratory tract infections are the second major problem, with an annual incidence of 1200 cases per 10,000, and third is diarrheal diseases. Finally, emerging or reemerging diseases, such as HIV and AIDS, epidemic meningitis, bacillary dysentery, and epidemic typhus, occurred at a time when the population had been weakened by 10 years of civil war. The World

Health Organization's (WHO) estimated prevalence rate for HIV/AIDS in adults ages 15 to 49 is 11.32%. The estimated number of children from birth to 15 years living with HIV/AIDS is 19,000. Since the report of the first AIDS case in Burundi, the progression of the disease has been extremely rapid. In 1989, seroprevalence was estimated at 11% in towns and 0.9% in rural areas. In 1996, estimates were 21% in towns and 6% in rural areas. In 1993, seroprevalence in female sex workers was 74.5%. About 40,000 people died from AIDS in 2000, and today it is the major cause of death in adults and a major cause of infant death. More than 70% of the beds in internal medicine wards of Bujumbura hospital are occupied by inpatients with AIDS, and the number of orphans created by the AIDS epidemic is estimated at 230,000. The loss of productivity caused by the death of people of reproductive age, some of whom received expensive educations, is significant. The HIV/AIDS epidemic is a new determinant of poverty for individuals, households, communities, and the entire country.

Health Team Relationships: Relationships between doctors and nurses are very hierarchical and independent of experience. The doctor dominates the interactions. In a country where the rates of those with secondary school and university educations are respectively 6.9% and 0.7%, the doctor has considerable power. In 2000 the country had only 323 medical doctors (with 42 specialists) and 1783 nurses (with only six specialists). Socially, doctors have a great deal of prestige, and patient satisfaction is always limited if a patient does not see a doctor. Unlike doctors who are difficult to approach outside the clinical setting, nurses are well integrated in their communities. Nursing education is inaccessible to the vast majority of people, so nurses are also well regarded. The nurses' capacity to heal, their counseling capabilities, and their presence in the community have maximized their roles as leaders. After the last elections, many nurses become deputies at the National Assembly.

Families' Role in Hospital Care: Traditionally, inquiring about someone's health indicates a person cares for another. Burundese show tremendous solidarity during times of illness. For example, when someone is seriously ill and cannot walk to the health center, one or more people will spontaneously carry the person on a traditional couch to the dispensary. This couch is used as an ambulance and hearse and is shared among families. People who are healthy and refuse to carry a sick person may have social sanctions brought against them. During hospitalizations, families and neighbors share the responsibility of patient care. Because the ill person often remains at home, the best sign of friendship and neighborly kindness is to visit and wish the person a quick recovery. Women ask if the sick person is eating well regardless of the person's age or sex and provide the person's favorite dishes. If the patient is a man, his companions give him drinks and chat with him if he is able to converse. These moments of companionship and empathy are often significantly therapeutic. If the disease persists or the person is too weak to resume labor, neighbors work for the person, and the women care for the person's children.

Dominance Patterns: Familial organization in Burundi is patriarchal. Close lineage includes husband, wife, and children. The enlarged patrilinear parenthood and allied families include relatives of wives and mothers. Other more extended links are related to the clan or neighborhood. The husband is the head of the household and responsible for providing for the family's essential needs. He makes important decisions in collaboration with his wife (who has the right to complain if he abuses his rights). The wife assumes responsibility for the family in case of the absence or death of the husband. Despite improvements, the Burundese women, especially in rural areas, are still exploited. They must produce many children and provide for the basic needs of the family by producing food and fetching wood and water. They are also in charge of the hygiene, health, and education of the children. They are the poorest, least educated, and least protected in terms of the society and law. Women have very little monetary power because the husbands determine the distribution of income and land for labor. When crops are plentiful, women can sell the surplus at the local market or exchange their production skills for other utilities. Higher income-producing commercial activities such as coffee growing are restricted to the husband, who harvests crops and sells them at public markets. This imbalance in the management of family income leaves women in a vulnerable position. They must often ask the man to pay for health care services when they or the children need it.

Eye Contact Practices: Culturally, eye contact is highly symbolic. A slight eye signal from a friend when in public means "beware of what you say." A Kirundi proverb says, "The enemy dissimulates his hate for you, and you dissimulate that you know his hate for you through the eyes." Direct eye contact is a sign of love among the young; however, the girl refrains from making direct eye contact with the boy because it is considered more romantic. The boy says that his lover has "the eyes of a young cow," a compliment because the cow has great symbolic value. It is strictly forbidden for young women to stare at their fathers-in-law; they must keep a certain distance and turn their heads slightly to prevent direct eye contact. This practice also applies to young men and their mothers-in-law. It is strictly forbidden to call in-laws by their names, regardless of their age or social status. Children must stay away or sit down when adults eat, and they cannot stare at an adult who is eating or look at the person's mouth, both of which are considered a sign of a bad education. Direct eye contact is not an issue in either traditional or modern health care settings, regardless of the sex of the patient or the caregiver.

Touch Practices: Physical contact is accepted but structured depending on what it conveys socially. Shaking hands for salutations is the most current practice but is based on rules. For example, to show utmost respect toward an older adult or other socially important individual, the person gives the individual the right hand and at the same time puts the left hand around the individual's right forearm. This gesture persists even with the growing Western influence on education and behavior. This form of salutation has variants. Older women put their hands on the shoulders of younger people and recite greetings and blessings. Younger women who have not met since their weddings hold each other and sing melancholy songs recalling their childhood years. Except for usual greetings, a father does not touch his daughter, and physical contact is limited between a son and his mother. Every gesture or word about sex or sexual relationships is scandalous and shameful for the whole family. The stability and functioning of the family is based on familial and social norms that include multiple interdictions and taboos and repression of deviant behaviors.

Perceptions of Time: In Burundi, use of the hour as a measure of time is an almost nonexistent practice outside of urban areas. The time indicators used in the countryside are *mu gitondo* (morning), *ku murango* (noon), *ku muhingamo* (afternoon), and *ku mugoroba* (evening). This division divides the day among productive (agriculture and other), domestic, and social activities. Time is not flexible except during social activities such as conversations or having drinks. Even in these situations, an appointment or invitation time is always respected. The most important occasions of Burundese life are political and administrative meetings and Sunday mass, and it is rare for people to arrive late to these events. People also use proxies such as the length of the shadow, position of the sun, or evolution of sleep (*mumikangura*). The other measure of time is the squawking of the chickens, first at dawn and then throughout the day until evening. Educated people have a tendency to be late unless coerced to be on time, so public events and meetings can be delayed for hours, without regard for poor peasants who arrived at the announced time. At night, time virtually stops. No activities take place out of the home. The family gathers in the living room, which is where traditional education (passing down of legends, herders' poems, history of the clan, moral principles) takes place. Religious rituals and incantations to placate ancestral spirits can transport participants to symbolic places such as rivers or caves.

Pain Reactions: Burundese culture tends to emphasize control of emotions. Showing pain overtly is synonymous with weakness, especially for adult men, who should never cry in public. It is acceptable for women to express their emotions when they are in physical pain (e.g., after being hurt in a domestic dispute) or emotional pain (e.g., when mourning the loss of a loved one). However, midwives reprimand women if they cry when giving birth.

Birth Rites: In Burundi a child is the best present God can give, so pregnancy is a period of hope and fear for the family. The dream of each woman is to have numerous children, because giving birth confers a highly desired social status. Sterile women are stigmatized by the family. Traditional members of society still believe in ancestral spirits, so pregnant women fear evil and wicked charms directed toward their babies. The women are therefore considered fragile and refrain from long walks and travel. They also use plants and personal hygiene practices to protect their own and the infant's health. Pregnant or breast-feeding women have no specific dietary limitations. The interdiction of game meat, chicken, or even eggs reported by people from Mugoyi is probably a local marginal phenomenon. Eating meat or any food hit by lightning is forbidden for all females, regardless of whether they are pregnant. Fewer than 20% of births are managed by health care professionals. In traditional practice, women give birth at home with help from local, essentially uneducated midwives. After the birth the husband and the mother sleep separately for the first week. On the eighth day after birth, a ceremony is held to honor the newborn and mother. This celebration has at least three meanings. First, it presents the infant to the family and neighbors, who represent the community and society. Second, it indicates that the woman may resume sexual relations with her husband. (In certain areas the couple is expected to have sexual relations on the eighth day but in other places, sexual relations do not resume until 3 or 4 weeks after the birth.) Third, the celebration means that the woman should resume her domestic work. Pregnant women are responsible for domestic activities as long as their health allows, but after giving birth they are exempt from performing all activities except for breast-feeding. Progressive return to work depends on family resources; in poor families, this may occur as soon as the eighth day. No significant differences in rituals for male and female infants exist. However, families prefer boys because they perpetuate the patriarchal lineage. A mother who has only daughters after many pregnancies is physically and psychologically harassed by her in-laws, which is a practice that can lead to divorce. Giving birth to twins is considered abnormal, and it is feared that the family will be exposed to evil influence or bad luck. Socioeconomic problems and the precarious public health situation are responsible for the high infant mortality rate. Twin births increase the likelihood of an infant dying in a family. The ritual after the birth of twins is very special and complicated to protect the family from bad luck. Parents and neighbors provide the family with many presents and help the parents as they face this risky situation.

Death Rites: In Burundi, death is defined by its cause and linked to its circumstances. Thus the cause of death is either an "accident" (an indirect expression that means "a violent death from civil war"), a "disease" (death from natural causes rather than from violence), or from "poisoning" (a reference to traditional beliefs). When a person from a rural area dies, the person is usually buried immediately. Because qualified personnel are not required to declare a person dead, tragic errors have occurred that have led to individuals in a comatose state being buried alive. The corpse is laid on a mat and taken to the local cemetery. After returning from the cemetery, all those who attended the burial perform ritual hand washing. The cemetery is a feared place because dead people's spirits are thought to be present; no one wants to be in a cemetery at night. Mourning is strictly observed for 1 week. Other than limited domestic work such as cooking, no other activities are permitted. Wearing black clothing is common in urban areas. During the mourning period, neighbors and friends continuously visit the deceased person's home to support the family. Members of the family shave their heads and recite incantations to calm the deceased person's spirit. Mourning is complete 1 year after the death.

Food Practices and Intolerances: Beans are the most common dish and are eaten at least once a day. Other basic foods are cassava, potatoes, banana, peas, and corn. Rice and white potatoes are becoming more common. Meat is reserved for wealthy people, and many families do not buy meat at all. The small fish of Lake Tanganyika are found all over the country. Sweet dishes are rare, so a meal rarely includes a dessert, even a meal in a city. Food taboos and interdictions exist, although young people rarely respect them. Few people eat meat from sheep, and it is forbidden for children to drink cow's milk after they have eaten peas. Herders are reluctant to eat their own animals, which is a sign of social status. At least 90% of people in Burundi eat with their hands. People wash their hands and then, according to age and occasionally gender, share a meal from the same plate. In general the father and the mother eat from the same plate in a separate room, and children share the same meal. Children are strictly forbidden to move around people when the people are eating. The habitants of Burundi enjoy drinking beer. *Brarudi*, a branch of the European brewery group Heineken, has been the most affluent company in the country for nearly half a century. People also make and sell a local banana-based beer called *urwarwa*. This drink has a major social role in that drinking urwarwa in a social group punctuates the rhythm of the day. *Impeke*, a drink made of millet, is also popular. During celebrations, people drink a lot of *urwarwa* and *impeke*.

Infant Feeding Practices: Almost all women in rural areas breast-feed their children. If for some reason they cannot breast-feed, their infant is fed with cow's milk (and in rare situations, another woman feeds the infant). Women in towns also breast-feed, often supplementing the breast milk with imported powdered infant formula or cow's milk. Mothers do not need to be isolated to feed their children, and feeding times are not limited or planned except by working women who must follow their employers' schedules. Maternal leave is about 3 months, but breast-feeding lasts about 2 years. Meanwhile, other nutrients are progressively introduced. If a breast-feeding woman becomes pregnant, she immediately stops breast-feeding.

Child Rearing Practices: Education of small children is the responsibility of the mother. She gives them guidance on hygiene, dressing, and good manners for their integration into society. The father's role is more associated with security; however, roles change during adolescence when the mother prepares her daughter for a woman's life and the son becomes closer to his father as he receives help preparing for his family life. Daughters and sons do not sleep in the same bed, but children of the same gender share beds. On certain occasions (e.g., visits, families serving as temporary hosts), adults of the same gender sleep together. Outside of urban areas, homosexuality is completely unknown.

National Childhood Immunizations: BCG at birth; DTP at 6, 10, and 14 weeks and at 18 months; OPV at birth and at 6, 10, and 14 weeks; measles at 9 months; and TT CBAW after first contact + 1 month. In 2000, reported cases of vaccine-controllable diseases were as follows: diphtheria, 0; measles, 18,383; neonatal tetanus, 16; pertussis, 72; polio, 0; and total tetanus, 33. The reported percentage of the target population vaccinated by antigen for 2000 was BCG, 80%; first dose of DTP, 74%; third dose of DTP, 64%; MCV, 57%; third dose of Pol, 64%; TT2 plus, 28%.

Other Characteristics: One of the consequences of the civil war in Burundi has been mass population movement. One out of six Burundese is displaced outside the country (in neighboring countries) or inside the country (in somewhere other than their areas of residency). Most left in the first days of killing and are still in camps protected by security forces because of the atmosphere of uncertainty and insecurity in the country. The living conditions of displaced people are daunting. In 76% of the camps, displaced people lack potable water, so they frequently get their water from polluted sources. Sanitation is nonexistent in most camps. Families have no means of recycling garbage and are exposed to the bites of insect and disease vectors such as mosquitoes, fleas, and rats. The diseases most frequently associated with poor hygiene in the camps are dermatological diseases (especially sarcoptosis), conjunctivitis, malaria, bacillary dysentery, measles, acute respiratory tract infections, exanthematic typhus, cholera, intestinal parasites, typhoid fever, and diarrheal diseases. Access to health services is still a major problem for displaced people in many regions. The people remain exposed to attacks by local terrorists, are malnutritioned, and have deplorable living conditions. Many reports indicate that the nutritional status of displaced Burundese is getting worse. This combined with transmissible diseases explains the high mortality rate in the camps.

BIBLIOGRAPHY

Abdul-Rasul TM: Le pluralisme thérapeutique en psychiatrieau quartier asiatique de Bujumbura au Burundi, *Bulletin des Médécins Suisses* 82:404–406, 2001.

Acquier J-L: *Le Burundi*, 1986, Éditions Parenthèses.

Arhin DC: The health care insurance scheme in Burundi: a social asset or a nonviable venture? Soc Sci Med 39: 861–870, 1994.

Baerts M, Lehmann J: L'utilisation de quelques plantes médécinales au Burundi, Belgium's Africa, *Gand* 21–23, Octobre 1999.

Center for Research on the Epidemiology of Disasters (1998): Burundi—priorités dans le secteur sanitaire. Document de travail no. 148. Retrieved February 14, 2002, from http://www.cred.be/centre/publi/148f/begin.htm

Chrétien JP: Burundi. In *Médecins sans Frontières: Populations en danger 1995. Rapport annuel sur les crises majeures et l'action humanitaire*, Paris, 1995, La Découverte.

Di Perri G et al: Tuberculosis among refugees and displaced people at the Burundi-Rwanda border, *Clin Infect Dis* 26:500–501, 1998.

Eono P, Migliani R, Philippe B, et al: Burundi: humanitarian mission (January-April 1994), *Med Trop (Mars)* 55(2):172–177, 1995.

Fournier AS et al: The management of severe malnutrition in Burundi: an ONG's perspective of the practical constraints to effective emergency and medium-term programmes, *Disasters* 23:343–349, 1999.

Hakizimana A: *La politique de santé reproductive et planification familiale au Burundi: contraintes issues de la contradiction entre communicatication et culture dans un contexte de développement*, thèse de doctorat, Montreal, Canada, 2001, Université de Montréal.

International Crisis Group: *Le Burundi après la suspension de l'embargo: aspects internes et régionaux*, Bruxelles, 1999, Author.

Isely BR: Experience in Africa. Findings keys to participation in varying socio-cultural settings. *Hygiene* 5:18–21, 1986.

Kalipeni E, Oppong J: The refugee crisis in Africa and implications for health and disease: a political ecology approach, *Soc Sci Med* 46, 1637–1653, 1998.

Lacopino V, Waldman R: War and health, *JAMA* 282, 1999.

Mahieu F-L (1997): Face à la pauvreté: stratégies universelles et recompositions africaines. In *Ménages et familles en Afrique*. Centre français sur la population et le développement, 1997.

Ministère de la Santé Publique: *Schéma d'intervention de salubrité dans les sites des personnes déplacées*, 1996.

Ministère de la Santé Publique du Burundi/OMS: *Profil épidémiologique du Burundi. Année 2000*. Retrieved on January 17, 2002, from http://mosquito.who.int/docs/country_updates/burundi.htm

Mworoha E: *Peuples et rois de l'Afrique des lacs: le Burundi et les royaumes voisins au 19ème siècle*, Paris, 1977, Les Nouvelles Éditions Africaines.

Ngarambe P, Vincke J: *Pragmatique de la terminologie de la parenté rundi. In La civilisation ancienne des peuples des Grands Lacs*, Paris, 1981, Centre de la Civilisation Burundaise, Khartala.

Ngendabanyikwa N, Nzisabira E: *Enquête d'évaluation auprès des bénéficiaires des services SMI-PF et IEC*, Ministère de la Santé Publique, Projet Santé et Population I, 1995.

Nzisabira E: *Étude sur les croyances, connaissances, attitudes et pratiques en matière de santé de la population burundaise*, Ministère de la Santé Publique, Projet Santé et Population II, 1996.

Office for the Coordination of Humanitarian Affairs—Burundi: *Update on the humanitarian situation*, August-September 2001.

République du Burundi: *Code des personnes et de la famille: décret-loi no 1/1 du 15 janvier 1980*.

Salama P, Spiegel P, Brennan R: No less vulnerable: the internally displaced in humanitarian emergencies, *Lancet* 357:1430–1431, 2001.

Stratégie Nationale Pour l'Environnement et Plan d'Action: *Documents de synthèse*, 1993.

Sydor G, Philippot P: *Conséquences psychologiques des massacres de 1994 au Rwanda. Santé mentale au Québec*, 21:229–246, 1996.

Thibon C: *L'évolution des ménages au Burundi. In Ménages et familles en Afrique. Centre français sur la population et le développement*, 1997.

Toole MJ, Waldman RJ: War, hunger and public health, *JAMA* 270:600–605, 1993.

United Nations Convention: The status of refugees. In Martin JP, Rangaswamy R, eds: Twenty-five human rights documents, pp. 57–76, 1994.

◆ CAMBODIA (KINGDOM OF)

MAP PAGE (867)

Chhan D. Touch

Location: A large, alluvial plain on the Indochinese peninsula in Southeast Asia, Cambodia is ringed by mountains and is bordered by Thailand on the west, Vietnam on the east, Laos on the north, and the Gulf of Thailand on the south. The total land area is 181,040 km² (69,900 square miles).

Major Languages	Ethnic Groups	Major Religions
Khmer/Cambodian	Khmer/Cambodian 90%	Buddhist
Chinese	Chinese 1%	(Theravada) 95%
Vietnamese	Vietnamese 5%	Muslim and other 5%
French	Cham and other 4%	
Other		

The majority of Cambodians speak Khmer. French is spoken by the educated and elite, and different dialects of Chinese are commonly spoken for business.

Health Care Beliefs: Acute sick care; magical-religious. Traditional health care beliefs are based on concepts of cause and effect. A serious illness after travel is thought to be caused by the wrong diet or violation of certain rituals or pledges. To resolve the problem, food and apologies are offered to the spirits. *Yin* (cold) and *yang* (hot) concepts widely influence the society. *Yin* (representing females, negative forces, the soul, the earth, the moon, the night, water, cold, and darkness) and *yang* (representing males, positive forces, day, fire, heat, expansion, and daylight) must be in absolute equilibrium for optimum health. Illness also may be caused by lack of equilibrium within the body force, known as *chi*. Restoring equilibrium cures the illness. Mental illnesses are often met with denial, and emotional disturbances may manifest themselves somatically because of the shame connected to mental illness. According to common beliefs, thinking too much (*kett-cha-roeun*), particularly during periods of stress, creates mental imbalance. Self-treatment strategies include suppressing and forgetting about sad thoughts, being sheltered and protected by family members, being encouraged to laugh, and not being left alone. It is common to take sleeping pills or drink alcohol, and suicidal ideology is not unusual. Posttraumatic stress disorder (PTSD) is common in older adults who lived through the reign of the Khmer Rouge. Alternative treatments, such as seeking help from a *shaman*, or *kru khmer* (traditional healer), or Buddhist monk, are frequently sought.

Predominant Sick Care Practices: Biomedical; traditional. According to traditional beliefs, illness is caused either by food and environment or supernatural causes (e.g., spells, gods, demons, evil spirits (*neak ta*) and by violation of certain religious codes. Some illnesses are treated with "cold" remedies such as herbal medicine, whereas others are treated with "hot" remedies such as Western medicine. During an illness or the postpartum period, cold and hot food consumption rules are strictly adhered to at home and in the hospital if possible. Certain illnesses are thought to be caused by "bad air" that is trapped in the body. Removing it (by vacuum-cup suction) allows the body to restore itself to its optimum state. Traditional treatments, such as skin pinching, coin rubbing, circular burning, therapeutic steam baths, acupuncture, alcohol treatment (to generate heat), and acupressure are also used, and some of these practices result in bruise marks or red lines on the skin. In Western countries, these practices are frequently misunderstood and considered a form of physical abuse. Cambodians believe in receiving medication each time they visit a doctor, preferably in the form of intramuscular injections with placebo solutions. They believe that injections are more potent than pills, and intravenous infusions of vitamin C or B complex are a favorite way to "gain energy" whether at home or abroad. Suffering is occasionally thought to be caused by past sins, so interventions (including medical treatments) may be considered inappropriate.

Endemic/Race Specific or Endemic Diseases: Endemic diseases include chloroquine-resistant malaria, hemorrhagic fever, HIV and AIDS, and hepatitis A. Cambodians are at risk for Japanese encephalitis, schistosomiasis, and PTSD. The World Health Organization's (WHO) estimated prevalence rate for HIV/AIDS in adults ages 15 to 49 years old is 4.04%. The estimated number of children from birth to 15 years living with HIV/AIDS is 5400. HIV/AIDS is the leading cause of death.

Health Team Relationships: Because doctors are considered to be experts in medicine and authority figures, neither nurses nor patients question their decisions. It is considered rude to question the integrity or credibility of a doctor. Patients are given little information, and they do not contradict doctors openly regardless of whether they intend to comply with the medical recommendations. An open show of impatience, non-compliance, or anger is culturally inappropriate, and remaining controlled protects the patients' self-esteem and the health professionals' status. Doctors are usually men, and nurses are usually women. Nurses are expected to be completely submissive to doctors, are not allowed to question orders, and are expected to carry files for doctors during rounds. A female patient may refuse care from a male health care provider, but her husband can override her decision.

Families' Role in Hospital Care: Family members are expected to provide support and comfort, including personal needs and food, during hospitalizations. The family is highly valued by patients, and asking family members about the best approach to use for a Cambodian patient creates positive patient-provider rapport.

Dominance Patterns: Women defer to men for decision making. The oldest member of the family is designated as the decision maker in medical matters, and male family members are given priority over females. Husbands are expected to answer all questions about their wife's health, including past medical history, although women are allowed to answer with their husband's consent. Husbands are responsible for earning money and providing what is necessary for family survival, and women are expected to manage household affairs, including raising the children. Everyone is expected to maintain and uplift family honor, and extended relatives and close friends are considered part of the family. Polygamy still exists, although it is illegal in Cambodia. Confrontations between legal wives and mistresses occasionally have devastating consequences. It is socially acceptable for married men to have extramarital affairs, but women who commit adultery are disowned and rejected by their families and society.

Eye Contact Practices: Direct eye contact is disrespectful and a sign of intentional confrontation. Cambodian patients attempt to avoid direct eye contact with health care professionals who are considered to be of higher social status, so this behavior should not be interpreted as dishonesty or an attempt to conceal information.

Touch Practices: The head, especially of a man, is considered to be the most sacred part of the body and is revered. Touching a child's head intentionally without parental consent may make parents or relatives angry and even physically violent. It is acceptable for parents to touch their children's heads, although touching in general is rare in most Cambodian families. Love and affection are expressed through simple acts such as massages, which are only done within the family. Hand-shaking has recently gained wide acceptance among men in the city; however, it is still not acceptable in the countryside for younger men to shake older men's hands. The *wai* gesture (placing both palms together and slightly bowing the head) is commonly used and acceptable among all ages and sexes. Physical contact during any greeting with a person of the opposite sex is strongly discouraged and prohibited.

Perceptions of Time: Time is irrelevant and flexible. Planning for the future and keeping appointments are not considered important, and tardiness should be expected. Setting a deadline for a certain task does not guarantee completion of the task. The concept of taking medication at a specific and set time is not well understood or practiced, so some Cambodians only take their medications if they feel ill.

Pain Reactions: Pain may be severe before relief is requested. Traditionally, pain has been thought of as a consequence of terrible deeds that were done in the past or a previous life *kama* (sin). Some prefer to endure pain so that they can reincarnate into a healthy life.

Birth Rites: Prenatal care is negligible for most because of the lack of good health care or finances for good health care. Prenatal care is available only for influential, well-educated, or wealthy families. Pregnancy is a private matter and rarely announced outside of the family. Because of concerns that prenatal vitamins increase the weight and size of the fetus and cause a difficult delivery, pregnant women sometimes reject them. They also diet during pregnancy to keep infants small. Childbirth is considered to be a "cold" process because excessive heat is lost during the delivery, so warmth is used to replenish the lost heat and energy and balance the yin and yang. Women who have just given birth may refuse cold baths, water, and foods. Hot drinks, extremely spicy foods, and heavy blankets are commonly used by patients to retain and replenish heat. Alcohol fermented with various herbs and animals' internal organs and blood are consumed because Cambodians believe that it will help regenerate and supplement lost heat. In the rural countryside, some women lie on mats over burning charcoal to regenerate heat. The family is expected to assume full responsibility of the newborn and mother. Certain tasks are restricted, such as getting up, walking, lifting, working, and self-care tasks. Certain foods are forbidden because of the potential for *torrs*, a form of food-induced illness. Praising a newborn is prohibited because it is considered a bad omen. A knife or weapon is placed above the infant's head to frighten away evil spirits and keep them from snatching the infant.

Death Rites: Life, birth, and *samsara* (the circle of life) are the main themes in Cambodian Buddhist culture. Good deeds in the current life ensure prosperity or rebirth into a beautiful image. Patients prefer to die at home rather than in the hospital and at the last moment of life, monks are invited to chant to help the spirit leave the body properly. Candles are lit to allow the spirit to see the path, and baskets of food, money, and other goods are placed at the foot of those who are near death—an offering to take to the next life. Neighbors join in the celebration and may bring small gifts of money. After death the family smears the person's face, palms, and soles with thick turmeric sauce. White clothes are placed on these areas to obtain physical imprints of the person, which serve as remembrances of the death. These imprints are also believed to have a protective function because the spirit of the deceased person will continually protect whoever carries or keeps these items. This process is most commonly followed when the deceased person is a parent, grandparent, or well-respected individual. The washing ceremony is carried out by the family as a way for them to pay their last respects and ask for forgiveness for wrongs unknowingly done to the deceased person while the person was alive. The body is ceremoniously stored in the house or temple for up to 7 days. Cambodians believe that the lost spirit may return and reenter the body. After the 7 days have passed, an elaborate ceremony and procession take place, and the body is prepared for cremation. Male family members are expected to shave their heads, and male and female family members must wear white with a black armband or a small piece of attached black cloth and wear no jewelry. Baskets of goods, food, and money are given to the Buddhist priest. A coin is placed inside the mouth of the deceased, and the favorite child finds this coin after cremation. Cremation in the temple is preferred, and the ashes are kept here for 7 days. After this period the ashes can be kept in an urn and placed in the temple or the family *stupa* (a small house that stores the ashes of dead ancestors). Some families prefer to bring the ashes home. Family members continue to wear white clothes during the 3-month mourning period, and elaborate decorations, celebrations, jewelry, or joyous activities are prohibited.

Food Practices and Intolerances: Families demonstrate love through food, and Cambodians enjoy several dishes at every meal. Meat, vegetables, and rice are the major parts of Cambodian diets, although meat is expensive and normally consumed only by wealthy individuals. Cambodians are frequently lactose intolerant.

Infant Feeding Practices: Breast-feeding is common practice and may continue until the child is 3 years. Formula is usually unavailable and expensive. Colostrum is considered dirty and is expressed and discarded. Solid foods are generally introduced at about 4 months. They are chewed by the mother, aunt, or grandmother before being given to the infant. In traditional families, boys may breast-feed for as many years as they desire to enhance their power and energy, whereas girls may be weaned at 2 years to prevent them from developing those male characteristics. Weaning from breast-feeding usually results in ending milk intake completely because no fresh milk is available in Cambodia. During weaning, spicy, salty, or bitter substances are smeared on the nipples to discourage the child from sucking.

Child Rearing Practices: The character and personality of an infant are thought to be determined by the time of the day, date, month, year, and season of birth. A girl is preferred as the first child, because it is thought that girls are more helpful to the mother than boys. Babies are frequently touched, cared for, and carried about by the mother or another woman in the family. Parents are relaxed and enjoy children younger than 6 years, but then the strict upbringing begins in which independence is discouraged and absolute obedience is demanded. To protest or question the demands of the parents is unacceptable and disgraceful. The oldest child, whether a boy or girl, is responsible for the younger siblings if the parents die, are old, or are ill. Large families are preferred, especially in poorer populations because more workers are available. Boys are encouraged to attend school and obtain an education, but when girls reach puberty they are discouraged from further learning. Between puberty and marriage, the traditional girl spends 1 month in seclusion and solitude, a practice known as *choul-ma-loup*. She observes many rites, eats a vegetarian diet, remains in her room in the dark, and is visited only by her mother. Her name may be changed to confuse potential evil spirits, and she is released only after she is married. The popularity of this practice is currently decreasing.

National Childhood Immunizations: BCG at birth; DPT at 6, 10, and 14 weeks; OPV at birth and 6, 10, and 14 weeks; measles at 9 months; vitamin A at 6 to 59 months, also for lactating women $\times$ 2 yearly; and TT after first contact $+4$ weeks, $+6$ months, $+1$, and $+1$ year.

Other Characteristics: Women do not assume their husbands' last name after marriage. Wrist strings or lead-wrapped waist strings are worn to prevent the soul from venturing outside the body. Infants may wear these strings around the neck, ankles, or waist. Speaking loudly, yelling, snapping fingers under the nose, pointing, beckoning with a finger, or holding hands outstretched with the palm up offends others.

BIBLIOGRAPHY

D'Avanzo C: Bridging the cultural gap with Southeast Asians, MCN, *Am J Matern Child Nurs* 17(4):204, 1992.

D'Avanzo C: The Southeast Asian client and alcohol and other drug abuse: implications for health care providers, *Subst Abuse* 15(2):109, 1994.

D'Avanzo C: Southeast Asians: Asian Pacific Americans at risk for substance abuse, *Subst Use Misuse* 32:829, 1997.

D'Avanzo C, Barab S: Depression and anxiety among Cambodian refugee women in France and the United States, *Issues Ment Health Nurs* 19:1, 1990.

D'Avanzo C, Barab S: Drinking during pregnancy: practices of Cambodian refugees in France and the United States, *Health Care Women Int* 21(4):319, 2000.

D'Avanzo C, Frye B: Research update: Stress and self medication in Cambodian refugee women, *Addictions Nurs Net* 4(2):59, 1992.

D'Avanzo C, Frye B, Froman R: Culture, stress and substance use in Cambodian refugee women, *J Stud Alcohol* 55(4):420, 1994.

D'Avanzo C, Frye B, Froman R: Stress in the Cambodian refugee family: perceptions reported by Cambodian women, *Image* 26(2):99, 1994.

Dunn JD: Educating sex workers in Cambodia, *Comm Nurse* 1(3):29, 1995.

Kelly BR: Cultural considerations in Cambodian childrearing, *J Pediatr Health Care* 10(1):2, 1996.

Lenart JC, St. Clair PA, Bell MA: Childrearing knowledge, beliefs, and practices of Cambodian refugees, *J Pediatr Health Care* 5(6):299, 1991.

Miller JA: Caring for Cambodian refugees in the emergency department, *J Emerg Nurs* 21(6):498, 1995.

Rasbridge LA, Kulig JC: Infant feeding among Cambodian refugees, MCN, *Am J Matern Child Nurs* 20(1):213, 1995.

World Health Organization (June 2000): *Epidemiological fact sheets by country*, Geneva. Retrieved March 1, 2002, from http://www.unaids.org/hivaidsinfo/statistics/june00/fact_sheets/index.html

World Health Organization (2001): *WHO vaccine-preventable diseases: monitoring system*, Geneva. Retrieved March 1, 2002, fromhttp://www.who.int/vaccines/

◆ CAMEROON (REPUBLIC OF)

MAP PAGE (862)

Abraham Ndiwane

Location: The Republic of Cameroon is a triangular-shaped independent country, covering approximately 475,000 km^2 (183,569 square miles) on the Atlantic coastline of West Africa. It is an independent and democratic country, occupying a central, strategic position in the African continent.

Major Languages	Ethnic Groups	Major Religions
English (official)	Cameroon Highlander 31%	Christian 53%
French (official)	Equatorial Bantu 19%	Traditional, animist 25%
African languages	Other African 13%	Muslim 22%
	Kirdi 11%	
	Fulani 10%	
	Northwestern Bantu 8%	
	Eastern Sudanic 7%	
	Other 1%	

As a result of the constitutional reforms of 1972, which were later reaffirmed in 1985, Cameroon became a bilingual nation. Cameroon is linguistically diverse, with more than 200 distinct dialects. The country also has 24 major native languages, predominantly of Bantu dialects.

Health Care Beliefs: Acute sick care; traditional. The people of Cameroon seek out Western medical practitioners and pay for the services themselves, especially in private and nonprofit health facilities. Like in other colonial African countries, the major emphasis of health care in Cameroon is on treating diseases rather than preventing them. Those who need services the most (predominantly poor, rural inhabitants) are the least able to afford them. The people recognize that health care should concentrate on primary health facilities for villages and rural inhabitants because practitioners at these facilities can respond to local demands and conditions.

Predominant Sick Care Practices: Biomedical; ethno-medical; magical-religious. Essential health services that are unavailable or difficult to access continue to present challenges to the health care infrastructure. Although government efforts to address regional disparities have improved, especially in rural areas, significant allocations of financial resources are needed to ensure adequate maintenance of medical services and good governance. For the 2000-2001 fiscal year, health expenditures increased by 48%, and it is anticipated that health and social services will significantly improve. In public or government-operated health facilities, health services are subsidized, but health facilities are usually not well equipped. Therefore patients may be referred to local drug stores and pharmacies for prescriptions, where they pay for the medications themselves. Traditional beliefs and value systems are strong and deeply rooted in the rich cultures and diversity of the people. Theories about the causes of certain diseases include witchcraft or the wrath of the gods (e.g., gods of river, forest, soil, rain, and stone), therefore people seek out interventions from a sorcerer, an herbalist, or a medicine man—a person believed to possess supernatural powers to cure and protect the sick through rituals or wearing amulets. Herbalists (who are often called *traditional doctors*) have gained national attention and acknowledgement from the Cameroon government for their ability to treat people who medical practitioners consider terminal. Although the scientific community dispels such outcomes as anecdotal, traditional herbalists in Cameroon have contributed significantly to health care delivery, particularly in rural communities where health services are not affordable. Particularly in the northwestern region of the country, herbalists are acknowledged for their ability to cure various ailments ranging from fevers and headaches to fractures, infertility, possession by evil spirits, and HIV and AIDS. People of all income levels, from all regions of the country, and of varying educational status use the services of herbalists. The coexistence of the biomedical and traditional models of care means that health care professionals must be nonjudgmental to facilitate the best possible treatment for the patient. Primary health care is a fairly new concept because essential health services are still lacking in most regions. A significant decline in the health infrastructure amidst budget cuts has led to poor-quality health services and management of health services, as well as the deterioration of health indicators such as infant mortality.

Ethnic/Race Specific of Endemic Diseases: Malaria, tuberculosis, childhood measles, and HIV/AIDS are significant health challenges. Although these diseases are preventable, they are the major killers of children and adults. The World Health Organization's (WHO) estimated prevalence rate for HIV/AIDS in adults ages 15 to 49 is 7.73%. The estimated number of children from birth to age 15 living with HIV/AIDS is 22,000. Although this rate is high, it is much lower than those of other southern African countries such as Botswana (36%) and Swaziland (25%). Unfortunately, programs to reduce disease may be thwarted by traditional beliefs, attitudes, and practices. For example, an attempt to reduce neonatal tetanus in females of child-bearing age was misinterpreted as a government attempt to sterilize women in retaliation for the people's launch of a new opposition party in the face of a ban on the creation of new parties. This politically charged rumor frightened women and virtually halted the initiative.

Health Team Relationships: Medical doctors command significant power in the relationships among patient, nurse, and primary care doctor. When patients seek health care, they usually prefer to be screened and treated by a doctor. Most patients also expect a knowledgeable doctor to prescribe oral or parenteral medications to address their underlying health concerns. Thus some patients are reluctant to follow instructions or medical advice when they do not receive medications. Although medical appointments for routine patient visits are not scheduled, patients usually prefer and in some cases request to be seen only by a doctor. Nurses with advanced training have an expanded role and work collaboratively with physicians to screen and treat patients, particularly in settings with few doctors, which are virtually all settings. Nurses are frontline caregivers, and they tend to have significant professional relationships with patients because they generally spend more time with them than the doctors, who are expected to address the more complex cases and have heavier work loads. Patients are gradually beginning to trust nurses and think of them as expert caregivers, particularly in health education at the primary prevention levels.

Families' Role in Hospital Care: Illness is a family business. It is common to find the immediate and extended family at a patient's bedside on a 24-hour basis. At times the numerous family members rallying at the bedside can be detrimental to care. However, family members generally cooperate with health care providers and observe visitation hours. Family visits are important because they provide a forum for family members to keep the patient updated about the community, and members bring home-cooked meals.

Dominance Patterns: The Cameroonian traditional, or rural, community is a closely knitted social structure composed of siblings and extended family members who live in compounds (large pieces of land headed by a patriarch). Although it is expected that adult siblings will leave their compounds of birth to create new ones, particularly when they are married, they are not expected to rush to do so, especially when illness and economic or financial constraints develop. Siblings who move out of their native compound live close by and can reconvene in the parent compound at a moment's notice in the event of an illness, a death, or a birth. Patients who are sick gain the respect, sympathy, and attention of all members, who strive to meet the needs of the ill. However, this is more difficult in urban communities because men and women have professional jobs, participate in the political structure of government, and are often dispersed throughout the country because of job assignments.

Eye Contact Practices: It is considered rude to stare at or maintain eye contact with an authority figure. Children may find it difficult to maintain eye contact with an authority figure during verbal disciplining even if they are told to look up at the person speaking; the general tendency of a person showing respect for authority is to look down. Health care practitioners must appreciate these underlying cultural differences when dealing with Cameroonians.

Perceptions of Time: Time is particularly important to those who have jobs because some are paid only for the time they actually spend working. Generally, punctuality is not a major concern, and people may be late for appointments and other commitments. Some keep time by approximation—for example, by looking at the direction and the intensity of the sun or the appearance and shape of the moon. Peoples' values and beliefs are strongly shaped and governed by past traditions handed down from one generation to another through nightly songs and stories when family members congregate.

Pain Reactions: It is generally expected that men should be stoical and not cry in public when feeling physical or emotional pain; however, women are free to express pain. In a rural community a person might hear a wailing woman half a mile away as she grieves the loss of a loved one, whereas the woman's husband would be disgustedly mopping tears from his face, ashamed that he is crying.

Touch Practices: Physical touching, such as traditional hugging or a handshake, is acceptable, but touching is also associated with rituals such as prayers and traditional healing practices. It is becoming more acceptable and common for members of the opposite sex to hold hands in public, particularly in the towns and cities, but this practice is rare in the rural villages, where traditional family customs are stronger.

Birth Rites: Pregnancy is regarded as a gift of nature to be nurtured, not a disease state. Parents of newlyweds are apprehensive if a couple has no children within a year or two of marriage or cohabitation. The woman is generally alleged to be the cause of infertility, but in some rare situations the man takes some of the blame. Infertile couples may seek the assistance of a traditional healer or a doctor. When a woman is pregnant, she is adored by her husband and relatives. She essentially gets everything she desires, and her husband makes every effort to accommodate her wishes. Similarly, the husband enjoys feelings of manhood and admiration from his peers. Some Cameroonians believe that labor and birth can be delayed until a mother can get to a birthing facility. For example, a woman in labor may leave her farm, walk 3 miles, and give birth almost immediately after arriving at the nearest birthing center. Women with these beliefs wear amulets or place a medicine leaf under their tongue, which is believed to offer guidance and protection for the mother and the unborn child until birth. Home births are rare, but they do occur. In such situations the mother and infant are taken to a medical facility for follow-up evaluations. Women who believe that pregnancy and birth are natural processes are reluctant to accept analgesics, which they believe interrupts nature's processes. A female relative or friend usually accompanies a woman in labor to a health facility. Husbands are not expected to be with their wives during labor or delivery because of the husbands' apprehension and discomfort with the process, a respect for the wife's privacy, and society's belief that the birthing process is best handled by women. These views are slowly changing through education that encourages husbands to get involved and participate in the birth of their children. Birth is a time of celebration marked by singing, dancing, and round-the-clock cooking and feasting. It is the perfect opportunity for grandparents and others to live with the family for an extended period and assist the new mother with chores. In the past, wealthy parents preferred to have sons so that they could one day be heir to the family fortune, whereas poor parents celebrated female children more because the family expected bridal gifts before marriage. However, these commodity-orientated perceptions have changed because more parents are sending their children to school, therefore the age of marriage tends to be older. The focus on education is the result of a joint effort by the government, missionary societies, and private initiatives to encourage literacy. Cameroon has one of the highest rates of school attendance in Africa, with 1994 data indicating that 93% of 6-year-old boys and 84% of 6-year-old girls were enrolled in primary school.

Death Rites: Death, like birth, is a family event and characterized by several days or weeks of mourning. If the deceased person is old or had attained some traditional status in the community, the death ritual and celebration tends to be more prolonged and elaborate than it is for the death of an infant. When the cause of death is poorly understood, people generally blame a dissenting family member or witchcraft rather than natural causes. The body may undergo special cleansing rituals by a traditional herbalist or someone believed to have supernatural powers. The body is buried quickly and far from commonly inhabited areas so that the ghost of the deceased does not return to hurt the living. Autopsies and organ donations are generally unacceptable and infrequently performed. In some communities the bodies of deceased Christians are washed and dressed according to local customs. A religious service is conducted by a priest or pastor before burial. If the deceased was a non-Christian or an atheist, traditional burial rites and celebrations take place.

Food Practices and Intolerances: Some men are slowly becoming involved in the kitchen duties, but the majority of these chores are the responsibility of women. In some traditional Cameroonian societies, a good wife is a woman who is able to prepare various dishes for her husband and his friends. However, a good husband should be able to work hard and provide the food for his wife and family. Food choices tend to vary according to regions of the country. For instance, in the northwest region a stable diet may consist of corn *fufu* (corn flour cooked into a paste) eaten with various vegetables that are mixed with well-spiced smoked meat or fish. A delicacy known as *achuh* is made from cocoyams (tuberous plants) that are cooked and pounded into a paste in a wooden vessel. *Achuh* is eaten with dried meat, "bush meat," or eggplant *njaniki* in a spicy pudding that is rich in sodium and potassium. *Fufu* and *achuh* are traditionally served on leaves, woven baskets, or wood dishes and eaten with the fingers. Foreigners are strongly encouraged to learn to eat liquid and semiliquid foods with their fingers according to traditional food rituals. Although other foods such as rice, beans, and plantains may be eaten sporadically, such foods may not be considered "real" foods because they do not leave people satiated for long periods unless they are supplemented with *fufu* or *achuh*. In the southwestern and coastal regions, a staple diet may include foods such as *kwacoco* (grated cocoyams cooked with palm-nut soup) and *minyado'oh* (fermented cassava tubers cooked and eaten with roasted fish.

Infant Feeding Practices: In the past, multinational companies advertised milk products and infant formulas to parents who could not afford them. In an attempt to increase the quantities of the expensive formulas, people ignored formula instructions and diluted them. This practice combined with poor sterilization techniques led to infant malnutrition and diarrhea. The Ministry of Health and private health facilities have recently begun emphasizing the importance of educating parents about the benefits of breast milk and the fact that it is the best source of nutrition for infants, particularly with regard to boosting the immune system. The duration of breast-feeding may span from birth to 18 months, although semisolid foods such as cornstarch *pap* cooked into a nectar consistency and fortified with sweeteners such as sugar or honey may be introduced at about 6 months. The consumption of poorly processed honey by children younger than 1 year of age has been associated with risk of botulism. Fruit such as bananas, pears, and avocados are mashed into a paste or made into porridge and fed to infants as young as 4 months.

Child Rearing Practices: Traditional communities are especially close, and almost all community members know one another well. Children rarely get away with criminal acts because the community participates in rearing the children, and corporal discipline such as spanking is the entire community's responsibility. In fact, some children are punished twice for the same crime—first by the person who observed the crime being committed and second by the parents. At an early age, children are taught moral codes of conduct involving obedience and respect for older adults. For example, children cannot carry on a conversation when older adults are talking. If an older person walks into a room, all children and young adults must rise and offer their seats, even when other seats are available. Disciplinary measures are primarily the responsibility of the father, but in some situations the mother is the dominant disciplinarian. Children are given daily tasks such as fetching wood and water for cooking after returning from school and assisting parents on the farm on days when they do not attend school. These chores encourage the development of a work ethic and inculcate a sense of skillfulness, autonomy, and civic responsibility important for later years.

National Childhood Immunizations: BCG at birth; DPT at 6, 10, and 14 weeks; OPV at birth and at 6, 10, and 14 weeks; measles at 9 months; and TT after first contact +1 month, +6 months, +1 year, and +1 year.

Other Characteristics: In spite of economic reforms, poverty is found throughout the country, although the effects are more significant in rural areas, where 86% of poor people live. However, Cameroon was ranked 134 out of 174 countries, indicating that it has better living conditions than most of its neighbors. Cameroonians think that the diverse cultures of its people characterize its identity, and cultural pride has tremendous significance for the people.

Acknowledgments: This work is dedicated to my beloved mother Magdalene Pekianze Ndiwane, also known as "Big Mami," the matriarch of the Ndiwane family, who died in Bangolan-Ndop, Cameroon at the age of 91 on October 22, 2001.

BIBLIOGRAPHY

Azevedo M, Prater GS, Lantum DN: Culture, biomedicine and child mortality in Cameroon, *Soc Sci Med* 32:1341, 1991.

Clark JI, Englebert P: *Regional surveys of the world, Africa south of the Sahara 2001,* ed 30, London, 2001, Europa Publications 2000.

Cutter CH: *The world today series. Africa 1999,* ed 34, Baltimore, 2000, United Book Press.

Defo BK: Determinants of infant and early childhood mortality in Cameroon: The role of socioeconomic factors, housing characteristics, and immunization status, *Soc Biol* 41(3–4):181, 1994.

DeLancey MW, Delancey MD: *Historical dictionary of the Republic of Cameroon*, ed 3, Lanham, Md, 2000, Scarecrow Press.

The Economist Intelligence Unit Limited: *Country profile, Cameroon*, London, 2000, Redhouse Press.

Feldman-Savelsberg P, Ndonko FT, Schmidt-Ehry B: Sterilizing vaccines or the politics of the womb: retrospective study of a rumor in Cameroon, *Med Anthro Quart* 14(2):159, 2000.

Muna BA: *Cameroon and the challenges of the 21st century*, Yaounde, Cameroon, 1993, Tama Books.

Ndumbe PM, Yenshu E: Cameroon: vaccination and politics, *Lancet* 339:8803, 1992.

Panford S et al: Using folk media in HIV/AIDS prevention in rural Ghana, *Am J Public Health* 91(10):1559, 2001.

Ross-Larson Human Development Report, United Nations Development Programme, New York, 1999, Oxford University Press.

UNAIDS and the World Health Organization: *Epidemiological fact sheet on HIV/*

AIDS and sexually transmitted infections: Cameroon (2000 update). Retrieved September 21, 2001, from http://www.who.int/emc_hiv/fact_sheets/pdfs/cameroon.pdf
World Health Organization (June 2000): *Epidemiological fact sheets by country*, Geneva. Retrieved March 1, 2002, from World Health Organization (2001): WHO vaccine-preventable diseases: monitoring system, Geneva. Retrieved March 1, 2002, from http://www.who.int/vaccines/

◆ CAPE VERDE (REPUBLIC OF)

MAP PAGE (862)

Félix Neto and Ana Veríssimo Ferreira

Location: The Republic of Cape Verde is in the North Atlantic Ocean, 600 km west-northwest of Senegal and west of West Africa's coast at Mauritania. Cape Verde has ten major islands and eight islets, all of volcanic origin. The total land area is 4030 km^2 (1556 square miles). The six inhabited islands, located more in the west, are characterized by mountainous landscapes, whereas the other three have long beaches. The islands are divided into two groups named after the trade winds from the African continent: windward (Barlavento) and leeward (Sotavento). The first group consists of the islands Santo Antão, São Vicente, Santa Luzia, Ilhéu Branco, Ilhéu Raso, São Nicolau, Sal, and Boa Vista. The second group, more to the south, comprises the islands of Maio, São Tiago, Fogo, and Brava. Cape Verde has a milder climate than neighboring countries at the same latitude, with a rainy season during August, September, and October. The east winds blowing from the African continent are extremely warm during January and February, making the climate tropical and dry. The standard temperature remains around 25° C, and fluctuations do not exceed 10° C because of the ocean's effects.

Major Languages	Ethnic Groups	Major Religions
Portuguese (official)	Creole (mulatto) 71%	Roman Catholic 80%
Crioulo (Portuguese and	African 28%	fused with
West African blend)	European 1%	indigenous beliefs
		Other or none 20%

Portuguese is used for formal communication in such fields as administration, teaching, literature, justice, and mass media. Crioulo (Creole) is used for informal communication. According to data from the National Statistics Institute of Cape Verde, the archipelago has 434,812 inhabitants, with 231,650 in urban and 203,162 in rural areas. Santiago is the largest island and the capital, containing about half of the total population. Santiago, São Vicente, Santo Antão, and Fogo together contain about 89% of the total population. The islands, which were initially uninhabited, were discovered and colonized by the Portuguese in the fifteenth century and became a trading center for African slaves. Most Cape Verdeans descend from both groups. Although independence was achieved in 1975, the vestiges of Portuguese culture are considerably more evident than are African, except in São Tiago, which has more people of African ancestry.

Health Care Beliefs: Acute sick care; traditional. Many challenges must be met for people to receive adequate health care in Cape Verde, namely developing a primary care system directed toward high-risk groups, a program of disease prevention and health promotion, and an efficient ambulance service that can transfer patients among islands. Health care access is particularly limited in socially and geographically underprivileged areas. Residents in these areas do not have balanced and sustained sanitary conditions because of problems with access to potable water and deficiencies in basic sanitation and sewer systems. It is common for people to either pray or wear amulets to ward off illnesses or bring about a cure. Mental heath has not been adequately addressed. People with mental illness are often found living on the streets and are assisted only by neighbors; people tend to believe that such disorders (epylepsis) are caused by evil spirits.

Predominant Sick Care Practices: Biomedical; magical-religious. Cape Verde is ranked fourth in Africa in the categories of health services, education, and quality of life. Patients seek help from doctors, as well as indigenous healers who use teas and treatments involving plants and oils. These two healing systems continue to coexist despite governmental efforts to promote and improve the Public Health Service and create more private services. Patients make appointments with doctors in either hospitals or smaller facilities called health units. Cape Verde has two central hospitals (Praia and Mindelo) and three regional hospitals (Santo Antão, Santa Catarina, and Fogo). All the islands have health units. In the official health service, people pay a hospital fee. In the private service, people pay about $35 per visit. Cape Verde has about 167 doctors and 300 nurses. The ratio of doctors to inhabitants is 1:2603, and the ratio of nurses to inhabitants is 1:1454, with more health professionals in urban areas. The average number of hospital beds in Cape Verde is about 626.

Ethnic/Race Specific or Endemic Diseases: Despite being near the African continent, Cape Verde has exemplary sanitary standards and good vaccination coverage on all islands. Until recently, no vaccinations were required to enter the country. However, since September 2001, local health officials have reported 66 cases of malaria, including one death from complications of cerebral malaria in Praia, São Tiago. Imported malaria from other countries in West Africa is believed to be the primary cause of the outbreak. In response the Ministry of Health and local public health officials are taking measures to reduce mosquito breeding sources and have increased malaria surveillance activities, including screening local residents and travelers from West African countries. Transmission of malaria on São Tiago has been reported as seasonal, peaking from

September to November. Health officials are greatly concerned about the spread of endemic diseases such as cholera, dysentery, meningitis, HIV and AIDS, and tuberculosis. Several projects are in progress to increase access to safe water and improve living conditions for the population. Heart disease registries did not exist in Cape Verde before 1989; however, it is clear that cardiovascular problems are increasing. Diarrheal and respiratory system diseases are the main causes of mortality in children younger than 5 years; malnutrition and perinatal infections are also major problems. With World Health Organization (WHO) assistance, the country is attempting to increase vaccination coverage and develop better screening for diseases. Increases in technical training and the introduction of new medical specialties are other methods being used to improve health care. WHO has no national statistics for HIV/AIDS rates, but some islands have implemented projects to increase awareness of the disease in addition to programs involving birth control and sexual education.

Health Team Relationships: Relationships among health care professionals (doctors, nurses, and others) and patients are excellent. Despite the lack of technical and human resources in hospitals and health care settings, health professionals form a team to assist ill people as best they can given their resources. Doctors and nurses work in cooperation in central, regional hospitals and in the health units of all the islands. The specialized services have many problems because of insufficient radiology, laboratory, instrumentation, and anesthesiology technicians. The country does have some specialists such as pediatricians, gynecologists, public health doctors, radiologists, and cardiologists. Although Cape Verde has a nursing school, health professionals urgently need more education.

Families' Role in Hospital Care: The traditional family is extended and includes children, grandparents, uncles, aunts, parentless godchildren, and homeless children. Family members are close and provide an important safety net when any members are sick. Family members frequently visit and bring food to hospitalized patients because the meals provided are inadequate. It is often common for families to provide other necessities such as sanitary products and diapers.

Dominance Patterns: Older adults have the most knowledge and experience and are still the most important and respected members of the families. The traditional culture also promotes the strict division of work according to sex. Boys are trained only to do chores that are considered men's work, and girls follow the example of their mothers. From preadolescence on, the roles of male and female are markedly different. Domestic violence against women such as spousal abuse is common. People rarely report crimes such as rape and spousal abuse to the police, and neighbors and relatives prefer to keep silent about such issues. Women's organizations are seeking legislation to establish a special family court to address crimes of domestic violence, but women are often reluctant to seek legal action. Despite constitutional prohibitions, sex discrimination continues. Technically, legal provisions delineate full equality, including equal pay for equal work. Women have difficulties obtaining certain types of jobs even though they are often paid less than men. The constitution prohibits discrimination against women in family and custody matters; however, most women are unaware of their rights largely because they are illiterate. The Organization of Cape Verdean Women alleges disparate treatment in inheritance matters despite laws calling for equal rights. Physical and sexual child abuse and mistreatment and juvenile prostitution are continuing problems, exacerbated by chronic poverty, large (unplanned) families, and the traditionally high levels of emigration of adult men. Neither females nor males are circumcised.

Eye Contact Practices: Direct eye contact is acceptable.

Touch Practices: Touch is acceptable even between members of the opposite sex. People are very gradually beginning to accept equality of the sexes as traditional ways begin to be replaced by modern ones.

Perceptions of Time: Cape Verdeans are not concerned with punctuality and consider it unimportant.

Pain Reactions: The people of Cape Verde are extremely expressive when in pain or grieving.

Birth Rites: In the last half of the 1970s, a program for maternal and infant protection and family planning was implemented in São Nicolau. The intent of this program was to educate the people on topics such as preventive medicine, pediatrics, birth control, and sexual practices that could lead to disease. Initial reactions to this program were negative, especially toward the concept of contraceptive use. Although some behaviors have been modified as a result of the program, the increasing trend of out-of-wedlock pregnancies has not abated. One third of all families are headed by single mothers, and first pregnancies often occur at a very young age. Women learn the art of being mothers from their families and must follow strict rules during pregnancy or risk being punished by supernatural forces. Mothers adhere to magico-religious traditions to protect themselves and their infants and facilitate childbirth. For example, it is believed that eating eggs during pregnancy causes an infant to be born with a big head, which makes childbirth difficult. People believe that pregnant women should not wear mourning clothes, go to funerals or cemeteries, see corpses, or be near children with disabilities because it could kill the fetus. Pregnant women are also never godmothers because they believe it will cause their child or the child being baptized to die. It is also believed that metallic objects near a pregnant woman's belly could cause the child to be born with the shape of the object on the body. Other than these interdictions, normal daily life goes on for pregnant women—carrying heavy objects on their heads, grinding corn, cooking, washing, getting water from the spring, fetching wood, and feeding animals—until very close to delivery. Abiding by three main superstitions is believed to help a woman have an easy delivery. She should walk around a church building three times, be faithful to her husband, and have all her wishes and cravings fulfilled. Midwives play an important social role. They deliver the infants, prescribe healing treatments of plants and herbs, say prayers, dress wounds, and assist with abortive measures. Childbirth involves rituals, prejudices, prohibitions, and taboos. Pregnant women give birth with the help of the midwife or female relatives or neighbors who have already given birth. Men wait and play cards, talk, and drink. If mother's labor is prolonged, the midwife prays to the protecting divinities and applies herbal remedies to facilitate the delivery. They also use infusions of plants (*Salvia officianalis*) and oils (ricinus and sweet almonds) for massage. Cape Verdeans believe that supernatural forces of evil can take possession of the fragile and immature bodies of children, causing weakness and death. Therefore rituals and ceremonies to protect the infant are performed. Immediately after birth, infants wear amulets to keep the evil spirits away; for example, a string around the neck, special beads, or charms inside a small pouch are believed to break the spell of the "evil eye" (causing a person harm just by looking at the person). In some islands, rites involve using the placenta to protect newborns. After cutting umbilical cords, they place them in the infants' mouth so that they can have some drops of blood (together with sulphur). Infants are then washed with urine. The goal of both of these procedures is protection from sorcery and the "evil eye." The cord and the placenta are buried to prevent bad spirits from influencing the child. Many Cape Verdeans say that they want to return to the place "where their navel was buried." It is accepted that birth and early infancy are dangerous periods for mother and child. The fact that many children die during the first week has influenced people to believe that potentially evil supernatural forces such as bewitching women and werewolves surround newborns in that first week, so they need the protection of family members. The *noite dos sete* (night of the seven) ritual is performed on the seventh day after birth. The family has a party with friends to celebrate the end of the isolation period and the infant's survival. During the period of sexual abstinence after the child's birth, women are symbolically considered virgins anew. Baptism comes a few months later, and godparents play an important role. They are chosen according to certain rules and are assumed to have potentially major responsibilities because they must raise the godchild if the parents die. Cape Verdeans also believe that godmothers can put curses on infants, so they must be the first person to cut the infant's nails.

Death Rites: Each culture has its own traditional funeral ceremonies. The moment a person seems close to death, a *cerimónia de perdão* (forgiveness ceremony) is held in the presence of a priest or a person representing him. In hospitals, autopsies may be performed after medicolegal forensic procedures have been followed. When a person dies at home, the body is prepared for a wake. It is washed with infusions of aromatic herbs, orange peels, and rosemary and dressed for the funeral. Three rites are performed to benefit the dead person. The vital elements of water, earth, and fire must be present. The body undergoes an immersion ritual associated with hiding the body in the earth when it is buried; candlelight must be part of the funeral. The funeral is Roman Catholic and performed by a priest, with songs being intoned. As the body is lowered into the grave, they play the "morna" *hour di bai* (hour of departure) as every person throws a handful of earth into the grave. After the funeral a procession of all the family members, who are crying and screaming out, return to the deceased person's house and have a meal together. The duration of the mourning period depends on who died. If the family members were very close to the person, they go into deep mourning; if the relationship was more distant, they practice half mourning. The rules are very specific regarding the time when the widow is allowed to leave the house (about 3 months). Death is associated with beliefs in ghosts, wandering souls, and many other superstitions.

Food Practices and Intolerances: Cape Verdean food is basically Portuguese, but some dishes are unique to the islands. One of the most unusual is *pastel com diablo dentro* (pastry with the devil inside)—a mix of fresh tuna, onions, and tomatoes wrapped in a pastry blended from boiled potatoes and corn flour, which is deep fried and served hot. Soups are also popular, one of the most common of which is *coldo de peixe* (fish stew). The national dish, *catchupa*, is a stew of hominy and beans with fish or meat. The people's daily foods are made more interesting by a diverse combination of popular foods—corn, beans, sweet potatoes, manioc, fish, and various meats—that are enriched by liqueurs and traditional sweets. The people have no religious bans on food or intolerances to particular foods.

Infant Feeding Practices: Mothers breast-feed their infants for about 1 year. The infant may also have a *mãe de leite*, another mother who feeds the infant when the actual mother is unable to do so. At about 4 or 5 months, mush and soup are introduced.

Child Rearing Practices: Children generally sleep with their parents or older brothers. Child rearing styles are quite permissive for young children. However, they are taught to obey and respect the older members of the family even though the children do not follow rigid rules.

National Childhood Immunizations: BCG at birth; DPT at 6, 10, and 14 weeks; OPV at birth and 6, 10, and 14 weeks; measles at 9 months; and TT after first contact, +4 weeks, +6 months, +1, +1 year.

Other Characteristics: The most common ways to become husband and wife are *amigarem-se* or *ajuntarem-se*, meaning to live in concubinage, and *tirar de casa* (eloping because of economic difficulties). Regardless of the method, the couple is considered by society to be a husband and wife worthy of respect. Later, they may legally marry, frequently during the time when their children or grandchildren are being baptized. Prewedding preparations start with family gatherings during which people offer water, wood, and corn, thus increasing friendship ties. The women prepare *pilagem do xerém* (maize meals), and men prepare capons and hens. When couples have not previously lived together, a common practice and an ancient tradition in the whole archipelago is the procedure of displaying the bride's virginity to wedding guests by showing them a stained towel. The girl's parents are congratulated for having taken such good care of their daughter. When a widow gets married, she has no celebrations. After the religious ceremony, the guests go home. The couple then proceeds to the cemetery where they both cry over the dead husband's grave so that his soul will not haunt them.

BIBLIOGRAPHY

The Africa Guide: 2002, http://www.africaguide.com/country/cverde/
Africana: Porto, Universidade Portucalense, 1993, Centro de Estudos Africanos.
Cape Verde Consular Information Sheet: March 2001, http://travel.stage.gov/cape-verde.html
Centers for Disease Control: http://www.cdc.gov/travel/other/cape-verde.htm
Destination Cape Verde: http://www.lonelyplanet.com/destinations/africa/cape-verde/
Filho JL: *Cabo verde. Retalhos do quotidiano*: Lisboa, 1995, Caminho, Col Universitária.
Filho JL: *Defesa do património sócio-cultural de Cabo Verde*, Lisboa, 1998, Ulmeiro.
Filho JL: Ilha de S. Nicolau de Cabo Verde: Mudanças Sócio-Económicas, *Cultura—Cabo Verde* 2: 202–215, 1998.
Fonseca M: Padronização do Alfabeto: sua importância. *Cultura—Cabo Verde* 2:98–107, 1998.
GEP/Ministério da Saúde, Estatísticas da Mortalidade, Praia, 2000.
Instituto Nacional de Estatística de Cabo Verde http://ine.cv/estatisticas-cv INE, 1990 e 2000—Censo 90 e 2000, Perspectivas demográficas de Cabo Verde—Horizonte 2020.
Política de saúde, de infância, e de juventude do Governo da República de Cabo Verde: http://www.governo.cv/Prog-Desenv-Social-Saúde.html,http://www.governo.cv/Prog-Desenv-Social-Infancia.html
Vaccination of the traveler to the African continent: Sub-Saharan Africa, http://www.saudepublica.web.pt/Infecções/Travel/africasubsahariantravel.htm
Veiga M: Implementação do ALUPEC, *Cultura—Cabo Verde* 2:94–97, 1998.

◆ CENTRAL AFRICAN REPUBLIC

MAP PAGE (862)

Patricia Laure Yepassis-Zembrou

Location: A landlocked republic 805 km (500 miles) north of the African equator, with an area of 623,000 km^2 (240,535 square miles), the Central African Republic is covered with tropical forest in the south and semidesert land in the northeast. The country shelters the geographical heart of Africa in Bakala (Ouaka). It shares boundaries in the north with Chad, east with Sudan, south with the Democratic Republic of Congo (formerly Zaire) and Congo (Brazzaville), and west with Cameroon. It has an extensive water system that flows all year long, including the Oubangui River, which runs south from east to west. It is one of the 25 poorest countries in the world.

Major Languages	Ethnic Groups	Major Religions
French (official)	Baya 34%	Protestant and Roman
Sangho	Banda 27%	Catholic 33%
Arabic	Mandjia 21%	Muslim 44%
	Sara 10%	Indigenous beliefs 23%
	Mboum, other 8%	

French is the official language used in school and all government administration, private, and business offices. Sango, the national language, is spoken nationwide and is the second official language. Though not yet taught in school, Sango is used by the media, at home, in church, and in public institutions. Arabic is mainly used in Muslim institutions such as mosques and Islamic schools. An additional 67 living languages are spoken by 83 tribes.

Health Care Beliefs: Acute sick care; traditional. The health system tends to involve traditional values perpetuated from generation to generation. Illness beliefs are rooted in supernatural incidents and belief in evil spirits. Traditional therapies involving abstinence from certain foods and use of laxative agents to ward off evil forces and wash off the core of the illness (*fa mama ti kobela*) are common. Minor illnesses are managed by the family, relatives, and neighbors through experienced-based procedures and are not regarded important enough to be treated in a health care facility. Therefore traditional rituals are used, occasionally with poor results. The government is targeting such practices through extensive weekly health education campaigns on rural and urban media channels. Herbal remedies are the first choice of therapy for ailments ranging from colds (*koro*) to diarrhea (sassa) to fractures (*herbal cast*). Despite the fact that 40% of the population lives in urban areas, traditional remedies such as suction-pad techniques using small horns to draw out illness are still used among ethnic groups. Mental disease is believed to originate from possession by evil spirits when an individual breaks a pact with ancestral spirits or black magic takes over. The society fears mental illness and marginalizes those who are possessed. AIDS is perceived as simply a misfortune, and people deny its actual cause. Hence AIDS treatment involves traditional healers and prayers rather than biomedicine. Prenatal care is insufficient outside of Bangui, and very few women comply with their full schedule of appointments. Most births in rural areas occur at home, and women prefer traditional birth attendants, relatives, or friends to hospital delivery rooms and midwives.

Predominant Sick Care Practices: Magical-religious, with biomedicine as a last resort. Traditional healers, witch doctors, and advice from older adults or neighbors from the community are the primary recourse for Central Africans because sickness is considered the result of fate or a spell. They seek out help from modern medical practitioners as the last resort if it is available. The government has recognized that traditional healers are a significant part of its effort to restore and promote the health of the population. Herbal remedies are the custom across the country. For example, a "sauna" of a boiling mixture of barks and leaves is used to heal illnesses ranging from malaria to measles. Scarification plays a dual role in prevention and cures. It is considered to be a shield against fate and sicknesses. The small, black, scarred areas on the arms or chest of patients, pregnant women, and children are common. Consultation with fortune tellers and wearing amulets are integrated practices of the society that are observed by Christians and Muslims. Although more people believe in the healing power of prayer and God's protective interventions, many still adopt mixed practices in which they rely on their talismans but also pray. Sunday is devoted to God, so very few patients go to health care facilities on Sundays, and most businesses are closed. Self-medication practices are also widespread despite efforts by the Ministry of Health to curtail the drug dealers, or boubanguere, many of whom are not qualified to give health advice or prescriptions.

Ethnic/Race Specific or Endemic Diseases: Malaria outbreaks rage nationwide throughout the year because of the extensive river network, hot and humid climate, and insufficient number of sewers to drain the rain—perfect conditions for mosquito breeding. The malaria strain is resistant to both chloroquine and sulfadoxine-pyrimethamine. Trypanosomiasis and schistosomiasis are rampant in some regions; the most recent trypanosomiasis outbreaks were reported in the High Mbomou area. Recent outbreaks of cholera and meningitis occurred in Kouango and Paoua, respectively. Although no yellow fever cases have been reported in the past decade, it is still a risk and vaccination is mandatory. Onchocerciasis is the main cause of blindness. Iodine deficiency disorders, especially goiter (*la perle de beauté*, or "beauty pearl"), are common among the Gbaya but occur in other regions also. The dry season is associated with acute respiratory tract infections, intestinal parasitic infestations, and diarrhea, which is one of the leading causes of death among children younger than 5 years. Childhood malnutrition is high at 23%. Overall infant and child mortality rates are, respectively, 93 and 156 per 1000 live births. Tuberculosis has run rampant as an opportunistic infection in patients with HIV. The Central African Republic is one of the 16 countries in the world with an HIV prevalence rate that reaches or exceeds 10% of the population. The World Health Organization's (WHO) estimated prevalence rate for HIV/AIDS in adults ages 15 to 49 is 13.84%. The estimated number of children from birth to 15 years living with HIV/AIDS is 8900. Transmission is essentially heterosexual. HIV prevalence among antenatal women was 10% in 1994 and 14% in 1996. Prevalence among sex workers was 16% in 1985 and 20% in 1989. The total number of children younger than age 15 who have been orphaned since the beginning of the epidemic is estimated to be 99,000; of those 69,780 were living at the end of 1999. One of the consequences of HIV has been a critical loss of teachers. Of the teachers who died between 1996 and 1998, 85% were infected with HIV. The life expectancy at birth, 45 years, is expected to decrease significantly because of the AIDS epidemic.

Health Team Relationships: Doctors head the health care system at the hospital level and are respected by nurses, midwives, and other health workers. The team relationship is well framed, and doctors' decisions are final. Complaints against doctors are not expressed openly because of fear of repercussions. The authority of the doctor stretches beyond the health facility to the community and into daily life. Midwives and the chiefs of health centers are the next level of authority and deference. Patients are not expected to openly disagree or discuss their health issues with doctors or health workers.

Families' Role in Hospital Care: The family assists the patient at all times, and family members, relatives, and friends take turns staying at the bedside. The family provides care, whereas the nurses provide the medical treatments. Each member of the family is required to visit the patient and contribute to his/her moral, physical, and financial support by visiting, bringing food, or paying for prescriptions because health insurance does not exist. Hospitals in Bangui serve at least one meal whereas in the provinces, hospitals cannot afford to provide food.

Dominance Patterns: The country has a patriarchal system. After marriage, wives yield their rights to their husbands and stay in the husband's family even after the husband's death. Family reunions are headed by fathers to maintain connections among members. Children are treated equally, although some ethnic groups believe it is preferable for the first-born child to be a boy. Girls are expected to help with and master the chores of a wife in preparation for her future life with her husband. A wife who cannot cook well or keep her husband's house neat is considered dishonorable. Although polygamy is legal (with a husband being allowed to have as many as four wives) and was instituted by former President Bokassa, not all men embrace the practice (although they may have multiple extramarital partners, and any resulting offspring bear the father's name).

Touch Practices: Touch is usual and natural. People of the same sex frequently walk holding hands or shoulders because they are friends or siblings. When two girls or women are chatting, they often touch. Adults also cuddle children as a sign of affection or appreciation. However, in some ethnic groups in southern areas such as the Gbaka and Yaloma, touching has rules. For example, a son- or daughter-in-law can never shake hands with or eat in front of parents-in-law.

Eye Contact Practices: Direct eye contact is considered impolite, disrespectful, and disobedient in some traditional ethnic groups such as Banda, Sara, and Gbaya. People are also expected to keep their eyes down when speaking to an older person or one in authority. This practice is not as important when among contemporaries.

Perceptions of Time: People in the Central African Republic are less concerned with punctuality than are people in the Western world. In rural areas, people judge time according to the solar cycle, and being on time is not extremely important. A person can show up any time after the scheduled hour. The *l'heure Africaine*, or "the African hour," method of time is used in urban areas and is well known by foreigners living in the country. In other words, people are expected to arrive later than scheduled for events or meetings. Recently, people have become more concerned with being on time. For example, people are more likely to be on time for work or government-related or medical appointments. Punctuality is extremely important in school, and children who do not arrive on time are either suspended for the day or have detention. The society mainly lives in the present.

Pain Reactions: Adults of all ethnic groups are expected to suppress external reactions to pain. Enduring pain is an important aspect of becoming an adult. Adults in intense pain may snap their fingers or nip certain body parts (e.g., legs, arms, abdomen). Men are not expected to express pain because it is a sign of weakness and womanhood. On the contrary, women are allowed to cry out in pain during childbirth or when bitten during a conjugal conflict. However, pain does not usually prevent women from completing household tasks. Children younger than age 10 are also allowed to express their pain loudly, but children who are 10 or older are reprimanded for not behaving like adults.

Birth Rites: In rural areas, mothers-in-law and close female relatives or friends assist with childbirth, whereas in urban areas they remain outside the delivery room. The crude birth rate is 37 live births per 1000 people. After birth the mother is given plenty of semiliquid food—usually soups made of fish, beef bones, or green vegetables and porridge made of rice, corn, or millet—to stimulate milk production. Muslim women usually add hot pepper to the porridge in the belief that it breaks up blood clots in the uterus after delivery. Members of some ethnic groups also drink alcoholic beverages such as beer and palm wine to stimulate breast milk production. To reduce postpartum morbidity and mortality, relatives and friends in some ethnic groups take care of the mother and help with the household duties for the first 3 months. It is not unusual to see the mother-in-law move into the new mother's home after birth. The maternal mortality rate is 700 women per 100,000 live births. In almost all ethnic groups, a new mother's care is based on traditional therapies, including squatting over or in a concoction of hot leaves, herbal massage, and wearing herbal pads. The baby shower takes place within the first month after the birth, and religious groups, co-workers, friends, and relatives bring gifts. Newborns undergo ethnic-specific rituals such as scarification identifying their ethnic group, application of makeup, head shaving, and use of amulets. The first-born son is highly celebrated in many ethnic groups because he bears the father's name and is expected to be the pillar of the family after the father's death. In rural areas, newborns are kept inside for at least a month to keep them from seeing the moon at night, which is believed to take away their beauty.

Death Rites: All ethnic groups consider the dead to be sacred. Bodies are only allowed to be buried in the ground; cremation and organ donations are unacceptable. Burial rituals and death rites differ according to religion (Christian or Muslim) and among ethnic groups. The common practice is for family members, friends, and relatives to spend several days and nights helping the mourning family. Most ethnic groups believe that after death the dead join their ancestors in the beyond, either in water or a traditional forest. Many groups (e.g., Gbaka, others) perform rituals to determine whether the dead person has arrived in the afterworld. A new generation of Christian theology focusing on living according to the Christian gospel has revolutionized traditional concepts of death and death rites. More frequently, Christian wakes are occurring across the country. Autopsies are rare and practiced in hospitals for legal purposes upon a doctor's request, rather than family demand.

Food Practices and Intolerances: Although great differences in food practices exist among ethnic groups, some foods are considered as "national" and offered to all visitors or strangers: *koko* (dark green, thinly chopped leaves that look somewhat like grass), ngouza (cassava or manioc leaves), and *gozo* (cassava root). The diet is well balanced, consisting of proteins (such as peanuts, beef, wild livestock, and fish), starch (such as *gozo*, banana plantains, corn, potatoes, yams, and millet), leafy vegetables, and tropical fruits that are in season. Milk is scarce in the north and northeastern regions where the *mbororos*, or nomad beef farmers, live. The northern ethnic groups such as the Banda, Sara, and Kaba consume more meat from wild livestock and starches such as *gozo* and millet; vegetables are a luxury and rarely available. Riverside ethnic groups such as the Ngbanziri, Gbaka, Mondjombo, Yakoma, and Sango ingest more fish, vegetables, plantains, yams, and corn. Forbidden foods are specific to each ethnic group. Some may not eat antelope, buffalo, or a certain kind of fish or vegetable that is considered a sacred ethnic totem. Food intolerances are uncommon. A two-meal eating pattern is the norm across the country. Rural families have one meal in the morning and the second in the evening, whereas urban families have one meal at noon and the next in the evening. People use their hands to eat in rural as well as urban areas. In many ethnic groups, it is only proper to use the right hand to eat when eating in a group. Men, women, and children have their own eating groups; in rural areas, these groups eat separately at mealtime and do not interact. In urban areas, this practice is less common. The father may eat with the boys and the mother with the girls. In some families, fathers use a spoon to eat, a practice that is increasing in urban areas. In some restaurants, people still eat with their hands, and the staff members provide water and soap.

Infant Feeding Practices: Breast milk is the first food given to infants at birth. Breast-feeding on demand is common and practiced by all women unless medical contraindications exist. Occasionally, the infant is bottle-fed water right after birth before the breast milk comes in. Colostrum is considered "dirty" milk that is bad for the infant, so it is purged and discarded for a couple of days. Exclusive breast-feeding is done only for a short period; however, the country has begun a national campaign, especially in urban areas, to promote breast-feeding. Supplementation with semiliquid cornstarch or millet porridge begins when the infant is about 3 months, but some women begin using supplementary foods with infants as young as 1 month. Bottle-feeding with formula is more common in urban areas and may begin at birth in addition to breast-feeding. Weaning begins at about 9 months or when the infant begins to walk. Some children are breast-fed until they are 2 years or older.

Child Rearing Practices: Child rearing is managed rigorously by parents, relatives, neighbors, and friends. Corporal punishment such as spanking is customary and still practiced in many elementary schools, although some parents object to spankings by school staff members. From early childhood, children are taught to respect their parents, older siblings, and adults. They are expected to refrain from raising their voice, grumbling, or raising their hands to older adults. Children perform chores according to their abilities. For instance, a 1-year-old boy who is asked to bring a cup or broom to his mother is expected to do it. A 7-year-old girl should be able to cook simple meals, prepare the *gozo*, and take care of her younger siblings, whereas a 7-year-old boy is expected to be able to fix a broken stool and run errands efficiently. Circumcision of boys is the norm and is performed either by trained men in the village, male nurses at home, or interns or doctors in a health facility. The procedure usually occurs when the boy is about to enter school, between ages 4 and 7, and according to his parents' request. Circumcision of girls is common among some groups such as the Bandas and carried out traditionally.

National Childhood Immunizations: BCG at birth or before 15 days; DPT at 6, 10, and 14 weeks; OPV at birth and 6, 10, and 14 weeks; measles at 9 months; and yellow fever at 9 months. The MMR and hepatitis vaccines are not automatically given and are provided if parents can afford them. Mothers are encouraged by peers, midwives, and birth attendants to bring their children for immunizations. In addition, the country has two National Immunization Days. The reported proportion of the target population vaccinated in 1999 was as follows: BCG, 62%; first dose of DPT, 55%; third dose of DPT, 33%; MCV, 37%; and Pol3, 36%. According to the United Nations Children's Fund (UNICEF), the percentages of 1-year-old children who were fully immunized between 1995 and 1998 were as follows: DPT, 46%; polio, 47%; and measles, 39%. In 2000, 3207 measles cases, 37 cases of neonatal tetanus, and 3 polio cases were reported.

BIBLIOGRAPHY

Adler MW, ed: Statistics from the World Health Organization and the Centers for Disease Control, *AIDS* 6(10):1229, 1992.

Bernet-Bernady P et al: AIDS and Aids: anthropological observations apropos the AIDS phenomenon in Lobaye, Central African Republic, *Bull Soc Pathol Exot Filiales* 82(2):260-266, 1989.

Dumas BM, Preux PM: Epilepsy and its impact in northwest region of the Central African Republic *Med Trop* 57(4):407-411, 1997.

Massanga M: Surveillance Sentinelle VIH/SIDA—Republique Centrafricaine, *OMS/ AFRO*, 1997.

Ministere des Finances, du Plan et de la Cooperation Internationale, Division des Stastistiques et des Etudes Economiques [Republique Centrafricaine]: *Annuaire statistique* 1993, Bangui, Republique Centrafricaine, 1994.

Ndamobissi R, Mboup G, Nguelebe EO: *Enquete Demographique et de Sante, Republique Centrafricaine 1994–95*, Calverto MD, Ministere de L'Economie et de la Cooperation Internationale Bangui, Republique Centrafricaine.

Sepou A et al: How is breast-feeding valued in the urban and semi-urban Central African milieu? *Sante* 11(2):85–89, 2001.

Sepou A et al: Prenatal care in a semiurban area of Central African Republic: frequency, influential factors, maternal and neonatal prognosis, *Med Trop* 60(3):257–261, 2000.

Somse P et al: Evaluation of an AIDS training program for traditional healers in the Central African Republic, *AIDS Educ Prev* 10(6):558–564, 1998.

UNAIDS (2000): *Fact sheets—HIV/AIDS and development*. http://unaids.org/ fact_sheets/files/Dev_Eng.html.

UNAIDS and the World Health Organization (2000): *Epidemiological fact sheet 2000 update (revised), Central African Republic*. http://unaids.org/hivaidsinfo/statistics/ fact_sheets/pdfs/Car_en.pdf

United Nations: *World population prospects: the 2000 revision*, New York, 2000, Author.

World Health Organization (2000): *Vaccines, immunization and biologicals— immunization profile, Central African Republic*, www.who.int/vaccines/

World Health Organization: Expanded programme on immunization (EPI). Immunization schedules in the WHO African region, 1995 erratum, *Wkly Epidemiol Rec* 22;71(12):90–94, 1996.

Wright J: Female genital mutilation: an overview, *J Adv Nurs* 24:251, 1996.

Yango A, Nganare KJ: *Recensement general de la population de decembre 1988*, vol 2, Rapport d'Analyse, tome 9: Langues parlees, Bangui, Ministere de l'economie, du plan, des statistiques et de la cooperation internationale, Division des statistiques et des etudes economiques, 1992, Republique Centrafricaine.

http://www.ethnologue.com/show_country.asp?name=Central+African+Republic

◆ CHAD (REPUBLIC OF)

MAP PAGE (862)

Lori Leonard

Location: Chad is the fifth largest country on the African continent, covering nearly 1.3 million km^2 (501,800 square miles). This landlocked country is in the northern portion of central Africa. Chad shares a border with Libya to the north, the Sudan to the east, the Central African Republic and Cameroon to the south, and Nigeria and Niger to the west. The country is generally divided into three climatic zones. The northernmost third of the country is part of the Sahara Desert and includes the Tibesti Mountains and the Ennedi Plateau. The central band, part of the Sahel, includes Lake Chad and the capital city of N'Djamena to the west. The southernmost tier is the primary agricultural region of the country and the site of a major oil exploration project that is currently underway.

Major Languages	Ethnic Groups	Major Religions
French (official)	Muslim groups 44%	Muslim 44%
Arabic (official)	Non-Muslim groups 56%	Christian 33%
Sara and Sango (in south)		Indigenous beliefs (primarily animism) 23%
More than 100 other languages and dialects		

Chad has a total population of slightly more than 6 million people. Most of the population lives in rural areas; only four cities have populations of 200,000 or more, including N'Djaména, Moundou, Koumra, and Kélo. There are more than 200 distinct ethnic groups, most of whom are Muslims. Muslim groups include Arabs, Toubou, Fulbe, Kotoko, Hausa, Kanembou, Baguirmi, Boulala, and Maba in the northern and central regions of the country. Most non-Muslims reside in the southern part of the country, groups such as the Sara, Ngambaye, Mbake, Goulaye, Moudang, Moussei, and Massa. More than 100 different languages and dialects are spoken in Chad, and the country has more than 200 different ethnic groups. Newspapers are generally printed in French and Arabic, and radio and television programs are broadcast in both languages.

Health Care Beliefs: Acute sick care; holistic. Health is defined holistically by many Chadians as a state that extends beyond physical well-being and includes harmony within the family and ethnic lineage. Health care practices reflect these beliefs and include use of a mixture of treatment modalities, including Western medicine and ritual and local healing practices.

Predominant Sick Care Practices: Biomedical where available; traditional. People seek health care from various sources. The public health care system is decentralized to provide basic services to as much of the population, which is mostly rural, as possible. An estimated 400 health centers function in rural areas of the country and are the primary point of care for most Chadians. People who cannot be treated at the health centers are referred to one of the approximately 36 district hospitals. Oversight of the public health care system is the responsibility of the Ministry of Health in N'Djamena, which has a health delegation in each of the country's 14 *prefectures*, or regional capitals. A plethora of traditional healers exist and are widely used in rural and urban areas. Medications, including antibiotics, are available in pharmacies and markets in urban centers but are less readily available in rural areas and are not affordable to all. Many families use plants and herbs to treat themselves for common ailments and do not consult a health care practitioner.

Ethnic/Race Specific or Endemic Diseases: Malaria, yellow fever, and schistosomiasis are endemic in Chad. The country also has frequent epidemics of cholera and meningitis. The first two cases of AIDS were documented in Chad in 1986. Since that time, the number of cases has risen rapidly. In 2000 a total of 1704 AIDS cases were reported. The World Health Organization's (WHO) estimated prevalence rate for HIV/AIDS in adults ages 15 to 49 is 2.69%. The estimated number of children from birth to 15 years living with HIV/AIDS is 4000. The rate of HIV infection is estimated to be between 9% and 10% for the entire population; rates are higher in some areas of the country and among specific population subgroups. For example, the seroprevalence rate among female sex workers in the southern city of Sarh was estimated to be 26.4% in 1997.

Health Team Relationships: In 1999 the Ministry of Public Health estimated that Chad had a total of 3228 active health care personnel. This number includes less than 250 doctors, most of who were practicing in urban centers. Rural health centers are largely staffed by nurses or nurses' aides. Working relationships in the health care sector vary from setting to setting; however, given the dearth of health care providers, many practitioners work without the support of a team.

Families' Roles in Hospital Care: Families play an important role in caring for the sick. They are responsible for preparing and bringing food to those who are hospitalized or receiving in-patient treatments. Most health care facilities allow and encourage visits. In some situations, family members sleep at the hospital with the hospitalized family member.

Dominance Patterns: The families of all ethnic groups in Chad are dominated by men. Living arrangements are also *patrilocal*, meaning that after women are married, they generally live in their husband's home or village. Children of parents who have been divorced or separated are generally raised by paternal aunts after the children have been weaned, although some exceptions to this practice exist, particularly in urban areas.

Eye Contact Practices: Young men and women are expected to show respect for older adults. Although eye contact is not expressly forbidden, it is uncommon among certain people (e.g., a young woman and her mother- or father-in-law. In the southern regions, no rules prohibit eye contact between the sexes.

Touch Practices: A handshake is the most common form of greeting in all parts of the country and is considered appropriate when greeting and bidding farewell to someone.

Perceptions of Time: Punctuality is becoming increasingly important, particularly in urban areas of the country.

Pain Reactions: In most ethnic groups in Chad, pain is something to be endured. With the exception of very young children, patients are often chastised for crying or complaining about physical discomfort.

Birth Rites: An estimated 88% of women give birth in their homes rather than in a clinic or other health care center. However, the percentage varies according to setting and other factors such as a woman's level of education. Women in urban areas are much more likely (35%) than women who live in rural areas (5%) to give birth in a hospital or other health care facility. Similarly, 53% of all women who had some high school education gave birth in a hospital or other health care facility, compared with 22% of women with a primary school education and 7% of women who had never been to school. Timing and characteristics of naming ceremonies for newborn children differ among ethnic groups.

Death Rites: Like birth rites, death rites vary widely among Chad's many ethnic and religious groups. Burials, rather than cremation, are the accepted practice. Among the Sara, Chad's largest ethnic group, families gather for 3 to 4 days to mourn. The mourning ceremonies include singing, dancing, and sleeping at the home of the relatives of the deceased person. Deaths are often announced on Radio Chad so that distant relatives are aware of family deaths. In recent years and in response to difficult economic times, these radio announcements have included messages asking relatives to stay at home to mourn.

Food Practices and Intolerances: Staple foods include millet, sorghum, rice, and corn, which are often consumed in the form of a paste called *boule* and eaten with a meat or vegetable sauce. Meals are communal, although children generally eat separately, as do men and women in some groups. Crops are generally harvested in December and January, a time when food is most plentiful. Planting season coincides with the onset of the rainy season in early June.

Infant Feeding Practices: Most mothers supplement breast milk with water and porridge when infants are several months old. Exclusive breast-feeding is uncommon; however, children continue to be breast-fed for extended periods—often until the mother's next pregnancy.

Child Rearing Practices: Children are raised by the extended family and often live with different members of the family, all of whom are responsible for providing for their education and upbringing. It is therefore not uncommon for children to live with aunts, uncles, grandparents, or cousins or to move from one household to another. This practice is especially common among school-age children who need to move from villages to larger cities to continue their studies.

National Childhood Immunizations: BCG at birth; DTP at 6, 10, and 14 weeks; OPV at birth and at 6 and 14 weeks; measles at 9 months; yellow fever at 6 months; and TT at 15 years or first pregnancy, +1 month, +6 months, +1 year, +1 year. Immunizations are provided as part of the national vaccination program.

BIBLIOGRAPHY

Bureau Central du Recensement: *Recensement general de la population et de l'habitat 1993. Tome 2: Etat de la population*, N'Djaména, 1995, Author.

DeCalo S: *Historical dictionary of Chad*, Metuchen, NJ, 1987, The Scarecrow Press.

Ministère de la Santé Publique: *Annuaire des statistiques sanitaires du Tchad: Tome A niveau national année 1999. N'Djaména, 1999*, Author.

Ouagadjio BK et al: *Enquete demographique et de sante, Tchad 1996–1997*, Calverton, Md, 1998, Bureau Central du Recensement and Macro International.

Programme National de Lutte Contre le SIDA/MST: *Tchad-Santé*, Année 1, Numéro 00, 2000.

World Health Organization: *Epidemiological fact sheets by country*, Geneva. Retrieved March 1, 2002, from http://www.unaids.org/hivaidsinfo/statistics/june00/fact_sheets/index.html

World Health Organization (2001): *WHO vaccine-preventable diseases: monitoring system*, Geneva. Retrieved March 1, 2002, from http://www.who.int/vaccines/

◆ CHILE (REPUBLIC OF)

MAP PAGE (859)

Barbara Carpio and Hugo Cardenas

Location: Chile fills a narrow, 2897-km (1800-mile) strip between the Andes Mountains and the Pacific Ocean. One third of Chile is covered by towering mountain ranges, and the southernmost city in the world is located at its tip. An 1127-km (a 700-mile) valley in Chile's center is densely populated, and the driest desert in the world, the Atacama Desert, is located in the north.

Major Languages	Ethnic Groups	Major Religions
Spanish (official)	European and Mestizo 95%	Roman Catholic 89%
	Indigenous 3%	Protestant 11%
	Other 2%	

The influence of Germans, Italians, and Arabs from Palestine and other Middle Eastern countries who emigrated to Chile is evident in different aspects of its cultural and political life. A large group of Chinese immigrants settled mostly in the north. Many of the groups have maintained their languages, and many bilingual schools exist. The resulting population mix is similar to the populations of Argentina and Uruguay and distinctly less racially mixed than the Caribbean and tropical Latin American countries. Only 3% of the population are indigenous. The primary indigenous group is the Mapuche, who live mostly in the rural central and southern regions. A few Aymara and Atacameños live in the north, and some Rapa Nui live on Easter Island. These indigenous groups speak their original languages but are taught Spanish in public schools. Although church attendance and other practices have declined in recent years, the legal system still reflects its strong Catholic influence. (For example, divorce and abortion are officially prohibited.) During the last 2 decades, numerous Protestant denominations have become more influential in daily life and politics.

Health Care Beliefs: Traditional; active involvement. Nutrition is believed to play an important role in health, so patients generally take an active role in retaining and regaining their health. In rural areas, traditional medicine is still an important part of the health belief system. Many Chileans in the urban sector also believe in homeopathy and herbal remedies, particularly in the form of teas (*hierbas*). A persistent belief rural Chileans share with many other Latin American and Caribbean countries is the belief of *mal de ojo*, or "evil eye." People with this "strong sight" who have evil intentions toward others can harm them. Patients are often taken to a healer—*curandera* or *cacique*—for treatments instead of or in conjunction with a Western allopathic practitioner. Religion is also incorporated into the traditional care system. For example, the process the *curandera* uses to heal is known as *santiguar*, a treatment of prayer and the burning of herbs. Although health services, especially the private-sector institutions that have developed during the past decade, are geared predominantly toward caring for people who are ill, primary disease prevention and health promotion are mandated by the National Health Services. National health education and treatment programs are being used to control traditional endemic illnesses (e.g., malnutrition, tuberculosis, diabetes), HIV and AIDS, and services for older adults (*tercera edad*). Health education is a strong component of the school curriculum. Discrimination against people with mental illness is a significant problem, although recent educational programs are trying to change this situation.

Predominant Sick Care Practices: Biomedical; traditional; religious. Chileans from the middle and upper classes have sick care practices that are similar to those used in mainstream North America, and all Chileans are eligible to receive care from doctors. Poor Chileans rely more on the public health system, which allows them to receive care from doctors working in the public *consultorios* and hospitals. In the last 10 years, numerous doctors emigrated from Cuba and other neighboring countries, and they now work primarily in private practice in low-income neighborhoods. Because these doctors charge substantially less than Chilean doctors, they are quite busy. Doctors, nurses, midwives, and other health care professionals receive a university education, so Chileans have confidence and pride in the system. People of European and indigenous descent continue to use some folk remedies. Prayer is a common adjunct to Western health care, reflecting the strong influence that religion, especially Roman Catholicism, has on Chilean daily life. Because of increased awareness of the influence of culture on health and sickness behaviors, patients are more willing to acknowledge that they combine folk or traditional practices with Western medicine. In South America, Chile has been a pioneer in its development of a universal health system modeled on Great Britain's system. In the past 2 decades an American-style mix of public and private health service delivery has emerged to provide alternative models of treatment and prevention. The public health system has a mandate to ensure coverage of all people unable to afford the high cost of private medical insurance. People with low incomes or who are older than 65 years have access to free health services through a nationally planned and regionally administered network of rural and urban clinics (*consultorios*) and public hospitals in all 13 regions of the country. In addition to providing preventive and curative services to these populations, the public system is the only one that provides free coverage for chronic and expensive illnesses such as cancer and HIV/AIDS. During the last decade a three-tiered system emerged. In addition to the public system, the National Health Fund (*Fondo Nacional de Salud; FONASA*) is an alternative for people with middle incomes. FONASA allows access to some levels of the private system and consists of three levels, all of which have a high deductible payment when used in the private system but very low costs when used in the public system. The private system, administered by insurance companies known as *ISAPRES (instituciones de salud previsional)*, is more expensive but provides a greater variety of services that occasionally are of higher quality that those of the public system. However, after the users reach age 65, the cost of the private system is too expensive for all but the very wealthy, and most people switch to FONASA.

Ethnic/Race Specific or Endemic Diseases: Cystic echinococcosis and trichinosis are endemic in rural areas of the southern and central valley. Typhoid and hepatitis A and E are endemic in most of the country, and Chagas' disease is endemic in the north. Diarrhea caused by *Shigella* organisms is frequent and in Chileans is self-contained, lasting about 24 hours; it is not usually treated with antibiotics. Visitors from other countries are encouraged to drink bottled or boiled water to avoid what is locally known as *chilenitis*, serious diarrhea caused primarily by shigellae and occasionally by *Escherichia coli* and resulting in loss of water and electrolytes. Because mosquitoes do not survive the Chilean winter and the weather is dry during summer, mosquitoes that are the vectors of dengue fever and malaria have not colonized the country. Therefore these diseases are rare except in visitors and Chileans coming back from other countries. The priority health problems in Chile parallel those of the developed world more than those of the Third World. The most common causes of illness and death are circulatory problems (high blood pressure and acute myocardial infarction), malignant neoplasms (of the stomach and respiratory system), injuries and poisoning (with prevalent alcoholism and the highest rate of liver cirrhosis in the region), and respiratory illnesses. The incidence of calculus in the gallbladder is one of the highest in the world, and some evidence suggests that it is related to diet. Because the incidence of cancer of the gallbladder is so high, standard medical practice is to remove the gallbladder after the first symptoms of calculus as a preventive measure. Respiratory illnesses in children are the major cause of illness and hospitalization, accounting for 60% of doctors' consultations for this age group. Malnutrition is found almost exclusively among poor children, with one study reporting a 9% incidence of goiter in school-age children (despite the fact that commercially available salt is iodized). During winters the flu is a problem of epidemic proportions, and the government provides free vaccination to those who are at risk, including infants and older adults. Children's health is considered a priority health concern. The government provides free powdered milk for infants during the first year of life, as well as breakfast and lunch programs for children attending public schools in economically disadvantaged communities. Obesity, alcoholism, smoking, and lack of exercise are health problems that the public is beginning to recognize and for which the Ministry of Health is designing preventive and educational programs. Digestive problems tend to increase during the summer, and fecal contamination of food in restaurants and public places is a problem. However, the public health system was able to effectively contain the spread of cholera from neighboring countries during an outbreak several years ago, and it never became a national problem (resulting in only a dozen reported cases). This success was more a result of public education regarding food handling and preparation than of immunizations. The World Health Organization's (WHO) estimated prevalence rate for HIV/AIDS in adults ages 15 to 49 is 0.19%. The estimated number of children from birth to 15 years living with HIV/AIDS is 260. Of the total number of people with HIV/AIDS, 89% are males, and 85% are men ages 20 to 49 years. Since 2000 the government has provided antiviral drugs to all people infected with HIV who are not able to afford the high cost of treatment. Public education programs are being developed, and hospice care is a newly emerging area of practice

Health Team Relationships: Relationships are doctor driven, so nurses are subordinate to doctors. The patient's attitude toward doctors and nurses is typically one of total faith and subordination. Until very recently, a doctor's attitude was one of total dominance, so much so that treatments were rarely discussed with the patient and family. This mindset changed enormously during the last decade, and many procedures that were previously done in public hospitals without the consent of the patient (such as sterilization and major surgeries) now require written informed consent from the patient. The Ministry of Health has implemented a local ethics committee in every hospital that reviews and approves or denies all the research procedures being evaluated in the hospital. One or two hospitals located in regions with high concentrations of indigenous people (e.g., the regional hospital of Temuco, capital of the IXth region) have instituted ethnoculturally responsive programs to orient patients and their families and assist them with accessing and understanding health care services. Nevertheless, indigenous and rural people have economic and cultural disadvantages in terms of their access to health care. Few professionally trained midwives and almost no physicians are Mapuche or Aymara.

Families' Role in Hospital Care: In public hospitals, families cannot stay with patients or bring them food, and visits are restricted to one or two relatives at a time from 2 PM to 5 PM. In private clinics, one relative can stay all day and night with a patient if so desired, but additional costs are incurred.

Dominance Patterns: Chile has a Latin culture with a strong male dominance. (This year the first woman was appointed to the Supreme Justice Court.) Men usually are paid more than women, and many companies prefer male employees so that they can avoid bearing the costs associated with childbirth. Needless to say, young women experience significant discrimination when applying for jobs in the public and private sectors. Since the racial mix is not as varied in Chile as it is in many other Latin American countries; social standing associated with racial or ethnic stereotypes is less evident in urban areas than in rural.

Eye Contact Practices: Chileans are usually open and frank in their interactions and look each other in the eye.

Touch Practices: Physical contact is much more prevalent in Chile than in North America, with both women and men shaking hands and kissing people on the cheek in greeting, even in professional settings. However, it is not appropriate for a health care provider to kiss patients. A handshake is always expected, and failure to extend a hand when greeting a person is interpreted as lack of acceptance of someone.

Perceptions of Time: Punctuality has less significance than in the United States or Germany, but it is significantly more important than it is in Mexico. People are typically 30 minutes late for most appointments and events.

Pain Reactions: People freely express their pain.

Birth Rites: The birth of a son is not more celebrated than the birth of a daughter. In some traditional families, it is considered important to have a male heir, but this preference is much less marked in people of the middle and upper income and urban classes. Almost all births (99.7%) occur in public hospitals and private clinics, with prenatal care and low-risk birth services being provided by university-prepared midwives. Recently, partners and other family members have begun to be permitted to attend hospital or clinic births. The public health system provides free surgical sterilizations for multiparous women who request the procedure. The most common contraceptives for women with low incomes are intrauterine devices. Adolescents primarily use oral contraceptives. Abortion is illegal, but rates are thought to be relatively high, particularly among young mothers with low incomes. Chile reportedly has the highest rate of abortions in the region, with 45 abortions per 1000 women of childbearing years. The provision of safe alternatives is a current subject of debate.

Death Rites: When possible, family members are present when a person dies. Organ donations are increasing because of strong educational campaigns launched on television and by other means by the Ministry of Health. Autopsies are mandatory after deaths at public hospitals and clinics when a physician cannot identify the cause of death. Chile has various religious groups, each of which has specific beliefs and practices regarding care of a body and interment after death. Cremation is becoming more accepted in the middle class.

Food Practices and Intolerances: Nutritional status relates to socioeconomic level. Nevertheless, the Chilean diet is firmly based on bread and butter, pasta, and rice, which contributes to the public health problem of obesity. Meat (beef and mutton) is the preferred source of protein, followed by poultry. Despite educational campaigns during the last 2 decades and the fact that the country has an extensive coastline with plenty of opportunities for fishing, fish has never become a primary source of protein in the Chilean diet. Eating with the hands is only acceptable at barbecues, but even then a fork, knife, and spoon are usually provided.

Infant Feeding Practices: In rural areas, breast-feeding is the norm for the first year of the infant's life. However, in urban settings and the middle class, the practice of breast-feeding more than the first few weeks is difficult for women who must return to work. National campaigns encourage a return to breast-feeding; however, the practice of providing formula and milk to mothers after birth persists. It is estimated that only 25% of mothers are still breast-feeding 6 months after delivery

Child Rearing Practices: While the mother is at work, infants primarily stay at nurseries under the care of university-trained child care workers called *parvularias*. In families with low incomes, mothers care for the children until they begin their formal education, which by law begins at 5 years. Child rearing is rather permissive compared with North American practices. Even very young children are part of the social activities of the family and attend parties in the evening, but the general expectation is that children should be respectful and obedient. The extended family, especially grandparents, also plays an important role in raising children. Most of the people value education as a means of promoting upward socioeconomic mobility and status; children are encouraged and rewarded if they do well in their studies. In families of the middle and upper classes, children have their own beds and do not sleep with their parents. Families tend to be more protective of their children than do families in North America. Living at home until marriage is common for young men and women.

National Childhood Immunizations: BCG at birth and 6 years; DPT at 2, 4, 6, and 18 months and 4 years; OPV at 2, 4, 6, and 18 months and 4 years; HIB at 2, 4, and 6 months; and MMR at 1 and 6 years. Immunizations are mandatory and provided free by the public health system; coverage has been enhanced through EPI initiatives. Periodically the Ministry of Health provides free vaccinations (e.g., against *Haemophilus influenzae*) for people who are at risk

BIBLIOGRAPHY

Araya R et al: Common mental disorders in Santiago, Chile: Prevalence and socio-demographic correlates, *Br J Psychiatry* 178:228, 2001.

Bell CW: Competition heats up in Chile. Healthcare reform proposals seek increasing role for nation's private sector, *Mod Health* 31(45):1262, 2001.

Ferreccio C et al: Epidemiologic patterns of acute diarrhea and endemic *Shigella* infections in children in a poor periurban setting in Santiago Chile, *Am J Epidemiol* 134(6):614, 1991.

Irart C, Merhy EE, Waitzkin H: Managed care in Latin America: The new common sense in health policy reform, *Soc Sci Med* 52(8):1243, 2001.

McArthur L, Pena M, Holbert D: Effects of socioeconomic status on the obesity knowledge of adolescents from six Latin American cities, *Int J Obes Relat Metab Disord* 25(8):1262, 2001.

Tanaka J: Hepatitis B epidemiology in Latin America, *Vaccine* 18(suppl 1):17, 2000.

Waitzkin H et al: Social medicine in Latin America: productivity and dangers facing the major national groups, *Lancet* 358(9278):315, 2001.

World Health Organization (June 2000): *Epidemiological fact sheets by country*, Geneva. Retrieved March 1, 2002, from http://www.unaids.org/hivaidsinfo/statistics/june00/fact_sheets/index.html

World Health Organization (2001): *WHO vaccine-preventable diseases: monitoring system*, Geneva. Retrieved March 1, 2002, from http://www.who.int/vaccines/

Gensalud@listserv.paho.org, November 19, 2001.

http://www.fonasa.cl

http://www.gobiernodechile.cl

http://www.minsal.cl

◆ CHINA (PEOPLE'S REPUBLIC OF)

MAP PAGE (865)

Zhao Yue, Wai-man Lee, and Frances Kam Yuet Wong

Location: The People's Republic of China is the world's third largest country and occupies the eastern part of Asia. The total land area is 9,596,960 km² (3,705,392 square miles). The northwestern part of China is mountainous and arid with high plateaus, whereas southeastern China has fertile agricultural land and river deltas. Tibet is part of the People's Republic of China, and the colonies of Hong Kong and Macao were returned to Chinese sovereignty in 1997 and 1999, respectively.

Major Languages	Ethnic Groups	Major Religions
Putonghua (Mandarin, official)	Han Chinese 92%	Zhuang, Uygur,
	Zhuang, Uygur,	Atheist (officially;
Cantonese	Hui, Yi, Tibetan,	however, elements
Local dialects	Miao, Manchu,	of Confucianism,
(six or more)	Mongol, Buyi,	Taoism, Buddhism,
	Korean 8%	Christianity,
		Islam can be found)

The Han group represents 92% of the total population, whereas other Chinese ethnic groups represent 8%. From an anthropological point of view, several hundred identifiable minority groups exist, of which 55 have been officially recognized.

Health Care Beliefs: Holistic; increasing interest in health promotion. Illness prevention and health promotion and maintenance are important to Chinese people. Children are taught at a very young age at home and school that it is necessary to be healthy and avoid damaging the body. Keeping the body healthy is considered an act of piety that pays respect to the parents. The Chinese attribute disease to a disruption in body energy. Health is believed to be a state of spiritual and physical harmony with nature. Health and illness are not considered separate but are thought of as part of a lifelong continuum. Some individuals avoid major surgery because they fear that qi, or the life force, may be disturbed. Chinese may resist attempts to draw blood because of the belief that sufficient amounts of blood keep the body strong and healthy, and insufficient amounts weaken it. Although Chinese people prefer natural therapies, they often choose dietary or herbal medical therapies in the form of tonics or pills to prevent disease. Stigmas are attached to mental illness, therefore a severe mental disturbance is the only criterion for entering the health care system. Chinese patients with psychiatric problems tend to somatize their problems and delay psychiatric consultations.

Predominant Sick Care Practices: Biomedical; traditional; passive involvement. The Chinese use a combination of traditional Chinese medicine

(TCM) and Western medicine; however, when both types of medicine are used in treatments, patients need to be advised of possible drug interactions. TCM is one of the oldest types of medicine practiced in the world; its theoretical base and diagnostic and treatment modalities are still in use. TCM includes acupuncture and moxibustion therapy, external treatments, massage therapy, pharmaceutical (herbal) therapy, and breathing exercises. Western medicine was introduced in China in the mid-1800s and during the past century, it has become widespread and has developed considerably. The introduction of Western medicine brought new medical practices that play an important part in health care. Since the end of the nineteenth century, Chinese medical experts have successfully been integrating TCM and Western medicine. The health care system is transitioning from a free system to an insurance system with an option for fee-for-service choices. According to TCM, people have five *zang* and six *fu* organs. The heart, liver, spleen, lungs, and kidneys have completely different connotations in TCM and Western medicine. For example, consider from a TCM perspective the liver and its numerous interacting physiological and psychological functions. The liver's physical functions include conducting and dispersing (i.e., dredging, smoothing, flowing, and dispersing life activity within the body), storing blood, promoting digestive functions, and regulating normal circulation of the *qi*, blood, and water. In addition, the liver helps regulate emotional activities. If the liver's visceral system is diseased, its ability to conduct and disperse decreases, and the functional activity of *qi* in the body stagnates. Therefore the person develops symptoms such as depression, sadness, moodiness, excessive worrying, belching, and sentimental sighing. Chinese medical practitioners use the *hot-cold* dichotomy to classify the energies of diets, physical constitution, disease, and symptoms. In the Chinese medical belief system, eating foods with "hot" energy (e.g., chili pepper, ginger, cinnamon bark) causes people to experience hot sensations, and foods with "cold" energy (e.g., tea, apple, bean curd) result in cold sensations. Therefore many Chinese try to have a balanced diet, with proper amounts of hot and cold foods as needed. They believe that people with a "hot" physical constitution should consume more cold-energy foods, whereas people with a "cold" physical constitution should consume hot-energy foods. The hot-cold dichotomy concept is applied to diseases, as well as symptoms. If a disease or symptom gets worse after exposure to cold surroundings, then it is a "cold" disease or symptom, and the same theory applies to hot surroundings. Therefore diseases and symptoms can be hot (e.g., constipation, hot rheumatism) or cold (e.g., cold vomiting, cold rheumatism). Chinese expect that when they are ill, others are obliged to care for them. This expectation reduces the active involvement of patients in improving their own health.

Ethnic/Race Specific or Endemic Diseases: Endemic diseases include fluorosis, endemic goiter, tuberculosis, thalassemia, and chloroquine-resistant malaria. Chinese are also at risk for viral hepatitis, Japanese encephalitis, schistosomiasis, and alpha-thalassemia. Neurasthenia (nervous exhaustion) is a common modern Chinese psychiatric disorder, and its psychological symptoms include anxiety, depression, and hypochondria. Cancer, cerebrovascular accidents (CVAs), cardiac disease, and tobacco-related diseases are the leading causes of death in cities. Respiratory diseases, cancer, and CVAs are the leading causes of death in rural areas. In 2001 the Chinese Health Department reported that more than 600,000 people were infected with HIV. The ratio of male to female HIV carriers is 5.2:1. Men and women ages 20 to 29 comprise about 56% of carriers, whereas men and women ages 30 to 39 comprise 24%. Experts predict that if no precautions are taken, China will have more than 10 million people infected with HIV by 2010. As Chinese society becomes more prosperous, obesity is becoming more prevalent, especially among young children.

Health Team Relationships: In 1999, China had about 1.24 million nurses and about 2.04 million doctors. Most nurses are women, and the men who are nurses usually work in emergency departments, intensive care units, or psychiatric services. Nurses supplement doctors. Because social assertiveness is usually not emphasized and because nurses and doctors are considered authority figures and experts, patients are not given much information about their illnesses, medicines, or diagnostic procedures. Today, the protection of patient's rights is of greater concern, which prompted the Law for the Protection of Consumer Rights. Patients do not like to express their concerns about prescribed interventions or treatments directly to their nurses and doctors. They express their thoughts politely, with restraint, and indirectly. The doctor or nurse is expected to understand their message. County hospitals, township hospitals, and village clinics form the health service network in rural areas in mainland China.

Families' Role in Hospital Care: Family members care take turns caring for older members who are hospitalized. Typically, at least one family member remains with a sick child or a severely ill adult during a hospitalization. The family supplies food and clean clothing and assists with feeding, bathing, and keeping the patient comfortable. In cases of serious illness, doctors often discuss the patient's condition and treatment in detail with the patient's family members. Family members make treatment decisions after discussions with the doctor, and the patient may not be involved in the decision-making process. Family reunions during significant festivals are important, so hospitalized patients may ask for home leave or to be discharged to celebrate a holiday such as the New Year during the Spring Festival.

Dominance Patterns: The family is more important than the individual. Marked role differences are based on generation, age, birth order, gender, and social status. When making decisions, the young defer to the old, and both parents make decisions about children. Older adults are not segregated from others and have a high status in the family and society. Older Chinese parents take pride in being supported and cared for by their children. Devotion to parents includes caring for them physically, psychologically, and socially. However, the migration of children for better work opportunities, China's "one child only" policy, and a decline in the number of multigenerational families that live together may be decreasing the frequency of this practice. The average number of family members decreased from 3.96 in 1990 to 3.44 in 2000. In China's patrilineal culture, father-son relationships are strong. In addition, women who marry become part of their husband's family.

Eye Contact Practices: Direct eye contact is common, but staring is inappropriate.

Touch Practices: Chinese do not like to be touched by strangers. Introductions involve a nod or a slight bow. However, personal space and confidentiality during caregiving do not seem to be as important in health clinics. Patients prefer health care professionals of the same sex.

Perceptions of Time: Chinese have a concept of time that is inexact, involves patience, and is broad. The language's past and present verb tenses are the same. The past is valued, so traditional approaches to healing are preferred when modern procedures or medications are in-effective. In the traditional Chinese calendar, the year is divided into four seasons with 24 solar periods. Wind, cold, summer heat, dampness, dryness, and fire are the "six evils" that are closely related to climate and seasonal change. The evils are occasionally considered causes of illness by TCM practitioners.

Pain Reactions: Strong negative feelings such as anger and pain are often suppressed. Chinese patients may be reluctant to report pain and may not interrupt health care professionals to ask for pain relief treat-ments, although analgesics and TCM such as acupuncture are available for pain control. Displays of emotion are considered a character weakness. Regardless, the Chinese language gives patients numerous descriptors to use for expressing pain, and women tend to describe pain more descriptively than men.

Birth Rites: Amniocentesis may be used to determine the sex of a fetus. The patrilineal culture and the government's one-child birth control policy can result in the abortion of female fetuses, especially in rural areas. A birthweight of less than 2500 g is considered low birthweight. In 2000 the maternal mortality rate was 53 per 100,000 live births, and the infant mortality rate was 32.6 per 1000. Acupuncture is used during labor induction, labor stimulation, and cesarean section. Fathers are not present in labor rooms, delivery rooms, or postpartum areas. Women in labor are fully clothed and deliver in the low lithotomy position. For 30 days after childbirth, mothers are particularly careful to avoid attacks by "cold" and "wind" because according to TCM, keeping warm is important. The mother may be advised not to bathe her body or shampoo her hair for the first few days after giving birth. When taking a shower, women use ginger to reduce the chance of being attacked by cold and wind. New mothers are confined for a month and eat certain foods to promote lactation. A celebratory feast takes place 1 month after the baby's birth. Mothers who already have a child use intrauterine devices, and national regulations forbid their removal.

Death Rites: The Chinese have an aversion to anything concerning death. Autopsies and disposal of the body are individual preferences; they are not prescribed by religion. Euthanasia is illegal, but organ donation is encouraged. Cremation is performed in urban areas and encouraged in rural areas. The oldest son is responsible for making all arrangements for a deceased person. The body is initially buried in a coffin but after 7 years it is exhumed and cremated, and the urn is reburied in a family tomb. White or yellow and black clothing is worn as a sign of mourning. Very traditional Chinese may hire professional criers for funerals. Relatives visit the tomb and pay their respects to deceased relatives at the Pure Brightness Festival and the Double Ninth Festival every year.

Food Practices and Intolerances: The traditional diet is changing. It is becoming higher in fat and concentrated sugar, and excessive amounts of soy sauce and dried and preserved foods contribute to high sodium intakes. Food is also used as therapy to help cure certain illnesses. The Chinese focus on different sorts of foods at different times of year to reflect the seasonal changing of the *yin-yang* balance. People are generally advised to avoid eating hastily or eating too much. The Chinese believe that soup is good for the body and helps to maintain health, especially for women who have given birth or those who are older or frail. Herbs are used with food; many kinds of food are believed to have medicinal qualities that can be used to treat symptoms, wounds, and diseases and maintain health. Hot and warm beverages are preferred. A typical meal consists of rice with meat, fish, and vegetables. The Chinese believe eating the animal organs that correspond to a human body part can improve the body part's functioning (e.g., eating a pig's heart, despite its high level of cholesterol, to revitalize cardiac functioning in the human).

Infant Feeding Practices: Breast-feeding is encouraged, continues for at least 1 year, and may continue for 4 to 5 years in rural areas. Manufactured infant formulas are being marketed and are becoming a popular albeit inferior alternative to breast milk. Weaning begins when the infant is 3 months old, with the introduction of rice soup cooked with fish or minced meat. Milk is used as a supplement.

Child Rearing Practices: Parents are permissive with young children and care for them constantly. Grandparents usually help rear children of working parents. Children are frequently tightly swaddled and warmly dressed. When children are old enough to understand authority, they are required to obey. They are encouraged to receive extra training after school, such as in painting, music, and sports. Until they are school age, children are placed in day care facilities or are cared for by older family members. Children are taught to show respect for parents and authority figures. Parents shame children or make them feel guilty as a form of discipline. Children learn to control their emotions; aggressive behavior is undesirable and suppressed. Children are taught to be unselfish and function competitively only in a group. Fathers are less involved in child rearing, and mother-son relationships are close and enduring. Child abuse is rare. Parents take an active role in influencing their children's educational choices and living environments.

National Childhood Immunizations: BCG at birth; DPT at 3, 4, and 5 months, and 1 1/2 to 2 years; TOPV at 2, 3, and 4 months and 4 years; MV at 8 months and at 7 and 12 years; and hep B at birth and at 1 and 6 months.

Other Characteristics: Chinese believe that illness needs to be drawn out of the body, therefore they may use coin rubbing for treatment. A coin that is heated or smeared with oil is vigorously rubbed over the body, producing red welts. It is believed that the red welts only appear if a person is ill. *Tai-chi chuan*, or "soft" exercise, is recommended for older adults and frail people because it does not strain or shock the body or result in painful muscles.

BIBLIOGRAPHY

Bechtel GA, Davidhizar R: A cultural assessment model for ED patients, *J Emerg Nurs* 25(5):377–380, 1999.

Bowman KW, Hui EC: Bioethics for clinicians: 20. Chinese bioethics, *CMAJ.JAMC* 163(11):1481–1485, 2000.

Chen YL: Conformity with nature: a theory of Chinese American elders' health promotion and illness prevention processes, *Adv Nurs Sci* 19(2):17–26, 1996.

Chan JY: Dietary beliefs of Chinese patients, *Nurs Stand* 9(27):30–34, 1995.

Chen RF: *A survey of China*, Shanghai, China, 1994, Shanghai Education Press.

Childhood immunizations: November 8, 2001, www.zichuan.gov.cn/bianmin/zcgk/ zcgk4.htm (in Chinese).

China Medicine: The number of tuberculosis patients in China is the second in the world, April 6, 2001, www.xinhuanet.com (in Chinese).

China Youth Daily: Tuberculosis has become one of the main killers among the infectious diseases, December 21, 2000, www.xinhuanet.com (in Chinese).

Chung WY et al: The use of Cantonese pain descriptors among healthy young adults in Hong Kong, *Anaesthesiologica Sinica* 36(4):S1–S11, 1998.

Enditem: *China spreads AIDS prevention knowledge among public*, November 13, 2000, www.xinhuanet.com

Enditem: *China has more HIV carriers*, October 31, 2000, www.xinhuanet.com (in Chinese).

Gao ZS: *The reformation of healthcare insurance system*, August 14, 2001, www.xinhuanet.com (in Chinese).

Holroyd E et al: A Chinese cultural perspective of nursing care behaviours in an acute setting, *J Adv Nurs* 28(6):1289–1294, 1998.

Hua LY, Ji XD: *Hepatitis is the "first killer" among the infectious diseases in China*, March 19, 2001, www.xinhuanet.com (in Chinese).

Kong P: *We are the consumers in hospital*, March 19, 2001, www.legaldaily.com.cn

Leininger M: Transcultural nursing research to transform nursing education and practice: 40 years, *Image* 29(4):341–347, 1997.

Li XY, Jiang ZZ, Jiang YZ: *Wenkang (the Minister of Health) spoke on the healthcare reform in China*, June 30, 2001, www.xinhuanet.com (in Chinese).

Lin T, Tseng W, Yeh E: *Chinese societies and mental health*, London, 1995, Oxford University Press.

Ma SL, Rou WJ, Li YR: Investigation on pain in 81 cases of late stage cancer, *Shangxi Nur J* 2:65, 1999.

The State Statistical Bureau of PRC: *The report of the fifth national population survey result, 2000*, March, 29, 2001, www.xinhuanet.com (in Chinese).

Wang ZG, Chen P, Xie PP: *History and development of traditional Chinese medicine*, Amsterdam, 1999, IOS Press.

Wang K: *Shouldn't be unconcerned with AIDS*, April 10, 2001, www.xinhuanet.com (in Chinese).

Wills B et al: Concerns and misconceptions about pain among Hong Kong Chinese patients with cancer, *Cancer Nurs* 22(6):408–413, 1999.

World Bank: *China: issues and options in health financing*, Washington, DC, 1996, China and Mongolia Department and Human Development Department, World Bank.

Wong FKY, Lee WM, Mok E: Educating nurses to care for the dying in Hong Kong: a problem-based learning approach, *Cancer Nurs* 24(2):112–121, 2001.

Wright F, Cohen S, Caroselli C: Diverse decisions. How culture affects ethical decision making, *Crit Care Nurs Clin North Am* 9(1):63–74, 1997.

Wuxi Daily: Dietary custom in China, May 28, 2001, www.xinhuanet.com (in Chinese).

Xinhua News Agency: The main religions and their characteristics of the minorities in our country, May 18, 2001, www.xinhuanet.com (in Chinese).

Xinhua News Agency: *The People's Republic of China yearbook 2000*, Beijing, China, 2000, Author.

Zhu Y: *A continual decline in the MMR and IMR in China*, July 24, 2001, www.xinhuanet.com

◆ COLOMBIA (REPUBLIC OF)

MAP PAGE (859)

Claudia Montilla

Location: Colombia is the only country in South America that borders the Atlantic and the Pacific Oceans. It is composed of low coastal plains along the oceans and three parallel mountain ranges that are part of the Andes and run north to south. The climate depends on the altitude. It is tropical along the coast and eastern plains and cooler in the highlands. Poverty levels are extremely high in Colombia. Migration from rural to urban areas has been heavy. The total land area is 1,138,910 km^2

(439,734 square miles). The urban populations increased from 57% of the total population in 1951 to about 74% by 1994, and 30 cities have a population of 100,000 or more.

Major Languages	Ethnic Groups	Major Religions
Spanish (official)	Mestizo 58%	Roman Catholic 90%
	White 20%	Other 10%
	Mulatto 14%	
	Black 4%	
	Mixed black and	
	Amerindian 3%	
	Amerindian 1%	

Most Colombian immigrants in the United States come from urban lower- or middle-class backgrounds. Colombia's ethnic diversity is a result of the intermingling of indigenous peoples, Spanish colonists, and African slaves. Only about 13% of the population is considered completely Indian on the basis of language and customs. Few foreigners have immigrated to Colombia, especially compared with the immigration numbers of several other South American countries. In addition to Roman Catholicism, other groups such as Anglican, Evangelic, and Mormon have altered the country's predominant religious preferences. The literacy rate was estimated in 1995 to be 91.3% of the total population age 15 and older: 91.2% for males and 91.4% for females.

Health Care Beliefs: Acute sick care predominates; traditional. It is believed that illness may be a punishment from God for transgressions. The Indians believe that people are controlled by their environment, nature can be dangerous, and nature is animated by the presence of spirits.

Predominant Sick Care Practices: Biomedical; magical-religious. Among Indian peoples, magical-religious practices are common, and shamans usually provide traditional remedies and care for the sick. During the past few years and in spite of deeply significant socioeconomic differences, an increasing number of urban and rural dwellers have gained access to medical services and social security coverage. Nevertheless, sociocultural and economic factors have allowed for the continued acceptance of folk healers (*curanderos*), who may be consulted in addition to biomedical practitioners. Most medications can be purchased in pharmacies over the counter.

Ethnic/Race Specific or Endemic Diseases: The primary endemic disease is chloroquine-resistant malaria. Colombians are also at risk for yellow fever, dengue fever, cholera, mild protein deficiency malnutrition, digestive tract parasitic diseases, malnutrition disorders, and iron deficiency anemia. The World Health Organization's (WHO) estimated prevalence rate for HIV/AIDS in adults is 0.31%. The estimated number of children from birth to 15 years living with HIV/AIDS is 900. Most infant and child deaths are linked to diarrheal diseases, digestive tract infections, nutritional disorders, and complications related to vaccine-preventable viruses. Many adult deaths result from "social pathologies," such as homicide and accidents. In addition, as their society ages, Colombians are experiencing a surge in diseases that are common in industrialized nations, such as coronary and heart disorders, hypertension-related illnesses, and cancer. Violent criminal attacks and homicides, referred to in Colombia as *blood deaths*, account for a significant percentage of the total number of deaths. The high rate of homicides and other violent deaths is associated with the structural problems of poor law enforcement, high levels of social and political violence, and criminal activities related to narcotics production and distribution. In the early 1980s, the most prevalent illnesses striking Colombians were respiratory infections, ophthalmologic and vision problems, digestive tract parasitic diseases, acute upper respiratory tract infections, peripheral vascular problems such as varicose veins, and malnutrition disorders. More than 14.2 million cases of individual illness were attributed to these diseases. The poorest people are affected the most by preventable and curable conditions and diseases such as gastrointestinal disorders and certain types of respiratory ailments, whereas the incidence of the degenerative and chronic diseases—conditions typical in urban dwellers and higher income earners—is relatively low in comparison. Tropical diseases are endemic to certain areas of the country. Because of the increased migration to the unexplored tropical hinterland, the incidence of diseases such as malaria, dengue, and yellow fever increased in the 1980s. During that time, malaria affected approximately 15% of the population, equivalent to roughly half of all rural inhabitants.

Health Team Relationships: Depending on education and socioeconomic levels, patients show enormous respect toward medical doctors, which can result in tentativeness and an extreme reluctance to ask questions. Patients may be very modest with care providers of the opposite sex. Hospitalized patients are expected to be passive, and family members provide for most self-care activities at home. The nurses' role in the relationship between the health team and patient is extremely important. They are responsible for establishing the first contact with patients when they arrive at the hospital (although in public hospital settings, they do so after a social worker has analyzed the patient's socioeconomic and cultural situation). They are also responsible for providing most of the care a hospitalized patient requires, such as prescription management and treatment process surveillance. When patients arrive at the hospital, the nurse asks questions and performs a preliminary examination to identify the patients' needs and health status. The nurse then refers them to the appropriate medical doctor. Chief nurses are usually highly specialized (at the graduate level) and have been trained to establish effective health team relationships. They are in charge of planning and coordinating patient care with the team. Nursing is a regulated profession in Colombia; curricula at state and private universities are controlled. However, because of deficiencies in the education received by nonprofessional auxiliary personnel, nurses are also in charge of supervising these workers. Because new regulations in the Colombian health system have resulted in a very tight schedule that allows medical doctors to devote only a modicum of time to their patients, nurses seem to be more accessible. They have more contact with patients because they spend more time with them. Consequently, patients trust and believe them. As one saying goes, "Doctors cure, and nurses care."

Families' Role in Hospital Care: Female family members may try to provide so much care that it becomes a hindrance to patients' resuming basic self-care activities. Mothers or older sisters might be expected to stay overnight. Commonly there are many visitors, bringing sweets, grapes, and flowers to the patient.

Dominance Patterns: Because of the high rate of migration from rural to urban areas, the growth of urban industrial centers, and accompanying socioeconomic developments, continued signs of change are evident in the traditional norms and patterns of family life. The decline of the patriarchal extended family structure has become more apparent in urban society as increased geographical and social mobility has weakened kinship ties and extended greater independence to young people. Nevertheless, the patriarchal pattern still prevails. In low- and middle-class environments, women are expected to be deferential to their husbands and follow their instructions overall. The father or older sibling is expected to be the spokesperson, and adult family members take part in most decision-making discussions, including those involving health issues.

Eye Contact Practices: Citizens of peasant and urban lower class origin may try to avoid making direct eye contact with authority figures or older adults or in awkward situations.

Touch Practices: Touch is important and used when giving bad news. Hugs are used to greet others. Handshaking is common, although some women may grasp the wrists of other women instead of their hands. In general, a narrow physical space is maintained between people, especially among close friends and relatives.

Perceptions of Time: Colombians have a relaxed and flexible sense of time. Short-term planning is more common than long-term planning. People may be a little late for appointments, and some appointments may be canceled at the last minute.

Birth Rites: During labor, pain relief is welcome but not expected by women in lower socioeconomic groups. The father or family members are not usually present during the delivery. Although abortion is illegal in

Colombia, many women, especially those in urban areas, seek out illegal abortion clinics to terminate unwanted pregnancies. Such actions put their lives at risk. The father's decision about continuing or terminating a pregnancy is usually the final word. Colombia has an impressive record for family planning and contraception, which are used by a significant portion of women. Although contraceptive methods for men are becoming more available, they are less popular because of the men's predominant *machismo* attitudes. In addition, although a significant number of women use contraceptives, sterilization is preferred. However, ample segments of the population, such as traditional Catholics, believe that abortion is a sin. Male circumcision is a personal (on the part of the parents) rather than a religious decision and is usually done at the time of birth. The infant mortality rate is 24.3 deaths per 1000 live births. The life expectancy at birth is 70.5 years, with men averaging 66.5 years and women 74.5 years.

Death Rites: Family members may want to view the body before it is taken to the morgue, and burials often take place within 24 to 36 hours. Cremation has become increasingly common in the last decade. Organ donations are not very common but are generally considered acceptable.

Food Practices and Intolerances: Breakfast is an important meal and usually includes freshly squeezed fruit juice, eggs, coffee with milk, and regional variations of cornmeal griddle cakes (*arepas*). The diet is mostly composed of starches—rice, potatoes, beans, plantain, and cassava— and the predominant meats are chicken, beef, and pork. Meats that are high in cholesterol are common. Although eaten more than they were in the past, salads that usually consist of lettuce, tomatoes, and onions are not considered a complete meal on their own. For most people, lunch, which often includes fruit, soup, a main course, and dessert, may be bigger than dinner. Sandwiches are considered a substitute for meals. Most Colombians drink coffee throughout the day. Fruit juice may be diluted with water or milk and primarily accompanies meals. Catholics may prefer fish on Fridays during the season of Lent.

Child Rearing Practices: Infants are mostly breast-fed. Depending on their socioeconomic status, mothers prefer to care for their children until they start school at 4 years. Children are very dependent on their parents and may live with them until they marry. In lower socioeconomic classes, punishment and threats, including the threat of being given an injection in a health facility, are used to influence behavior. Children are expected to be obedient, respectful, and quiet in the presence of adults. Rearing practices may vary from region to region.

National Childhood Immunizations: BCG at birth; DPT at 2, 4, 6, and 18 months and 5 years; OPV at birth, at 2, 4, 6, and 18 months, and

5 years; hep B at birth and at 2 and 6 months; HIB at 2, 4, and 6 months; MMR at 1 and 10 years; yellow fever before 1 year in at-risk areas; and TT CBAW at +4 weeks, +6 months, +1, and +1 year.

Other Characteristics: Injections of oil are used to treat infections and create hard lumps under the skin. Indicating a person's height by extending the arm with the palm down is an insulting gesture. A drink made of unprocessed sugar and water (*agua de panela*) is believed to help cure respiratory problems and influenza. The city of Bogotá created international interest in its "kangaroo care" system of treatment for premature (low birthweight) infants.

BIBLIOGRAPHY

de Lima L, Bruera E: Palliative care in Colombia: program in "La Viga," *J Pall Care* 10(1):42, 1994.

de Orjuela ML: Evolution of nursing: Its influence and commitment in the social development of Colombia, *J Prof Nurs* 5(6):330, 1989.

de Pheils PB: Colombians. In Lipson JG, Dibble SL, Minarik PA: *Culture and nursing care: a pocket guide*, San Francisco, 1996, UCSF Nursing Press.

Library of Congress, Federal Research Division, Country Studies, Area Handbook Series (1988): *Colombia*. Retrieved February 23, 2002, from http://lcweb2.loc.gov/frd/cs/cotoc.html

Pan American Health Organization Country Profile (1998): *Colombia*. Retrieved February 23, 2002, from http://www.paho.org/English/SHA/prflhcol.htm

Stewart EC, Bennett MJ: *American cultural patterns: a cross-cultural perspective*, rev ed, Yarmouth, Me, 1991, Intercultural Press.

Virgin C, Jacobsen U: *More female warmth and less high technology*. Paper presented at the Fifth International Council on Women's Health Issues, Copenhagen, 1992.

◆ COMOROS (FEDERAL ISLAMIC REPUBLIC OF THE)

MAP PAGE (863)

Location: The three volcanic islands of Comoros—Grand Comore (Njazidja), Anjouan (Nzwami), and Moheli (Mwali)—are located in the Mozambique Channel of the Indian Ocean between Madagascar and southeast Africa. It is a mountainous developing nation, and the total land area of the three islands is 1862 km² (719 square miles), about 12 times the size of Washington, DC. The island shores are rocky with many offshore islets and a steeply sloping seabed. The capital is Moroni. The total population is 596,202, and 67% of the population lives in rural areas. The daily temperature usually does not exceed 30° C (85° F), and the country has two seasons: one dry and one rainy. The gross domestic produce (GDP) per capita is $725. Comoros also claims a fourth island, Mayotte

(375 km², or 146 square miles), but Mayotte is still a dependency of France. Its population is 88,000, and the capital is Mamoudzou. Despite the many cultural groups in Comoros, it has few strong ethnic divisions.

Major Languages	Ethnic Groups	Major Religions
Arabic (official)	Antalote	Sunni Muslim (state
French (official)	Cafre	religion) 98%
Comoran (blend of Swahili	Makog	Roman Catholic 2%
and Arabic)	Oimatsahu	
	Sakalava	

Predominant Sick Care Practices: Acute sick care. Medical facilities are poor, and prescription drugs and preventive medicine are in short supply. When the country gained independence in 1975, French medical teams were withdrawn and the very rudimentary health system that was in place deteriorated rapidly, creating crisis conditions. Medical assistance later came from other sources such as the World Health Organization (WHO) and again from the French. However, Comoros continues to face myriad public health problems, as do other developing economies. The World Bank estimated in 1993 that the country had one doctor per 6582 people (up from one per 13,810 in 1983). Life expectancy, infant mortality, and the overall quality of medical care are still poor by Western standards. About 80% of the people live within an hour's walk of a health facility of some sort, and it is usually staffed by a trained nurse. Many facilities are in poor condition and have very few paramedical staff members.

Ethnic/Race Specific or Endemic Diseases: The major endemic disease is chloroquine-resistant falciparum malaria. It is believed that 80% to 90% of the population is affected by malaria. Tuberculosis, leprosy, and parasitic diseases also are endemic. The World Health Organization's (WHO) estimated prevalence rate for HIV/AIDS in adults ages 15 to 49 is 0.12%. WHO has no estimates for children from birth to 15 years. No evidence of HIV infection among antenatal women in Moroni was reported between 1991 and 1996. In 1994, 57% of sex workers tested in Moroni were infected with HIV. In 1994 a World Bank report highlighted the high prevalence of sexually transmitted diseases and infrequent use of condoms as a significant health threat to the spread of HIV/AIDS.

Dominance Patterns: Polygyny, a form of polygamy in which a man has more than one wife, is practiced if a man can afford it. Each wife has her own house and is given large amounts of gold jewelry, which provides her with some measure of financial security. Most women wear the *chirumani*, a traditional cotton dress. The principal community celebrations are associated with marriage, especially the first marriage, called the *grand marriage*. If the family is wealthy, these celebrations can last for weeks and include public and private ceremonies accompanied by a concert with traditional musicians called a *twarab*. Divorce is easy for men, but custom allows the divorced wife to retain her home. Under Islamic law, only men can inherit and own land. However, certain land holdings called *magnahouli* are inherited by women and controlled through the female lineage in accordance with a surviving matriarchal African tradition. Women married to farmers or laborers often have more freedom than the more elite women because they have more flexibility in movement (e.g., working in fields, selling produce at stands). Women in Mwali have more freedom because Islamic values are less pronounced. According to the World Bank, about 67% of girls in Comoros attend school, compared with 82% of boys. Literacy rates are 64.2% for males, and 50.4% for females. Female merchants in Mahore have been active in the movement for continued political association with France and separation from Comoros. Despite this, women's roles in the political realm are quite limited, with women being relegated to family and agricultural roles.

Birth Rites: According to studies in the country, women prefer to wait much longer between births than they do in practice. However, they often have little control over their fertility and reproductive choices, which affects maternal mortality and childhood nutrition, subsequent morbidity, and death. Maternal mortality rates in 1990 were 950 per 100,000 births. The birth rate is 39.52 births per 1000 people. The infant mortality rate is 84.07 deaths per 1000 live births; the rate was 89 in 1991 and 113 in 1980. Life expectancy at birth is 58.2 years for men and 62.68 for women, a considerable increase from 1990 rates (51 years combined). The total fertility rate is 5.32 children born per woman.

Death Rites: Autopsies are uncommon because the body must be buried intact. Cremation is not permitted. For Muslim burials the body is wrapped in special pieces of cloth and buried without a coffin in the ground as soon as possible after death (often within 24 hours).

Food Practices and Intolerances: Staples are corn, cassava, rice, bananas, vegetables, fish, and poultry. However, the islands depend heavily on imported food (which comprises 40% of their sustenance). Njazidja, the largest island, has virtually no topsoil for growing crops, although it has dense rain forest on the slopes of the active Karthala volcano. The two smaller islands have fertile soil, but cash crops take up most of the best land.

Child Rearing Practices: About 43% of the population is between infancy and 14 years of age, and children continue to be malnourished. Their generally poor diets tend to be particularly deficient in protein because of a belief that fish is unhealthy for children. Children are also most susceptible to contracting intestinal parasites because of the scarcity of safe drinking water.

National Childhood Immunizations: BCG at birth; DTP at 6, 10, and 14 weeks; OPV at birth and 6, 10, and 14 weeks; measles at 9 months; and TT CBAW. The reported percentage of the target population vaccinated is as follows: BCG, 90; first dose of DPT, 85; MCV, 70; Pol3, 70; and TT2 plus, 40. In 1989, these rates (except for TT) were closer to 50%, so they have improved markedly.

Other Characteristics: Comoros is prone to political insurrection and coups and has had 19 coups since gaining independence from France in 1975. The island of Anjouan (Nzwani) has moved to secede from Comoros. Although home-grown narcotics are not a problem in Comoros, the islands are used as a transit site for drugs from Madagascar.

BIBLIOGRAPHY

Ahmed A et al: Influence of HIV infection on presentation of Kaposi's sarcoma, *Trop Doc* 31(1):42, 2001.

Imwong M et al: Association of genetic mutations in *Plasmodium vivax dhfr* with resistance to sulfadoxine-pyrimethamine: geographical and clinical correlates, *Antimicrob Agents Chemother* 45(11):3122, 2001.

Rafalimanana H, Westoff CE: Potential effects on fertility and child health and survival of birth-spacing preferences in sub-Saharan Africa, *Stud Fam Plan* 31(2):99, 2000.

http://encarta.msn.com/find/Concise.asp?ti=03948000

http://lcweb2.loc.gov/frd/cs/kmtoc.html

http://travel.state.gov/comoros.html

◆ CONGO (DEMOCRATIC REPUBLIC OF)

MAP PAGE (863)

Jean-Claude Mwanza

Location: With 2,345,000 km² (905,170 square miles), the Democratic Republic of Congo (DRC) is the third largest country in Africa. Located in Central Africa, it is surrounded by the following countries: the Central African Republic and Sudan to the north; Uganda, Rwanda, Burundi, and Tanzania to the east; Zambia and Angola to the south; and the Republic of Congo to the west, with a narrow opening of about 35 km to the Atlantic ocean. The country can be roughly divided into three main geographical regions: the central Congo basin, a large depression occupying about one third of the country and covered by one of the world biggest forests; hills and plains of savannah with woodlands; and an eastern region covered by high mountains with large lakes. The climate is tropical with a rainy and dry season. Overall, the country is extremely rich because of abundant mineral and forest resources, fertile soil, and the enormous hydroelectric potential of the Congo River.

Major Languages	**Ethnic Groups**	**Major Religions**
French (official)	Mongo (Bantu), Luba	Roman Catholic 50%
Lingala	(Bantu), Kongo	Protestant 20%
Kiswahili	(Bantu), Hamitic	Kimbanguist 10%
Kikongo	(Mangbetu and	Muslim 10%
Tshiluba	Azande) 51%	Syncretic sects and
	Sudanic, Pygmy,	traditional beliefs 10%
	other 49%	

Syncretic sects have been well known in the country since the 1920s. The most common are *Kimbanguism* (The Church of Christ on Earth by Simon Kimbangu), inspired by the "prophet" Simon Kimbangu (an originate of the Bas-Congo region), who is very famous in Kinshasa and the Bas-Congo region; *Peve ya longo*, *Bima*, *Kitawala* (which first appeared in the Katanga region before spreading to South Africa), whose followers support the existence of a black God; and the *Jamaa* movement, which originated from the Roman Catholic church. The number of syncretic sects has rapidly increased during the last 5 years. A substantial number of people also have traditional religious beliefs. It has been estimated that more than 200 different languages are spoken within the country, some of which are very similar. In addition to French, the people have shown enormous interest in learning English. Although no updated census has been carried out since the 1980s, the size of the population is between 50 and 55 million, with about 48% of the population younger than the age of 15. Life expectancy is estimated at 50 years for men and 53 years for women. Approximately 65% of the population lives in rural areas. The literacy rate is 84% for men and 61% for women.

Health Care Beliefs: Acute sick care; passive role. Mental illness is greatly feared because of the belief that even when treated it never disappears forever. Most think that mental illness is caused by curses from a jealous person or is a punishment from God. Other grave or fatal diseases may be viewed in the same context, with people believing that the ill individual has done something very wrong (e.g., stolen something, murdered someone) to someone else and is receiving God's justice. Others believe in fate—that good and bad events happen to all people regardless of whether they are good or bad. Such attitudes inhibit the people from understanding the origin of diseases. Prevention of disease and heath promotion are the tasks of the Ministry of Health. Although the country has a *Bureau National* (national office) responsible for the prevention and eradication of each commonly encountered infectious disease (malaria, trypanosomiasis, tuberculosis, onchocerciasis, HIV/AIDS, schistosomiasis, diarrheal diseases, leprosy), such activities are hampered by the size of the country, poor roads, and the poor financial state of the country. Disease prevention is currently limited to free vaccinations of children (where possible) against measles, tetanus, diphtheria, tuberculosis, pertussis, and poliomyelitis. It is assumed that people going abroad are vaccinated against numerous diseases before leaving the country, but officials from the Ministry of Health occasionally verify a person's vaccination coverage for a fee at the airport even though the person has not received the vaccines. The country has an effective program against tuberculosis, with a case detection rate of 70% to 75% and a treatment (which is almost free) success of 75% in Kinshasa. After the recognition of the first cases of AIDS, people in Kinshasa reacted negatively by calling HIV the *syndrome inventé pour décourager les amoureux*, meaning "pure fiction and designed to discourage lovers." Some years later, well-known individuals such as actors and musicians were among the first to die from the disease, and then relatives, friends, and neighbors began to die. People quickly recognized AIDS was more than fiction and changed their sexual behavior. These factors and an effective national AIDS program resulted in a reduction in HIV prevalence. Health promotion is not being carried out at the governmental level, but some private attempts have been made by journalists to use the media to promote disease prevention; unfortunately, only people in urban areas are reached by such activities. Information on HIV/AIDS has been made available in antenatal clinics since the start of the pandemic. However, better methods such as the use of modern technology need to be used to affect disease prevention and health promotion outcomes.

Predominant Sick Care Practices: Traditional healing; biomedical when available and religious. Only about 35% of the total population has access to health care. Available hospitals and health centers have collapsed, and no medications or equipment are available. Under these conditions, it is not surprising that the majority of people primarily use traditional health care practices, especially people in rural areas. Although in cities, people are usually treated in health centers, Congolese of all social and intellectual levels consult traditional healers. It is also common for people to consult a doctor and traditional healer simultaneously for the same problem. In some cases, hospitalized individuals continue to combine modern and traditional methods without their medical doctor's knowledge. Traditional healers are so abundant that they have recently asked for official recognition by state authorities, an idea supported by the Ministry of Health primarily because traditional medicine is the first source of health care for about 80% of the population. This issue continues to be debated because the Congolese Medical Council does not support this type of liberalization in medical practice unless precautions are taken to ensure patient safety. Plants and herbs are commonly used, such as *kongo bololo* (which has a bitter taste and is believed to have the same effect as quinine) for malaria, *tangawisi* (ginger) to cure diseases and back or hemorrhoid pain and sexual impotence (for which the cola nut is used as well), and avocado leaves for anemia. Because of the collapse of the biomedical health system, it is becoming common for sick people to avoid seeking care in health facilities and instead spend time in churches (syncretic sects) waiting and hoping to be cured miraculously by God through a prophet or priest. When the expected miracle cure does not come, the priest or prophet tries to convince the sick believers that what is important is "that they be accepted by Lord in his kingdom, in paradise, because life has no meaning on earth."

Ethnic/Race Specific or Endemic Disease: Malaria, onchocerciasis (river blindness), and trypanosomiasis (sleeping sickness) are major public health problems because of their socioeconomic impact on the country. Onchocerciasis is endemic in almost the entire country. The DRC has the highest percentage of African trypanosomiasis cases (70% of all cases) because of poor surveillance and lack of vector control. Angola and Sudan also have numerous cases. However, extensive community-based programs for eradication of these diseases have shown encouraging preliminary results. Certain diseases are specific for some regions. Goiter and cretinism are endemic in the Kivu and Equator regions because of iodine insufficiency in the soil and water. Konzo is a neurological disease associated with repeated intake of cyanide-producing compounds from consumption of poorly processed bitter cassava and the low intake of sulfur amino acids from animal protein; it is found in the Yaka (Bandundu region). Glaucoma is more prevalent in the *Mongo* ethnic group, and albinism is prevalent among Luba people. The grave economic deterioration in the country in the last 10 years, resulting from constant political instability and war, as well as deliberate poor management of available resources, has led to gradual disintegration of the health system. Consequently, diarrheal diseases, meningitis, polio, and others are common, with children being the most affected. The World Health Organization's (WHO) estimated prevalence rate for HIV/AIDS in adults ages 15 to 49 is 6.43%. The estimated number of children from birth to 15 years living with HIV/AIDS is 4000. In contrast, the 1999 report by the *Bureau Central de Coordination du Programme National de Lutte contre le SIDA/MST* (Central Office for Coordination of the National Program against AIDS/STD) indicated an overall HIV prevalence of 4.3%. At the end of 1999, 95,000 deaths were attributed to AIDS, and 680,000 children younger than age 15 had experienced the death of either one or both parents because of the disease. Heterosexual transmission accounts for 77% of cases.

Health Team Relationships: Doctors are not considered superior to nurses even though the health care system is doctor driven. Doctors and nurses have friendly relationships and in remote rural areas without doctors, a nurse often is the highest authority in the region. Nurses and doctors are very low paid. For example, after 11 years of work at a university hospital in Kinshasa, I (the author of this chapter, a specialist in ophthalmology) earned approximately $19 U.S. dollars (paid irregularly) for clinical, academic, and research tasks. In addition, it is not unusual for nurses to earn higher salaries than doctors. Despite these frustrations, doctors and nurses have good relationships and are trusted by patients.

Families' Role in Hospital Care: The role of the family in hospital care varies with the facility and services available. Because of lack of transportation to medical facilities and poor pay, nurses are not available to do tasks that were once nursing duties. Hospital pharmacies also lack sufficient medications. Therefore the family plays an important role in taking care of sick relatives. One or several members usually spend time at the hospital, buy and cook food in the hospital from the nearest market, change and wash clothes and bedding (which belong to the family), and occasionally administer pills prescribed by the doctor. When the medical team needs a particular drug, a family member is ready to go elsewhere to buy it, and another stays with the patient. In private health centers, which are primarily those run by Roman Catholic churches, only one family member is allowed to stay if needed, and no cooking at the hospital is allowed. The family then brings food from home. Because of the current state of the health care facilities, it is rare to find an inpatient without a relative staying permanently at the bedside. The role of the family when a person is hospitalized is vital to the sick person.

Dominance Patterns: According to state law, the society is patriarchal, so children belong to the clan of the father and only the father receives allowances for children. In most of the country's ethnic groups, married woman are entirely dominated economically by their husbands. For example, he has the right to ask his wife's employer to withdraw her work responsibilities. Although men are primarily dominant, some matrilineal ethnic groups exist, primarily the *Kongo* people in the western part of the country. Among the Kongo the women's family, especially the *noko* (maternal uncle), controls the power, including over a woman's marriage. However, gender-based discrimination is less common in public life, and women are found at high levels in the government and hospital administration.

Eye Contact Practices: Although eye contact is no longer an important issue, it is still thought that making direct eye contact with parents when being scolded is impolite. The child is expected to look down.

Touch Practices: Touching is not an important issue for most Congolese. However, in some religious sects (e.g., Branhamism) it is forbidden for men to embrace (hug) any women other than their wife during greetings.

Perceptions of Time: It general, very little value is attached to punctuality. It is uncommon for events (e.g., national day ceremonies, meetings, academic graduation ceremonies, parties in connection with weddings or concerts) to start on time. Any invitation to attend a given ceremony is usually followed by the comment, "*à la zaïroise or à la congolaise*," meaning that the ceremony will start in the Zairian or Congolese way, or very late. In public administration the costs of such delays have caused the current chaotic state of the public administration in the country. Time is regarded as only existing in the present and is not used for planning the future. Time can be thought of as a function of the profit someone expects to get from an appointment. Therefore people tend to be on time for highly important matters such as written examinations, job interviews, or consultations about health problems. Those who have been educated in Christian-based colleges (mainly Roman Catholic) and been taught the importance of punctuality are usually more punctual.

Birth Rites: Birth is an occasion for rejoicing, especially after the birth of the first child. The first event after birth is the naming of the child, which usually takes place immediately after birth and is generally not accompanied by a special ceremony. The names, one for a boy and another for a girl, are usually known by the parents before the child is born. The name choice is always determined within the clans from the names of grandparents, parents, and relatives of the father and mother. The child is either named with a given name (from the clan) followed by the father's names, or all the children of the same family have a common first name (the father's), followed by another from the clan. In addition, a third name, usually a French name, is given according to the tradition acquired from the colonization. In many ethnic groups, names have significance and are chosen according to the circumstances surrounding the birth of the child. Special names are given to twins depending on the ethnic groups. Among Luba, the first twin is named Mbuyi and the second Kabanga, among Kongo they are named Nsimba and Landu, Mbo and Mpia by those in Bandundu region, and Songe Mbo and Mukonkole. In general, no special ceremony follows a birth today because of the country's significant change in attitude toward life and death. Many of the rites are no longer practiced, and birth has become an occasion to pray and thank God. The infant mortality rate is 130 per 1000 live births.

Pain Reactions: Although high pain tolerance is common in men and women, men are expected to express pain less, a sign of manhood. Adults also are expected to be more tolerant than children of pain. Pain expression may depend on whether expression is considered normal for a certain circumstance. For example, women who think that dysmenorrhea is normal pain keep it private and do not express it. Pain after a spontaneous fall is expressed moderately, whereas pain from a punch or kick from a husband tends to be expressed vigorously.

Death Rites: Death rites vary among those in urban cities, but cremation is not done. In the second largest city, the burial ceremony takes place 1 or 2 days after death, and the corpse is taken directly from the mortuary to the cemetery. In Kinshasa, 2 or more days may pass between death and burial. One day before burial, the corpse is taken home for the last time and memorialized by the family, friends, and acquaintances. Most traditional rites have disappeared; instead, people recite prayers and sing religious songs. Usually a final religious service is held at the home, and a funeral procession consisting of hundreds of people continuously singing or crying accompany the body to the burial. After the cemetery a representative of the family thanks people for their support and announces the end of mourning. People are then given mild alcoholic drinks and food. During the weeks after the death, the family of the deceased person receives visitors. Autopsies are rare, and organ donation does not exist because of cultural beliefs and a lack of services needed to perform transplantation.

Food Practices and Intolerances: Cassava (*Manihot esculenta*) is the staple crop for the majority of Congolese, providing at least 60% of their total energy intake. Cassava flour is not eaten alone; it is mixed with corn flour to make ugali (= *fufu* = *nshima*), a kind of pasta. Rice is widely consumed, especially by Tetela people. Plantains are the main staple food in the Province Orientale, and beans are widely available as well. Among vegetables, cassava leaves remain the most widely consumed, but sorrel, sweet potatoes, and gourd leaves are also eaten. Because of the socioeconomic collapse of the country, most people eat only one meal daily.

Infant Feeding Practices: Approximately 35% of newborns are exclusively breast-fed until 3 months. About half of infants from 6 to 9 months also receive supplementary food. Breast-feeding may continue up to 2 years, particularly in rural areas. Television and radio programs encourage mothers to breast-feed as long as possible.

Child Rearing Practices: Raising children is the responsibility of both parents. Educated women do not carry their children on their backs, but this is a common practice in rural areas and among uneducated women in rural and urban areas. Children are expected to be respectful and polite to older adults. The parents' friends, as well as any other mother or father, are called *papa* and *maman*, and older brothers and sisters are called *yaya*. Any child who refers to an older person by the person's name is considered ill-mannered. Grandparents are usually very kind and very permissive; they like to "spoil" the grandchildren. Children are not usually present when parents entertain guests. Girls are initiated into doing "women's work" at a young age, tasks that include helping the mother in the kitchen, cooking, serving food to the father and her brothers, removing and washing the dishes after meals, washing clothes, cleaning the house, taking care of younger siblings, buying food at the market, and returning home earlier in the evening than boys. The boys are expected to do the hard-labor chores at home, but they are usually away playing football or other games with friends and only return for meals and bedtime. Girls tend to be authoritarian when it comes to kitchen matters, an attitude encouraged by parents. It would not be unusual to hear a girl saying to her brothers in the kitchen, "What are you doing here? This is not your place!" or "Do you want to be a girl?" In general, parents are more demanding with girls. It is rare for girls to achieve early independence, except in rich families. Girls usually live with parents until they have the chance to get married; if they do otherwise, they dishonor the family. Education is encouraged because it is believed to be the only path to a better future. However, it is generally accepted that boys should continue their education as long as possible, whereas girls' education is discouraged. The majority of parents who are able send boys overseas for a better, more thorough education. Even when educated, girls are expected to get married as soon as possible.

National Childhood Immunizations: BCG at birth; DTP at 2, 3, 4, and 16 months; OPV at birth and 2, 3, 4, and 16 months; measles at 9 months; and TT after first contact, +1 month, +1 year, +1 year, and +1 year. According to recent United Nations Children's Fund (UNICEF) statistics, the percentages of fully immunized children up to 1 year of age are as follows: BCG, 22%, and poliomyelitis (three doses), 16%. Recent immunization campaigns have endeavored to reach all 321 health zones in the country, including those areas under rebel control.

BIBLIOGRAPHY

Ekwanzala M et al: In the heart of darkness: sleeping sickness in Zaire, *Lancet* 348:1427–1430, 1996.

Kingsolver B: *The poisonwood bible*, New York, 1998, HarperCollins.

Maertens K: Onchocerciasis in Zaïre, *Int Ophthalmol* 14:181–188, 1990.

Mudimbe VY: *The rift*, Minneapolis, 1993, University of Minnesota Press, 1993 (Translated by M. De Jager).

Mulanga-Kabeya C et al: Evidence of stable HIV seroprevalence in selected populations in the Democratic Republic of Congo, *AIDS* 12:905–910, 1998.

Mwanza JCK, Kabasele PM: Corneal complications of local ocular traditional treatment in the Democratic Republic of Congo, *Med Trop* 61:500–502, 2001.

United Nations Children's Fund Statistics: *Africa 2000*.

UNPOP: *The Human Development Report, 2000*.

World Health Organization (June 2000): *Epidemiological fact sheets by country*, Geneva. Retrieved March 1, 2002, from http://www.unaids.org/hivaidsinfo/statistics/june00/fact_sheets/index.html

World Health Organization (2001): *WHO vaccine-preventable diseases: Monitoring system*, Geneva. Retrieved March 1, 2002, from http://www.who.int/vaccines/

◆ CONGO (REPUBLIC OF THE)

MAP PAGE (863)

Location: Not to be confused with its neighbor Zaire, which recently changed its name to the Democratic Republic of Congo, this western Central African nation (formerly the French Congo) lies astride the equator between Gabon and Angola bordering the southern portion of Atlantic Ocean. It is covered by thick rain forests. Its climate is tropical, with a rainy season (March through June) and a dry season (June through October). Temperatures and humidity are constantly high. The total land area is 342,000 km^2 (132,012 square miles), slightly smaller than Montana. The population is 2,894,336. The capital is Brazzaville, and 70% of the population lives within this city. Congo is a developing country with a gross domestic product (GDP) per capita of $1100.

Major Languages	Ethnic Groups	Major Religions
French (official)	Kongo 48%	Christian 50%
Lingala (trade language)	Sangha 20%	Indigenous beliefs 48%
Monokutuba (trade language)	Teke 17%	Muslim 2%
Kikongo	M'Bochi 12%	
Local languages and dialects	European 3%	

Predominant Sick Care Practices: Acute sick care. Ethnic violence in Congo has virtually destroyed the infrastructure of the country, including its health facilities. Since 2000, considerable reconstruction has taken place. However, in July 2000, United Nations (UN) teams found significant needs for shelter and health care. For example, the UN cited that children younger than 5 years had high rates of morbidity and mortality because of the departure of qualified medical personnel and the destruction of primary care services. According to the UN, Medecins Sans Frontières (Doctors Without Borders) has increased its public health and training initiatives in the country. The International Red Cross has also provided medicines to 18 health clinics. Other relief agencies have also expanded their health services in the country. Although still insufficient, these efforts have provided some relief to the struggling health sector.

Ethnic/Race Specific or Endemic Diseases: Endemic diseases include chloroquine-resistant malaria, schistosomiasis (from *Schistosoma mansoni* and *S. intercalatum*), poliomyelitis, sleeping sickness (which has experienced a resurgence in the last decade), TT virus (TTV), hypothyroidism, gonococcal infections, tinea capitis and corporis, *Loa loa* microfilaraemia, and protein energy malnutrition in children. Congolese are at risk for histoplasmosis, tuberculosis, glucose-6-phosphate dehydrogenase (G6PD) deficiency, plague, and human T-cell lymphoma (HTLV). Congo had a major outbreak of Ebola virus in 1995 and a Marburg virus epidemic from 1998 to 2000. Malnutrition is common, particularly in children, because of war. Tap water is not potable and is polluted from dumped raw sewage, which increases the threat of water-borne illnesses. The World Health Organization's (WHO) estimated prevalence rate for HIV/AIDS in adults ages 15 to 49 is 6.43%. The estimated number of children from birth to 15 years living with HIV/AIDS is 4000. During 1999, approximately 8600 people died of AIDS, and 53,000 orphans have resulted from the epidemic (i.e., children whose mother or both parents have died of AIDS). In 1987 (the last year these statistics were computed), 50% of the sex workers tested in major urban areas were infected with HIV. About 86,000 people currently have HIV/AIDS in the Congo.

Dominance Patterns: Numerous girls and women were raped during the war; a serious problem in that in many ethnic groups, virginity is a requirement for a suitable marriage.

Birth Rites: According to the UN, the maternal mortality rate is estimated at 810 per 100,000 live births, one of the highest in the world. The birth rate is 38.24 births per 1000 people, and the infant mortality rate is 99.73 deaths per 1000 live births. The total fertility rate is 5 children born per woman. About 42% of the total population is between infancy and 14 years of age. The life expectancy is 44.38 for males and 50.85 for females.

National Childhood Immunizations: BCG at birth; DTP at 2, 3, 4, and 16 months; OPV at birth and 2, 3, 4, and 16 months; measles at 9 months; TT after first contact, +1 month, +1, and +1 year. The reported percentages of the target population vaccinated are as follows: BCG, 50; third dose of DTP, 33; MCV, 34; and TT2plus, 39.

Other Characteristics: Ethnic-based political violence has destabilized the Congo for about 10 years. In addition to the many Congolese who became refugees in Gabon and the Democratic Republic of Congo, as many as 30,000 are displaced within the borders of their own country (internally displaced). By 1999, about 20,000 Congolese had died as a result of the violence, and about 800,000 had been displaced.

BIBLIOGRAPHY

Adler MW, ed: Statistics from the World Health Organization and the Centers for Disease Control, *AIDS* 6(10):1229, 1992.
Paverd N: Crimean-Congo haemorrhagic fever: a nursing care plan, *Nurs Rsa Verpleging* 3(4):33, 1988.
http://www.odci.gov/cia/publications/factbook/geos/cf.html
http://www.refugees.org/world/countryrpt/africa/congobrazzaville.htm

◆ COSTA RICA (REPUBLIC OF)

MAP PAGE (857)

Jorge Azofeifa

Location: Costa Rica, the southernmost of the Central American republics, extends 51,700 km² (19,962 square miles) from northwest to southeast. It shares borders with Nicaragua in the north and Panama on the southeast. The two coastlines are defined by the Caribbean Sea on the east and northeast and by the Pacific Ocean on the west and southwest. The land area is crossed by three major mountain ranges, the Cordillera de Talamanca, Cordillera Volcánica Central, and Cordillera de Guanacaste— all of which are "geographical accidents" that have created a tropical climate and vast biological diversity. Politically, the country is divided into seven provinces: Alajuela, Cartago, Guanacaste, Heredia, Limón, Puntarenas, and San José.

Major Languages	Ethnic Groups	Major Religions
Spanish (official)	White 95%	Roman Catholic 85%
Jamaican dialect	Black 3%	Evangelical Protestant 14%
	Indian 1%	Other 1%
	Chinese 1%	
	Amerindian 1%	

Costa Ricans, like Americans, have a multiethnic population. A genetic study estimated that the ancestry of the Costa Rican gene pool is 61% white (mainly Spanish), 30% Amerindian, and 9% black. Almost all Costa Ricans speak Spanish, but English is also spoken because it has been taught in most private kindergartens and schools since the 1970s. English is obligatory in all high schools. A variant of the Jamaican dialect of English is also spoken, because people living in the black community of Puerto Limon on the Caribbean coast were originally from Jamaica. Amerindian languages belonging to the Chibchan Stock are also spoken: Bribri, Cabecar, the Guaymi languages Ngäwbere, and Buglere. Two others, Guatuso and Boruca, are almost extinct. The National Population Census reports a total population of 3,810,179.

Health Care Beliefs: Active involvement; health promotion important. Western medicine and disease prevention are given priority and accepted by the people, who tend to seek out doctors and medical teams for care. However, other medical practices such as homeopathy, acupuncture, and traditional indigenous medicine are also used by some.

Predominant Sick Care Practices: Biomedical and traditional. Costa Rica has a national health care system with a Western approach. After the abolition of the army in 1948, the government invested resources in two socially important areas: education and health. The national health system is led by the Ministry of Health and has established prevention programs into practice through the Primary Health Care and Rural Health Programs. In addition, the Costa Rican Social Security Program (*Caja Costarricense de Seguro Social, or CCSS*) developed clinical and hospital services that provide universal coverage to the population. Both institutions have been responsible for joint improvements in environmental sanitation such as water purification and piping, waste water disposal in urban areas, latrines in rural areas, and a vaccination program for almost the entire population. These steps have resulted in dramatic progress in terms of the national health profile. Since the 1970s, Costa Rica has had health statistic profiles similar to those of other developed countries. Infectious diseases are no longer the major cause of morbidity and mortality, but the relative significance of chronic diseases has increased. More recently the Ministry of Health and the CCSS transformed the primary health care system by implementing the Basic Teams of Integral Health Attention (*Equipos Básicos de Atención Integral en Salud, or EBAIS*). These teams consist of a doctor, nurse, nutritionist, and health assistant. By March 2001, 706 of these teams had been created and were treating 76% of the population in 89 health areas of the country. In addition, private medical practice has gained importance in the last 2 decades among wealthy people desiring more timely and expert care. Despite the availability of excellent health care, some Costa Ricans continue to consult healers for health problems and sentimental issues. People consulting healers because of health problems are primarily those with incurable or intractable diseases.

Ethnic/Race Specific or Endemic Diseases: Infections of the upper respiratory tract are the main cause of illness except in older adults, whose major health problem is arterial hypertension. Parasitic infections are also a significant problem. Rates (per 100,000) for reportable diseases in 2000 were as follows: diarrhea, 4175; dengue, 124.5; malaria, 47.6; hepatitis, 44.1; gonorrhea, 33.4; tuberculosis, 24; syphilis, 18.9; leptospirosis, 4.86; AIDS, 3.2; rubella, 2.2; measles, 0.6; pertussis, 0.5; non-gonococcal urethritis, 0.024; and other sexually transmitted diseases, 0.011. The main causes of death (rates per 10,000) were as follows: diseases of the circulatory system, 12.4; tumors, 8.1; external causes, 4.8; diseases of the respiratory system, 3.9; and diseases of the gastro-intestinal system, 2.7. The World Health Organization's (WHO) estimated prevalence rate for HIV and AIDS in adults ages 15 to 49 is 0.54%. The estimated number of children from birth to 15 years living with HIV/AIDS is 290. The first AIDS cases were reported in 1983 and were only found in people with hemophilia during the next 4 years. The first cases in homosexuals were documented in 1985; in the 1990s, heterosexual and vertical transmission from mother to infant emerged. Life expectancy is 80.29 for women and 74.81 for men.

Health Team Relationships: Relationships among health professionals are hierarchical, with doctors being the most dominant. This situation is accepted, and working relationships are generally good. All health professionals are respected and appreciated by the society.

Families' Role in Hospital Care: Visits to the hospitals of the CCSS are allowed once a day at scheduled times. Food cannot be brought to the patients. Food is provided as directed by nutritionists depending on the special medical needs of patients. In certain cases and with permission, favorite foods may be brought from home. Family members rarely interact with doctors. In private hospitals and clinics, visits are permitted during the day, and a relative or friend of the patient is allowed to stay overnight if necessary.

Dominance Patterns: Traditionally, Costa Rica has had a male-dominated society. During the last 3 decades, more women have gained access to higher education, and literacy rates are high for both sexes (95.7% for women and 95.5% for men). More women are now professionals, and they have promoted campaigns for sexual equality, activity that in 1990 resulted in the Law of Social Equality of Women. Still, some obstacles to equity remain. For example, women continue to be excluded in the decision-making process, are limited in the exercise of power, and have unequal access to resources. Women assume the main caring role when a family member is sick; however, decisions regarding treatments and therapies are discussed by the entire family.

Eye Contact Practices: Direct eye contact is customary when talking with or greeting someone of the same or opposite sex.

Touch Practices: Shaking hands is the usual way to greet people. In comfortable situations or when greeting relatives, kissing one cheek and embracing are also customary. Touching is more common among women.

Perceptions of Time: Punctuality is not an important concept for Costa Ricans. The expression *hora tica*, or Costa Rican time, refers to the fact that delays of 30 minutes are accepted and tolerated. However, in certain situations such as academic and official situations, being on time is more of an issue. People live in the present but do not forget traditions; planning for the future is not unusual.

Pain Reactions: No cultural rules exist regarding pain aside from the stereotypical belief that men should tolerate pain better. Pain reactions primarily depend on the physiological threshold of each person, therefore pain reactions range from stoical to very expressive.

Birth Rites: As a Western Christian society, no particular birth rites are observed by the general population. Given the facilities offered by EBAIS, most women (89% in 2000) receive prenatal care, instruction, and assistance during childbirth. If a newborn is unhealthy and may die, Catholics baptize it as soon as possible. The Bribri Amerindians of the Cordillera de Talamanca follow traditional practices related to childbirth. For example, when labor begins, the woman leaves the house and gives birth alone in a hut in the woods (ideally near a creek with calm water) that was previously built for this purpose. After the birth the mother lives in a small hut adjacent to the lodge in the village and stays there with the child for nearly a month. Mother and infant are "cleansed" through a series of rituals, after which they go back to their home. In 2000 the infant mortality rate in Costa Rica was 10.2 per 1000 live births, the lowest in the history of the country.

Death Rites: Because most of the population is Christian, no specific death rites are observed other than the wake and church ceremonies. Extended families and friends usually participate. Death is perceived as an unfortunate and sad fact of life. The Talamancan Bribri still participate in some ceremonies that involve purification of close family members and "packing" the body before the burial. Organ donation is acceptable. When the cause of death is suspicious or unexplainable, autopsies are mandated by law.

Food Practices and Intolerances: Costa Ricans eat the three usual main meals: breakfast, lunch, and dinner. Costa Rica has a great variety of foods, and diet depends on the socioeconomic status and geographical (urban or rural) location of the family. Breakfast in the rural areas usually consists of coffee or *agua dulce* (a beverage made by diluting sugar cane molasses with hot water), *gallo pinto* (fried rice with black or red beans), tortillas, and fresh cheese or eggs. In urban areas, coffee or tea, bread or tortillas with cheese or sour cream and eggs, and honey or marmalade is common. Cereal with milk is becoming more popular among children, adolescents, and young adults in urban areas. For lunch and dinner, rice, beans, and tortillas are common. Potatoes; cassava; plantains (cooking bananas); beans such as chickpeas, peas, and kidney beans; and pasta are also major components of these meals. Meat includes beef, pork, chicken, and fish, and salads are generally made with tomatoes, cabbage, or lettuce. A wide variety of fruits are cultivated in the country, such as oranges, lemons, grapefruit, watermelons, papayas, melons, pineapples, mangos, blueberries, bananas, and strawberries. They are eaten as fruit or consumed as juices and drinks with meals. During the last decades, many Costa Ricans have become vegetarians, so vegetarian restaurants are not difficult to find. International cooking has also become popular, and Chinese and Italian fast food restaurants are booming. Use of a fork, knife, and spoon is the norm. Eating with the hands is permitted only when eating certain dishes such as tortillas or pizza.

Infant Feeding Practices: Both breast- and bottle-feeding are common. Bottle-feeding gained popularity during the 1960s through the 1980s, but campaigns initiated in the early 1980s promoted breast-feeding. Breast-feeding has become so popular that the decrease in infant death rates observed in 2000 was attributed to this practice.

Child Rearing Practices: Familial ties are very important, and children usually live with their parents until they marry. The concept of family includes parents, grandparents, aunts, uncles, and cousins. Traditionally, women remained at home and took care of the children, and this is still common in rural areas. However, in urban areas, many more women have careers and work outside of the home, and children remain with their grandmothers or sisters. Therefore disciplining children is mainly the task of women. Respect and obedience are valued qualities in children. If a family can afford a house with several rooms, children sleep in their own rooms because sleeping with parents is considered a bad habit.

National Childhood Immunizations: BCG at birth; DTP at 2, 4, and 6 months, and at 2 and 4 years; OPV at 2, 4, 6, and 15 months and 4 years; hep B at birth and 2, 4, and 6 months; HIB at 2, 4, 6, 8, and 15 months; MMR at 15 months and 6 years; and DT school, adult × 2. In 2000 the mean vaccination coverage for children younger than 1 year reached 86.5%: BCG, 95.3%; third dose of DPT, 88.00%; MMR, 82.10%; and third dose of OPV, 79.6 %.

BIBLIOGRAPHY

Bozzoli ME: *Birth and death in the belief system of the Bribri Indians of Costa Rica*, doctoral dissertation. Athens, Georgia, 1975, University of Georgia.

Centro Centroamericano de Población, Universidad de Costa Rica: http://ccp.ucr.ac.cr

Centro Centroamericano de Población, Universidad de Costa Rica: http://censos.ccp.ucr.ac.cr/cgi-bin/login.pl

Constenla-Umaña A: *Las lenguas del área intermedia. Introducción a su estudio areal*, San José, Costa Rica, 1991, Universidad de Costa Rica.

Estado de la Nación en Desarrollo Humano Sostenible: *Sétimo Informe 2000, 1ª edición*, Proyecto Estado de la Nación 2001, San José, Costa Rica.

Mata L, Ramírez G, Quesada J: HIV/AIDS in Costa Rica: epidemiological and sociological features, *Cell Mol Biol* 41:S53–S63, 1995.

Mata L, Rosero L: *National health and social development in Costa Rica: a case study of intersectoral action*. Technical Paper No. 13, Washington, DC, 1988, Pan American Health Organization.

Meléndez C, Duncan Q: *El Negro en Costa Rica*, ed 6, San José, Costa Rica, 1979, Editorial Costa Rica.

Mohs E: Infectious diseases and health in Costa Rica: the development of a new paradigm. *Pediatr Infect Dis* 1:212–216, 1982.

Morera B, Barrantes R: Genes e historia: el mestizaje en Costa Rica, *Rev Hist* 32:43-64, 1995.

Nacional de Estadísticas y Censos Instituto (2001): *IX Censo Nacional de Población y V de Vivienda del 2000: resultados generales*, San José, Costa Rica, http://www.inec.go.cr/INEC2/censo2000.pdf

Observatorio del Desarrollo: *Costa Rican development trends. Chronological series 1985-2000*, versión 2001, compact disc, San José, Costa Rica, 2001, Universidad de Costa Rica.

Pan American Health Organization: *Costa Rica. Country profile. Data updated for 2001*, 2002. http://www.paho.org/English/SHA/prflCOR.html

Solano-Salazar E: *El estudio de grupos étnicos a través del IX Censo Nacional de Población y V de Vivienda, 2000. Población indígena*, San José, Costa Rica, 2001, Instituto Nacional de Estadísticas y Censos http://www.inec.go.cr/INEC2/Estudio Etnias.pdf

◆ CÔTE D'IVOIRE (IVORY COAST)

MAP PAGE (862)

Michael Zimmerman

Location: The Côte d'Ivoire borders the Gulf of Guinea in West Africa. Its neighbors are Liberia and Guinea to the west, Mali and Burkina Faso to the north, and Ghana to the east. The total land area is 322,460 km² (124,470 square miles), making it slightly larger than the state of New Mexico. Other than low mountains in the northwest, the country is mainly flat with undulating plains. The 515-km coastline has heavy surf and no natural harbors. Estimates of land use include 9% arable land, 4% permanent crops, 9% meadows and pastures, and 26% forest and woodland. Southern Côte d'Ivoire has a tropical climate. Temperatures vary from 22° C (72° F) to 32° C (90° F), and the heaviest rains fall from April to July and in October and November. During the rainy season, torrential flooding of rivers is common. In the northern savanna, temperatures are more extreme, with nighttime lows dropping in January to 12° C (54° F) and daytime highs in the summer rising above 40° C (104° F). Annual rainfall is 210 cm (83 inches) on the coast and 120 cm (48 in) on the central plain. The total population was estimated to be 16.4 million in 2001. Nearly half the population is between infancy and 14 years old, and the population growth rate is 2.5%. The population per square kilometer was estimated at 50.2, with 46.4% of the population living in urban areas. Côte d'Ivoire has the largest population and economy of the West African Economic Monetary Union.

Major Languages	Ethnic Groups	Major Religions
French (official)	Foreign Africans, mostly	Christian 34%
60 African	Burkinabe and Malians 27%	Muslim 27%
languages and	More than 60 ethnic groups 25%	None 21%
dialects, with	Malinke, Juula and Bambara 17%	Animist 18%
Dioula most	Senoufou 10%	
widely spoken	Baoule 15%	
	Bété 6%	

More than 60 indigenous ethnic groups exist, but they are usually grouped into four major ethnic clusters: the East Atlantic (primarily Akan), West Atlantic (primarily Kru), Voltaic, and Mandé. They share common environments, economic activity, language, and overall cultural characteristics. The East Atlantic and West Atlantic cultures are found in the southern half of the country, separated by the Bandama River, and the people each constitute one third of the total population. The Voltaic peoples in the northeast and Mandé in the northwest together make up the remaining one third of the indigenous population. Because its present boundaries reflect colonial rule, each of Côte d'Ivoire's large cultural groups has more members outside the country than within, and many Ivoirians have strong cultural connections with people in neighboring countries. For example, the Akan peoples of the East Atlantic culture are descendants of eighteenth-century immigrants from the kingdom of Asante. Both Ghana and Togo have much larger Akan populations. Akan regions are mainly organized into farming communities and have a history of highly centralized chiefdoms that descend through maternal links. However, in the region that is now Côte d'Ivoire, they did not form large empires like the Asante of Ghana. The largest group of the Akan peoples is the Baoulé, who make up 15% of the total population. Smaller groups live in the southeastern lagoon region, where they depend on fishing and subsistence farming and are not politically organized above the village level. The West Atlantic group includes the Kru, the oldest of Côte d'Ivoire's current ethnic groups. Traditionally organized into villages relying on hunting and gathering, they traced descent through male ancestors and did not form large centralized chiefdoms. The largest Kru group is the Bété, who make up about 6% of the population. In the north, cultural differences are more accentuated than in the south. The Voltaic peoples live in the northeast. The largest group, the Sénoufo, make up about 10% of the total population. The Mandé ethnic group occupies northwest Côte d'Ivoire and northern Guinea and Mali. These people—including the Malinké, Juula, and Bambara groups—make up 17% of the population of Côte d'Ivoire. In 1998, it was estimated that non-Ivoirian Africans, Lebanese, Asians, and Europeans made up 27% of the population. Entrenched stereotypes among ethnic and cultural groups place blame for social ills on other rival ethnic groups and immigrants more than on socioeconomic forces. The Baoulé tend to hold high political offices and are therefore perceived by critics as dominant and arrogant. Akan groups, perhaps because of their history of hierarchical organization, are perceived as elitist toward other groups. Groups that tended to avoid politics, such as the Bété, Lobi, and Senoufu, are stereotyped as unsophisticated. Within the large immigrant work force, Africans from neighboring countries are often resented and suspected of taking jobs and wealth from those born in Côte d'Ivoire. More than 60 native dialects are spoken, corresponding roughly to number of ethnic groups. Dioula is the most widely spoken, followed by Baoulé. A variation of Mandé-kan is used throughout the country as a common commercial language. The majority of foreign migratory workers are Muslim (70%) and Christian (20%).

Health Care Beliefs: Acute sick care; traditional. Ivoirians in rural areas have a widespread belief that illness can be drawn out by traditional methods, which include magical, religious, and herbal aspects. Mental illness is greatly feared and poorly understood. Family elders are often sought out for advice on traditional health care.

Predominant Sick Care Practices: Magical-religious primary; biomedical where available. During the past several decades, economic progress has outpaced improvements in general health status, despite increased public health expenditures. Traditional healers continue to provide health care for the majority (as many as 70%) of the rural population. The country has sharp urban and rural as well as regional imbalances in the delivery of health care. Western medical care is available for middle- and upper-class urban households; however, even in the larger cities, shortages of equipment and medicines are common.

Ethnic/Race Specific or Endemic Diseases: Food-, insect-, and water-borne diseases are the leading cause of illnesses, including diarrhea and vomiting (from *Escherichia coli*, salmonella, cholera, and parasites), fever (from malaria, typhoid fever, and toxoplasmosis), and liver damage (from yellow fever and hepatitis). Dengue, filariasis, leishmaniasis, schistosomiasis, onchocerciasis, and trypanosomiasis (sleeping sickness) are also common. In 2001, life expectancy at birth was 45.3 years (men, 43.6 years; women, 46.3 years), up from 39 years in 1960. But national statistics mask sharp regional and socioeconomic differences. In the mid-1980s, life expectancies ranged from 55 years in Abidjan to 48 to 50 years in rural areas of the south and 38 to 40 years in rural areas of the north. The World Health Organization's (WHO) estimated prevalence rate for HIV/AIDS in adults ages 15 to 49 is 10.76%. The estimated number of children from birth to 15 years living with HIV/AIDS is 32,000. In 1987, when the government began testing programs for HIV, 250 AIDS cases were detected nationwide, most of them in Abidjan. By 1999 the HIV/AIDS adult prevalence rate was 10.8%, the number of people infected with the virus was estimated to be 760,000, and 72,000 deaths from AIDS had been recorded. Public health programs are in place to discourage spread of HIV and include an emphasis on condom use. However, many men do not consider use of a condom masculine and are resistant to the practice. In addition, discussion in rural areas of HIV disease is typically avoided, and a person infected with or suspected of being infected with the virus is shunned.

Health Team Relationships: Health team relationships tend to be doctor driven, and doctors hold a superior and respected position. They generally maintain good working relationships with nurses and auxiliary workers. Because access to health care workers is so limited, rural Ivoirians highly respect all members of the health care team, including doctors, pharmacists, nurses, and health aides. Health services have severe shortages of nurses and auxiliary health care personnel, particularly in rural areas of the north. In the late 1980s the country had 6.5 doctors, 0.7 dentists, 10.9 midwives, 24.9 nurses, 11.2 auxiliary workers, and 158 hospital beds (120 of which were for maternity care) per 100,000 people. In the north and particularly the northeast, these ratios are lower.

Families' Role in Hospital Care: Family members nearly always accompany patients to the hospital and remain with them for the duration of their hospital stay. Although food is usually provided by the hospital, portions are meager and usually supplemented by food from home.

Dominance Patterns: Nearly all aspects of Ivoirian culture are male dominated, particularly in rural areas. The status of women is significantly lower than that of men. Women tend to direct all aspects of child rearing and food preparation and many other aspects of the household except for household financial matters. Educational opportunities for women seem to be improving, and a substantial minority of students at the university level are women. The number of salaried women in the work force is increasing. Women make up approximately one third of the civil service and are employed in medicine, law, business, and university teaching jobs, positions that were previously only held by men. The illiteracy rate is 45% for men and 61% for women older than 14 years. The percentage of school-age children enrolled in primary school is 55%, with 47% of school-age girls attending primary school.

Eye Contact Practices: People usually make eye contact during greetings. Eye contact may be avoided when two adults of very different social status greet one another.

Touch Practices: Among family members and close friends, physical touching is acceptable and encouraged. Among acquaintances, females exchange kisses with females on both cheeks, males exchange kisses with females on both cheeks, but males only touch the foreheads of other males. Among new acquaintances and people who do not know each other well, people shake hands.

Perceptions of Time: Strict punctuality for meetings and appointments is not emphasized, and arriving for an appointment up to 30 minutes late is not unusual.

Pain Reactions: Pain reactions range from stoical to expressive. In general, men tend to be more stoical than women.

Birth Rites: In the early 1960s the infant mortality rate was 127 deaths per 1000 live births. This rate has decreased steadily, and by 2001 the infant mortality rate was 94 deaths per 1000 live births. In 2001, it was estimated that the total fertility rate was 5.7 children born per woman, and the birth rate was 40.4 births per 1000 population. Traditionally, after a baby is born the new parents organize a small celebration of greetings and congratulations. Particularly in rural areas, sons are generally preferred to daughters. Parents feel privileged when a son is born because he can carry on the name of the family. In addition, sons are thought of as having greater potential and the ability to make more important decisions later in life. In 2001 the mortality rate for children younger than 5 years was 180 deaths per 1000 live births. Nearly half of all deaths in the Ivoirian population were infants and children younger than the age of 5. Infectious diseases—mainly gastrointestinal and respiratory infections, malaria, measles, and tetanus—account for most illness and death in infants and young children. Unsanitary conditions and poor maternal health also contribute to deaths of infants and preschool-age children. Maternal Health Care (MHC) centers teach classes aimed at reducing maternal and infant mortality.

Death Rites: In 2001 the death rate was estimated to be 16.6 deaths per 1000 people. Almost always, numerous family members and close friends are present when they think a person may die. Organ donation procedures are not performed because most people die in rural areas under the care of a traditional healer. For the same reason, autopsies are rarely performed. It is usually clear to the family and friends who is responsible for the death of a deceased person. Alternatively, the relatives of the deceased person believe that an autopsy is unnecessary because the deceased has simply been "taken by God."

Food Practices and Intolerances: In the northern and western regions of Côte d'Ivoire, cereals such as rice, millet, corn, and sorghum are the main staples. In the central region of the country, yams are the staples, and in the south, cassava and plantain are the primary foods. In the urban centers, particularly Abidjan, various foods are eaten by different ethnic groups depending on the people's place of origin, and some imported foods are available from other West African countries and industrialized countries. In rural areas and many urban households, people eat with their hands. Families in the middle and upper socioeconomic levels use forks, knives, and spoons. In the mid-1980s, it was estimated that the food energy supply was generally adequate, averaging 110% to 115% of the minimum daily requirement. However, inequalities in seasonal, regional, and socioeconomic factors produce widespread malnutrition in the northern regions and poorer sections of cities. Deficiencies of iron and vitamin A are common among infants, children, and women of child-bearing age.

Infant Feeding Practices: Breast-feeding is universal in the rural areas and almost universal in the larger cities. Most women have no choice about feeding methods because they cannot afford formula. Breast-feeding mothers avoid or consume various foods based on whether they think the foods reduce or promote breast milk production. Breast-feeding is done openly, and most breast-fed infants are weaned at around 10 to 12 months. In poor rural areas, close spacing of births contributes to high rates of malnutrition in the first 2 years of life, because weaning foods tend to be of poor quality.

Child Rearing Practices: Until children marry or are about age 15, they usually sleep close to their parents. Child rearing tends to be strict. The father and the mother discipline sons, but usually only the mother disciplines daughters. Obedience to parents and respect for older adults are emphasized. The oldest family members often meet to settle disputes and prescribe or enforce rules of etiquette and marriage. They also pressure individuals to conform to socially accepted standards. Ritual circumcision of girls and boys during early adolescence is widespread in certain ethnic groups, particularly those in the north.

National Childhood Immunizations: BCG at birth; DTP at 6, 10, and 14 weeks; OPV at birth and at 6, 10, and 14 weeks; measles at 9 months; YFV at 9 months; and TT after first contact, +1, +6 months, +1, and +1 year. WHO and the United Nations Children's Fund (UNICEF) assist in programs to vaccinate children and pregnant women through widespread and effective national immunization campaigns.

Other Characteristics: Marriage, particularly in rural areas, is a family affair. The family of the groom pays a "bride price" to the family of the bride to compensate for the loss of their daughter. This payment legitimizes any future children of the marriage, who are considered members of their father's lineage; their mother retains her place in her father's lineage. Although not recognized by Ivoirian law, dual marriages by men in rural areas (particularly in Bété societies) are relatively common. They provide a man who can afford it the potential advantages of more children, more sexual experiences, and increased prestige. After a divorce the children retain their father's lineage, although they continue to live with their mother.

BIBLIOGRAPHY

Centers for Disease Control and Prevention: http://www.CDC.Gov/travel/wafrica.htm
Central Intelligence Agency: *The world factbook*, http://www.odci.gov/cia/publications/factbook/geos/iv.html
Ghys PD et al: Increase in condom use and decline in HIV and sexually transmitted diseases among female sex workers in Abidjan, Côte d'Ivoire, 1991-1998, *AIDS* 16:251–258, 2002.
Jackson RH, Rosberg CG: *Personal rule in black Africa*, Berkeley, Ca, 1982, University of California.
Library of Congress, Federal Research Division: http://lcweb2.loc.gov/frd/cs/citoc.html
Larsen U, Yan S. Does female circumcision affect infertility and fertility? A study of the Central African Republic, Côte d'Ivoire, and Tanzania, *Demography* 37:313–321, 2000.
Levine JA et al: The work burden of women, *Science* 294:812, 2001.
Oppong C, ed: *Female and male in West Africa*, Boston, 1983, Allen and Unwin.
Reinhardt MC, Lauber E: Maternal diet, breast feeding and infants' growth. A field study in the Ivory Coast (West Africa), *J Trop Pediatr* 27:229–236, 1981.
World Bank, *World Bank participation sourcebook*, http://www.worldbank.org/html/edi/sourcebook/sbxa0107.html
Zimmermann MB et al: Persistence of goiter despite oral iodine supplementation in goitrous children with iron deficiency anemia in the Côte d'Ivoire, *Am J Clin Nutr* 71:88–93, 2000.

◆ CROATIA (REPUBLIC OF)

MAP PAGE (860)

Andrea Cvitković Kuzmić and Boris Brkljačić

Location: The Republic of Croatia (Republika Hrvatska) is located in central and southeastern Europe, bordering the Adriatic Sea, Slovenia, Hungary, Yugoslavia, and Bosnia-Herzegovina. The country consists of Mediterranean coastline with more than 200 islands, mountain areas, and a fertile agricultural area. The total land area is 56,542 km² (21,825 square miles), and the border with the Mediterranean is 31,067 km². Land borders are 2028 km and 932 km with Bosnia-Herzegovina, 501 km with Slovenia, 329 km with Hungary, and 206 km with Yugoslavia. The lowest point is the Adriatic Sea, and the highest is Mount Dinara, 1830 m. The population is estimated to be 4.5 million, but the official results of the 2001 census are as yet unpublished. The capital is Zagreb, with a population of 770,000. Other major cities include Split, Rijeka, Osijek, Zadar, Dubrovnik, Pula, and Sibenik. Croatia was part of the Austrian Empire until 1918. From 1918 until World War II, it was the Kingdom of Yugoslavia, and from 1945 to 1991 it was one of the republics of Socialist Federative Yugoslavia. Independence was declared on October 7, 1991; the Republic of Croatia is a parliamentary democracy. The literacy rate is 99%.

Major Languages	Ethnic Groups	Major Religions
Croatian	Croat 78%	Roman Catholic 77%
Minor Languages	Serb 12%	Orthodox 11%
	Bosniak 1%	Slavic Muslim 1%
	Hungarian 0.5%	Protestant 1%
	Slovenian 0.5%	Other 10%
	Italian 0.5%	
	Other 8%	

Health Care Beliefs: Active involvement; holistic; prevention important. The attitude of the population toward official medicine and alternative medicine (e.g., macrobiotics, homeopathy) is similar to that of other central European countries, so alternative approaches are becoming more popular and accepted. Prevention programs are promoted through a strong net of primary health care practices under the auspices of the School of Public Health. Awareness of the risks of smoking is increasing, and programs of cancer screenings for breast and prostate cancers have recently been proposed. Attitudes toward mental illness are similar to those of people in other central European countries. A specific and very significant problem in Croatia is posttraumatic stress disorder (PTSD) in soldiers, a result of the war from 1991 to 1995.

Predominant Sick Care Practices: Biomedical and alternative. The health care system provides coverage for all citizens, and the state health system is a combination of public and private practice. The health care system employs 66,221 people, of whom 45,586 (71%) are health care personnel and 19,635 are administrative. Croatia has 10,436 medical doctors (with 7873 working in the public health care system and 2563 working in private practice and private institutions). The number of medical doctors increased between 1990 and 1999 by 2.7%. Croatia also has 2833 doctors of dentistry and 2077 pharmacists. The country has 23 general hospitals, 2 university hospital centers, and 29 specialized hospitals (e.g., psychiatric, pulmonary, orthopedic); 4 rehabilitation medical institutions; 120 local health community centers; and 5610 private units (e.g., private doctors' offices, dentistry practices, laboratories).

Ethnic/Race Specific or Endemic Diseases: The major endemic disease is endemic nephropathy, which affects people living adjacent to the Sava River in East Croatia. The same disease is well known in river areas of the neighboring countries of Bosnia and Serbia. The most common causes of mortality are cardiovascular diseases, which are responsible for 52% of all deaths, and cancer, which is responsible for 22% of deaths. In 1997, 20% of all deaths were from malignant diseases, and 11,046 people (6650 men and 4396 women) died of cancer. The most common cancers in men (in descending order) are lung, stomach, prostate, rectum, colon, urinary bladder, pancreas, and brain. In women, they are breast, uterus, colon, stomach, rectum, ovary, cervix, and pancreatic cancer. In 1999, 2949 people were treated for drug addiction; the most common type of drug addiction is to morphine. The World Health Organization's (WHO) estimated prevalence rate for HIV/AIDS in adults ages 15 to 49 is 0.02%. The estimated number of children from birth to 15 years living with HIV/AIDS is less than 100. The number of adults living with HIV/AIDS in Croatia is estimated to be 350. Life expectancy is 70.3 years for men and 77.7 for women.

Health Team Relationships: Education of health professionals, both doctors and nurses, is good. Health team relationships are similar to those in other central European countries (e.g., Slovenia, Austria, the Czech Republic), and responsibilities of doctors and nurses are clearly defined.

Families' Role in Hospital Care: Family members may visit and bring gifts and food to hospitalized patients during visiting hours. Family members are informed regularly about medical procedures performed on patients. Parents have to give their informed consent for procedures performed on children, and they may stay with the children in the hospital (although this practice is limited because of lack of space). In the last few years, it has become more common for husbands or partners to be in the labor room during childbirth.

Dominance Patterns: Male and female dominance largely depends on the area of the country and the educational level of the residents. Male dominance was very common until 30 or 40 years ago. This has clearly changed in Croatia as it has in other central European countries, particularly in cities where women are just as likely to be employed as men. In agricultural areas the traditional lifestyle has been retained, and male dominance is the norm.

Eye Contact Practices: Direct eye contact is acceptable between sexes and among people of various social classes. Not maintaining eye contact with someone who is talking is considered impertinent.

Touch Practices: When friends or relatives meet after a long separation, it is customary for them to kiss both cheeks twice. People usually greet each other by shaking hands. An embrace represents a close relationship or affection, and couples on the street commonly hug each other or hold hands while walking, which is socially acceptable. The sight of couples kissing in public is not unusual. Greetings among those in professional relationships are limited to shaking hands.

Perceptions of Time: Being late to a business appointment is considered rude. It is expected that individuals will be punctual for business appointments, but this differs regionally. As a rule, punctuality is considered more important in the northern and western parts of the country than in the southern regions.

Pain Reactions: Pain reactions are quite individual in Croatia, and no rules delineate what is acceptable. People living in the southern regions near the Mediterranean tend to be more expressive, whereas people living in northern areas are more likely to hold back their feelings.

Birth Rites: In recent years, it has become more common for husbands or partners to be present in the labor room during childbirth, but it is still not a widespread practice. Male circumcision is not routine except in minority religious groups. Employed mothers are granted a 12-month leave from work to take care of their child, and fathers usually take a week off. In rare situations, fathers take the leave of absence rather than the mothers. It is very common for grandparents to take care of small children while the parents are working. The number of single parents is increasing. Mothers are encouraged by medical personnel to breast-feed their children. Generally, sons are not celebrated more than daughters, although this varies by educational level and region of the country. In regions that are less developed and in families with less education, sons tend to be more valued. The birth rate is 9.9 births per 1000 births, and the infant mortality rate is 7.7 deaths per 1000 live births.

Death Rites: The majority of families bury the dead according to the rites of the Roman Catholic Church, and people of other religions follow their own customs. Bodies are usually buried in caskets, but in the last few decades cremation has become more popular. Bodies are not exposed in the caskets during the funeral. It is customary to bring flowers, and a funeral procession usually goes to the cemetery. Organ donations are acceptable and being encouraged by the press and medical institutions. Organ donation cards are being issued and public awareness is increasing, resulting in regular heart, kidney, and liver transplantations. Permission for autopsies of hospitalized patients who have died or people who died under specific circumstances is regulated by law.

Food Practices and Intolerances: The usual Croatian practice is to eat with a fork, knife, and spoon; eating with the hands is considered impolite. The diet in the northern parts of the country is mostly continental, and in the southern parts it is Mediterranean, with abundant fish and seafood. Bread is part of most meals, and potatoes and rice are also common. Croatians consume beer and wine, and many good wines are produced throughout the country. All kinds of meat are eaten and because of increasingly pressured lifestyles, the number of fast food restaurants has grown rapidly during the last 10 years.

Infant Feeding Practices: In 1994 a national plan and program was implemented to promote breast-feeding in Croatia, and awareness of breast-feeding among women who have just given birth is high. Bottle-feeding is also a common supplement to breast-feeding.

Child Rearing Practices: Children are usually treated very affectionately, and grandparents play an important role in caring for them. Working families enroll their children in kindergarten programs that are usually very well organized. Grade-school education is compulsory for all children, and every child has to complete at least the 8 years required by law. The number of homeless children is very low, and they are cared for in specialized institutions. More people are becoming interested in being foster parents, but this process is strictly regulated by law.

National Childhood Immunizations: BCG at birth and 1, 8, and 14 years; OPV at 3, 4 to 5, and 6 months and at 1 and 3 years; hep B at 12 years; Per at 3 and 4 to 5 months and at 1 and 3 years; MMR at 1 year; DT at 3, 4 to 5, and 6 months and at 1 and 3 years; and Td at 7, 14, and 18 years.

BIBLIOGRAPHY

Croatian health-statistics annals for 1999.
Croatian Institute for Public Health publications 1999–2002.
Croatian Institute for Statistics.
The Registry of Health Care System Employees.

◆ CUBA (REPUBLIC OF)

MAP PAGE (XXX)

Angel Arturo Escobedo Carbonell

Location: Cuba is the largest and most varied island of the Caribbean Sea—a long and narrow archipelago, sometimes compared to a big lizard. It is located 90 miles south of the southern tip of Florida and is separated from Florida by the Straits of Florida. Cuba's territory includes the Island of Youth and several cays and coastal islets. The total land area is 110,860 km^2 (42,803 square miles).

Major Languages	Ethnic Groups	Major Religions
Spanish (official)	Mulatto 51%	Roman Catholic 85%
	White 37%	Other or none 15%
	Black 11%	
	Chinese 1%	

Spanish is spoken throughout the island. Roman Catholicism is considered the principal religion and has a great number of followers, but numerous Cubans simultaneously practice a form of African worship known as *Santería*, a syncretism of Catholic rites with elements of African roots. More Cubans are beginning to attend Protestant services.

Health Care Beliefs: Traditional; health promotion important. Health care beliefs in Cuba are strongly linked to Cuban history. They are superimposed over indigenous customs—Spanish and African traditions—that have become the foundation for today's Cuban health beliefs. Beliefs are influenced by Chinese, North American, French, Haitian, and Arabic cultures. Supernatural forces, such as the "evil eye" (being able to look at people and make them ill or curse them), are thought to cause some illnesses. Therefore treatments must involve ethnic treatments or magic spells in addition to treatment by doctors. It is not unusual for people in a doctor's office, especially babies and children, to be wearing amulets on a bracelet or necklace or pinned to clothing to help protect them against the "evil eye." "It's better to prevent than to cure" is a common phrase in Cuba, where health promotion is a part of daily life. Since 1959, successful disease control programs have been in place and have had a significant emphasis on community involvement and participation. The health and medical system guarantees unrestricted access to health care services for the entire population.

Predominant Sick Care Practices: Biomedical; magical-religious. A syncretism between the Catholic and African religions affects sick care practices and health beliefs. Herbalists treat common disorders and are specialists in the treatment of "evil eye"; supernatural forces such as those involved in the evil eye must be cured by use of ethnic treatments or magic spells and concurrent biomedical treatment. Ill people may seek the aid and advice of a "godfather" who is a member of the *Santería*. The cure often involves becoming *santo*; they may have to perform a certain ritual, wear white clothes for a year, obey some food restriction in food intake, or not shake hands for a period of time. The advice of family and neighbors is also considered during times of illness, and they play an important role in health beliefs and health-seeking behavior. Occasionally they evaluate the disease according to their experience and recommend medication or herbal treatments, even when the person has consulted a doctor. The Cuban government places a great deal of emphasis on health, and the easy and free access to the health care system has contributed to dramatic improvements in people's health status. Although the use of some alternative therapies has increased, Western medical treatment is usually preferred to treat illness. People living in rural areas have the same access to health care and other benefits as urban dwellers. Health care coverage includes the entire spectrum of services, from vaccinations to sophisticated interventions such as organ transplants. Other social services available to the Cuban population include maternity, sickness, disability, work, injury benefits, and old age and survivors' pensions. Cuba's health statistics are similar to those of most developed countries.

Ethnic/Race Specific or Endemic Diseases: Many of the tropical diseases have been eliminated. Cuba has no poliomyelitis, malaria, diphtheria, or filariasis. Other diseases such as leprosy and tuberculosis are controlled by health programs. As in most developed nations, the major health risks in Cuba are chronic diseases. Cuba has some cancer prevention programs, such as for breast cancer. Preventive measures have been implemented to decrease risk factors related to lifestyle and behaviors, factors such as smoking, alcohol consumption, poor nutrition, and lack of physical exercise. These measures are crucial because of their relation to many chronic, noncommunicable diseases. The World Health Organization's (WHO) estimated prevalence rate for HIV and AIDS in adults ages 15 to 49 is 0.03%. The estimated number of children from birth to 15 years living with HIV/AIDS is less than 100. Cuba has an efficient HIV/AIDS control program. With a population of almost 11 million inhabitants, the country has one of the lowest rates of HIV infection. Public education campaigns have been introduced to the general population and those with a high risk of infection. As in most parts of the world, the majority of new infections are in young people, and prevention programs emphasize the risks of unprotected sex and benefits of condom use. Transmission of the virus is mainly through sexual intercourse. Women need to feel empowered so that they can have control over their sexual relationships and know how to negotiate the use of condoms with their sexual partners. Antenatal care with blood screening of parents is done to avoid transmission of HIV from mother to child. Interventions with men have been based on education and promoting their participation in efforts to be responsible for their own and their partners' sexual health.

Health Team Relationships: Doctors are the primary authority in hospitals and community settings; nurses are subordinate. In situations in which nurses are the only health care professionals available (e.g., in schools, day care centers, ships), they are more respected. The family doctor (a general practitioner) and the nurses live in the same community, frequently in the same building, and are available at all times. They share prevention responsibilities in the community and visit the homes of ill and healthy clients.

Families' Role in Hospital Care: A member of the family or close friend of the family stays in the hospital to help the patient. The member may provide extra food and basic hygiene if necessary. Visitors are expected, and in some families one of the healthy members notes the people who visit. Parents can stay in the hospital the entire day and care for hospitalized children. Patients assume a passive role and expect care to be provided by the family, such as bathing and feeding, if at all possible.

Dominance Patterns: Cuba is traditionally a male-dominated culture with strong interdependent family networks for love, emotional support, material assistance, and overall well-being. Mothers are considered the primary parent, offering security and constancy, although the father's role is important. Parents do not care for girls and boys differently. Women also have occupations once traditionally considered to be men's positions, such as professionals, politicians, electricians, drivers, and doctors.

Eye Contact Practices: Direct eye contact is considered polite. Tenderness, affinity, and confidence are shown by direct eye contact between parents and children, between doctors and subordinates, and among clients. Looking away may be interpreted as a sign of disrespect, dishonesty, or lost of interest.

Touch Practices: Close contact and touching are acceptable. Doctors may put their arms on a patient's shoulder in a show of sympathy and support. Shaking hands and hugs are common among men.

Perceptions of Time: In general, punctuality is an important value and is considered good manners. For some Cubans, being late is a sign of elegance or glamour; people who arrive late do so intentionally. For some meetings, people are asked to arrive earlier than the actual starting time.

Pain Reactions: "Men don't cry" is one of the most frequent Cuban expressions, and it is used to discourage boys from crying. Another common phrase is, "You will deliver your baby with pain." Verbal expressions of pain are acceptable.

Birth Rites: Mothers are included in an antenatal program to help them understand the pregnancy, childbirth, and the postpartum periods. They have prenatal consultations with family doctors, gynecologists, psychologists, and any other health care professionals that are necessary. Topics such as family planning and correcting nutritional deficits are discussed with women who are planning to become pregnant. Almost 100% of births occur at hospital facilities, which decrease deaths of women and newborns. During pregnancy, loud noises, looking at people with deformities, and talking about deformities are avoided. If possible, the woman's mother and husband are present during labor and delivery. In traditional families, the new mother moves to her parents' house for 41 days after the delivery. New mothers are not allowed to wash their hair until this "quarantine" is complete. Relatives and close friends go to the hospital to meet the newborn, and most husbands celebrate the infant's arrival with male friends. Older women say that malts with milk increases breast milk production. Six weeks before and 1 year after a birth, women are able to take a leave of absence from their jobs.

Death Rites: Fear of death is common, and people do their best to be close to their family when a death is expected. When a person dies, relative and friends remain with the body through the night. The burial takes places within 24 hours. If someone, especially a close relative, is out of the city or the country, they make considerable efforts to be present before the burial. Cremation is uncommon.

Food Practices and Intolerances: The majority of people usually eat three times a day, but the largest meal is dinner because this is the meal when all the members of family meet around the table. Drinking juice is considered healthy. The adult diet tends to be high in fat, cholesterol, sugar, and fried foods and low in vegetables and fiber. Occasionally Cubans make comments such as, "this is grass and is for cows," a reference to their preference for meat rather than salads and vegetables. Regardless, attempts have been made to change this attitude and promote healthier dietary habits. Milk is available only for pregnant women, older adults, ill people, and children younger than 7 years old, unless people are able to purchase it with dollars. Rice and beans are common, especially with pork, and the intake of sweets is high. Food taboos include drinking coffee with bananas and eating unripe mangoes.

Infant Feeding Practices: During the first moments after birth, mothers make their best effort to breast-feed their infants so that the children can benefit from the colostrum. A national program promotes exclusive breast-feeding for the first 4 months. Breast-feeding may cease as early as 3 months, at which time solid foods are introduced according to medical criteria.

Child Rearing Practices: Crying is undesirable because a happy, contented child is thought to be a quiet child. Physical punishment is less common than it was in the past. When adults are speaking, children are expected to be quiet. The majority of children stay in day care centers during the day from ages 1 to 5 years. Children usually sleep in their parents' room until they are about a year old. After 1 year, they sleep in another room if possible. Parents have many ways to boost self-confidence and encourage a sense of responsibility in their children. The school system provides health education and assumes much of the child rearing responsibilities. Children may remain dependent on their parents long after they are the legal age of independence.

National Childhood Immunizations: BCG at birth; DPT at 3, 4, 5, and 17 months; anti-*Haemophilus influenzae* type b at 2, 4, 6, and 15 months; anti-tifoidic at 9, 12, and15 years; MMR at 12 months; DT at 6 years; anti-meningococcal at 3 and 5 months; tetanus toxoid at 13 years; and anti-poliomyelitis through vaccination campaigns. Adults are also vaccinated according to risk (e.g., against leptospirosis).

BIBLIOGRAPHY

Gonzalez E et al: Economic and social impact of the National Tuberculosis Control Program (NTCP) on the Cuban population, *Cad Saude Publica* 16(3):687–699, 2000.

Landen MG: Latino mortality rates, *Am J Public Health* 90(11):1798–1799, 2000.

Sedane J: *El folclor médico de Cuba*, ed 1, Havana, Cuba, 1987, Editorial de Ciencias Sociales.

Warman A: Living the revolution: Cuban health workers, *J Clin Nurs* 10(3):311–319, 2001.

◆ CYPRUS (REPUBLIC OF)

MAP PAGE (864)

Theano Kalavana

Location: Cyprus is on the outer border of Europe in the northeastern corner of the Mediterranean close to the Asia Minor and Syrian coasts. It is the third largest island in the Mediterranean (after Sicily and Sardinia) and has a total land area of or 9250 km^2 (3572 square miles).

Major Languages	Ethnic Groups	Major Religions
Greek	Greek 78%	Greek Orthodox 78%
Turkish	Turkish 18%	Muslim 18%
English	Armenian, other 4%	Other 4%

The majority of Cypriots are Greeks who speak the Greek language. English is also widely spoken because the island was a British colony for many years. The estimated total of the Greek-Cypriot population is more than 700,000. It is difficult to estimate the number of Turkish-Cypriot inhabitants who now live in the northern occupied sector, which is about 37.5% of the total area of Cyprus. The Turkish-Cypriots are Muslims, speak the Turkish language, and comprise about 18% of the population. Minorities such as Armenians and Maronites are mainly Catholics who speak Greek as well as their own language.

Health Care Beliefs: Acute sick care; passive role; selective traditional. Disease prevention and health promotion are not very common among Cypriots. The Ministry of Health has made a few positive steps in the last decade regarding disease prevention and health promotion. Every year, they print leaflets with information about different diseases and how people can protect themselves from infections. In addition, campaigns to decrease the most frequent illnesses of the century occur at specific times each year. The major problem with this approach has been the lack of input from health care professionals other than doctors, such as psychologists, social workers, and nurses. Thus the information has comprised detailed medical information and little information to help people change their health habits. Most Cypriots have not established consistent health habits designed to prevent illness. For example, in 1997 the Cyprus Ministry of Health created mass screening programs for mammography and Pap tests. A study on cervical cancer screening in Cyprus and the importance of social cognition models in preventive health indicated that women who are married undergo cervical cancer screenings, whereas women who are not married but have active sexual relationships do not. Moreover, numerous married women had their first Pap test after giving birth and because their gynecologist requested the test. In the past, Cypriots heated cups and placed them on the back of an ill person to draw out the illness. They also applied a special type of alcohol made from grape kernels (*zivania*) to the back of an ill person. Rubbing painful areas with hot olive oil was also common. Today, these beliefs and habits exist only in small villages and among older people. However, even these individuals first go to a doctor for care; they then practice their traditional beliefs as additional therapy.

Predominant Sick Care Practices: Biomedical; magical-religious. Greek Cypriots usually go to doctors for treatment, use Western medicine, and try to take care of their health. Most Cypriots believe in God (*Theos*) and pray. Older adults tend to go more often to churches to pray for their health and the health of their relatives and friends. They believe that aside from doctors, God helps them recover from illnesses and maintains their health. They also frequently make vows to churches and specific saints. For example, if a man has a problem with his foot, he may offer the church or a saint a wax candle shaped like a foot. This practice is also common when a newborn baby is very ill and in danger of dying. The parents offer a likeness of a baby made of wax and pray that God will save their child's life. Cypriots often wear small amulets, usually made of gold, in the shape of a cross or the Virgin Mary, as well as blue stones that may have the image or be in the shape of an eye. These amulets protect them from evil that can harm their health and bring misfortune or bad luck.

Ethnic/Race Specific or Endemic Diseases: Thalassemia (mesoyiaki anaemia) is a group of hereditary anemias occurring in people who live along the Mediterranean Sea. People with thalassemia have problems with their circulatory systems and blood. The disease is becoming rare because of prenatal testing. Cyprus Health Statistics reported the following disease data in 1999: injury, poisoning, and other external causes are responsible for the most illness (16.2% of the total 54,457 patients); diseases of the digestive system affected 11.4%; diseases of the respiratory system affected 10.5%; diseases of the circulatory system affected 10%; complications of pregnancy, childbirth, and the puerperium affected 8.4%; neoplasms affected 7.7%; and diseases of the genitourinary system affected 7.4%. All other disease categories accounted for the remaining 28.4% of patients. Certain viral and respiratory system diseases develop primarily among those in younger age groups, whereas other diseases such as malignancies and diseases of the eye and adnexa, circulatory system, and respiratory system were found among older people. Digestive system diseases and injuries, poisoning, and consequences of other external causes were equally distributed among the various age groups. The World Health

Organization's (WHO) estimated prevalence rate for HIV/AIDS in adults ages 15 to 49 is 0.10%. The estimated number of children from birth to 15 years living with HIV/AIDS is less than 100.

Health Team Relationships: Nurses and doctors have good working relationships. However, doctors have a higher social status. Nurses are very respectful to doctors and do not feel that they are equals. Patients are also very respectful to doctors. They consider them to be intellectual authorities who can relieve them of pain and make them healthy. Patients tend to complain about pain to nurses more than to doctors and believe that nurses are there to help them follow the doctors' orders.

Families' Role in Hospital Care: Families, especially the wives and mothers of patients, usually stay overnight with hospitalized patients. Fathers and husbands usually do not stay, perhaps because they consider caring for an ill person to be a woman's job. It is also occasionally easier for women to get permission for time off from work. Families tend to disobey the rules of hospitals and clinics. For example, they may bring food to patients, ignore posted visiting hours, or use mobile phones in the hospital (which is prohibited).

Dominance Patterns: Males are still dominant in Cyprus. In the past, men and women in traditional Cypriot society had different roles and obeyed different rules. Women had two basic obligations: to maintain the family's honor and take care of family members' physical and emotional needs (e.g., food, cleanliness, comfort). The men's role was to protect the family, provide the means for the family's survival, and represent the family in the community. The woman's role was obviously passive and subordinate, and the man's role was active. Women were not supposed to work outside the home. If they had to do so for economic reasons (especially if they had to work for a person who was not a family member), it reflected poorly on the good name of the man of the house and damaged his reputation as a provider. Today things have changed. Men, although still dominant, are less dominant than they were in the past. Powerful positions in society still tend to be held by men, whether they are related to jobs, organizations, or politics. However, women are much more independent, work outside the home, and are obtaining more powerful positions in many disciplines. Cypriots still believe that certain jobs are for men, and certain jobs are for women. Many men still believe that domestic activities (e.g., shopping, cooking, cleaning) and raising children are women's responsibilities. Men think of themselves as the "hard" workers—the people who work all day to provide the family income—whereas women are responsible for the "soft" duties. A small percentage of women do not seek employment. Both men and women in Cyprus are well educated, and most have graduated from universities or colleges. Both are treated equally, and discrimination on the basis of gender is not allowed. Women go to doctors much more often than men and seem to be much more supportive and caring when a family member is ill. Public and private hospitals employ many female doctors in various areas of medical specialization.

Eye Contact Practices: Direct eye contact between patients and doctors is common. Direct eye contact is also usual when people are greeting one another or talking. In the past, women avoided eye contact because they were expected to behave demurely outside their homes. Women did not work outside the house, thus any contact with unfamiliar people, especially men, reflected badly on the good name of the family. Women were not allowed to visit coffee shops or socialize with strangers, so during unexpected meetings with unfamiliar people or men, they would be bashful. In contemporary society, direct eye contact is quite common among members of both sexes.

Touch Practices: Physical touching is acceptable, and handshaking, hugging, and kissing on the cheeks is the norm among friends. In terms of health care, physical touch is acceptable during examinations. However, very personal examinations are sometimes difficult for women. For example, some women are too embarrassed to have a Pap test.

Perceptions of Time: Punctuality is not a significant issue in Cyprus. It is generally expected that guests will arrive late and public performances may not start on time. People must have an appointment to visit a doctor, but only a few of them get to their appointments on time; therefore doctors have a hard time maintaining schedules. In the past, traditional Cypriots tended to focus on the present because events happened very slowly; rushing things was considered unnatural. This emphasis on the present did not seem to pose serious problems at the time, but it became an issue when the structure and dynamics of the society changed and thinking ahead became necessary for social advancement. Even though the social rules have changed, Cypriots are still somehow focused on the present and tend to do things slowly, with the exception of young professionals, who tend to focus on the future.

Pain Reactions: Women are much more expressive than men regarding pain. The society still believes that "real men don't cry," and men are symbols of power. Men, especially the older men, are stoical and try to hide their pain.

Birth Rites: During childbirth the husband is encouraged to be with his wife. In the past, mothers delivered their babies at home with the help of midwives, and the husbands were at coffee shops, drinking coffee and talking with their male friends. When a husband was informed about a birth, he would offer a drink to everyone in the coffee shop if the baby was a boy. If the baby was a girl, the father would say nothing and just accept the "sad" event. The other men in the coffee shop may not have even congratulated a man whose wife had given birth to a baby girl. A son was celebrated more because he continued the family name, represented the family in public, and provided family income. Today, boys and girls are equally welcomed by parents and relatives. Children are often named after their parents, with boys being named after the husband's father and girls after the woman's mother. If a baby has a serious illness, the parents offer vows to the church and Saint Stylianos (*Ayios Stylianos*) or St. Marina (*Ayia Marina*), the saints who are considered the guardians of babies. Mothers do not avoid bathing or certain foods and carefully follow the doctor's advice about child care. The infant mortality rate per 1000 live births is 6%. The birth rate per 1000 people is 12.8%.

Death Rites: Death is a very personal matter between parents and offspring, husbands and wives, loving neighbors and friends, and God and the dying person. The death of a family member is a most upsetting and dreaded event, because the death of a loved one is a more terrifying prospect than a person's own death or illness. Family members are always present when a beloved relative is dying. They are very expressive and show their grief by crying or even screaming; females are more expressive than males. Grieving may go on for months or years. Close relatives of the dead person usually wear black clothes for 40 days or even 6 months. Parents of a dead child may wear black clothes for years; fathers may not shave and may grow long beards for months or years, whereas mothers may stop using makeup or taking care of their appearance. Cypriots believe that when people die, their souls go to God (*Theos*) in heaven. If the deceased person is a child, the soul becomes an angel. According to traditional Cypriot culture, death is a process by which the soul travels from this world to heaven, so a series of ceremonies led by a priest take place to aid in this process. Funeral events start from the house of the dead person, where close relatives and friends go to support the rest of the family. A service takes place in a Christian Orthodox Church and is followed by the burial. Cremation is generally unacceptable; the corpse's eyes are closed and the body is buried in a coffin. After the funeral, all the relatives and friends eat a piece of bread, which may be accompanied by black olives, goat cheese, and coffee. Organ donations and autopsies are acceptable in Cyprus. Autopsies are allowed when the cause of death is suspicious.

Food Practices and Intolerance: The phrase "your eyes are bigger than your stomach" perfectly characterizes Cypriots' eating habits. They like to have massive amounts of food on their table. In fact, every Christmas and Easter, people go to the emergency room with digestive problems because of the enormous amount of food they have eaten. Digestive system problems were the cause of 21.3% of the surgical operations in 1999. Cypriots use very unhealthy cooking methods such as frying and using a great deal of oil because they believe that oil makes food tasty. Meat consumption is high and includes pork, chicken, rabbit, beef, lamb, liver, and animal intestines. Despite the fact that Cyprus is an island, fish is not eaten regularly, and many fatty dairy products such as cheese and yogurt are consumed. Salad and bread are usually served with meals, and vegetables and legumes are eaten twice a week. The basic foods are meat, potatoes, and salads. Cypriots have many favorite foods: soups such as *avgolemono* (boiled chicken pieces or chicken stock in egg and lemon broth with rice) and *trahana* (dry wheat with milk stock); pasta (*pastichion*) such as *makoronia tou fournou* (baked pasta with minced-meat filling and bechamel sauce) and *pourgouri* (crushed wheat rice with spaghetti); meats such as *souvlakia kebabs* (small pieces of meat on skewers cooked over charcoal and served with salad in pita bread), *sheftalia* (marinated minced meat made into sausage and cooked over charcoal), *souvla* (large pieces of meat cooked over charcoal), *kotopoulo psito* (chicken, potatoes, tomatoes, and oil baked in an oven), *koupepia* (vine leaves stuffed with minced meat, tomato, rice, and onions), and *keftedes* (minced lamb that is rolled and fried); fish such as *kalamaria* (squid cut into rings or small pieces and fried); and cheeses such as *halloumi* (white cheese made from goat's milk). It is acceptable and common to eat certain foods with the hands, although knives, forks, and spoons are preferred.

Infant Feeding Practices: Breast-feeding is common. About 50 years ago, Cypriot mothers became interested in the baby food industries of Western countries and replaced their own milk with formula. Fortunately, this practice soon ended.

Child Rearing Practices: Child rearing tends to be very permissive and may be inconsistent. Most parents know little about disease prevention but may become overprotective in children's daily activities. Children are allowed to sleep in the same bed with their parents if they have nightmares or are not feeling well. The majority of children's time is spent with mothers and grandparents, and discipline is the mother's responsibility. Although, children spend less time with their fathers, they are generally obedient and respectful to them.

National Childhood Immunizations: DPT at 2, 4, 6, and 18 to 24 months and at 5 to 6 years; Td at 14 to 15 years; OPV at 2, 4, 6, and 18 to 24 months and at 5 to 6 years; measles at 15 months; and hep B at birth, 1 and 5 months, and at 5 to 6 years.

BIBLIOGRAPHY

Attalides M: *Social change and urbanization in Cyprus: a study of Nicosia*, Nicosia, Cyprus, 1981, Social Research Centre.

Georgiou SN: Family dynamics and school achievement in Cyprus, *J Child Psychol Psych* 36(6):977–991, 1995.

Health Statistics: *Cyprus statistics for health and hospitals*, Series I, Report No. 20, 1999, Printing Office of the Republic of Cyprus.

Kalavana T: *Screening for cervical cancer in Cyprus: applying the health belief model and multi-dimensional health locus of control scale*, master's thesis, 1999, United Kingdom, University of Surrey.

Loizos P: *The Greek gift: politics in a Cypriot village*, Oxford, England, 1975, Basil Blackwell.

World Health Organization (June 2000): *Epidemiological fact sheets by country*, Geneva. Retrieved March 1, 2002, from http://www.unaids.org/hivaidsinfo/statistics/june00/fact_sheets/index.html

World Health Organization (2001): *WHO vaccine-preventable diseases: monitoring system*, Geneva. Retrieved March 1, 2002, from http://www.who.int/vaccines/

◆ CZECH REPUBLIC

MAP PAGE (860)

Joseph Dolejs and Tomas Morcinek

Location: The Czech Republic is situated approximately in the geographical center of Europe and has a total land area of 78,866 km^2 (30,442 square miles). It is a landlocked country 326 km from the Baltic and 322 km from the Adriatic. It shares borders with Germany (810 km), Poland (762 km), Austria (466 km) and Slovakia (265 km). The capital is Prague (Praha) with a population of 1,213,800. Population density is 131 inhabitants per square kilometer. The Czech Republic is a parliamentary democracy.

Major Languages	Ethnic Groups	Major Religions
Czech (official)	Czech 94.4%	Atheist 39.8%
Slovak (minority language)	Slovak 3%	Roman Catholic 39.2%
	Polish 0.6%	Protestant 4.6%
	German 0.5%	Orthodox 3%
	Roma (gypsy) 0.3%	Other or none 13.4%
	Hungarian 0.2%	
	Other 1%	

Of the 4.6% who claim Protestant as their religion, 1.9% are in the Czech-founded Hussite Reform Church, 1.6% in the Czech Brotherhood Evangelic Church, and 0.5% in the Silesian Evangelic church. In addition, many foreign churches have been introduced since 1989 and have established small parishes around the country. A small Jewish community of 10,000 still exists.

Health Care Beliefs: Active role; health promotion important. There are many rubrics in newspapers and magazines that discuss healthy life-styles. Health is an important topic on television. The major focus of health prevention in the media is on restricting saturated fats and controlling cholesterol, and increasing exercise through sports. Mental hygiene, or a focus on good mental health is stressed in prevention programs, even for people without psychological problems. Serious mental health disturbances requiring psychiatric care can cause one's social status to be lowered, due to stigma against mental disorders. Therefore, the majority of people are reluctant to admit that they have a problem, and avoid diagnosis and treatment if at all possible. In general, people think that the consumption of hard drinks and smoking are not particularly dangerous, and they are reluctant to change these risk factors. Folk medicine practices such as healing illness by means of heated coins or cupping no longer have credence. Wearing amulets as objects to prevent illness is not a habitual practice, whereas praying for health is common for part of population.

Predominant Sick Care Practices: Biomedical; alternative. Western medical treatment is regularly used in hospitals and polyclinics. Some physicians offer alternative treatment such as homeopathy or acupuncture. Some people consult home-based herbalists if they are not satisfied with the doctor's diagnosis and recommended treatment. Nevertheless, seeking out the help of indigenous healers and folk medicine practices are rather limited. The system of health care is based on compulsory insurance. Insurance from employers is compulsory, while the government is responsible for children, students, pensioners, the unemployed, and the disabled. The majority of medicines are free of charge, and medical care is free of charge. Some stomatological care and extraordinary medicines are the exceptions, and require payment from the patient. Alternative medical care (homeopathy, acupuncture) is not covered by medical insurance, so requires self-payment.

Ethnic/Race Specific or Endemic Diseases: Racial and ethnic diversification of the society does not exist in the practical sense. The leading cause of deaths is diseases of cardiovascular system: these diseases caused 56% of all deaths in the period from 1986–1993. Malignant neoplasms caused 22% deaths in this period. The World Health Organization's (WHO) estimated prevalence rate for HIV/AIDS in adults 15–49 is 0.04%. The estimated number of children 0–15 years living with HIV/AIDS is <100. By May 2001, there were a total of 514 HIV-infected persons registered in the Czech Republic. Of this number, 151 persons have already developed the clinical stage of AIDS: 90 people have so far died of the disease. Intravenous drug-dependent individuals are considered at highest risk for HIV/AIDS in the Republic.

Health Team Relationships: Physicians in the Czech Republic are the dominant group in health care units: they are responsible for health care. Nurses are required to follow physician instructions. Nurses and physicians, however, tend to work in teams in some health care settings (for example, psychiatry), and nurses are valued members of such teams. The relations of clients to physicians are very submissive, with clients usually afraid to ask for information regarding their diseases and health care. Clients are not partners with physicians when decisions need to be made regarding health care: this is usually the decision of the physician only. This is presently in transition, with efforts being made to provide a better working partnership between client and physician. Relationships between clients and nurses are more informal, more natural and less ceremonious compared to the relation between physician and nurse.

Families' Role in Hospital Care: Families are not responsible for preparing food or attending to personal hygiene for their hospitalized family members. Involvement of family members is not particularly welcomed in the hospital setting, with the exception being overnight accommodations for mothers of sick children. Family members visit hospitalized people frequently when family relations are good. When they are not good families seldom visit. Visits can range from half an hour to 2 hours, and families bring snacks, fruits, mineral water, and juice for patients. Hospital rooms are generally shared by at least two other, and sometimes as many as eight, patients.

Dominance Patterns: Male dominance is not a large issue in the Czech Republic. In general, people are afraid of even simple ideologies, such as feminism. During communism the women had to work in factories, and their role in taking care of children was forcibly reduced. The situation is better now, and after childbirth mothers can be at home for 7 months, during which time her employer has to pay 90% of her previous salary. If she has a second child the government will pay her half of the minimal state salary for 4 years. Despite this system, it has not resulted in increased numbers of pregnancies. Many people today would prefer to have more money and individual comforts, rather than to have more children.

Eye Contact Practices: Direct eye contact is a generally used and is the expected method of interpersonal communication in various relations. Differences in eye contact involve time and circumstances of its use. For example, in relations between a man and a woman close and frequent eye contact is usually perceived as a sign of affection.

Touch Practices: Touch is commonly socially acceptable in non-sexual ways, depending on the age and the gender of the persons involved, the range and character of relations between participants, and the professional context in which it occurs. Greeting another person with a handshake is common.

Perceptions of Time: People usually attach considerable importance to punctuality. Differences in how punctuality is perceived result from place of residence—rural dwellers attach smaller importance to this feature than people living in big cities; kind and character of professional activity—people working as policemen, professional military officers, bank workers pay more attention to punctuality.

Pain Reactions: It is not very acceptable to verbally demonstrate that one is in pain. Pain sensation is shown by facial expressions, grimace, body position, body stature, and limited activity and this will be interpreted by the health professional. People suffering pain usually use medical methods for relieving it. The health care system upholds the principle that, whatever the cause, individuals should not and cannot suffer pain and that the role of health professionals is to relieve it.

Birth Rites: As a rule, children are delivered in hospitals. The delivery procedures are usually typical of Western practice with the woman lying down with her legs elevated on leg rests, but some hospitals offer different postures. Home delivery is very rare and not accepted by physicians. It is common for fathers to be present in the maternity ward, but not for other family members. Fathers are increasingly interested in using this option. Mothers can usually choose whether she wants to stay with her newly delivered baby in one hospital room (rooming-in) or to have the baby go back to the nursery after feedings. Mothers bathe themselves and their babies, usually every day, in the first month of the newborn's life. In the breast-feeding period mothers avoid certain foods in their diet; for example, beans, peas, cabbage. Instead they eat other vegetables and fruit. In general, there are no differences in celebrating the birth of a son or a daughter, although fathers are especially happy when a son has been born. For those who are Christians, an inseparable element connected with birth of a child is the baptism ceremony. Life expectancy at birth in 2001 was 74.73 years for the total population: 71.23 years for males and 78.43 years for females.

Death Rites: The majority of people die in hospital without family members present. In villages, sometimes people die in their homes, but it is rare. Recent surveys show an increase in cremation worldwide. The highest ratio in Europe is in the Czech Republic, where over 72% of those dying are cremated. Britain is at 71%, and the United States at 27%. Organ donation and autopsy is possible where there is agreement of family members.

Food Practices and Intolerances: The consumption of meat is very high. Although reducing the amount of fat in the diet is strongly promoted, attention is given to this concept only by a small part of society. There are some vegetarians, but they are the exception to the rule. The Czech kitchen is traditional and it plays an important role in life. The national meal is pork with dumplings and boiled cabbage. Eating with the hands is not done, except for sandwich-type foods. Knives and forks are necessary: it is not considered polite to eat only with a fork. It is also not common to use a plastic fork and knife. Meals are usually prepared at home, even when a celebratory one. Visits to restaurants are infrequent.

Infant Feeding Practices: Physicians recommend breast-feeding, and it is an important focus of the national health system. Mothers try to continue to breast-feed as long as possible. Bottle-feeding is also common, but it is considered as a substitution for breast milk.

Child Rearing Practices: It is commonly thought that strict upbringing with positive reinforcement is the best way. The time that children spend watching television is less than in the United States, but the tendency is that the new generation spends more time with electronic entertainment than previous generations. The school system is not ideal for talented children. In basic school the majority of teachers are women due to the low income of teachers. Children are quantitatively evaluated from the first class (from the age of 6 years), and everyone is educated to read and write. Even mentally retarded children are educated in special schools. The highest level of education in mathematics in the world exists in the Czech Republic, but the last statistical survey showed that there is intense antipathy to math. Grandparents play a more important role in the life of grandchildren than in the United States, in that frequently people live in one city their whole lives and family relations are very intense. Having more money is not considered as a reason to change one's living arrangements.

National Childhood Immunizations: BCG birth; DTP 3, 4, 5, 18 months; OPV 3, 5, 15, 24 months, 14-15 years; MMR 15, 21-24 months; DT 5-6 years. The vaccination program in the Czech republic is free of charge. There is compulsory vaccination for all children in the population. In addition, those people who have dangerous employment relative to certain infections not necessarily covered by initial vaccinations are also vaccinated free of charge according to a special program. For example, dentists are vaccinated without cost against hepatitis B and influenza, and those who work with animals receive rabies immunization. Except for persons covered because of their employment, individual citizens must pay for vaccines for influenza, hepatitis B, and streptococcal pneumonia. Tetanus is part of the standard treatment after a lesion.

REFERENCES

1. *Statistical yearbook of the Czech Republic*, 1990, Czech Statistical Office.
2. World Health Organization: *The international classification of diseases-9* (revision), 1977.
3. WHO Mortality Database: http://www.who.int/whosis/mort/download.htm
4. *History of cremation*: 605 Pine Street, Manchester, NH 03104, 603 622–2829.
5. Czech Citizenship Vaccination Identity Card.
6. Twenty-sixth Special session of the general assembly on HIV/AIDS, New York, 27 June 2001, Statement by H. E. Mr. Bohumil Fizer, Head of the Delegation, Minister of Health of the Czech Republic.

◆ DENMARK (KINGDOM OF)

MAP PAGE (860)

Helle Ussing Timm (Consultant: Nana Thrane)

Location: Denmark is a part of Scandinavia and the northernmost part of Europe. It is the smallest and most level of the Scandinavian countries, with its highest point only 174 m (570 ft) above sea level. Greenland and the Faroe Islands are a part of Denmark but have very different landscapes. The Kingdom of Denmark has 5.3 million inhabitants. The total land area is 43,070 km² (16,629 square miles).

Major Languages	Major Ethnic Groups	Major Religions
Danish	Scandinavian	Danish National
Faeroese	Eskimo	Evangelical Lutheran
Greenlandic	Faeroese	85%
(Inuit dialect)	German	Roman Catholic 2%
German		Muslim 3%
		Other 10%

Danish is the primary language. Children are required to attend grades 1 through 9 in school, where they learn English, as well as German or French. In the Faroe Islands a local dialect and Danish are spoken. In Greenland an Inuit (Eskimo) dialect is spoken in addition to Danish.

Health Care Beliefs: Active involvement; health promotion important. In daily life, explanations of poor health, illness, and disease can be numerous and complex and far beyond the rational explanations of health care professionals. In the professional health care system the biomedical model is dominant, and the biomedical understanding of the body, health, and illness is becoming more "medicalized." Denmark has a significant emphasis on health promotion and disease prevention, an emphasis that has been intensified by the fact that life expectancy in Denmark has stagnated and is now among the lowest in Europe. The Danish government has established the Health Promotion Program (for 1999 to 2008) to prevent "too-early-death" among middle-aged Danes and prevent social inequalities in health care. Health promotion and prevention of illness and disease are thought to be closely related to lifestyle choices, especially smoking and drinking alcohol, eating unhealthy food, and a lack of exercise. Critical research on daily Danish life is being carried out as well. For example, research is being conducted on the consequences of working long hours—90% of Danish women work outside of the home, the highest percentage of working women in the world. It has been documented recently that the incidence of mortality from cancer is higher than in other Scandinavian and northern European countries. In addition to lifestyle factors, this incidence is believed to be related to inefficient cancer treatments. Since the 1980s the Danish welfare program, including the professional health care system, has been undergoing substantial reforms. Part of this modernization program involves an emphasis on cost-effectiveness and better management of resources. The focus in the hospital system is on quality assurance, evidence-based medicine, and patient satisfaction. At the same time, an ideology revolving around the home has dominated health care; people are thought to be better at home than in health care institutions when possible.

Predominant Sick Care Practices: Biomedical and alternative. The Danish health care system consists of three parallel systems: the system of daily life, the alternative system, and the professional system. Many common problems of health and illness are solved by people in their daily life. Laypeople also seek help in the alternative system, and some alternative practices such as chiropractic treatment and acupuncture are being integrated into the professional system. The professional health care system is part of the public welfare system, which plays a major role in Scandinavian countries. The public welfare system is characterized by three distinct features: universality (free access for everyone), tax financing (which is free), and a strong public sector that supports social welfare and the health of its citizens. The professional health care system is divided into a primary sector at a local community level, with the general practitioner as the lead professional, supplemented by specialist doctors (consultants), physiotherapists, chiropractors, and home care services and a secondary sector at regional and national levels, primarily consisting of specialized hospitals. Denmark also has a few private hospitals and hospices.

Ethnic/Race Specific or Endemic Diseases: Most Danes (95%) live to be older than 45 years of age, and 79% live to be older than 65 years old. Most deaths are related to diseases and conditions of old age. The most common medical causes of death are cardiovascular diseases (40%), cancer (26%), and pulmonary diseases (8%). The increase in lung cancer incidence in women is among the largest in the world, and musculoskeletal diseases and psychiatric disorders are common. The World Health Organization's (WHO) estimated prevalence rate for HIV/AIDS in adults ages 15 to 49 is 0.17%. The estimated number of children from birth to 15 years living with HIV/AIDS is less than 100.

Health Team Relationships: Collaborative relationships among health care professionals have changed during previous decades. The dominance of the medical profession by doctors has weakened, and paramedical groups such as groups of nurses, therapists, and others have grown. Interdisciplinary teamwork is the ideal, as is patient empowerment; patients' rights have been legalized. Health team relationships are rather relaxed and informal; however, they are still hierarchical, and the power of the professionals dominates the layperson's perspective. In clinical practice, doctors are the final authority, and in health care research the biomedical research models and methods are still dominant.

Families' Role in Hospital Care: The role of relatives in hospital care has changed significantly during the previous decades. Close family members are thought of as health care participants when a member is hospitalized, therefore visiting hours have become quite liberal. Parents can normally stay with a child during the child's hospitalization. Family members are not expected to take care of hospitalized relatives, but occasionally they do because they want to or think they need to.

Dominance Patterns: Denmark is characterized by a tradition of democracy and an ideology of equality regardless of class, gender, ethnic background, or age. Regardless, it is a society built on capitalism, industrialization, and social control; social inequality and inequality in health care are increasing. Women's rights are well established in Denmark, although men still dominate positions of power in society and women do most of the domestic chores. The current public debate involves equality and its relationship to ethnic background and minorities; the rights of emigrants and refugees have been reduced. Youth is preferred to old age.

Eye Contact Practices: Direct eye contact symbolizes interest and is expected during conversation, but the eyes shift back and forth from time to time. If eye contact is held for a longer period, it can symbolize power or intimacy.

Touch Practices: Touching involves intimacy. Touch practices vary according to social class, gender, ethnicity, and age. Some people never do more than shake hands with someone outside the family. Others consider it quite normal to exchange hugs.

Perceptions of Time: Punctuality is an issue. It is considered important to get to appointments on time, although short delays are acceptable if a person has an explanation. Mainstream culture focuses on the future—to get on with life, be busy, and have a lot to do.

Pain Reactions: In general people are expected to react stoically to pain, but it is acceptable for children and adults in great pain (physical or psychological) to react more expressively (e.g., wail or cry).

Birth Rites: Pregnancy and birth are thought of as natural events. Women can work until the end of a pregnancy or can begin their leave a month before birth. Pregnant women are advised to refrain from smoking or drinking alcohol but otherwise to live their normal lives. Most children are born in the hospital, and it is common for fathers to be present during delivery. The mother can stay in the hospital for a few hours or days if she prefers. Within the first few days, close relatives and friends come and visit to celebrate and see the baby. Breast-feeding is the norm, and women are instructed to avoid chocolate, strawberries, very strong food, and alcohol.

Death Rites: Despite the fact that death is ever present (e.g., in the newspaper, on television, in computer games, in movies), a person's own death is still a taboo subject in Denmark. Danes try not to acknowledge the fact that they are all going to die until they are personally confronted with death through a serious illness, accident, or sudden death. Most Danes (80%) die in hospitals or care homes. For the last 10 years the hospice movement, which focuses on palliation, has expanded in Denmark, meaning more attention is being given to death and dying. Usually family members are present when a family member is close to death, but some people die alone. Organ donations and autopsies are accepted, but Denmark has the chronic shortage of organs common in most countries.

Food Practices and Intolerances: It is normal to eat three meals a day and enjoy different kinds of refreshments in between such as coffee, fruit, or sweets. Breakfast may consist of cereal, oatmeal, or bread and cheese or jam, tea, coffee, and milk. Lunch may consist of open-face sandwiches. The main meal is dinner between 6 and 7 pm and is normally hot food—meat with potatoes, pasta, or rice and salad. Forks, knives, and spoons are used for most meals, but it is acceptable to use the hands to eat sandwiches and fast food. The evening meal has an important function because the family members gather together. In recent years, fast food has become more common, especially among younger people. Food allergies in children are becoming increasingly common. Danes drink quite a lot of coffee, and alcohol consumption in some population groups is high.

Infant Feeding Practices: Breast-feeding is the ideal, and it is encouraged and common. After a couple of months, breast-feeding is supplemented with other kinds of food and normally ends when the mother has to resume work (after 5 to 12 months).

Child Rearing Practices: Children are regarded as autonomous human beings with a personality and a will of their own; they are respected as such and learn to participate in decision making quite early. Almost all children spend the day in some kind of care center.

National Childhood Immunizations: DTP at 3, 5, and 12 months; HIB at 3, 5, and 12 months; IPV at 3, 5, and 12 months; MMR at 15 months and 12 years; and Td at 5 years.

BIBLIOGRAPHY

Andrews MM, Boyle JS: *Transcultural concepts in nursing care*, ed 2, Philadelphia, 1995, Lippincott.
Axelsen M: Midwifery in Denmark, *Birth Gazette* 12(1):26, 1995.
Gamborg H, Madsen LD: Palliative care in Denmark, *Supp Care Cancer* 5(2):82, 1997.
Henry B, Hamran G, Lorensen M: Nursing management in the Nordic countries: a health system perspective,
Intern Nurs Rev 42(1):11, 1995.
Houshian S, Poulsen S, Riegels-Nielsen P: Bone and joint tuberculosis in Denmark: increase due to immigration, *Acta Ortho Scand* 71(3):312, 2000.
Melbye M, Biggar RJ: A profile of HIV-risk behaviors among travelers—a population based study of Danes visiting Greenland, *Scand J Soc Med* 22(3):204, 1994.

◆ DJIBOUTI (REPUBLIC OF)

MAP PAGE (862)
Location: Formerly French Somaliland (and from 1961 to 1977, the Territory of the Afars and Issas), this small, sparsely populated, developing country is in northeast Africa bordering the Gulf of Aden at the southern

entrance to the Red Sea. The area is hot, dry, and sandy, and made up of coastal plains, volcanic plateaus, and mountains (in the north). In the cool season the temperature is an average of 77° F, and in the hot season is 112° F. Djibouti shares borders with Ethiopia, Somalia, and Eritrea, and is slightly smaller than Massachusetts. The total land area is 22,000 km^2 (8494 square miles). Djibouti is the capital, where about 70% of the population lives. Outside of the capital city the primary economic activity is nomadic subsistence. The country has few natural resources and little industry. The population is 460,700, and the gross domestic product (GDP) per capita is $1200.

Major Languages	Ethnic Groups	Major Religions
French (official)	Somali 60%	Muslim 94%
Arabic (official)	Afar 35%	Christian 6%
Somali and Afar	French, Arab, Ethiopian,	
(widely used)	Italian 5%	

The Somalis are the predominant group in the south, and Somali is the most widely spoken language, including in the capital city. More than 50% of Somalis belong to the Issa clan. The Afar is the predominant group in the north, where the Afar language is widely spoken.

Predominant Sick Care Practices: Acute sick care; traditional. Medical facilities are very limited, and medications are often unavailable. When ill, the only option for most individuals is reliance on traditional practices.

Ethnic/Race Specific or Endemic Diseases: Diseases endemic in Djibouti are malaria, especially the falciparum form (including reported chloroquine-resistant strains); yellow fever; rabies; cholera; typhoid; polio; hepatitis A, B, and E; and vitamin A deficiencies. The country recently had an epidemic of dengue fever. People in some geographical areas are at risk for meningococcal meningitis and for bilharzia in fresh-water lakes. Land-mine accidents are a constant source of potentially fatal injuries. Risk of injuries from motor vehicle accidents is also high because of poor road conditions. The World Health Organization's (WHO) estimated prevalence rate for HIV/AIDS in adults ages 15 to 49 is 11.75%. The estimated number of children from birth to 15 years living with HIV/AIDS is 1500. About 3100 adults and children died of AIDS during 1999, and the number of children whose mothers or both parents have died of AIDS since the beginning of the epidemic is 7200. At the end of 1999, the country had 5901 living orphans. In 1999, approximately 37,000 people were living with HIV/AIDS; in 1998, 28% of the sex workers tested were infected with HIV.

Birth Rites: The birth rate is 40.66 births per 1000 people, and infant mortality rates are high, 101.51 deaths per 1000 live births. The total fertility rate is 5.72 children born per woman. Life expectancy at birth is 49.37 for males and 53.1 years for females.

Death Rites: Autopsies are uncommon because the body must be buried intact. Cremations are not permitted. For Muslim burials, the body is wrapped in special pieces of cloth and buried in the ground without a coffin as soon as possible.

Food Practices and Intolerances: The soil is poor, and droughts are common. Djibouti has virtually no arable land, so the people depend almost entirely on food imports. Typical foods are fish (especially Red Sea fish in spicy sauce), fried meat or chicken with lentils or other vegetables, and flat bread. Because Djibouti is a Muslim country, alcohol is not readily available. Locals frequently chew qat, a mild stimulant that is sold daily in the markets under wet cloths. Less than half of the population has access to safe drinking water. Water mains in the city are normally heavily chlorinated but can cause gastrointestinal problems. Outside of the cities the water is usually contaminated and causes various water-borne illnesses, especially in children. Milk is unpasteurized and occasionally a source of illness.

Child Rearing Practices: Almost all females are circumcised. Approximately 43% of the population is between infancy and 14 years of age, and only about 39% of primary-school-age children attend school. The literacy rates are 60.3% for males and 32.7% for females.

National Childhood Immunizations: BCG at birth; DTP at 6, 10, and 14 weeks; OPV at birth and at 6, 10, and 14 weeks; measles at 9 months; and TT at first pregnancy, +1, +6 months, +1, and +1 year. The reported percentages of the target population vaccinated are as follows: BCG, 34; first dose of DTP, 66; third dose of DTP, 46; MCV, 50; third dose of Pol, 46; and TT2 plus, 15.

Other Characteristics: The government's record of human rights is extremely poor. Political opponents have reportedly been beaten, raped, and tortured. Land mines are known to be present in the districts of Tadjoureh and Obock in the north.

BIBLIOGRAPHY

Adler MW, ed: Statistics from the World Health Organization and the Centers for Disease Control, *AIDS* 6(10):1229, 1992.

Cholera in 1997, *Weekly Epidemiol Rec* 73(27):201, 1998.

Djibouti, *Microsoft Encarta Online Encyclopedia 2001*, Microsoft, http://encarta.msn.com

Hatem MM: Health development in Djibouti, *World Health Forum* 17(4):390, 1996.

Rodier GR et al: Epidemic dengue 2 in the city of Djibouti 1991-1992, *Trans Roy Soc Trop Med* 90(3):237, 1996.

Rodier GR et al: Recurrence and emergence of infectious diseases in Djibouti city, *Bull WHO* 73(6):755, 1995.

Wright J: Female genital mutilation: an overview, *J Adv Nurs* 24:251, 1996.

http://travel.state.gov/djibouti.html

http://www.wtg-online.com/data/dji/dji080.asp

◆ DOMINICA (COMMONWEALTH OF)

MAP PAGE (858)

Robert Kohn, Liris Benjamin, and Griffin Benjamin

Location: Dominica is one of the largest of the Windward Islands, located between the French islands of Guadeloupe and Martinique in the Eastern Caribbean. The total land area is 750 km² (290 square miles). It has a population of more than 71,000, of whom 16,000 reside in Roseau, the capital. Dominica, a former British colony that gained independence in 1978, is only 29 miles (47 km) long and 16 miles (26 km) wide. Its mountainous terrain makes access to the capital difficult for most of the villagers. The only surviving indigenous Carib population, estimated to be 2000 people, lives in this country. In 1903, they were assigned a 3700-acre territory in the northeast.

Major Languages	Ethnic Groups	Major Religions
English (official)	Black 89%	Roman Catholic 70%
Kwéyòl	Mixed 7%	Protestant 14%
	Indigenous 2%	Other or none 16%
	White 1%	

The majority speak Kwéyòl, a French Creole, in addition to English. A 1995 poverty assessment survey in Dominica showed that 27% of households are in poverty. The unemployment rate is estimated to be approximately 9.9%.

Health Care Beliefs: Both active and passive involvement; selective health promotion.

The definition of mental illness is narrow. Other than psychosis, behavioral disturbances are not considered by the general public or professionals to be mental illness or serious problems. Most disconcerting is the lack of knowledge revealed on surveys about attitudes toward mental illness among those directly involved in care: nurses, teachers, and police officers.

Predominant Sick Care Practices: Biomedical. A well-developed primary care system serves each of the 10 parishes. The system has a network of seven health centers and 44 clinics throughout the island. The care in the public health centers and clinics is free. Each health district has a network of type I clinics that serve approximately 600 people in an 8-km (5-mile) radius. Type II and III clinics offer comprehensive services. Hospital care, including inpatient psychiatric treatment, is primarily provided through Princess Margaret Hospital, which has 195 beds. The country has 2.6 hospital beds per 1000 people. Private health care is limited to outpatient services.

Ethnic/Race Specific or Endemic Diseases: Typhoid fever, dysentery, tuberculosis, and gastroenteritis in children are the most common infectious diseases. The incidence rate for tuberculosis is 7 per 10,000. Dengue fever is the only vector-borne disease of significance in Dominica. In 1995, 297 cases were caused by the *Aedes aegypti* mosquito. In 1994, diabetes was found in 4% of the population and hypertension in 18%. A more recent survey revealed the rate of diabetes to be closer to 3%. Obesity is found in 8.7% of the population. Only 31% of 12 year-old-children in a 1990 national study were free of dental caries. A study of the prevalence of medical disorders in 123 older adults found that 20% were dependent on others relative to activities of daily living. Hypertension was noted in 40% of the population, diabetes mellitus in 15%, impaired visual acuity in 20%, and evidence of glaucoma in 10%. More than half of the older adults used their medications more than prescribed. Substance use disorders are a major concern as well. Approximately 9% of inpatient psychiatric admissions were a result of alcoholism, 8% a result of cannabis psychosis, and 2% of result of cocaine abuse. A national mental health report found that 90% of the patients in the prison psychiatric clinic had a history of drug abuse. The island frequently has hurricanes, but the mental health impact of disasters on the island has not been studied. The principal cause of death is related to circulatory system diseases (37.6%) among adults. Neoplasms accounted for 20% of the recorded deaths. The leading causes of death among children younger than the age of 5 were caused by congenital abnormalities, premature births, and respiratory distress syndrome. About 77.5% of households have direct access to piped and treated water, but 25% of the homes do not have an approved sewage disposal system, a fact that has obvious health implications. More than half of the cases of AIDS are in people ages 20 to 29, and the prevalence is three times higher in males. Currently, 15 cases of AIDS have been registered. The estimated annual AIDS incidence rate in 1997 was 211.3 per million.

Health Team Relationships: District nurses are the basis of the primary health care services and are primary health personnel in type I clinics. Types II and III clinics are staffed with a health officer and a district nurse midwife. Evaluations for hypertension, diabetes, pregnancy, and immunizations account for 40% of appointments with nurses in type I clinics. Only about 20% of patients are referred to the district medical officer. Dominica has 4.9 physicians, 41.6 nurses, and 0.6 dentists per 10,000 inhabitants.

Families' Role in Hospital Care: Families are usually supportive. Although meals are available in hospitals, relatives frequently feel it is their duty to prepare meals and do laundry for their hospitalized family members.

Dominance Patterns: The nuclear family is prevalent in Dominica; however, in the rural areas the extended family is prevalent, a pattern that may be related to the high number of older adults. Dominica has numerous residents who are 100 years or older. (Ma Pampo Israel, a Dominican who is currently alive, is 127 years old.) Fathers are usually the head of the household; however, single-parent families are increasing in number.

Eye Contact Practices: Direct eye contact is common among members of the same or opposite sex.

Touch Practices: In general, Dominicans are very courteous. It is common to shout out a greeting to a friend while driving or walking. Occasionally, people even stop their vehicles in the middle of the road to exchange greetings, which does not seem to annoy the other people held up in the resulting traffic. Handshaking and hugging are common.

Perceptions of Time: People are usually on time for work. However, concerts may start 30 to 45 minutes after the scheduled time.

Pain Reactions: Pain perceptions and thresholds are not based on cultural issues.

Birth Rites: Dominica is primarily a Christian society, and most Christian residents are Catholics. Other religions include Seventh-Day Adventist, Methodist, and Pentecostal. Birth is a time of celebration. Babies are usually carried to church for a blessing, and the ceremony is considered a special occasion. Catholic and Methodist parents choose godparents, who are expected to play a special role in the care and nurturing of the child. On special occasions such as birthdays, godparents usually give gifts to their godchildren and as the children get older, they bond with the godparents. Pregnant women have universal access to health care, yet according to 1995 statistics only 36% of women receive prenatal care by the 16th week of pregnancy. Nearly all births are attended by trained personnel. Birth control is used by 38% of women of child-bearing age (ages 15 to 44). The 1991 fertility rate was reported as three children per woman, and the mean age of childbirth was 26.8 years. The crude birth rate in 1992 was 25.5 per 1000 people. The infant death rate was 28 per 1000 live births. Life expectancy was estimated to be 66.7 years.

Death Rites: Dominicans rally around families and friends at the time of death. On the night of a death, many friends from the community gather at the home of the bereaved family for a wake. At this time, condolences are offered, religious hymns are sung, food is prepared, and coffee, ginger tea, and wine are drunk. Burial is usually within the first 5 days after the death.

Food Practices and Intolerances: Dominicans enjoy a wide variety of local dishes. Local breakfasts include *farine* (a coarse cassava flour) and pear, as well as *ackra* (small pancakes made from special tiny fishes called *titiwi*). Citrus juices, especially grapefruit, and passion fruit, which are grown locally, are very popular. Fish broth, a soup made with fish, pickled pig snout, bananas, and yams, is a favorite for lunch and parties. Another favorite is *dasheen callaloo*, a soup made from young dasheen leaves, coconut milk, potatoes, dumplings, and occasionally crabs. Codfish and roasted breadfruit with cucumber salad is extremely common. Vendors blow conch shells to announce a sale of fish such as dolphin, jacks, and balahoo on the roadside or seaside.

Infant Feeding Practices: Nearly 10% of all newborns are born with a low birthweight. No cases of severe malnutrition among children were reported in 1995.

Child Rearing Practices: Families generally have more than one child, with three to four children being the norm. Working parents employ a babysitter and take their children to day care centers. Grandparents and relatives also play a role in child rearing. Although the country has no compulsory education program, 91.6% of the population between the ages of 5 and 19 was registered in school in 1993. A majority (67.1%) of the population has completed primary school. The functional illiteracy rate is estimated to be 10.5%.

National Childhood Immunizations: BCG at 3 months; DTP at 3, 4 1/2, and 6 months; OPV at 3, 4 1/2, and 6 months and at 3 and 11 to 13 years; hep B at 1 month; MMR at 1 year; DT at 3 to 5 years; and Td at 11 to 13 years. Immunization coverage among infants is almost 100% for DPT, the third dose of OPV, BCG, and measles. Other than measles, vaccine-preventable diseases have been eradicated in Dominica. The country has approximately one or two measles cases per year.

BIBLIOGRAPHY

Kohn R et al: Attitudes towards mental illness in the Commonwealth of Dominica, *Rev Panam Salud Publica* 7:148–154, 2000.

Kollman PM et al: District nursing in Dominica, *Int J Nurs Stud* 35:259–264, 1998.

Leake JL et al: The dental health of 12-year-old children in Dominica: a report of a survey using WHO methods *J Can Dent Assoc* 56:1025–1028, 1990.

Pan American Health Organization. *Volume II: Health conditions in the Americas*, Scientific Pub No. 569, Washington, DC, 1998, Author.

Sattenspiel L, Powell C: Geographic spread of measles on the island of Dominica, West Indies. *Hum Biol* 65:107–129, 1993.

Sharma D, Nasiiro R: *Prevalence of alcoholism in a rural community in Dominica*, paper presented at the Commonwealth Caribbean Medical Research Council, Trinidad, 1996.

Tull ES et al: The use of capture-recapture methods to monitor diabetes in Dominica, West Indies, *Rev Panam Salud Publica* 3:303–307, 1998.

Tull ES et al: Should body size preference be a target of health promotion efforts to address the epidemic of obesity in Afro-Caribbean women? *Ethn Dis* 11:652–660, 2001.

van der Veere CN Luteyn AJ, Sorhaindo BA, et al: Obstetrical condition and neonatal neurological outcome in Dominica, the Caribbean: a comparative study, *Trop Geogr Med* 44:338–345, 1992.

Veen-de Vries NR et al: Health status of the elderly in the Marigot Health District, Dominica, *West Ind Med J* 48:73–80, 1999.

◆ DOMINICAN REPUBLIC

MAP PAGE (858)

Teresa L. Lynch and Joseph D. Lynch (Consultant: Leon Fay)

Location: The Dominican Republic occupies the eastern two thirds of the Caribbean island of Hispaniola—the second largest island in the Caribbean—with Cuba being the largest. Hispaniola consists of the Dominican Republic and Haiti. The island lies just west of Puerto Rico, is southeast of Cuba and Florida, and is slightly smaller than South Carolina. The total land area is 48,730 km^2 (18,815 square miles). The population is approximately 8,600,000.

Major Languages	Ethnic Groups	Major Religions
Spanish	Mixed 73%	Roman Catholic 90%
English (widely spoken)	White 16%	Other, none 10%
	Black 11%	

English is often taught as a second language. The majority of the people are mixed European (predominately Spanish) and African descent. Approximately 25% of the population is considered to live below the poverty line. Internal migration and external emigration, primarily to the United States, has been heavy since the 1970s. The primary industries include tourism, industrial duty-free zones, sugar processing, tobacco, ferrous nickel and gold mining, and cement production. The economy is quite dependent on outside forces such as the price of oil and coffee. The Dominican Republic is the home of merengue and bachata, and music is an integral part of their culture. Environmental issues include water shortages, soil erosion into the sea, deforestation, damaged coral reefs, energy pollution, and air pollution. The climate is moderate year round; hurricane season is in the fall.

Health Care Beliefs: Acute sick care; traditional. Preventive health care is emphasized in the public health sector but is ineffective because of the limited resources of the country. Superstitious rituals are not widely practiced, although in some areas, healers (*curanderos, santeras*) are still consulted occasionally, and some people believe that a person with *mal de ojo* ("the evil eye") can harm others, especially young children. It is believed that the evil eye can cause almost any symptom and is often counteracted by a procedure called *ensalmo*, which includes blessing, massaging, and bathing the child. The "hot-cold" theory of health is occasionally encountered and is based on the concept that a healthy body is the result of balance between hot and cold, and illness is the result of a hot-cold imbalance. Other health beliefs are occasionally encountered, such as *viento*, which involves pain caused by air entering a muscle or another part of the body—a process that is initiated by exposure to cool air. *Empacho* is based on the idea that something spoiled (e.g., food, milk, saliva) can get stuck in the body as a mass or bolus and cause abdominal discomfort, vomiting, and weight loss. Treatment may include various teas and the help of a folk healer. Herbal and folk medicines are common, particularly in rural areas. Examples include garlic (*ajo*) for hypertension, gas, headaches, and cholesterol control; coconut juice for urinary tract infections, cleansing the kidneys, and constipation; orange leaves (*ojas de naranja*) in teas for colds, toothaches, and dizziness and applied directly for headaches; and aloe (*sabila*) for colds, tuberculosis, dry skin, and diabetes. Other customs include bathing for "cleansing" purposes or drinking water from the first rain in May (*primera agua de mayo*) for youth and good health. Some spiritually based approaches (e.g., *santeria*) may be used alone or in combination with the help of a healer to address health or other needs, especially psychological or interpersonal relationship problems or lasting illnesses.

Predominant Sick Care Practices: Biomedical and magical-religious. When available, doctors' clinics and hospitals are preferred, although poverty and lack of availability often results in self-care because of limited services. The population tends to be quite religious so prayer is common, particularly in the rural areas. Communicable diseases are the most common causes of death in preschool children. Cardiovascular diseases, cancer, and accidents are the most common causes of death in the adult population. Tuberculosis is the second most common cause of death in women ages 15 to 44. Antibiotics and most other medications can be purchased without a doctor's prescription. Nearly all health indexes have improved significantly in recent years because of widespread government and nongovernmental organization efforts. Currently, the government is emphasizing improving maternal and child health. Life expectancy has risen from 53.6 years (1960 to 1965) to 71 years in 1998 (69 for men and 73 for women). Since 1992, state public health policy has mandated that health care is a right of all people, and priority should be given to those who are the most disadvantaged. Lack of adequate funding has left this noble goal unfulfilled.

Ethnic/Race Specific or Endemic Diseases: Malaria exists, but the risk is low except in the Haitian border areas or where construction or similar projects have attracted large numbers of foreign workers. Malaria is responsive to chloroquine. Malaria, dengue fever, rabies, and hepatitis B are considered endemic. Giardiasis and bilharziasis (schistosomiasis) are also a risk. Sexually transmitted diseases are a significant problem but have been decreasing recently. Haitian bateys (areas where Haitian workers live, often for years) are particularly underserved. The World Health Organization's (WHO) estimated prevalence rate for HIV/AIDS in adults ages 15 to 49 is 2.8%. The estimated number of children from birth to 15 years living with HIV/AIDS is 3800. The annual incidence rate for AIDS in the Dominican Republic is 30.7 per million people for males and 20.9 per million for females. HIV is primarily transmitted heterosexually.

In 2000 a limited outbreak of poliomyelitis occurred in rural Dominican Republic and Haiti. The cases were well documented and were the first cases of polio attributed to wild polio virus in the Americas since 1991. The affected people had acute flaccid paralysis and fever and were living in an area of very low vaccine coverage. Three rounds of mass vaccinations have been performed and seem to have successfully stopped the outbreak in the country. However, all visitors to the Dominican Republic should be completely vaccinated against polio, and the disease should be considered in visitors from the Dominican Republic.

Health Team Relationships: Patients are generally deferential toward health care professionals and are quite accepting of the limitations of health care. Accessibility to doctors is limited among the poor and in rural areas. The country has a marked shortage of nurses.

Families' Role in Hospital Care: Families are very supportive and tend to stay with hospitalized patients. In public hospitals, patients and family members may have to purchase medications before they can be provided. Private hospitals generally include the cost of medications in the total bill.

Dominance Patterns: The country has a male-dominated, "machismo" culture, although women's rights groups are active and advances have been made in recent years. Women generally direct activities in the home and tend to be the caretakers of the family.

Eye Contact Practices: Eye contact is generally accepted among people of similar status and education. As in most cultures, individuals who are poor or have a lower social status are less likely to initiate or maintain eye contact.

Perceptions of Time: The Dominicans are warm and affectionate. Greetings with hugs (*abrazos*) and cheek touching among all ages and both sexes are common. Dominicans have a smaller "personal space" than people in some other countries (e.g., the United States). Punctuality is much less important in the Dominican Republic, particularly in the rural areas, than it is in the United States and can be confusing—or funny—in various situations. However, among businessmen and similar individuals, punctuality is expected. As in other countries, the poor are forced to live day by day, although many traditions are greatly respected such as the importance of families, religious rites, and Carnaval.

Pain Reactions: The authors are unaware of any credible data on pain reactions in Dominicans. Occasionally, pain and other complaints are loudly and dramatically expressed, but generally the people seem somewhat stoic and accept pain as part of life.

Birth Rites: Prenatal care and birthing procedures are quite advanced. Approximately 97% of all pregnant women have some form of prenatal care from doctors, and 95% of all births take place in medical facilities. Even 82% of women who are illiterate give birth in medical centers. Consequently, superstitions and ill-advised practices are uncommon. The births of sons and daughters are both celebrated, particularly in the rural areas. Parents are happy to have a son who will help in the fields with manual labor, but they are happy to have a daughter who will be able to help with the chores in a home without modern conveniences. The birth rate is typical of other Latin American countries at 21.6 per 1000 people (2003 estimate), but it has been decreasing. It is still significantly higher than the birth rate of the United States, which is 13.2 per 1000 people (2003 estimate). Approximately half of females of child-bearing age practice some type of birth control, and sterilization is the most common form (64%). Contraceptive pills (taken by 20% of females) are free from the state. More than 40% of Dominican women are or have been pregnant by age 20.

Death Rites: Death is accepted because most Dominicans believe in an afterlife. Family-centered funerals and burials are the norm. There is generally no embalming, especially in the rural areas, and the body is buried within 24 hours. The casket is usually handmade and carried in public accompanied by family and friends to the grave. Widows and widowers often have a long mourning period—up to 1 year or more—during which they are not allowed to participate in festivities. Nine-day novenas with daily gatherings for prayers, food, and conversation are common.

Food Practices and Intolerances: Malnutrition is found among the poor and is estimated to affect 6% of those younger than age 5 and as many as 20% of people in the rural poor areas such as the southeast near the Haitian border. The food staple is rice and beans, also referred to as *la bandera Dominicana* ("the Dominican flag"). Favorite foods include plantains, mangos, yucca, sweet potatoes, eggplant, and chicken. Soups such as *sancocho*, which may include meat or chicken, and *asopo*, which also includes rice, are also popular. In the poorer areas the diet primarily consists of starch and little meat or protein.

Infant Feeding Practices: The government has established a campaign to promote breast-feeding during the first 6 months. Most women are given 12 weeks of maternity leave from their jobs. The first foods, which are often bean broth and plantain broth, are frequently introduced between 4 and 5 months. Although some recent changes have taken place, mothers in the rural areas primarily breast-feed, partly for economic reasons. In the city or more wealthy areas, bottle-feeding is more common, although the recent emphasis on the benefits of breast-feeding has increased its popularity. *Campesinos* (children in rural areas) may breast-feed for a long time, perhaps until age 4 or 5 if the mother does not become pregnant.

Child Rearing Practices: Rural, or *campesino*, areas tend to be stricter with children, and discipline and obedience are expected. Small children often sleep with parents, especially in the poor or rural areas. Dominicans tend to treat their children with much love and are demonstratively affectionate, but many children, especially the girls, have to take on many responsibilities in the household and raise the younger children. The boys often work in the fields at a young age. Mothers are usually responsible for daily discipline, but fathers often handle more serious problems.

National Childhood Immunizations: BCG at birth; DPT at 2, 3, 4, 15, and 59 months; OPV at birth and 2, 3, 4, 15, and 59 months; hep B at birth and at 1 and 6 months; HIB at 2, 4, 6, and 15 months; measles at 9 months; MMR at 12 and 59 months; and vitamin A at 6, 12, 18, 24, and 30 months. Recent countrywide immunization campaigns for have been generally successful.

ACKNOWLEDGMENTS: We would like to express our appreciation to Leopoldo Carretero, Ramon Antonio DeLeon, and Mandy Gittler for their assistance. We would especially like to thank Leon Fay for sharing his enthusiasm for and knowledge about Dominican culture and folk medicine.

BIBLIOGRAPHY

Centers for Disease Control and Prevention: www.cdc.gov
Harvey S: *Dominican Republic: the rough guide*, London, 2000, The Rough Guides.
Health in the Americas, vols I and II, Washington, DC, 1998, Pan American Health Organization.
Pan American Health Organization: www.paho.org
Smith RP, Sears SD: Travel medicine. In *Blackwell's primary care essentials*, Malden, Mass, 2002, Blackwell.
U.S. State Department: www.state.gov/www/services.html
World Fact Book: www.odci.gov/cia/publications/factbook/
World Health Organization: www.who.int

◆ ECUADOR (REPUBLIC OF)

MAP PAGE (859)

Fernando Alarçon

Location: Ecuador is a member of the Andean Community of Nations. It is named after the equator, which crosses the country, so a small part is in the northern hemisphere and the rest is in the southern hemisphere. Ecuador is bound on the north by Colombia, on the south and east by Peru, and on the west by the Pacific Ocean. The total land area is 283,560 km^2 (109,483 square miles). The country's mainland territory is divided into three well-defined regions: the coastal region on the Pacific Ocean, the highlands of the Andes, otherwise known as the *sierra*, and the Amazon region, with its tropical vegetation and rain forest, also known as the *Oriente*. The country's island territory comprises the Galápagos Islands, which are 1000 miles away from Ecuador's shoreline

Major Languages	Ethnic Groups	Major Religions
Spanish (primary)	Mestizo (mixed) 70%	Catholic 90%
Quecha	Indigenous 20%	Other 10%
English	White 8%	
	Black 2%	

Health Care Beliefs: Acute sick care; traditional. To prevent children from being spooked or hexed, mothers tie an amulet with a red string around the wrist of their children. When children have been spooked by the "evil eye," they lose weight, are sad and listless, and have no appetite. To cure the children, a raw hen's egg has to be passed over their body for 3 days. When children have been frightened and cannot get past their fear, a raw hen's egg that has been dipped in medicinal waters is also passed over their body. Other ways of curing spooking is suddenly spraying of water or liquor on a child's face. In certain communities, people with epilepsy are considered as endowed with superhuman force and godly powers. When patients have a severe illness and little chance of recovering after hospitalization and treatment by a doctor, it is not unusual for them to resort to traditional healers (*curanderos*) or Catholic shrines.

Predominant Sick Care Practices: Magical-religious; alternative and biomedical when available. Ecuador has many popular health-related customs. *Muyuyo* flower tea or milk boiled with garlic is popular for coughs. Homemade syrups consisting of diced red onions with sugar that are kept outside all night are also quite common. Compresses of *tomate de árbol* (a fruit called *tree tomato*) or honey mixed with liquor are used for sore throat. Among blacks, a cure for a migraine is a band tied around the head. To prevent children from becoming dumb, their hair is not cut until after they are at least a year old. Women prevent ovarian problems by not walking barefoot. In the Amazon region, a wide variety of natural herbs and plants, which are being studied by several countries for their special properties, are used to cure diseases. The climate and humidity foster the growth of a broadly diverse collection of plants, trees, and animals, from which medicinal substances are obtained. An analgesic that is stronger than morphine can be extracted from certain varieties of frogs. Other medicinal uses can be found in plants such as *sangre de drago*, which is effective for healing wounds, and *ayahuasca*, known since ancestral times for its strength-giving properties and which has now also been recognized for its brain dopaminergic properties. Natural medicines in the Ecuadorian sierra are widely used in all strata of society—natural herbs such as *matico*, which has antiinflammatory and antiseptic properties, and valeriana and *pasiflora*, which have hypnotic powers and are taken as tranquilizers. Cobwebs and the inner shell membranes of eggs are commonly used to treat surface wounds; they are placed on the open wound and effectively heal tissue. Chieftains, priests, or shamans think they must impress fellow men by demonstrating supernatural powers, effects that can usually be obtained from hallucinogenic plants such as the coca leaf. The frequent use of certain plants deemed to be sacred by the shamans may inadvertently lead to psychiatric and neurological disorders. Some Amazon communities still use curare for muscle relaxation. The tip of an arrow is dipped in curare and then shot out by a blowpipe to hunt wildlife or paralyze enemies. Ecuador has several institutions that focus on health: the Ministry of Public Health, the Social Security Institute, the armed forces, the police force, the municipal authorities, and nongovernmental organizations, each of which functions independently. This situation has prevented the development of a national health plan providing standardized coverage. The Ministry of Health has attempted to set up a national health plan, but it works only partially. At the grassroots level, this system relies on *puestos de salud*, which are local health units that can be found even in the smallest villages. At the other end of the spectrum are the highly specialized public hospitals in the country's largest cities—Quito, Guayaquil, and Cuenca—to which patients with difficult cases are referred for treatment or diagnosis. The social security system has a similar system, albeit smaller. Hospitals and services provided by the Ministry of Public Health focus on the lower income sector of the population. The country's social security hospitals are for the workers who are affiliated with the social security system and the *campesinos* (agricultural workers) who are part of the Campesino Insurance Program. For a small monthly stipend, rural workers are permitted to use social security services. Nongovernmental organizations, the hospitals of the armed forces and the police force, and private practices meet the health needs of the rest of the population. Because of low salaries, most public health professionals also have their own private practice, which are primarily for the middle- and upper-class sectors of society. In the country's modern private hospitals, state-of-the-art technology is available.

Ethnic/Race Specific or Endemic Diseases: In the Amazon region, known as the *Oriente*, the climate is tropical, and diseases such as yellow fever are typical of this tropical climate. The inhabitants live in temporary makeshift huts made of local plants. They subsist by fishing and hunting and rely on rivers—tributaries of the Amazon River—for communication and transport. The Ecuadorian coastal region has hot and humid tropical weather. A large part of the population in the northwestern province of Esmeraldas is black. The absence of proper medical care, clean water supply systems, and sanitary education are the major endemic causes of malaria, onchocerciasis, and dengue fever (including hemorrhagic dengue, which is more severe). Ecuador also has endemic diseases such as leishmaniasis in certain areas of the country's northern coastline. Infections, malnutrition, and dehydration are the main causes of death among children in Ecuador. In the southern part of the country near the Peruvian border is a famous valley, Vilcabamba, which is noteworthy for the longevity of its dwellers. This valley has been the focus of in-depth studies by many universities around the world. Transmission of AIDS is still fairly low in Ecuador. The World Health Organization's (WHO) estimated prevalence rate for HIV/AIDS in adults ages 15 to 49 is 0.29%. The estimated number of children from birth to 15 years living with HIV/AIDS is 330.

Health Team Relationships: The health care system is dominated by doctors, who are unquestioned, well-respected figures of authority. Patients do not have the confidence to express themselves to, complain to, or request explanations from doctors because of this power balance. Practitioners from other regions of the country are obliged by law to provide service for 1 or 2 years in rural areas. However, these rural doctors are viewed as outsiders and mistrusted by rural inhabitants, which undermines the relationship between doctor and patient. In contrast, traditional healers (*curanderos*) are widely accepted in the family and communities because they usually build up a special, holistic relationship with patients, and involve family members and friends in the healing process. This has encouraged the government to incorporate traditional healers into the public health care system, although as yet these efforts have only been successful with the traditional birth attendants, or midwives (*parteras*), who receive training from the Ministry of Public Health. Patients prefer practitioners of the same sex and older practitioners.

Families' Role in Hospital Care: The family of a hospitalized patient actively helps care for and feed a relative who has been admitted to a hospital. They often help other patients who have no relatives, participate in cleaning chores in the hospital, and are generally willing and ready to cooperate. In the health services of the Ministry of Public Health, families are required to cover all the expenses for hospitalization, tests, and medication that the patient might need. A government commission regulates the prices of medicines. Because of high prices, attempts are being made to introduce locally produced generic medicines as an alternative to high-cost imports.

Dominance Patterns: The family structure is patriarchal, with men dominating family decision making. Still, women have become more independent, especially those in middle-class families. Women play a major role in taking care of the household, especially in situations involving health and disease. Mothers provide homemade remedies, ensure cohesion of the extended family (especially when taking care of the ill and the older relatives), and decide when to resort to using a doctor or health care service.

Eye Contact Practices: In rural sectors, direct eye contact is avoided, especially with women and children because of their vulnerability to being spooked or bewitched (from *mal de ojo*, or evil eye). Otherwise, the traditional downcast gaze of rural dwellers is gradually disappearing, especially in the cities.

Touch Practices: Closeness and touching are common among family and friends and especially with children, who are believed to receive protection from the evil eye through physical contact. Kissing and embracing are also frequent in all strata of society and among all ages to express trust, friendliness, and affection, although rural Andean dwellers tend to be more reserved, less expressive, and even brusque.

Perceptions of Time: Traditionally time has been extremely elastic and imprecise. People arrive late for appointments and social gatherings. "Yesterday" may sometimes mean "several weeks ago" and "tomorrow" may mean "tomorrow," "in a week," "next year," or "never." A person greeting a friend after a long separation is likely to say, "Call me so we can get together" or "I'll be calling you." Often, no phone call follows. However, during the last few years, urban life has required all people—of all ages and social classes—to be more punctual. Nevertheless, people in low-income groups continue to postpone seeking medical care until their disease is quite severe.

Pain Reactions: Because people traditionally delay seeking medical care in the hopes that homemade remedies or time will heal them, they generally show great resistance to pain. They also feel uncomfortable expressing their discomfort or pain to doctors or health care personnel. However, during childbirth, women are accustomed to screaming and shouting, although they usually do so at regular intervals with rhythmic breathing that helps relieve the pain. However, these reactions are only common among rural or marginal urban people.

Birth Rites: In the most remote villages, births are attended by traditional birth attendants, or midwives, who are usually women who live in the village and receive periodic training from the Ministry of Public Health of Ecuador.

Death Rites: When a patient is dying, family members take turns keeping the person company 24 hours a day. After the person's death, the family often cries loudly, screams, shows expressive gestures of grief, and may even show hyperkinetic behavior and have seizures, although these reactions prevail mostly among people in rural or lower-income urban groups. Mourning lasts overnight and often is an opportunity for friends and family to get together and tell jokes, gossip, and talk about politics while drinking coffee or a hot cinnamon beverage with liquor, rum, or whisky, a practice that is common among all social classes. All Souls' Day is a holiday for remembering the dead and visiting the tombs of dead relatives in cemeteries or church vaults.

Food Practices and Intolerances: In the sierra the diet is composed mainly of beef, pork, or chicken. Guinea pigs, a typical delicacy, are also eaten. On the coast the staple foods are fish, rice, plantains and bananas, tuna, and shrimp, which are also the country's major agricultural export products. The Ecuadorian sierra has an abundance of potatoes, corn, and vegetables. An ancestral food combination, which modern nutritional experts have stated to be highly nutritional because it increases protein intake, is a mixture of cereals and legumes, such as rice with lentils or beans, grilled corn kernels (*tostado*) with edible lupine seeds (*chochos*), and specially prepared maize kernels (*mote*) with broad beans (*habas*). These dishes have been part of the Andean diet for millennia. Some farms are highly developed and produce high-quality meat and dairy products.

Infant Feeding Practices: Breast-feeding is the norm among all social classes and frequently lasts until the child's first birthday.

Child Rearing Practices: Birth control methods are widely used by all women except for the poorest rural dwellers. Children are expected to be obedient and listen to their parents, older adults, and older brothers and sisters. Boys have more freedom than girls, who are usually expected to lead more sheltered lives.

National Childhood Immunizations: BCG at birth; DPT at 2, 4, and 6 months and 1 to 4 years; OPV at 2, 4, and 6 months and 1 to 4 years; hep B at birth and at 2 and 6 months; measles at 9 to 11 months; MMR at 12 to 23 months; YFV at 1 and 10 years; and Td after first contact CBAW, +4, +1, +6 months, and +2 years.

Other Characteristics: Ecuador is a developing country with a highly imbalanced distribution of wealth; 20% of the population has 60% of the wealth, and more than 20% have access to only 2% of the wealth. Ecuadorian archaeology is the oldest in the Andean region. The oldest culture is the Valdivia culture, which developed between 3990 and 2300 BC. It is noteworthy for its two-headed sculptures, which are believed to represent hallucinations induced by the consumption of various plants. During the period known as *Regional Development* between 500 BC and 700 AD, the peoples who had settled in Ecuador produced a wide variety of ceramics, providing impressive evidence of the magical and religious beliefs of the time and indications of how health and disease were viewed. They believed the head was the center of all intellectual powers and magical forces, therefore deformation of the cranium, head shrinking, and trepanation were common. Head shrinking was initially practiced by the people of the Tolita culture, but now only a few ethnic groups in the Amazon region practice this custom, which is mostly used with the heads of animals. The shrunken heads (referred to as *tzantzas*) are used as ceremonial ornaments or war trophies.

BIBLIOGRAPHY

Cruz M: Historia de las Neurociencias en América. In Salvador DO, ed: *Salud: historia y cultura de América*, pp 152–157, Quito, Ecuador, 1992, Editorial Abya Ayala.

Normas Técnico Administrativas del Programa Ampliado de Inmunización, Ministerio de Salud Pública, Quito, Ecuador, 1989.

World Health Organization (June 2000): Epidemiological fact sheets by country, Geneva. Retrieved March 1, 2002, from http://www.unaids.org/hivaidsinfo/statistics/june00/fact_sheets/index.html

World Health Organization (2001): *WHO vaccine-preventable diseases: monitoring system*, Geneva. Retrieved March 1, 2002, from http://www.who.int/vaccines/

◆ EGYPT (ARAB REPUBLIC OF)

MAP PAGE (862)

Khaled Ahmed Nagaty

Location: Egypt is in the northeast corner of Africa on the Mediterranean Sea. The total land area is 1,001,450 km^2 (386,660 square miles). It is bordered on the west by Libya, on the south by Sudan, and on the east by Israel and the Red Sea. Most of its citizens reside in the Nile River Valley because 97% of the country is desert.

Major Languages	Ethnic Groups	Major Religions
Arabic	Eastern Hamitic 99%	Sunni Mouslim 94%
English	Other 1%	Other 6%
French		

Health Care Beliefs: Passive involvement; traditional. The belief that Allah dictates health promotes a passive and sometimes contradictory situation because a patient may do the opposite of what a doctor advises. Islamic teachings coexist with modern medical practices. The concept of disease prevention is becoming more accepted.

Predominant Sick Care Practices: Biomedical and magical-religious. Egyptians accept the biomedical model of illness, and Western medical practices are well accepted. However, they also accept magical-religious explanations for ill health such as "the evil eye" (the power of a person to harm others merely by looking at them), although Islam prohibits it. For example, a common traditional treatment to treat illness is the practice of using a new razor blade (new to prevent transmission of blood diseases) to make scratches on the back and then heating cups and applying them to the skin to extract "bad blood." During another traditional practice, a person makes a doll from a piece of paper. The person makes holes in the doll while mentioning the names of the people who envy the person. The doll is then burned. This practice is considered magic; Islam strictly prohibits it and considers its practitioners infidels. Injections and intravenous fluids are perceived as more effective than oral medication, and self-medication is the norm. Pharmacists can prescribe drugs without a physician's consent. Amulets inscribed with verses of the Koran, turquoise stones, hanging a baby's shoe in a car where it can easily be seen or on a key chain, or placing a horseshoe on the door of a house are believed to provide protection from the "evil eye". Though the government combats such traditions, even educated people seem to at least partially believe in them. Expressions such as "this is God's will," "the great God," or "touch wood" or carrying a charm of a hand with five fingers are believed to enhance one's protective powers against the evil eye. Mental illness is particularly feared. The biomedical and the traditional views are both well ingrained and are important to consider when providing health care. Hope, optimism, and the positive advantages of treatment should be stressed when discussing outcomes.

Ethnic/Race Specific or Endemic Diseases: Chloroquine-sensitive bilharzia is an endemic disease. In villages, peasants wash their cattle in canals, and children swim in these canals, which contain stagnant and polluted water. Women who are not aware of the health consequences of using the polluted canal water also wash their kitchen utensils or family clothes in it. This leads to widespread infection in the countryside with these harmful worms. Egyptians are also at risk for schistosomiasis. The World Health Organization's (WHO) estimated prevalence rate for HIV/AIDS in adults ages 15 to 49 is 0.02%. WHO has no estimates for children from birth to 15 years living with HIV/AIDS.

Health Team Relationships: When health practitioners are assessing patients, they should clarify the reasons they are asking personal questions. In addition, patients do not openly express their feelings to doctors when an illness is emotional or sexual in origin. Men may refuse care by female doctors or nurses, especially if their problem is a sexual one. Women also may refuse care for intimate health problems by male doctors. It is not considered a serious issue if a patient discontinues treatment with a particular health provider on the basis of gender. Patients' rights are respected, but it is customary for family members to inform their loved ones when a patient's diagnosis is grave. Occasionally, a family will not tell a patient about serious diagnosis to protect the person from fear and pain. Physicians are the primary decision makers. Nurses do not diagnose illnesses or prescribe treatments. The role of the nurse is to take care of the patient and provide prescribed treatments. The government supports health care, but people with sufficient incomes prefer to seek more adequate health services in private hospitals or Western countries. Wealthy citizens have built charity clinics and small hospitals in the mosques for poor people. Some of these clinics are more advanced than others and have radiography and surgery services.

Families' Role in Hospital Care: In Egypt, family and friends visit patients as often as possible to ensure that health care personnel care for the patients properly. In Islam culture, it is common for a close family member to stay with and care for a patient, especially at night. In villages in particular or in public hospitals in the city, food may be brought to hospitalized patients to ensure they are well fed. It is not uncommon for family members to be present during patient interviews and examinations, and they may answer questions addressed to the patient. Health care professionals should include in discussions the oldest family member present. Taking individual responsibility for health actions and signing informed consent forms are usually reserved for those with the most knowledge, therefore the patriarch of the family or another respected individual rather than the patient may give consent to the surgeon.

Dominance Patterns: Egypt has a patriarchal and male-dominated society. However, women have access to higher education and professional careers. Though the law that mandated wearing a veil was overturned decades ago, many women still choose to wear one. Some women retain their surname after marriage. It is common for wealthy families to have one or more maids in their homes.

Eye Contact Practices: It is common for Egyptians to observe and evaluate the eyes of others at close range (approximately 2 ft) during conversations. Dilation of the pupil is equated with interest in the conversation, whereas contraction is interpreted as dislike. Religious individuals only make direct eye contact with members of the same sex.

Touch Practices: Although touch is an important part of communication in Egypt, it is limited to members of the same sex. Men and women may shake hands, but religious women may wear gloves, cover their hands with their veils, or refuse to shake hands with men.

Perceptions of Time: A verse in the Koran says, "Do not say for a thing that 'I'll do this tomorrow' except if God wills." Time is oriented to the present because planning ahead could be in defiance of God's will. Talking about the future must be preceded or ended with the expression "if God wills," as dictated by the Koran.

Pain Reactions: Except during childbirth or after extensive surgery, pain is usually expressed privately or in the company of close relatives or friends. Pain medications may be taken because pain is anticipated and feared, so hospitalized patients may persistently request drugs and expect immediate relief. This practice does not mean that a patient is addicted. In addition, patients believe that exertion when ill impedes recovery, so they rely on considerable assistance from their nurses and may be reluctant to perform self-help activities. Long-term therapies are often not well received by Egyptian patients.

Birth Rites: Newborns are swaddled and dressed in a shirt called a *jalabiya* that is made by relatives, and the grandmother stays close to the mother during the mother's hospital stay. A celebration that is sponsored by the grandparents is held on the seventh day after birth, and males are circumcised on the seventh or fortieth day.

Death Rites: Hope is valued; confronting a patient with a grave diagnosis shatters hope and creates mistrust. It is believed that only God knows a patient's true prognosis, so people are not supposed to speak of death. Health care professionals may be asked to keep a patient who has a terminal illness from knowing the truth. Near the time of death, Muslims help the patient recite the Declaration of the Faith (i.e., the *Monatism*: "There is no God but God, and Muhammad is God's messenger.") Although expressive and vocal wailing is traditional and acceptable, it has recently become inappropriate because Islam prohibits it. One of the family members may stay in the room with the body and recite versus of the Koran. God is asked to forgive the deceased and allow the person to go to heaven. The family also reflects on the person's accomplishments. It is common for women to give their condolences at the house of the deceased for at least 3 days after the death. Men give their condolences at the funeral or the next night at a specified place. Family members wash the body according to Islamic tradition. Organ donations and transplants are allowed, and Muslim doctors may recommend transfusions to save lives. Autopsies are uncommon except for forensic reasons because the body must be buried intact; cremation is not permitted. After the funeral, Muslim burial practices involve wrapping the body in special pieces of cloth (preferably white) and burial without a coffin in the ground.

Food Practices and Intolerances: The evening meal is eaten at approximately 10 pm, and pork, carrion, and blood are forbidden. Food tends to be spicy. During Ramadan, except for those who are sick, children, and travelers, people traditionally fast between sunrise and sunset. Charity food tables are set up in the country and cities for the poor during Ramadan. Common foods include *tamiya* (beans fried in oil), *foul* (beans), *koshary* (a mixture of rice, pasta, and lentils), and *molokai* (from a green plant whose leaves are cooked as soup). Hands are used to eat food that is in a loaf, and rice, *koshary*, and pasta are eaten with spoons. Forks, spoons, and knives are used in restaurants and at banquets.

Infant Feeding Practices: Breast-feeding is extremely common and continues for 2 years in villages; in the cities, weaning occurs sooner. When a child refuses to transition to normal foods, several methods may be used to discourage the desire to breast-feed, such as covering the nipples with a bitter substance or putting hair on them. Sugar water and more recently glucose is introduced at a young age, with the introduction of hot beverages such as anise, peppermint, caraway, cinnamon, and *tillio* as soon as 40 days after birth. Soft foods such as yogurt with honey; apple, pear, and orange juices; and corn flakes with milk are introduced after 4 months. After 6 months, well-cooked pieces of chicken and soup with vegetables are introduced.

Child Rearing Practices: Child rearing tends to be permissive. The hymen is viewed as the ultimate proof of virginity, and female circumcision is believed to decrease a teenage girl's lust for sex. The practice is widespread in villages and remote areas (90%) and less so in cities (2%).

The procedure is generally done when a girl is 7 or 8 years old or 1 year after menarche begins. A law prohibiting this practice was passed in 1996, and doctors in cities are forbidden to do the procedure. However, in villages it may be done secretly in private clinics.

National Childhood Immunizations: BCG by 3 months; DPT at 2, 4, 6, and 18 months; OPV at 2, 4, 6, 9, and 18 months; measles at 9 months; MMR at 18 months; hep B at 2, 4, and 6 months; and TT for pregnant women.

Other Characteristics: When making contracts, a verbal consent is equal to a written consent. Pressing for written consent suggests mistrust of a verbal contract and is an insult.

BIBLIOGRAPHY

Fullerton JT, Sukkary-Stolba S: Advancing the status of nursing in Egypt: the project to promote the development of the High Institutes of Nursing, *Int J Nurs Stud* 32(5):518, 1995.

Galanti GA: *Caring for patients from different cultures*, ed 2, Philadelphia, 1997, University of Pennsylvania Press.

Harrison GG et al: Breastfeeding and weaning in a poor urban neighborhood in Cairo, Egypt: maternal beliefs and perceptions, *Soc Sci Med* 36(8):1063, 1993.

Mansour E et al: Integration of hepatitis B immunization in the expanded program on immunization of the child survival project, *J Egypt Public Health Assoc* 68(5–6):487, 1993.

Younis TA, el-Sharkawy IM, Youssef FG: Prevalence of intestinal parasites in filariasis endemic areas in Egypt, *J Egypt Soc Parasitol* 27(1):291, 1997.

www.unaids.org/hivaidsinfo/statistics/june00fact_sheets/index.html

www.who.int/vaccines/

◆ EL SALVADOR (REPUBLIC OF)

MAP PAGE (857)

Mary-Elizabeth Reeve (Consultant: Erin Conrad)

Location: The smallest of the Central American countries, El Salvador is situated along the Pacific coast. The total land area is 21,040 km² (8,124 square miles). Much of the land is fertile volcanic plateau. The country is divided into 14 departments, the most densely populated of which is San Salvador, where 30.7% of the population lives. Because of its geographical position and geology, El Salvador has frequent natural disasters such as hurricanes, floods, and earthquakes. El Salvador sustained tremendous damage and loss of life from Hurricane Mitch in October 1998 and two major earthquakes in January and February 2001.

Major Languages	Ethnic Groups	Major Religions
Spanish	Mestizo 90%	Roman Catholic 75%
Indigenous languages	Amerindian 7%	Protestant and other 25%
	White 3%	

Indigenous languages include Kekchí (Mayan), Lenca, and Pipil (Uto-Aztecan); Lenca and Pipil are nearly extinct. A high percentage of people are young; 37% are younger than 15 years of age. The literacy rate among men is 81.6% and among women is 76.1%. The recent history of El Salvador has been marked by a civil war that lasted from 1980 to 1992. During this time, more than 80,000 people died or disappeared, and more than 1 million became refugees.

Health Care Beliefs: Acute sick care; traditional, with increasing focus on prevention. Local health promoters carry out preventive care in many rural areas. Where access to local health promoters and local health centers is limited, preventive care does not exist. Mental illness is not feared, nor is it particularly stigmatized. Mental disorders are a significant cause of mortality, with alcoholism being the most common disorder.

Predominant Sick Care Practices: Biomedical and magical-religious. Health care practice is predominantly biomedical. However, in the rural areas, folk remedies, curers (*curanderos*), and massagers (*gente que soban*) continue to be important sources of care. For every 10,000 inhabitants, El Salvador has 9.1 physicians, 5.4 midwives, 3.8 nurses, and 2.1 dentists. Approximately 60% of all doctors, nurses, and dentists are concentrated in the capital city, San Salvador. The Ministry of Public Health and Social Welfare services include 16 hospitals, 14 health centers, 313 health units, 32 health posts, 11 community posts, 8 dispensaries, and 33 rural nutrition centers. Approximately 80% of the population is assigned to the ministry, although actual usage is less. About 17% of the population has access to social security (ISSS) health services. In 1994 to 1997, it was estimated that 56% of pregnant women received some prenatal care, and trained personnel attended 62% of deliveries. Because access to health care services is more limited in rural areas, rural inhabitants may rely more on traditional medical practices.

Ethnic/Race Specific or Endemic Diseases: Diseases of special concern in the country include dengue, malaria, tuberculosis, and AIDS. An epidemic of dengue occurred in 1995, with 9529 cases of dengue fever and 129 cases of dengue hemorrhagic fever. Malaria is predominantly chloroquine-sensitive *Plasmodium vivax*. The latest available Pan American Health Organization (PAHO) statistics (2001 update) report an annual malaria parasitic index of 0.3. In 1996 the malaria incidence rate was 29 per 100,000. Tuberculosis continues to be a serious health problem, and a total of 1623 registered cases were reported in the PAHO 2001 update. In 1995 the tuberculosis incidence rate was 29 per 100,000. In general, indigenous populations in Latin America are the most underserved, and rural inhabitants have less access to health care than those living in urban areas. Disparities in basic sanitation also exist. For El Salvador as a whole, 53% of the population has access to the public water supply and 69% to waste disposal. In urban areas, 86% of the population has access to a public water supply, 57% to a sewage system, and 25% to latrines. In rural areas, only 17% of the population has access to a public water supply, and 56% of the population depends on latrines. HIV and AIDS are an increasing threat. The 2001 PAHO update reported 425 registered cases of AIDS for the year. The World Health Organization's (WHO) estimated prevalence rate for HIV/AIDS in adults ages 15 to 49 is 0.60%. The estimated number of children from birth to 15 years living with HIV/AIDS is 560. The annual incidence of AIDS has been increasing since the early 1990s. The predominant route of HIV transmission is sexual contact, with more than 75% of cases resulting from heterosexual exposure. UNAIDS estimated the total number of men and women ages 15 to 49 with HIV infection to be 19,000 at the end of 1999. The estimated number of deaths from AIDS in 1999 was 1300. For the population as a whole, mortality rates from diseases of the circulatory system, external causes, and communicable diseases are the highest. Mortality under registration was estimated at 21% in 1994.

Health Team Relationships: Doctors retain a superior role, although information is shared between doctors and nurses. In rural and urban areas, people do not trust the medical capabilities of doctors or nurses.

Families' Role in Hospital Care: Families are not allowed to stay with sick patients in public hospitals and may only visit during visiting hours (although they do bring food to hospitalized family members).

Dominance Patterns: Men are dominant, particularly in the public sphere.

Eye Contact Practices: No particular eye contact avoidance patterns exist.

Touch Practices: In rural areas, physical touching is uncommon, even in couples.

Perceptions of Time: People are generally very punctual, particularly for appointments such as medical appointments.

Pain Reactions: All people in El Salvador, both men and women, tend to have a high tolerance for pain and discomfort.

Birth Rites: Treatment varies depending on whether the birth takes place with a midwife (*partera*) in a hospital or clinic. Women observe special dietary restrictions during the *dieta* after the birth of a child. The infant mortality rate is estimated to be 35 per 1,000 live births. A higher rate of postneonatal mortality exists in rural versus urban areas. The most common cause of death is reported to be conditions originating in the perinatal period. The mortality rate of children younger than 5 years is estimated to be 38.5 per 1000. Acute respiratory tract infections and intestinal infectious diseases are the most common causes of death for children younger than 5 years. The leading cause of outpatient medical appointments for infants and children younger than 5 is acute respiratory tract infection, followed by intestinal parasitic diseases. Almost half of deaths among adolescents are from external causes, with the second leading cause being diseases of the circulatory system. The maternal mortality rate is 120 per 100,000 live births.

Death Rites: When a family member dies, the family normally "accompanies" the dead person during a celebration. Organ donation is not a widely accepted practice.

Food Practices and Intolerances: Principal foods include rice, beans, and tortillas. Protein sources include small quantities of meat, eggs, cheese, and cream. Sugary drinks are popular with children.

Infant Feeding Practices: Women prefer to breast-feed their infants; however, those with jobs outside the home are forced to rely more on bottle-feeding. About 25% of infants are exclusively breast-fed in the first 4 months, and more than 75% are given complementary foods between 6 and 9 months. More than half of all infants breast-feed for 12 to 15 months, and 40% of infants breast-feed until they are 2 years of age.

Child Rearing Practices: Children make important economic contributions to the household, particularly in rural areas and extremely poor urban neighborhoods. Parents tend to be strict with children, and children are obedient. Children share sleeping quarters with their siblings and parents.

National Childhood Immunizations: BCG at birth; DTP at 2, 3, 4, and 15 months and a4 to 5 years; OPV at birth and 2, 3, 4, and 15 months and 4 to 5 years; hep B for high-risk children only; measles at 9 months; and MMR at 15 months to 2 years. Vaccination coverage rates are high for children younger than 1 year. In the mid-1990s, 98% of children younger than 1 year were being vaccinated against poliomyelitis and 97% against measles; 100% received BCG and DPT in 1995. As of 1997, three national vaccination campaigns were being carried out each year.

BIBLIOGRAPHY

El Salvador. In Health in the Americas: Vol II, Pan American Health Organization Scientific Publication No. 569, Washington, DC, 1998, PAHO.

Ethnologue report for El Salvador: languages of El Salvador. Retrieved February 15, 2002, from http://www.ethnologue.com/show_country.asp?name=El+Salvador.

International Planned Parenthood Federation country profile: El Salvador. Retrieved June 7, 2000, from http://www.ippf.org/regions/countries/slv/index.htm.

Pan American Heath Organization country health profile: El Salvador. Retrieved February 15, 2002, from http://www.paho.org/English/SHAprflELS.htm.

Personal communication, Erin Conrad, San Salvador, El Salvador, January 2002.

Salud de los pueblos indígenas: orientación de los marcos jurídicos hacia la abogacía en salud de los pueblos indígenas: Pan American Heath Organization: División de Desarrollo de Sistemas y Servicios de Salud, Washington, DC, 1998, PAHO.

UNAIDS and the World Health Organization epidemiological fact sheet, 2000 update: El Salvador: Retrieved February 21, 2002, from http://www.unaids.org/hivaidsinfo/statistics/fact_sheets/pdfs/Elsalvador_en.pdf Accessed 2-21-02.

USAID Center for International Health Information: *Country health statistical profile for El Salvador*. Retrieved June 7, 2000, from http://www.cihi.com/PHANstat/EL_SALVADOR.

USAID Center for International Health Information: *El Salvador country health profile report, December 1996*, Washington, DC, 1996, USAID.

World Health Organization: *WHOSIS basic health indicators: El Salvador*. Retrieved June 7, 2000, from http://www3.who.int.whosis/reported/reported_process.cfm?path=statistics,basic,reported,endpoint&language=english.

◆ EQUATORIAL GUINEA (REPUBLIC OF)

MAP PAGE (863)

Location: Equatorial Guinea is on the western coast of Africa between Cameroon and Gabon, where coastal plains give rise to interior hills. The Gulf of Guinea is to the west. The mainland area of Equatorial Guinea is called Mbini, which is on the western coast, and its principle city is Bata. The country also has the coastal islets of Corisco, Elobey Grande, and Elobey Chico, as well as the islands of Bioko (where the capital, Malabo, is located) and Annobon in the Gulf of Guinea. The total land area is 28,051 km^2 (10,831 square miles), slightly smaller than Maryland. The country has hot, humid, rainy, tropical weather and thick vegetation. The population is about 486,060, and about 75% of the people make their living by subsistence agriculture supplemented by hunting and fishing. About 43% of the population is between infancy and 14 years. Barter is a way of life. Equatorial Guinea is a developing country and poverty is severe, with a gross domestic product (GDP) per capita of $2000.

Major Languages	Ethnic Groups	Major Religions
Spanish (official)	Fang 83%	Roman Catholic 85%
French (official)	Bioko (primarily Bubi)	Traditional African 15%
Pidgin English	Rio Muni (primarily	
Fang, Bubi, and	Fang)	
Ibo	Europeans (mostly	
	Spanish)	

Fang, a Bantu language, is the most widely spoken indigenous language. Literacy rates are 89.6% for males and 68.1% for females. Most government control resides with the individuals of the majority Fang tribe. Many people are believed to be living abroad because of the unstable political conditions.

Health Care Beliefs: Acute sick care; traditional. The Fang people hold strongly to traditions such as black magic. Sorcerers are important community members. Ceremonies such as the *abira* ceremony are used to cleanse the community of evil. Traditions strongly influence conceptions about the causes and treatment of illness, and traditional methods may be used before modern medical practices.

Predominant Sick Care Practices: Magical-religious; biomedical treatment limited. Many economic aid programs, which were greatly beneficial for the health care infrastructure, have been cut off because of gross corruption and mismanagement by the government—creating considerable impediments to health care access and specific programs of disease prevention. Medical facilities are extremely limited. Pharmacies in Malabo and Bata are well stocked, but medications are often impossible to obtain in many other areas. The country has no trauma center, so travelers in the country who have serious accidents or illnesses are evacuated to another country if possible.

Ethnic/Race Specific or Endemic Diseases: Chloroquine-resistant falciparum and plasmodium malaria are hyperendemic in Equatorial Guinea. Other endemic diseases include HIV type 1, yellow fever, cholera, schistosomiasis, *Loa loa*, hepatitis (A, B, and E), and onchocerciasis (river blindness). People are at risk for trypanosomiasis (sleeping sickness), meningococcal meningitis, rabies, tetanus, polio, typhoid fever, dysentery from *Giardia* and other parasites, fungal infections, tuberculosis, diphtheria, and typhus. Injury and death from vehicular accidents are also a threat because roads are poorly maintained. Visitors who are involved in an accident with a local person may receive "village justice," putting them in danger of immediate physical retribution. The World Health Organization's (WHO) estimated prevalence rate for HIV/AIDS in adults ages 15 to 49 is 0.51%. The estimated number of children from birth to 15 years living with HIV/AIDS is less than 100. WHO estimates that 120 adults and children died of AIDS in 1999, and about 1000 were living with HIV/AIDS. In 1996, 1% of women who went to an antenatal clinic in Malabo and Bata were infected with HIV, and 3% and 29% of patients who went to a clinic for sexually transmitted diseases in Malabo and Bata, respectively, were infected.

Birth Rites: Equatorial Guinea has 37.72 births per 1000 people, and the infant mortality rate is 92.9 deaths per 1000 live births. The total fertility rate is 4.88 children born per woman. Life expectancy at birth is 51.89 for males and 56.07 for females.

Food Practices and Intolerances: Cassava (tapioca) and sweet potatoes are the staple foods. Other frequently consumed items are coffee, cocoa, and bananas. The tap water is not potable.

National Childhood Immunizations: BCG at birth; DTP at 6, 10, and 14 weeks; OPV at birth and 6, 10, and 14 weeks; measles at 9 months; and TT CBAW for pregnant women. The reported percentages of the target population vaccinated are as follows: BCG, 34; first dose of DPT, 39; third dose of DTP, 32; MCV, 19; Pol3, 32; and TT2 plus, 30.

Other Characteristics: The discovery and exploitation of large oil reserves has contributed to rapid economic growth in recent years.

BIBLIOGRAPHY

Basaras M et al: Seroprevalence of hepatitis B and C, and human immunodeficiency type 1 viruses in a rural population from the Republic of Equatorial Guinea, *Trans Roy Soc Trop Med Hygiene* 93(3):250, 1999.

Boussinesq M, Gardon J: Prevalences of *Loa loa* microfilaraemia throughout the area endemic for infection, *Ann Trop Med Parasitol* 91(6):573, 1997.

Mas J: Prevalence, geographical distribution and clinical manifestations of onchocerciasis on the Island of Bioko, *Trop Med Parasitol* 46(1):13, 1995.

http://encarta.msn.com/find/Concise.asp?ti=04AF6000

http://www.odci.gov/cia/publications/factbook/geos/ek.html

http://travel.state.gov/equatorial_guinea.html

http://www.wtgonline.com/data/gnq/gnq080.asp

◆ ERITREA (STATE OF)

MAP PAGE (862)

Thomas Tolfvenstam and Tesfaldet Tecle

Location: Eritrea is located on the horn of Africa, covering a total land area of 121,000 km² (46,862 square miles) on the Red Sea coast, neighboring Ethiopia and Sudan to the west and Djibouti to the south. The central part of the country is mountainous with fertile agricultural valleys, whereas the coastal lowlands are hot, semiarid deserts. Eritrea is the youngest country in Africa and gained independence from Ethiopia in 1993 after 30 years of struggling. The country's population was estimated to be 4.3 million in 2000, and 20% of the population lives in urban areas. Partly because of the many years of civil unrest, the country is poor, with a gross domestic product (GDP) per capita of only $710. Eritrea is governed by the National Assembly, which was established as a transitional legislature in 1993, and also by the assembly-elected president. The constitution was ratified in 1997.

Major Languages	Ethnic Groups	Major Religions
Tigrinya (official)	Tigrinya 50%	Islam 50%
Arabic (official)	Tigre 25%	Eritrean Orthodox
English	Kanama 15%	Christianity 50%
	Afar 4%	
	Saho (inhabitants of Red Sea coast) 3%	
	Other 3%	

English is used in schools after the sixth grade. Some Italian is also used, a result of the Italian colonization from 1890 to 1941. The native languages belong to three distinct groups: Semitic languages such as Tigrinya (50%) and Tigre (25%), both closely related to Ethiopian Amhar written by the ancient Geez characters; Cuschitic languages such as Afar, Beja, and Saho, spoken by the ethnic groups of the same names; and Nilotic langages such as Kunama and Baria. Eritrea is a multiethnic nation with nine major ethnic groups. The Tigrinya dominate politics and culture, and the Tigre populate the northern highlands. The smaller ethnic groups include the Afar, Kunama, Bilen, Saho, Hadarb, Nara, and Rashaida. Christianity includes primarily Muslims and orthodox Christians, as well as a few Roman Catholics and Protestants. Christianity is the religion of the Tigrinya ethnic group, whereas Islam is the primary religion of the other ethnic groups. A few rural tribes still practice traditional African religions.

Health Care Beliefs: Acute sick care; traditional. Traditionally, a uvulectomy is performed to prevent respiratory diseases. Scarring of the skin around the eyes is thought to prevent eye infections. Men and women are both circumcised, and genital mutilations have been reported in 95% of Eritrean women. Afflictions or illnesses may be attributed to transgressions against God or sorcery motivated by envy.

Predominant Sick Care Practices: Biomedical and ethnic-medical beliefs. People predominantly tend to seek medical care from doctors or practitioners at local health care clinics. The country has few medical doctors (1 per 35,000 inhabitants), therefore minor medical assistance is provided by local nonprofessional knowledgeable individuals whose therapeutic arsenal may include such treatments as traditional herbs.

Ethnic/Race Specific or Endemic Diseases: Infectious diseases dominate the disease panorama in Eritrea; malaria, tuberculosis, and hepatitis B are widespread. Studies of the Rashaida minority tribe have revealed a particularly low seroprevalence of rubella and varicella, a fact that could be important when isolated tribes are incorporated into the society. Furthermore, malnutrition, anemia, intestinal parasites, and respiratory disorders are common. The World Health Organization's (WHO) estimated prevalence rate for HIV/AIDS in adults ages 15 to 49 is 2.87%, which is lower than the rate in many other parts of Africa. WHO has no reported estimates for children. The seroprevalence of HIV type 1 in female sex workers was reported to be 26%, whereas no HIV was found among the secluded Rashaidas. Life expectancy has increased in recent years because of better medical facilities and health care information campaigns and has been estimated to be 56.18 years.

Health Team Relationships: The doctor dominates the health care team. Because the time spent on consultations is limited because of the shortage of doctors, patients' attitudes can be repressive.

Families' Role in Hospital Care: Hospitals provide food and staff to help with the patients' general sanitary needs in the major cities. In rural areas, hospital care depends on the families, who provide food and support for the patients' basic needs during hospitalizations.

Dominance Patterns: Eritrean families are traditionally patriarchal, and the women are primarily responsible for domestic duties. However, during the long war, women fought side by side with men, so attitudes toward women became more permissive. (Women comprised a third of the country's 100,000 soldiers.)

Eye Contact Practices: Eritreans avoid direct eye contact with strangers, authority figures, and older people.

Touch Practices: Strangers of both sexes shake hands, and touching practices are liberal among friends. Men may greet each other by hugging and women by reciprocal kisses on the cheeks.

Perceptions of Time: Perhaps because of the long war, the Eritreans anticipate the future. Public communications are fairly punctual, and punctuality in general is not disregarded.

Pain Reactions: Stoical reactions to pain are common. For instance, in the Afar culture, men are judged by the bravery with which they bear the pain of circumcision.

Birth Rites: Midwives and traditional birth attendants from within the community assist in childbirth. If a newborn is a boy, he is celebrated on the third day after birth (or on the seventh day if a girl) by friends, neighbors, and relatives, who bring presents to the mother and child. Traditionally, *gheat*, a dough made of flour and water and served with butter, spices, and sour milk, is served during the celebration. The infant mortality rate is still high: 74.14 deaths per 1000 live births.

Death Rites: Twelve days of mourning are usual. Friends, relatives, and neighbors pay their condolences. Both organ donations (which are very rare) and autopsies are accepted but require the consent of close relatives.

Food Practices and Intolerances: Food is traditionally served on a big platter on the center of the table, and people eat from it with their hands. *Ingera*, a type of pancake, is often used to scoop up the food from the platter. The diet varies depending on religious beliefs. For example, Muslims do not eat pork.

Infant Feeding Practices: Infants are usually breast-fed for 1 or 2 years.

Child Rearing Practices: Children have a strict upbringing. Physical punishment is used, primarily by the father. Children are expected to obey their parents, respect older adults, and help at home without being asked.

National Childhood Immunizations: BCG at birth to 11 months; DPT at 6 weeks to 11 months × 3; OPV at birth and at 6 weeks to 11 months × 3; measles at 9 to 11 months; and TT for pregnant women and CBAW. Immunization coverage reported in 1999 was as follows: BCG, 98%; DPT, 93%; polio, 93%; and measles, 88% fully immunized 1-year-old children.

BIBLIOGRAPHY

CIA: *The world factbook—Eritrea: 2002*. www.odci.gov/cia/publications/factbook/geos/er.html

Eritrea: epidemiological fact sheets on HIV/AIDS and sexually transmitted infections, revised, 2000 UNAIDS and the World Health Organization.

Ghebrekidan H et al: Prevalence of herpes simplex virus types 1 and 2, cytomegalovirus, and varicella-zoster virus infections in Eritrea, *J Clin Virol* 12(1):53–64, 1999.

Ghebrekidan H et al: Prevalence of infection with HIV, hepatitis B and C viruses, in four high risk groups in Eritrea, *Clin Diag Virol* 9(1):29–35, 1998.

Tolfvenstam T et al: Seroprevalence of viral childhood infections in Eritrea, *J Clin Virol* 16(1):49–54, 2000.

UNICEF statistics—Africa: 2002, www.unicef.org/statis.html

World Health Organization: *Women's health 2002*, www.who.int/frh-whd/

◆ ESTONIA (REPUBLIC OF)

MAP PAGE (861)

Laima M. Karosas

Location: Bordering on the Baltic Sea to its north and west, Estonia is mainly a lowland country with numerous lakes in northeastern Europe. Lake Peipus is Estonia's largest lake and important for the shipping and fish industries. It is bordered on the north and northeast by the Gulf of Finland, on the southeast by the Russian Federation, on the southwest by Latvia, and on the northwest by the Baltic Sea. The total land area is 45,100 km^2 (17,413 square miles).

Major Languages	Ethnic Groups	Major Religions
Estonian (official)	Estonian 62%	Lutheran 78%
Russian	Russian 30%	Orthodox Christian 19%
	Ukrainian 3%	Other or none 3%
	Belorussian 2%	
	Finn 1%	
	Other 2%	

Health Care Beliefs: Acute sick care; traditional. Although the need for prevention is understood, resources are first allocated to crisis care and inpatient services.

Predominant Sick Care Practices: Biomedical, holistic, and magical-religious. The majority of people go to traditional practitioners, although biomedical, holistic, and magical-religious therapies are used. Older adults are more likely to consult folk healers.

Ethnic/Race Specific or Endemic Diseases: Cardiovascular disease is the biggest killer, but people are at risk for tuberculosis, nutritional deficiencies, hepatitis, influenza, and thyroid disorders. The World Health Organization's (WHO) estimated prevalence rate for HIV/AIDS in adults ages 15 to 49 is 0.04%. The estimated number of children from birth to 15 years living with HIV/AIDS is less than 100.

Health Team Relationships: Patient care is doctor directed, with increasing nursing content identifiable in schools or practice. Nurses and doctors are predominantly women, and nurses follow doctors' orders. Nursing is emerging from 50 years of Soviet influence. Asking questions of the health care provider is becoming more common, and many people try to diagnose their own illnesses. Patients address health care professionals by title and last name. Patients may offer gifts to health care providers to ensure quality care.

Families' Role in Hospital Care: Family members are no longer expected to assist with bathing, feeding, comforting, and elimination. All health care needs are provided by doctors and nurses.

Dominance Patterns: Traditionally, the men assume a slightly more dominant role; however, the men and women share responsibilities in decision making. Women have taken on a more prominent role as their economic status has increased.

Eye Contact Practices: Direct eye contact is preferred in conversations between health care providers and patients.

Touch Practices: Touching is infrequent even within families. A handshake is common at the beginning and end of an interaction in a professional situation.

Perceptions of Time: People in health care are focused on the present and crisis management. Previous traditions, including how older adults healed illnesses, are important. Younger people are more future oriented. If a patient is not present when called for an appointment, the health provider calls the next patient; however, the patient may return to the line and be called later.

Pain Reactions: Pain tolerance is valued, although pain relief is both desired and requested. Verbal expressions of discomfort signify more severe pain. Although during labor some women may express their pain, many still attempt to keep silent and be stoical. Because of short supplies, pain medications may be limited or unavailable in the hospital.

Birth Rites: Almost all births occur in hospitals and are attended by doctors and possibly a midwife who may or may not be a nurse. The father may choose to be present during the delivery and is permitted to coach the mother's labor. Courses for natural childbirth and prenatal and postpartum care are becoming more popular. Circumcision is not practiced.

Death Rites: If an illness is fatal, the family of the patient is told; they decide whether the patient should be told. After death, an open coffin permits people to view the body for up to 3 days. Burial occurs on the third or fourth afternoon. Grief may be verbally expressed, and crying in public is acceptable. Cremation is not practiced.

Food Practices and Intolerances: The preferred main meal is lunch. Potatoes, seasonal vegetables, bread, meat, and soups are common. Large quantities of milk and other dairy products, tea, and coffee are consumed.

Infant Feeding Practices: Breast-feeding is encouraged more than bottle-feeding. Some women may choose not to breast-feed or will breast-feed for a short time to regain their prepregnancy physical condition more quickly. Foods are introduced at 4 to 5 months.

Child Rearing Practices: Children are cooperative and reared using disciplinary styles ranging from logical reasoning to authoritarian. The grandmother may have a valued position in child rearing, especially in rural and suburban single-parent families or families in which both parents work. Some children may have chores to do at home or be taught to rely more on their parents. Women are entitled maternity leave at 32 weeks gestation and may lengthen the leave until the child is 3 years old. Maternity leave wages are only a percentage of a woman's regular rate, therefore many choose to return to work sooner.

National Childhood Immunizations: BCG at birth and 8 years; DPT at 3, 4 1/2, and 6 months and 2 years; OPV at 3, 4 1/2, and 6 months and at 2 and 7 years; hep B at birth and at 1 and 6 months; MMR at 12 months and 13 years; and DT at 7, 12, and 17 years. The reported percentages of the target population vaccinated are as follows: BCG, 100%; third dose of DTP, 93%; MCV, 93%; and Pol3, 93%.

BIBLIOGRAPHY

Kalda R et al: Family planning and family doctors in Estonia, *Adv Contracept* 14(2):121–130, 1998.

Kalnins I: Pioneers in academia: higher education for nurses in Estonia, Latvia, and Lithuania, *Nurs Outlook* 43(2):84, 1995.

Levin A: The mother-infant unit at Tallinn Children's Hospital, Estonia: a truly baby-friendly unit, *Birth* 21(1):39, 1994.

Nadisauskiene RJ, Padaiga Z: Changes in women's health in the Baltic republics of Lithuania, Latvia and Estonia during 1970-1997, *Int J Gynaecol Obstet* 70(1):199–206, 2000.

Puska P: Health promotion challenges for countries of the former Soviet Union: results from collaboration between Estonia, Russian Karelia and Finland, *Health Promot Int* 10(3):219, 1995.

◆ ETHIOPIA (FEDERAL DEMOCRATIC REPUBLIC OF)

MAP PAGE (862)

Vered Kater

Location: Ethiopia is located in the northeastern horn of Africa, bordered by Eritrea to the north, Djibouti and Somalia to the east, Kenya to the south, and Sudan on the west. Ethiopians and Eritreans are similar cultural groups because Eritrea was an Ethiopian province that gained independence in 1993.

Major Languages	Ethnic Groups	Major Religions
Amharic (the official language only spoken by 60% of the population)	Oromo 35%	Muslim (Sunni) 33%
	Amhara 30%	Orthodox Christianity (Coptic) 50%
	Tigrean 12%	Animist, other 17%
Tigrinya	Somali 6%	
Oromo	Sidamo, Afar, Guraghe, other 17%	
40% speak in 70 different tongues		
Guraghe, other		

Health Care Beliefs: Acute sick care; traditional. Health promotion and disease prevention do not exist in Ethiopia. Many nongovernmental organizations teach prevention of HIV and AIDS and provide free condoms, but little attention is paid to this or other prevention strategies. Vaccinations are virtually the only preventive care that is sought. Many illnesses are believed to be caused by someone with "the evil eye" (i.e., the power to harm others by looking at them). Fresh air may be considered dangerous because it is believed to cause *mitch*, a general name for mental illness. Attitudes toward mental illness are unclear because Ethiopians believe all illnesses are physical. They think that bad food, wet feet, or the wrong type of thinking can all cause disasters. Ethiopians have the basic assumption that every human individual has a personal spirit, referred to as *qole* or *wegabi*. It is easy to offend or insult this spirit, and the result is a variety of physical or spiritual ailments. Mystical and physical healing are often combined in Ethiopia. Care for acute illnesses is frequently sought from the family first, followed by traditional healers, and then as a last resort, a modern doctor.

Predominant Sickness Care Practices: Traditional, magical-religious and Western. Traditionally, healers use Western as well as magical-religious methods. Local practices include prophylactic uvulectomy to prevent throat infections, extraction of the lower incisors to prevent diarrhea, and amulets and tattooing to drive away pathogenic agents. Modern medicine combined with traditional therapy, such as white onions with alcohol and butter, is used as treatment for malaria. Ethiopia has no system of health insurance, and each item used by the doctor is paid for separately. Even when a woman is hospitalized for childbirth, the gloves used by the midwife are brought by the expectant mother.

Ethnic/Race Specific and Endemic Diseases: Active and endemic diseases include typhoid, dysentery, trachoma, scabies, and HIV-related diseases such as tuberculosis. In the lowlands, endemic diseases include malaria, trypanosomiasis, onchocerciasis, yellow fever, schistosomiasis, and leishmaniasis. Ethiopians are at risk for measles complications, malnutrition, intestinal parasites, diarrhea, eye infections, and vitamin A and B deficiencies. The World Health Organization's (WHO) estimated prevalence rate for HIV/AIDS in adults ages 15 to 49 is 10.63%. The estimated number of children from birth to 15 years living with HIV/AIDS is 150,000. Prevalence of HIV increased from 8% in 1987 to 38% in 1992. In 1998 a median of 9% of antenatal women tested in Addis Ababa were infected with HIV. Few individuals have access to AIDS treatments, resulting in an unwillingness to be tested.

Health Team Relationships: Ethiopians highly respect health care professionals, so much so that patients often visit several healers and follow all of their advice simultaneously, even when this advice is contradictory. Patients tend to demand injections because of the widespread belief that pills will not influence their symptoms.

Families' Role in Hospital Care: Families move into the hospital and help with patients' physical care. Patients do not want to be left alone, especially if they are gravely ill. In the hospital the family has to bring food to the patients and take care of their hygienic needs. Care for patients with chronic conditions is provided by the extended family, and older adults usually live at the home of one of their children.

Dominance Patterns: Fathers are traditionally the authority figures, and men are responsible for handling family contacts with the world outside the home. The woman's role is defined in terms of household management and matrimonial duties.

Eye Contact Practices: Many Ethiopians do not make direct eye contact with doctors and nurses because of the perceived higher status of health professionals.

Touch Practices: Handshaking is customary, and it is polite to simultaneously shake both hands of older adults. Greetings do not include kissing, but people touch cheek to cheek four times when meeting close friends. Family members touch in public, and holding hands with someone of the same sex is not unusual.

Perceptions of Time: Time is not as important as it is in Western cultures. A common saying is that "each hour has 500 minutes." In addition, many people work according to a local time that is actually 6 hours ahead of the official time.

Pain Reactions: Individuals have a high pain tolerance but eventually accept pain medication when and if it is offered.

Birth Rites: Sex is not discussed. Women have no preparation for childbirth, and rectovaginal and vesicourinal fistulas are common complications of delivery. Pregnancy is considered a dangerous time because of the potential for damage from the evil eye and sorcery against the fetus. It is believed that unfulfilled cravings can cause a miscarriage, malformation, or prematurity. Childbirth is attended by a traditional birth attendant or a female family member, and the woman assumes the side-lying position. Traditionally, fathers do not participate in labor or delivery. About 1000 women die from pregnancy-related causes per 100,000 live births. The mother remains confined for 12 days, and the newborn stays within the confines of the home for at least 40 days because sun rays are believed to cause severe illnesses. More then half of the total admissions involving obstetric problems are caused by illegal, frequently septic abortions.

Death Rites: Ethiopia does not have a systematic birth and death registration process. Autopsies are uncommon because of the belief that the body must be buried intact. Cremation is not permitted. For Muslim and Fallasha burials, the body is wrapped in special pieces of cloth and buried without a coffin in the ground. Loud wailing is a normal grief reaction for men and women, and the mourning period varies from a few days to a month.

Food Practices and Intolerances: Many children younger than 5 years suffer from some degree of malnutrition—about 60% of them are 80% or less than the expected weight. Daily caloric supply per capita is estimated to be 76% of the recommended daily intake. The food is always very spicy, causing a high incidence of stomach ulcers. *Injera*, a flat, round bread made from *teff* grains that is high in iron, is the main staple and eaten three times a day with other foods that are pureed and placed on top. The dish is eaten with one hand without utensils. Many cups of black coffee and sweet tea are consumed during the day. Some people do not eat the meat of wild animals, pigs, dogs, horses, and shellfish. Ethiopians have numerous fasting days. On some of the days, people are allowed to eat before sunrise and after sunset; on other days, they are not allowed to eat animal products or are allowed no food or water for 24 hours.

Infant Feeding Practices: Water with butter is given to the infant immediately after the delivery because it is believed that it softens the voice of the baby. This practice frequently causes aspiration pneumonia. Breastfeeding continues for several years, and solid food is not introduced until the child can walk. When an infant has diarrhea, Ethiopians believe that withholding food and fluids will cure the child.

Child Rearing Practices: Children are raised in a highly protective, indulgent atmosphere until they are about 3 years. Obedience and politeness are the goals of upbringing. Children who are ill may be kept lying in one place until they get better. Approximately 90% of boys are circumcised, and the procedure is performed between birth and 5 years. Some girls in certain groups are still circumcised.

National Childhood Immunizations: BCG at birth; DPT at 6, 10, and 14 weeks; OPV at birth and 6, 10, and 14 weeks; measles at 9 months; and TT CBAW. The reported percentages of the target population fully vaccinated are as follows: BCG, 80%; polio, 64%; measles, 53%; and TT 35%.

BIBLIOGRAPHY

Hodes RM: Cross-cultural medicine and diverse health beliefs: Ethiopians abroad, *West J Med* 166(1):29, 1997.

Hodes RM, Befekadu T: Traditional beliefs and disease practices of Ethiopian Jews, *Israel J Med Sci* 32(7):561, 1996.

IPAS: *African reports,* http://server2.netenterprises.com

Kassaye T et al: Prevalence of vitamin A deficiency in children aged 6-9 years in Wukro, northern Ethiopia, *Bull WHO* 79(5):415, 2001.

Kater V: A tale of teaching in two cities, *Int Nurs Rev* 47(2):121, 2000.

Menachim S, Portugheiz E: Uvulectomy and blue gingiva tattoo among Ethiopian immigrants in Israel, *Harefuah* 132(2):128, 1997.

Reiff, M, Zakut H, Weingarten MA: Illness and treatment perceptions of Ethiopian immigrants and their doctors in Israel, *AJPH* 89:1814, 1999.

Whaley LF: *Nursing care of infants and children,* ed 6, St Louis, 1999, Mosby.

www.unaids.org

www.who.org

www.wube.net/language.html

◆ FIJI (REPUBLIC OF)

MAP PAGE (856)

Location: Fiji is made up of more than 800 islands and islets (about 100 of which are inhabited) in the southern Pacific, and is mostly mountainous and of volcanic origin. Only about 10% of the land is arable. It is about 2000 miles (3218 km) east of Australia and about 600 miles (965 km) from Vanuatu, its nearest neighbor. The climate is tropical marine, with only slight seasonal temperature variations. The total land area is 18,270 km² (7054 square miles), slightly smaller than New Jersey, and the capital is Suva. About 65% of the land area is forest and woodland. Fiji has a developing economy; 41% of the population is urban and 59% is rural. The total population is 844,300, and 63% are between the ages of 15 and 64. The gross domestic product per capita is $7300.

Major Languages	**Ethnic Groups**	**Major Religions**
English (official)	Fijian 51%	Christian 52%
Fijian	East Indian 44%	Hindu 38%
Hindustani	European other 5%	Muslim 8%
		Other 2%

Fijians are predominantly Melanesian with a Polynesian mixture. The Fijians are primarily Christian, the East Indians are primarily Hindu, and the Muslims are the minority. Literacy rates are 93.8% for males and 89.3% for females.

Health Care Beliefs: Acute sick care; traditional; increasing emphasis on prevention. Strides toward disease prevention are being made as the population adopts more sedentary Western lifestyles and has higher rates of obesity. For example, a recent program in a village used a combination of Western smoking cessation methods combined with indigenous traditional rituals (rapid inhalation ceremony and a tabu formalized by means of a kava ceremony). This approach was so successful that the village is now known as "the village that gave up smoking."

Predominant Sick Care Practices: Fiji has a system of free care, but the facilities are barely adequate for even routine medical problems. Emergency and outpatient services are available in Suva, the capital (at Colonial War Memorial Hospital), and Lautoka (at Lautoka Hospital). Other facilities such as clinics are very limited. Most medical emergencies of visitors to the area are referred to facilities outside of the country.

Ethnic/Race Specific or Endemic Diseases: As diet and exercise patterns transition away from more traditional patterns, mortality from cardiovascular disease has risen dramatically. Obesity and diabetes with diabetic retinopathy and nephropathy are also steadily increasing. Driving is hazardous, and automobile accidents are a frequent cause of morbidity. Sugar cane workers have illnesses associated with pesticide use. Fiji's East Indian population has unacceptably high rates of suicide, particularly among young women. Iron deficiency anemia is common in young children. Lung cancer rates are lower in Fiji than in other South Pacific countries, despite similar smoking rates. Researchers have suggested an association between lower cancer incidence and consumption of *kava* as a beverage. Endemic diseases include dengue fever, typhoid fever, hepatitis A, and lymphatic filariasis. Fijians are at risk for diarrheal diseases and hepatitis B. The World Health Organization's (WHO) estimated prevalence rate for HIV/AIDS in adults ages 15 to 49 is 0.07%. WHO has no estimates for children from birth to 15 years. Life expectancy at birth is 65.83 years for men and 70.78 for women.

Birth Rites: Fijians have a strong love of family. A particular postpartum somatic illness known as *na tadoka ni vasucu* occurs among ethnic Fijian women and is associated with a lack of social support. Although physical symptoms are relatively minor, this syndrome helps the new mother get the increased social surveillance and care she needs. The birth rate is

23.33 births per 1000 people. The maternal mortality rate is 90 per 100,000 live births, and the total fertility rate is 2.86 children per woman. The infant mortality rate per 1000 live births is 14.08.

Food Practices and Intolerances: Fijians have experienced drastic dietary changes during the past 50 years and have decreased their consumption of traditional foods. Intake of cereal and sugar has increased dramatically, as has the consumption of butter, margarine, and oil for frying. Cassava, bread, and sugar are consumed daily as the main sources of carbohydrates, and fish and meat are eaten daily. Sweet tea with whole milk is also consumed. Coconut cream and lamb flaps increase the saturated fat content of the diet.

National Childhood Immunizations: BCG at birth; DTP at 2, 3, and 4 months; OPV at birth and 2, 3, and 4 months; hep B at birth and at 2 and 5 months; HIB at 2, 3, and 5 months; measles at 9 months; and rubella for girls younger than 11 years. The reported percentages of the target population vaccinated in 1998 were as follows: BCG, 95; third dose of DPT, 86; third dose of hep B, 98; MCV, 75; and Pol 3, 88.

Other Characteristics: It is considered impolite to raise the arms while talking to someone. Talking with the arms crossed over the chest is a sign of respect.

BIBLIOGRAPHY

Andy TC: The utilisation of a primary health care centre on an isolated island: Cicia, Fiji, *Cent Afr J Med* 36(10):246, 1990.
Becker AE: Postpartum illness in Fiji: a sociosomatic perspective, *Psychosomat Med* 60(4):431, 1998.
Groth-Marnat G, Leslie S, Renneker M: Tobacco control in a traditional Fijian village: indigenous methods of smoking cessation and relapse prevention, *Soc Sci Med* 43(4):473, 1996.
Lako JV: Dietary trend and diabetes: its association among indigenous Fijians 1952 to 1994, *Asia Pacific J Clin Nutr* 10(3):183, 2001.
Le-Marchand L et al: An ecological study of diet and lung cancer in the South Pacific, *Int J Cancer* 63(1):18, 1995.
Szmedra P: The health impacts of pesticide use on sugarcane farmers in Fiji, *Asia Pacific J Pub Health* 11(2):82, 1999.
Steiner GG: The correlation between cancer incidence and kava consumption, *Hawaii Med J* 59(11):420, 2000.
http://www.cia.gov/cia/publications/factbook/geos/fj.html
http://travel.state.gov/fiji.html

◆ FINLAND (REPUBLIC OF)

MAP PAGE (860)

Marja Kaunonen, Katja Rask, and Hilkka Sand

Location: Finland is one of the Nordic countries and stretches about 1126 km (700 miles) north and south from the Arctic Circle to the Gulf of Finland, with Sweden along its western border and Russia along its eastern border. The total land area is 337,030 km² (130,127 square miles). It is the second northernmost country in the world, but the climate is relatively mild because of the influence of the North Atlantic current, the Baltic Sea, and more than 100,000 lakes. The landscape of southern Finland is characterized by its lakes and forests, and northern Finland, which is called *Lapland*, by its *fjelds* and wilderness areas. Lapland is north of the Arctic Circle and has unique summers during which the sun does not set and winters during which the sun does not rise. Finland has one of the highest standards of living in the world.

Major Languages	**Ethnic Groups**	**Major Religions**
Finnish (official)	Finnish 94%	Evangelical Lutheran 89%
Swedish (official)	Swedish, Lapp,	Greek Orthodox 1%
Lapp	other 6%	Other 10%
Russian		

About 6% of the Finns speak Swedish as their first language. In addition, Finland has two ethnic minorities, Sami (7000 people) and Roma (10,000 people). In 2000, Finland had about 91,000 immigrants and refugees. Finns study two to three foreign languages in school, and their command of English and Swedish is good.

Health Care Beliefs: Active involvement; high levels of health promotion. Active involvement in health care and health promotion is considered important. Health is considered a subjective sense of well-being and an absence of physical complaints.

Predominant Sick Care Practices: Biomedical and alternative. Biomedical sick care practices are predominant. Legislation provides the right to good health care and related treatments, the right to be informed, and the right to self-determination. Public health care services are mainly financed by relatively high income taxes. In addition, health care services are provided by the private health care sector. In the private sector, a person can directly make an appointment with a specialist at a specified time, which is different from the "first come, first serve" approach of the public sector. Private doctors are paid for in cash, but the Social Insurance Institution compensates for part of the payment. Certain forms of alternative medicine such as acupuncture have become more common and to some extent accepted by the medical profession.

Ethnic/Race Specific or Endemic Diseases: Finns are at genetic risk for numerous congenital diseases such as nephrosis, generalized amyloidosis syndrome, and polycystic liver disease. Cardiovascular diseases, cancer, stroke, musculoskeletal disorders, alcohol abuse, and mental disorders are common illnesses in Finland. Lifestyle diseases and depression are emerging as serious public health problems. Despite these issues the life expectancy at birth is 77.6 years. Suicide rates are quite high in Finland.

The suicide rate per 100,000 inhabitants was 24.3 in 1996. However, Finland was the first country to fully implement a nationwide suicide prevention project through multisectoral cooperation from 1986 to 1996. In 1996 the number of suicides in Finland had decreased by 18% from 1990. The World Health Organization's (WHO) estimated prevalence rate for HIV/AIDS in adults ages 15 to 49 is 0.05%. The estimated number of children from birth to 15 years living with HIV/AIDS is less than 100.

Health Team Relationships: Health care is doctor driven. Nursing education is offered at polytechnic schools, and graduate and postgraduate training in nursing education and administration is offered at five Finnish universities. In recent years, research in and implementation of family nursing programs have attracted increasing attention in Finland. Family nursing reinforces family strategies and resources, improving the response to changes in family structures. Finland has several examples of successful research activities and implementation of family nursing in child welfare clinics and in the care of older adults. Nurses and doctors work closely in outpatient clinics and school health services. Patients want strong, interactive relationships with nurses and doctors, and patient motivation is linked to good compliance, especially among adolescents. Successful nurse and patient collaboration involves active commitment of both parties.

Families' Role in Hospital Care: Most hospitals prefer open visiting hours, and family members and volunteers help feed patients. It is not unusual for family members to participate in the care of a hospitalized child and stay overnight.

Dominance Patterns: Men and women are considered equals, and both contribute to making health care decisions for children. Most Finnish women work outside the home.

Eye Contact Practices: Finns greet guests and friends by shaking hands; kisses on the cheek are less common. Direct eye contact is considered polite and necessary especially when greeting a person, but it is intermittent. Regardless of age, a confidential connection between health care personnel and patients must involve eye contact.

Touch Practices: Hugs and kisses for children in the family are common, but touch practices among adult family members depend on familial culture. Regardless of age or gender, touching is considered natural by health care professionals. Nurses have their own distinct patterns of interaction. The frequency of touching in nursing care situations increases with very sick patients. In the nursing care of older patients, nurses use three main types of touch: touch used to perform a physical nursing procedure, touch used to help a restless patient relax for a nursing procedure, and touch used to comfort a patient. Because of the nature of their professional role, doctors have less overall physical contact with patients.

Perceptions of Time: People are usually punctual and may be irritated by tardiness. The impact of postmodernism and individualism on Finnish culture is characterized by the preference of a career rather than a family. On the other hand, laypersons in Finland have an increasing interest in genealogy. In addition, Finnish culture has some significant traditions, such as the celebration of Christmas and Midsummer. (Finland is known as the home of Santa Claus.)

Pain Reactions: Finns respect pain, and it is common for them to discuss it. Finns are accustomed to expressing their pain in detail but in a matter-fact-of-fact way. Extreme pain and suffering are often experienced tacitly. The consumption of medication for pain is relatively high, but other treatments such as massage, physical therapy, and psychotherapy are also used. Benefits from the Social Insurance Institution and insurance companies compensate for part of the treatment costs. Hospitalized patients in pain are often reluctant to reveal their discomfort. Thus nursing and medical staff members must pay attention to nonverbal messages, changes in conduct, and certain somatic complaints such as dizziness and nausea. The subjective experience of pain is composed of physical and emotional reactions such as fear, anxiety, and guilt. In hospitals, pain is measured with different self-rated assessment forms. Doctors of all specialties treat patients with pain, but all the university hospitals and numerous other hospitals have pain clinics researching and treating chronic pain.

Birth Rites: The average age of the primigravida woman is 27.6 years. Having one or two children is common, and births of sons and daughters are celebrated equally. Any woman living permanently in Finland who has a doctor's examination before the end of the fourth month of her pregnancy is entitled to the "one-off" maternity benefit. This bonus is granted in the form of either a maternity package (containing basic clothing, linens, and other necessities for a newborn) or cash. The cash alternative amounts to 140 tax-free Euro per child, but the value of the package is almost three times the amount of money. Midwife-assisted hospital births predominate and are associated with one of the lowest infant mortality rates in the world. Positive childbirth experiences as perceived by first-time mothers are strongly related to the positive characteristics and professional skills of the attending midwife and positive attitude of the spouse toward the pregnancy. Most fathers participate in the delivery and consider their presence important for their growth into fatherhood. Infant "rooming in" (i.e., infants staying in the mother's hospital room) is prevalent in Finnish hospitals. Parental involvement with sick infants is encouraged, and the hospital has open visiting hours for siblings. "Kangaroo care" is used, and breast-feeding is the feeding method of choice.

Death Rites: Most Finns die in a hospital setting. The first hospice in Scandinavia, Pirkanmaan Hoitokoti in Tampere, Finland, opened in 1987.

Currently, Finland has three hospices. Family members typically want to participate in and follow the care of their ill family members. Study findings indicate that when a patient's condition deteriorates, the family's need for information increases. Family members often want to be at the bedside of the dying person to pay their final respects. Organ donations and autopsies are both acceptable in Finnish culture. Funeral rituals are important for grieving people because they allow them to express their grief, especially as the old mourning customs such as wearing black clothing or black veils (for widows) have begun to disappear during the last decades. Funeral directors assist the family with postmortem care. Burial is common, but cremation is becoming more frequent. The funeral takes place 1 to 3 weeks after the death, and a memorial service is usually held following the burial. The death is announced in newspapers either after the burial or before it, when the obituary serves as an invitation to the funeral. Family members often attend a church service the day after the funeral. Even though 58% of Evangelical Lutheran parishes offer bereavement support groups, only 4% to 17% of bereaved family members participate in these groups. Family members and friends are the most important source of social support for grieving people.

Food Practices and Intolerances: Finnish people eat much of the same food as other Europeans. Coffee, meat and cheese sandwiches, and porridge or cereal are common for breakfast. Lunch is the main meal. A small meal of coffee and sandwiches is eaten after work.

Infant Feeding Practices: Breast-feeding is common in Finland. Whether the mother successfully breast-feeds is related to whether she has a positive experience breast-feeding in the maternity ward and whether she has emotional and concrete support from her social support network. In addition, whether a first-time mother successfully copes with childcare is related to her success with breast-feeding.

Child Rearing Practices: Child rearing practices are relatively permissive in Finland. Children express their opinions freely to their parents at home and teachers in school. The family may have only one children's room, which is shared by boys and girls. Finland has ratified the United Nations convention on the Rights of the Child, and corporal punishment is forbidden by law. Family structures have undergone changes in the recent years. Single-parent families are relatively common and constitute 19% of all families with children. However, many single parents have joint custody, and the child meets with the other parent regularly. Mothers receive 263 working days of maternity allowance, the last 158 of which can be used by the mother or the father. In addition, fathers receive 18 days of paid paternity leave. The mother's job is secure until the child is 3 years old—or 7 years old if the mother works only 6 hours a day. Each child living in Finland receives a paid child benefit until 17 years of age. Free dental care is provided until age 18, and free health care from birth to school age. One full meal is offered to children at school. Compulsory military service begins for boys at the age of 19 and lasts 6 to 12 months. Military service is voluntary for girls.

National Childhood Immunizations: BCG at birth; DPT at 3, 4, and 5 months and 20 to 24 months; OPV not in use, but polio given at 6 and 12 months, 20 to 24 months, 6 and 11 years, and 16 to 18 years; HIV at 4, 6, and 14 to 18 months; and MRR at 14 to 18 months and 6 years. Since 1941, the BCG vaccination has been included in the national vaccination program in Finland. More than 99% of children received the BCG vaccination at birth or soon thereafter. The BCG vaccination may cause a positive reaction to the intradermal Mantoux tuberculin test.

BIBLIOGRAPHY

Åstedt-Kurki P et al: Family member as a hospital patient: sentiments and functioning of the family, *Int J Nurs Prac* 5:155, 1999.

Friedemann M-L: The concept of family nursing, *J Adv Nurs* 14:211, 1989.

Harmanen E: *Pastoral care in grief counseling groups—a study from the viewpoint of group leader in the Evangelical Lutheran Church of Finland*, academic dissertation, 1997, Helsinki, Finland, Suomen teologisen kirjallisuusseuran julkaisuja 207

Hyrkäs K, Kaunonen M, Paunonen M: Recovering from the death of a spouse, *J Adv Nurs* 25:775, 1997.

Kaunonen M: *Support for a family in grief*, academic dissertation, Tampere, 2000, Acta Universitatis Tamperensis 731.

Kuuppelomäki M: *The suffering experience of patients with incurable cancer and their coping with cancer*, academic dissertation, 1996, Turku, *Annales Universitatis Turkuensis* Series C, Vol 124.

Kyngäs H, Hentinen M, Barlow JH: Adolescents' perceptions of physicians, nurses, parents and friends: help or hindrance in compliance with diabetes self-care? *J Adv Nurs* 27(4):760, 1998.

Paavilainen E, Åstedt-Kurki P: The client-nurse relationship as experienced by public health nurses: toward better collaboration, *Pub Health Nurs* 14(3):137, 1997.

Perhehoitotyön kehittäminen yliopiston, ammattikorkeakoulujen ja terveydenhulto-organisaatioiden yhteistyönä Seinäjoella, Porissa ja *Tampereella. In Paavilainen E et al*, eds: *Tampereen yliopiston hoitotieteen laitos, Perhekeskeisen hoidon tutkimus- ja opetuskeskus, julkaisuja 1*, 1999.

Råholm M, Lindholm L: Being in the world of the suffering patient: a challenge to nursing ethics, *Nurs Eth Int J Health Care Prof* 6(6):528, 1999.

Routasalo P, Lauri S: Expressions of touch in nursing older people, *Euro Nurse* 3(2):95, 1998.

Tarkka M-T, Paunonen M, Laippala P: First-time mothers and child care when the child is 8 months old, *J Adv Nurs* 31(1):20, 2000.

Tarkka M-T, Paunonen M, Laippala P: Importance of the midwife in the first-time mother's experience of childbirth. *Scand J Caring Sci* 14(3):184, 2000.

Tarkka M-T, Paunonen M, Laippala P: What contributes to breastfeeding success after childbirth in a maternity ward in Finland? *Birth* 25(3):175, 1998.

Upanne M, Hakanen J, Rautava M: Can suicide be prevented? The suicide project in Finland 1992-1996: goals, implementation and evaluation. Helsinki, Finland, 2002, STAKES (National Research and Development Centre for Welfare and

…d January 8, 2002, from http://www.stakes.fi/verkkojulk/pdf/…9.

…en K, Liukkonen A: Fathers' experiences of childbirth, *Midwifery*…

…ietop/ 01-05-2002
http://www.ktl.fi/oppaita/roko/ 01-05-2002
http://www.mil.fi/varusmieheksi2001/ 01-08-2002
www.unaids.org/hivaidsinfo/statistics/june00/fact_sheets/index.html

◆ FRANCE (FRENCH REPUBLIC)

MAP PAGE (860)

Catherine Bungener

Location: As Benjamin Franklin once said, "Every man has two nations, and one of them is France." France is the second largest European nation, with a total land area of 551,000 km² (214,890 miles). The English Channel lies to the northwest, the Atlantic Ocean to the west, and the Mediterranean Sea to the south. France shares borders with Germany, Luxembourg, Belgium, Switzerland, and Italy.

France has 96 *départements* (administrative units) within the country, four overseas *départements* (Guadeloupe, Martinique, French Guinea, and Réunion), three overseas territories (French Polynesia, New Caledonia, and Wallis and Futuna), and two territorial collectivities (Saint Pierre et Miquelon and Mayotte). The French Alps include the highest peak in Europe, Mont Blanc (4800 m, or 15,750 ft). The climate is predominantly temperate with mild winters, except in mountainous areas and the northeast. The Atlantic has a profound impact on the western part of the country, where the weather is characterized by high humidity, often violent westerly winds, and a lot of rain. The northeast has a classic continental climate with fairly hot summers and cold winters. The southern area has a Mediterranean climate, and cold frosts are rare. Spring and autumn downpours are sudden but brief, and summer is hot with no rain.

Major Languages	Ethnic Groups	Major Religions
French	Celtic	Roman Catholic 54%
	Latin	Protestant 2%
	Teutonic, Slavic, North	Jewish 1%
	African, Indochinese,	Muslim 6%
	and Basque	Other (e.g., Buddhist,
	minorities	Hindu, Orthodox) 2%
		Unaffiliated 35%

France has a population of 59 million: 94% French, 3% Northern African, and 3% from other foreign countries. The capital is Paris, which has a population of 13 million. Although 99% of the population speaks French as their first language, the country has numerous rapidly disappearing dialects, such as Provencal, Alsatian, Breton, Creole, Catalan, Corsican, and Basque. The unemployment rate is 12.3%.

Health Care Beliefs: Active involvement; strong health promotion. People are paying more attention to their health. They tend to eat healthier foods such as fruits and vegetables and try to avoid saturated fats. They are encouraged to participate in sports regularly, and smoking, drinking, and taking drugs are strongly discouraged. The government has many initiatives in place for health promotion activities. For the most part, religion does not influence health care beliefs in France, except among some minority populations. Because treatments with herbs, homeopathic, or chiropractic measures are not considered to be scientifically based, the costs of these treatments are not paid by national health insurance.

Predominant Sick Care Practices: Biomedical. The French are great consumers of pharmacological treatments. When they are sick, they go to their doctors, who are either in a private practice or in a hospital. They can freely choose their doctor or hospital. If they choose a private hospital or doctor, only a part of the cost is reimbursed. All French people are affiliated with the *Sécurité Sociale*, which gives access to free medical care in all public hospitals. Everyone who is employed or has a parent or spouse who is employed is covered by this health and accident insurance, contributions to which are automatically taken out of the salary.

Ethnic/Race Specific or Endemic Diseases: Cardiovascular diseases and cancer are the two major causes of death. The World Health Organization's (WHO) estimated prevalence rate for HIV/AIDS in adults ages 15 to 49 is 0.43%. The estimated number of children from birth to 15 years living with HIV/AIDS is 1000. France has approximately 130,000 people infected with HIV, and about 2000 deaths from AIDS occur each year. The disease remains a significant health problem, particularly for foreigners living in France. In fact, many Africans come to France to be treated for HIV infections. Life expectancy is 78 years: 74 for men and 82 for women.

Health Team Relationships: Doctors remain at the top of the hierarchy in the hospital, followed by physiotherapists, psychologists, social workers, and then nurses. The hierarchical domination of doctors over nurses is intact in all hospitals. Doctors study for 6 years to graduate and 4 more years to become specialists. Psychologists graduate after 5 years. Nurses begin patient care at the end of 4 years of study at the baccalaureate level.

Families' Role in Hospital Care: The mother of a child or a spouse is allowed stay overnight at a hospital when a patient is severely ill. Otherwise, specific visiting times are set. Food and treatments are always provided by the hospital, so families do not have to assume this responsibility.

Dominance Patterns: The father remains dominant and the head of the family. However, more single-parent families are evolving, and in most cases the mother becomes the head of the family. More women are working, so moral and financial responsibilities are divided between both parents. Now fathers as well as mothers are entitled to parental leave for the education of the children.

Eye Contact Practices: As a sign of respect, the French maintain direct eye contact when talking to someone. Facial expressions and gestures tend to be quite expressive.

Touch Practices: The French touch frequently, especially in the southern part of the country where people prefer closeness during conversation. Handshaking or giving a kiss on each cheek when greeting or leaving a person is the norm. Carrying on a conversation with the hands in the pockets is impolite. When meeting people, protocols are observed and behavior is polite. Titles and status are important. First names should not be used. Engaging in general conversation to establish social contact is acceptable. When working with patients, giving logical, sequential explanations for health-related actions is important to ensure compliance. Rules and regulations may be circumvented to reach a goal.

Perceptions of Time: Strictly adhering to schedules is not routine, and changing plans at the last minute is acceptable. However, the French are becoming more time oriented with regard to their schedules. Long waiting times are common in all public administration settings, including public hospitals.

Pain Reactions: Pain is usually expressed by saying, "aïe!" or "ouille!" Women express pain and emotions more freely than most men. During the last several years, pain control has become a major concern in France. Every university hospital has a pain treatment department, and analgesics are freely given to patients who need them. Previously, pain tended to be underestimated and not treated correctly. Much remains to be done to improve the treatment of pain, especially for patients outside the larger cities.

Birth Rites: During pregnancy, regular doctor's visits are prescribed, as are a minimum of three ultrasound scans. Many parents want to learn the sex of the baby as soon as possible rather than wait until birth. An amniocentesis is performed on all mothers age 38 or older. Cesarean sections are common and suggested to the mother when the position of the infant is anticipated to make the delivery difficult. Epidural anesthesia and episiotomies are the norm for all mothers unless they refuse them. Terminations of pregnancy are authorized until the twelfth week of pregnancy. Most women give birth in a hospital, where they stay from 1 to 5 days. They usually keep their infants with them at all times. If a mother is particularly tired or is ill, infants stay in a nursery for the first few nights. Although religion does not play a very significant role in birth rituals, it is customary for infants to be baptized some time during the first year. Maternity leave begins 6 weeks before the birth and ends 8 weeks after. Fathers now have 10 days of leave after the birth of their children. For a third child, the mother has a maternity leave of 6 months.

Death Rites: Most people die in a hospital, and close family members are generally present. After a death the French Christians usually have a ceremony in a church. On November 1, chrysanthemums are brought to all the cemeteries, and families visit their parent's graves. Organ donations and autopsies are performed if the patient or the family has given consent.

Food Practices and Intolerances: French place great importance on food, and they are very fond of fine food and wines. At breakfast, bread with butter and jam or croissants is served with juice and tea or coffee (black coffee or coffee with cream). Lunch and dinner are full meals and include a first course, main course (meat or fish and vegetables, rice, or pasta) that is often accompanied by a green salad, cheese if it was not served as first course, and dessert. Bread is always served with meals; the typical baguette remains the favorite, although recently new kind of breads with grains or different types of flour have become quite popular. People regularly drink wine with their meals. After the dessert, small cups of black coffee are frequently served. *Foie gras* (goose liver) and seafood, especially oysters and snails, are considered very fine food. The French eat a lot of meat, especially red meat. Frog's legs are not as popular as in the past, but they are served in some restaurants. Every region has its own specialties: *choucroute* (sauerkraut) in Alsace; *crêpes* in Bretagne; *foie gras* and *cassoulet* in the southwest; bouillabaisse (fish soup) or courses with tomatoes, garlic, and basil in the south; cheese meals in the Alps (*fondue, raclette,* or *tartiflette*); and seafood near the sea. France has more than 300 different kind of cheese.

Infant Feeding Practices: After childbirth, about 60% of women breast-feed their babies; about 30% do so after the first 2 or 3 weeks. Relatively few mothers breast-feed their children for many weeks. In the hospital the trend is toward bottle-feeding, and breast-feeding is not particularly encouraged unless the mother insists on it.

Child Rearing Practices: Child rearing practices are increasingly more permissive. Children usually have their own rooms and do not typically sleep with parents unless they are sick.

National Childhood Immunizations: The only two compulsory vaccinations are BCG before 6 years and DPT at 2, 3, and 4 months. Vaccination for

ROR (measles, mumps, and German measles) and pertussis are strongly recommended.

Other Characteristics: The French are very fond of sports, and more people every year practice a sport regularly. Football, rugby, and cycling are the most popular and are watched on television. The French are often considered by foreigners to be chauvinists. They do a lot of walking in the countryside or the mountains and ski during the winter. They often spend their vacations in France; the beaches of the Mediterranean Sea, the Atlantic Ocean, and the French Channel are very popular during summer holidays. Most people take their vacations during August.

BIBLIOGRAPHY

Giger JN, Davidhizar RE: *Transcultural nursing: assessment and intervention*, ed 2, St Louis, 1995, Mosby.

Goscinny R, Uderzo A: *Le tour de Gaule d'Asterix*, Neuilly-sur-Seine, 1965, Darguad.

Hall ET, Hall MR: *Understanding cultural differences: Germans, French and Americans*, Yarmouth, Me, 1990, Intercultural Press..

Spector RE: *Cultural diversity in health and illness*, ed 4, Stamford, Conn, 1996, Appleton & Lange.

Storti C: *The art of crossing cultures*, Yarmouth, Me, 1990, Intercultural Press.

INSEE: *National Institute of Economic and Epidemiology survey*, 1999.

www.France-culture.fr.

◆ GABON (GABONESE REPUBLIC)

MAP PAGE (863)

Francine Ntoumi

Location: This central African country sits astride the equator along the Atlantic seaboard. Most of the total land area of 267,667 km^2 (103,319 square miles) is covered by dense tropical forests and savannahs. The country is bordered by Cameroon and Equatorial Guinea to the north and Congo-Brazzaville to the east, with a long common border. The climate is tropical—always hot and humid. Gabon is a developing nation but is one of the more prosperous Black African countries. It has a per capita income four times that of most nations of sub-Saharan Africa: $6300. The population estimate is 1,221,175. Libreville is the capital.

Major Languages	Ethnic Groups	Major Religions
French	Fang 25%	Christian 60%
Fang	Bapounou 10%	Muslim 1%
Myene	Other 65%	Indigenous, other 39%

The distribution of the different tribes in the country is as follows: Fang: 34.5%, Aduma: 17%, Bakota: 14%, Eshira: 10.5%, Banzabi: 7.5%, Bakélé: 7%, Okanda: 4.5%, Pongwe: 3%, and Pygmee: 1%.

Health Care Beliefs: Acute sick care. The common perception is that mental illness has an occult origin. It is believed that enemies can use an evil spell to disturb the mind because of jealousy or for other reasons. The first reaction to having mental illness is to go a traditional healer, who uses plants, incantations, and prayers to chase away the evil spirits from the body.

Predominant Sick Care Practices: Biomedical; traditional; magical-religious. The people seek out doctors at hospitals and local dispensaries. Medical facilities and access to medication in Gabon's major cities are limited but generally adequate for routine or basic needs. Medical services in rural areas are generally unavailable. The most vulnerable populations—those with low incomes—go to the dispensary only after treatment with traditional medicine has failed; the treatments are less expensive than those imported from Europe. No prescription is required for buying medicines at the pharmacies. Because oral medications are the most common, people often share medicine if they think they have the same ailments, a practice that is common in the country. Whether a person is dealing with a physical or mental illness and even if a doctor is consulted, traditional healers are also used and herbal treatments are common. Traditional healers often use an exorcism ceremony to treat patients.

Ethnic/Race Specific or Endemic Diseases: Endemic diseases include malaria, schistosomiasis, and yellow fever. People are at risk for loiasis, leptospirosis, onchocerciasis, hemorrhagic fevers, sleeping sickness, intestinal parasites, and hepatitis B and C. Gabon had two large outbreaks of Ebola virus in 1996; Ebola is approximately 70% fatal. The World Health Organization's (WHO) estimated prevalence rate for HIV/AIDS is 4.16%, lower than many neighboring countries. The estimated number of children from birth to 15 years living with HIV/AIDS is 780. During 1999, about 2000 deaths from HIV/AIDS were recorded, and approximately 8600 children have lost either their mother or both parents to the epidemic. It is estimated that 23,000 people are living with HIV/AIDS today. Life expectancy at birth is 48.7 years for men and 50.75 years for women.

Health Team Relationships: The relationships between the people and medical personnel are as good as can be expected given the shortages of personnel and equipment. Hospitals need medical equipment, supplies, and reagents, so it is common for patients to bring these items with them. Supplies necessary for surgical operations, such as gloves, cotton, and bandages, also must be supplied by the patients or their families.

Families' Role in Hospital Care: It is always recommended that the family stay with the patient in the hospital. The family is responsible for the physical care of the patient and also supplies needed food.

Dominance Patterns: Men are dominant in the family and make all of the important decisions. However, mothers raise the children.

Eye Contact Practices: Gabon has no restrictions relating to direct eye contact between sexes or people of different ages.

Touch Practices: Touching is not only acceptable, it is used to communicate. Hand movements punctuate discussions and are usually expressive.

Perceptions of Time: Punctuality is not an issue. People tend to be more punctual for administrative appointments. Time is never an issue for private appointments, and being late is acceptable. The people tend to focus on historical traditions such as respect for ancestors and older adults.

Pain Reactions: Reactions to pain vary among ethnic and socioeconomic groups. In general, it is more acceptable for women and children to express pain.

Birth Rites: It is uncommon for the father to assist his wife at his child's birth. A female member of the family generally assists. The celebration of the birth is the same regardless of the infant's gender, but the celebration of twins (either girls or boys) is particularly special and important. The hair of the child is not cut until a certain time passes after the birth, usually at the celebration of the first birthday. Gabon has the lowest fertility index in sub-Saharan Africa, with 3.69 children per woman; a link seems to exist between bilharzial diseases and infertility and ectopic pregnancies in Gabon. Schistosomiasis from *Schistosoma haematobium* occurs, with an incidence of 8% to 55% of the adult population. In addition, studies show that 14% of pregnant women recently tested had either gonococcal infections, chlamydial infections, or both, which affects the spread of other sexually transmitted diseases such as HIV/AIDS. The birth rate is 27.42 births per 1000 people, and the infant mortality rate is high at 94.91 deaths per 1000 live births.

Death Rites: All members of the family are expected to be present for the death of a relative, and relatives living in another country generally come back to attend the burial ceremony. To encourage the presence of all family members at the funeral, friends of the family gather donations to provide the funds needed for people to return to the country. Organ donations and autopsies are unacceptable.

Food Practices and Intolerances: People use knives, forks, or spoons to eat, although some food such as cassava is eaten with the hands. Meals with sauce containing peanuts, served with rice and cassava, are commonly eaten.

Infant Feeding Practices: Breast-feeding is the most common form of infant feeding because of its health advantages and the high cost of formula. In addition, when water supplies are unclean, bottle-feeding increases the risk of the infant contracting parasites and other organisms.

Child Rearing Practices: Education is considered to be important for children. Children are taught to obey all adults, and they consider all adult women and men to be mothers and fathers. It is considered improper to contest the decision of an older person. Literacy rates are 73.7% for males and 53.3% for females.

National Childhood Immunizations: BCG at birth; DPT at 6, 10, and 14 weeks; OPV at 6, 10, and 14 weeks; measles at 9 months; hep B at birth and at 1 and 6 months; yellow fever 12 months; and TT CBAW ×5, pregnant women ×2. The reported percentages of the target population vaccinated are as follows: BCG, 48; first dose of DTP, 24; third dose of DTP, 10; MCB, 27; Pol3, 52; and TT2 plus, 16.

BIBLIOGRAPHY

Anonymous: *Outbreak of Ebola haemorrhagic fever in Gabon, communicable disease report, CDR Weekly* 6(9):75, 1996.

Bourgeois A et al: Prospective evaluation of a flow chart using a risk assessment for the diagnosis of STDs in primary healthcare centers in Libreville, Gabon, *Sex Trans Inf* 74(suppl 1):128-132, 1998.

Ville Y et al: Tubal schistosomiasis as a cause of ectopic pregnancy in endemic areas?: a report of three cases, *Eur J Obstet Gynecol Reprod Biol* 42(1):77, 1991.

Wahl G, Georges AJ: Current knowledge on the epidemiology, diagnosis, immunology, and treatment of loiasis, *Trop Med Parasitol* 46(4):287, 1995.

http://www.odci.gov/cia/publications/factbook/geos/gb.html

http://travel.stat.gov/gabon.html

◆ GAMBIA (REPUBLIC OF THE)

MAP PAGE (862)

Location: Referred to as "The Gambia," this country, the smallest in western Africa, is located on the Atlantic coast and bordered by Senegal. The country is primarily savannah with some low hills and is bisected by the wide Gambia River. The climate is tropical with a hot, rainy season from June to November and a cooler dry season from November to May. The total land area is 11,300 km^2 (4362 square miles), slightly less than twice the size of Delaware. The capital is Banjul. The total population is 1,411,205. Many people live at a subsistence level in bush villages. The major export is peanuts and peanut products, and the gross domestic product (GDP) per capita is $1100.

Major Languages	Ethnic Groups	Major Religions
English (official)	Mandinka 42%	Muslim 90%
Mandinka	Fula 18%	Christian 9%
Wolof	Wolof 16%	Indigenous beliefs 1%
Fula	Jola 10%	
Other	Serahuli 9%	
	Other 4%	
	Non-African 1%	

Health Care Beliefs: Health promotion is important. The country's primary health care plan is an excellent model for other developing countries.

Predominant Sick Care Practices: Biomedical; magico-religious and traditional. Medical facilities are limited and not up to European or North American standards. Common medications are frequently unavailable. Most of the major health care facilities are located in areas south of the Gambia River, so people to the north are at an even greater disadvantage relative to health care access.

Ethnic/Race Specific or Endemic Diseases: Water-borne diseases are prevalent. Endemic diseases include chloroquine-resistant malaria (throughout the year, including in urban areas), trachoma, syphilis, tuberculosis, hepatitis B, and histoplasmosis. People are at risk for loiasis, tick-borne illnesses, cholera, hepatitis A, meningitis, schistosomiasis, typhoid fever, and yellow fever (regional). Most young children are pneumococcus carriers. Both *Streptococcus pneumoniae* and *Haemophilus influenzae* type B (HIB) frequently cause meningitis in children, a major cause of morbidity and mortality. Those who survive meningitis often have hearing loss, mental retardation, motor abnormalities, and seizures. The Gambia had an outbreak of Ebola hemorrhagic fever in 1995. The World Health Organization's (WHO) estimated prevalence rate for HIV/AIDS in adults ages 15 to 49 is 1.95%. The estimated number of children from birth to 15 years living with HIV/AIDS is 520. An estimated 1400 people died of AIDS in 1999, and about 9500 children have lost either their mother or both parents to AIDS since the beginning of the epidemic. About 13,000 people are currently living with HIV/AIDS.

Dominance Patterns: Polygamy is practiced by some. Traditionally, the man occupies one house, and his one to four wives and their children occupy another house.

Birth Rites: The total fertility rate is 5.68 children born per woman, and the birth rate is 41.76 births per 1000 people. Infant mortality rates are high at 77.84 deaths per 1000 live births. Life expectancy at birth is 51.65 years for men and 55.58 years for women. Trained midwives deliver a large percentage of the infants, particularly because of the shortage of doctors. Outside of cities, most children are born with the assistance of traditional birth attendants; however, even in cities traditional attendants may be preferred. Squatting or supine positions are used for childbirth. Some believe that the father must provide the razor blade used to cut the umbilical cord. A special naming celebration with drums and dancing is held on the eighth day after birth. A witch doctor *(maribou)* provides holy verses in small leather pouches that are fastened on a string and worn around the infant's neck for protection.

Death Rites: Some Muslims forbid organ donations or transplants, although transfusions may be recommended as life-saving procedures. Autopsies are uncommon because the body must be buried intact. Cremation is not permitted. For Muslim burials the body is wrapped in special pieces of white cloth and buried without a coffin in the ground as soon as possible after death.

Food Practices and Intolerances: Rice is the dietary staple. Peanuts are grown for export and frequently used in traditional dishes.

Infant Feeding Practices: The newborn is given only warm water the first day. Breast-feeding starts the second day. Weaning foods such as *sanyo,* a local millet, tend to be low in energy and protein. Families often have goats, but their milk is not commonly used in infant food preparation.

Child Rearing Practices: About 45% of the population is between infancy and 14 years. Literacy rates are 58.4% for males and 37.1% for females. Family planning may not be acceptable. Female circumcision and excision is widespread in some groups.

National Childhood Immunizations: BCG at birth; DTP at 2, 3, and 4 months, and +1 year; OPV at birth and 2, 3, 4, 9, and 18 months; hep B at birth and at 2 and 4 months; HIB at 2, 3, and 4 months; measles at 9 months; vitamin A from 6 months; YFV at 9 months; and TT after first contact and at +1 and +6 months, and +1, +1 year. The reported percentages of the target population vaccinated are as follows: BCG, 97; first dose of DTP, 89; third dose of DTP, 83; third dose of hep B, 91; third dose of HIB, 83; MCV, 88; Pol3, 89; TT2 plus, 90; and YFB, 85.

BIBLIOGRAPHY

Campbell H, Byass P, Greenwood BM: Acute lower respiratory infections in Gambian children: maternal perception of illness, *Ann Trop Paediatr* 10(1):45, 1990.

Daly C, Pollard AJ: Traditional birth attendants in The Gambia, *Midwives Chron* 103(1227):104, 1990.

Goetghebuer T et al: Outcome of meningitis caused by *Streptococcus pneumoniae* and *Haemophilus influenzae* type B in children in The Gambia, *Trop Med Int Health* 5(3):207, 2000.

Ho E: Midwifery training and practice in The Gambia, *Midwives Chron* 100(1191):109, 1987.

Hoare K: Tackling infant malnutrition in The Gambia, *Health Visit* 67(3):102, 1994.

Mwanatambwe M et al: Ebola hemorrhagic fever (EHF): mechanism of transmission and pathogenicity, *J Nippon Med School* 68(5):370, 2001.

Wright J: Female genital mutilation: an overview, *J Adv Nurs* 24:251, 1996.

http://www.fco.gov.uk/travel/countryadvice.asp?GA

http://www.odci.gov/cia/publications/factbook/geos/ga.html

http://travel.state.gov/gambia.html

◆ GEORGIA (GEORGIAN REPUBLIC)

MAP PAGE (861)

Robert O'Donovan and Manana Sopromadze

Location: Part of the former Soviet Union, Georgia is located northeast of Turkey on the eastern shore of the Black Sea. The total land area is 67,700 km² (26,911 square miles). Snow-capped mountains, dense forests, fertile valleys, and turbulent rivers that provide abundant hydroelectric power characterize Georgia's topography.

Major Languages	Ethnic Groups	Major Religions
Georgian (official)	Georgian 70%	Georgian Orthodox 65%
Russian	Armenian 8%	Russian Orthodox 10%
	Russian 6%	Armenian Orthodox 8%
	Azeri 6%	Muslim 11%
	Ossetian 3%	Other 6%
	Abkhaz 2%	
	Other 5%	

Health Care Beliefs: Acute sick care; traditional. Common colds, especially among children and older adults, are generally believed to be caused by exposure to drafts. Infants and very small children are often swaddled in many layers to protect them from such drafts. Upset stomachs and headaches are often treated with a glass of *Borjomi* mineral water. Girls and women are actively discouraged from sitting directly on cement or stone, because Georgians believe that their reproductive systems will be damaged by the "cold" radiating out of those materials. Nearly all newborns wear an eye-shaped amulet on the wrist or have one hung near their crib to ward off the "evil eye" (the ability of a person to harm others by simply looking at them). Fevers are occasionally treated by wiping vodka or rubbing alcohol on a patient's entire body or placing a vinegar compress on a patient's forehead.

Predominant Sick Care Practices: Biomedical, alternative, and magical-religious. Western medical treatment is regularly sought in hospitals and polyclinics. However, many people first consult with a home-based herbalist because the treatment costs are lower. Georgians also may consult an herbalist if they are not satisfied with their doctor's diagnosis and recommended course of treatment. Informal, surreptitious monetary and nonmonetary payments are the norm and constitute a significant portion of income generated by medical staff. Costs of medications may be considerable. Children younger than 5 years are taken to a doctor for regular examinations. Children older than 5 years and adults usually visit a doctor only in the case of illness. Abortion is relatively common in Georgia, as it is throughout the former Soviet Union. One 35-year-old woman estimated that her married female friends had each undergone four or five abortions. The topic of abortion is not openly discussed, but there is no question about whether a woman is allowed to choose to have an abortion. Persons with a nagging cough often do not seek out professional health care. They ask a neighbor or co-worker for their recommendations and may experiment with a wide variety of medications before they consider visiting a doctor.

Ethnic/Race Specific or Endemic Diseases: Malaria and fasciola hepatica are endemic. Recent health risk appraisals indicated that Georgians were in the "very high risk" category because of lack of seat belt usage and stressful lifestyles, in the "high risk" category because of lack of exercise, and in the "moderate risk" category because of blood pressure and smoking. Body weight was comparable to American statistics, but the total cholesterol was lower than American values. The estimated prevalence rate for HIV/AIDS in adults ages 15 to 49 is 0.01%. The estimated number of children from birth to 15 years living with HIV/AIDS is less than 100. Homosexuality is discussed primarily in private and considered a taboo subject. Many homosexuals are married to members of the opposite sex and have children with them. Alcoholism is a problem in Georgia but has yet to be addressed seriously.

Health Team Relationships: Nurses are expected to take care of health maintenance tasks such as giving injections or changing surgical dressings. Doctors are responsible for providing a diagnosis, recommending a course of treatment, and administering delicate or complicated treatments. During the Soviet period, nurses provided home care for women who had recently given birth or individuals who had undergone serious surgeries. These services were provided as part of the health care system, and only nominal fees were charged. It is possible to access a similar level of care in the capital city despite the fact that the health care system is in disarray, but such services are too expensive for most people. Nurses are educated in 3-year programs in technical colleges.

Families' Role in Hospital Care: Families are responsible for preparing food for their hospitalized family members. They are also responsible for cleaning the patients and their bedpans. Because the health insurance industry is still in its infancy in Georgia, families are required to cover the full cost of medications, especially families in rural regions. At least one family member is always in a patient's room unless the patient is in the hospital to give birth. Women about to give birth are largely isolated from their families. Families visit pregnant women by communicating through a window that is usually closed. Hospital rooms are generally shared by at least two and sometimes as many as ten patients.

Dominance Patterns: The head of the family and the central decision maker in most Georgian families is the father or patriarch. In social situations, men often dominate group conversations while pairs of women quietly discuss other issues.

Eye Contact Practices: It is customary for men and women to make eye contact except with individuals that they are trying to avoid, such as beggars on the street.

Touch Practices: Georgians greet each other with handshakes, hugs, and kisses on the cheek. While waiting in line, Georgians do not hesitate to bump into or occasionally shove the person ahead of them.

Perceptions of Time: Punctuality is not highly valued in Georgia. In many instances, people's ability to arrive on time does not affect their access to health care. Many doctors do not require an appointment; patients simply show up, get in line, and wait. As long as patients meet with a doctor and obtain written confirmation of the appointment *(spravka)*, they are not penalized at the workplace.

Pain Reactions: Many women (one woman estimated 60%) cry out loudly during labor. This is considered normal behavior, and women who are not particularly loud concern health professionals.

Birth Rites: Primarily, Georgian women deliver their infants in a hospital. The delivery procedures are typical of Western practices, with the woman lying down and her legs elevated on leg rests. The pain of delivery is not usually eased with local anesthesia. Family members are not allowed into the maternity ward, and newborns are separated from their mothers except for three or four daily feedings. Both of these practices are to maintain a sterile environment for the infant and mother. Women and their infants remain in the hospital for 5 to 7 days, barring any unusual circumstances.

Death Rites: Most people die at home and are embalmed and prepared for viewing in the home. If a person is ill and dies in a hospital, the embalming and preparation of the body is conducted in the hospital. In either situation the deceased individual is dressed in nice clothes that are provided by the family and lies in state in the home, usually in the living room. If the death was unexpected, the family orders a coffin and the body is displayed on a makeshift wooden couch. Once the coffin arrives, the body is placed inside, and family and friends of the person come and visit during the next 3 or 4 days. Often a few personal effects of the deceased are placed in the coffin (e.g., jewelry, shaving implements, watches, glasses, writing implements, cigarettes) and eventually buried with the person. However, a previously selected item is placed in the coffin and then withdrawn just before the coffin is finally nailed shut. This item is said to bring good luck to the family. No pictures of the person's family members are allowed to be put in the coffin because Georgians believe that the people in the photograph would die shortly after the burial. The deceased person is buried on the fifth or seventh day after death. The body is removed from the home in a procession that can be quite short (e.g., for an older person—from the home to a waiting hearse on the curb) or very long (e.g., up to 2 km for a young person or for a person whose death was particularly tragic). When the procession concludes, the coffin is placed in the hearse and taken to a nearby cemetery. The coffin is placed on the ground next to the place where it will be buried, and family and friends have an opportunity to say their final farewells. The family of the deceased person goes first and then leaves the site shortly thereafter so that they will not have to watch the actual burial. During the final farewells, it is expected (particularly in rural areas) for family members to cry out loudly to show how much they miss the dead person. In fact, professional "wailers" are hired sometimes to increase the show of the family's loss. The family hires employees of the cemetery to bury the coffin.

Food Practices and Intolerances: Most people eat three times a day and have the largest meal in the evening. The staples of the Georgian diet are bread and various cheeses. Vegetables and fruits are available seasonally, including tomatoes, cucumbers, eggplant, corn, carrots, potatoes, strawberries, raspberries, oranges, and grapes. Many Georgian dishes feature chicken or turkey in sauces made with spices and ground walnuts. Georgians believe that eating raspberries or raspberry jam is beneficial for people with a fever.

Infant Feeding Practices: Breast-feeding is typical, and most women recognize that it is healthy for an infant to receive its mother's milk. Breast-feeding is not done in public; however, if breast-feeding is impossible for medical reasons or a woman chooses not to breast-feed, formula is available.

Child Rearing Practices: Parents are responsible for naming their children. They often name them after their own parents and tend to choose the paternal grandparents' names.

National Childhood Immunizations: BCG at birth; DTP at 2, 3, 4, and 18 months; OPV at 2, 3, 4, and 18 months and 5 years; measles at 12 months; DT at 5 months; and Td at 14 years. The reported percentages of the target population vaccinated are as follows: BCG, 95%; third dose of DTP, 98%; MCV, 97%; and Pol3, 98%.

BIBLIOGRAPHY

Imnadze P: Malaria in Georgian Republic, *Med Parazitol I parazitarnye bolezni* 1:20, 2001.

Kiladze M et al: Obstruction of common bile duct caused by liver fluke-Fasciola hepatica, *Sbornik lekarsky* 101(3):255, 2000.

Sabatinelli G: The malaria situation in the WHO European region, *Med Parazitol (Mosk)* 2:4, 2000.

Schengelia R: Georgia, country of ancient medical traditions, *Vesalius Acta Internationals Historiae Medicinae,* 6(1):64, 2000.

Wold JL, Williams AM, Kobaladze A: Health risks of health care workers: health risk appraisal results from the newly independent country of Georgia, *AAOHN* 47(4):151, 1999.

kiss in public. At the same time, public touching among members of the same sex (e.g., holding hands while walking or conversing) is common and not assumed to have sexual overtones.

Perceptions of Time: Time perception is Ghana is typically event oriented rather than time oriented. Continuing social interactions until an event is complete is considered more important than being punctual for another event.

Pain Reactions: In a health facility, commodity shortages may result in a complete lack of analgesics or use of an available but suboptimal analgesic. Outside of health facilities, self-diagnosis and self-treatment, often combined with advice from traditional healers, family, friends, or market sellers, may result in the use of inappropriate or ineffective analgesics.

Birth Rites: A little more than half of the births in Ghana take place at home, whereas the remainder take place in some kind of health facility. About 40% of deliveries are attended by traditional birth attendants, some of whom have had rudimentary training and some of whom have not. Of the deliveries in health facilities, most are attended by nurse midwives. Doctors are present at less than 10% of all deliveries and are usually called for in emergency situations. Newborns are typically kept inside for a period after birth until they prove they are healthy and have the will to live. At this point, usually 8 days after the delivery, the infant is brought outdoors and formally presented to the gods, the spirits of the ancestors, and society. This ceremony often includes a naming ritual.

Death Rites: Deaths in Ghana are typically followed by burial. Funerals are an occasion for mourning but also an opportunity to celebrate the life of the deceased person. Funerals are often colorful affairs and may last for days. Family and friends gather and have food and libations. Preparation of the body for burial is usually the responsibility of the deceased person's female relatives. In parts of Ghana, custom-made caskets representing some significant aspect of the deceased person's life are commissioned. The costs of funerals can be high, but even the poorest families usually collect the funds to provide a decent burial. Even if a costly funeral means incurring significant debt, it is preferable to risking the wrath of the ancestors. Anniversaries of deaths are also important and may be marked by remembrance events.

Food Practices and Intolerances: The Ghanaian norm is to eat three meals per day, with the evening meal being the most important. Common Ghanaian foods include staples such as cassava, yams, millet, corn, plantains, and rice. Most Ghanaians appreciate spicy foods such as pepper sauce. Meat, fish, and vegetables are commonly part of Ghanaian meals, and fresh fruit is often served as a dessert. Generally, the right hand is used to eat because the left hand is used to wipe the body after elimination. Malnutrition is widespread, especially among young children. In some situations, females have less access to food than males. Overall, access to safe water has improved in recent years and is available to approximately 75% of the population, although an urban (90%) and a rural (60%) differential remains.

Infant Feeding Practices: Breast-feeding for the first 18 months is nearly universal. About a third of all infants are exclusively breast-fed for the first 3 months. Neither formula nor milk is commonly used as a supplement, but use of other liquids such as juice and sugar water is widespread and they are introduced at a young age. Seven out of ten infants from 6 to 7 months old are breast-fed and supplemented with foods made out of grains, tubers, or animal products. Breast-feeding steeply declines at about 2 years, and less than 10% of children are still breast-feeding at age 3.

Child Rearing Practices: In Ghana the extended family is the primary socialization core and passes down traditional values to children through numerous informal mechanisms such as music, stories, and rituals. In general, society considers acts by individuals to reflect the values of the family. Consequently, child rearing tends to emphasize compliance with group norms rather than displays of independence and individuality. Despite a 1994 ban on the practice, female genital cutting continues to be practiced among some groups in the northern region of the country.

National Childhood Immunizations: BCG at birth; DPT at 6, 10, and 14 weeks; OPV at birth and 6, 10, and 14 weeks; measles at 9 months; YFV at 9 months; and TT for pregnant women and CBAW. The percentages of Ghanaian children who are fully immunized by age 1 are as follows: BCG, 85.9; third dose of DPT, 67.6; third dose of polio, 67.1; measles, 60.9; and all, 50.5. About 40% of 1-year-olds are immunized for yellow fever. Approximately 18% of mothers are not vaccinated against tetanus.

BIBLIOGRAPHY

Central Intelligence Agency: *The world factbook—Ghana.* Retrieved January 28, 2002, from www.cia.gov/cia/publications/factbook/geos/gh.html

Ghana Statistical Service and Macro International: *Demographic and health survey: Ghana, 1998,* Maryland, 1999.

Sarpong P: *Ghana in retrospect: some aspects of Ghanaian culture,* Accra, 1974, Ghana Publishing Corporation.

U.S. Department of State (February 1998): *Background notes: Ghana,* Office of West African Affairs/Bureau of African Affairs. Retrieved January 28, 2002, from www.state.gov/background_notes/ghana_0298_bgn.html 1/28/2002

USAID Global Health: *HIV/AIDS in Ghana,* www.usaid.gov/pop_health/aids/Counties/africa/ghana.html

World Health Organization (2001): *WHO vaccine-preventable diseases: monitoring system,* Geneva. Retrieved March 1, 2002, from http://www.who.int/vaccines/

World Health Organization: *Country statistics—Ghana.* Retrieved February 9, 2002, from www.unicef.org/statis/Country_1Page67.html

◆ GREECE (HELLENIC REPUBLIC)

MAP PAGE (860)

Elisabeth Patiraki-Kourbani

Location: Greece is on the southern border of the Balkan Peninsula in southern Europe. The country is surrounded by the Mediterranean Sea and has an archipelago of about 2000 islands. It shares borders with Albania, Bulgaria, and Macedonia to the north, Turkey to the northwest, the Aegean Sea to the east, the Mediterranean Sea to the south, and the Ionian Sea to the west. Its terrain is mostly mountainous, with ranges extending into the sea as peninsulas or chains of islands. The total land area is 131,940 km^2 (50,942 square miles).

Major Languages	Ethnic Groups	Major Religions
Greek (official)	Greek 98%	Greek Orthodox 98%
English	Turkish 1%	Muslim 1.3%
French	Other 1%	Other 0.7%

The number of residents who speak other languages such as Pakistani and Bulgarian is steadily increasing.

Health Care Beliefs: Acute care; traditional. The health culture tends to focus on acute care rather than prevention and is occasionally saturated with religious elements. The Greek Orthodox religion can be very influential in the sense that Greeks strongly believe that God gives health and allows illnesses for a reason. Therefore it is believed that illness may be cured through atonement and forgiveness. Some believe that health is promoted by eating certain foods, wearing amulets to protect against the "evil eye" (i.e., the power of a person to harm others simply by looking at them), prayer, good nutrition, and wine. Once quite common, the belief in the protective power of traditional blue beads is becoming less usual, but wearing a Christian cross is common. Many Greeks still use various folk healing practices and home remedies for treating particular diseases. Homemade preparations of numerous herbs are used as medications, elixirs, ointments, beverages, and plasters. Roots, leaves, flowers, and seeds are used according to their special qualities (e.g., as diuretics, soothers, neuroleptics, stimulants, analgesics). Common preparations include peppermint for stomach pain; chamomile as a soother; cinnamon, zeylanicum, and cloves for the common cold; poultices made with acorus, calamus, and alcohol for alleviation of arthritic pain; willow leaves for constipation; and eucalyptus for bronchitis. Approximately 30 years ago, mental illness was associated with significant social stigma, and attitudes toward it were more negative. Today, people with mental illness are easily accepted in social and economic life.

Predominant Sick Care Practices: Biomedical, alternative, and magical-religious. The biomedical view toward illness is replacing the more traditional, magical-religious views. Illness is attributed to pathogenic etiologies, but outside of the scientific community divine punishment and moral transgressions are traditionally considered causes of illness. Although medical care follows the Western model, Christian beliefs are also strong shapers of traditional caring practices. Greeks tend to withhold diagnoses of serious illness from patients to prevent anxiety, and relatives are informed before patients about their diagnosis. Greeks avoid saying the word "cancer" and prefer to refer to it as "the disease" or "the bad illness." Visiting sacred Christian sites and monasteries is common among people with chronic and serious illnesses and is combined with established medical practices. People may also use massage, wear talismans or charms to discourage evil, and use healing rituals and prayers. Use of over-the-counter drugs, especially vitamins and antibiotics, is widespread.

Ethnic/Race Specific or Endemic Diseases: Greeks are at risk for Mediterranean-type G6PD deficiency, β-thalassemia, and familial Mediterranean fever. Common health problems are cardiovascular diseases, traumas from automobile accidents, hypertension, diabetes mellitus, obesity, cancer, and smoking-related diseases. The increasing incidence of cancer and cardiovascular diseases in the last 30 years may be attributed to the dietary shifts of a great percentage of Greeks toward Western-style eating. The World Health Organization's (WHO) estimated prevalence rate for HIV/AIDS in adults ages 15 to 49 is 0.16%. The estimated number of children from birth to 15 years living with HIV/AIDS is less than 100. A cumulative total of 2163 AIDS cases were reported in Greece through December 2000, of which 32 (1.5%) were children. Out of a total of 21.31 adults and adolescents with AIDS, 86.9% are males and 13.1% are females. Greece seemed to have lower HIV incidence rates in 2000 than Switzerland, the United Kingdom, Luxembourg, Italy, Ireland, Denmark, and Belgium.

Health Team Relationships: Health care is doctor driven and centered. Doctors and administrators in the professional environment are usually dominant over nurses. The concept of a health team is practically non-existent because the authority and expertise of nurses for clinical decision making is not recognized, and nursing needs of patients receive low priority. Multiprofessionalism is still an aspiration rather than a reality in many clinical settings as is individualized holistic care. Poor multi-professional teamwork is a significant barrier to nursing professionalism. Conflict also occurs among nurses because of the many different educational preparation levels.

Families' Roles in Hospital Care: Hospitals have long visiting hours, and patients receive extensive care from family members and friends. Because of a nursing shortage, family members are allowed to stay at the hospital to provide practical, social, and psychological support. When a person is seriously ill, a peer or family member stays with the patient constantly. Family members bring in food that satisfies nutritional needs and meets dietary restrictions.

Dominance Patterns: Family unity and cooperation are important. Although primarily patriarchal, Greek families also have patterns of strong Mediterranean matriarchy. The accepted social norm is to fall in love with a member of the opposite sex, get married, and establish a family. Only 28% of older adults live alone. Love of family and respect for elders are strong values, and extended family relationships are close and supportive. Given the great respect for older adults, most Greeks would never consider institutional care for aging relatives. Regardless, the expanding population of older adults can create many family problems. Strong familial ties are also developed with non-family peers from churches and neighborhoods. Family lineage is respected, and children may be named after their grandparents. As in many European countries, marriage rates have decreased, divorce rates have increased slightly, and more women have entered the labor market. However, the traditional household structure has not changed as much as is has in other European countries because family solidarity is still very much the norm. Nearly half of all private households consist of couples with dependent children, whereas only 6% of households are single-parent households, the lowest in Europe.

Eye Contact Practices: Staring in public is acceptable, and direct eye contact denotes interest in and care for the speaker.

Touch Practices: Close physical proximity is maintained during conversations. Patients tend to prefer nurses of the same sex.

Perceptions of Time: Health care providers consider a delay of 5 to 10 minutes for an appointment to be acceptable. For social occasions, it is expected that people will be "fashionably late," or about 30 minutes late.

Pain Reactions: Expression of emotions when in pain are allowed and even encouraged. Most Greeks freely express their discomfort using facial grimaces and moaning, but some are quiet and stoical. It is often assumed that someone who does not express pain is not in a great deal of pain. Passive reactions to pain may be common among men who were taught that open and free expressions of pain are not masculine. However, it is often women who do not express their suffering in an attempt to spare their families from worry.

Birth Rites: Doctors deliver the majority of infants in hospitals. Some Greeks still celebrate the birth of a son more than the birth of a daughter because of the desire to pass on the family name.

Death Rites: People who are dying may be physically isolated from the outside world, and knowledge of their terminal diagnosis may be withheld. Close relatives travel vast distances to visit a dying person or attend a funeral. Dying at home is preferable, and friends, relatives, and family members visit and gather at the bedside to pray before a person's death. Icons depicting the saint after whom a person was named or one associated with the local church are commonly placed near the dying person. Folk culture instills a dread of death, and death rites maintain a social relationship with the deceased person. Children may be excluded from the rituals. Traditionally, a relative or older woman washes the body with water or wine. After cleaning, the body is wrapped in white cloth and placed in a coffin. When a young girl dies, it is common for her to be dressed as a bride for the burial. Coffins are often left open in church, and the face of the deceased person may be kissed by friends and family. Burial is preferred, preferably in a family's traditional burial grounds. Most bereaved women wear black after a death, but the length of time they wear it varies. Rural women usually wear black for the rest of their lives. Men do not wear black clothing but do wear an armband or black tie for 40 days and may not shave. Rituals are not concluded until the body has been exhumed 5 years later and the bones have been placed in an urn or vault. Grief is displayed openly and volubly. The traditional view is that death is not the end of life but the last ceremony in the present life. Bereaved family members receive sustained support from relatives and friends. If a sick child may die, the child is usually baptized quickly. In the case of sudden death, last rites are administered as quickly as possible. Organ donation is legal and receiving greater acceptance by the community. Some pagan (ancient Greek) traditions such as food offerings blend with Christian traditions; however, traditional grieving and mourning practices are becoming more affected by the influence of modern society.

Food Practices and Intolerances: Greeks typically eat three meals a day. Most Greeks have a light breakfast with coffee or milk and cookies. The main meal is lunch (at about 3 PM), and dinner is usually between 8 and 9 PM. Fasting during certain periods of the year is practiced for religious reasons; for example, on certain holy days Greeks do not consume meat, fish, milk, or eggs. During religious holidays the extended family is usually invited to the grandparents' home for a meal. Greeks still follow the typical Mediterranean diet, characterized by numerous grains, vegetables, and fruit and a low intake of saturated fats. Although overall sugar and fat intakes have increased, most increases in fat are in the form of mono-unsaturated olive oil. Adults traditionally consume alcohol in moderate quantities during recreational activities and meals.

Infant Feeding Practices: Most children are delivered in maternity hospitals, where about 77% of mothers begin breast-feeding. It is estimated that 47% continue breast-feeding at the end of the first month, 23% at the end of the third month, and 5% by the end of the sixth month. Introduction of foods depends on the infant's growth but usually starts at the sixth month, with fruits, vegetables, meat, eggs, and fish being introduced sequentially during the next few months. Mothers feel it is an obligation to breast-feed their children.

Child Rearing Practices: Parents are frequently overprotective of daughters; all children depend heavily on their families. After 40 days, infants are moved from their parent's bedroom into their own. Child rearing is permissive, and spanking is not allowed. However, parents may occasionally threaten to hit their children or lose their tempers and slap them. Mothers are responsible for most of the discipline.

National Childhood Immunizations: BCG between 6 and 7 years; DPT at 2, 4, 6, and 18 months; DT/Td at 14 to 16 years; OPV at 2, 4, 6, and 18 months and 4 years; MMR at 15 months and 6 years; ACT; HIB; and hep B at 2, 3, and 8 months.

BIBLIOGRAPHY

Andrews MM, Boyle JS: *Transcultural concepts in nursing care,* ed 2, Philadelphia, 1995, Lippincott.

Lofvander M, Papastavrou D: Clinical factor, psycho-social stressors and sick-leave patterns in a group of Swedish and Greek patients, *Scand J Soc Med* 18(2):133, 1990.

Madianos MG et al: Changes in public attitudes towards mental illness in the Athens area (1979/1980-1994), *Acta Psychiatr Scand* 99:73–78, 1999.

Ministry of Health and Welfare: Half yearly edition of Hellenic Centre for Infectious Diseases Control (HCIDC), *HIV/AIDS Surveillance in Greece,* No. 12, December 2000.

Rosenbaum JN: Cultural care of older Greek Canadian widows with Leininger's theory of culture care, *J Transcultural Nurs* 2(1):37, 1990.

Rosenbaum JN: The health meanings and practices of older Greek-Canadian windows, *J Adv Nurs* 16(11):1320, 1991.

Spector RE: *Cultural diversity in health and illness,* ed 4, Stamford, Conn, 1996, Appleton & Lange.

Stevens Mich M: Care of the dying child and adolescents: family adjustment and support. In Derek D, Hanks GWC, MacDonald N, eds: *Oxford textbook of palliative medicine,* ed 2, pp 1057–1075, Oxford, 1998, Oxford University Press.

Taylor R: Relaxation in the Peloponnese, *Midwives* 108(1228):152, 1995.

Willet WC et al: Mediterranean diet pyramid: a cultural model for healthy eating, *Am G Clin Nutr* 61:14024–65, 1995.

◆ GRENADA

MAP PAGE (858)

Cheryl Cox Macpherson

Location: Grenada is one of the Windward Islands at the southern end of the Caribbean. Within a 100-mile radius are the neighboring islands of Barbados to the east, St. Vincent and the Grenadines to the north, Trinidad to the south, and the Venezuela and Guyana coastlines to the west. Grenada is 35 km long (22 miles), with a total land area of 340 km^2 (131 square miles) and has a population of about 95,000. Most Grenadians live in and around the capital of St. George's at the southern end of the island. Areas outside of St. George's are more rural and often referred to as "the country." Many Grenadians immigrate to the United

States, Canada, or the United Kingdom for higher education and employment. Many of them return to Grenada regularly or when they retire. Grenada's main industries are tourism and export of fruits and spices. Socioeconomic levels range from households with incomes of approximately $3000 (U.S. dollars) per year to middle- and upper-class households and lifestyles. Most homes have a telephone and television and access to programs from the United States and Britain. The literacy rate is 98%.

Major Languages	Ethnic Groups	Major Religions
English (official)	Mainly Black African descent	Roman Catholic 64% Anglican 21% Other Protestant 15%

Health Care Beliefs: Traditional; health promotion increasing. It is widely believed that hot, cold, and wet conditions cause illnesses that may lead to death. Grenadians avoid rain and do not let children play in the rain. Many avoid exposure to such conditions and do not touch water (which is cold and wet) after ironing (which is hot) until the next day.

Predominant Sick Care Practices: Biomedical, religious, and traditional herbal medicine. Biomedical clinics are free in each parish or community. They are staffed primarily by community nurses, and doctors attend weekly. All medical facilities in Grenada are limited by financial and other resources, so they provide a different standard of care than in the United States. For example, Grenada currently has no intensive care or dialysis available. The main hospital is being extensively expanded and modernized but is not yet in service. Many doctors work for the government and in private practice; the majority of Grenadians prefer to attend private practices or clinics if they can afford to. When possible, patients with serious illness go abroad for treatment. The government pays for a few patients, whereas others assume bank loans to cover the cost; a few are able to afford it themselves. Traditional herbal medicine is called *bush medicine;* local plants are boiled into "teas" and consumed. People learn about these remedies from older relatives and community members. The Windward Islands Research and Education Foundation (WINDREF) at St. George's University is identifying and documenting the plants used for the various treatments and investigating their effectiveness. Some Grenadians avoid bush medicine for fear of pesticide contamination or because they do not know anyone who can instruct them on its proper use. Others use it to manage temporary and chronic illness including colds, flu, and hypertension or to supplement biomedical treatments. A drink said to be made from the bark or root of a local tree *(bois bande)* is used as an aphrodisiac, and occasionally patients have emergencies related to genital symptoms caused by large doses.

Ethnic/Race Specific or Endemic Diseases: Sickle cell anemia, rheumatic fever, dengue fever, rabies, toxoplasmosis, intestinal protozoan diseases, hypertension and diabetes, and human lymphotropic T cell virus

(HTLV-1) are all endemic diseases. The prevalence for sickle cell trait is 9.3%. The very first documented case was a 20-year-old Grenadian dental student in Chicago. He returned to Grenada and is buried in a cemetery at the north end of the island. The incidence of rheumatic fever is 20 cases per 100,000 people per year. An eradication project is underway through a collaborative program between the WINDREF, the Grenada Heart Foundation, the Grenadian Ministries of Health and Education, and Rockefeller University. The seroprevalence for dengue type 2 is about 93%. In late 2001, dengue type 3 was introduced and identified in Grenada for the first time. Rabies is present among wildlife, and humans are occasionally exposed (most recently, in 2001). The seroprevalence of toxoplasmosis in pregnant women younger than age 40 is 50%; it is 30% in cats. The prevalence of intestinal protozoans is 4% in conjunction with *Cryptosporidium* species and 30% in conjunction with *Giardia* and *Entamoeba* organisms. Hypertension and diabetes are major contributors to morbidity and mortality. HTLV-1 causes tropical spastic paresis and severe morbidity. It is fatal and transmitted vertically, with a prevalence of 3.9% in the general population (comparable to other Caribbean islands) and 7.7% in pregnant women. Although the World Health Organization (WHO) has no estimated prevalence rates for HIV/AIDS, local statistics indicate that the seroprevalence in pregnant women is about 0.5% (similar to recent data from the neighboring island of St. Vincent). The first Grenadian AIDS case was reported in 1984. By 1999 a total of 174 cases had been reported. Grenada has a national AIDS foundation and an AIDS unit within the Ministry of Health. (Existing programs encourage condom use.)

Health Team Relationships: The health care team consists primarily of doctors and nurses but is generally headed by doctors. Social services and technical staff are very limited because of scarce resources. Nurses are trained locally in a 3-year clinically based program of education.

Families' Role in Hospital Care: Families often supplement food, drink, bed linens, and toilet paper for hospitalized patients. For the most part, the nursing staff accepts family members' involvement in care.

Dominance Patterns: Women are often heads of households, but men are dominant in relationships.

Eye Contact Practices: Direct eye contact is acceptable among anyone.

Touch Practices: Greetings may include a handshake or other forms of touch. Kissing when greeting someone is uncommon.

Perceptions of Time: In businesses and workplaces, people are generally on time. Social events and parties start 1 or 2 hours later than scheduled. Grenadians are relaxed about time. One widely used phrase is "just now," which translates to Americans as "later" (sometimes hours later).

Pain Reactions: Strong narcotics are seldom prescribed; those with chronic pain turn to prayer and spirituality for comfort. Some patients with terminal diseases refuse pain medications to avoid side effects or because they believe that suffering is part of life and spiritually cleansing.

Birth Rites: Midwives are involved in hospital births, and work compatibly with local obstetricians. Obstetricians encourage hospital deliveries. Some infants are delivered in "maternity homes"—houses in which women give birth with the help of a midwife and allowed to stay overnight. Anecdotally, only one midwife promotes and facilitates home births; she calls an obstetrician if difficulties arise.

Death Rites: Many people choose to die at home with family or friends as their caregivers. Little or no medical or social support is available for patients who die at home or their caregivers. Patients seek comfort from family, friends, and spiritual connections.

Food Practices and Intolerances: Grenadians are relying more on fast and junk foods, which are readily available. Some children treated for intestinal "worms" say that the worms come from eating too many "corn curls" (a snack resembling American cheese puffs). Grenada has a local Food and Nutrition Council, and government standards govern the sale of fresh meat and fish. Common foods include *calaloo* (which resembles spinach), *provision* (root vegetables), *oil down* (a stew of local vegetables with coconut and dried fish or meat), and *buljol* (dried fish prepared like tuna salad).

Infant Feeding Practices: The Ministry of Health encourages breast-feeding during the first year of life, and most women breast-feed for at least that amount of time. When women say they are giving their infants "tea," they usually mean a bottle or a feeding (but occasionally mean sugar water, so it is best to ask for clarification). Bottle-feeding with formula or breast milk is common. A dilute solution of cereal in formula is sometimes introduced at 2 or 3 months. Solid foods are usually introduced at 4 or 5 months and consist of mashed produce (typically bananas, potatoes, *calalloo,* or pumpkin).

Child Rearing Practices: Extended families often involve homes with half-siblings and cousins living together with one parent. Grenadians have conventional marriages and families, as well as common-law marriages that last for years. Many women are single parents who raise several children who have different fathers, and some children in one family may also have different mothers. What Americans consider child abuse is common in Grenada, and spanking is an acceptable form of discipline. Corporal punishment is the norm in schools, where children are expected to speak only when spoken to. Older children learn public speaking in school.

National Childhood Immunizations: DTP at 6 weeks and 3, 5, and 18 months; OPV at 6 weeks, 3, 5, and 18 months, and 4 years; hep B at 6 weeks and at 3 and 6 months; HIB at 6 weeks and at 3 and 5 months; MMR at 12 and 18 months; and DT at 4 years. About 85% of all children are immunized in accordance with U.S. schedules and standards.

BIBLIOGRAPHY

Cox C, Macpherson CNL: Modified informed consent in a viral seroprevalence study in the Caribbean, *Bioethics* 10(3):222–232, 1996.

National HIV/AIDS Surveillance Program: Ministry of Health of Grenada Epidemiology Unit, 1999. Caribbean Epidemiology Center (CAREC), Trinidad and Tobago, www.carec.org

Pan American Health Organization: *Health in the Americas.* Scientific Pub No. 569, Vol II, pp 285–293, 1998, www.paho.org

Voelker R: HIV/AIDS in the Caribbean: big problems among small islands, *JAMA* 285(23), 2001.

Windward Islands Research and Education Foundation at St George's University: True Blue Campus, St George's, Grenada, www.sgu.edu

---

◆ GUATEMALA (REPUBLIC OF)

MAP PAGE (857)

Location: Bordered on the north and west by Mexico, on the east by Honduras and Belize, and on the south by El Salvador, Guatemala is the northernmost of the Central American nations. The country is primarily mountainous, with narrow coastal plains and a rolling limestone plateau. The climate is tropical—hot and humid in the lowlands and cooler in the highlands. The total land area is 108,890 km² (42,042 square miles). The population is approximately 12,974,361, with Spanish-speaking Ladinos more concentrated in urban areas and the indigenous Amerindian (Mayan) population primarily concentrated in the western highlands. About 42% of the population is between infancy and 14 years. Guatemala is a developing economy with wide income disparities: 60% of the population (mostly indigenous peoples) lives below the poverty line. The gross domestic product (GDP) per capita is $3700.

Major Languages	Ethnic Groups	Major Religions
Spanish (official)	Ladino (mixed	Catholic 88%
Amerindian languages	Spanish and	Protestant,
	Amerindian) 55%	indigenous
	Amerindian/	Mayan beliefs 12%
	Mayan 43%	
	White, other 2%	

Guatemala has 23 dialects of Amerindian languages, and the major dialects are Quiche (with approximately 300,000 speakers) and Cakchiquel,

Kekchi, Xinca, Mam, and Garifuna (with approximately 100,000 speakers each). The population structure of Guatemala is unique in that it has almost as many *indigenas* (those with a traditional Mayan lifestyle and languages) as Ladinos (Hispanics and individuals of Mayan descent with a Western lifestyle and who speak Spanish). Many people have a combination of Roman Catholic and indigenous Mayan beliefs and may seek favors from patron saints of villages using a combination of incense (Catholic in origin) and alcohol (Mayan in origin).

Health Care Beliefs: Acute sick care only. Measures to cure acute problems are valued and linked to preventive measures by some health care practitioners. Particularly in the rural areas, which have a higher concentration of indigenous peoples, Guatemalans prefer homemade remedies, such as verbena for a cough. At least a part of these traditional preferences are related to the lack of availability of other medications or treatments because of distance or cost. Traditional healers, or *curanderos,* serve the health needs of this population. Traditional peoples in particular may use a health system that categorizes medications and illnesses as either "hot" or "cold." According to this system, "hot" medications must be used to cure cold illnesses. Therefore, penicillin (which is considered "cold") could be used to cure a fever (which is "hot") but not pneumonia, a "cold" illness. Ladinos tend to seek modern Western, biomedical treatment, which is available in the city.

Predominant Sick Care Practices: Biomedical; alternative; traditional. Traditional herbs are incorporated into some health care treatments. *Nervo forza* is a popular liquid vitamin taken to promote health. Injections may be considered more effective than oral medications. A full range of medical care is available in Guatemala City. With more than 2 million people, it is the largest city in Central America. Although public hospitals are free, they often face serious shortages of basic medications and equipment. Care in private hospitals is generally adequate for most routine injuries and illnesses but must be paid for by the patient. Although they charge fees, Guatemalans many prefer private doctors to public facilities. Medical care outside the city is limited, although small towns generally have health clinics. Health workers also go into rural areas regularly to provide immunizations. They generally have no appointment system, and many drugs such as penicillin are available without a prescription.

Ethnic/Race Specific or Endemic Diseases: Endemic diseases include falciparum malaria, filarial, leishmaniasis (cutaneous and mucocutaneous), coccidioidomycosis, dengue fever, leprosy, Chagas' disease, polioviruses, onchocerciasis, parasitism, respiratory scleroma, and protein calorie malnutrition. Young children are at risk for lower respiratory tract infections and measles. Vitamin A deficiency is the most common cause of childhood blindness. Fatal automobile accidents are common, making driving hazardous. The World Health Organization's (WHO) estimated prevalence rate for HIV/AIDS is 1.38%. The estimated number of children from birth to 15 years living with HIV/AIDS is 1600. It is estimated that about 73,000 people in the country are living with HIV/AIDS. The estimated number of adults and children who died of AIDS in 1999 is 3600. The estimated number of children who have lost their mother or both parents because of AIDS is 5200.

Families' Role in Hospital Care: The family may care for all personal needs and sleep on mats around the patient's bed. Older relatives are usually cared for by the family. The concept of putting older people in institutions is strongly frowned on.

Dominance Patterns: Family life is important to Guatemalans, and families tend to stay close—emotionally and physically. The mother is the most important source of emotional support throughout her lifetime. Social functions include everyone in the extended family and create a sense of strength and solidarity. A double standard for husbands and wives exists, and women tend to ignore the extramarital affairs of their husbands. Men spend much time socializing with other men during the week, an important part of the culture. The literacy rate is 68.7% for males and 58.5% for females, with lower rates in indigenous populations than Ladino.

Touch Practices: Guatemalans are expressive in their touch practices. Touching is an important part of physical examinations and treatment by *curanderos* and Western practitioners. If a person's head hurts, it is expected that the *curandero* or doctor will touch the head. If the doctor does not, diagnosis and treatment may not be accepted.

Perceptions of Time: Punctuality is not valued in the Western sense. However, in cities and among Ladinos, being on time is more important than it is in rural areas. The concept of time is more relaxed for indigenous peoples. Traditions of the past are important among all groups and passed on through numerous festivals throughout the year.

Birth Rites: Traditional midwives with little or no training attend the births of more than 80% of indigenous Mayan women. Studies have shown that these midwives do not understand basic aseptic techniques and are unfamiliar with basic lifesaving skills, putting their patients at great risk. The birth rate is 34.61 births per 1000 people, and the infant mortality rate is 45.79 deaths per 1000 live births. The total fertility rate is 4.58 children born per woman. Life expectancy at birth is 63.85 years for men and 69.31 for women, with lower longevity in indigenous populations.

Death Rites: Funeral practices usually follow either Roman Catholic or Mayan traditions or a combination of both. November 1 is the *Day of the Dead,* when people return (if possible) to their birthplace to put food, alcoholic beverages, and flowers at the graves of family members and friends.

Food Practices and Intolerances: Three meals a day are the rule. Breakfast may be coffee and porridge or beans and eggs. Frequently the first meal is the midday meal, or *almuerzo*—a large meal of soup, meat, rice, vegetables, and salad. A lighter meal is eaten in the evening about 8 PM and consists of beans, bread, or leftovers from lunch. Fruits such as mameys, pitahayas, mangoes, and jocotes are popular. In rural areas, breakfast often consists of coffee, tortillas, and black beans. The mid-morning snack may be a drink or corn or rice mixed with sugar and cinnamon. The midday meal is large and similar to what is eaten in urban areas. At about 4 PM, it is common to have coffee and pastry, and the evening meal may be beans and tortillas, perhaps with eggs and onion. Corn and beans are the foundation of Mayan food practices. A *tamal* is cornmeal wrapped in a banana leaf and steamed, and a *chuchito* is cornmeal steamed in corn husks. Cornmeal mixed with lime is grilled to make tortillas. *Bunuelos,* enjoyed by all Guatemalans—particularly on feast days—are small doughnuts glazed with honey and sprinkled with cinnamon.

Child Rearing Practices: Rural children are at a disadvantage in terms of obtaining an education. Rural areas have fewer schools, and many children must stop their schooling to help support their families. In larger towns and villages, schools may be more available, but because students must pay for books and uniforms, school may still be unaffordable. More affluent people send their children to private schools. At age 15, a major party called a *quinceanos* is held to celebrate the attainment of adult-hood. The party is accompanied by feasting and breaking of *piñatas,* hollow containers of pottery or paper that hold candy and treats. The celebrants are blindfolded and given sticks to break the *piñatas,* which are usually hung from rafters. Most children do not leave the family home until they are to be married, regardless of their age. Living together before marriage is uncommon.

National Childhood Immunizations: BCG at birth; DTP at 2, 4, 6, and 18 months; OPV at 2, 4, 6, and 18 months; MMR at 12 months; vitamin A_6 before 35 months; DT at 6 to 15 years; and Td 1st contact older than 6 years, +1, +6 months, +1 year. The reported percentages of the target population vaccinated are as follows: BCG, 97; first dose of DTP, 94; third dose of DTP, 95; MCV, 88; Pol 3, 95; TT2 plus, 22; and vitamin A, 49.

Other Characteristics: Guatemala has one of the highest crime rates in Central America. Armed robbery, kidnapping, rape, armed assaults, and murder, especially of foreigners, have increased. Guatemala is a transit country for cocaine and heroin and a minor producer of opium poppy and cannabis for the international drug trade. Its proximity to Mexico makes it a major staging area for drugs (cocaine and heroin) intended for other parts of the world.

BIBLIOGRAPHY

Krauthahn K, Basarsky L: People of the corn: a nursing student experience in Guatemala, *Alberta Assoc RN* 51(4):18, 1995.

Lang JB, Elkin ED: International exchange. A study of the beliefs and birthing practices of traditional midwives in rural Guatemala, *J Nurse Midwife* 42(1):25, 1997.

Luecke R: *A new dawn in Guatemala,* Prospect Heights, Ill, 1993, Waveland Press.

Richards F et al: Knowledge, attitudes and perceptions (KAP) of onchocerciasis: a survey among residents in an endemic area in Guatemala, *Soc Sci Med* 32(11):1275, 1991.

Rowell M: Eradication of vitamin A deficiency with 5 cents and a vegetable garden, *J Ophthalmic Nurs Tech* 12(5):217, 1993.

Stewart EC, Bennett MJ: *American cultural patterns: a cross-cultural perspective,* rev ed, Yarmouth, Me, 1991, Intercultural Press.

http://www.cia.gov/cia/publications/factbook/geos/gt.html

http://cwr.utoronto.ca/cultural/english2/Guatemala/guatemalaENG.htm

http://travel.state.gov/guatemala.html

◆ GUINEA (REPUBLIC OF)

MAP PAGE (862)

Mohamed Sakho

Location: The Republic of Guinea covers 245,857 km^2 (94,925 square miles) and is situated along a 320 km (198 miles) coastline with the Atlantic Ocean in West Africa. Guinea-Bissau, Senegal, Mali, Côte d'Ivoire, Liberia, and Sierra Leone are its neighboring countries. Guinea has a tropical climate with two seasons: wet season from May to November with the heaviest rainfall occurring in July and August and dry season from December to April. Guinea is divided into four great natural areas: lower, middle, upper, and forest Guinea.

Major Languages	Ethnic Groups	Major Religions
French (official)	Peuhl 35%	Muslim 85%
Tribal languages	Soussou 30%	Christian 8%
(Peuhl, Malinke,	Malinke 25%	Indigenous beliefs 7%
Soussou, Kissi,	Guerze, Toma 9%	
Guerze, Toma)	Others 1%	

The population is estimated at 7,165,750 million with an annual population growth of 2.9%, and it still remains one of the poorest countries of the world. Although French is the official language, it is spoken only by 15% to 20% of the literate population.

Health care beliefs: Acute sick care; traditional. The national health program is based on the principles of primary health care and includes an extensive program of immunization and essential drugs. Since its inception, it has played a central role in disease prevention and health promotion. Mental illness is feared by the population, and thought to be the "work" of evil spirits, such as marabouts and djinna. A marabout is an erudite person with knowledge of the Holy Koran, who may use his knowledge in both good and bad ways to influence a person's destiny. A djinna is thought to be a powerful and invisible human living in the midst of other persons who may perform either good or bad acts. Given the supposed influence of these beings, it is believed that indigenous healers are more capable of treating certain diseases. Therefore, when patients seem not to be responding to treatment in a hospital, family members often remove them so that indigenous healers may treat them.

Predominant Sick Care Practices: Magical-religious and biomedical where available. Because of poverty and strong traditional beliefs, modern medicine is often used late; after traditional care practices have been unsuccessful. Despite the fact that the Guinean health system is known to be one of the best in West Africa, the predominant sick care practice continues to be herbal medicine that is used by *"tradipraticiens"* or indigenous healers. Their acceptance is so strong that there is a Department of Traditional Medicine within the national health program that coordinates traditional activities throughout the country. The use of different amulets in the shape of a neck, hand, or leg worn under a belt or other clothing is found in all the ethnic groups. People also believe that the evil spirits spread diseases, but that marabouts can counteract them by writing cabalistic formulas on wood in a liquid medium. This liquid is collected and used as a talisman by drinking it, or spreading it on the body. This is thought to prevent and heal numerous ailments. Scarification and deeper incisions are made by certain tribes to drain "bad blood" or to cut the invisibles ropes put there by witches in order to retain the patient in the sickness. When a woman is infertile, it is believed that throwing sheep's blood at her, followed by symbolic whipping, will chase away the cause of her infertility.

Ethnic/Race Specific or Endemic Diseases: The most deadly diseases in childhood are malaria followed by respiratory diseases. Tuberculosis and leprosy are major public health concerns in Guinea, but there are no specific diseases affecting only one ethnic group. Geography appears to be a factor, in that sickle cell disease is predominant in Middle Guinea due to a high rate of intrafamilial marriage in this population. High levels of goiter are found in Upper Guinea because of a lack of seafood rich in iodine, in addition to poverty. Upper Guinea is also in the onchocerciasis belt, a disease that is responsible for high levels of blindness in this population. Forest Guinea has high levels of Schistosomiasis. Guinea is host to Africa's second largest population, including 130,000 Liberians and 330,000 from Sierra Leone. This displaced population has worsened the status of health in Guinea for over a decade. These populations, who do not live strictly within camps, as well as those who interact with them in Forest Guinea, are in great need. Outbreaks of cholera and shigellosis raise the death rate periodically. They often start in the tiny islands disseminated along the coastline in Lower Guinea where there is no running water. Recently, a series of yellow fever outbreaks have resulted in the deaths of hundreds of people, primarily children. Lassa fever is an endemic hemorrhagic fever, with a seroprevalence of 14%. The World Health Organization's (WHO) estimated prevalence rate for HIV/AIDS in adults 15 to 49 is 1.54%. The estimated number of children 0 to 15 years living with HIV/AIDS is 2,700.

Health Team Relationships: People generally show respect and confidence toward physicians in particular, and to the medical corps in general. Since there is also great confidence in the skills of traditional healers, this same positive relationship is also noted towards *tradipraticians*. Nurses are in a subordinate role, and usually work in good relationships with physicians, faithfully executing their recommendations.

Families' Role in Hospital Care: The notion of family is very broad, and family ties are extremely strong in Guinea. For example, grandparents are part of the family structure, and their advice is prized. They usually have more knowledge of traditional medicine than everyone else, and advise family members on the treatment of illness. This often explains why herbal medicines are used initially, rather than sending the sick as soon as possible to the hospital. If a person is hospitalized, many people visit the patient and bring food. This is important in Guinean culture, since it is the responsibility of everyone in the neighborhood to visit the person. They are expected to contribute money to help the patient pay hospitalization fees, and to cover the cost of food and drugs. This is particularly important as health costs rise, and the people continue to live in poverty. Patients also may receive talismans, herbal medicines, and amulets in secret during their stay.

Dominance Patterns: The elderly have the most power in all ethnic groups, and males are dominant over females. This pattern remains unchanged regardless of the circumstances.

Eye Contact Practices: Rules regarding direct eye contact have a great deal to do with status. If an elderly person is speaking it is impolite to maintain eye contact, and looking down is considered to be a sign of good education.

Touch Practices: Physical touching, such as hugging and shaking hands, is acceptable in general among friends and relatives, where there is no risk of any sexual connotation. Tradipraticiens touch their patients in the process of healing ceremonies to chase away pain or illness. Physicians are allowed to touch patient of both sexes, but within the professional context. The patient's permission must be sought, especially if the patient is of the opposite sex.

Perceptions of Time: The fact that people are paid little for the time spent in the workplace is one of the reasons why the notion of time is not strongly considered in the population. Since punctuality is not a major issue, when someone needs to arrive at a particular time one must constantly insist that it is important to do so.

Pain Reactions: Reactions to pain vary, depending upon the cultural context. It is generally acceptable for girls to exhibit pain more than boys. Different cultural groups also have rules as to what is acceptable in terms of pain expression or not. For example, when a *Peulh* woman is delivering a baby, since culturally this group is more introverted, she is expected to handle the pain quietly. When a *Soussou* woman is delivering, her cries alert the entire neighborhood.

Birth Rites: Having a child after marriage is the greatest wish of all women. When a woman is unable to have a child this is often interpreted in negative ways. The infertile woman may be thought to be unfaithful or a witch. If she continues to be infertile, the husband may take a new wife, since polygamy is accepted and the culture authorizes up to four wives. Pregnant women avoid bathing in the evening to avoid giving birth to a Mongolian or deformed child. In Lower and Forest Guinea, in particular, but also in other ethnic groups, when a child has conditions such as spina bifida or a frank and early expression of chromosomal aberration (Djinnna or Se yinye) they are frequently sent away, and the medicine man/woman will give them a deadly mixture. In general, a son is more celebrated than a daughter, and at the hospital there is an extra fee when the baby is a male. During the pregnancy certain activities and foods are avoided, which is believed to save the baby from malformations or adopting animal behaviors. Future mothers eat special meals that contain medicinal herbs. Whenever someone is cooking she is offered food: thought to prevent black marks on her baby's skin.

Death Rites: Death is perceived as a definitive physical separation, and as such it is a sad event. The dead body is not exposed to view after being cleaned by two or three respectable and trusted individuals, and is then buried. Children are often taken away to be disposed of without formal burial. Organ donation is not approved of since it would make the family uncomfortable, and because culturally, the body is supposed to leave the earth intact as it arrived the first day of birth.

Food Practices and Intolerances: Most people avoid eating pork and other animals in which the blood has not been completely drained. However, Forest Guineans eat all kinds of game. The basic food throughout the country is rice. It is crushed so that the outside hull and subsequent vitamins are removed, before being washed and cooked. Therefore an important vitamin source is lost. The most important source of protein is seafood, and this is afford-able by almost everyone. Generally, people eat with their hands.

Infant Feeding Practices: Breast-feeding is always practiced except in rare cases of sickness. Certain nongovernmental organizations (NGOs) and the ministry of Health actively encourage it until children are at least over 6 months old.

Child Rearing Practices: All adults in the same family and even siblings have the right to educate their children the same manner as did their parents. Certain tribes (Tomah, Guerze) send their child to the "sacred forest." This is a secret and strong traditional institution where children receive their final education over a period of years far removed from their parents. Males and females usually are circumcised before 13 years of age. Corporal punishment is acceptable and the basis of education.

National Childhood Immunizations: BCG birth; DPT 4, 6, 10 months; OPV birth, 4, 6, 10 months; Measles 9 months.

REFERENCES

Sakho M: Des Anopheles dans la paume de Dieu, *Med Trop* 56(4):416, 1996.
Sakho M: Villages d'Endemie, *Med. Trop* 57(4): 346, 1997.
Sakho M: Emergence dans le Tropic, *Med. Trop* 59: 4, 1999.
Ter Meulen J, Lukashevich I, Sidibe K, et al: Hunting of peridomestic rodents and consumption of their meat as possible risk factors for rodent-to-human transmission of Lassa virus in the Republic of Guinea, *Am J Trop Med Hyg* 55(6):661, 1996.
World Health Organization: *Epidemiological fact sheets by country,* 2000, Geneva. Retrieved March 1, 2002, from
http://www.unaids.org/hivaidsinfo/statistics/june00/fact_sheets/index.html
World Health Organization: *WHO vaccine-preventable diseases: monitoring system,* 2001, Geneva. Retrieved March 1, 2002, from http://www.who.int/vaccines/

◆ GUINEA-BISSAU (REPUBLIC OF)

MAP PAGE (862)

Malene Kongsmark Flanding and Anja Poulsen

Location: The Republic of Guinea-Bissau is one of West Africa's smaller countries. It has a total land area of about 93,600 km² (36,000 square miles), which is approximately the size of Switzerland. Much of the coastal part of the country is mangrove, whereas the interior of the country is either cultivated or wooded savannah. Guinea-Bissau gained independence from Portugal in 1974. In 1998 and 1999 a military revolt evolved into a complex emergency. The country is still politically and economically unstable.

Major Languages	Ethnic Groups	Major Religions
Portuguese (official)	African 99%	Indigenous
Criolo	European, mulatto 1%	(animist) 56%
Numerous African		Muslim 35%
languages		Christian 9%

Guinea-Bissau has approximately 1.2 million inhabitants, of which approximately a third live in the capital of Bissau. Almost all of the population is of African descent. The main ethnic groups are Balanta (30%), Fula (20%), Mandinka (14%), Manjaco (13%), Papel (7%), and others (16%). Each ethnic group has its own language, but in the urban setting of Bissau, it is Creole—a mixture of Portuguese and indigenous languages—the most commonly used language. The beliefs in witchcraft and sorcery and other forms of spiritual entities are usually intertwined with whatever religion people practice. Guinea-Bissau is one of the world's poorest countries; the gross national product (GNP) per capita was estimated to be $250 in 1996. The country ranks 164th out of 174 nations using UNDP's human development index. The economic state of the country has deteriorated because of the war in 1998 and 1999. Adult literacy rates are 68% for males and 42.5% for females.

Health Care Beliefs: Acute care; traditional. Three health sectors exist: professional, folk, and popular. They are all complementary and used in combination, particularly in the urban setting of Bissau. The folk sector consists of various types of traditional healers, whereas the popular sector involves "home medicine," which includes self-diagnosing and self-medicating (e.g., treating malaria with chloroquine) because drugs are sold without prescriptions in pharmacies and local markets. The popular sector also includes the use of homemade medicines consisting of fruits, spices, herbs, and roots. Wearing amulets for health protection is a widespread practice throughout Guinea-Bissau, as is finding causes for illnesses in the world of the ancestors and spirits or attributing illness to witches or sorcery.

Predominant Sick Care Practices: Biomedical where available; self-treatment and magical-religious. Although access to the professional sector (i.e., hospitals, trained doctors, Western medicine) is very available in Bissau, it is much more difficult to obtain adequate Western medical care in rural areas. Because of the high mortality rates resulting from poor biomedical health care access, most people who are getting ill tend to quickly seek advice either at a health center from an indigenous healer or at the local pharmacy. Whether a person seeks help at a health center from an indigenous healer or just at the pharmacy depends on where in the country the person lives, the type of disease the person has, and the person's financial status. In the rural areas, Western medical care is often difficult to obtain and most villages have a "witch doctor." In the capital the health centers are popular. Indigenous healers are often preferred for treating chronic diseases and psychiatric disorders. The wealthier families in the capital go to private clinics. Health centers are placed in bigger towns and villages all over the country and in the different suburbs of the capital. In the countryside the medical staff normally includes an analyst and a nurse; in the capital, most of the centers have a medical doctor as well. One general problem is the lack of essential drugs and equipment because of the poor medical infrastructure (which has become especially problematic since the war). Adults can officially be charged a small fee for the consultation. According to health authorities, treatment of children and pregnant women is free; however, it is common for them to be charged. This practice is accepted in many places because the public wages for health personnel are very low. Drugs, needles, and dressings are normally purchased at the local pharmacies or paid for at the health centers. In the countryside a few smaller hospitals exist, but in the capital, the hospital Simao Mendes receives patients from all over the country. Currently the hospital lacks essential equipment (e.g., oxygen, needles, medicine) and electricity. It is generally accepted that patients should pay for the treatments and medicine, often directly to the health staff. About 41% of the population has access to health services.

Ethnic/Race Specific or Endemic Diseases: Malaria is highly endemic and can be resistant to chloroquine. Information campaigns to prevent spread of the disease are currently arranged by the health authorities. Tuberculosis is common in children and adults. Both tuberculosis and AIDS have an attached stigma, which makes communication about these diseases difficult among doctor, patient, and family. In the 1990s, large outbreaks of cholera and meningitis occurred. Other endemic diseases include human rabies, hepatitis B and A, and measles. Childhood mortality for all ages is among the highest in the world. The most frequent causes of death are malaria, diarrhea, acute respiratory tract infections, and malnutrition. Only about 60% of the population has access to safe water, a factor in the spread of disease. AIDS is a serious health problem. In contrast to many other African countries, the human immunodeficiency virus type 2 (HIV-2) is still more common than HIV-1, and about 10% of people older than 35 years of age are infected with HIV-2. Individuals with HIV-2 have higher mortality rates than those who are uninfected, but the development of AIDS is slower than AIDS caused by HIV-1. Compared with other countries, the incidence of HIV-1 is low. The World Health Organization's (WHO) estimated prevalence rate for HIV/AIDS in adults ages 15 to 49 is 2.5%. The estimated number of children from birth to 15 living with HIV/AIDS is 560. These figures are expected to rise as a result of the recent war. In 2000, 4% of women who gave birth in the country's largest hospital were infected with HIV.

Health Team Relationships: After independence from Portugal in 1974, the country had very few doctors. At the hospital in the capital, doctors were primarily Cuban and Portuguese. At many health centers, nurses or assistant nurses have for many years been responsible for all medical treatment. During the 1980s and 1990s, more Guinean doctors finished their education either in Guinea-Bissau or abroad. Although the health system is hierarchical, nurses and doctors normally collaborate without any major problems. The patient is expected to be submissive and respectful toward the doctors and nurses. The nurses and doctors do not usually show empathy toward sick patients. Patients always expect a prescription for oral medications, or even better (from he patients' perspective), medication injections. If Guineans have a nurse or a doctor in the family, they normally seek their advice first. Although the government has clear rules for payment, it is common for health personnel to charge the ill person lesser or greater amounts for the consultation than outlined.

Families' Role in Hospital Care: Families assume responsibility for care of their hospitalized family member. Not only do they assume financial responsibility (e.g., pay for medicine and syringes), but they also care for the patient in terms of their food, water, and hygiene.

Dominance Patterns: Guinea-Bissau is a patriarchal society. Still, in practice, the head of a household can be a woman, who assumes responsibility should someone in the household become ill. The relationship between men and women also varies according to ethnic group, social status, and whether the people are in an urban or a rural setting. Age is also an important factor in relationships; people must be respectful of anyone who is older.

Eye Contact Practices: Direct eye contact is not an issue between sexes or among people from different age or social groups.

Touch Practices: Physical contact between men and women is very rarely seen in public settings, whereas physical contact (e.g., holding hands) among members of the same sex is quite common. Women in urban settings may greet each other by kissing on the cheek, whereas men shake hands. A man may hold the wrist of a woman in a firm grip. This form of touch does not have sexual connotations but can be a way of conveying that the man has a matter he would like to discuss.

Perceptions of Time: Punctuality is not usually an issue among friends and family members although if a person is employed, punctuality is more important. Wearing a watch is a sign of status, so it is not uncommon for some young people to wear watches even when the watches do not work. The intensity and position of the sun is widely used as a way to assess the time of day, particularly among people of older generations.

Pain Reactions: Telling a person to *sufri,* or suffer, is common when the person is in any kind of pain. "Controlling the head"—displaying self-control—and controlling emotional expressions are behavioral ideals in the society. Words are considered powerful, therefore verbal expressions of pain are not always accompanied by the body language Westerners might expect. Being able to express pain verbally and in a controlled way is considered sufficient in many respects. This does not mean that peoples' reactions to pain are never expressed verbally or with body language; it does mean that when people are in pain, others often try to calm them in a way that may seem rather harsh (e.g., by telling them to suffer or stop crying). It is more accepted for women and children to cry, whereas men are expected to suffer quite stoically. Women often react to pain and show pain by tying a piece of cloth tightly around their forehead *(mara kabeca).*

Birth Rites: Birth is considered a preoccupation and concern for women, not men. If a woman is giving birth at home, an old woman from the family and a local midwife assist her. In the capital city, half of the deliveries occur at the hospital or at health centers; only the midwife assists, and the family must wait outside the room. Traditionally the mother and the child were expected to stay inside the house for the first week to avoid harm from the wind (or evil spirits); however, this tradition is not strictly practiced today. Some ethnic groups have a feast for the child on the seventh day after birth. The infant receives gifts and is celebrated—and is finally considered a "real" child. Muslims circumcise boys before they begin school. Several of the other ethnic groups perform circumcisions when the boys are 7 to 14 years of age. Men of the Balanta ethnic group have to prove that they are real men before their circumcision, so often a man has several children before the procedure. Traditionally, the circumcision is performed after a period of isolation in the forest, where the rituals of the ethnic group are taught. Girls are normally not circumcised, although Muslims may perform the procedures in rural areas. The mortality rate for children younger than 5 is 27 per 1000 live births, which is the sixth highest in the world; life expectancy at birth is 43.4 years.

Death Rites: The body is usually buried within 24 hours. If an older person dies, the death is regarded as a happy event, and the family has a feast celebrating the person's long life. The feast lasts for at least a week, and it is the responsibility of the family to provide food and beverages. Funerals are extremely important social events (and in some cases are business events) where contacts are maintained or created. It is important for people to attend a funeral if they know any of the deceased person's family members. When a child or a young person dies, it is an unhappy event, and no large feast is arranged. Roman Catholics have a mass at a church, and other ethnic groups perform the appropriate ceremonies, in some instances a year later. The size of the funeral represents the prosperity of the family and can be very costly for members of a poor society such as Guinea-Bissau. Muslims normally do not have long funerals. Autopsies and organ donations are generally unacceptable.

Food Practices: Breakfast is not a main meal, and often a little leftover rice from the day before is eaten. If the family has enough money, they may make porridge or fried eggs or buy bread and margarine. Rice is the main staple throughout Guinea-Bissau. In the morning, the women go to the market to shop for the day's meals and usually buy either a bit of fish, chicken, or meat. Lunch, which is the main meal of the day, can be eaten anytime between 1 and 4 in the afternoon. A person who is sitting and eating lunch invites anyone who passes to come and eat. This is more of a polite greeting than a real invitation. Different members of the household do not always eat at the same time. They may take turns, and the whole household is divided up according to who eats from the same bowl—divisions that are made according to age, gender, or both. People usually eat with spoons or their hands. If people eat in the evening, the meal is light. Children may be given some boiled potatoes or soup with spaghetti or porridge. Fruits such as mangoes, oranges, and bananas are eaten as snacks, as are peanuts and cashew nuts.

Infant Feeding Practices: Infants are breast-fed for an average of 22 months. Length of breast-feeding varies considerably according to ethnicity. The Balanta breast-feed for the longest period and the Muslims for the shortest. The Balanta often regard the colostrum as "bad" milk. In the capital of Bissau, bottle-feeding is a symbol of social status but is seldom used. Supplementary food normally is introduced at 4 to 6 months, although the age varies according to ethnic group. The most common semiliquid food is made of rice or corn.

Child Rearing Practices: Children spend most of their time in or around their family's home. The use of a local form of adoption *(criacon)* is common, so children do not always live with their mother or father. It is common for older siblings to take care of younger siblings, and children, especially girls, perform various chores in the house. Children usually sleep in the same room and bed with family members of their own age group until they are in their teens, at which time they sleep only with children of the same age, not the same sex.

National Childhood Immunizations: BCG at birth; DTP at 2, 3, 4 months; OPV 2, 3, and 4 months; measles at 9 months; and TT CBAW. Mothers in Guinea-Bissau are generally very positive about immunizations. In Bissau a high percentage of children are vaccinated, whereas vaccine administration in rural areas has been irregular (especially after the war) because of logistic problems, resulting in low immunization coverage in certain areas.

BIBLIOGRAPHY

Aaby P et al: *Child mortality in Guinea-Bissau. Malnutrition or overcrowding,* 1978.
Forrest JB: *Guinea-Bissau. Power, conflict, and renewal in a West African nation,* 1992, Westview Press.
Larsen OD: *Epidemiology of retroviral infections in Guinea-Bissau,* doctoral dissertation, 1998.
Godtfredsen U: *Disease perceptions and therapy strategies,* Interim Report No 2, Guinea-Bissau, 1995, Projecto Saude de Bandim, Bissau.
Kovsted J, Tarp F: *Guinea-Bissau: war, reconstruction and reform,* Working Papers No 168, Helsinki, Finland, 1999, UNU World Institute for Development Economics Research.
www.ui.se/fakta/afrika/guineabi.htm

◆ GUYANA (COOPERATIVE REPUBLIC OF)

MAP PAGE (859)

Consultant: Narinee Persaud

Location: Formerly a colony of Britain (British Guiana), the country is located on the northern coast of South America. The North Atlantic Ocean is to its north, Suriname to the east, Brazil to the south, and Venezuela and Brazil to the west. Guyana has rolling highlands, a low coastal plain, and savannah in the south. An extensive network of rivers runs from north to south. The climate is tropical—hot and humid, moderated by northeast trade winds. Guyana has two rainy seasons: May through mid-August, and mid-November to mid-January. The total land area is 214,970 km^2 (83,000 square miles), slightly smaller than Idaho. The low coastal areas are inhabited by 90% of the total population of 679,286. The capital is Georgetown. Guyana is a developing nation with a gross national product (GNP) per capita of $4800. About 62% of the population lives in rural areas.

Major Language	Ethnic Groups	Major Religions
English	East Indian 51%	Christian 50%
Amerindian dialects	Black African 30%	Hindu 33%
Hindi	Mixed 14%	Muslim 9%
Urdu	Amerindian 4%	Other 8%
	European and Chinese 1%	

African slaves were brought to Guyana to work the sugar plantations, followed by workers from the Indian subcontinent. These groups make up the majority of the population. Each ethnic group has retained its own culture and lifestyle and has strong African and Indian traditions. Guyana more closely resembles the islands of the West Indies rather than South America in terms of history, culture, and economic characteristics. Guyana is tolerant of religious diversity. For example, Indians may be baptized as Christians and continue to participate in Hindu rituals.

Health Care Beliefs: Acute sick care; traditional; limited prevention. Some prevention procedures are practiced, such as blood pressure checks for individuals with hypertension. However, most visits to doctors are because of sickness. People believe in the "evil eye" as a cause of illness (the power of a person to harm others merely by looking at them), especially regarding infants and children. A particular brownish yellow soaplike substance or oil is also rubbed on the clothes of infants; the strong smell is thought to keep illness away. When adults believe they may have been affected by the evil eye, they frequently go to a priest (if they are Hindu), who tells them which prayers they should recite to thwart the evil actions. An amulet in the shape of the number three with another inverted three on top is also held or worn to prevent evil or sickness.

Sick Care Practices: Limited biomedical and magical-religious. The government provides a considerable amount of social assistance in the form of old-age pensions, relief for older adults, and relief for destitute or infirm children. The public health system has been successful in eradicating malaria as an endemic disease. Medical care is available for minor health conditions, but the individual must pay for doctor's visits and hospital care. Emergency care for major medical illnesses or surgery is available but limited because of a lack of appropriately trained specialists, outdated diagnostic equipment, and poor sanitation. Ambulance service is substandard and may not be available when needed for emergencies. Some prescription medicines (mostly generic) are available in the country, but many cannot be obtained.

Ethnic/Race Specific or Endemic Diseases: Endemic diseases include filariasis, dengue fever, American cutaneous leishmaniasis, and intestinal parasites. Chloroquine-resistant malaria has recently been eliminated as an endemic disease but remains a risk. People are also at risk for diabetes mellitus, yellow fever, and leprosy. Water pollution from sewage and agricultural and industrial chemicals poses a health risk. The World Health Organization's (WHO) estimated prevalence rate for HIV/AIDS in adults ages 15 to 49 is 3.01%. The estimated number of children from birth to 15 years living with HIV/AIDS is 140. About 900 children and adults died of AIDS in 1999, and 1100 children have lost either their mothers or both parents to AIDS since the epidemic began. HIV prevalence in antenatal women ranged from 4% to 7% between 1992 and 1997, and 44% of sex workers tested in Georgetown in 1997 were infected with HIV. In addition, in 1997 25% of males and 18% of females in clinics for sexually transmitted diseases were infected with HIV. It is estimated that 15,000 people are currently living with HIV/AIDS.

Health Team Relationships: Doctors and nurses seem to respect each other. Most people, especially those outside of cities, see private doctors rather than go to hospital clinics because of the distance to health care facilities. Doctors head the health care team, and nurses primarily provide personal care and specified treatments.

Families' Role in Hospital Care: Family members visit often and may stay with friends or family near the hospital so that they can be there early in the morning to assist their relative. It is common to bring in homemade food even though the hospital provides food, and provisions are made to heat or cool food as necessary. Families make an effort to consult with the health personnel so that they can bring food appropriate for the patient's medical condition.

Dominance Patterns: Men are considered the head of the household, but most consult with their wives about important decisions. Most women do not work outside of the home and assume the major responsibilities for the children and household.

Eye Contact Practices: Although children have much respect for their parents, direct eye contact is usual and acceptable. Children may also maintain direct eye contact with older adults. When children meet older adults on the street, they are expected to greet the adults politely (rather than ignore them) out of respect, regardless of whether they know them.

Touch Practices: People who know each other well commonly kiss each other in greeting or hug or shake hands. It is common for men and women to shake hands, and a handshake is the usual greeting when meeting someone for the first time.

Perceptions of Time: People look to the future, but past traditions are very important.

Pain Reactions: It is acceptable for men and women to express pain. Men are not usually as open about the pain they are experiencing and seldom cry out. Regardless, many individual variations exist. Some women are quite stoical and silent about pain, and some men are very expressive.

Birth Rites: On the first day of an infant's birth, Hindu families go to a priest and tell him the day and time of the infant's birth. Consulting a book, the priest picks a name for the infant. A bracelet of black and white beads is put on the infant's ankle as quickly as possible to protect against the evil eye. A small black dot may also be put on the forehead of the infant for extra protection. Mother and infant usually stay at home in the bedroom and rest for 9 days while either a sister or older family member takes care of them. Although the mother stays in bed much of the time, family and friends are allowed to visit. On the ninth day, the mother says prayers privately, and mother and child go outdoors for the first time for a party with friends and family.

Death Rites: Family members (who are able) gather to say their final goodbyes to a person who is dying. During and after the dying process, Christians and Hindus stay up most of the night singing hymns and saying prayers to sympathize with the family. As a rule, Hindus favor cremation and Christians favor burial, but some Hindus bury and some Christians cremate their loved ones. When a person dies in the hospital, the funeral home is called to take the body for immediate cremation or to the person's home. If the body is brought home, a special metal coffin with a clear plastic area over the head is obtained from the funeral home. The climate is hot, and embalming is not done. During the several days while the body is viewed at home, ice is put under and around the person regularly by the funeral home staff, and the melted water is drawn off. Hindus obtain permission to publicly cremate their loved ones in an open area such as the beach. Wood and other materials are gathered, and family and friends gather to observe the ceremony. Afterward, those attending stay together for a meal. Prayers are then recited for 12 days. On the twelfth day, family and friends have a large service and recite additional prayers in memory of the person.

Food Practices and Intolerances: Chicken fried rice, spicy dishes, curried chicken, yellow peas, and *dholl-puri* (a special bread) are very popular among those of East Indian descent, although people of Black African descent like these foods as well. Black Africans especially like the *pepper pot,* a combination of beef, vegetables, and rice, or *brown stew,* which is a combination of peas and rice with meat. Cooking is done on stoves or outside over open fires. It is common for people to have concrete squares with burners on top and a place for burning wood below, which makes practical sense in this hot country, even for people who live in cities.

Infant Feeding Practices: Breast-feeding is very common and varies greatly in terms of duration—from 1 month to years. It is also common to breast-feed part of the time and bottle-feed part of the time. As foods begin to be introduced, it is common to make porridge out of green plantains (which are similar to bananas). The plantains are dried and brought to the mill to be ground into flour that is mixed with cow's milk or formula and occasionally sugar to form a thin gruel. Barley seeds are processed in the same way for infant food. The infant mortality rate in Guyana is 38.72 deaths per 1000 live births, and the total fertility rate is 2.1 children born per woman. Life expectancy at birth is 60.52 for males and 66.24 for females.

Child Rearing Practices: In 1995, 100,300 pupils were enrolled in 422 elementary schools, and 62,000 were attending either technical, secondary, or teacher education programs. The one source for higher education in Guyana is the University of Guyana in Georgetown. Literacy rates are 98.6% for males and 97.5% for females (a 1995 estimate).

National Childhood Immunizations: BCG at birth; DPT at 3, 4, 5, and 17 months and 3 to 4 years; OPV at 3, 4, 5, and 17 months and 3 to 4 years; MMR at 12 months and 3 to 4 years; YFV at 1 and +10 years; DT at 5 years, +1, +6 to 12 months, and 11 years; and TT for pregnant women, +1 month. The reported percentages of the target population vaccinated are as follows: BCG, 93; first dose of DTP, 97; third dose of DTP, 88; MCV, 86; Pol3, 78; TT2plus, 81; and YFV, 83.

Other Characteristics: Severe drought and political turmoil caused a decline in economic expansion in 1998. In 2000 the situation reversed, and Guyana resumed a pattern of economic growth. It is a transshipment point for narcotics from South America, primarily from Venezuela, to Europe and the Untied States. It is also a producer of cannabis.

BIBLIOGRAPHY

Palmer CJ et al: HIV prevalence in a gold mining camp in the Amazon region, Guyana, *Em Infect Dis* 8(3):330, 2002.

Rawlins SC et al: American cutaneous leishmaniasis in Guyana, South America, *Ann Trop Med Parasitol* 95(3):245, 2001.

http://www.cia.gov/publications/factbook/geos/gy.html

http://encarta.msn.com/

http://travel.state.gov/guyana.html

◆ HAITI (REPUBLIC OF)

MAP PAGE (858)

Bette Gebrian and Jean Claude Tabuteau (Consultant: Kathleen Clerie)

Location: Located in the West Indies of the Caribbean, Haiti occupies the western one third of the island of Hispaniola, which it shares with the Dominican Republic. The total land area is 27,750 km² (10,714 square miles). Much of the mountainous northern soil is denuded. Haiti is known as the poorest nation in the Western Hemisphere.

Major Languages	Ethnic Groups	Major Religions
French	Black 95%	Catholic 80%
Creole	Mulatto and	Protestant 16%
	European 5%	Other 4%
		Voodoo (Regardless of their religion, as many as 90% of Haitians believe in voodoo.)

Health Care Beliefs: Passive and somewhat fatalistic role; acute sick care only. Traditional individuals may evaluate their illness according to symptoms previously experienced by close relatives. Families play an important role in health beliefs and health-seeking behavior. Herbal infusions are used for various common complaints such as upset stomach *(te zebaklou),* heat rash *(amidon and clarin),* and many others. Teas and infusions are used to a much greater extent than they are in the traditional U.S. culture. Abortion is never openly discussed, although hundreds of herbal concoctions reportedly induce abortions. Untrained people regularly do abortions, and the resulting death rate is unknown. Many Haitians prefer injected medications rather than oral, believing that injections are more effective in curing illness. Prevention is not a strong concept but can be integrated into family health care with empirical evidence of importance (e.g., rehydration during episodes of diarrhea). In some cases, AIDS is considered to be caused by supernatural forces and unrelated to individual behavior.

Predominant Sick Care Practices: Biomedical and magical-religious. Western medical treatment is sought (including in rural areas) more often than traditional medicine is used. Belief in voodoo is important, as is the belief in prayer and the healing power and protection of God against misfortune. Illnesses that are perceived to originate supernaturally or magically can be treated with voodoo medicine only. Ethnomedical beliefs about disease are based on maintenance of a hot/cold equilibrium within the body. Herbalists treat common disorders and specialize in the treatment of the "evil eye" *(maldyok,* or the power of a person to harm others merely by looking at them).

Ethnic/Race Specific or Endemic Diseases: Chloroquine-sensitive falciparum malaria is endemic, and dengue fever is also frequently found in Haiti, although it is only indirectly diagnosed. Vitamin A deficiency is the most common cause of childhood blindness, and umbilical hernias are common. The rate of childhood malnutrition is the highest in the Western hemisphere, and as many as 20% of the children younger than 5 years have some degree of undernourishment. The overall contraceptive prevalence rate of women in relationships in Haiti is 28%. The World Health Organization's (WHO) estimated prevalence rate for HIV/AIDS in adults ages 15 to 49 is 5.17%. The estimated number of children from birth to 15 years living with HIV/AIDS is 5200. Homosexuality is discussed primarily in private, and many homosexual people are married to people of the opposite sex and have children. In the capital city, people are attempting to promote others to openly discuss homosexuality and sexual practices to decrease the spread of HIV.

Health Team Relationships: The doctor is the primary authority in hospital settings, and nurses are subordinate. If nurses are the only health care professionals available, they are afforded more respect. Patients believe that expert authority should dictate care, but in some cases the "expert" is an untrained paraprofessional who has set up a thriving practice because doing so is inexpensive and easy. Disapproval with a health care professional is not outwardly expressed, but contact is severed.

Families' Role in Hospital Care: The family is required to stay with the patient, provide food, and help with basic hygiene. Some may wait to be told how they can help. *Family* is a loose term that encompasses close friends. Visiting the sick is expected, and friends and families rally around people in need.

Dominance Patterns: Haiti has a matriarchal society. The family is a mutual support system and siblings remain close, even after marriage. Unlike in some cultures, girls and boys receive equal medical attention. Girls are expected to be more proficient in homemaking skills than boys. Haiti has women professionals and politicians.

Eye Contact Practices: It is customary to maintain eye contact with everyone except authority figures and the poor. Children are not supposed to look their parents in the eye and are expected to look down.

Touch Practices: Shaking hands is the customary greeting. Haitians have adopted the French custom of kissing on both cheeks when greeting a friend (but not a stranger); children kiss one cheek of an adult when they greet them in any situation. It is considered rude for a young man to touch a woman (e.g., put his hand on her arm or shoulder). When a child or adult has a fever or a cold, families warm freshly made castor oil ($15 [U.S. dollars] per gallon) and rub it on one side of the body one day and on the other side the next day. This process is repeated as many times as necessary. When a woman is in labor, the midwife rubs her belly with homemade Haitian soap to advance labor.

Perceptions of Time: Punctuality is not an important value. A formal social system of publishing starting times exists in which the real starting time is later than the published time. Hope for the future promotes a future-oriented view; however, the society is oriented predominantly to the present.

Pain Reactions: A high tolerance for pain and discomfort exists, although some sources indicate that Haitians have a low threshold. Loud verbal expressions may be heard during labor.

Birth Rites: Some women believe they must continue sexual intercourse during pregnancy to keep the birth canal lubricated or that they must avoid exposing themselves to cold air. Purgatives are regularly taken during pregnancy to cleanse impurities from the fetus, primarily from its blood and stomach. A newborn or child may receive laxatives to foster health and strength. Most infants are delivered at home with the mothers in a squatting or semi-seated position. Believers in voodoo have the delivery performed under a sheet, because bright light during delivery is feared. Traditionalists may bury the placenta beneath the doorway at the birth site or burn it at a corner of the home. Infants are not named until after a confinement month. If they die during confinement, burial is done without ceremony. Women who have given birth do not usually leave the home after dark for the first month. However, postpartum confinement practices are becoming less common. Some also have continued the practice of squatting over a pot of boiling herbs to "close the birth canal," and burns can result. According to the hot/cold equilibrium theory, the postpartum period is the hottest state the body can reach, so mothers do not eat "hot" foods. Some women eat foods that are thought to increase milk production for nursing. Women believe that the postpartum period should be calm, because strong emotions spoil breast milk, resulting in premature weaning unless traditional infusions are taken. Nutmeg, castor oil, or spider webs are placed on the umbilical cord and contribute to neo-natal tetanus. Belly bands are commonly used because of the endemic problem of umbilical hernias. Haiti has one of the highest infant mortality rates in the world at 89.4 per 1000 births.

Death Rites: Death is believed to be from either natural (i.e., caused by God) or supernatural (caused by the spirits) factors. Relatives and friends expend considerable effort to be present when a person is near death. The family does not express grief out loud until most of the deceased person's possessions have been removed from the home, at which point the wailing and crying begins. People who are knowledgeable about Haitian customs wash and dress the body and place it in a coffin. A priest may be summoned to conduct the burial service. Burial usually takes place within 24 hours and does not include embalming. Autopsies are not routinely performed, which increases speculation about a person's cause of death. A popular local belief alleges that witch doctors use herbal substances to make people appear dead so that they can bring them back to life later and enslave them. Because of this popular story, people may doubt whether a person is truly dead or merely appears dead. White clothing represents death. During mourning, some may assume the symptoms of the deceased person's last illness. Cremation is unacceptable.

Food Practices and Intolerances: The majority of people eat once a day. If they eat more than one meal the largest is often at lunch, and water is consumed only after the meal is finished. Some women avoid drinking cold orange juice or pineapple while menstruating. The diet is spicy, with rice, beans, and plantains as staples; being plump is considered healthy. Iced drinks are never consumed during highly emotional times, because strong emotions are associated with a "hot" condition.

Infant Feeding Practices: Colostrum is considered bad milk. It is often used as a purgative (instead of castor oil) to rid the infant's body of meconium. Some mothers stop breast-feeding if the infant develops diarrhea because they believe that breast milk causes diarrhea or intestinal parasites. Breast-feeding is more common in rural areas and may be continued for 9 to 18 months. A national program promotes exclusive breast-feeding for the first 6 months of life. A plantain porridge supplement is introduced as young as 2 months. A fat child is believed to be a healthy child. Haitian infants and children do not routinely suck on their fingers or use pacifiers.

Child Rearing Practices: It is customary to treat children harshly and strictly and use corporal punishment such as spanking. Children who ask questions or seek information from parents are considered disrespectful. When adults are speaking, children are expected to remain quiet. Bottle-feeding is sometimes used as a pacifier to keep children quiet. Many children have multiple caretakers (relatives or friends). Grandmothers are considered appropriate caretakers for children, and children can be left indefinitely with grandparents or other relatives while parents seek employment or go to school. In cases of extreme poverty, children work after school to help support the family. Haitians are reluctant to discuss sex education or reproduction with health care professionals who are not Haitian. Male circumcision is not encouraged. Bladder and bowel control is expected by between 3 and 5 years of age; however, enuresis is not considered a situation warranting professional help. Enuresis is said to run in families and is not considered an abnormal developmental event. Early independence is promoted, and very young children help with daily chores.

National Childhood Immunizations: BCG at birth; DPT at 6, 10, and 14 weeks; OPV at birth and $1\frac{1}{2}$, $2\frac{1}{2}$, and $3\frac{1}{2}$ months; measles at 9 months; and TT CBAW at 15 to 49 years. BCG leaves a scar on the right upper arm. Some children may test positive for PPD because of the BCG vaccine and not because they have active tuberculosis. The rate of vaccine completion in Haiti for children 12 to 59 months of age is 19%. Polio has not yet been eradicated in Haiti.

BIBLIOGRAPHY

Adler MW, ed: Statistics from the World Health Organization and the Centers for Disease Control, *AIDS* 6(10):1229, 1992.

DeSantis L: *Bridging the gap: cultural diversity in nursing,* Unpublished manuscript, 1990.

DeSantis L, Tappen RM: *Preventive health practices of Haitian immigrants.* Paper presented at the West Virginia Nurses Association research symposium, Sulphur Springs, W Va, 1990.

DeSantis L, Thomas JT: Childhood independence: views of Cuban and Haitian immigrant mothers, *J Pediatr Nurs* 9(4):258, 1994.

DeSantis L, Thomas JT: Health education and the immigrant Haitian mother: cultural insights for community health nurses, *Public Health Nurs* 9(2):87, 1992.

DeSantis L, Thomas JT: The immigrant Haitian mother: transcultural nursing perspective on preventive health care for children, *J Transcultural Nurs* 2(1):2, 1990.

DeSantis L, Ugarriza DN: Potential for intergenerational conflict in Cuban and Haitian immigrant families, *Arch Psychiatr Nurs* IX(6):354, 1995.

Kirkpatrick S, Cobb A: Health beliefs related to diarrhea in Haitian children: building transcultural nursing knowledge, *J Transcultural Nurs* 1(2):2, 1990.

Rowell M: Eradication of vitamin A deficiency with 5 cents and a vegetable garden, *J Ophthalmic Nurs* 12(5):217, 1993.

St. Hill PF: *Acceptability and use of family planning services by refugee Haitian women in Miami,* doctoral dissertation, San Francisco, 1992, University of California, San Francisco.

Thomas JT, DeSantis L: Feeding and weaning practices of Cuban and Haitian immigrant mothers, *J Transcultural Nurs* 6(2):34, 1995.

◆ HONDURAS (REPUBLIC OF)

MAP PAGE (857)

Arthur Engler

Location: Honduras is part of the north central section of Central America. Honduran coastlines include the Caribbean Sea and the Pacific Ocean. The total land area is 112,090 km^2 (43,278 square miles). Although Honduras is primarily mountainous, it also has fertile plateaus, a river valley, and a narrow coastal plain. Honduras has eight culturally differentiated ethnic groups: the Lencas, Pech, Garifunas, Chortis, Tawahkas, Tolupanes or Xicaques, Miskitos, and an English-speaking Black population (approximately 6% of the total population). The areas populated by indigenous people are among the most severely underserved in terms of health care.

Major Languages	Ethnic Groups	Major Religions
Spanish	Mestizo 90%	Catholic 97%
Indian languages	Native American 7%	Protestant, other 3%
	Black 2%	
	White 1%	

Health Care Beliefs: Acute sick care; traditional. The use of herbs in home remedies is common, especially among the poor, who constitute the majority of the population. Most villages have a layperson who is knowledgeable about herbs and provides basic care for common ailments. Mental illness is not a generally accepted concept by health care professionals or laypeople. Two national psychiatric hospitals are located in Tegucigalpa. San Pedro Sula has a psychiatric care clinic that refers patients to one of the two hospitals in Tegucigalpa. Each general hospital (of which Honduras has 28) has two or three beds available for patients with psychiatric problems. Preventative practices are not widespread because most Hondurans live in such poverty that funds for such care are not readily available. The state does not provide preventative services, with the exception of the very successful immunization programs.

Predominant Sick Care Practices: Biomedical where available and herbal treatments. The country has significant herbal resources and a wealth of traditional knowledge about herbal medicine, and its combination of herbal and Western therapies is of interest to other countries. Honduras is one of the poorest countries in the Western hemisphere, and health promotion practices are not a high priority to the average person. In the last 10 years the Honduran government reports it has been focusing on changing public health attitudes and practices through educational communication. The availability of hospitals and clinics varies throughout the country. Public hospitals are understaffed, poorly maintained, and lack most basic supplies and equipment. Private clinics and hospitals are preferred but only available to those who can pay for their services. The larger cities have specialized hospitals and clinics such as ophthalmological clinics. At such clinics a full ophthalmological exam including and eye ultrasound costs approximately $20 (U.S. dollars). However, even this relatively low cost is unaffordable for the vast majority of Hondurans.

Ethnic/Race Specific or Endemic Diseases: In 1990 the five leading causes of death in the general population were ischemic and hypertensive diseases, diseases of pulmonary circulation, and other forms of heart disease (19%); accidents and violence (13%); diseases of the respiratory system (9.5%); intestinal infectious diseases (9%); and malignant neoplasms (8.2%). The leading causes of infant mortality in 1990 were intestinal infectious diseases (28.2%), diseases of the respiratory system (21.8%), and certain disorders originating in the perinatal period (20.6%). The number of cases of malaria increased to nearly 75,000 in 1996, infecting inhabitants primarily in the country's northern and southern areas, which accounted for 52% of the cases reported in 1996. Honduras had nearly 8000 cases of dengue fever in 1996, primarily in the central and northern areas of the country. In 1993 and 1994, most cases of dengue fever occurred in females, and more than 50% were in females older than 15 years. No cases of poliomyelitis have been reported since 1989. The number of cases of neonatal tetanus has been reduced by 50% since 1994. Subclinical vitamin A deficiency affects 13% of the population ages 1 to 3 years, particularly in rural areas in the western and northern regions and in several urban areas. Iron deficiency is prevalent and in 1996 affected more than 30% of children ages 1 to 3 years. The age at which young people begin to use tobacco and alcohol has decreased and ranges from 10 to 16 years. The World Health Organization's (WHO) estimated prevalence rates for HIV/AIDS in adults ages 15 to 49 is 1.92%. The estimated number of children from birth to 15 years living with HIV/AIDS is 4400. The numbers of people infected with HIV (regardless of whether they have developed symptoms of AIDS) are as follows: adults 58,000; women 29,000; and children 4400. The estimated number of adults and children who died of AIDS during 1999 was 4200. The estimated number of children who have lost their mother or both parents to AIDS (while the children were younger than age 15) since the beginning of the epidemic is 19,000. The estimated number of children who have lost their mother or both parents to AIDS and who were alive and younger than age 15 at the end of 1999 is 13,599. The modes and rates of HIV transmission are as follows: 57.6% heterosexual contact, 9.3% homosexual or bisexual contact, and 0.1% injectable drugs.

Health Team Relationships: The National Autonomous University of Honduras (UNAH) is responsible for the education of health professionals. From 1992 to 1996, an average of 19 nurses, 41 dentists, and 272 physicians graduated each year. In 1990, nurse specialists in maternal and perinatal health were recognized as a distinct category of health professional. On average, Honduras has 0.2 dentists, 2.4 professional nurses, and 6.5 doctors per 10,000 people. The public sector has insufficient human resources for the majority of health professions. In addition, Honduras has a severe imbalance in geographical distribution of resources, with some communities having a job market saturated with health personnel and others (usually the most remote) having many vacant positions. The public sector employs 69% of all health workers in the country.

Families' Role in Hospital Care: Female family members generally provide whatever health care is possible for as long as possible to avoid dealing with the health care system. Home remedies are common, as is assistance from lay midwives in the villages.

Dominance Patterns: Men dominate most areas of domestic and public life. In rural areas in particular, women are expected to remain indoors and be silent when business matters are being discussed. Approximately 500,000 women are physically abused by men. Many marriages are informal because of the expense of weddings and the dearth of priests. Men often desert their wives for other women, and extramarital affairs and having sexual relations with prostitutes is expected. However, despite such attitudes and conditions, women are becoming more active in Honduran public life, including in politics and business.

Eye Contact Practices: Among many groups, particularly the poor and less educated, making direct eye contact is considered impolite. Women who make direct eye contact with men are thought to be inviting the men to introduce themselves and solicit a date. Honduran women occasionally catch the eye of North American men and introduce themselves, a practice that would not occur with Honduran men.

Touch Practices: It is common to shake hands when meeting friends or acquaintances.

Perceptions of Time: Hondurans generally do not watch the clock. For example, it is acceptable for a Honduran to arrive late to a scheduled meeting, but it is rude for a North American to do so.

Pain Reactions: In general, children and adults bear pain stoically and treat it as a normal part of life. Even mild analgesics are not widely available to the majority of the population because of their cost, but they are available in most pharmacies.

Food Practices and Intolerances: Hondurans eat a light breakfast after waking, a moderate midday meal (usually between noon and 2 PM), and supper (between 6 and 8 PM). Depending on socioeconomic status, a typical meal might consist of a chunk of beef accompanied by fried plantain, beans, marinated cabbage, rice, a piece of salty cheese, and a dollop of sour cream. Saffron rice might be served instead of plain rice, well-prepared beans instead of canned refried beans, or yucca instead of plantain. Tortillas, usually corn, are served on the side. Near the coasts, seafood plays an important role in daily diets.

Infant Feeding Practices: The percent of exclusively breast-fed infants (from birth to 3 months) rose from 26.7% in 1991 to 42.4% in 1995. Among infants 6 to 9 months old, 69.2% were being breast-fed with supplemental feeding, and among children 20 to 23 months old, 45.4% continued to breast-feed. Breast-feeding continues for an average of about 2 months. Unfortunately, bottle-feeding is also common; mothers often use contaminated water for formula preparation, resulting in frequent and serious episodes of diarrhea.

Child Rearing Practices: In 1996, 54.3% of the population (estimated to be 5.6 million) was comprised of children from infancy to 19 years of age. Life expectancy at birth in 1996 was 71 years for women and 66 years for men. Families must pay for their children's uniforms and books even when the children attend public schools, so children of poorer families often receive little or no formal education. It is common for children of 4 or 5 years of age to carry buckets of sand or water on their heads or bundles of firewood in their arms.

National Childhood Immunizations: BCG at birth and at 7 and 2 years; DPT at 2, 4, and 6 weeks; OPV at birth and 2, 4, and 6 weeks; and measles at 9 months and 1 to 14 years. According to the Pan American Health Organization, 93% of infants younger than 1 year in 1996 had updated immunizations, 93% had received their third dose of DPT, 94% had received their polio vaccine, 99% had received BCG, and 91% were had their current measles vaccine. However, in some areas of the country only 80% have received all needed vaccinations.

BIBLIOGRAPHY

Humphrey C: *Honduras,* Emeryville, Ca, 2000, Avalon Publishing.
Pan American Health Organization Country Profile (2000): *Honduras.* Retrieved October 16, 2001, from http://www.paho.org/English/SHA/prflhon.htm
Pan American Health Organization (2001): *Honduras.* Retrieved October 6, 2001, from http://www.paho.org/english/sha/honrstp.htm
UNAIDS and the World Health Organization (2000): *Epidemiological fact sheet on HIV/AIDS and sexually transmitted infections: 2000 update.* Retrieved October 5, 2001, from http://www.unaids.org/hivaidsinfo/statistics/june00/fact_sheets/pdfs/honduras.pdf

◆ HUNGARY (REPUBLIC OF)

MAP PAGE (860)

Bettina F. Piko

Location: Hungary is a landlocked country in Central Europe and is characterized by fertile plains and mountains of medium height, with a famous freshwater lake called Balaton that serves as a major tourist attraction. It is bordered by the Czech Republic, Slovakia, Ukraine, Romania, Serbia, Croatia, Slovenia, and Austria. The total land area is 93,030 km^2 (35,919 square miles).

Major Languages	Ethnic Groups	Major Religions
Hungarian	Hungarian 94%	Catholic 66%
	Gypsy 5%	Calvinist 21%
	German, Romanian, Croatian,	Lutheran 4%
	Slovak, and other	Other 4%
	(e.g., Serbian, Slovenian) 1%	Not reported 5%

Health Care Beliefs: Acute sick care; traditional; alternative. Health care beliefs are dominated by Western culture, and people believe in the omnipotence of biomedical science and doctors. When Hungarians are disappointed in biomedical health care, they often turn to alternative healers. Older people living in the country who are involved in agriculture also have a greater tendency to believe in the strength of herbs; moreover, they have the knowledge of how to use them. It is also a custom for many Hungarians to start the day with a small glass of brandy (or *pálinka,* such as the world famous apricot brandy *barack pálinka*) because they attribute cleansing and purifying effects to this spirit. Hungarian people are generally more concerned with illness treatment than with prevention. They are less interested in actively preventing disease through changes in dietary habits or regular exercise. However, this mindset is beginning to change as prevention programs are being introduced to children in school. Social reactions to mental illness are rather controversial and dominated by fear. Labeling those with mental illness is common, and it is difficult for people who have recovered from mental illness to free themselves of the label. To change these negative attitudes, a positive approach toward mental health prevention (called *mental hygiene*) is being promoted.

Predominant Sick Care Practices: Western health care and medical treatments are dominant. Health care services can be found at three levels: primary health care, involving family doctors or general practitioners with a primary health care team consisting of district nurses and assistants; outpatient care, involving polyclinics where specialists provide service for outpatients; and hospitals, which are staffed by clinical specialists who treat hospitalized patients. Children younger than age 18 are treated by primary pediatric health services managed by pediatricians. Health care is financed by the National Social Insurance Company, and contribution payments are compulsory for all employees. Medications are partially subsidized by insurance and partially by patients. Although the biomedical health care system is dominant, many individuals turn to alternative healing practices, although the costs are not covered by social insurance. Doctors may recommend alternative healing practices for prevention. Alternative healers are required to be licensed to practice.

Ethnic/Race Specific or Endemic Diseases: Various types of cancer and diseases of the circulatory system are the leading causes of death in Hungary. Alcoholism-related diseases such as cirrhosis of the liver and smoking-related diseases such as lung cancer are also common, as are mental health problems and rheumatism (which is caused by the cold, damp weather in autumn and winter). Hungary's suicide rate is one of the highest in the world. Gypsies are a special minority group and have particular health care needs. Their birth and mortality rates are much higher than those of the majority population. Because of social and cultural problems such as lower levels of education and higher unemployment rates, their health care needs are often not met because they are generally less health conscious and do not seek medical care. HIV and AIDS are relatively rare in Hungary, and statistics reveal a stable, unchanging situation. The World Health Organization's (WHO) estimated prevalence rate for HIV/AIDS in adults ages 15 to 49 is 0.05%. The estimated number of children from birth to 15 years living with HIV/AIDS is less than 100. Anonymous tests are available for everyone. Schools have nationally supported anti-AIDS program networks for primary and high school students. Surveys show that students are usually well educated about HIV and

AIDS. Homosexuality is often considered a taboo subject because Hungarians are very conservative. People tend to conceal homosexuality except in larger cities, where liberal views are more common.

Health Team Relationships: Doctors are dominant in the health care system and responsible for the overall treatment of patients. The paramedical staff consists of nurses, assistants, midwives, community nurses, social workers, and psychologists. The relationship between nurses and doctors is often guided by a hierarchical approach; doctors are in charge, and nurses follow orders. The patient-doctor relationship is often similar in that patients are expected to follow the orders of the doctor without much input regarding their opinions about the course of treatment.

Families' Role in Hospital Care: Because hospital care is provided by health care services and paid entirely by social insurance, the role of family members toward their relatives is mostly as providers of psychological support rather than direct care. When children are hospitalized, parents are allowed to stay in the hospital with their children in a special room for parents; it is more common for the mother to stay. Caring for family members in the home is difficult in Hungary as it is in most Western countries, because often the husband and wife work full time. If they can afford it, families may employ a private nurse to care for infirm or older family members in their homes.

Dominance Patterns: The dominance patterns of social groups vary greatly. In well-educated families the responsibility for decision making is often shared by husband and wife. In working-class or farming families, it is more common for the father to be the head of the family and the central decision maker. Despite changes recognizing the equality of women during the last few decades, the leading positions in the workplace are often dominated by men. Moreover, as a result of cultural conditioning, women often think they are not competent to take part in management tasks.

Eye Contact Practices: Eye contact plays an important communicative role in Hungary, and it is customary to make eye contact during conversation. If another person avoids eye contact, it may be interpreted as embarrassment or that the two people speaking have a poor social relationship.

Touch Practices: Touching and hugging during greetings or conversation is only accepted among very close friends or family members. Hungarian people tend to prefer a large personal space so when individuals outside of their family or circle of friends get too close, the experience may be interpreted as threatening.

Perception of Time: Time perception is rather controversial in Hungary. People who work according to Western management rules usually insist on punctuality. Outside of the work environment, people often do not make extensive future plans or adhere to strict time tables. This discrepancy between work habits and everyday patterns sometimes causes conflicts among individuals.

Pain Reactions: Hungarian people tend to be stoical about pain and think that not revealing suffering is a sign of strength. Even during childbirth, women in labor tend to avoid crying out loudly.

Birth Rites: Hungary has a low birth rate, and the population is steadily decreasing. Although Hungarian people value family and children greatly, they want to provide well for their children in a material sense. Therefore Hungarians often have only one or occasionally two children. It is unusual to have more than two children, except in Orthodox religious families. Most deliveries take place in hospitals and include obstetricians and midwives. Pregnant women usually choose one doctor who takes care of her during pregnancy and helps during delivery. Delivery is typically in the back-lying position favored by those in many of the Western countries. However, this position is receiving criticism, and some women are now choosing alternative positions such as sitting. Female obstetricians are rare, and men receiving high salaries fill the specialty. After birth, most hospital stays are less than a week unless the mother or infant has complications. After discharge from the hospital, a district pediatric nurse makes a home visit within 24 hours. Traditionally, infants are separated from their mothers in the hospital, but recently more hospitals use the "rooming-in" system, in which infants and mothers stay together at all times. Another new tendency is to allow fathers in labor and delivery rooms. ("Labor with fathers" is *"apás szülés"* in Hungarian.) Fathers now often cut the umbilical cord after delivery. Although delivery at home is popular in some families, it is strongly discouraged by doctors who declare that it increases the probability of complications.

Death Rites: Most people die in hospitals, often without family members present. Death and dying are not discussed in Hungary. Health care providers generally have little knowledge about appropriate care of the psychological aspects of dying people. Recently the hospice movement has been introduced in an increasing number of hospitals, with the major goal of providing appropriate medical and psychological care for patients who are terminally ill. After death and an autopsy (which is usually recommended if a person dies in the hospital), the deceased person is placed in a coffin and buried. Cremation is being done more frequently, although older adults generally disapprove of the practice. Burial is usually accompanied by religious services. Organ donations are acceptable from an ethical point of view, but approval is strictly regulated by the legal system. Older village people continue to follow socially patterned rituals of death and mourning, such as covering mirrors immediately after a person's death or wearing special black dresses or suits during the mourning period. It is still customary after the funeral for the family members and other relatives to come together and share a meal called the "funeral feast" *(halotti tor)*. This custom is based on a belief that the deceased people are watching from paradise, seeing their beloved together, loving one another. This helps the deceased accept the reality of death and leave their lives behind.

Food Practices: Traditional foods are usually high in carbohydrates and animal fat (e.g., meat with fried potatoes or stuffed cabbage—*töltött káposzta*—which contains minced meat and rice and is a national food). Eating salad during meals is rare but gaining in popularity among young people. Hungarian people usually eat three to five times each day. Usually, lunch is the main meal and is typically eaten in small restaurants or workplace canteens. Lunch always begins with various soups, and meals are usually followed by coffee. Breakfast is often light, and dinner is typically heavy. Tea or coffee breaks with cookies and pastries or tea or coffee and fruit or cereal are eaten between the main meals. Breaks are also a time of social support for close relatives. Vegetarian and so-called "body-control diets" emphasizing carbohydrates or proteins are preferred by some and considered either fashionable or part of recent health promotion movements. Vegetables and fruits are now available year round in the markets for those who can afford them. Most families have gardens in which they raise vegetables for themselves as a hobby.

Infant Feeding Practices: Breast-feeding is highly encouraged by pediatricians and district pediatric nurses. Although some time ago breast-feeding usually ended at 6 months, many mothers now prefer to continue for a year or more. About 2 weeks after birth, lemon and orange juice and then apple juice are introduced in small spoonfuls between breast-feedings. Mashed fruit is introduced at 6 weeks, and mashed vegetables, primarily potatoes and carrots, are added at 4 months. Between the seventh and twelfth months, animal protein, primarily chicken and cow's milk, are added. Infants who do not breast-feed receive cow's milk or other formulas as a substitute for their mother's milk.

Child Rearing Practices: Mothers who prefer to stay at home with their infants after birth are allowed a maternity allowance of 3 years. Fathers are also entitled to this subsidy, which is paid by the social insurance company. However, to preserve their jobs, many parents go back to work after 1 year or even sooner, preferring to pay for a private day nursery. Child rearing practices are rather permissive because parents want their children to have a better life than their own. This approach occasionally results in an emphasis on material items and less concern with psychological strength and emotional security.

National Childhood Immunizations: BCG at birth or within 42 days; DPT at 3, 4, 5, and 36 months and 6 years; IPV at 3 months; OPV at 4, 5, and 15 months and 6 years; MMR at 15 months and 11 years; HIB at 2, 4, and 5 months; hep B at 14 years; and DT at 11 years.

BIBLIOGRAPHY

Andorka R: *Introduction to sociology,* Budapest, Hungary, 1997, Osiris.

Delvaux T et al: Barriers to prenatal care in Europe, *Am J Prev Med* 21(1):52, 2001.

Gergely L: *Medical microbiology,* Budapest, 1999, Semmelweis University

Hungarian Statistical Office: *Census data,* Budapest, 1990.

Hungarian Statistical Office: *Statistical yearbook of Hungary 2000,* Budapest, 2001.

Kopp MS, Skrabski A, Szedmak S: Psychosocial risk factors, inequality and self-rated morbidity in a changing society, *Soc Sci Med* 51(9):1351, 2000.

Pikhart H et al: Psychosocial work characteristics and self rated health in four post-Communist countries, *J Epidemiol Community Health* 55(9):624, 2001.

www.who.int/vaccines

www.unaids.org/hivaidsinfo/statistics/june00/fact_sheets/index.html

---

◆ ICELAND (REPUBLIC OF)

MAP PAGE (860)

Elín M. Hallgrímsdóttir

Location: Iceland is Europe's westernmost country, a little more than 3 hours by air from London or Paris. It is the second largest island (103,000 km² or 39,758 square miles) in the North Atlantic, about the same surface area as Ireland or the state of Virginia. Iceland is sparsely populated, with only 3 people per km² who live primarily along the coast. The interior of the country contains stunning contrasts. Iceland is largely an arctic desert, punctuated with mountains, glaciers that cover more than 11,922 km² (or 4,601 square miles—11.5% of the total land area), volcanoes, and waterfalls. Most of the vegetation and agricultural areas are in the lowlands close to the coastline.

Major Languages	Ethnic Groups	Major Religions
Icelandic (official)	Descendants of Norwegians and Celts	Evangelical Lutheran 88%
		Other Protestant and Roman Catholic 11%
		No affiliation 1%

The ethnic groups that account for about 97.8% of the Icelandic nation are a homogenous mixture of descendants of people of Nordic and Celtic origin. The number of immigrants is increasing. For example, in the rural areas of the western part of the country, immigrants from approximately 38 countries make up 6.7% of the population (58% of which is Polish).

Health Care Beliefs: Active involvement; health promotion important. According to the Ministry of Health and Social Security Act of 1990, all inhabitants have the right to access to the best possible health service at any given time for the protection of their mental, social, and physical health. Health promotion and illness prevention is stressed, with an emphasis on accident, tobacco, and drug prevention. The primary health care centers have the responsibility for general treatment and care, examinations, home nursing, and preventive measures such as family planning, maternity care, child health care, and school health care. Many people in Iceland have considerable interest in alternative medical practices such as acupuncture and naturopathic or homeopathic medicine. However, Icelandic law only permits medical doctors to diagnose illness. Regardless, the use of alternative approaches is currently being revised in the Icelandic parliament. The use of prayer is common among older adults in particular, although many others probably pray but simply do not discuss it.

Predominant Sick Care Practices: Biomedical and alternative. The health service in Iceland is primarily financed by the central government and is based on taxes. About 85% of bills for care at ambulatory care centers, primary health care centers, and emergency departments is covered. Users pay a service fee (copay) of about 15%. The country is divided into health regions, each with its own primary health care center— some of which are run jointly with local community hospitals. The biomedical model is predominant, but numerous unorthodox options in alternative medicine may be used, such as aromatherapy and herbs (biological-based methods), meditation (mind-body interventions), massage (manipulative and body-based methods), and therapeutic touch (energy therapies). Availability of these therapies has increased in recent years in response to greater emphasis on holistic health, which is the preservation of mental, social, and physical health.

Ethnic/Race Specific or Endemic Diseases: Heart and coronary diseases, stroke, cancer, and accidents cause most deaths. Cardiovascular disease incidence has been decreasing since 1980, and research has shown that it is a result of fewer cases of hypertension and the decreased consumption of high-fat foods. Obesity is an increasing problem in children as well as adults and is attributed to lack of exercise and the increased consumption of unhealthy foods such as soft drinks and deep-fried foods, items that are especially popular among young people. Many argue that accidents are the country's most serious health problem and the primary cause of death of children and young people. Accidents are expensive and devastating for the society and families, because many survivors need expensive life-long care and treatment. Cancer and respiratory diseases are still increasing. Smoking cigarettes was very common among people born between 1950 and 1965, so they have increased rates of chronic obstructive pulmonary disease (COPD). Average life expectancy at birth for women is 81.3 years and for men is 76.5 years. The World Health Organization's (WHO) estimated prevalence rate for HIV/AIDS in adults ages 15 to 49 is 0.14%. The estimated number of children from birth to 15 years living with HIV/AIDS is less than 100. By the end of 2001 a total of 154 HIV cases had been reported, of which 52 patients have developed AIDS and 35 have died from the disease. Most reported cases in recent years are among heterosexuals. Blood donors and people who are being treated for drug addiction are systematically tested for HIV infection.

Health Team Relationships: Working relationships in health care teams are usually good, and collaboration among different groups is increasing. Only medical doctors have the permission to diagnose and order treatment for illness, but in-patient hospital wards are directed by nurses. Nurses comprise the majority of the health care staff, which gives them a powerful position in the health care system. Therefore admission and discharge of patients are based on collaborative decisions between nurses and doctors. The relationships between patients and nurses or doctors are generally open and friendly. Since 1986, all nursing education in Iceland has consisted of 4-year bachelor of science programs at the universities. The Ministry of Health and Social Security Act of 1997 states that patients are responsible for their own health—as they are able and if their physical condition permits. They are to participate actively in the treatment to which they have consented. Patients have the right to obtain information regarding their state of health, the proposed treatment and its risks and benefits and other possible remedies, the consequences of lack of treatment, and the possibility of seeking the opinion of another specialist as appropriate regarding treatment, condition, and prognosis. The rights of patients to decide whether they accept treatment are respected.

Families' Role in Hospital Care: Patients have the right to receive support from their family, relatives, and friends during their treatment and hospital stay. Furthermore, the patients and their closest relatives have the right to spiritual, social, and religious support. Visiting hours are fairly liberal. Parents who have custody of children must give their consent for treatment of a patient younger than 16 years of age. If a parent who has custody of a child refuses to consent to treatment for a sick child in need of acute life-sustaining measures, the child's health is the determining factor and the necessary treatment is started immediately. The good of the child overrides objections of the parents (e.g., refusal of blood transfusions for religious reasons) if the child's condition is sufficiently serious. Sick children are consulted when possible (although they cannot refuse treatment) but always if they are older than 12 years of age. Sick children staying in a health institution are entitled to the presence of their parents or other close relatives, who are provided with facilities when possible. Sick children of school age are provided with in-hospital education suited to their age and state of health. Surroundings and care of sick children in health institutions is matched to their age, maturity level, and condition.

Dominance Patterns: According to the Act on the Equal Status and Equal Rights of Women and Men, all individuals have an equal opportunity to benefit from their own enterprise and develop their skills regardless of gender. Employers and labor unions make systematic efforts to equalize the participation of the sexes in the labor market, and women and men who are in the service of the same employer receive equal pay and enjoy equal terms for equal value and comparable work. In reality, men often have more prestigious titles and earn more than women, even when they do the same work. Some women have sued their employers because of this situation and received reimbursements for damages. According to a new survey, the average wage differential between men and women is about 12% to 14%. The fact that people live geographically close to one another fosters large, extended family connections. Decision making is cooperative between parents, but mothers still have more influence and responsibility in the area of child rearing and housework. Women also help family members who are sick or have disabilities more than men.

Eye Contact Practices: As in other Western European societies, people are generally comfortable with direct eye contact.

Touch Practices: People in Iceland do not use touch extensively. Women touch each other more than men do, but men and women are comfortable touching and kissing small children. Friends and family members shake hands or kiss each other on one cheek, but the masculine greeting is to shake hands. Hand holding (e.g., between nurses and patients) is considered a supportive gesture.

Perceptions of Time: People are rather punctual, but a 5- to 10-minute delay at an appointment is accepted. People are present and future oriented, but the ability to tell stories and describe events from the past is considered a sign of wisdom by older adults.

Pain Reactions: People do not express their pain loudly. Patients do not complain much and often do not want to bother a nurse by asking for pain medication even when they are in considerable pain.

Birth Rites: Almost all births occur in hospitals, and the semiseated position is common. The father or a family member is usually present during delivery, and a shower is permitted for mothers soon after the baby is born. Most midwives are nurses because for many years people had to be a nurse before being admitted into a midwifery program. Midwives handle normal deliveries, and hospital stays range between 1 and 5 days. Infants "room in" (i.e., stay with their mothers at all times) in the hospital. Mothers who want to go home within 36 hours after birth receive follow-up visits in their homes by midwives during the first few days after discharge. Otherwise, health visitors (nurses in the health service) make follow-up home visits once a week the first 4 or 5 weeks (or more often when needed). Infant mortality is among the lowest in the world: 5.5 per 1000 live births.

Death Rites: Most people die in health institutions and are surrounded by close family members. A funeral is conducted with a pastor and choir and is followed by a burial. Usually, the individual is buried in a wooden casket about 1 week after death, but cremation is also practiced. Autopsies are acceptable if needed to confirm the cause of death, and organ donations are acceptable. A unique Icelandic practice is decorating churchyards and cemeteries with festive lights during Christmas and the New Year celebrations.

Food Practices and Intolerances: Breakfast may consist of yogurt products, cereals, bread with cheese or ham, milk, juice, and coffee or tea, and daily consumption of cod liver oil is considered very healthy. Most people have a light lunch, such as sandwiches, salad, soup, or yogurt. The main meal is eaten in the early evening, consisting mainly of meat or fish that is boiled or fried with potatoes. Having rice, spaghetti or pasta, bread, and salad instead of potatoes is becoming more popular, and young people increasingly favor fast foods such as pizza. Eating a meal with the bare hands is unacceptable, and a fork, knife, and spoon are the usual eating implements. The Icelandic Nutrition Council advises people to consume less fat and salt but eat more vegetables, fruit, and corn.

Infant Feeding Practices: Breast-feeding is encouraged and very common for 4 to 6 months after birth. Only in special cases does a woman not breast-feed, such as when she is giving up an infant for adoption or is not producing any breast milk. Formula is used when breast-feeding alone is not enough for an infant, and pacifiers are common. The recommended practice for introducing foods is to start with porridge at the age of 6 months and then add vegetables and fruits. From the age of 4 weeks, A and D vitamins are given. Sleeping outside on the balcony once or twice a day is believed to be healthy for infants, even when it is very cold.

Child Rearing Practices: Of women ages 25 to 54, 88.2% are in the workforce, compared with 96.1% of men of the same age. Maternity leave is 3 months for each parent, in addition to 3 months shared by both parents. Of children from infancy to 2 years old, 21.6% are in nurseries, and of children 3 to 5 years old, 91% are in nurseries (with a daily attendance of 4 to 9 hours). Both parents maintain discipline, but child rearing practices are permissive. Children are allowed to participate in decision making that involves them, and they generally have a great deal of autonomy. Of children from birth to 17 years, 20.6% are living with one adult. School is compulsory for children between ages 6 and 16 years.

National Childhood Immunizations: DPT at 3, 4, 6, and 14 months; DT at 6 to 7 years; HIB at 3, 4, 6, and 14 months; OPV at 6, 7, and 14 months and 4, 9, and 14 years; Morbilli-MMR at 18 months; and rubella for girls with low titer at the age of 12.

Other Characteristics: Each member of the nuclear family can have a different last name. For example, a girl uses as her last name her father's first name with "*dóttir*" added, a boy uses his father's first name with "*son*" added, the mother keeps her maiden name, and the father uses his own last name.

BIBLIOGRAPHY

Allansson JG, Edvardsson IR, eds: *Community viability, rapid change and socio-ecological futures: papers from the Conference on Societies in the Vestnorden Area,* Akureyri, 2000, Alprent.

Bender SS: Attitudes of Icelandic young people toward sexual and reproductive health services, *Family Plan Persp* 31(6):294–301, 1999.

Blöndalc T et al: Nicotine nasal spray with nicotine patch for smoking cessation: randomized trial with six year follow up, *Brit Med J* 318:285–288, 1999.

Kristjansdóttir G: Perceived importance of needs expressed by parents of hospitalized two- to six-year-olds, *Scand J Car Sci* 9(2):95–103, 1995.

Magnusson A et al: Lack of seasonal mood change in the Icelandic population: results of a cross-sectional study, *Am J Psych* 157:234–238, 2000.

Ministry of Education, Science, and Culture: *The educational system in Iceland,* Reykjavík, Iceland, 1998, Oddi.

Ministry of Health and Social Security: http://heilbrigdisraduneyti.is/interpro/htr/htr.nsf/pages/forsid-ensk

Ministry of Social Affairs: http://felagsmalaraduneyti.is/interpro/fel/fel.nsf/pages/english-index

Statistic Iceland: http://www.statice.is/

Thome M, Adler B: A telephone intervention to reduce fatigue and symptom distress in mothers with difficult infants in the community, *J Adv Nurs* 29(1):128–137, 1999.

◆ INDIA (REPUBLIC OF)

MAP PAGE (866)

Santanu Chatterjee

Location: The Indian subcontinent is the seventh largest country in the world. It covers three distinct geographical regions—the Himalayan ranges in the north, the flat alluvium plains in the central region, and the peninsula in the south. The mainland covers a total land area of 387,273 km^2 (149,487 square miles), with a land frontier of 15,200 km (9,446 miles), accounting for 2.47% of the world's surface area but sustaining 16.7% of the world's population. The Himalayas form a great arc and comprise three almost parallel ranges interspersed with plateaus and valleys. The northern plains extend across the country, stretching to approximately 2400 km (1491 miles) in length and up to 320 km (198 miles) in breadth and supporting one of the world's greatest stretches of flat alluvial soil. This area forms the basins of three distinct river systems, the Ganges, Indus, and Brahmaputra, which support one of the most densely populated areas in the world. The rivers are primarily snow fed, originating in the Himalayas and ending in extensive deltas to the sea. In the south the area is mostly flat plateau flanked by the *ghats,* or low-lying hills running parallel to the eastern and western coasts. The climate, though broadly tropical monsoon, ranges from almost equatorial in the south to Mediterranean in the north. India has four distinct seasons—winter, hot summer, rainy monsoon, and post-monsoon.

Major Languages	**Ethnic Groups**	**Major Religions**
Hindi (national)	Indo-Aryan 72%	Hindu 82%
English	Dravidian 25%	Muslim 12%
Other official languages (13);	Mongol, other 3%	Christian 2%
at least 24 languages		Sikh 2%
spoken by a million or		Buddhist, Jain,
more; numerous other		and others 2%
languages and dialects		

India has unparalleled cultural diversity, with 325 languages expressed in more than 2000 dialects and 25 scripts. Each region has an individual character with its own unique social, ethnic, and linguistic characteristics. The coexistence of the traditional and the contemporary and the extreme contrasts of affluence and poverty are striking. Cities have modern amenities and a stressful lifestyle. Life in rural areas is more relaxed and traditionally agriculture based with low productivity. Agriculture remains the single most important economic activity and employs 64% of the workforce. Poverty and unemployment in rural regions prompt increasing urban migration contributing to periurban slums and strains on urban infrastructure. India's population is about 1 billion 27 million, with an urban population of 285 million. As the second most populous country in the world, the subcontinent adds 16 million people each year to its population (equivalent to the population of Australia). This increase accounts for a fifth of the annual increase in global population. The population density was 324 per square kilometer in 2001, but the statistics vary widely from state to state. West Bengal is the most densely populated state (with a population density of 904 people per square kilometer), compared with Arunachal Pradesh in the northeast region (with 13 people per square kilometer). Decades of population stabilization efforts have demonstrated that fertility decline is a dynamic process with multiple forces acting as causes and consequences. Increased availability and awareness of contraception, improved literacy rates, reduced infant mortality, and better economic prospects all typically drive declines in fertility. The numerous people in the reproductive age group contribute an estimated 58% to the population growth in India, and marriages of young girls promote the typical reproductive pattern.

Health Care Beliefs: Acute sick care; traditional. Diseases are believed to be caused by an upset in body balance. Generally, acute sick care is practiced; however, traditional medicine practices are important. Yoga, an ancient system of physical exercises and breathing techniques designed to maintain a healthy body and mind, is practiced. Ayurveda, the knowledge of life and longevity, is not merely a medical knowledge system, it is a way of life. Ayurveda involves not only the problems of the body and mind but also of the human spirit and consciousness. These biomedical and traditional practices focus on disease prevention. Spiritual values permeate most aspects of life and death. Allopathic medicine may be used in almost all rural communities, but poor Indians use more informal or traditional systems of medicine. Mental illnesses have a social stigma, and concepts of insanity are culturally rooted in the community. Urban environments lead to higher levels of psychoneuroses, but the incidence of psychoses is low and predominantly benign. The tendency for chronic psychoses is lower as well, possibly because of the permissive and tolerant attitude of the social milieu toward such behavior. Like psychoneuroses, psychoses are more common among people in urban areas. High stress levels combined with urban complexities contribute to high levels of anxiety and depression. Believing that a person in a dissociative trancelike condition is possessed by a supernatural force (e.g., spirits, demons, ghosts, gods) is particularly common in rural settings. Emotional problems are frequently expressed as somatic symptoms in the form of headaches, sleep disturbances, or ill-defined body pain. Praying and giving offerings to religious places of worship to alleviate illness and suffering are common. Given their changing sex roles, women are more susceptible to mental illnesses. The social milieu fosters a sense of extreme insecurity and helplessness in women even though they have the greater share of family responsibilities. Migration to the city, disruption of the village lifestyle, and subsequent urbanization contribute to increases in emotional morbidity.

Predominant Sick Care Practices: Biomedical; traditional Indian; magical-religious. The Indian systems of medicine have been practiced in the country for centuries. Such systems include Ayurveda, Siddha, Unani, and drugless therapies such as yoga, naturopathy, and homeopathy. Each has its own individual philosophy, merits, and strengths and offers a safe and cost-effective alternative to modern medicine. The government has recognized these strengths and understands that "health for all" cannot be achieved by the allopathic system alone. Efforts have been made to develop these indigenous systems of medicine under an institutional framework—the Indian Systems of Medicine and Homeopathy (ISM&H)—and integrate them with allopathy to address the health care needs of the population. The infrastructure under ISM&H consists of 2854 hospitals, 22,735 dispensaries, 9496 pharmacies and manufacturing units, and 587,000 practitioners. Certain goals have been identified as priorities: improving educational levels by continuing education, reorientation training programs for teachers and paramedics, minimum educational norms and curriculum, evolving accreditation procedures for the institutes, standardization and quality control of drugs, ensuring sustained availability of raw materials, and providing grants for research and training. Medical services are provided through an integrated system involving the state and central government with nongovernmental, voluntary, and private institutions. In rural areas, health services function through a network of health and family welfare systems offering prevention, promotion, curative, and rehabilitative services as part of a primary health care approach. Hospitals at district and subdivisional levels are being developed to assume responsibility for referral services, thereby reducing the burden on the urban health infrastructure. As of 1999, hospitals numbered 15,533 and served a population of 63,177 per hospital. Private health care is booming and experiencing a steady increase in consumer spending on nongovernmental medical treatment. Recent studies reveal a higher dependence (59%) on private health care providers as household incomes increase and for treatment of acute, out-patient illnesses. Public health care facilities are more frequently used (60%) for cases requiring hospitalization. The overall expenditure on health is 6% of the gross domestic product (GDP). Recent liberal economic policies have advocated "cost-effective" strategies, leading to an overall decreased investment in health and less state intervention in public health. This step has created less access to health care for the poor. Most regions in the country have adopted a mixed approach of public and private sector participation. Life expectancy at birth is 62.3 years for men and 65.27 for women.

Ethnic/Race Specific or Endemic Diseases: Endemic diseases include malaria (chloroquine resistant) and visceral leishmaniasis. Indians are at risk for viral hepatitis types A, B, C, and E; Japanese encephalitis; tuberculosis; dengue fever; typhoid fever; rabies; ascariasis; hookworm infection; amoebiasis; lymphatic filariasis; poliomyelitis; measles; mumps; diphtheria; trachoma; and anemia in women. Vitamin A deficiency is the most common cause of childhood blindness. Communicable diseases are still a major cause of morbidity and account for 14.5% (rural) and 13.3% (urban) of all the reported illnesses. The country is in the midst of an epidemiological transition because it is currently contending with communicable and noncommunicable diseases. This transition is primarily attributable to the aging population, a shift from rural to urban lifestyles, changes in dietary intake, increases in sedentary living, and increases in smoking and alcohol consumption. Cardiovascular diseases are the leading cause of noncommunicable diseases. The prevalence of diabetes is increasing in rural regions from 2% to 5% and in urban areas from 8.2% to 11.6%. The effect of urbanization on such prevalence seems more profound among men. The major health problem in rural India is pneumonia. Pulmonary tuberculosis is also a problem, especially in the states of Bihar, Madhya Pradesh, Rajasthan, and Uttar Pradesh. Bronchitis and asthma remain the major noncommunicable conditions causing premature mortality. Cancer is a health problem in all Indian states. Automobile accidents top the cause of death list in Rajasthan and Haryana, and suicide is a major issue in Andhra Pradesh. The prevalence of cardiovascular diseases among men has risen to 4.5 (rural) and 9 (urban) per 1000 people. Neuropsychiatric conditions are a close second on the list of major noncommunicable diseases, especially unipolar depression among women ages 15 to 44 years. An estimated 68 million people are older than 60 years; multiple chronic illnesses, frequent acute illnesses, and hearing and vision deficits are the major health and functional problems in this group. The National Family Health Survey II (1998 to 1999) revealed that 46.7% of 2-year-olds are underweight. Micronutrient deficiencies, especially of vitamin A and iodine, are another health problem. The World Health Organization's (WHO) estimated prevalence rate for HIV/AIDS in adults ages 15 to 49 is 0.70%. The estimated number of children from birth to 15 years living with HIV/AIDS is 160,000. An estimated 3.97 million people are living with HIV/AIDS, with the highest number of people living in the states of Tamil Nadu and Maharashtra. The point estimate for 2000 was 3.31 million HIV infections among adults ages 15 to 49 years. Given a 20% variability for un-accounted people who use intravenous drugs and people in other age groups, a working estimate of 3.97 million HIV infections was estimated. The HIV epidemic is predominantly heterosexual with equal distribution in both sexes. The majority of infected individuals are in the economically productive age group (15 to 49 years). Patterns indicate that the epidemic is spreading from urban to rural areas and from individuals displaying high-risk behavior to the general population. The prevalence is increasing among people with tuberculosis. Awareness levels of HIV/AIDS, other sexually transmitted diseases, and sexual behavior vary greatly among the different states. In most instances, females and rural residents are less educated about the topics. One third of males (33.6%) and one fourth of females (26.6%) reported consistent use of condoms during sex with people who were not their regular partners. Most people in rural areas have insufficient access to condoms. The median age for the first sexual encounter is 21 for men and 18 for women; the wide interstate variations range from 16 years in Bihar to 21 years in Goa among urban females and 19 in Andhra Pradesh to 25 in Assam among urban males. Awareness of sexually transmitted diseases (32.1% awareness) and their association with HIV (20.7% awareness) is consistently low. Large-scale labor migration, low levels of literacy among potentially high-risk groups, and unsafe blood transfusion practices have led to the proliferation of HIV/AIDS.

Health Team Relationships: Nurses usually work under medical supervision and have little direct influence on health care decisions. However, nursing is increasingly gaining importance, and nurses are an integral part of the health care team. Patients' attitudes toward members of the health team are generally appreciative and encouraging. Language proficiencies and communication skills are key issues for acceptance and success in such interactions. India has 400,000 registered allopathic doctors and 560,000 million nurses, with 0.75 beds per 1000 people.

Families' Role in Hospital Care: Some women are uncomfortable when examined by male health practitioners. Health care professionals find it difficult to discuss terminal illnesses with patients; however, they may be discussed with the patients' relatives. Adults do not enter into the decision-making process if older parents are present.

Dominance Patterns: In India's patriarchal society the dominant figure is the father or male surrogate. Hierarchies are built within the family according to age, sex, and familial relationships or within the community based on caste, lineage, education, wealth, occupation, and relationship with the ruling power. Values and habits are rooted in external realities that are diverse and complex. The social structure is hierarchical and based on the culture of superior and subordinate relationships, with a clear distinction of rights and duties. However, once the hierarchy is established, individuals support each other regardless of their position in the group. Unquestioned obedience to older adults is expected. In extended family households, older adults are often considered indispensable because of their experience and wisdom. Close relationships among generations is still one of the foundations of Indian families. Boys are especially desired. The concept of a husband owning his wife is quite pervasive and may allow men to abuse women in certain situations. Women depend on men, more so in traditional families, and they remain more vulnerable than men to exploitation and subjugation. Sex role differentiation and ideological assumptions about women's roles are linked to the unequal distribution of resources. Their lower status decreases women's access to resources because of lack of autonomous decision making, control over time, and parenting responsibilities. Women, especially in urban areas, often delay marriage and having children to complete their formal education. Nutritional deficiencies are common in aging women. The cumulative effects of undernutrition in childhood combined with poor dental care, consumption of food of low nutritional value, chronic parasitic infestations, domestic chores such as carrying loads of water long distances, and indoor air pollution from smoky kitchens contribute to the lower health status of the rural poor. The recent globalization process has affected women significantly. Urban, educated, and relatively affluent women have benefited from more opportunities for work and training, particularly in global software and information technology arenas. In comparison, poor and relatively uneducated women from the rural areas have been adversely affected because globalization has promoted conservative monetary and fiscal policies that have further reduced their income and employment opportunities. Women of reproductive age and children constitute 62% of the population. Maternal mortality is unacceptably high at 407 per 100,000 live births. Adolescent girls comprise 27% of females, and 10% of all reported births are to girls younger than 20. Reproductive health issues of adolescents in rural and urban school settings are closely related to violence, poor mental health, and risky behaviors such as substance abuse. Women also comprise a significant part of the workforce; 90 million (22.73%) of the total 407 million women are registered as workers. In rural areas, 87% are predominantly employed in the agriculture sector as laborers and cultivators, whereas 80% of those in urban areas are employed in sectors such as household industries, petty trading, and construction. In the organized employment sector, women comprise only 16.4% of the workforce. Iron deficiency anemia is the most common form of malnutrition, and Indian women account for half of world's women with anemia. The prevalence of anemia among pregnant women is approximately 88% and no appreciable decreases have been noted, even though strong antenatal programs promoting iron and folic acid supplementation are in place. The preference for having boys is particularly strong in rural north India and influences decision making in pregnancies and contributes significantly to fertility rates. During previous Vedic times, history reveals that women were adored, respected, and recognized as having their own identities. Today, dominance patterns are undergoing great changes because of India's greater access to the media and the increasing influence of Western ideas and attitudes. Moreover, increased education and decision making among women is having an influence as well. Marriage arrangements are becoming more diverse, and individual independence within marriage is being emphasized more. Female literacy rates have increased from 39.29% in 1991 to 54.16% in 2001, compared with 64.13% in 1991 to 75.85% in 2001 for males. In working environments, dependency is a cultural characteristic. Subordinates tend to seek attention, support, and advice from others, even in situations in which they are fully capable of making decisions. Work relationships are perceived as part of a social relationship, and co-workers tend to relate directly to one another. Such emotional affinity and preference for personalized interactions are common. People tend to accept ambiguity in emotions, ideas, and relationships, with a low-key tolerance for contradictory impulses and feelings. Trust and friendliness, readiness to form attachments, and expectations of reciprocal familiarity are typical Indian character traits.

Touch Practices: Men shake hands with other men but not with women. Instead, men place their palms together and bow slightly to women. Educated upper-class men and women mingle freely and have less regard for adherence to social strata rules. Modesty in dress is typical, and bare upper arms or shoulders are considered indecent. Public displays of affection are rare, and body contact is uncommon. Embracing is acceptable among social acquaintances, especially among men or within families. People touch the feet of older adults as a sign of respect or to seek blessings. It is unacceptable to touch another person with the feet, so apologies are offered in cases of such inadvertent contact. The right hand is used for all social interactions, especially when giving or receiving money.

Perceptions of Time: Perceptions of time are relaxed, especially in rural areas. People are more oriented to the past. The concept of time is closely related to the Indian concept of an infinite universe of unending cycles that extend beyond birth, life, and death. Respect for tradition is an integral part of society.

Pain Reactions: Patients generally quietly accept pain but accept pain relief measures.

Birth Rites: Voluntary sterilization of males is encouraged through monetary incentives and prizes. Prenatal sex determination by diagnostic procedures is prohibited by law and strictly enforced. Although abortion is legal, unhygienic and unsafe abortions are a major cause of maternal mortality (8.9%). Surveys reveal that 33% of births occur in institutions, and 42% of mothers giving birth receive assistance from trained health professionals. Major regional differences exist, and some mothers are assisted by untrained traditional birth attendants or relatives at home. Cravings during pregnancy are satisfied because they are thought to be those of the unborn child. Pregnancy is a time for rest and care, and expectant mothers may return to their mother's home for the delivery. Pregnancy marks the beginning of a process that establishes a woman as an adult and garners respect and consideration from society. In extended families, responsibilities for the care of a pregnant woman are shared among the older adults in the family. Pregnant women avoid sun, heat, and certain foods that are considered "hot" and therefore unsuitable. In villages, celebration of a son's birth may include the beating of drums or blowing of conch shells, and the midwife is paid a reward. Infants are nurtured in an environment of tolerance, emotional vitality, and protectiveness. The infant mortality rate is 70 per 1000 live births, and the maternal mortality rate is 407 per 100,000. The total fertility rate is 2.9 children per woman.

Death Rites: Often because they are accepting God's will, patients may make indirect references to their own deaths. A patient's desire to be lucid as death approaches must be considered in the medical treatment plan. A time and place for prayer is essential for family members and patients because prayer helps them handle anxiety and conflict. In Hindu society a priest reads from the holy Sanskrit books. Some priests tie strings (signifying a blessing) around the neck or wrist. After death the son pours water on the mouth of the deceased person. Blood transfusions, organ transplants, and autopsies are permitted. Cremations are preferred. Reincarnation is a Hindu belief.

Food Practices and Intolerances: Hindus do not eat beef, but it is freely available in Muslim restaurants. Rice and corn comprise the staple cereals. Breakfast, lunch, and dinner are the three main meals, and dinner is served late. Strict vegetarianism is confined primarily to southern India. Pork is generally available in areas with large Christian communities (e.g., Goa) or in the Tibetan and Nepalese communities in the hills. Regional variations in food are common. Northern Indians consume more meat and emphasize spices and breads. Rice is preferred by southerners, and the curries are liberally spiced with chilies. Fish is a favorite in the coastal areas and the eastern regions. Lentils are consumed throughout the country. Curd, or yogurt, is usually a side dish. Although seasonal, fruits such as mangoes, melons, bananas, pineapples, oranges, pomegranates, and grapes are fresh and widely available. People usually eat with their right hand because the left hand is considered unclean. Using the personal spoon to serve more food from a buffet is considered rude.

Infant Feeding Practices: Breast-feeding on demand is the norm and may continue for 3 years. National surveys on infant feeding practices reveal that 50.9% of mothers exclusively breast-feed for up to 3 months, and 26.4% breast-feed for 4 to 6 months. One third of the children receive regular, supplementary feedings between 6 and 9 months, and introduction of other foods starts between 6 and 12 months. Inadequate feeding practices rather than lack of food are often a cause of malnutrition (which affects 53% of children younger 5 years). Traditional Indians support breast-feeding, but certain practices undermine the process. It is believed that colostrum is undesirable, and prelacteal feedings of sweetened water, goat's milk, or diluted cow's milk are commonly given in the first 2 or 3 months. Economic resources influence breast-feeding, and decreased rates are noted among working women. Low-income urban women often think that they do not have enough breast milk when their infants cry a lot, so this is commonly cited as reason for supplementation.

Child Rearing Practices: The country has approximately 157.86 million children younger than 6 years (15.37% of the population). The Integrated Child Welfare Scheme offers a package of services to children and expectant or nursing mothers through the *Anganwadi* centers. The package involves supplementary nutrition, immunizations, health check-ups, and preschool education. The focus of the scheme is to reduce social and gender inequalities; it serves 22.36 million beneficiaries and provides supplementary nutrition to 18.2 million children. On average, every child has 1.6 episodes of diarrhea per year for the first 5 years of life. Every year a total of 25 million infants are born, of which 1.2 million die within 28 days. Most newborn deaths occur among infants who had a low birth weight (i.e., less than 2500 g). Lack of care at birth and subsequent infections contribute to the high infant mortality. The predominant theme in child rearing is protective nurturing and extreme permissiveness. The child is indulged, cuddled, and remains intimately attached to the mother until age 3 or 4. Toddlers usually sleep with parents until 4 or 5 years and are not pushed into toilet training. Discipline in late childhood includes scolding and light spanking. Children are rarely praised for doing what is expected of them because praise may cause them to be susceptible to the "evil eye." Care practices and resources vary tremendously among families. Traditional knowledge is valuable, and widespread changes in families caused by urbanization and the greater economic role of women in society have led to certain adaptations in care practices. Girls are less preferred in certain sociocultural settings, therefore they are less likely to receive appropriate health care. More than 80% of home health care is performed by women, particularly mothers.

National Childhood Immunizations: BCG at $1\frac{1}{2}$ months; DPT at 6, 10, and 14 weeks and 16 to 24 months; OPV at birth, 6, 10, and 14 weeks and 16 to 24 months; measles at 9 months; vitamin A at 9 months and then every 6 months until 3 years; DT at 5 years; and TT at 10 and 16 years and first dose as soon as possible during pregnancy, +1 month. The reported percentages of the target population vaccinated are as follows: BCG, 99; third dose of DTP, 94; MCV, 89; Pol3, 95; and TT2 plus, 80. More boys receive immunizations than girls.

Other Characteristics: The Sikh religion forbids cutting or shaving any body hair. Older women enjoy heightened social prestige. No expression for "thank you" exists; a social act is a fulfillment of an obligation or a duty and requires no verbal acknowledgment. The head motions for "yes" and "no" are opposite of those used in the United States. Modern children and adolescents often follow the Western customs rather than traditional practices regarding life choices such as premarital sex, establishing nuclear families, and choosing their own spouses. Social change has been gradual and bearable. Political and demographic pressure to abandon the cultural emphasis on the emotional and aesthetic qualities of life is increasing, as is the pressure for families to share responsibilities for daily chores.

BIBLIOGRAPHY

Aggarwal A, Arora S, Patwari AK: Breast-feeding among urban population of low socio-economic status: factors influencing introduction of supplementary feeds before four months of age, *Ind Pediatr* 35:269-273, 1998.

Asma S, Jha P: *Counting the dead in India in the 21st century,* Proceedings of the International Workshop on Certification on Causes of Death, Mumbai, India, 1999, Centers for Disease Control.

Balaji LN, Abdullah D: Nutrition scenario in India: implications for clinical practice, *J Ind Med Assoc* 9:536-542, 2000.

Becktell PJ: Endemic stress: environmental determinants of women's health in India, *Health Care Women Int* 15(2):111, 1994.

Burton B, Duvvury N, Varia N: Domestic violence in India: a summary report of a multi-site household survey, *ICRW* 3:1-34, 2000.

Central Bureau of Health Intelligence, Directorate General of Health Services, Ministry of Health and Family Welfare: *Health information of India 1994,* New Delhi, 1996, Government of India.

Chakravorty A: *Social stress and mental health—a social-psychiatric field study of Calcutta,* New Delhi, 1999, Sage Publications.

Davis CF: Culturally responsive nursing management in an international health care setting, *Nurs Adm Q* 16(2):36, 1992.

Deen JL: Health transition in India: implications for health policy, *Natl Med J India* 12:197-198, 1999.

Department of Women and Child Development, Ministry of Human Resource Development, Government of India: *Twenty years of the ICDS,* New Delhi, 1995.

Gillespie SR: Major issues in the control of iron deficiency anaemia, Ottawa, *Micronutrient Initiative,* 8-9, 1998.

Haddad L, Hoddin HJ, Alderman H, eds: *Intrahousehold resources allocation in developing countries: methods, models and policy,* Baltimore, 1996, Johns Hopkins University Press.

Haq M, Haq K: *Human development in South Asia: the education challenge,* Karachi, Pakistan, 1999, Oxford University Press.

Human development in South Asia 2001: globalisation and human development, Karachi, Pakistan, 2002, Oxford University Press.

Indrayan A et al: Estimates of the years-of-life-lost due to the top nine causes of death in rural areas of the major states in India in 1995, *Natl Med J India* 15:5-13, 2002.

International Institute for Population Studies: *National Family Health Survey (NFHS-II): key findings,* Mumbai, Inida, 2001.

International Institute for Population Studies: *National Family Health Survey (MCH and Family Planning),* Mumbai, India, 1992–1993.

Marriot M: Changing identities in South Asia. In David KA, ed: *The new wind: changing identities in South Asia,* Chicago, 1977, Aldine.

Ministry of Health and Family Welfare, Government of India: *National family health survey,* New Delhi, 1993, Author.

Ministry of Health and Family Welfare, Government of India: *Prevention and control of anaemia,* New Delhi, 1989, Ministry of Health and Family Welfare and the United Nations Children's Fund.

National AIDS Control Organisation: *Changing epidemiology of HIV/AIDS in India. Country scenario,* New Delhi, 1997, NACO.

National Nutritional Anaemia Prophylaxis Programme, Indian Council of Medical Research: *Task force study,* New Delhi, 1989, ICMR.

Patel NR: Nursing in India, *Nurs Adm Q* 16(2):72, 1992.

Patel V, Andrew G: Gender, sexual abuse and risk behaviour in adolescents: a cross-sectional survey in Schools in Goa, *Natl Med J India* 14:263–267, 2001.

Patel V, De Souza N: School drop-out: A public health approach, *Natl Med J India* 13:316-318, 2000.

Paul VK: The newborn health agenda: need for a village-level midwife, *Natl Med J India* 13:281-283, 2000.

Pethe S: Changing socio-cultural value impact on family, *Nurs J India* 86(2):39, 1995.

Population Research Centre: People's perspective and reproductive behaviour in Northwest India: an interdisciplinary field study of eight districts in Haryana, Himachal Pradesh and Uttar Pradesh, Chandigarh, 1993, Centre for Research in Rural and Industrial Development.

Ramachandran A et al: Rising prevalence of NIDDM in an urban population in India, *Diabetologia* 40:232-237, 1997.

Reissland N, Burghart R: The quality of a mother's milk and the health of her child: beliefs and practices of the women of Mithila, *Soc Sci Med* 27:461– 9, 1998.

Rowell M: Eradication of vitamin A deficiency with 5 cents and a vegetable garden, *J Ophthalmic Nurs Tech* 12(5):217, 1993.

Salunke SR et al: HIV/AIDS in India: a country responds to a challenge, *AIDS* 12:S21-S23, 1998.

Sandal V ed: *Reducing malnutrition: a call for urgent action,* New Delhi, India, 1-10, 1995, United Nations Children's Fund.

Viswanathan H, Rohde J: *Diarrhoea in rural India—a nationwide study of mothers and practitioners—all India summary,* New Delhi, India, 1990, Vision Books.

◆ INDONESIA

MAP PAGE (867)

Tjandra Yoga Aditama

Location: The Indonesian archipelago lies between Southeast Asia and Australia, stretching from the Malay peninsula to New Guinea. It is bordered by the South China Sea on the north, the Pacific Ocean on the north and east, and the Indian Ocean on the south and west. Indonesia consists of 13,700 islands, approximately 6000 of which are inhabited. The total land area is 741,097 square miles (1,926,852 km^2), with a coastline of 34,006 miles (54,715 km). The mountains and plateaus in the major islands have a cooler climate than the tropical lowlands.

Major Languages	Ethnic Groups	Major Religions
Bahasa Indonesian (official)	Javanese 45%	Muslim 88%
English (official)	Sundanese 14%	Protestant 5%
Dutch	Madurese 8%	Catholic 3%
Local languages, such as	Coastal Malays 8%	Hindu 2%
Javanese	Other 25%	Buddhist 1%
		Other 1%

Health Care Beliefs: Acute sick care; traditional. Magical religious beliefs are significant in many aspects of life in Indonesia, but adherence to these traditional beliefs is greatest in rural areas of the country. The *adat* (or "way of the ancestors") governs rituals performed at births and funerals, as well as many other aspects of behavior. During the seventh month of pregnancy a traditional ceremony is held for the protection of the mother and infant. In villages, pregnant women often carry scissors to symbolize cutting the cord when the infant is born. In some regions of the country, Indonesians believe that they can receive blessings from the dead in graveyards.

Predominant Sick Care Practices: Biomedical and infrequent magical-religious. Modern medicine is widely practiced in Indonesia through approximately 7000 health centers distributed throughout the country up to the sub-district level. Each health center is responsible for at least 30,000 people and has at least one medical doctor, as well as other health care personnel. The villages have sub-health centers, village midwives, or both. Indonesia has more than 1000 hospitals around the country to which people can be referred. The availability of private practitioners enhances the health-seeking behavior of the people. Large hospitals are located in big cities and can have as many as 2500 beds. More than 30,000 medical doctors are available in Indonesia and include general practitioners, specialists, and super-specialists. Most people seek modern medical care from a doctor or health staff member when they get sick. Very few people go to traditional healers, and those who do live primarily in very remote areas where no health staff members are available.

Ethnic/Race Specific or Endemic Diseases: Indonesia has the double burden of infectious and noninfectious diseases; cardiovascular diseases and certain infections such as cholera are major causes of death. Chloroquine-resistant malaria is endemic, but generally no risk exists in major cities. People are at risk for Japanese encephalitis and schistosomiasis. Vitamin A deficiency is the most common cause of childhood blindness. The World Health Organization's (WHO) estimated prevalence rate for HIV/AIDS in adults ages 15 to 49 years is 0.05%. The estimated number of children from birth to 15 years living with HIV/AIDS is 680.

Health Team Relationships: Patients may consider medical titles more important than names. Working relationships between doctors and nurses are generally good. Like in many countries, medical doctors graduate from the faculty of medicine after 6 years of study beyond senior high school. Most nurses in Indonesia still graduate from basic nursing school at the high school level rather than university level. A government movement is promoting university-based nursing education for all nurses.

Families' Roles in Hospital Care: Strong family ties exist in Indonesia. Community and family support is strong in decision making concerning care of the sick, people with disabilities, and older adults. Hospitalization or institutionalization is a last resort. Visiting the sick, bringing food to the hospital, and keeping a sick person company on the ward are the norm. Family members take turns spending the night with and helping hospitalized relatives.

Dominance Patterns: In daily life the roles of men and women are relatively equal, as they are in many Western countries. However, for some, particularly Muslims, the roles of men and women are guided by their interpretation of the Koran; therefore the husband may make all of the decisions, and the wife is expected to agree.

Eye Contact Practices: Direct eye contact is considered improper and disrespectful. This is particularly true if a man is looking directly at a woman.

Touch Practices: Shaking hands is generally acceptable, but touching the bodies of others is generally unacceptable.

Pain Reactions: Reactions to pain are not defined by the culture, rather they depend on the amount of pain a person has. When pain is extreme, it is acceptable to express it by crying or screaming. Conversely, pain that is less severe is tolerated as well as possible.

Birth Rites: Having many children is valued, even though in many areas the concept of family planning is widely accepted. Children lend support and are a source of security for their parents in old age. Free birth control supplies are available from the government and distributed through health stations and in small shops. Male circumcisions are usually performed between the ages of 6 and 15 years. Occasionally they are performed as young as at birth or as old as at 20 years. Female circumcisions are usually not performed.

Death Rites: Organ donations and transplantations are not widely practiced, with the exception of cornea donations and kidney transplantations. Blood transfusions are acceptable and widely used as needed for medical emergencies. Autopsies are uncommon and used only when required for forensic reasons, because the deceased body must be buried intact according to Muslim rituals. For Muslim burials the body is wrapped in special pieces of cloth and buried without a coffin in the ground. Cremations are not permitted.

Food Practices and Intolerances: The staple food for Indonesians is rice, although the diet consists of a large variety of foods. Rice is eaten with meat, fish, poultry, and vegetables. Pork, carrion, and blood are forbidden for Muslims. Fruit is served as dessert. During Ramadan, the Islamic month of fasting, breakfast must be eaten before dawn. Breakfast is followed by a ritual washing to prepare for morning prayers, which must coincide with sunrise. During the day, eating and drinking are forbidden for all except children, older adults, and those who are sick. At dusk after the fourth ritual prayer of the day, the fasting concludes.

Infant Feeding Practices: The majority of mothers breast-feed their infants. Mixed feeding (combined breast- and bottle-feeding) usually starts when mothers resume working. Indonesians believe it is best to breast-feed for 18 months or longer. Solid foods are introduced as young as 4 months of age. Rice-milk porridge is a common infant food.

National Childhood Immunizations: BCG at birth to 11 months; DPT at 2 to 11 months ×3; OPV at birth to 11 months ×3; hep B birth to 11 months ×3; measles 9 to 11 months ×1; vitamin A 6 to 59 months; DT at grade 1; TT at 7 years; CBAW, pregnant women.

Other Characteristics: Indonesians are always addressed by the first part of their name, so many use only one name professionally and socially. Most Indonesians do not have a family name, so names of fathers, mothers, and children may all be different. Men are allowed to have up to four wives simultaneously, although in practice polygamy is fairly limited. Carrying on a conversation with the hands in the pockets is considered rude, and standing with the hands on the hips is perceived as defiance. The gesture of curling the index finger inward is used for calling animals only, not people.

BIBLIOGRAPHY

Hull V, Thapa S, Pratomo H: Breast feeding in the modern health sector in Indonesia: the mother's perspective, *Soc Sci Med* 30(5):625, 1990.

Lickiss JN: Indonesia: status of cancer pain and palliative care, *J Pain Symptom Manage* 8(6):423, 1993.

Rowell M: Eradication of vitamin A deficiency with 5 cents and a vegetable garden, *J Ophthalmic Nurs Tech* 12(5):217, 1993.

U.S. Agency for International Development: Indonesia lowers infant mortality, *Front Lines* 31(10):16, 1991.

Wikan U: Bereavement and loss in two Muslim communities: Egypt and Bali compared, *Soc Sci Med* 27(5):451, 1988.

◆ IRAN (ISLAMIC REPUBLIC OF)

MAP PAGE (864)

Majid Sadeghi

Location: The Islamic Republic of Iran (also known as *Persia*) is located in the Middle East between the Caspian Sea and the Persian Gulf. Its neighboring countries are Armenia, Azerbaijan, and Turkmenistan to the north; Afghanistan and Pakistan to the east; and Iraq and Turkey to the west. The country has mountains to its north and west, large deserts in its central region, and fertile lands in its northern, northwestern, and southwestern regions. Iran's total land area is 1,648,000 km^2 (636,294 square miles).

Major Languages	Ethnic Groups	Major Religions
Farsi (Persian)	Persian 51%	Shi'a Muslim 89%
Turkic (Azerbaijani)	Azerbaijani 24%	(official)
Kurdish	Gilaki and	Sunni Muslim 10%
Other (English)	Mazandarani 8%	Baha'i, Jewish, Christian,
Arabic (Arab)	Kurd 7%	Zoroastrian
	Arab 3%	
	Lur 2%	
	Baloch 2%	
	Turkmen 2%	
	Other 1%	

Health Care Beliefs: Active health promotion; traditional. Prevention and health promotion are the major components of the health care system, and Iran has a widespread primary health care program. Although mental illness can be stigmatized, mental health care is also integrated into the health system. Emotional problems are frequently expressed in somatic forms (e.g., headaches, gastrointestinal problems, difficulties sleeping). Beliefs that illness may be caused by a person with the "evil eye" (a person who can harm others merely by looking at them) or imbalances in "hot/cold" temperaments or foods are common and coexist with more modern medical concepts. The integration of these concepts must be considered by health care professionals when they are providing care.

Predominant Sick Care Practices: Biomedical and magical-religious. Most people go to medical facilities when they become ill, but traditional healers are also consulted, especially by those in rural areas. Patients seldom visit doctors alone; they are usually accompanied by one or more people who would are present during the interview, listen very carefully, and often answer questions directed to the patient. It is common for parents to attach amulets to their infant's clothes to prevent the effects of the evil eye, and prayer is common during times of illness.

Ethnic/Race Specific or Endemic Diseases: Endemic diseases include chloroquine-resistant malaria (although no risk exists in urban areas) and cardiovascular diseases. Indonesians are at risk for schistosomiasis. The World Health Organization's (WHO) estimated prevalence rate for HIV/AIDS in adults ages 15 to 49 years is less than 0.01%. WHO has no reported estimates for children from birth to 15 years.

Health Team Relationships: The doctor is usually the leader of the health team and is dominant to co-workers such as nurses. Patients' attitudes toward health professionals is respectful, submissive, and obedient. Men may refuse care by female doctors and nurses. Conversely, women may also refuse care from male doctors and nurses.

Families' Role in Hospital Care: If a woman or child is hospitalized, family members (such as a husband) are likely to remain with them. If staying overnight is impossible, relatives visit them every day. Families frequently are extremely concerned and pay significant attention to the patient, and bad news may be kept from the patient.

Dominance Patterns: The family and their position in society take precedence over individuals. Indonesia has a patriarchal society, and the dominant figure in the family is the father or his male surrogate (e.g., grandfather, oldest son). This is the usual pattern in extended families in small cities and rural areas, whereas in larger cities and nuclear families it is becoming more common for authority to be distributed between both parents. Traditional girls may wear a veil at about age 9. Boys and girls usually play together until the end of primary school; restrictions on boy-girl relations are usually in place after this age and are established by adolescence. Discipline of boys tends to be less strict than of girls.

Although women are not equal to men in Iran, the social status of women is considerably better than it is in some neighboring and similar countries. Women are members of parliament, and some are celebrated doctors, university teachers, and researchers. Women comprise 62% of university students. Many women work outside the home and do not have to be accompanied by a male relative. Iranian women wear a scarf over their hair (a practice that is more prevalent in larger cities such as Tehran), the traditional Iranian Islamic veil *(chador),* or both when they are outside of the home.

Eye Contact Practices: As a sign of respect or possibly shame, a person of lower social status avoids direct eye contact when confronting a person of higher status. Women are expected to be modest and do not make direct eye contact with men who are not family members.

Touch Practices: Shaking hands and embracing are acceptable parts of social encounters during greetings and farewells. Women usually avoid shaking hands with men in public.

Perceptions of Time: Iranians are not generally very punctual, and being on time is not particularly important. However, keeping promises is very important and serious. Not keeping a promise means that a person is unreliable. Being respectful of past traditions is a major characteristic of Iranian people.

Pain Reactions: Reactions to pain are usually quite expressive and accompanied by crying and screaming. Such behaviors are particularly acceptable by women. Emotional problems and neuroses often take somatic forms.

Birth Rites: Some Iranian families, especially in rural areas, prefer to have boys so that they can help the father and eventually replace him and take care of the family. A boy is considered a gift from God, but it is also believed that girls bring health and wealth to a family. Boys and girls receive equal medical treatments when they are sick. Some months before birth the family prepares the infant's clothing and utensils. In the last month of pregnancy, it is recommended that the mother eat lightly and refrain from lifting heavy objects. When the delivery is impending, mothers avoid gas-producing foods. In cities, doctors and educated midwives assist in deliveries, which primarily occur in hospitals. In many rural areas, mothers give birth at home with the assistance of a local (practical) midwife, who is often an old and experienced family member. Some Iranians believe that bathing too early (less than 40 days after birth) may cause puerperal infections, but sponge baths and showers are allowed. Some mothers give their infants an herbal product *(shir khest)* mixed with butter to clean out the intestines in the first few days after birth. After the birth an older male family member (usually a grandparent) whispers *Azan* (an Islamic prayer) into the infant's ear, claiming that the child has been born a Muslim and believes in Allah and his prophet Muhammad. The family member then writes down the time and place of the infant's birth on the back cover of the Koran. The infant's name is usually chosen on the sixth day after birth and may be Iranian or Islamic (Arabic). If an Iranian name is chosen, an Islamic nickname is chosen as well. Circumcisions are usually performed before 6 years and usually immediately after birth. The circumcision is followed by a party. All family members are invited, and they bring gifts for the child.

Death Rites: According to Islamic beliefs a deceased person continues to live after death in another world. Family members are usually present at the time of death, but they do not express their emotions in the presence of the dying person. However, after death, mourning is loud and expressive. The dead body is washed and wrapped in a special cloth *(kafan)*. A clergyman *(rowhani)* prays for the deceased person, and the body is buried in the ground without a coffin. The third, seventh, and fortieth days after death are important dates, because family members and friends participate in ceremonies in the home of the deceased person or a mosque and express condolences to the grieving family. A clergyman speaks to the mourners about the nature and philosophy of death in Islam and asks Allah to accept the deceased person, forgive sins, and place the person in Heaven. Anniversary ceremonies of the death also occur. Autopsies are acceptable, and organ donations are performed as permitted by the religious leaders and the Supreme Leader.

Food Practices and Intolerances: Breakfast, lunch, and dinner are the three main meals, with the midday meal being the most important. Dinner is usually served late in the evening. Basic foods are rice with meat, vegetables, stew, wheat bread, dairy products, and broth. Fresh vegetables, fruit, yogurt, or sherbet may be served as dessert. Tea and nonalcoholic beverages are widely used, and food is usually eaten with a spoon, fork, and knife. Pork and alcohol are forbidden. Total fasting is practiced in Ramadan between sunrise and sunset, so an early meal is often eaten before sunrise. The Ramadan fast is not obligatory for children, those who are sick, or pregnant women.

Infant Feeding Practices: In general, Iranians prefer to breast-feed for up to 2 years. Some mothers also bottle-feed, especially mothers who work outside the home and do not have enough time to feed their infants. Mothers may also work part time or may breast-feed at their workplace during established "feeding hours." Nursing mothers usually avoid foods that might change the taste of the milk, but generally they have no restrictions during the breast-feeding period. The two most common liquid and semiliquid foods introduced between the third and sixth months are made from almonds and rice, which are boiled in hot water and then filtered through a smooth, clean cloth. The resulting juice is combined with sugar and given by bottle or spoon. The juice is nourishing and helps gradually wean the infant.

Child Rearing Practices: Until preschool the education of children is entirely the mother's domain. The upbringing of boys and girls is clearly defined by tradition, and behaviors for each sex are distinct and well differentiated. From the age of reason, a girl is supposed to act like her mother. She performs tasks such as helping with the housework and preparing for her father's return home from work, thus she fully identifies with her mother. Among boys the oldest son is the one who identifies the most with the father and is the "man of the family" during the father's absence. In most parts of the country, child rearing is rather strict, and the father is the main authority figure. Children are expected to do what their parents say, but especially what the father says, regarding life choices such as selection of a job, choice of a spouse, and choice of a place to live. Children still obey their parents even after becoming adults and having their own children. In recent years, child rearing has become more flexible, especially in larger cities and in educated families. A growing number of parents complain that compared with their own parents, they have become so permissive that their children actually rule the family.

National Childhood Immunizations: BCG at birth; DTP at birth, at 6 weeks, at 3, 4 1/2, and 15 months, and at 4 to 6 years; OPV at birth, at 6 weeks, at 3, 4 1/2, and 15 months, and at 4 to 6 years; measles at 9 and 15 months; hep B at birth, 6 weeks, and 9 months. DT only if DTP is unavailable; and Td at 14 to 16 years and every 10 years.

Other Characteristics: Two books are found in every Iranian home: the Koran and the *Diwan* (poems) *of Hafiz.* Hafiz was a great Iranian poet who lived in the fourteenth century AD.

BIBLIOGRAPHY

Djazayery A, Pajooyan J: Food consumption patterns and nutritional problems in the Islamic Republic of Iran, *Nutr Health* 14(1):53, 2000.

Ghods AJ, Ossareh S, Khosravani P: Comparison of some socioeconomic characteristics of donors and recipients in a controlled living unrelated donor renal transplantation program, *Transplant Proc* 33(5):2626, 2001.

Obermeyer CM: Reproductive choice in Islam: gender and state in Iran and Tunisia, *Stud Fam Plan* 25(1):41, 1994.

Sarraf-Zadegan N et al: The prevalence of coronary artery disease in an urban population in Isfahan, Iran, *Acta Cardiol* 54(5):257, 1999.

Shahri J: *A social history of Tehran in the last century,* Tehran, 1990, Rasa Publications.

Singh RB et al: Hypertension and stroke in Asia: prevalence, control and strategies in developing countries for prevention, *J Hum Hyperten* 14(10–11):749, 2000.

Willis EA, Taghipour J: Effects of prolonged war and repression on a country's health status and medical services: some evidence from Iran, *Med War* 8(3):185, 1992.

World Health Organization (June 2000): *Epidemiological fact sheets by country,* Geneva. Retrieved March 1, 2002, from http://www.unaids.org/hivaidsinfo/statistics/june00/fact_sheets/index.html

World Health Organization (2001): *WHO vaccine-preventable diseases: monitoring system,* Geneva. Retrieved March 1, 2002, from http://www.who.int/vaccines/

◆ IRAQ (REPUBLIC OF)

MAP PAGE (864)

Fawwaz Shakir Mahmoud Al-Joudi

Location: Iraq is located in Southeast Asia and occupies the valleys of the Tigris and Euphrates Rivers. Northern Iraq is mainly mountainous, the central portion consists of plains, and river valleys extend south and west and fade gradually into desert. The country has a total land area of approximately 438,317 km² (169,235 miles²) and has a population of about 22 million people.

Major Languages	Ethnic Groups	Major Religions
Arabic (official and major)	Arab 75%	Shi'a Muslim 60%
Kurdish (official in northern Iraq)	Kurdish 17%	Sunni Muslim 38%
Kildani (old Assyrian)	Other 8%	Christian 2%
Turkish (Turkmani)	Armenian, Turk, Sabi'a, Yazidia (Turkmanis), and minor groups such as Chechnians, Sharkas, and Daghastanis	

Health Care Beliefs: Traditional; health promotion important. People say that "Good health is a blessing from Allah, the Creator." This general belief pervades the Iraqi mentality, and people are expected to maintain the invaluable gift of health. Iraqis have a predominant belief that health care can be achieved by avoiding harmful or potentially harmful practices. A general awareness of disease has developed even in rural communities, although to a lesser extent than in urban areas. Traditional beliefs and practices prevail, such as regular prayers for health or healthy children. The importance of good hygiene and cleanliness are highlighted in religious instruction. However, many individuals are not aware of the role contaminated water, soil, fruit, vegetables, and other foods play in the transmission of harmful, unseen factors such as microbes. Nevertheless, the relationship between microbes and illness is becoming better understood by the people. Since the introduction of vaccination programs in Iraq approximately 50 years ago, it has become common for women to wait in line with their children at health centers for the children's vaccines. Even in remote areas, people now understand the role of vaccinations in reducing illness, although illness is also partly attributed to the influence of fate. Mental defects are the most feared; in the Iraqi community, those with mental illnesses or disabilities are considered cursed creatures who extend their curse to their families. Not only are they a burden to their families, but they are considered somewhat shameful. Such individuals are generally sent to mental institutions for treatment and isolation.

Predominant Sick Care Practices: Biomedical; alternative; magical-religious. The majority of people receive medical care at government institutions. Some, especially those in rural communities, consult traditional healers and practitioners. Traditional medicine includes herbal medicines based on old recipes and use of local and imported herbs. People also consult *sheikhs,* who are usually old men or women who claim to have special powers. Sheikhs provide those who are ill with amulets called *doa. Doa* (meaning "to invite" or "to ask") repel evil spirits and ask God for help—for care, a cure, forgiveness, or peace. Desperate individuals often seek such healers as a last resort—when conventional medicine has failed to cure a difficult or incurable disease. Traditional medical practices were supplemented by modern medical care until the 1990s, when shortages of drugs and medical supplies increased.

Ethnic/Race Specific or Endemic Diseases: Endemic diseases include chloroquine-sensitive malaria (primarily in northern Iraq), cutaneous leishmaniasis (in the Baghdad area), visceral leishmaniasis (in the eastern regions), hepatitis B, and cystic hydatidosis (throughout Iraq). Iraqis are at risk for schistosomiasis (*Schistosoma haematobium,* the urinary type), amoebiasis, cyclosporiasis, tuberculosis, cryptosporidiosis, trachoma, measles, and pertussis (whooping cough). Iraq had a pertussis outbreak in 1996 and a poliomyelitis outbreak in 1999. Zoonotic diseases include brucellosis and toxoplasmosis (in addition to hydatidosis). Other problem diseases are gonorrhea and syphilis. Iraq's major organic diseases are cardiovascular diseases and cancer. The World Health Organization's (WHO) estimated prevalence rate for HIV/AIDS in adults ages 15 to 49 years is less than 0.01%. WHO has no estimates for children from birth to 15 years.

Health Team Relationships: In health care settings the doctor is the primary authority, and nursing is a woman's profession and associated with a low status. Patients generally abide by doctors' instructions. Men may refuse care by female doctors and nurses. Medical services are primarily state sponsored and include central hospitals, peripheral hospitals, and clinics distributed throughout the country. However, the availability of basic care may differ among centers. Midwifery is still widely practiced in rural and remote areas. Midwives are generally professionally trained, but most of them lack the skills required for complicated deliveries.

Families' Role in Hospital Care: A patient may be accompanied by one or more people who would like to be present during examinations and answer questions for the patient. Occasionally they perform some of the nursing tasks such as washing patients and positioning them in bed. They also bring food for the patient unless it is forbidden for medical reasons, and the food may be shared by other patients and the hospital staff. Older adults expect to be treated with respect, and the role and expectations of the family are fulfilled through the extreme concern for and attention paid to family members. Reading verses from the Koran to very ill people is common among Muslims, who believe that it cleanses the soul, prepares the individual for meeting God, and may bring mercy to the suffering person.

Dominance Patterns: Iraq has a patriarchal society. Official regulations state that Iraqi women (women who carry an Iraqi passport) who are younger than 45 years must travel with a first-degree male relative (husband, father, or son) or have written approval from their husbands (if married) or fathers (if unmarried) when leaving the country. Generally, women have made progress outside the domestic arena; they are achieving professional status in medicine, teaching, engineering, law, and even the political sectors. Women are somewhat autonomous in the domestic arena; within the family, women usually assume responsibility in the absence of men.

Eye Contact Practices: Socially and religiously, members of the opposite sex generally avoid direct eye contact, even when conversing. Eye contact between members of the same sex is the norm.

Touch Practices: Shaking hands is the formal method of greeting, whereas hugging and kissing are more intimate welcomes that are practiced among closely related people. In these instances, people may touch each other's cheek in a show of affection and tenderness. On arrival and departure, shaking hands, hugging, and kissing are common among family members of both sexes but only between those of the same sex when greeting people outside the family. Because of religious beliefs, many women refrain from shaking hands with men who are not family members.

Perceptions of Time: Punctuality practices vary according to location. Rural communities have so much extra time that punctuality is almost irrelevant; thus the concept of keeping an appointment is relative. However, the situation is different in urban communities, where time has become an important commodity now that business practices have set in. Planning ahead is similar; the horizons of thinking and aspirations dictate the dimensions of plans. (In colloquial language, Iraqis say, "God asked us to be assiduously determined, and only then he would support us.")

Pain Reactions: Iraqis generally have a high pain threshold; however, those in severe pain expect immediate relief, and they may persistently ask for pain medication. Therapy involving exertion contraindicates the Iraqi belief in energy conservation for enhancing recovery. Pain is usually expressed privately or only to close relatives and friends. However, during labor and delivery, pain may be expressed freely and vehemently (as it is in most cultures). The use of analgesics and tranquilizers is usually kept to a minimum to ensure the health and safety of the newborn.

Birth Rites: During the early days of pregnancy, pregnant women are encouraged to satisfy their cravings for desired foods. If cravings are denied, Iraqis believe the infant will be born with a birth sign *(wiham)*. Access to antenatal care is increasing. Many pregnant women prefer to have ultrasounds, primarily to discover the sex of the infant. Clothes, bedding, and food needed by the infant are usually ready at the time of delivery. An infant boy is preferred to an infant girl and is the pride of his family, particularly when he is the first infant. After birth, mothers bathe as they normally do, but they are considered to be in the puerperal period *(nifas)* for 40 days and are treated as rehabilitating patients. They are encouraged to eat nutritious foods to regain their normal health status and strengthen them for breast-feeding. Family gatherings to welcome the new infant are common. To keep their bones straight and begin training them for restraint, infants are wrapped with two layers of cloth. The inner layer is wrapped around the chest, abdomen, and legs. The second layer is a large, triangular cloth that covers every part of the body except the head. Underneath this layer is absorbent material such as cloth, cotton, or commercial disposable diapers (which are very expensive and not affordable for every mother).

Death Rites: Cutting a dead human body is forbidden by the Muslim religion; therefore autopsies are uncommon because the body must be buried intact. Organ donations and transplants from a deceased person for the purpose of saving a life is allowed but requires special approval by the authorities. If an autopsy must be performed (e.g., for forensic reasons), the body must be sutured back into one piece before it is taken to the family and buried. In Muslim burials the body is thoroughly washed with water, wrapped in special pieces of white cloth, and buried without a coffin in the ground. Cremation is not permitted.

Food Practices and Intolerances: Pork, carrion, and blood are forbidden foods. Food tends to be spicy. Rice, bread, meat, and vegetables are the staple foods. Except for children and those who are sick, people fast during Ramadan between sunrise and sunset. Surveys by the United Nations Children's Fund (UNICEF) in 1999 in cooperation with the government of Iraq and local authorities in the "autonomous" (northern Kurdish) region provide reliable estimates of infant and child mortality, which are closely related to food supply. In the autonomous region, better food and resource allocation during the oil-for-food program has contributed to a decrease in childhood mortality. However, childhood mortality clearly has increased in the south central region of Iraq under United Nations sanctions. UNICEF maintains that in-country management of the oil-for-food program did not take into account the special requirements of children ages 1 to 5.

Infant Feeding Practices: Traditionally, mothers breast-feed their infants to increase the mother-child bond, and they may continue breast-feeding until almost the second year of the child's life. Some working mothers stop breast-feeding, although they are allowed a 1-year paid leave after delivery. The Iraqi government is currently carrying out a campaign to encourage mothers to breast-feed their infants. In the past, when the mother did not produce enough milk, "foster mothers" were used. Bottle-feeding is now an alternative, although the comparatively high cost makes this option unaffordable for many families. Infants are introduced to other foods after a few months, and they gradually consume regular meals as they finish their first year.

Child Rearing Practices: The father has the final word in disciplinary situations, and children must have their father's permission to travel. Muslim boys are usually circumcised during childhood, and the procedure is performed at home or in a hospital. Circumcision is celebrated as the first step toward manhood. In Iraq, very few Christians circumcise their infant boys. In accordance with Iraqi law, any child whose father is an Iraqi citizen is also considered an Iraqi citizen, even though their names are written in the mother's foreign passport.

National Childhood Immunizations: BCG at birth; DPT at 2, 4, 6, and 8 months and 4 to 6 years; OPV at birth, at 2, 4, 6, and 18 months, and 4 to 6 years; hep B at birth and at 2 and 6 months; measles at 9 months; MMR at 15 months; and Td at 7 years.

Other Characteristics: The economic sanctions imposed on Iraq since 1990 have severely affected the health and welfare of the country, change that is clearly reflected in the country's health and educational standards.

BIBLIOGRAPHY

Ali MM, Shah, IH: Sanctions and childhood mortality in Iraq, *Lancet* 355(9218):1851-1857, 2000.

Andrews MM, Boyle JS: *Transcultural concepts in nursing care,* ed 2, Philadelphia, 1995, Lippincott.

Dixon J: A global perspective on statutory Social Security programs for the sick, *J Health Soc Policy* 13(3):17-40, 2001.

Garfield R: Studies on young children's malnutrition in Iraq: problems and insights, 1990-1999, *Nutr Rev* 58(9):269-277, 2000.

Kandela P: Medical services continue to decline in Iraq, *Lancet* 353(9167): 1861, 1999.

www.state.gov/www/global/human_rights/1998_hrp_report/iraq.html
www.unaids.org/hivaidsinfo/statistics/june00/fact_sheets/index.html
www.who.int/vaccines/

◆ IRELAND (REPUBLIC OF)

MAP PAGE (860)

Erin O'Donnell Miller

Location: The Republic of Ireland is located west of England and sits between the Irish Sea and the North Atlantic Ocean. It occupies all but the most northeastern territory of the island, which is still part of the United Kingdom. Ireland encompasses 26 of the 32 counties on the island. The total land area of the republic is 70,280 km^2 (43,671 square miles), of which 1390 km (864 miles) are water. Rugged hills and low mountains run along most of the island's perimeter, whereas the inland areas are flat and undulating. Ireland has 1448 km (900 miles) of coastline. Nearly 70% of the land is permanent pastures. More than 40% of Ireland's 3,840,838 people live within 97 km (60 miles) of Dublin, the capital city.

Major Languages	Ethnic Groups	Major Religions
English	Celtic	Roman Catholic 93%
Irish Gaelic	English minority	Anglican (Church of Ireland) 3%
		None 1%
		Other 3%

On average, Ireland has 142 people per square mile, with the majority of the population (57.5%), residing in urban areas. In the last few years, Ireland has had an influx of Eastern European and African immigrants. The indigenous language of the Celtic people of Ireland is Irish, also known as Gaelic, but most people speak English as their first language. In the far west and areas of the southwest, some people speak Irish.

Health Care Beliefs: Active involvement; traditional. Ireland has a rich tradition of paganism. Although largely modernized and Catholicized, many of Ireland's inhabitants still heed the superstitious words and traditions of their ancestors—just in case. Many of the Irish remain at least partially steeped in a culture of oral tradition that carries with it magical explanations and remedies. Irish fairy legends carried on for generations are said to reveal "a whole complex of stored information about land and landscape, community relations, gender roles, medicine, and work in all its aspects: tools, materials, and techniques" (Bourke, p 33). Many fairy legends deal with death and illness and continue to reflect some contemporary health care beliefs. Oral legends reveal that fairies often had a hand in death and illness, hence remedies required something equally magical. Although less common today, herbs may be used in a ritual manner to cure illness (e.g., picking St. John's wort at sunrise on June 23, St. John's Eve, and then giving it to a sick person). *Hyoscyamus niger* (*gafann* in Irish) has been used as a pain killer and sedative. New cow's milk, which is the first milk from a cow after calving, that was boiled with herbs was believed by many to thwart illness. Today, charms and word-for-word recitation of prayers are also believed to provide protection against illness, as well as curing powers. Prayer is a very powerful aspect of the health care beliefs in Ireland, albeit less than it was 20 years ago. Prayers are said to particular saints to prevent and relieve sickness, and some believe that sickness is punishment or preparation for an event.

Predominant Sick Care Practices: Biomedical and magical-religious. Until very recently, the absence of prevention and wellness programs resulted in people relying on secondary rather than primary care, thereby overwhelming the system and causing great delays. Ireland is moving toward an interdisciplinary, team-based type of primary care. Micheál Martin, Minister for Health and Children, explains that the process of harnessing public and private health care will gradually help to phase in the new system. Under the new scheme, primary and secondary care will be linked more efficiently. The new program is proactive, and prevention and wellness are both aims of the plan. People are beginning to rely more on professional care than self-help measures. Primary care teams made up of interdisciplinary provider members will each serve between 3000 and 7000 people. It is estimated that 600 and 1000 teams will be necessary to meet the needs of the population. Primary care teams will, at a minimum, consist of the following professions: general practitioners, nurses, midwives, health care assistants, home helpers, physiotherapists, occupational therapists, social workers, receptionists, clerical officers, and administrators. Primary care networks will consist of the following: a chiropodist, community welfare officers, community pharmacists, dentists, dieticians, psychologists, and speech and language therapists. The goal of this new health care approach, as announced by *Taoiseach* (Irish President) Bertie Ahern on November 26, 2001, is to gradually increase the expedience and accessibility of medical services to all. This new Treatment Purchase Fund will provide expedited treatment to public patients who have had to wait for more than 3 months for care from the time of the initial referral. The Department of Health and Children hopes to decrease the waiting period from a maximum waiting period of 12 months for adults in 2002 to 3 months by the end of 2004. Children will be guaranteed care within 6 months in 2002 and within 3 months by the end of 2003. Free medical care service is provided to less fortunate patients. The Department of Health is currently establishing a new means test to determine eligibility for a medical card, increasing the proportion of people who will have access to state provided medical assistance. Pressure is increasing within the health care profession to provide medical care cards (i.e., free coverage) to all children younger than 18. Also, in July of 2001, 85% of general practitioners, represented by the Irish Medical Organization (IMO), voted to extend medical care coverage to all adults over the age of 70, regardless of means. Nearly 31% of the Irish population has medical cards, which entitles them to obtain all medical services free; the consumer price index is examined yearly to adjust the levels of income necessary to qualify. However, the Department of Health provides medical cards to those who may exceed the "means test" if an individual has a medical condition that requires frequent care. Those without medical cards are entitled to certain services for statutory charges. These services include but are not limited to services from publicly funded hospitals and public consultant treatment.

Differential coverage for hospitals for primary care is a distinctive feature of the Irish public health care system. Mental health care eligibility is determined by geography; people must be residents in a mental hospital's district to obtain care. However, an effort is being made to remove this prerequisite. People not eligible for medical cards often have private health insurance (PHI); in fact, approximately 1.5 million people (about 42% of the population) have PHI. PHI entitles people to beds designated specifically for private care in public hospitals, which can result in beds being given to people solely on the basis of having PHI rather than on the basis of who is most in need of care. The care and the expediency with which that care is received is often far superior for PHI holders than for those who have medical cards. These factors have been a driving force behind reorganizing the health care system in Ireland.

Ethnic/Race Specific or Endemic Diseases: Heart diseases account for 23% of the mortality rate, strokes for 8.2%, other circulatory diseases for 10.8%, and cancer for 23.9%. Diseases of the circulatory system have been the leading cause of death among the Irish at least since 1968; nevertheless, the percentage dying from these diseases has been steadily decreasing. Smoking-related diseases were estimated to be the cause of 23% of all male and 16% of all female deaths in 1995. The World Health Organization's (WHO) estimated prevalence rate for HIV/AIDS in adults ages 15 to 49 years is 0.10%. The estimated number of children from birth to 15 living with HIV/AIDS is 170. As of June 2000, 2364 reported cases of HIV have been reported, and 169 new cases have been detected since December 1999. Those who use intravenous drugs make up the largest portion (41%) of those infected, and homosexuals account for 22.4%. Heterosexuals and those whose risk has not been determined total 19.5%. Children, people with hemophilia, and others comprise the remaining 17%. The number of AIDS cases decreased dramatically from 1996 to 1997 and increased only slightly in 1998.

Health Team Relationships: Doctors occupy the dominant role on health care teams and are more respected than other health care professionals. Nevertheless, the autonomy of nurses within the team is increasing as nurses' educational levels increase. Nurses in Ireland can hold various types of degrees. A general diploma in nursing requires full-time study at a university or nursing school for 3 years. This 3-year diploma often entails taking one class each of the social and biological sciences and spending the remaining time in the nursing wards after they have passed these classes. After nurses with their diplomas register with the nursing board, they may then attempt to obtain a bachelor in nursing (BNS), which requires 1 additional year of study. Ireland is moving toward a 4-year nursing degree program that involves 3 years of classes rather than 1. The fourth year of education would be exclusively in the hospital. A graduate diploma in nursing (GDN) is also available through the collaboration of clinical partners and institutions. This program usually focuses on specializations in nursing practice, education, and management. Throughout the GDN program, students focus on research, innovation, theory, ethics, and policy, and five major modules are supplemented by three specialization modules. This program is usually completed within 2 years, after which students may decide to pursue a master of science (MSc) degree, which includes a 15-unit research dissertation and an advanced research and training module. The number of nurses has decreased sharply because of emigration and fewer people training to be nurses. Irish nurses are among the most respected and in demand around the world and as a result, many have left; today, many of the nurses in the Irish health care system are not Irish. Master's degrees enable many nurses to further their careers by allowing them to become nurse practitioners, providing increased autonomy. Nurse practitioners can admit and discharge patients and write prescriptions. The National University of Ireland registered its first two doctoral students in nursing in 1997. Ireland is optimistic about preventing the development of a two-tier nursing system that could result from disparities in education, and opportunities for existing nurses to improve their skills are being provided. The increasing number of immigrants to Ireland is also changing the shape of the profession. Nurses are increasingly conscious of the need to incorporate multicultural practices into their nursing care.

Families' Role in Hospital Care: Until recently, health care in Ireland did not focus on the family, not even during a patient's recovery. A lack of available hospital space and beds makes it difficult not only for patients to obtain beds but also for their families to visit for extended periods. The people most likely to visit hospitalized patients are mothers and siblings. Ireland has made a concerted effort to develop separate health care facilities for children, who have previously been housed in adult wards. When children are hospitalized, especially for cancer and other life-threatening illnesses, the family plays a key role in recovery; more hospitals are focusing on the emotional support of the family. By reshaping parenting techniques, the Department of Health and Children in Ireland is moving toward a more family-friendly environment for patients and visitors. They are increasing their efforts to attend to the emotional and psychological needs of those with sick family members. A main goal of the shift to a dual system of primary and secondary care is to facilitate the support of the family in times of illness.

Dominance Patterns: Before the Great Irish Potato Famine, which began in 1845, Ireland was predominantly a matriarchal society. The mass exodus of emigrants resulting from the famine began to alter the role of women. A gradual shift toward male dominance began to occur in the 1840s and was well established by 1940. The economic boom in the 1990s, known as the *Celtic Tiger,* began to alter the patriarchical society. More women are beginning to work outside of the home, and 26% of all households are headed by women.

Eye Contact Practices: Direct eye contact is expected because it indicates respect and honesty.

Touch Practices: A firm handshake is preferred. The Irish have a strong sense of personal space. They may feel comfortable with physical contact with members of their family or very close friends, but acquaintances and casual friends are not usually embraced.

Perceptions of Time: Although traditionally oriented to the past, the Irish have two interpretations of modern time: professional time, which applies to work and education settings, and recreational time. The Irish are expected to arrive on time and be prepared for work or school events. Punctuality in social interactions is far different. Most social events generally start 20 to 30 minutes late, or on "Irish time," as some people say.

Pain Reactions: The Irish seldom exhibit or vocalize pain because of their stoical nature.

Birth Rites: The majority of the Irish are Roman Catholic and have their children baptized on the day of a child's birth or approximately 40 days after. The priest pours holy water over the infant, which symbolically initiates the infant into Christianity and the mother and father into parenthood.

Death Rites: In an attempt to thwart evil spirits from entering the body, the Irish have long kept vigil over the dead. The associated ritual was maintained throughout the rise and triumph of Christianity and is referred to as "waking the dead." Friends and family congregate in the home of the deceased person, where they celebrate the individual's life and celebrate the person's passage into the next life. Participants comfort one another and dance, sing, and tell stories during this celebration.

Food Practices and Intolerances: Potatoes are still a large part of the Irish diet. Fish and chips (French fries) are also a very common dish. Chips are also served in abundance with many other meals. Irish soda bread is a favorite of tourists and natives alike. Vegetables such as carrots, turnips, parsnips, and cabbage are also a large part of the Irish diet. Roast beef or lamb is usually broiled after it is marinated with spices and herbs, and duck and goose are also enjoyed. Puddings of custard, fruit, meat, or vegetables are popular as well.

Infant Feeding Practices: According to a recent survey, approximately 30% of mothers in Ireland breast-feed their children. The percentage decreases with the birth of each additional child, and 4 out of every 10 women have stopped breast-feeding by the time the infant reaches 6 months of age. Breast-feeding and education seem to be correlated because mothers who are more highly educated are more likely to nurse their children. In addition, the more professional the husband's career, the more likely his wife is to breast-feed. Most mothers (59%) bottle-feed their infants with formula, perhaps because almost 50% of all Irish mothers work and approximately 50% of children are born to single mothers.

Child Rearing Practices: Most Irish still believe that mothers are the experts on raising children. The mother functions as the primary parent; the father is secondary and focuses more on being a support system for the mother. However, more recent studies show that modern fathers participate in domestic and child care duties more than previous generations of fathers, although mothers still carry the bulk of those responsibilities. More frequently Irish fathers are being expected by others and themselves to be nurturing and emotionally involved with their children. Parenting styles of a husband and wife are often similar and depend largely on the economic, social, and educational status of the family. Fathers are the main child care providers when the mothers are working. The Department of Health is taking proactive steps toward preventing physical and psychological abuse of children. All parents have access to the "Parents Plus Programmes," which provide videotaped parenting courses designed to teach parents to cope with and solve disciplinary issues of children and adolescents. The style of parenting the government is advocating is to refrain from acting out of anger and be firm about the rules that have been set. In 1998 a committee on the rights of the child expressed alarm about the level of violence in many Irish households and the absence of mandatory reporting legislation. Ireland banned corporal punishment in schools in 1982; in 1997, corporal punishment in schools was made a criminal offense. In the same year the Parliamentary Select Committee on Social Affairs recommended that the existing defense for chastisement of children by parents, teachers, and person having lawful control of them should be abolished. However, Ireland opted to reduce and prevent physical punishment through education rather than legislation.

National Childhood Immunizations: BCG at birth and 10 to 14 years; Dtap (diptheria) at 2, 4, and 6 months and 4 to 5 years; tetanus (T) at 2, 4, and 6 months and 4 to 5 years; acellular pertussis (aP; whooping cough) at 2, 4, and 6 months and 4 to 5 years; IPV at 2, 4, and 6 months and 4 to 5 years; HIB at 2, 4, and 6 months; meningitis C at 2, 4, and 6 months and 4 to 5 years; and MMR at 15 months and 4 to 5 and 11 years. After completion of high school, young adults should obtain Dtap and T vaccines.

BIBLIOGRAPHY

Bourke A: *The burning of Bridget Cleary,* New York, 1999, Viking Press.
Central Intelligence Agency (2001): *The world factbook 2001.* Retrieved January 2002 from http://www.cia.gov/cia/publications/factbook/index.html
Department of Finance and Personnel, Belfast (2001): *Physical punishment in the home—law inadequate says Minister Durkan.* Retrieved March 21, 2002, from http://www.northernireland.gov.uk/press/dfp/010911f-dfp.htm

Department of Health and Children, Dublin (1999): *White paper: private health insurance.* Retrieved March 24, 2002, from http://www.doh.ie/pdfdocs/phi.pdf

Department of Health and Children, Dublin (December 2001): *Fathers and families: research and reflection on key questions.* Retrieved March 19, 2002, from http://www.doh.ie/pdfdocs/fathers.pdf

Department of Health and Children, Dublin (2001): *Minister announces degree level education for nurses.* Retrieved March 20, 2002, from http://www.doh.ie/pressroom/pr20011101a.html

Department of Health and Children, Dublin (January 2001): *Minister for children, Mary Hanafin TD, launches parents plus, families and adolescents programme.* Retrieved March 19, 2002, from http://www.doh.ie/pressroom/pr20010125.html)

Department of Health and Children, Dublin (2001): *New health strategy to focus on people, quality, and fairness.* Retrieved March 28, 2002, from http://www.doh.ie/pressroom/pr20011126.html

Department of Health and Children, Dublin (2001): *Primary care model: a descripton.* Retrieved March 20, 2002, from http://www.doh.ie/hstrat/primcare/part_two.html

Department of Health and Children, Dublin (2001): *2001 primary care: a new direction: quality and fairness—a health system for you.* Retrieved February 2, 2002, from http://www.doh.ie/pdfdocs/primcare.pdf

Department of Health and Children, Dublin (2001): *Report of the consultative forum sub group on eligibility.* Retrieved March 18, 2002, from http://www.doh.ie/hstrat/repel.pdf

Department of Health and Children, Dublin (2001): *Statistics on HIV and AIDS.* Retrieved January 30, 2002, from http://www.doh.ie/pdfdocs/stats_hivaids.pdf

Dublin City University (2001): *School of nursing.* Retrieved March 18, 2002, from http://www.dcu.ie/nursing/

Dublin City University: *MSc: Graduate diploma in nursing, online prospectus entry 2002.* Retrieved March 20, 2002, from http://www.dcu.ie/prospects/prospectus/mdn.html

Galanti G-A: *Caring for patients from different cultures,* ed 2, Philadelphia, 1997, University of Pennsylvania.

Giger JN et al, eds: *Transcultural nursing: assesment and intervention,* ed 3, St Louis, 1999, Mosby.

Ireland Department of Health and Children, Information Management Unit, Stationery Office (2001): *Health statistics 1999.* Retrieved January 30, 2002, from http://www.doh.ie/statistics/health_statistics/healthst.pdf

Irish Nurses Organisation (1999): *Child health—the role of the sick children's nurse.* Retrieved March, 24, 2002, from http://www.ino.ie/news_detail.php3?nNewsId=1440&nCatId=228

Irish Times (1999): *Department code on discipline urged.* Retrieved March 19, 2002, from http://www.corpun.com/iesc9904.htm

Irish Times, in association with The Royal College of Surgeons in Ireland: *Nursing a revolution from TLC to a degree.* Retrieved March 20, 2002, from http://www.ireland.com/special/supplements/surgeons/story14.htm

McKeown K (2001): *Fathers and families: research and reflections on key questions,* Limited Social and Economic Research Consultants. Retrieved February 2, 2002, from http://www.doh.ie/pdfdocs/fathers.pdf

Merriman B, Miriam M, Wiley MW: *Women and health care in Ireland: knowledge, attitudes and behaviour,* Dublin, 1996, Oak Tree Press.

Population Reference Bureau (2002): *Population data sheet.* Retrieved February 3, 2002, from http://www.data.worldpop.org/prjprbdata/wcprbdata.asp?DW=DR&SL=

United Nations (2000): *Report on the global HIV/AIDS Epidemic—June 2000*. Retrieved March 26, 2002, from http://www.hc-sc.gc.ca/hpb/lcdc/osh/info/hivaids_e.html

United Nations High Commissioner for Human Rights, Centre for Europe's Children (1998): *Concluding observations of the committee on the rights of the child: Ireland 1998*. Retrieved March 18, 2002, from http://eurochild.gla.ac.uk/Documents/UN/StatePartyReports/ConcludingObservations/IrelandCO.htmorhttp://www.hri.ca/fortherecord1998/vol6/irelandtb.htm

University of Nevada Las Vegas Department of Hotel Administration: *European cultural practices and influences*. Retrieved January 31, 2002, from http://www.unlv.edu/Tourism/audreych4-333.ppt

University of Louisville, Ekstrom Library Government Publications (2001): *Ireland: health and vital statistics*. Retrieved February, 1, 2002, from http://www.louisville.edu/library/ekstrom/govpubs/international/ireland/irehealth.html

UTV, U1993: *Keeping the party going: Irish wakes*. Retrieved March 19, 2002, from http://www.network-irl-tv.com/10000033.html

Vihihealthe: a wealth of health online: *What vaccines does your child need?* Retrieved February 2, 2002, from http://www.vihealthe.com/calculators/vaccine/vaccine.jsp#nohref

---

◆ ISRAEL (STATE OF)

MAP PAGE (864)

Vered Kater

Location: Israel is located at the eastern end of the Mediterranean Sea with Lebanon to the north, Syria to the northeast, Jordan to the east, and Egypt to the southwest. The total land area is 20,770 km² (8,019 square miles). The coastal plain is fertile, and the southern region is primarily desert.

Major Languages	Ethnic Groups	Major Religions
Hebrew (official)	Jewish (Israel born) 82%	Jewish 82%
Arabic (official for Arab minority)	European, American, and Oceanian born 20%	Sunni Muslim 14%
English (widely spoken)	African born 7%	Christian 2%
Yiddish (ultra orthodox and Ashkenazim immigrants from Europe)	Asian born 5% Non-Jewish, mostly Arab 18%	Other (including Druze) 2%

The total population in December 2001 was 6.5 million, including 60,192 immigrants (44,233 from the former Soviet Union and 2201 from Ethiopia).

Health Care Beliefs: Active involvement; prevention important. Israelis believe in the value of health prevention and promotion, as well as curative care. The majority of individuals younger than 50 are very active in self-care and complementary and alternative health care activities.

Naturopathy and Feldenkrais methods, acupuncture, and homeopathy are accepted forms of treatment. Vitamins and over-the-counter food supplements are frequently used. Preventive medical examinations are not routine. The medical establishment sends notices for mammograms but not for yearly examinations with family doctors or gynecologists. Mental health care is under the Ministry of Health, and 5.8% of the health budget goes to this service. In 1995, Israel instituted obligatory reporting of all mental health cases. Today, 148,000 cases are registered; 5589 beds are available in 20 hospitals, and an additional seven centers for day care have the ability to treat 1300 clients. Religious beliefs do not affect attitudes toward people with mental health problems; however, families prefer not to acknowledge such problems because it may decrease their children's marriage prospects.

Predominant Sick Care Practices: Biomedical, alternative, and religious. Israel has a widespread public health system with broad insurance coverage, so all citizens have government-provided medical insurance. All citizens have to be members of one of the "sick funds," and soldiers are insured by the army. The country has a basic package of health services, but 30% of costs are paid by the patients. The average Israeli is willing to spend money for complementary health care. Immigrants from the former Soviet Union often prefer to go to a healer first; if the healer cannot cure them, they go to their general practitioner. The use of religious objects, pictures, prayers, and booklets is common when someone is ill, and red string bracelets are still placed on some newborn infants to protect them. Before signing a medical consent form, most religious families ask their leader (a rabbi) for his opinion and abide by his decision, even if a medical practitioner does not agree.

Ethnic/Race Specific or Endemic Diseases: Glucose-6-phosphate dehydrogenase (G6PD) and lactose deficiency are common. Eastern European Jews have a high occurrence of the *BCRA* gene, which is associated with a high incidence of breast and colon cancers. Tay-Sachs disease is now rare because of prenatal testing, and infantile Niemann-Pick disease is now uncommon as well. Familial Mediterranean fever is ethnicity specific. Adult Gaucher's disease, diabetes, and atherosclerosis are prevalent, and salmonellosis is much more prevalent then shigellosis (3543 versus 5695 cases in 2000). Incidence of drug-resistant tuberculosis, HIV, and AIDS has increased because of the immigration of large numbers of Ethiopians and Russians. The World Health Organization's (WHO) estimated prevalence rate for HIV/AIDS in adults ages 15 to 49 years is 0.08%. The estimated number of children from birth to 15 years living with HIV/AIDS is over 100.

Health Team Relationships: Israel has a high level of health care with high doctor-patient ratios and has 180 nurses per 100,000 inhabitants. A nursing law setting a legal framework for the profession has not been passed, although discussions have been ongoing since the 1970s. Perceptions of overwork, low income, and lack of control contribute to dissatisfaction within nursing. Nursing education in Israel is 3 years for a registered nurse and 4 years for a nurse with a bachelor of arts. Both types of nurses must take state board examinations. Israel has two schools of nursing where nurses with bachelor's degrees can obtain a master's degree in nursing. Nurses who want to continue and obtain their doctoral degree in nursing can do so at universities in Tel Aviv and Jerusalem. Israel has no nurse practitioners, so nurses with a clinical nurse specialty master's degree from the United States are not allowed to open an independent practice in Israel. Immigrant nurses must be recognized by the Ministry of Health to be qualified to work, and many have to retake the state board exams. Almost all schools of nursing have reschooling courses for immigrant nurses, typically allowing them to qualify for state board exams in 1 or 2 years. In general, nurses are considered professionals but are not thought of as independent workers.

Families' Role in Hospital Care: Most hospitalized patients are accompanied by family members, and one person is allowed to stay with the patient at all times. The family often wants to bring food to patients, but it is not allowed because of the dietary laws. In reality, the family often does find a way to provide their hospitalized relatives additional food. The meals in the hospitals are sound and sufficient, but patients do not always like the taste. Personal care is occasionally but not frequently provided by the family. Every patient is washed daily and the bed linens are changed (although exceptions exist, such as in homes for older adults).

Dominance Patterns: Approximately 230 Israeli communities are known as *kibbutzim*. These communal living areas began at the turn of the century as agricultural cooperatives protected by armed settlers. Property is shared equally and although residents do not receive a salary, they are provided housing, pocket money, and necessities such as medical care and education. Women do the same work as the men. Originally, the children lived in a separate house near their parents, but today the children spend their days with other children and only eat and sleep in their parents' quarters. Another form of communal living is the *moshav*, in which each family owns their own land and house but purchasing and selling are both cooperative. The community often has communal farming equipment and marketing policies. Israel has a reputation of being an egalitarian society, especially because of its common military service. Men and women are compelled to join, but women only serve 21 months, whereas men serve 38. Israel is a religious state, so religion is part of its politics. The religious authority *(rabbinate)* rules on personal and family issues. Marriage must be contracted religiously, and no civil marriages are allowed. A couple can only obtain a divorce through the rabbinical offices. Polygamy is prohibited by civil law but not by religious authorities (either Jewish or Arab). Dispensations can be granted for men to take a second wife, but this is rare today. Some religious groups arrange marriages, and authorities tend to ignore the practice. Israel has a low (20%) divorce rate, and the average number of children per family is three. Only 1% of families are headed by a single parent. The ideal woman is a wife and mother and is considered the cornerstone of the family. Israelis undergo more fertility treatments than any country in the world, and the treatments are subsidized by the government. The education levels of men and women are equal, but women still work for lower wages. In 2001 the average salary was 6.113NIS (about US $1346) for a man and 3.235NIS (about US $673) for a woman. The average yearly income is about 73,332NIS (US $17,600). Wage differentials exist even for men and women with the same job. Unemployment rates are higher for women as are poverty rates, but women tend to accept the situation. The ultra orthodox Israeli women are in the worst position, although they claim to be happy with the status quo. Organizational arrangements of communal living (with at least three different kinds of *moshav* and four kinds of *kibbutz* systems) have produced more equality between men and women. However, Israel remains patriarchal, with men making major decisions for their families—a fact that is true for all groups, not just for the ultra orthodox. It is important for health care personnel to realize that men and women who are not related by blood are not allowed to be alone in a room together. Therefore when a male nurse or doctor is talking to a woman, the door to the room must be left open. Women belonging to ultra orthodox groups have defined roles and restrictions. They must obey their husbands without questioning the rationale behind their orders. According to Jewish religious law, husbands have total control over the marital relationships and can grant or deny a divorce. Many women are considered *agunot* (meaning "chained"); they want a divorce and but their husbands refuse to consent.

Eye Contact Practices: Israelis maintain direct eye contact when meeting and talking with others.

Touch Practices: Handshaking and hugging are common practices among friends. First names are used with superiors and strangers. Among religious Jewish males (whether in Israel or elsewhere), a man never shakes hands with or touches a woman because she may be menstruating, and contact during this period is not allowed. Female nurses should recognize the importance of this tradition and never touch male patients until they have confirmed their religious beliefs. Other females are allowed to touch or comfort children and women.

Perceptions of Time: Focus on the future decreases with age, and focus on the past increases—as it does in every society. Because of the increase in terrorist activities in 2001 and 2002, many Nazi Holocaust survivors need mental health assistance. For these older adults, recurring nightmares, tension, and an inability to cope are significant problems.

Pain Reactions: Patients can be very demanding so if a doctor does not do what they want, patients may invent additional symptoms and exaggerate pain to receive the drugs they believe they need. Often patients' friends tell them to take a particular drug for a certain ailment. Patients frequently ask for second and third opinions and consider numerous invasive and expensive tests to be very important and desirable.

Birth Rites: Many orthodox Jews will not utter the name of an infant until the infant is born for fear of inviting the "evil eye" *(ayin hara)*. Traditionalists believe that no one should buy anything for the infant or decorate the nursery before the birth because it may attract the evil eye or bad energy. Families rarely have baby showers, although many Jews order items before the birth and have the store send them after the infant is born. In orthodox families, no man is allowed to touch any female (including a wife or daughter) during menstruation. During the delivery the husband is encouraged to be near his wife, and often he sits with his back to the birth and makes eye contact with his wife. The newborn is believed to be susceptible to evil influences during the first week of life, so a talisman such as a prayer book or knife is often put next to the infant. Jews perform circumcision on the eighth day after birth, and Muslims perform the procedure on the fortieth day. Orthodox Jews may be heard reading prayers together even at the height of the labor pains, a practice that adds a uniquely Jewish dimension to an intensely physical experience. These prayers can be thought of as mantras. Frequently used prayers repeat a sentence from the *Amida* (a daily prayer): *"Adonai sifatai ʲftach uʼfi yagid tehilatecha,"* ("Gd open up my lips and my mouth will declare your praise" [the name of God is never written with the letter "o"] and *"Aneni"* ("answer me"), which is a priestly benediction from the days of the temple. The healing process after the delivery ends with the immersion in the ritual bath *(mikvah)* after termination of vaginal bleeding. Only after bleeding ends is the woman allowed to rejoin her husband in his bed. This ritual also is repeated after each menstrual period.

Death Rites: According to Jewish custom, it is disrespectful to leave a dying person alone, so a relative remains with a dying person to ensure that the soul does not leave the body. Rituals may start before a death has occurred. Embalming and the use of cosmetics are forbidden by the orthodox. Autopsies are forbidden except for forensic reasons in the case of a suspicious cause of death. Many rabbis, including orthodox, encourage organ donations. The family asks their permission, and few refuse. Rabbis even encourage organ donations by the extreme religious in the media. Burial is in the ground in a shroud, and only casualties of war or people who had an accidental death are buried in a coffin. Jewish law requires burial within 24 hours of death unless the Sabbath intervenes. The eyes of the deceased person are to be closed at death, and the body is left covered and untouched until a family member or Jewish undertaker is contacted for ritual proceedings. Seven days of mourning and an official leave from work are observed after the funeral.

Food Practices and Intolerances: Observant Jews are allowed to eat animals with hooves that chew their cud, and only fish with scales are considered fit for consumption. In addition to food, utensils must also be kosher. Milk and meat are not eaten at the same meal. Many religious people bring their own utensils and food when eating in countries other than Israel. Food preferences differ vastly among the various population groups in the country. Eastern Europeans have a tendency to sweeten their food even when eating fish dishes. Asians add many hot spices and enjoy garlic, even for breakfast.

Infant Feeding Practices: Breast-feeding is encouraged in all hospitals and La Lèche groups are common. Approximately 86% of all women begin breast-feeding after birth. Among Jewish women of higher educational levels, breast-feeding is increasing, whereas the opposite is occurring in Arab populations. In orthodox Jewish and Arab communities the period of breast-feeding is slightly longer than it is in other groups. The average duration of breast-feeding is 26 weeks for Jewish and 37 weeks for Arab women. Breast-feeding begins immediately after delivery unless the new mother specifically states that she does not want to try it. Mothers are entitled to 12 weeks of paid maternity leave.

Child Rearing Practices: At age 13 for boys and 12 for girls, Jewish children celebrate becoming full members of the community with a ceremony of bar mitzvah (for boys) or bat mitzvah (for girls). At age 18, all must join the armed forces (although some exemptions are allowed). Joining the military is the true rite of passage into adulthood. Education is rather permissive, and children are the center of the family. Religious families tend to be stricter. Children begin religious schooling at the age of 3 or 4 years, and the routine of daily prayers and intensive bible study adds several extra hours of lessons to the day. Education is obligatory until the age of 16 years and free until age 18; however, many educational items are actually bought by parents who can afford them.

National Childhood Immunizations: DTP at 2, 4, and 6 months and 1 year; OPV at 4 and 6 months and 1, 6, and 13 years; hep B at birth and 1 and 6 months; HIB at 2, 4, and 6 months and 1 year; IPV at 2 and 4 months and 1 year; hep A at 18 months and 2 years; MMR at 1 and 6 years; and Td at 7 and 13 years. The reported percentages of the target population vaccinated in 2000 were as follows: first dose of DTP, 97%; third dose of DTP, 96%; third dose of hep B, 97%; third dose of HIB, 94%; MCV, 94%; and Pol3, 92%.

Other Characteristics: Israelis classify themselves as "religiously observant Jews" or "not religiously observant Jews." Observant Jews cannot travel, write, or turn on electric appliances on the Sabbath (Saturday). American rabbis of conservative or reformed denominations may not be recognized by the Israeli chief rabbinate. Religion is not a major part of daily life for a significant proportion of the population. Israelis are becoming increasingly concerned about cocaine and heroin abuse involving drugs from Lebanon and increasingly from Jordan. They are also becoming more concerned about alcoholism resulting from the recent waves of immigration from the former Soviet Union. Terrorists are a constant threat to the region's stability and safety.

BIBLIOGRAPHY

Cohen I: Nursing care in the multicultural society, *Nurse Israel* 164:14-17, 2001

Callister LC: Cultural meanings of childbirth, *J Obstet Gynecol Neonatal Nurs* 24(4):327, 1995.

Ehrenfeld M: Social correlates of satisfaction and stress among Israeli nurses within intensive care units (ICCUs), *Int J Nurs Stud* 28(1):39, 1991.

Gilad J et al: Epidemiology and ethnic distribution of multidrug-resistant tuberculosis in southern Israel, *Chest* 117(3):738, 2000.

Malach-Pines A: Nurses' burnout: an existential psychodynamic perspective, *J Psychosoc Nurs Ment Health Serv* 38(2):23, 2000.

Musgrave C: Rituals of death and dying in Israeli Jewish culture, *Eur J Palliat Care* 2(1):83, 1995.

Orpaz R, Korenblit M: Family nursing in community-oriented primary health care, *Int Nurs Rev* 41(5):155, 1994.

Svarts S, Frenkel DA: Nurses in Israel: the struggle for regulating the profession, *Clin Excellence Nurse Pract* 2(6):376, 1998.

http://lcweb2.loc.gov/cgi-bin/query/frd/cstdy@field

◆ ITALY (ITALIAN REPUBLIC)

MAP PAGE (860)

Giorgio Tamburlini

Location: The Italian peninsula extends into the Mediterranean Sea in southern Europe and includes Sicily and Sardinia. It is bordered by Austria and Switzerland on the north, Slovenia on the northeast, the Adriatic Sea on the east, the Ionian Sea on the southeast, the Mediterranean Sea on the west, and France on the northwest. The total land area is 301,230 km^2 (116,305 square miles). The Po River flowing from the Alps provides alluvial plains. Italy is a prosperous country with a per capita income of $21,400.

Major Languages	Ethnic Groups	Major Religions
Italian	Italian 98%	Roman Catholic 98%
German	Other 2%	Muslim 2%
French		
Slovene		

German is spoken in the Trentino-Alto Adige, French in Valle d'Aosta, and Slovene in Trieste-Goriza. The majority of the population is ethnic Italians, but Italy also has clusters of German, French, Greek, Slovene, and Albanian Italians, as well as Sicilians and Sardinians.

Health Care Beliefs: Active involvement; some traditional beliefs. In general, the great majority of the Italian population no longer has superstitions or a sense of fatalism linked to health or health care. Still, many people still go to or bring their ill relatives to holy places such as Lourdes (in Spain) or S. Giovanni Rotondo (in southern Italy), hoping that the healing powers of the Madonna and the saints will prove curative. In most cases, these practices are officially approved by the Roman Catholic Church. Traditional healers and practices are still found in some places. By far, consultation with traditional healers is more common in southern Italy and among older adults and uneducated people.

Predominant Sick Care Practices: Biomedical primarily, with Western medicine sought for illness. Some people may still follow practices such as hanging garlic or onions in the home or on the body to prevent illness, but this is uncommon and generally done by older adults or uneducated individuals. Although not necessarily practicing Roman Catholics, some people turn to the Madonna or saints during times of illness.

Ethnic/Race Specific or Endemic Diseases: Italy's population risk for chronic diseases is not different from most industrial countries. Cardio-vascular diseases (although somewhat less prevalent than in northern Europe because of the healthier Italian diet) and cancer are by far the most prevalent chronic diseases. Like in other Western countries, obesity and lack of activity are resulting in a higher incidence of diabetes, and tuberculosis is an emerging problem, particularly among new immigrants. Endemic diseases include goiter (in Calabria), Lyme borreliosis (in north-eastern Italy), tick-borne encephalitis (TBE), and hepatitis delta virus (in southern Italy). Italians are at risk for malaria imported by foreigners from countries in which it is highly endemic—although it was endemic in the Sibari plain until recently. They are also at risk for hepatitis C (especially older people) and Toscana virus. No single diseases are highly specific for Italy, with the possible exception of β-thalassemia, which is Mediterranean rather than Italian and has almost disappeared because of prenatal diagnosis methods. Hepatitis B has almost disappeared because of the mass vaccination campaigns. Statistics show that Italians are among the healthiest people in the world and live longer than most. The World Health Organization's (WHO) estimated prevalence rate for HIV/AIDS in adults ages 15 to 49 is 0.35%. The estimated number of children from birth to 15 years living with HIV/AIDS is 700. HIV incidence was increasing until 1995. Because of prevention programs, fewer cases have been reported in adults, and almost no new cases have been reported in children.

Health Team Relationships: Patients often complain about lack of communication between themselves and health professionals. Doctors in particular are slowly developing communication skills and awareness that communication is an important part of their profession. The topic has been completely ignored by medical schools but is increasingly being incorporated into continuing medical education programs (e.g., counseling skills for family doctors, specialists, and oncologists). Nurses are generally more aware of the importance of communication, and the topic is included in their education. As nurses have achieved higher educational degrees, their professional status has increased. Teamwork is the exception rather than the rule and depends on the hospital, particularly the departmental leaders. Pediatric hospitals are leading a movement toward child-friendly hospitals, and a network of pediatric wards is working on building team-based relationships.

Families' Role in Hospital Care: Many families are close and provide moral support to their relatives during hospitalizations.

Dominance Patterns: Italian society is fairly egalitarian, although women may take the major responsibility for keeping the house and rearing children, whereas men assume the major responsibility for economical support of the family.

Eye Contact Practices: Direct eye contact is preferred.

Touch Practices: Touch is common among Italians, who tend to be warm and outgoing. Shaking hands and hugging and kissing between members of the same or opposite sex are common and acceptable. It is common for women to walk arm-in-arm. Recently, practices based on touching such as shiatsu and massage have become popular. Also popular are various forms of direct contact such as massage for pregnant women, especially by midwives in preparation for delivery. Direct skin-to-skin contact with small, premature infants is being recommended and practiced more frequently although it is not being used in the majority of hospitals yet.

Perceptions of Time: Italians' perceptions of time cannot be characterized in a particular way. Punctuality practices are very similar to those of other European countries. Italy has had a historical trend toward attention to the present—a part of the general hedonistic trend in the Western world.

Pain Reactions: Pain relief has become an important therapeutic concept, with increased attention being given to patient groups such as older adults, women who are giving birth, and people with chronic diseases. Pain control is regulated by the medical system, and patients have few concerns about possible addiction if the reasons for administering analgesia are sound. The Roman Catholic culture does not influence pain management. Avoiding unnecessary pain and trying to alleviate it is now common in all spheres of Italian medicine and for all ages of patients including newborns.

Birth Rites: Traditional rites have gradually disappeared. Increasingly, fathers are present in delivery rooms, but they are still in the minority because of policy restrictions in some maternity units. More frequently, mothers, sisters, or friends are present at childbirths as well. Circumcisions are uncommon except among Jewish children. Religious ceremonies such as baptisms are arranged later, after the infant is several weeks old.

Death Rites: The rite of *estrema unzione* (the blessing by a priest when death is impending) is still common among all Roman Catholics. Funeral and burial practices generally follow the rites of the church, with burial being most common. About 70% to 80% of Italians define themselves as Roman Catholic, but only a minority of them are practicing Catholics. The Muslim population follows the rites of Islam, with the body being wrapped in white cloth and almost immediate burial without a coffin in the ground. Organ donations are permitted and encouraged, and all citizens have a card declaring their option for organ donation in case of death. Most people are in favor of organ donation.

Food Practices and Intolerances: Most Italians follow a typical Mediterranean diet, which includes fish, vegetables, fruits, and grains and less emphasis on red meat. Heart-healthy red wine with meals is common. However, as in other Western countries fast and foods and foods that are high in saturated fat are becoming more popular, especially among the young.

Infant Feeding Practices: Breast-feeding prevalence has increased during the last decade, mainly because of changing attitudes among health care professionals and consequently the public. Prevalence of exclusive breast-feeding after discharge from the hospital now ranges from 85% to 95%. By 4 months after delivery, 35% to 45% of women are still breast-feeding. The rates are highest among educated women in higher socio-economic classes. The government mandates a 6-month leave for those who have just given birth. However, many mothers do not receive this benefit because of private or informal work activities, therefore the need to return to work is still one of the main reasons for ending breast-feeding.

Child Rearing Practices: Child rearing styles vary significantly. The role of fathers has changed considerably, and fathers are much less authoritarian than they have been in the past. In most families the father no longer makes all the rules. Currently, child rearing practices are receiving much consideration in Italy. After the previous period of permissiveness, parents have again begun considering the value of establishing clear rules and boundaries. Particularly among educated people and those in more northern parts of the country, men are taking on many traditionally female roles and activities within the family, such as food preparation and caring for children. The southern part of the country is still more traditional.

National Childhood Immunizations: DPT at 3, 5, and 11 to 12 months and 5 to 6 yrs; OPV at 11 to 12 months and 3 years; hep B at 3, 5, and 11 to 12 months; HIB at 3, 5, and 11 to 12 months; IPV at 3 and 5 months; MMR at 12 to 15 months; and Td at 11 to 12 and 14 to 15 years.

BIBLIOGRAPHY

Callister LC: Cultural meanings of childbirth, *J Obstet Gynecol Neonatal Nurs* 24(4):327, 1995.

Ciceroni L et al: Isolation and characterization of *Borrelia burgdorferi* sensu lato strains in an area of Italy where Lyme borreliosis is endemic, *J Clin Microbiol* 39(6):2254, 2001.

Costante G et al: Iodine deficiency in Calabria: characterization of endemic goiter and analysis of different indicators of iodine status region-wide, *J Endocrinol Invest* 25(3):201, 2002.

De Silvestri A, Guglielmino CR: Ethnicity and malaria affect surname distribution in consenza Province (Italy), *Human Biology* 72(4):573, 2000.

Jaussaud R et al: Tick-born encephalitis, *Rev Med Interne* 22(6):542, 2001.

Romi R, Sabatinelli G, Majori G: Malaria epidemiological situation in Italy and evaluation of malaria incidence in Italian travelers, *J Travel Med* 8(1):6, 2001.

http://www-nt.who.int/vaccines/globalsummary/sGS2000.cfm

http://www.unaids.org

◆ JAMAICA

MAP PAGE (858)

Steve R. Weaver

Location: The island of Jamaica covers a total land area of 10,991 km² (4,242 square miles) and is 885 km (550 miles) south of Miami, Florida, and 145 km (90 miles) from Cuba. It is the largest English-speaking Caribbean island and the third largest in the region. The island is divided into 14 parishes and has two major urban centers: Kingston, the capital, on the southeast coast and Montego Bay on the northwest coast. Jamaica has been an independent state of the Commonwealth since 1962 and is governed by a parliamentary system of democracy based on the Westminster/ Whitehall model. Traditionally the economy has been based on agriculture, with sugar cane, bananas, and citrus fruits as the main export crops. During the 1960s, bauxite mining surpassed agriculture, and today tourism has replaced bauxite as a major foreign-exchange earner.

Major Languages	Ethnic Groups	Major Religions
English	Black 91%	Church of God 21%
Creole/Patois	Mixed 7%	Seventh-Day Adventist 9%
	East Indian 1%	Baptist 9%
	White, Chinese,	Pentecostal 8%
	other 1%	Anglican 6%
		Roman Catholic 4%
		Other, including
		spiritualist cults 43%

Health Care Beliefs: Acute sick care; traditional. Health is described in various ways, but most people interpret a lack of obvious disease or infirmity as good health. Although Jamaicans recognize they can have an illness that does not manifest itself, they consider themselves healthy if they are able to carry out their daily activities. People are also considered to be healthy if they are physically fit and have extra energy and vitality, hence the reliance on herbs and homemade tonics to maintain a state of health. Illness is divided into two categories: natural and unnatural. Natural illness is perceived to be the result of physical changes in the individual caused by an interaction with the natural environment (e.g., traumatic injuries, coughs, colds). The "hot/cold" theory of illness is applicable in Jamaica; some illnesses are believed to be the direct result of exposure to unfavorable environmental conditions such as drafts that cause colds. Getting wet in the rain after being in a warm environment is also thought to contribute to illness. Home treatments for illness involve the use of "hot" and "cold" remedies, and it is believed that natural products are superior to pharmaceutically prepared medications (e.g., hot *bush teas,* a common remedy for many kinds of illness). Bush teas are made from the leaves and roots of various herbs that are steeped or boiled in water. The tea is served sweetened with sugar or honey. Some types of plants such as marijuana *(ganja)* are used extensively in rural areas to treat many illnesses. *Ganja* is considered a "hot" treatment and is usually soaked with other herbs in overproof alcohol called *white rum* and used to treat colds. Religion plays an important role in how illness is interpreted. It is believed that natural illness can be the physical manifestation of spiritual factors, transforming it into an "unnatural" illness. Jamaicans strongly believe that some people have the power to make others ill. The *Obeah* men and women are usually thought to have the ability to cause others to become ill. They are reputed to have a well-developed system of supernatural knowledge that is used to cause good or evil at the request of individuals in the community. To cause an unnatural illness the Obeah man or woman sends a spirit, or *duppy,* to the person who is to be made ill. The ill person must consult another Obeah person to be released from this spiritual influence. Obeah men and women seem to have an inherent dichotomy; some specialize in using their spiritual knowledge to do good, whereas others do harm. The prevention and treatment of illness depends on the ability of the individual to determine the etiology of the illness through its signs and symptoms. People take preventative measures to maintain health by consulting Western medical practitioners available within the extensive system of health care facilities in the country. Particularly in rural communities, this type of preventative service is complemented by the use of the traditional practices. Some preventative rituals include healing, cutting and clearing, and baptism ceremonies. The healing ceremony involves intercessional prayers, ritual washing with herbs and chemicals that are purchased from specialized pharmacies, and the invocation of spiritual protection. The cutting and clearing ritual involves sacrifices of goats, chickens, and pigeons and is performed to ensure the safe conduct of business and continued good health. Baptism is believed to be a spiritual cleansing that ensures good health, prosperity, and healthy social interactions between the baptized and the community. It is also a preventative measure to protect against spiritual attacks by others. The Bible is considered a very potent object and is usually kept open to various psalms and placed at open windows and under the pillow of people who may be ill. Some people wash the floors of their homes with special substances purchased at special pharmacies and recommended by traditional practitioners. Incense mixed with other ingredients such as grated goat's hoof and horn with sulfur is used to prevent spirits, or *duppies,* from entering a home. In many communities, people plant strong-scented herbs such as basil to alert them to spiritual forces that may be entering the home. It is believed that the presence of a spiritual force causes the herb to produce its odor, thus alerting the occupants to its presence. When an illness is believed to be unnatural, Jamaicans have many magico-religious rituals that can be used to cure the individual. Many of these rituals involve the use of the churches as holy ground, as well as rivers and springs considered to have special healing properties. The use of water in rituals is common.

Predominant Sick Care Practices: Biomedical and magical-religious. The health care system is divided into two components and superimposes Western biomedical services with the more traditional magical-religious practices. Many of the latter practices have their roots in the influence of the West African tribes brought to Jamaica as slaves. Both components of the health care system receive endorsement from the general populace, who make decisions about which type of care is appropriate for their health condition. The key to this decision-making process is for individuals to decide whether an illness is natural or unnatural. The term *unnatural* has strong spiritual connotations and requires special intervention from traditional practitioners. If the illness is perceived to be *natural,* the individual either uses homemade herbal preparations or consults Western medical practitioners. In some instances, they may use both strategies. In some cases, although the illness is considered unnatural, the individual first consults a Western medical practitioner and then continues treatment with a traditional practitioner. The individual uses three classes of information to make this decision about the illness. The first type of information is the signs and symptoms of the illness, including its severity and suddenness. If the illness comes on suddenly and its symptoms are severe, people seek immediate help from Western medical practitioners. Second, if the symptoms are not sudden or severe, people wait for a while before taking action, paying attention to any "divine cues" in the form of omens or dreams. Prophetic dreams are important as a guide to health care behaviors. It is believed that some dreams are sent by divine messengers seeking to assist individuals. The third category of information is social cues derived from interactions with other members of the community. Others are observed within the context of their personal health-related experiences and offer advice regarding health behavior.

People who perceive that they may have health problems use these three categories of information to make a decision regarding their subsequent health behaviors. Having made a decision about the nature of the illness, people select between Western medical practitioners and traditional practitioners. The traditional health care provider can be divided into three groups: herbalists, healers, and Obeah men and women. The herbalists are usually farmers who have obtained their knowledge by apprenticeship with another herbalist, and they are able to ply their trade legally. The healers and Obeah men and women are all considered illegal practitioners because they are in contravention of the Obeah Act of 1898, which is still enforced in Jamaica. Many traditional healers are members of the Revival faith, a Christian sect; therefore fasting and praying play a major role in the type of treatment provided for their patients. Protection from spiritual influences is important, and amulets called *guards* are used to protect the believer. The guards are divided into two types: internal and external. The external guards are usually made in the form of a small cloth bag about 2 × 2 inches and contain herbs and pages of the Bible folded into small squares. Occasionally *guard rings* are specially made with a hollow base for the insertion of herbs. The internal guards are usually concoctions made by the traditional practitioner and ingested by the patient. These internal guards are made from herbs, and a substance called *alum* is often a part of the substances ingested. The latter guards are used to protect the individual from "bad food," or food that has been physically or spiritually contaminated. Some individuals do not fully trust Western practitioners because they do not believe that they are capable of dealing with all their illnesses. In rural communities, medical doctors are held in high esteem when they are willing to refer patients to traditional healers. When seeking Western medical care, individuals in rural communities frequently consult a doctor and use the prescribed medication for a short period, hoping for a symptomatic response. After 2 days of using the medication without immediate relief, they discontinue the medication and consult another medical practitioner. After following this pattern with three doctors, they consult a traditional practitioner.

Ethnic/Race Specific or Endemic Diseases: In 1999 the population of the island was 2,576,300 million, with an annual growth rate of 0.9%. The age distribution shows that the population is essentially a youthful one, with 30% younger than 30 years. In 2000 the crude birth rate was 23 per 1000, the crude death rate was 5.2 per 1000 people, and life expectancy at birth was 73 years for women and 70 years for men. The five leading causes of death per 100,000 people are as follows: cerebrovascular disease, 78.2; diabetes mellitus, 51.05; ischemic heart disease, 53.25, and other heart diseases, 34.11; and hypertension, 33.99. In all cases, more women die of these diseases than men. The World Health Organization's (WHO) estimated prevalence rate for HIV/AIDS in adults ages 15 to 49 years is 0.71%. The estimated number of children from birth to 15 years living with HIV/AIDS is 230. From 1982 to June 2001, 5547 AIDS cases had been reported in Jamaica. An estimated 1.5% of the adult population is living with HIV/AIDS. All parishes are affected by the epidemic; however, the two major urban parishes, which are the Kingston and St. Andrew metropolitan areas and St. James, have reported the most cases. Reported AIDS cases range from 76.3 per 100,000 people in St. Elizabeth to 501.2 per 100,000 people in St. James. HIV/AIDS is the second leading cause of death in children ages 1 to 4 years. Seroprevalence rates among high-risk groups are as high as 25% among men who have sex with men and 20% among female commercial sex workers. The HIV infection prevalence rate among pregnant women in the parishes ranges from 0.5% to 2.6%, with the highest infection prevalence rate recorded among women ages 15 to 19 and 25 to 29 years. The group most affected by AIDS is 15-year-olds to 19-year-olds, and the link between having had previous sexually transmitted diseases and having HIV/AIDS is strong. The mode of transmission in Jamaica is primarily heterosexual; the HIV transmission rate through homosexual and bisexual relations is only 7%. HIV/AIDS infections affect members of all occupational and social classes.

Health Team Relationships: In most instances, members of the health team have a good working relationship; however, the doctors are generally at the top of the social status hierarchy. Nurses have worked hard during the years to develop and maintain professional standards, which is reflected in their interpersonal relationships with others on the health team. Nurses continue to make a pivotal contribution to health care in spite of the chronic shortage of registered nurses. Some doctors still cling to the idea of being superior to nurses in the working environment, but their numbers are dwindling. Nurses are now obtaining higher levels of education, including master's and doctoral degrees, thus balancing the educational and social equations between health professionals. Patients hold Western medical practitioners, including nurses, in high esteem to a certain extent because patients recognize the efficacy of Western biomedical sciences.

Families' Role in Hospital Care: Families play an unofficial part in the hospital care of patients. In hospitals with a severe shortage of nursing staff members, relatives are allowed to assist with patients' personal needs. Food is an important social variable, and patients complain that the taste of the hospital food does not meet their standards. Families consider the role of providing food for their hospitalized relatives to be very important, despite the fact that the patients may be on a special diet. The physical nature of in-patient facilities does not allow for relatives to remain with their hospitalized family members. However, pediatric hospitals that are infant friendly allow parents, usually mothers, to stay overnight with their children.

Dominance Patterns: The Jamaican culture is one of overt male dominance, although in practice it has a matrifocal tendency. The ideal is to have a man as the head of the household, but in reality approximately 43% of all households are headed by women. Similarly, the ideal is to be married, but sexual relationship and courtship patterns show a tendency for relationships to begin as visits, proceed to common-law relationships, and later in life after all the children have been born conclude in marriage. Under normal circumstances, men assume dominant sexual roles. They sire children with many different women, who are referred to as their *baby mothers,* a practice that gives them social status among their peers. Knowledge about health-related matters tends to be passed on from mothers to daughters, and the power roles between men and women are reversed during times of illness. At these times women, particularly the older mothers and grandmothers, have the power to control the actions of the men. They dictate the sick roles in the household and make decisions about health behaviors.

Eye Contact Practices: In general, eye contact is common among peers, but it is avoided with authority figures unless a nonverbal challenge is being issued. Women who are in a courting relationship and want to seem demure avoid eye contact with their suitor. However, as the relationship proceeds, eye contact can be used as a warning signal or an invitation. Among men in the lower social classes, eye contact is used to challenge strangers but among friends and peers is an acknowledgment.

Touch Practices: Jamaicans are very expressive, and they greet each other with hugs and handshakes. The culture is very homophobic, so men do not normally embrace each other except in prescribed situations such as church ceremonies. Among men from the lower social classes, a common greeting is to touch the closed fists by placing one fist on the top of the other and then reversing the action. Women embrace when they greet each other, particularly if they are close friends.

Perceptions of Time: Punctuality is considered the ideal, but in reality people are not always on time for their social activities.

Pain Reactions: Individuals are very expressive in their reactions to pain, whether it is physical or emotional. At funerals, loud weeping and moaning is expected from relatives.

Birth Rites: Many pregnant women give birth at hospitals and therefore must conform to the standards of care prescribed by Western medicine. Many cultural practices are followed for births at home. In some rural communities a *nana,* or traditional birth attendant, performs many deliveries even though the community has midwives. The nana is culturally acceptable because she stays with the mother before and after delivery. When the mother feels that she is ready, she sends her partner or oldest child to call the nana, who usually lives in the village. When the nana arrives, she examines the mother and begins to prepare the birth room. All cracks and crevices are sealed with old newspapers, and the windows are closed and covered with heavy cloth to ensure that the mother does not develop a "baby cold" from drafts in the room. The bed is prepared by laying down several sheets of old newspaper to protect the mattress. Extra sheets of newspapers are usually collected for this purpose before the labor and delivery. After the nana examines the mother, she gives her an enema made of soap and water. If the mother is having an unusually long labor, the nana usually offers her some thyme tea to hasten the process. After the baby is born, it is wiped clean, preferably with clean flannel cloth. Visitors are not allowed to enter the room immediately for two reasons—they may carry infectious agents such as the common cold, and they may unwittingly bring spirits into the room, and the infant is thought to be susceptible to these influences. The infant is usually protected with warm clothes for protection from drafts, and special attention is paid to its "mold"—the unclosed suture line at the crown of the head. It is important to ensure that the infant does not develop a "mold cold," a type of cold that manifests as frequent discharges from the eyes and nose. The infant is usually given a warm sponge bath the second day after delivery. In many instances a Bible opened to Psalm 23 is placed under the pillow of the infant. Occasionally an open pair of scissors is placed under the mattress of the infant's cot to ward off evil influences. The infant is given a small external guard made with *asafetida,* a pungent substance used to keep away spirits. A red string, usually in the form of a bit of clean red cloth, is tied to the wrist of the newborn. Red is the color of power and is used to ward off any supernatural influences. In rural communities where possible, the parents of a newborn bury the umbilical cord and plant a fruit tree on the spot. A typical Jamaican saying states that people may travel to distant places, but they always return to the place where their "navel string is buried." This implies that people have a permanent commitment to their relationship with their ancestral home and family. After the birth the mother is allowed to sit on a pail to collect the afterbirth and attend to personal hygiene matters. The mother does not have a full bath until 9 days have passed. In cases in which mothers have help or the nana stays, mothers do not leave the birthing room for the entire 9 days unless it is very important that she does so. During this time, she wears a belly band, which is a piece of cloth tied around her abdomen. She continues to wear this until all bleeding has ceased. If the nana feels that the mother is bleeding excessively, she boils cobwebs collected from the house and leaves the drink to cool overnight. The mother drinks the mixture as a tea. During the 9-day period of confinement the mother's diet is restricted to corn porridges and thin soups. The perinatal mortality is 30.2 per 1000 births, the infant mortality is 24 per 1000 live births, and the maternal mortality is 10.2 per 10,000 women.

Death Rites: Death is a very important time because of its implications for the living. The culture has strong aspects of ancestor worship. During celebrations, it is customary for people to pour a little of their beverages on the floor for "those who are not here," a way for the living to pay homage to those who have passed on. In concept, the dead can also assist the living in maintaining land tenure. Land owners seek and obtain permission to be buried on their property, and the land is then referred to as "family land." It cannot be sold and must be passed on in trust from one member of the family to another. When a person dies, a definite number of activities must be carried out systematically. If a person's death was expected, people have a less overt emotional response. However, if a death is unexpected—or worse, a child dies—Jamaicans overtly express their grief. When young people or children die, the mothers express their grief the most vocally. They hold their bellies and bend over at the waist while crying out loudly. A common expression heard by mothers experiencing this kind of grief is, "Me belly bottom hurt me." After the initial stages of grief the family begins to prepare for the funeral. Funerals are occasionally delayed as much as a week to accommodate relatives overseas. The family has a wake and provides food and entertainment. The wake involves family, friends, and the general community sitting up all night for approximately 3 nights with the family. It is customary for the family to provide coffee, salted biscuits, and alcohol in the form of white rum, or *whites*. The type of entertainment depends on the religious affiliation of the family. If they are members of the more established religious groups (e.g., Anglican, Adventist, Pentecostal), they tend to sing more hymns and drink less alcohol. If the family is in the Revival religious community, they play drums and sing hymns and other songs related to their religion. Trained individuals care for the body at a funeral home, the body is prepared for *churching,* or the transport of the casket to the church for the ceremony before burial. The body is removed from the home feet first so that the person's spirit, or *duppy,* knows it cannot return. When the body is removed from the house, the curtains are removed from the windows. While the body is at the church, the tomb is prepared, which is usually a $6 \times 6 \times 4$ foot hole in the ground with concrete bricks for its sides and a concrete slab for the top. When the body leaves the church, it is usually followed by a procession of people walking and singing hymns if the funeral is in a rural community. In an urban setting the hearse is usually followed by a motorcade that takes people to the cemetery, where the rest of the formal ceremony takes place. The family pays people to seal the coffin into the tomb at the grave site after the ceremony. At the home the family cleans the house, turns mirrors around, and leaves the house with no curtains for 3 days. Although autopsies are acceptable, it is felt that removing parts of the body makes the *duppy* restless, therefore organ donation is unacceptable. It is very important to ensure that the *duppy* be allowed to rest because it is believed that these restless spirits can return and harm those who did not follow the prescribed methods of laying them to rest, resulting in possession by the spirit and loss of good fortune.

Food Practices and Intolerances: Food is an important factor in the social life of Jamaicans. From a cultural perspective, foods can be divided into "good food" and "bad food." Good foods are fresh, healthy, and nourishing for the body, but the term also involves the mode of preparation and storage. Good food refers to food that is prepared in a prescribed manner, is clean, and is served at the correct temperature. Processed foods such as white rice are considered to have little or no nutritional value because the processing robs the food of its value. Bad food refers to foods that are prepared and stored inappropriately or have been purposely contaminated to harm the person eating them. The average Jamaican likes yams and green bananas, which are given the general name *food* in the common parlance. These foods are considered to be strengthening and are appropriate for a working person who needs extra energy. They are prepared by boiling and can be served hot with a side dish at any meal of the day. A typical breakfast may consist of boiled yams, boiled green bananas, and wheat flour made into dumplings, with mackerel cooked in coconut oil. The meal is served with hot teas made from cocoa or one of the common varieties of mint. Another common breakfast consists of *ackee* fruit cooked with salt fish and wheat flour dumplings that are fried in oil and served with hot tea. *Ackee* and codfish is the national dish of Jamaica. The *ackee* is a fruit that grows in a red pod on tall *ackee* trees; when ripe, the pod opens to expose a delicate pink fruit with a black seed. The seed is removed, and the deep pink center of the pod removed. The fruit is then boiled until it becomes soft, and the water is removed. The remaining fruit, which at this point resembles scrambled eggs, is then fried with the codfish and tomatoes. It is extremely important that the *ackee* is properly prepared because it contains a potent water-soluble hypoglycemic agent. Jamaicans often think that they should have something hot in the morning to remove the gas from their stomach, so breakfast must include hot teas. In rural communities that had limited access to refrigeration, people used salt to preserve their foods. As a result, some salted meats and fish became known as *saltin,* and the word is still used in reference to salted fish, pork, and beef used to flavor foods. Meat *patties* are a favorite snack food throughout the country. A *patty* is a pastry filled with seasoned ground meat, usually beef, and eaten hot. The most common form of protein is chicken. The chickens that are reared by mass production methods are considered healthier than those reared at home. The latter must be caught and allowed to cleanse their systems before being eaten. The segment of the population that is Seventh-Day Adventist does not eat pork. The Rastafarian religion also prohibits pork consumption. These religions consider pork to be unclean because of the references in the Bible. However, pork prepared in the way of the Maroons (African slaves who escaped from their plantations and formed communities in the hilly areas of Jamaica) is called *jerk pork* and considered a delicacy by the segments of the population that consume this type of meat. The jerked pork is prepared using special herbs and seasonings and cooked slowly over a smokeless fire made of pimento wood, which provides the distinctive flavor in the meat. In rural communities the women usually prepare the food, but when it is being prepared in bulk for festivities, men play a part in preparations. The goat plays a major role in many rituals and festivities. Curried goat and a soup made from the goat's tripe and testes are delicacies regularly offered at functions. Jamaicans tend to avoid eating foods from strangers because they do not know about the food's preparation and storage; therefore they could accidentally consume bad food. This practice is especially important for men because they tend to have polygamous relationships. A man may fear that a woman may give him food that has been prepared in a way that will compel him to stay with her, a practice known as *tying* the man. It is thought that occasionally women put their menstrual blood into stewed red peas to force men to stay with them. Another method that men fear is the *sweating* of rice, a practice in which women are reputed to stoop over boiling rice and allow the steam to condense on their genitalia and then fall back on the rice. To protect themselves from these assaults, men tend to use internal guards, which are expected to negate the effects of any bad food.

Infant Feeding Practices: A very strong public health campaign has promoted breast-feeding. This campaign seems to have been successful because breast-feeding is widely accepted at the present time over bottle-feeding. However, breast-feeding is not necessarily exclusive, and many mothers also give their infants water and fruit juices. Mothers have been resistant to breast-feeding because bottle-feeding with formula is a status symbol and shows that the mother can afford to purchase formula. Many mothers do not mix the formulas properly, and the infants may become malnourished. Mothers also have concerns about the physical changes in their breasts that are caused by breast-feeding. Today, mothers are discouraged from using bottles when they attend well-infant clinics. Anthropometrical measures show that among children who are between infancy and 59 months 5.4% show signs of overweight, 5.1% have low weight for age, 4.2% have low height for age (stunting), and 2.2% have low weights for height (wasting).

Child Rearing Practices: Parents can be very strict with their children, and corporal punishment is still a method of discipline in schools. Many people in the society support corporal punishment. Children are still expected to be seen but not heard, especially when adults are having a conversation. In many instances the father is used as a threat for children who misbehave; the care giver says, "Wait till yuh father come home." However, it is actually the women who provide the daily discipline for their children, particularly because so many households are headed by women.

National Childhood Immunizations: BCG at birth; DTP at 6, 12, and 20 weeks, 18 months, and 3 to 6 years; OPV at 6, 12, and 20 weeks, 18 months, and 3 to 6 years; MMR at 1 year; and TT for pregnant women, +4 to +6 weeks. Malaria, hemorrhagic dengue fever, tuberculosis, and typhoid continue to be a threat to the Jamaican population. Among children ages 6 to 59 months, approximately 93.9% receive OPV, 93.8% receive the DPT/DT vaccine, 97.5% receive the BCG vaccine, and 91.3% receive the MMR vaccine.

BIBLIOGRAPHY

Chevannes B: *Rastafari—roots and ideology,* Jamaica, 1995, Syracuse University Press and The Press University of the West Indies.

Ministry of Health, Jamaica: *Jamaica HIV/AIDS/STI national strategic plan 2002–2006. Time to care, time to act,* Jamaica, 2001, The Ministry.

Pan American Health Organization: *Health in the Americas,* Scientific Pub No 56, Vol II, Washington, DC, 1998, The Organization.

Planning Institute of Jamaica and Statistical Institute of Jamaica: *Jamaica survey of living conditions, report 2000,* Jamaica, 2001, The Institute.

Sobo E: *One blood—the Jamaican body*, New York, 1993, State University of New York Press.

Statistical Institute of Jamaica: *Statistical year book of Jamaica, 2000,* Jamaica, 2000, The Institute.

Wedenoja W: *Religion and adaptation in Jamaica,* University of California, 1978, Ph.D. dissertation.

◆ JAPAN

MAP PAGE (865)

Sachiyo Murashima

Location: Japan is in East Asia and is separated from the eastern coast of Asia by the Japan Sea. It is an arc-shaped country, consisting of four major islands and more than 7000 small islands spread over 3500 km (2175 miles). Most people live in densely populated urban areas. The country has many volcanoes and is often shaken by earthquakes. The population of Japan is about 126 million, and recently the number of foreigners increased to 0.7% of the population. The features of the population pyramid of Japan are the rapid increase in the number of older adults and decrease in the number of children. The average life expectancy of Japanese men and women is 77.10 and 83.99 years, respectively. The percentage of population of the various age groups are as follows: children (birth to 14 years), 14.8%; working-age individuals (15 to 64 years), 68.5%; and older adults (65 and older), 16.7%. The population in Japan is aging more quickly than the populations of other

Western countries, and it is estimated that one of four people will be older than 65 in 2025. The total fertility rate in 1999 was 1.34 children per woman, which is far lower than the level needed to maintain the current population numbers, and this figure is decreasing every year.

Major Languages	Ethnic Groups	Major Religions
Japanese	Japanese 98%	Shinto Buddhist 89%
	Korean, others 2%	Christianity 2%
		Other 9%

Health Care Beliefs: Acute sick care; traditional. Today, people know that illness can be caused by working too hard and factors such as smoking, high-fat diets, and stress; however, health promotion and disease prevention concepts are only slowly being integrated into the health care system, and people are reluctant to change their habits.

Predominant Sick Care Practices: Biomedical and alternative. Western medicine is predominant, but Eastern medical practices, such as acupuncture and herbs, are also used. Japan has universal medical care insurance; however, people are required to pay from 10% to 30% of their medical expenses. Generally, if Japanese feel ill or have a health concern, they consult a doctor in a clinic or a hospital or buy medicine in a pharmacy.

Ethnic/Race Specific or Endemic Diseases: The three main causes of death in Japan are malignant neoplasms, heart disease, and cerebrovascular diseases. The main causes of death have shifted from infectious diseases to lifestyle-related chronic diseases. In addition, emerging and reemerging infectious diseases are major concerns. Epidemics of *Escherichia coli* 0157 have been problematic and were a particular problem in 1996. The World Health Organization's (WHO) estimated prevalence rate for HIV/AIDS in adults ages 15 to 49 years is 0.02%. The estimated number of children from birth to 15 years living with HIV/AIDS is less than 100. A total of 7855 HIV/AIDS cases had been reported as of May 2000, with the highest prevalence in foreign female sex workers (2.7%). Most reported cases during the early phases of the epidemic were caused by blood transfusions. However, as of 1999, about 70% of diagnosed HIV infections seem to have been acquired through sexual contact.

Health Team Relationships: In hospitals the health care team consists of doctors, nurses, pharmacists, dietitians, clinical laboratory technicians, and radiology technicians. Under certain circumstances, physical therapists, occupational therapists, and speech therapists are available. Certified social workers are not paid for by health insurance, limiting their availability to the general population. Respect for social rank is pervasive in the system, with doctors at the top of the hierarchy. As in most cultures the doctor is responsible for medical treatment, and nurses serve as caregivers. Most patients follow decisions made by their doctor, and it is uncommon to request or receive a second opinion by another doctor. Patterns of thought are expressed indirectly; the listener is expected to get the point of a conversation without being explicitly told what it is. A person may divert the subject away from an embarrassing topic or avoid direct confrontations, and individual verbal agreements do not imply compliance. The family is generally consulted before medical decisions are made; however, informed consent is stressed more today because it is the doctors' duty to explain the meaning of *consent*. The patients' right to know their diagnosis and treatment options is gradually becoming an accepted concept in the health care system.

Families' Role in Hospital Care: In the past the family was expected to take care of their hospitalized family members. Today, nurses are responsible for care of in-patients, and the role of the family is primarily one of support; however, it is still common for mothers to care for their hospitalized children.

Dominance Patterns: The traditional Japanese perspective in the past was that men should work outside the home and women should take care of family affairs. However, the values of individuals have changed because of Western influences, the changing structure of society, and the improving economic power of women who work outside the home. Since the Equal Employment Opportunity Law for Men and Women was established, working environments for women have improved; however, it is still very difficult for women to get jobs after having children because of concerns that their work will be interrupted by family responsibilities or future pregnancies. Traditionally, children take care of their aging parents, but this has been changing as the number of women who work has increased. Workers can take a leave from work so that they can care for their parents. In addition, since the establishment of long-term care insurance in 2000, it has become easier to receive assistance for the care of frail, aging parents.

Eye Contact Practices: In the past, direct eye contact was considered disrespectful. In modern Japan, this mindset has diminished, and direct eye contact has become more common between the sexes and with older adults. In very traditional families, it is still considered more polite to avert the eyes when speaking with older adults and other respected adults.

Touch Practices: Bowing is the customary greeting among Japanese, although handshakes are also acceptable. A pat on the back is unacceptable and considered rude. Lovers may greet each other with a kiss to express tender feelings.

Perceptions of Time: Punctuality is important, and being on time for appointments is valued. Many Japanese spend much of their time working, so work becomes a source for some social activities.

Pain Reactions: The majority of patients believes it is important to tolerate pain, so they are embarrassed to complain of discomfort. Crying out because of pain is considered somewhat shameful and not something one would want others to hear. However, the concept of pain relief as an accepted form of medicine has recently become more widely accepted, and the use of analgesics for pain is becoming the norm.

Birth Rites: Japan has one of the lowest infant mortality rates in the industrialized world. The infant mortality rate in 2000 was 3.2 per 1000 live births. A newborn with a birth weight of 2300 g is considered premature. People readily comply with prenatal care and health promotion advice. Women in labor are silent and even eat during labor; most give birth in a hospital or clinic. Recently, more husbands have attended the birth of the children. Women may be assisted by midwives or doctors. After birth the mother enjoys long periods of rest and recuperation and may stay in the hospital or clinic for 5 to 7 days and indoors for as long as 2 months. Nurses recommend taking a shower several days after birth. When an infant is 1 month of age, the grandmother takes the infant to a shrine to pray for healthy growth.

Death Rites: The crude death rate in 1998 was 7.5 per 1000 people, and the rate has been increasing because of the increase in numbers of older people in the population. The Japanese tend to control public expressions of grief. Relatives and close friends attend a wake, and then a funeral ceremony is performed. In the past the ceremonies were performed according to the religion of the family, with the majority of funeral ceremonies being Buddhist. More recently, Japanese have been more flexible about funerals and usually follow the wishes of the deceased person. For example, ceremonies may be performed with no vestiges of religion but many flowers. It is customary to give the family an obituary gift of money. Usually half of the gift is returned with green tea and cakes after 49 days—one of the customs of the funeral ceremony used to recognize those who attended. Cremation is widely practiced in Japan.

Food Practices and Intolerances: Most people enjoy raw fish and mushrooms. Traditional foods (such as tofu, which is made from soybeans) are very light and not greasy. Western-style food such as bread and meat has spread throughout Japan, but many Japanese are returning to traditional diets that are low in fat and include numerous vegetables because of the health benefits.

Infant Feeding Practices: Approximately 40% of mothers breast-feed, and weaning generally begins about 3 months after birth. Children are then bottle-fed with formula and begin receiving semiliquid foods.

Child Rearing Practices: The mother-child relationship is strong. Boys were traditionally considered more important than girls and were more likely to receive a higher education. Today, this distinction and favoritism is decreasing, providing better opportunities for women. The Tango Festival, in which people pray for boys to grow up safely, is held on May 5; the Doll Festival, celebrated on March 3, also includes prayers for the safety of girls. Decreases in the fertility rates and an emphasis on nuclear rather than extended families have meant that some new mothers, especially those in urban areas, cannot find an experienced mother or consultant to guide her in child rearing practices. Without social support, some mothers feel trapped, which occasionally causes them to mistreat their children. The community is being warned to be aware of signs of abuse and help to raise the children; however, many middle-age women are working, and the society has an insufficient number of adequate day care centers. The percentage of students who go on to a university or college is approximately 34% for men and 46% for women, so it is clear that the culture no longer considers it unimportant for women to have an education. Students spend long hours preparing for school entrance examinations; this is a period that is particularly competitive and stressful for them because of the influence admission has on their future prospects.

National Childhood Immunizations: BCG at 3 to 12 months and if negative, revaccination at 8 to 12 years; polio ×2 at 3 to 90 months; DPT ×3 at 3 to 12 months, once at 18 to 30 months, then once at 11 years; measles at 12 to 24 months; rubella at 12 to 36 months or at 11 years; and Japanese B encephalitis ×3 at 3 to 4 years, once at 9 years, and once at 14 years.

Other Characteristics: Most Japanese are fond of comparatively long, hot baths and take them in the winter and the summer; the bath is often followed by a shower. People who are ill do not take baths and showers. People rarely use nonverbal expressions to display their feelings. About 54% of men and 15% of women smoke cigarettes, and smoking rates of teenage girls are increasing.

BIBLIOGRAPHY

Anders RL, Kanai-Pak M: Karoshi: death from overwork, *Nurs Health Care* 13(4):186, 1992.

Anders RL: An American's view of nursing education in Japan, *IMAGE: J Nurs Sch* 26(3):227, 1994.

Asahara K et al: Long-term care for the elderly in Japan, *Ger Nurs* 20(1):23-26, 1999.

Engel NS: An American experience of pregnancy and childbirth in Japan, *Birth* 16(2):81, 1989.

Galanti GA: *Caring for patients from different cultures,* ed 2, Philadelphia, 1997, University of Pennsylvania Press.

Ikegami N: Public long term care insurance in Japan, *JAMA* 278(16):1310-1314, 1997.

Japan Ministry of Health and Welfare: *Statistical abstract on health and welfare in*

Japan 2000, Tokyo, 2000, Statistics and Information Department Minister's Secretariat Ministry of Health and Welfare.

Kagawa-Singer M: Ethnic perspectives of cancer nursing: Hispanics and Japanese-Americans, *Cancer Nurs Perspect* 14(3):59, 1987.

Kawabuchi K: Diversified needs and aging. In *Introduction to health care economics in Japan,* pp 19-34, Tokyo, 1998, Yakuji Nippo.

Kayama M, Zerwekh J, Thornton KA, Murashima S: Japanese expert public health nurses empower clients with schizophrenia living in the community, *J Psychosoc Nurs* 39(2):40-45, 2001.

Kobayashi M: Promoting breast-feeding: a successful regional project in Japan, *Acta Paediatr Jpn* 31(4):404, 1989.

Kolanowski RJ: Japan's gold plan emphasizes home care and the consumer, *Caring Magazine* 16(4):38-40, 1997.

Minami H: Support workers in Japan. *Int Nurs Rev* 38(6):176, 184, 1991.

Murashima S et al: Around-the-clock nursing care for the elderly in Japan, *IMAGE: J Nurs Schol* 30(1):37-41, 1998.

Murashima S et al: The meaning of public health nursing: creating 24-hour care in a community in Japan, *Nurs Health Sci* 1:83-72, 1999.

Okamoto Y: Health care for the elderly in Japan: medicine and welfare in an aging society facing a crisis in long term care, *BMJ* 305:403–405, 1992.

Shand N: Culture's influence in Japanese and American maternal role perception and confidence, *Psychiatry* 48(1):52, 1995

Tashiro J et al: Long-term care for the elderly in Japan, *IMAGE: J Nurs Schol* 31(2):133–134, 1999.

Trommsdorff G: Value change in Japan, *Int J Intercult Relations* 7:337, 1983.

Yoshikawa A, Utsonomiya O: Japan's health insurance system: from cradle to grave. In Okimoto DI, Yoshikawa A, eds: *Japan's health system: efficiency and effectiveness in universal care,* pp 21–44, New York, 1993, Faulker & Gray.

◆ JORDAN (HASHEMITE KINGDOM OF)

MAP PAGE (864)

Ismat Fayez Mikkey

Location: Formerly known as the Amirate of Transjordan (East Bank), the Kingdom of Jordan is located in the Middle East and is bordered on the west by Israel and the Dead Sea, on the north by Syria, on the east by Iraq, and on the south by Saudi Arabia. It is now known as the Hashemite Kingdom of Jordan, with a total land area of 91,880 km^2 (35,465 square miles), most of which is arid desert. In 2000 the population of Jordan was estimated to be 5.04 million; 43% of the population is younger than 14 years and only 2.6% is older than 65. Three fourths of the population lives in three major cities: Amman, Zarq'a, and Irbid.

Major Languages	Ethnic Groups	Major Religions
Arabic (official)	Arab 98%	Sunni Muslim 93%
English	Circassian 1%	Christian 5%
	Armenian 1%	Other 2%

Non-Arab minorities (e.g., Circassians, Armenians) also speak Arabic, and English is widely understood among middle and upper classes. Jordanians distinguish between Tranjordaninas (citizens of the Amirate of Transjordan which existed from 1921 to 1948) and Palestinians (citizens of the British-mandated territory of Palestine, which existed from 1922 to 1948, who comprise 55% to 60% of the population). Non-Arab ethnic groups include Circassians, Shishans, Armenians, and Kurds. In addition to Sunni Muslims, about 2000 Shia also live in Jordan, and other small religious groups such as Druze and B'hai exist.

Health Care Beliefs: Fatalistic; traditional. The use of nontherapeutic drugs such as heroin or marijuana is strictly forbidden. People smoke cigarettes despite strong prohibitions by many Islamic scholars. It is the most predominant unhealthy behavior (50%) among male Jordanians; Jordanians often offer cigarettes to guests as a form of hospitality. Few women (10%) smoke because the habit is less socially acceptable for them. Water-pipe smoking has become a widely practiced habit, and almost every home has at least one pipe. Special coffee shops have even been opened for water-pipe smoking. Because religion permeates all aspects of life, Arabs face adversities and terminal illnesses with faith in God's (Allah's) mercy and compassion. This practice leads to a more fatalistic than activist approach to illness and greater dependence on the family during illness than is common in many Western societies. Psychiatric disorders are the major source of stigma in Arab countries, and they are often attributed to the "evil eye" (i.e., the power of a person to harm others merely by looking at them), evil spirits, and sorcery. Psychiatric services are often delayed while traditional and religious modalities that are less stigmatizing are sought. Another general reason people consult traditional therapists is because of consistency between people's beliefs and the healers' cultural explanations of disease.

Predominant Sick Care Practices: Biomedical and magical-religious. The number and distribution of health care facilities has increased in rural areas since the adoption of the primary care concept—recognizing that the expense and inconvenience of travel hinders rural people from seeking advanced medical care and attention. In major cities, modern medicine is the primary choice, and alternative healing is usually thought of as a last resort when other treatments fail. Institutions with advanced medical equipment are located in major cities such as Amman, Irbid, Ramtha, Az Zarqa, and As Salt. The majority of tribal citizens living in rural areas and the desert consult indigenous healers and wear amulets as an adjunct to modern medical care. Traditional healers such as those who use the Koran for healing also may be consulted. For example, people with fertility problems seek the advice of a doctor as well as a religious person *(shykh)* to obtain amulets. Traditional infertility treatments include "closing the back." A woman healer rubs the woman's pelvis with olive oil and places suction cups on her back. Also used are abdominal and external ovarian massage and herbal vaginal suppositories. Traditional health practices are the domain of women who are known in their communities to possess skills in treating certain injuries and disorders. The most prevalent practice is massaging children with warm olive oil. Within the family, women assume responsibility for nutrition and treatment of illness. Beliefs in the efficacy of traditional healing practices occasionally prevent or postpone appropriate medical attention.

Ethnic/Race Specific or Endemic Diseases: Jordanians have water shortages and inadequate sanitation, which contributes to many health problems. However, as conditions have improved, the incidence of diseases related to these issues has significantly decreased. Meningitis, scarlet fever, typhoid, and paratyphoid have notably decreased, although some increases in infectious hepatitis, rubella, mumps, measles, and schistosomiasis have been noted. Thalassemia is a prevalent disease because of the high rate of intermarriages within families (50% of all marriages). Cardiovascular diseases and cancer are increasing and associated with changes in diet and lifestyle. Being overweight is a serious health problem in Jordan and is especially prevalent among women, possibly because of lifestyle issues and fewer overall activities outside of the home that provide more exercise. In 2000 the average life expectancy was 69.8 years. The World Health Organization's (WHO) estimated prevalence rate for HIV/AIDS in adults ages 15 to 49 years is 0.02%. WHO has no estimates for children from birth to 15 years.

Health Team Relationships: Doctors dominate the health care environment, so nurses' knowledge and expertise are often discounted. Nurse-doctor interactions are very limited and occur during rounds (in the morning and evening) or when a nurse is calling a doctor to assess patients' needs. Because nurses are not recognized as knowledgeable professionals, patients do not seek information from them. Doctors' representation on national committees and councils of nursing practice continues to be the norm in some nursing programs.

Families' Role in Hospital Care: Family and kinship are the main sources of social support in areas where relatives live close to each other. Children are socialized to be obedient and loyal to their families, and individual interests are secondary. Families assume many roles when a member is ill: patient advocates, counselors, or long-term care providers if necessary. At the time of hospital admission, close relatives accompany the patient for support and to answer questions for the patient. Most people are suspicious about the quality of food served in government hospitals, so relatives often prepare foods such as meat, vegetables, and rice. Nurses rely on family members to provide basic care for their relatives and for assistance with bathing, eating, walking, and changing clothes. Visitors bring food, chocolate, biscuits, or fruit. Close relatives who stay most of the day show their hospitality by serving visitors coffee, candy, or fruit. Visitors tend not to comply with visiting hours, and special security personnel control the influx of visitors, who can interfere with routine or emergency care.

Dominance Patterns: Jordan is a male-dominated society in which greater value is placed on boys because they perpetuate the family name and maintain economic security for their aging parents (although Islamic teachings promote gender equity). The father is the head of the family and its breadwinner, whereas the mother raises the children and takes care of the house. However, many educated women occupy positions in health, educational, and other institutions, so taking care of the children becomes the responsibility of grandmothers. A mid-1980s study documented that boys received more immunizations and were taken to see doctors more frequently at earlier stage of illness than girls, contributing to higher infant mortality for girls. However, boys and girls are equally likely to receive adequate care today. The poor health status of some Arab women is attributed to marriage at a young age, repeated childbirths, limited access to health care, ignorance, and poverty. Their poor health manifests as work-related fatigue, anemia, malnutrition, and numerous chronic conditions. Men's reluctance to participate in household or child care tasks is attributed to the societal ideology that these are purely women's responsibilities. The adult literacy rate for females is 81.2% and 92.5% for males. Young educated women sometimes encounter difficulties accessing modern health care when they reside in extended family households. Older women usually are entitled to more authority and given a greater voice than the mother in making decisions related to child health care, nutrition, and health expenditures.

Eye Contact Practices: It is considered impolite and unacceptable for women to make direct eye contact with men or children to make direct eye contact with parents, grandparents, or other older adults. People from the Middle East who are of the same gender are likely to stand quite close to each other, but men and women maintain a greater distance.

Touch Practices: Jordanians behave conservatively in public. They communicate modestly, and displays of affection are highly private. Displays of affectionate feelings between spouses (such as kissing or hugging) do not occur in public areas and are considered inappropriate social behavior. It is unacceptable for men and women to shake hands with strangers (i.e., people who are not close relatives) of the opposite sex. It is preferable for patients to be treated by health professionals of the same sex. Islam prohibits male-female touching except in an emergency or when no competent health professional of the same sex is available.

Perceptions of Time: Schedules, deadlines, and punctuality are cornerstones of Arab life. Arabs often begin their meetings with chatting and social activities. Showing hospitality by serving tea or coffee and inquiring about people's health and families precedes attending to business at hand. Arabs are more tuned to the past and present than the future. Although they do think ahead and have plans for the future, financial and economic constraints are major barriers to focusing on the future.

Pain Reactions: Jordanian patients tend to attribute wellness and illness to God's will, therefore they tend to use prayers and other religious practices as ways of coping. They face adversities with patience and endurance because they believe that they are God's purpose, and their suffering will be remembered in the afterlife. Jordanians may believe that they ought to please their health care providers so that they can be labeled "good" patients—in other words, patients who do not complain. Men in particular avoid overt displays of emotions because they are considered weak, and enduring pain is regarded as masculine. This behavior is rooted in the socialization process of Arab boys and girls. Sons are usually taught to be strong and protect their sisters, whereas daughters are taught to be sources of love and emotional support. It is more acceptable for females than males to request pain medication.

Birth Rites: When a woman gives birth to a new infant, relatives, friends, and neighbors congratulate her and bring her gifts. Most families believe that a mother should stay home for 40 days after birth, during which time she is cared for by her mother and sisters and occasionally by her husband's family. Circumcision is the norm for boys and is often performed during the first week after birth but occasionally occurs years later. At the time of birth, some traditional Jordanians rub the infant's gums with chewed dates and use *kohl*, a charcoal-like powder, to dilate the pupil of the infant's eye. Swaddling the infant with a blanket and rope is still common and believed to strengthen the infant's muscles, prevent deformities such as scoliosis, and control movements of the hands that might scare the infant during the night. Infants sleep in cribs close to the mother. During the postpartum period the mother is not allowed to perform religious rituals (i.e., recite prayers, fast during Ramadan) or have sexual intercourse until all postpartum discharge is gone. She is encouraged to consume special drinks such as boiled cinnamon sticks and boiled fenugreek *(hilbah)* seeds, which are believed to accelerate discharge and increase milk production. In some families, it is customary to shave the infant's head, estimate the weight of the hair, calculate the price of an equivalent weight of gold or silver, and give this amount as charity. Parents frequently slaughter a goat or lamb and invite relatives and friends to eat as a show of gratitude to God and so that all can welcome the infant. The total fertility rate is 3.6 children per woman. This high fertility rate is attributed to the value parents place on children as a source of security in old age. Religious beliefs have a strong influence on Jordanian women's contraceptive behavior. Islam approves of family planning for child spacing but not to limit the size of the family, thus sterilization is strictly prohibited for men and women. Many Jordanians have the misconception that oral contraceptives cause cancer, weight gain, and headaches.

Death Rites: For patients with brain death whose body organs or systems are being artificially maintained, it is acceptable to discontinue artificial prolongation of life or to take organs for transplantation for a patient who is in jeopardy. Thus saving a life outweighs preserving the integrity of a body because injuring the donor body is considered less evil than allowing a patient to die. Autopsies are permissible if conducted for the right purpose, such as determining the cause of death in cases of suspected foul play or for educational purposes. Most people are reluctant to have autopsies performed on deceased loved ones because it is more common to bury the dead without delay. The body is washed, wrapped in white cloth (but not placed in a coffin), taken to the mosque for prayer, and then taken to the cemetery for burial. Relatives accept condolences for 3 days. If death occurs overseas, it is preferable to bring the body home. Cremation is forbidden.

Food Practices and Intolerances: Food consumption patterns among Jordanians have changed during the last 30 years as the consumption of sugar, fat and oil, meat, and poultry have greatly increased. Pork and alcohol are strictly prohibited. In Jordan, thyme and olive oil are an integral part of breakfast. *Shawarma* (gyro) made with lamb or turkey is a very popular fast food and served in almost all restaurants. Gyro is served as strips of meat in an Arabian loaf of bread with different salads and dressings. *Kunafa,* a two-layer dish of finely or coarsely shredded dough stuffed with sweet white (whole-milk) cheese is the most popular type of dessert. Once out of the oven, the sweet syrup is trickled on the top of the hot tray. The stuffed *maamoul* is also very popular and made of mixed flour and semolina (cream of wheat) stuffed with dates or nuts. People like to prepare large amounts of *maamoul* to celebrate the two major feasts for Muslims: the Al-Fiter Eid feast (the morning of the next-to-last day of the Ramadan fasting month) and the Al-Adha Eid feast (on the tenth day of the pilgrimage month in which people travel to Mecca). Muslims fast during the month of Ramadan, abstaining from food, drink, and sexual intercourse between sunrise and sunset. Fasting is not mandatory for patients or older adults for whom it could have negative consequences. Jordan's national dish is *mansaf,* a whole stewed lamb cooked in a yogurt sauce and served on a bed of rice. *Maglouba* is a meat, fish, or vegetable stew served with rice and fried vegetables (sunflower, eggplant, or both) on the bottom, and *musakhan* is chicken that is cooked with onions, olive oil, and pine nuts and baked on a thick loaf of Arabic bread. Also popular is Middle Eastern *sheish kebabs,* skewered pieces of marinated lamb or chicken, tomatoes, and onions that are cooked over a charcoal fire. Nutritional deficiencies are not uncommon, particularly in rural areas. Most foods are eaten with spoon and fork.

Infant Feeding Practices: Breast-feeding is preferred. In urban areas, people are more flexible about bottle-feeding because of the increasing number of women who work and must leave their infants with a close relative all day. In rural areas, mothers breast-feed their infants according to traditional beliefs and because of advice about its benefits. Infants begin eating solid foods at about 9 months. Anemia is common among young children in Arab countries and is attributed to mothers' practice of offering children bread soaked in tea in the morning.

Child Rearing Practices: Children may sleep in their parents' room until they are 3 to 4 years, then all young children may sleep in one room. Mothers take on more responsibility for discipline, and children perceive fathers as more strict. Older adults live in their older son's (or daughter's if they have no sons) home with respect and dignity and may assume some responsibility for disciplining children even when it interferes with the mother's role. Deviant behaviors by one family member affect the reputation and honor of the entire family.

National Childhood Immunizations: DTP at 2, 3, 4, and 18 months; OPV at 2, 3, 4, 10, and 18 months and 6 years; hep B at 2, 3, and 4 months; measles at 10 and 18 to 24 months; DT at 2, 3, 4, and 18 months; Td at 6 and 15 years; and TT after first contact, +1, +6 months, 1 to 3 years, and 1 to 5 years later.

BIBLIOGRAPHY

Al-Hassan M, Alkhalil M, Ma'aitah R: Jordanian nurses' roles in the management of postoperative pain in the postanesthesia care unit, *J Perianesth Nurs* 14(6):384-389, 1999.

Abu Gharbieh P, Suliman W: Changing the image of nursing in Jordan through effective role negotiation, *Int Nurs Rev* 39(5):149-152, 1992.

http:www.dist.maricopa.edu/eddev/intledev/exer5&6.html

http://islamicity.com/science/organ.shtml (viewed Sep. 18, 2001).

http://lcweb2.loc.gov/cgi-bin/query/r?frd/cstudy:@field (DOCID+jo0004-56)

http://www.ourdialogue.com/p17.htm

http://www.traderscity.com/abcg/culture1.htm

◆ KAZAKHSTAN (REPUBLIC OF)

MAP PAGE (861)

Robert O'Donovan and Manana Sopromadze

Location: The Republic of Kazakhstan, part of the former Soviet Union, is in Central Asia with Russia to the north, China to the east, and the Caspian Sea to the west. Kazakhstan is the second largest country in the Commonwealth of Independent States and is the ninth largest country in the world with a total land area of 1,049,151 square miles (2,717,300 km^2). Vast, often deserted steppes and dramatic mountain peaks dominate the country's topography. Horses and sheep are common pastoral animals.

Major Languages	Ethnic Groups	Major Religions
Kazakh (Qazaq, official)	Kazakh (Qazaq) 48%	Muslim 47%
Russian (official)	Russian 35%	Russian Orthodox 44%
	Ukrainian 4.9%	Protestant 2%
	Uzbek 2%	Other 7%
	Tatar 2%	
	German 1%	
	Other 7%	

Kazakhs are a majority of the population because of their higher birth rates and emigration of other groups such as the Germans. Kazakh is spoken by more than 40% of the population of Kazakhstan, and two thirds speak Russian, the language used in everyday business.

Health Care Beliefs: Acute sick care; traditional. Common colds, especially among children and older adults, are generally believed to be caused by exposure to drafts, so infants and very small children are often swaddled in many layers. Upset stomachs and headaches, even those not associated with drinking in excess, are occasionally treated with a shot of vodka. Fevers may be treated by rubbing vodka on the forehead and neck. Drinking cold beverages or drinks with ice is thought to cause sore throats. Girls and women are actively discouraged from sitting directly on cement or stone because they believe that their reproductive systems will be damaged by the cold radiating out of the material. Nearly all Kazakh newborns either wear an amulet or have one hanging near their crib. The amulet may be a sheep's vertebra wrapped in cloth and tied with a ribbon, an amulet that signifies the hope the child will have a strong neck throughout its life. Abortions are relatively common in Kazakhstan as they are throughout much of the former Soviet Union. Many women have had more than two abortions. The topic of abortion is not openly discussed, but it is well known that it is a woman's right to choose to have an abortion.

Predominant Sick Care Practices: Biomedical when available and magical-religious. Political upheaval has created economic difficulties that have affected the health care system. The old Soviet health system emphasized specialist hospitalizations with long stays and unnecessary admissions. Care that would normally be considered out-patient treatment often occurred in a hospital. Western medical treatment continues to be regularly sought out in hospitals and polyclinics. Informal, surreptitious monetary and nonmonetary payments are the norm and are a significant portion of the income generated by medical staff. Costs of medications may be considerable. People recognize that the health care system in Kazakhstan needs to be restructured into a system of primary care that will better serve the health needs of the population. A movement toward a model based on medical insurance is developing.

Ethnic/Race Specific or Endemic Diseases: The country and its water supplies are contaminated in the region around Semey (formerly Semipalatinsk) in northeast Kazakhstan, where repeated above-ground nuclear tests took place during the 1950s and 1960s. Recent studies have reported a noticeable increase in the number of cases of Hashimoto's thyroiditis and thyroid cancer. The area around the Aral Sea is contaminated and because the Aral is shrinking, sediments heavily contaminated with fertilizers are exposed to the prevailing winds, subsequently exposing people to the dust, which is laden with toxic chemicals and heavy metals. The contamination has also translated into high levels of organochlorine pesticides in breast milk, posing a risk to newborns. Nutritional surveys of children younger than 3 years have reported significant undernutrition among Kazaks, children in southern and central regions, and rural children. The country has occasional outbreaks of cholera in the larger cities, particularly Almaty. The incidence of congenital abnormalities and cancers is 30% to 50% higher than it is in Western countries. The World Health Organization's (WHO) estimated prevalence rate for HIV/AIDS in adults ages 15 to 49 is 0.04%. The estimated number of children from birth to 15 years living with HIV/AIDS is less than 100. Studies in the region indicate dramatic increases in the number of HIV infection among users of injected (nonmedical) drugs.

Health Team Relationships: Nurses are generally in a subordinate role to doctors in hospitals and are expected to take care of health maintenance tasks such as giving injections and changing surgical dressings. During the Soviet period, nurses provided home care for women who had recently given birth or individuals who had undergone serious surgeries. These services were provided as part of the health care system, and only nominal fees were charged. Although it is possible to access a similar level of care in Almaty and other large cities despite the disarray of the health care system, such services are unaffordable for most people. Nurses are educated in 3-year programs in technical colleges.

Families' Role in Hospital Care: Families are responsible for preparing food for and cleaning their hospitalized family members and their bedpans. Because the health insurance industry is still in its infancy in Kazakhstan, families are required to cover the full cost of medications, especially families in rural regions. At least one family member is always in a patient's room unless the patient is in the hospital to give birth. Women about to give birth are largely isolated from their families and visited by one, usually female, relative at a time. Hospital rooms are generally shared by at least two and occasionally as many as ten other patients.

Dominance Patterns: The youngest woman in Kazakh families has the lowest position in the family and is responsible for serving tea, preparing meals, and waiting on the patriarch of the family, other family members, and guests.

Eye Contact Practices: It is customary for men to make eye contact with everyone except people they want to avoid such as beggars on the street. Girls and young women often do not make eye contact with strange men. Kazakh men often shake hands, hug, and kiss each other on the cheek during greetings, whereas Russian men tend to just shake hands. These greeting patterns apply to friends and strangers, but the greeting and physical contact is warmer with friends. Both Kazakh and Russian women tend to greet friends with a hug but do not make physical contact when greeting women they do not know well.

Perceptions of Time: Punctuality is not particularly valued in Kazakhstan. Much more emphasis is placed on maintaining relationships. If a person is late for an appointment with a health care professional, little if anything is lost.

Birth Rites: Kazakhstani women prefer to give birth in a hospital. The delivery procedures are typical of those of Western nations, with the woman lying down with her legs elevated on leg rests. The pain of delivery is not usually eased with local anesthesia. No family members are allowed into the maternity ward, and newborns are separated from their mothers except during three or four daily feedings. Women and their infants remain in the hospital for 5 to 7 days, barring any unusual circumstances.

Death Rites: Most people die at home regardless of their ethnic background. Kazakhs do not embalm the body of the dead. The body is cleaned and then wrapped tightly in white cotton cloths; members of the family often perform these duties. An *imam* (Muslim clergyman) is summoned to the home, and he conducts a series of prayers with the men, often outside the home. A group of mourners then gathers loosely outside of the main entrance to the home, and the body is carried out. The mourners, especially the women, wail loudly and cry profusely. Women who do not wail loudly or with sufficient sincerity may be criticized after the funeral for being unfeeling. The body is often placed in an uncovered coffin or wrapped in a rug so that it can be more easily transported by hearse to the cemetery. Only men follow the body to the cemetery. A special burial arrangement is made at the cemetery—a 2-m deep grave is dug, and a small burial chamber is created off the bottom of the grave. The wrapped body is carefully lowered into the small burial chamber, and the men take turns filling in the grave. A short dinner follows the men's return to the deceased person's home. Another memorial meal is held 40 days and then 1 year after the death.

Food Practices and Intolerances: Most people eat three times a day and have the largest meal in the evening. The staple of the Kazakh diet is mutton. Various vegetables and fruits are available seasonally, including tomatoes, cucumbers, onions, potatoes, watermelons, and cantaloupes.

Infant Feeding Practices: Breast-feeding is typical. Most women recognize that it is healthy for an infant to receive its mother's milk. However, breast-feeding is not done in public. If breast-feeding is impossible for medical reasons or if a woman chooses not to breast-feed, formula is available.

Child Rearing Practices: As Muslims, ethnic Kazakhs circumcise their male children; however, Russians and other Slavic people often do not.

National Childhood Immunizations: BCG at birth and at 4, 6 to 7, and 11 to 12 years; DTP at 2, 3, 4, and 18 months; OPV at birth and 2, 3, and 4 months; hep B at birth and at 2 and 4 months; measles at 12 months and 6 to 7 years; and mumps at 12 months and at 6 to 7 and 12 years.

BIBLIOGRAPHY

Britt TW, Adler AB: Stress and health during medical humanitarian assistance missions, *Mil Med* 164(4):275, 1999.

Dehne KL et al: The HIV/AIDS epidemic in Eastern Europe: recent patterns and trends and their implications for policy making, *AIDS(London)* 13(7):741, 1999.

Ensor R, Savalyeva L: Informal payments for health care in the former Soviet Union: some evidence from Kazakstan, *Health Pol Plan* 13(1):41, 1998.

Ensor R, Thompson R: Rationalizing rural hospital services in Kazakstan, *Int J Health Plan Mngmnt* 14(2):155, 1999.

Hooper K et al: Analysis of breast milk to assess exposure to chlorinated contaminants in Kazakstan: high levels of 2,3,7,8-tetrachlorodibenzo-p-dioxin (TCDD) in agricultural villages of southern Kazakstan, *Env Health Perspect* 106(12):797, 1998.

Sawyer D: Tucson nurses making a difference in Kazakhstan, *Ariz Nurse* 48(4):5, 1995.

Sharmanov T-Sh et al: Nutritional status of early age children in Kazakhstan, *Voprosy Pitaniia* 4:23, 1997.

Zhumadilov Z et al: Thyroid abnormality trend over time in northeastern regions of Kazakhstan, adjacent to the Semipalatinsk nuclear test site: a case review of pathological findings for 7271 patients, *J Rad Res* 41(1):35, 2000.

◆ KENYA (REPUBLIC OF)

MAP PAGE (863)

Sam Kariuki

Location: Kenya is located on the equator on the East Coast of Africa and borders part of Somalia and the Indian Ocean to the east, Uganda and Lake Victoria to the west, Ethiopia to the north, and Tanzania to the south. Kenya is largely arid and semiarid in the north, whereas the Great Rift Valley and Highlands to the east are the major farming regions. The total land area is 582,650 km^2 (224,962 square miles). The Great Rift Valley, which extends north to south, is flanked by high mountain ranges and contains important fresh water lakes including Lakes Turkana, Baringo, Bogoria, Nakuru, and Naivasha.

Major Languages	Ethnic Groups	Major Religions
English	Kikuyu 22%	Protestant 38%
Swahili	Luhya 14%	Catholic 28%
Other	Luo 13%	Indigenous beliefs 26%
	Kalenjin 12%	Muslim 8%
	Kamba 11%	
	Other 28%	

English is the official language in all government and private business transactions, but Swahili is the national language. In the workplace and most service occupations, individuals communicate in Swahili or English. Kenya has about 42 other languages corresponding to each of the 42 ethnic groups.

Health Care Beliefs: Traditional; health promotion important. The Ministry of Health has put great emphasis on preventive health care, therefore much education involves use of the mass media. Mental illness is misunderstood and greatly feared among all the ethnic groups of Kenya. They have a general belief that mental illness is brought about by demon possession, possibly as a result of an angry ancestral spirit that must be appeased. Most ethnic groups believe that witch doctors have the ability to remove these spirits, so they pay the doctors a fee in cash and live-stock. Because more of the population is attaining some formal basic education, the attitude toward mental illness is gradually changing, especially in urban populations. Groups such as the Turkana, Kisii, and Luo perform scarification, using hot metal rods to draw out illness by draining "bad blood" from the sick person. Induced vomiting is used to remove disease from the gastrointestinal tract and was common among the Kikuyu, although the practice is slowly dying out.

Predominant Sick Care Practices: Traditional, magical-religious, and biomedical when available. Currently, about 70% of Kenyans in rural areas seek medical attention from traditional healers. Traditional medicine is also being promoted by the government so that it can be legally considered a complement to official government health services. Among people in rural areas, it is common to see amulets worn by most of Kenya's 42 ethnic groups, particularly by children. It is generally believed amulets ward off evil spirits that cause illness. Prayer is common for Christians (who comprise 80% of the population, and Muslims (17%). Sunday is revered as a Christian day of prayer and church attendance is heavy; therefore most businesses are closed. Main prayers for Muslims occur on Friday.

Ethnic/Race Specific or Endemic Diseases: Certain epidemic disease outbreaks are associated with geographical location, lifestyle choices, and preference for particular foods. For example, cholera is endemic along the Lake Victoria region, which has perennial flooding. Kenya has had numerous recent outbreaks of typhoid fever in urban centers, which are thought to be a result of a poor and an inadequate health infrastructure, resulting from the rapid increase in population and overcrowding as people flock to cities to seek employment. Malaria is the most predominant disease and is common along the coast and lake region, where the hot and humid climate favors mosquito breeding and transmission of the disease. Acute respiratory tract infections, intestinal parasitic infestations, and diarrheal diseases (in decreasing order of importance) are the other major diseases. More recently, HIV and AIDS and their associated opportunistic infections have become a major problem, and in some public hospitals almost half of the beds are occupied by patients with HIV/AIDS. Rates of HIV/AIDS vary from one region of the country to another. The World Health Organization's (WHO) estimated prevalence rate for HIV/AIDS in adults ages 15 to 49 is 13.95%. The estimated number of children from birth to 15 years living with HIV/AIDS is 78,000. Adult prevalence varies from region to region, from 18% in major urban centers to 4% to 6% in most rural areas.

Health Team Working Relationships: Working relationships in the health care sector depend primarily on the setting. In the main public hospitals, care is doctor driven. In the dispensaries that provide primary health care, nurses and paramedics are the main players. In all health care settings the doctor-nurse relationship is fairly well defined in terms of roles and responsibilities. Patients highly regard health care workers and usually take advice promptly and without question.

Families' Role in Hospital Care: Families are usually encouraged to visit patients, and most would visit without being prompted. It is traditionally believed in Kenya that family members are responsible for caring for their sick. Most hospitals offer food, but family members still bring food to patients, especially fruit and drinks. No family members stay overnight with the patients in the hospital unless the patients are children. However, this is unnecessary in high-cost private children's hospitals because they have more nurses and attendants. In rural settings that are served mainly by sub-district hospitals, relatives may take food and other necessities to the patient as a matter of routine.

Dominance Patterns: The culture is male dominated in all tribes in Kenya. During times of illness the mother takes on the major role as caregiver for the children. Mothers are also responsible for keeping the home clean, obtaining water and wood for fuel, preparing food, and feeding the children. Girls in the home may also help with these chores when they return from school. Although issues of discipline are generally the responsibility of the father, the mother may discipline the children when the father is away.

Eye Contact: Eye contact is generally unacceptable except between people of the same gender. For example, among the Masai, a girl cannot make eye contact with her father and mother-in-law, whereas among the Teso, the girl cannot make eye contact with her brother-in-law. Avoiding eye contact is considered a sign of respect among people of different age groups and sexes.

Touch Practices: Touch is acceptable. For example, males hold hands as sign of friendship and affection. Adults may also touch children on the forehead as a greeting and to show respect.

Time Perceptions: In urban areas, punctuality is important in the work arena, and people are expected to be on time for appointments. Children are expected to be on time for school. For less important matters, being on time is of little concern. In rural areas, punctuality is not an issue; the traditional belief is that time is unlimited, so people only approximate the time using the sun as a guide. Level of education, as well as tradition, are the major factors that influence people's attitude toward time.

Pain Reactions: In all the ethnic groups, adults generally react to pain stoically. It is rare to see adults express pain because it is a sign of weakness. For example, adult women with severe back pain from excessive manual labor are still expected to carry out household chores as usual. However, children are allowed to express pain freely and are excused from chores and activities if they complain of being in pain.

Birth Rites: After birth the mother is cared for by women friends from the neighborhood, who help with cooking and other household chores for at least a month. In no ethnic group is the mother advised to avoid bathing or certain foods. During the first 3 months after birth, the mother's diet is supplemented with high-protein foods such as traditional soup made from bones, roots from special herbs, black beans, and milk. In most of the ethnic groups, the birth of a son is more celebrated than the birth of a daughter. A son is valued as a recipient of the family's inheritance and an extension of the family. It is argued that because daughters usually get married and leave home, they are not able to receive an inheritance and carry on the family name. If the first-born in a family is a boy, the birth of a second son is not celebrated as much.

Death Rites: Because most Kenyans believe death is a continuation of life and the spirit naturally joins its ancestors in a different world, they have a sense of immortality. However, modern Christian and Muslim teachings are changing traditional attitudes toward death because they teach that doing good deeds on earth is the only way to open the entrance to heaven; all sinners go to eternal hell. Family members may be present at a person's death if a relative becomes ill at home. In most ethnic groups in Kenya, an older adult who is about to die calls all his family members to bless them and reveal their inheritance. Organ donation is not practiced by any of the ethnic groups in Kenya. Autopsy is common and acceptable in hospital settings but is requested only for legal reasons and hence is not the general practice.

Food Practices and Intolerances: Food consumption varies considerably among ethnic groups. People in the country rely heavily on plant proteins supplemented with meat protein, whereas those living around the lake region survive on fish and starches, especially cornmeal, or *ugali*. Those who live in the highlands depend mostly on beans and corn as their staple foods. Most traditional diets are well balanced (e.g., *githeri* [boiled corn and beans], *ugali,* kale, and a protein source). Milk is consumed in different forms: fresh, fermented, or—among Masia—mixed with blood. Most individuals in rural communities use their hands to eat, but they generally wash them before meals. In more recent years, spoons have become common. In restaurants, spoons and other utensils are available.

Infant Feeding Practices: Breast-feeding is acceptable in all communities and religiously promoted and practiced. It is almost taboo for a mother not to breast-feed unless she has medical reasons. However, bottle-feeding with formula is gaining popularity among working mothers, especially those in urban areas.

Child Rearing Practices: Child rearing is generally strict, with instant discipline (e.g., spanking) being the most common method. Young children usually sleep with parents until age 4. It is the role of the women to discipline young children and keep them quiet and obedient, especially when visitors are in the home. Female circumcision and excision is common in some groups; however, the government and several lobbying groups in the country have recently launched a major educational campaign to discourage Kenyans from practicing female genital mutilation, and the effort seems to be working.

National Childhood Immunizations: BCG at birth; DPT at 6, 10, and 14 weeks; OPV at birth and 6, 10, and 14 weeks; measles at 9 months; and TT for pregnant women ×2 and for the next pregnancy. Numerous rural people do not understand the preventive nature of immunizations, but the government has been aggressively promoting immunization through health care education in hospitals and the mass media.

BIBLIOGRAPHY

Cronk L: Parental favoritism toward daughters, *Am Scientist* 81:272, 1993.
Dean NR: A community study of child spacing, fertility and contraception in West Pokot district, Kenya, *Soc Sci Med* 38(11):1575, 1994.
Fonck M et al: Healthcare-seeking behavior and sexual behavior of patients with sexually transmitted diseases in Nairobi, Kenya, *Sex Transm Dis* 28(7):367, 2001.
Haaland A, Vlassoff C: Introducing health care workers for change: from transformation theory to health systems in developing countries, *Health Policy Plann* 16(suppl 1):1, 2001.

Kaler A, Watkins SC: Disobedient distributors: street level bureaucrats and would-be patrons in community-based family planning programs in rural Kenya, *Stud Fam Plann* 32(3):254, 2001.

Littlewood R: Psychotherapy in cultural contexts, *Psychiatr Clin North Am* 24(3):507, 2001.

Macintyre K, Brown L, Sosler S: "It's not what you know, but who you knew": examining the relationship between behavioral change and AIDS mortality in Africa, *AIDS Educ Prev* 13(2):160, 2001.

Mpoke S, Johnson KE: Baseline survey of pregnancy practices among Kenyan Massai, *West J Nurs Res* 15(3):298, 1993.

Nyambedha EO, Wandibba S, Aagaard-Hansen J: Policy implications of the inadequate support systems for orphans in western Kenya, *Health Policy* 58(1):83, 2001.

Wright J: Female genital mutilation: an overview, *J Adv Nurs* 24:251, 1996.

www.unaids.org/hivaidsinfo/statistics/june00/fact_sheets/index.html

www.who.int/vaccines/

◆ KIRIBATI (REPUBLIC OF)

MAP PAGE (856)

Location: Kiribati, formerly the Gilbert Islands, is an archipelago of approximately 30 low-lying coral *atolls* (ring-shaped islands with central lagoons) surrounded by extensive reefs. It is part of the division of Pacific Islands known as Micronesia. Kiribati includes sixteen Gilbert Islands, eight Phoenix Islands, eight Line Islands, and Banaba. Located in the mid-Pacific, it is the largest atoll state in the world. Most islands are low lying with erratic rainfall. Kiribati's nearest neighbors are Nauru to the west and Tuvalu and Tokelau to the south. The total land area is 811 km² (313 square miles), about four times the size of Washington, DC. The low levels of some of the islands make them very sensitive to changes in sea level. Kiribati was declared a "least developed country" by the United Nations. The gross domestic product (GDP) per capita is $850, one of the lowest in the Pacific.

Major Languages	Ethnic Groups	Major Religions
English (official)	Micronesian 99%	Roman Catholic 53%
Gilbertese	Other 1%	Protestant (mostly Congregational) 41%
		Other 6%

Predominant Sick Care Practices: Acute sick care; traditional, and some biomedical. Kirbati has a system of public health in place with dispensaries employing doctors, nurses, and village health workers. The distance to dispensaries creates access problems. Health facilities are not on par with American health standards.

Ethnic/Race Specific or Endemic Diseases: People are at risk for dengue fever and leprosy. Hepatitis C is endemic, and about 55% of the population has the antibody for the hepatitis C virus. Hepatitis B is also endemic, and 69% to 81% of individuals infected with hepatitis B also have antibodies to the hepatitis delta virus. Kiribati has a strong hepatitis B immunization program in place that focuses on infants. Vitamin A deficiency is a public health problem, resulting in xerophthalmia in about 15% of the population. Prevalence of coronary heart disease is increasing. High levels of impaired glucose tolerance are found in urban male Micronesians in Kiribati (28%). Public transportation and road conditions are not safe, increasing risk for automobile accidents. The World Health Organization's (WHO) has no estimated prevalence rates for HIV/AIDS for adults or children on Kiribati.

Dominance Patterns: In this egalitarian society, boasting or considering oneself to be better than another is unacceptable.

Perceptions of Time: Life moves at a slow, deliberate pace.

Birth Rites: The total fertility rate is 4.36 children born per woman. The infant mortality rate is 88 per 1000 live births. Life expectancy at birth is 60.2 years: 57.25 for men and 63.22 for women. Women make up 33% of those who are formally employed in the workforce. Social life is centered primarily on the churches.

Food Practices and Intolerances: Kiribati has no arable land. The sandy soil limits vegetation, so the islands are insufficient for food production and the people rely heavily on imported foods. However, marine life thrives around the islands, and an abundance of fish is consumed. Access to safe water and sanitation is good in urban areas, where about a third of the population resides. Breadfruit boiled or fried in butter is a staple.

National Childhood Immunizations: BCG at birth; DPT at 6, 10, and 14 weeks; OPV at birth and at 6 and 14 weeks; measles at 9 months; vitamin A at 6 to 12 months and 1 to 6 years; and TT for pregnant women. The reported percentages of target population vaccinated are as follows: BCG, 80; first dose of DTP, 95; third dose of DTP, 90; hep B, 90; MCV, 80; Pol3, 90; and TT2 plus, 50.

Other Characteristics: People are friendly and inquisitive about others and may seem somewhat bold. Most live with extended families, especially in the rural areas, where two thirds of the population live. People tend to be involved primarily in subsistence activities and live in traditional houses of wood and coconut leaves. In southern Tarawa, more Western influences predominate; families are smaller, and people have more modern housing facilities.

BIBLIOGRAPHY

Daulako EC: Population screening and mass chemoprophylaxis in Kiribati, *Int J Leprosy Mycobact Dis* 67(4): S23, 1999.

King H, Rewers M: Global estimates for prevalence of diabetes mellitus and impaired glucose tolerance in adults, *Diabetes Care* 16(1):157, 1993.

Schaumberg DA, O'Connor J, Semba RD: Risk factors for xerophthalmia in the Republic of Kiribati, *Eur J Clin Nutr* 50(11):761, 1996.

Schaumberg DA et al: Vitamin A deficiency in the South Pacific, *Public Health* 109(5):311, 1995.

Tibbs CJ: Delta hepatitis in Kiribati: a Pacific focus, *J Med Virol* 29(2):130, 1989.

http://www.odci.gov/ciapublications/factbook/geos/kr.html

http://travel.state.gov/Kiribati.html

◆ KOREA, NORTH (DEMOCRATIC PEOPLE'S REPUBLIC OF KOREA)

MAP PAGE (865)

Sung Ok Chang

Location: The Democratic Republic of Korea occupies the northern part of the 966-km (600-mile) Korean peninsula off of eastern Asia and is bordered by China, South Korea, and Russia. The total land area is 120,540 km^2 (46,541 square miles). North Koreans call the country *Choson*. Most of the Democratic Republic of Korea is covered with hills, mountains stretching from north to south, with narrow valleys and small plains between them.

Major Languages	Ethnic Groups	Major Religions
Korean	Korean 99%	Atheist, unaffiliated 95%
	Other 1%	Buddhism, Confucianism, syncretic Chondogyo 5%

Chondogyo, a synthesis of Confucian, Buddhist, shamanistic, Daoist, and Catholic influences, is considered one of the new religions. Very few people practice any form of religion.

Health Care Beliefs: Biomedical; holistic; traditional. Acupuncture, acupressure, herbal medicines, and cupping are common therapies. Western and traditional treatments, as well as Eastern and Western medicines may be used at the same time. The cause of an illness may be attributed to disturbance of the body's vital energy, *ki*. Health can be regarded as balanced and strong *ki*. Illness is considered a pattern of disharmony in which *ki* is not in balance because it is blocked or weak. Physical symptoms may be based on psychological determinants.

Predominant Sick Care Practices: Alternative and biomedical when available. Because of continuous economic hardships, health care in North Korea is far below the standards of most Western countries and continues to deteriorate. Hospitals in Pyongyang and other cities may lack medications, food, heat, and basic supplies and have frequent power outages. The flow of international food aid is critical for meeting basic food needs. Malnutrition rates are among the world's highest, and mortality estimates are in the hundreds of thousands as the direct result of starvation or famine-related diseases.

Endemic/Race Specific or Endemic Diseases: Localized air pollution is a significant problem and is attributable to inadequate industrial controls. Water pollution and inadequate supplies of potable water are instrumental in disease. *Hwa-byung* is a Korean folk illness label that was categorized into a Korean culture-bound syndrome in the fourth edition of the *Diagnostic and Statistical Manual of Mental Disorders (DMS-IV)*. It translates as "anger syndrome." Because of the continuing deterioration of the health care infrastructure, no accurate data regarding disease incidence or prevalence are available. The World Health Organization's (WHO) estimated prevalence rate for HIV/AIDS in adults ages 15 to 49 is 0.01%. WHO has no estimates for children from birth to 15 years living with HIV/AIDS.

Health Team Relationships: The medical system is in chaos, although ostensibly the country has a system in which doctors cover particular districts. In reality, access to health care is either very poor or nonexistent. Doctors receive training for a period of 3 to 6 years and have the dominant role on the health care team. Nurses are poorly educated at the technical level. Neither doctors nor nurses have an adequate infrastructure in which to work.

Dominance Patterns: In general the ages of 30 and 31 for men and 28 and 29 for women are considered the proper ages for marriage. Women's labor is important in the society, constituting about 48% of the labor force. A system of public nursery schools makes it possible for women to work. At age 60 (for men) and age 55 (for women), older adults earn the status of "elder" and can retire.

Touch Practices: Hand holding and touching among friends of the same sex is acceptable.

Perceptions of Time: Punctuality is considered basic etiquette in formal and informal interpersonal meetings.

Death Rites: North Koreans are experiencing a trend toward more secular, rather than religious (Confucian), funerals. Funerals usually last 3 days and burial, rather than cremation, is preferred.

Food Practices and Intolerances: In traditional families the father, using chopsticks or a spoon, may dine alone. After meals, which usually consist of rice, fish, soup, and vegetables, the family gets together for conversation. The diet is healthy, with the exception of a high sodium intake. The usual dessert is fruit.

National Childhood Immunizations: BCG at birth; DTP at $1\frac{1}{2}$, $2\frac{1}{2}$, and $3\frac{1}{2}$ months; OPV at $1\frac{1}{2}$, $2\frac{1}{2}$, and $3\frac{1}{2}$ months; hep B at birth and at

$2\frac{1}{2}$ and $3\frac{1}{2}$ months; measles at 9 months; vitamin A at 6 to 59 months, $+6$ months; and TT at 3 months and 6 months gestation.

Other Characteristics: Both hands are used to hand something to another person. The legs are not crossed during prayer and singing at religious ceremonies. Sunglasses are removed when speaking to others. It is acceptable for males to urinate on the side of the road and children to run around without clothing. Family names are placed in the following order: the family name first, the generation name second, and the personal or first name last. A woman does not change her name when she marries. The fertility rate is 2.3 children born per woman.

BIBLIOGRAPHY

Galanti GA: *Caring for patients from different cultures,* ed 2, Philadelphia, 1997, University of Pennsylvania Press.

Joo KH: *North Korean living ways for 50 years,* Seoul, 2001, Minzokwon.

http://www.famnetkorea.com

http://oneness.pe.kr/study/soc

http://www.odci.gov/cia/publications/factbook/geos/kn.html

See also South Korea bibliography.

◆ KOREA, SOUTH (REPUBLIC OF)

MAP PAGE (865)

Sung Ok Chang

Location: The Republic of Korea (South Korea) is on a peninsula jutting off of Manchuria and China in eastern Asia. Eastern Korea is mountainous, and the west and south have many mainland harbors and offshore islands. The total land area is 98,480 km² (38,023 square miles).

Major Languages	Ethnic Groups	Major Religions
Korean	Korean 99%	Atheist or other 54%
	Chinese 1%	Protestant 20%
		Buddhist 18%
		Roman Catholic 8%

Cheondo-kyois, a synthesis of Confucian, Buddhist, shamanistic, Daoist, and Catholic influences, is generally regarded as the first of Korea's "new religions." Other major new religions include *Taejonggyo* (worship of Tangun, the legendary founder of the Korean nation), *Chungsanggyo* (which emphasizes magical practices), and *Wonbulgyo* (Won Buddhism), a combination of traditional Buddhist doctrines and modern concern for social reform. However, in reality, very few people practice religion.

Health Care Beliefs: Active involvement; health promotion. The mind-body interaction is considered essential for good health. The cause of illness may be attributed to a disturbance of the body's vital energy, or *ki*. Health can be regarded as balanced, strong *ki*. Illness is considered a pattern of disharmony in which *ki* is unbalanced because it is blocked or weak. Physical symptoms may be based on psychological factors, and improvement is frequently evaluated in terms of functional ability.

Predominant Sick Care Practices: Biomedical (Western), holistic, and traditional therapies. Acupuncture, hand acupuncture, acupressure, herbal medicines, and cupping are traditional treatments that are used often. Eastern and Western medicine may be used simultaneously. The implementation of health insurance for the entire nation has increased the demand for health care. Medical services are provided by general and educational hospitals and clinics established and operated by national or local governments or private clinics, hospitals, and individuals. Private institutions (primarily concentrated in urban areas) comprise more than 91% of all medical facilities, employ 88.8% of doctors, and account for 91% of total beds. Koreans have access to two systems of care: Western medicine, which is the mainstream form of care, and Oriental medicine. No referral system between the two systems has been established. Oriental (traditional Korean) medicine differs fundamentally from Western in its principles and characteristics and has a history of excellent success. The Oriental Medicine Bureau was established as one of the major bureaus of the Ministry of Health and Welfare in 1996 to fulfill the public demand for Oriental medicine nationally and internationally. Korea's health insurance plan was introduced in 1977 and expanded in 1988. Coverage gradually included workplaces with more than five employees, rural residents such as farmers, and the self-employed. By 1989 a compulsory health insurance program for the entire population was in place. All insurers are members of the National Federation of Medical Insurance (NFMI). On behalf of its members, NFMI designates medical care institutions to provide service to the insured and reviews and pays all claims under the guidance and supervision of the Ministry of Health and Welfare. Major financial contributions to the system are paid by the insured and their employers and supplemented by government subsidies.

Ethnic/Race Specific or Endemic Diseases: *Hwa-byung* is a Korean folk illness label, and it was categorized into a Korean culture-bound syndrome in the fourth edition of the *Diagnostic and Statistical Manual of Mental Disorders (DSM-IV)*. It is considered an anger syndrome. Korea is now experiencing an epidemiological transition. During the last few decades the incidence of infectious diseases has decreased while the incidence of chronic degenerative diseases has constantly increased. Korea has a notification system for all infectious diseases and a laboratory surveillance system for diseases such as influenza, Japanese encephalitis, typhoid fever, and vibrio infections. If an epidemic outbreak occurs, a special investigation is conducted. Prevalence rates for major chronic diseases present in the population are hypertension, 44.73; diabetes mellitus, 22.38; cardiac disease, 18.29; liver disease, 17.04; palsy, 6.48; and stomach cancer, 0.85. The World Health Organization's (WHO) estimated prevalence rate for HIV/AIDS in adults ages 15 to 49 is 0.01%. The estimated number of children from birth to 15 years living with HIV/AIDS is less than 100.

Health Team Relationships: Since the end of the Korean War, the number of health care professionals in South Korea has risen dramatically. In the past, doctors and nurses were considered authority figures and treated with great respect. People generally did not disagree with them. Today, this is changing. Patients are more vocal about participating in health care decisions, and in hospitals patients' rights are receiving more emphasis.

Families' Role in Hospital Care: When a family member becomes sick the family prefers to do personal care, and to be guardians for the sick family member. Therefore, patient education performed in the hospital settings must involve family members in treatment plans.

Dominance Patterns: Parent-child relationships are more highly regarded than husband-wife relationships, and the oldest son inherits the patriarchal position. The father is dominant and makes decisions for all family members. As the head of the household he is responsible for all its economic needs. The mother is the homemaker in charge of the domestic and emotional needs of the family. In addition to the traditional role of tending the home and raising children, women are responsible for managing the family's health; many women spend a considerable portion of their time handling this issue. Men have more legal advantages than women in terms of rights to children because children traditionally belong to the husband's family. In less traditional families, decision making is more family oriented. At age 65, older adults earn the status of "elder" and can retire.

Eye Contact Practices: Status determines whether direct eye contact is avoided or maintained briefly. When a person is avoiding eye contact, the eyes are turned to the side—not turned up or down.

Touch Practices: Hand-holding among good friends of the same sex is acceptable. In health care situations, touching related to *ki* such as massage and acupressure (which are considered therapeutic modes in Oriental medicine) is used to treat illness.

Perceptions of Time: Punctuality is basic etiquette in formal and informal interpersonal interactions.

Pain Reactions: South Koreans tend to be stoical.

Birth Rites: From conception, the mother starts prenatal training *(taegyo)*, which is the care pregnant women provide for themselves and their fetus. After delivery, mothers are expected to avoid exposure to cold, including air conditioning, and consume no iced drinks—only warm foods. *Sanhujori*, a period of 7 weeks after delivery, is a prevailing tradition among Korean women. *Sanhujori* involves recovering strength by warming the body and avoiding exposure to cold. It is expected for women to eat warm and soft food; avoid salty, spicy, sweet, and sour foods; and attend to personal hygiene while their body is restored to its prepregnancy condition. As is true in China, cultural attitudes affect family planning. Koreans still prefer sons. According to the Confucian value system, the sons carry on the family name and must care for parents in their old age. Parents with daughters may continue to have children until they have a son, although government campaigns urge couples to have only one child because of a projected critical increase in the population size.

Death Rites: Family members are summoned to observe a dying person's last breath and may respond with loud wailing and intense displays of emotion. Death rites may differ according to religious affiliation and death orientations. More simplified death rituals occur today compared with the elaborate rituals of Confucian funerals in the past. The funeral generally lasts for 3 days, and burial, not cremation, is preferred.

Food Practices and Intolerances: The Korean diet is essentially healthy, with the exception of its high sodium content, which may contribute to the high prevalence rates of hypertension in the country. Rice is the basic food, and many meals include *kimchi,* or pickled cabbage. Fruit snacks are frequently eaten, and dessert is usually fruit. Chop sticks and a large spoon are used to eat. Hot soup or stew is preferred at all meals, whereas cold liquids are not usually consumed.

Child Rearing Practices: The mother tends to be careful, permissive, and affectionate, whereas the father tends to be strict. Breast-feeding is recommended for the health of the mother and child, but the length of time mothers breast-feed varies significantly. "Examination hell," or the pressure created by the need to excel on college entrance examinations, is blamed for the occasionally grim lives of some adolescents and their high suicide rate. Entrance examinations are thought to determine the fate of Korean students.

National Childhood Immunizations: BCG at 4 weeks; OPV at 2, 4, and 6 months and 4 to 6 years; hep B ×3, start up before third month; JapEnc at 12 to 25 months +12 months and at 6 and 18 years; DtaP at 2, 4, and 6 months; MMR at 12 to 15 months and 4 to 6 years; and DT at 4 to 6 years.

Other Characteristics: Koreans have three names: the family name is written first, the generational name second, and the given name last. Given names are used only by family members and intimate friends. A woman does not change her name when she marries. When first offered, food and drinks are refused out of politeness, regardless of how much they are desired; the offer must be repeated. Both hands are used to hand something to another person.

BIBLIOGRAPHY

American Psychiatric Association: *Diagnostic and statistical manual of mental disorders,* ed 4, pp 843-849, Washington, DC, 1994, American Psychiatric Association.

Chang SB et al: *Factors of the 'Taegyo' of Korean pregnant women,* The proceeding book of the International Nursing Research Conference, Seoul, Korea, 1996.

Chang SO: The meaning of *ki* related to touch in caring, *Holistic Nurs Pract* 16(1), 2001.

Chang SO: The meaning of physical touch in caring, doctoral dissertation, 1996, Yonsei University.

Choi EC: A contrast of mothering behaviors in women from Korea and the United States, *J Obstet Gynecol Neonatal Nurs* 24(4):363, 1995.

Choi EY, Kim JS, Lee WB: *Health care system in Korea,* Seoul, 1998, Korea Institute for Health and Affairs.

Choi SD: *Modern society and family,* Masan, 1986, The Foundation of Social Welfare.

Dusan encyclopedia, Seoul, 2001, Dusan Publishing.

Gallup Korea-the children and mother, Seoul, 1991, Gallup Polls.

Gallup Korea-the Korean religions and religious rituals, Seoul, 1998, Gallup Polls.

Jeoung GH, Kim SJ: The pregnant women's decision-making process about their infant feeding method, *J Korean Acad Women's Health Nurs* 6(2):203-216, 2000

Kim SJ: *Death orientation of the Korean elderly,* doctoral dissertation, Seoul, 1994, Seoul National University.

Korean Pediatric Association: *The guideline of booster,* ed 4, Seoul, 1997, Eui Hak Moon Hwa Sa.

Lee KH et al: *Women's health nursing,* Seoul, 1996, Hyun-Moon Sa.

Lee SD: A study on the philosophical background and health concept in Oriental Medicine, *Korean J Health Promo* 2(1):88-98, 2000

Park JH: Nursing administration in Korea, *Nurs Adm Q* 16(2):78, 1992.

http://www.nso.go.kr

◆ KUWAIT (STATE OF)

MAP PAGE (864)

Salim M. Adib

Location: Kuwait is located in the northwestern corner of the Persian Gulf. Its total land area is 17,818 km² (about 7000 square miles). The surface of the country slopes down gradually from west to east, with a few hills scattered in the eastern parts, where the country becomes primarily desert. Temperatures may be rather low during winter nights; the absolute low record was –4° C (30° F) in 1964. Temperatures can soar to amazing highs on summer days, often exceeding 50° C (120° F).

Major Languages	Ethnic Groups	Major Religions (Kuwaitis only)
Arabic (official)	Kuwaiti 45%	Sunni Muslim 68%
English (widely spoken)	Other Arab 35%	Shi'a Muslim 30%
Iranian	South Asian 9%	Other 2%
Hindi	Iranian 4%	
Urdu	Other 7%	

The population is estimated to be 2.5 million, including non-Kuwaiti expatriate residents (60%), who are transient and primarily include Arabs and Southeast Asians. The majority of Kuwaitis claim an affiliation to large Bedouin tribes, and about 30% are original urban dwellers (and known as the "city dwellers" or "*dira* families"). About 20% of the Kuwaiti population is of Persian origin. Tolerance of non-Kuwaiti religions is mandated by Kuwaiti law. (Approximately 98% of Kuwaitis are Muslim.) Kuwait currently has at least eight declared Christian churches in the country.

Health Care Beliefs: Acute sick care; traditional. In a survey of Kuwaitis, about 55% agreed that *djinns* (evil spirits) play a role in making people sick, and an additional 29% were unsure. For example many believed in the "evil eye"—that certain people with special powers can harm others merely by looking at them. Of those surveyed, 65% believed some diseases can only be healed by faith-related practices. In addition to reading Koranic verses, various healers ask patients to drink "blessed" water that is occasionally mixed with saffron to eat blessed honey or dates, or to massage a painful area with blessed oil. Almost half of 428 patients surveyed indicated having used herbal preparations in the previous year. Patients may be massaged by a practitioner who has spit in his hands to ensure passage of Koranic powers from his reciting mouth to his massaging hands. Patients may be told to play tapes of specific healing verses continuously until their problem vanishes. Some powerful spirits can only be driven out by some degree of physical violence, ranging from slight slapping of the hands and face to serious beating with sandals and sticks. More worrisome is that in recent years, some healers have even begun giving electrical shocks to patients to cure their ailments.

Predominant Sick Care Practices: Biomedical and magical-religious. Modern medicine in Kuwait began in 1904 with the arrival of an Indian doctor hired by the British delegation to open a new clinic within the walled city. Since then, modern medicine has gradually supplanted traditional health practices. After the discovery of oil, resources were allocated by the state to create a public health system that was accessible and free to all. In 1999, user fees were introduced for non-Kuwaitis. A private care system exists, but the majority of people use the public system. Although the overwhelming portion of medical care is sought within the formal care system, some traditional practices persist, albeit in combination with modern medicine. Traditional health practices still found in Kuwait include "Islamic" or "Koranic" healing practices performed by primarily self-taught "practitioners" acting with almost no control or regulation. Those practitioners tend to be consulted when patients or their families suspect than an evil spirit is contributing to their ill health. A recent survey of a random sample of 376 Kuwaiti civil servants revealed that people still use these types of practitioners. About 56% of those surveyed had used the services of Koranic faith healers, and 18% had done so in the previous year. A previous survey in 1997 found that 15% of those surveyed (400 patients in primary health care clinics) had used the practitioners in the previous year. Until recently, cauterization was a traditional procedure most often practiced by Bedouins. Traditional parts of the body of the affected person are marked with a hot iron or a heated wooden rod, a practice that is believed to draw out the offending illness. The most common areas for cauterization are the foot and belly, and the most commonly treated conditions are fevers, diarrhea, epilepsy, and headaches. A survey of 300 individuals randomly selected from primarily Bedouin sectors found that up to 43% had experienced cauterization. However, it is very likely that the national rate is much lower. Among 400 patients surveyed in the capital city area, only 8% indicated having had an experience with cauterization. Of cauterized individuals, 37% had been most recently cauterized after their twentieth birthday. Of all surveyed, 31% believed the practice to be useless or harmful; among those who had been cauterized, 16% believed the practice to be useless or harmful. Belief in the efficacy of herbal treatments has been channeled through the Islamic Center for Herbal Medicine since the mid-1980s. The center ensures that herbs utilized by the public are not harmful.

Ethnic/Race Specific or Endemic Diseases: Kuwait is a country in social, cultural, demographic, and epidemiological transition. Although still maintaining many features of more traditional, less advanced societies, it has recently acquired many similarities to more advanced nations. For example, infectious diseases have ceased to be a public health concern. Currently, the most prevalent diseases in Kuwait are diabetes (15% of the population) and asthma (13% of 9- to 12-year-old school children). Of concern is the increase in the prevalence of tobacco smoking, especially among young men. Other risks include obesity and anemia. Drug abuse incidence is reported to be increasing among young adults. Infant mortality rates have been decreasing steadily for the past 30 years and are now about 11 per 1000 live births (comparing favorably with 9 in the United States). The low infant mortality in Kuwait is largely a result of the massive, mandatory free childhood immunization program that has been in place since the mid-1980s. As of 2002 the program included vaccinations against measles, mumps, rubella, diphtheria, whooping cough, tetanus, hepatitis B, poliomyelitis, *Haemophilus influenzae,* bacterial meningitis, and tuberculosis (BCG vaccine). The main causes of death in Kuwait are similar to those in the United States, with cardiovascular diseases heading the list, followed by various cancers. Injuries from automobile accidents have been increasing during the past 10 years, although the fatality rate seems to have reached a plateau. Accidental deaths are the third most common cause of death. HIV and AIDS are rare, and no more than 100 cases have been reported since 1984. HIV infections were reported primarily from 1984 to 1986 while the screening tests for blood and blood products were being established. Non-Kuwaitis are required to have a negative HIV test before obtaining permanent residency. The World Health Organization's (WHO) estimated prevalence rate for HIV/AIDS in adults ages 15 to 49 is 0.12%. WHO has no estimates for children from birth to 15 years.

Health Team Relationships: Until recently the medical field in Kuwait was dominated by men. However, more women are graduating from the only faculty of medicine in the country. A more gender-collaborative medical environment is expected to emerge. Nursing is not held in high esteem by the locals. The only program graduating registered Kuwaiti nurses was closed in 1999 because of a lack of students.

Families' Role in Hospital Care: Family and friends are expected to be with hospitalized patients as much as possible. Families are demanding of health care personnel to ensure that the patients receive adequate care and attention. Food services are generally highly rated in public hospitals and often include daily treats of baked goods and fresh juices. Nevertheless, gifts of sweets and chocolates (and occasionally flowers) are generally expected from visitors. News of a serious diagnosis or poor prognosis is normally delivered to families. Doctors normally do not relay this type of information directly to the patient if the family prefers, providing that this lack of disclosure does not affect a patient's therapeutic course.

Dominance Patterns: By law, men and women are supposedly equal. The remaining areas of gender inequality involve the right to vote and polygamy. Despite an attempt at changing the laws in 1999, women have not yet obtained the right to vote. Polygamy is a right reserved to men by Islam. However, less than 9% of those who are married practice polygamy. Polygamy is slowly being replaced by serial marriages, as indicated by the increasing rate of divorce in the 1990s. In 1999, one divorce occurred for every marriage and by age 50, 95% of all Kuwaitis have been married at least once. Being single is considered undesirable. In practice, Kuwaiti society remains highly patriarchal, and women are not expected to have prominent public or leadership roles. In many Kuwaiti families the surviving grandmother plays an essential role as the hostess of family events and remains the center of conflict resolution within the family. Norms of public behavior for women differ greatly with respect to traditional dress. It is common to encounter women who are wearing very modern and trendy clothes walking next to women totally covered with a dark chador. Many Kuwaiti women have prominent positions in academia, business, and diplomacy arenas.

Eye Contact Practices: Eye contact is expected during a conversation; however, when men and women converse, it is preferred that the eye contact be brief. Many women are uncomfortable with direct eye contact.

Touch Practices: Touching is not encouraged between the sexes. A man is not expected to shake hands with a woman if she does not take the initiative by stretching out her hand. If a man is uncomfortable about shaking hands with a woman, he discreetly touches his chest as a signal to the woman.

Perceptions of Time: Kuwaitis tend to glorify past traditions as reflections of a blessed time when life was simpler and social ties stronger and warmer. When these attitudes are studied, most recognize that the "good old times" were also very harsh times, when life was often precarious and survival often a matter of sheer luck. The rapidity with which modern prosperity and convenience have overtaken Kuwaitis may have reinforced the tendency to dwell on the past and the present with a fatalistic eye and confidence in Allah's providence. This attitude is projected into the future. It is uncommon to hear any public debate involving serious concerns about the future. Nevertheless, in recent years, growing numbers of people are saying that maintaining the same standard of living in the future will be more difficult and may require more effort.

Pain Reactions: It is preferred that pain be expressed only privately or with close relatives and friends. However, pain can be, and is expected to be, expressed loudly during labor and delivery.

Birth Rites: As in most traditional cultures, the birth of a boy is generally considered a more joyous event than the birth of a girl, especially if the infant is a first-born child. Childless women are generally regarded with sorrow and pity. Studies indicate that the preferred number of children among young Kuwaitis is five, with three boys to two girls. After delivery, women are considered impure for up to 40 days, during which time they must not pray, fast, or engage in sexual relations. According to tradition, they cannot be visited by new brides. Kuwaiti mothers of Bedouin and Iranian origins eat traditional foods after delivery, most of which include a mixture of spices to help the body shed excess fluids and promote lactation. The median age of marriage has increased in the past 20 years. In 1996, it was 18 years among women ages 45 to 49 and 21 years among those ages 25 to 29. The fertility rate is 4.12 children per woman.

Death Rites: When a person dies, friends and relatives are not expected to show too much grief because it is contrary to the religious belief that the person has moved on to a better place. Autopsy is uncommon because the body must be buried intact according to Muslim tradition. For Muslim burials the body is wrapped in special pieces of cloth and buried without a coffin, usually within 1 day of death. Cremation is not permitted. Family members receive condolences for 3 days from relatives and friends, with separate venues for men and women. Organ donations have been allowed in Kuwait since 1983 in accordance with current interpretations of Islamic regulations. The kidney transplant unit in Al-Sabah Hospital has already conducted hundreds of kidney and other organ transplant operations. A nongovernmental organization, the Kuwait

Transplant Society, has been urging citizens since the mid-1980s to become organ donors by signing an organ donation card.

Food Practices and Intolerances: The staple food in Kuwait is rice, and fish is abundant. Kuwaiti cuisine is heavily influenced by Indian and Iranian cuisines, and they particularly enjoy lamb meat. However, all types of ethnic and international food, as well as fast food chains, can be found all over the country. Pork, carrion, blood, and alcohol cannot be consumed by Muslims. These items are not imported, sold, or served in public in Kuwait. Public observance of Ramadan fasting is mandatory for all adults. The ceremonial collective meal consisting of a mound of spiced saffron rice topped with a whole lamb and eaten from a dish on a carpet is still common among more traditional Bedouin families, particularly during special social events such as weddings and the end of the period of condolences. Eating with the hands is common, especially during collective meals in which using the right hand for eating is the norm.

Infant Feeding Practices: Breast-feeding is still the norm for most women in Kuwait. It can last for up to 18 months, with lactation periods decreasing with increasing numbers of children.

Child Rearing Practices: Child rearing is relatively permissive, and parents tend to rely on the abundant and cheap domestic servants that are available to provide daily personal care and supervision of children. Despite this assistance, physical abuse is common and tends to occur randomly. A 1997 survey of Kuwaiti parents found that 86% agreed that physical punishment is a legitimate way to discipline children. Public denigration of children is preferred rather than praise because of fear of the evil eye. Children older than 1 year rarely sleep with their parents. Formal schooling of children begins at age 4.

National Childhood Immunizations: BCG at 4 to 5 years; OPV at birth and 2, 4, 6, and 18 months; hep B at birth and 2 and 6 months; DTPHiB at 2, 4, 6, and 18 months and 3 1/2 years; MMR at 12 months and 4 to 5 years; rubella at 12 years for girls; DT at 10 and 18 years; and TT at fourth and seventh month of pregnancy.

BIBLIOGRAPHY

Al-Awadi E, Al-Hashel J, Al-Hajeri D: *Quranic faith-healing practices in Kuwait,* Department of Community Medicine, Health Sciences Center, Kuwait University, 1999, Kuwait City.

Al-Enezi A et al: *Postpartum beliefs and practices among Kuwaiti women,* Department of Community Medicine, Health Sciences Center, Kuwait University, 1999, Kuwait City.

Al-Mutairi MMF et al: *Traditional healing by cauterization in Kuwait,* Department of Community Medicine, Health Sciences Center, Kuwait University, 1998, Kuwait City.

Al-Rashoud RH, Adib SM, Farid SM: *Reproductive health in Kuwait: findings from the 1996 Family Health Survey.* Paper presented at the Fourth International Epidemiological Association-East Mediterranean Region Meeting, Tunisia, 1998.

Buresly SM et al: *Use of alternative medicine among Kuwaiti patients visiting polyclinics in the capital governorates,* Department of Community Medicine, Health Sciences Center, Kuwait University, 1997, Kuwait City.

Harrison A: Comparing nurses' and patients' pain evaluations: a study of hospitalized patients in Kuwait, *Soc Sci Med* 36:683-692, 1993.

Kuwait University Health Sciences Center: The history of medicine in Kuwait. In *The faculty of medicine memorial book,* 1997, Kuwait University Publishing Services, Kuwait City.

Meeting Al-Owaish: We are not immune to the AIDS threat, *Al-Anbaa* (daily Arabic newspaper), Kuwait, January 5, 2002.

Memon A et al: Epidemiology of smoking among Kuwaiti adults: prevalence, characteristics and attitudes. *Bulletin WHO* 78:1306-1315, 2000.

Ministry of Planning: *Annual statistical abstract,* ed 37, Kuwait, 2000.

Qasem FS et al: Attitudes of Kuwaiti parents toward physical punishment of children, *Child Abuse Negl* 22:1189-1202, 1998.

World Health Organization (June 2000): *Epidemiological fact sheets by country,* Geneva. Retrieved March 1, 2002, from http://www.unaids.org/hivaidsinfo/statistics/june00/fact_sheets/index.html

World Health Organization (2001): *WHO vaccine-preventable diseases: monitoring system,* Geneva. Retrieved March 1, 2002, from http://www.who.int/vaccines/

◆ KYRGYZSTAN (KYRGYZ REPUBLIC)

MAP PAGE (861)

Gunay Balta

Location: Kyrgyzstan declared its independence from the former Soviet Union in 1991. It is located in northeast Central Asia and has a total land area of 198,000 km^2 (76,428 square miles). Most of the territory lies within the Tien Shan mountain range, which is covered with perennial snow and glaciers. Kyrgyzstan is remarkable for its natural beauty. It is a country of sunshine, snow-covered mountains, deep gorges cut by swift rivers, and 1923 mountain lakes. The country occupies a strategic location on the Silk Road between the markets of the former Soviet Union and Europe, the Middle East, South Asia, and China. Kyrgyzstan's cosmopolitan population of 4,832,000 is a unique mix of over 80 ethnic groups.

Major Languages	Ethnic Groups	Major Religions
Kyrgyz	Kyrgyz 61%	Muslim 75%
Russian	Russian 15%	Orthodox Christian 20%
	Uzbek 14%	Other 5%
	Ukrainian 2%	
	Other 8%	

The Kyrgyz culture has been greatly influenced by its nomadic heritage, which is reflected in the way a household is run and in the country's customs and rituals. The masterpiece of folk creation is the Kyrgyz tent *(yurta),* which is easy to assemble and transport from place to place.

Today, the *yurta* is popular with shepherds *(chabans)* who spend their summers in the high pastures. The Kyrgyz are one of the most ancient nationalities in the world. Much of Kyrgyz history has been learned from the epic story of *Manas* written in the nineteenth century. The work contains 500,000 lines of poetry that have been transmitted orally through generations. The work is the longest epic poem in the world. The Manas legend gives insight into all aspects of traditional life of the Kyrgyz—their origin, customs, morals, general knowledge, and language. Many places and things in Kyrgyzstan bear the name of this ancient hero. The Kyrgyz Republic has maintained a high educational standard and almost universal literacy. Compulsory primary school lasts for 9 years. Additional education is available free at one of 1922 secondary schools and 23 universities and institutes. In addition to the state sector a tuition-charging private education sector is developing at all levels. Kyrgyzstan has low-cost laborers, and the average monthly salary is less than $20 (U.S. dollars).

Health Care Beliefs: Acute sick care; traditional. Because of their very low incomes and often neglect, people seek professional help only when they are seriously ill. However, for mild illnesses they often use alternative treatments based on their beliefs and experiences. For example, they may apply melted lamb fat over their chest and stomach to treat respiratory or stomach illnesses. Childhood vaccinations play a major role in disease prevention. Disease is perceived as a part of life and not a punishment from God.

Predominant Sick Care Practices: Biomedical and alternative. Like other former Soviet Union countries, health care is delivered through a hierarchy of services. Primary care is given by *feldsher*—midwifery posts in villages, doctors' clinics in small towns, and polyclinics in urban areas. The extensive system of hospitals range from village hospitals to central district hospitals, regional and national hospitals, and numerous specialized hospitals. However, because of the present economic situation of the country, the health care system is not responding effectively or efficiently to the health needs of the population. In principle, health services are free and accessible to everyone. In reality, health care services are no longer free because of the limited state resources. Informal, out-of-pocket payments are increasing. Copayments or full payments for any kind of health service and unofficial surreptitious payments to doctors, particularly to specialists, are very common. Most of the drugs (90%) are imported, and foreign loans and grants are used to supply emergency drugs in particular. Drugs donated from foreign countries are another source. Despite improvements in drug supplies in recent years, part of the population cannot afford required medications because of poor living standards and the unregulated high prices of drugs. However, this situation began improving after the establishment of the Mandatory Health Insurance Fund. Except for certain drugs, prescriptions from doctors are not mandatory; therefore people search for the lowest price at numerous pharmacies.

Ethnic/Race Specific or Endemic Diseases: A specific problem in recent years is the gradual increase in the frequency of iron deficiency anemia and iodine deficiency disorders. Mortality from noncommunicable diseases such as heart disease and stroke is increasing. The incidence of communicable diseases such as tuberculosis and syphilis is also increasing. The epidemiological situation in the country is characterized by the increasing prevalence of morbidity from pertussis, brucellosis, echinococcosis, viral hepatitis, and gonorrhea. The World Health Organization's (WHO) estimated prevalence rate for HIV/AIDS in adults ages 15 to 49 is 0.01%. The estimated number of children from birth to 15 years living with HIV/AIDS is less than 100.

Health Team Relationships: As is true in most Western countries, doctors are the principal authorities on most health issues. Nurses, who have lower levels of education, play a supporting role. In addition, *feldshers* and midwives provide primary care in the villages.

Families' Role in Hospital Care: Families are responsible for finding and purchasing all medications and needed medical supplies for hospitalized family members. They also may make full or partial payments for various services and laboratory tests. Many of the most popular medications are not readily available, so families often have difficulties finding specific prescribed medications.

Dominance Patterns: Kyrgyzstan has a conservative, male-dominated society, and male and female roles tend to be quite traditional. Although women are found in nearly all areas of the workforce, women primarily focus on the family. Their position in the household is important and respected. The family is a mutual support system, and siblings remain close even after marriage. Families are expected to care for their aging parents; therefore parents often move in with one of their children as they become less able to live on their own.

Eye Contact Practices: Direct eye contact is acceptable and the norm.

Touch Practices: Men usually shake hands when greeting, but men and women rarely shake hands. Women usually greet other women by kissing on one side of the face. While greeting, people of the same sex tend to hold each other by the shoulder, although hugging is uncommon except among close relatives. Women and couples often walk arm-in-arm in public.

Perceptions of Time: Generally, punctuality is not important in daily life, and people do not rush. However, some professionals, especially those working for foreign companies, must be prompt.

Pain Reactions: Kyrgyz people are calm when faced with physically or emotionally painful situations, and they usually bear misfortune with stoicism.

Birth Rites: Birth rites are based on religion and culture. An interesting feast—*Djengek Toi*—celebrates the birth of an infant. Another interesting ritual is the celebration day *(Tyshoo Kesuu)* for an infant who has just learned to walk, in which invited young children participate in a competition or race. Before the race the infant's feet are tied with a black and white string. The child who wins the race is allowed to cut the infant's strings. It is believed that after being released from the strings, the infant will be healthy and live confidently.

Death Rites: Kyrgyz people participate in religious and cultural rituals at the time of death. Relatives and friends gather at the home of the deceased person. Even in the cities, they build a *yurta* (traditional tent) right next to the house on the same day of death, in which they place the body on a special bed. Close relatives, especially the women, sit inside the *yurta,* pray to God, and express their sorrow. Usually they sacrifice a horse, and traditional dishes are prepared from its meat and served to the visitors in memory of the dead person. The body is usually buried 3 days later. Cremation is not allowed. All of the belongings of the deceased person are distributed to the relatives in memory of the person.

Food Practices and Intolerances: Dinner is the largest meal of the day and is a time when all family members come together. Meat (often lamb, but occasionally horse meat or beef), including entrails, and pastries are the most common ingredients of Kyrgyz dishes. *Beshbarmak* ("five fingers") is the most popular traditional dish. Vegetables are often included in traditional dishes. The most festive soup, *shorpo,* is prepared with meat broth, vegetables, and spices. Bread, potatoes, and fruit are also important components of the daily diet. Dessert is very rare in Kyrgyz cuisine, but milk and milk products are often consumed. The favorite drinks are *kumys*—mildly alcoholic fermented mare's milk—and *maksim*—boiled and fermented wheat. Tea is the most common beverage and is served at any time and place. However, coffee is uncommon. The people of Kyrgyzstan love to entertain; therefore they like to celebrate every occasion. They congregate, usually at homes, whenever possible, have a large meal, and drink and dance until late at night. Most Kyrgyz like to drink alcohol—at least with guests—and vodka is popular. Hospitality is an important part of life in Kyrgyzstan; people are very friendly and generous and share whatever they have with others.

Infant Feeding Practices: Infants are always born at hospitals and kept at least for 7 days for general examinations and vaccinations. During this period, infants whose mothers are unable to produce breast milk are fed with breast milk from other mothers. Breast-feeding is considered to be the best form of nutrition for newborns, so most new mothers attempt it. Formula is used if a mother is unable to produce enough milk. Mashed fruit, vegetables, creamed cereals, rice, and potatoes supplement breast milk or formula when the infant is about 6 months of age.

Child Rearing Practices: As the primary caregivers for children, mothers are allowed by law to take a maternity leave of up to 3 years after the birth of an infant. Maternity leaves are unpaid, so the ability of the woman to stay home with her infant depends almost entirely on her financial ability to do so. It is becoming increasingly more common for mothers to take short leaves because most families depend on the income they normally earn. It is fairly common for mothers to return to work several weeks after delivery. Grandparents are most frequently called on to care for children whose mothers have returned to work.

National Childhood Immunizations: BCG at 3 to 4 days and 7, 11 to 12, and 16 to 17 years; DTP at 2, 3, and 4 1/2 months and at 2 to 3, 9, and 16 to 17 years; OPV at 3 to 4 days and 2, 3 to 4, 5, 16, and 18 months; measles at 12 months; hep B at birth and at 2 and 5 months; mumps at 18 months; DT at 5 to 6 years; and Td at 11 to 12 and 15 to 16 years.

Other Characteristics: One of the most important family events is a wedding. The celebration includes *kalym* payment, various clothes that are exchanged between the bride and bridegroom's parents, expensive dowries, farewell wailing, and an animal sacrifice for the couple. Kyrgyz men and women are very unlikely to marry outside their people, but women are free to choose their spouse. People get married at a young age and have relatively large families. Wedding customs are very interesting, especially the tradition of kidnapping the bride. Usually the man plans the day of the kidnapping beforehand, and his friends and relatives help him. Relatives gather at his home, set tables, and cook a festive dinner. One corner of a room is curtained off *(koshego)*. When the woman is brought to the house, her head is covered by a kerchief as a symbol of virginity, and she is placed behind the curtain. This custom is still practiced in Kyrgyzstan today.

BIBLIOGRAPHY

Beishenova D: Personal communications, April 9-21, 2002, Faculty of Medicine, Department of Obstetric and Gynecology, Hacettepe University, Ankara, Turkey.

Glinyenko VM, Abdikarimov ST, Firsova SN, Sagamonjan EA, et al: Epidemic diphtheria in the Kyrgyz Republic, 1994-1998, *J Infect Dis* 181:1S98-S103: 2000.

Weeks RM, Svetlana F, Noorgoul S, Valentina G: Improving the monitoring of immunization services In Kyrgyzstan, *Health Policy Plan* 15(3):279-286, 2000.

World Health Organization Regional Office for Europe: *Health care systems in transition,* Kyrgyzstan, 2000.

◆ LAOS (LAO PEOPLE'S DEMOCRATIC REPUBLIC)

MAP PAGE (867)

Location: Laos is located in southeastern Asia in the northeastern part of the Indochinese peninsula. Myanmar is to the northwest, China to the north, Vietnam to the east, Cambodia to the south, and Thailand to the west. The climate is tropical monsoon with rainy (May through November) and dry (December through April) seasons. The land is mountainous (especially in the north), with dense forests and jungle. The total land area is 236,800 km^2 (91,429 square miles), slightly larger than Utah. The capital is Vientiane, which is on the border of Thailand. The population is estimated to be 5,635,967. Laos is a developing country with a communist government. The gross domestic product per capita is $1200.

Major Languages	Ethnic Groups	Major Religions
Lao (official)	Lao Lum 68%	Buddhist 60%
French	Lao Theung 22%	Animist, other 40%
English	Lao Soung (including	
Ethnic languages	Hmong and Yao) 9%	
	Ethnic Vietnamese	
	and Chinese 1%	

Laos has approximately 67 different ethnic groups.

Health Care Beliefs: Acute sick care; traditional. Because of the poor state of the health care system and lack of prevention programs other than immunization, crisis care is the norm. Unhealthy air currents or bad winds are thought to cause illness. Pinching or scratching an area affected by these winds produces marks or red lines and is believed to release the bad "wind: from the body, thus restoring health. Strings around the neck, ankles, or waist prevent "soul loss," which is thought to cause illness. Blood that is lost is considered irreplaceable, so having blood drawn is perceived with some trepidation. Because of stigmas against mental illness, emotional disturbances may be manifested somatically.

Predominant Sick Care Practices: Biomedical, magical-religious, and traditional. Traditional health practices are closely linked to religious traditions. The Lao believe that 32 spirits inhabit the body and govern its functioning. Herbal medicine is an important traditional practice and is classified as "cool treatment," whereas most Western medicine is considered "hot." Traditionally, illness is handled through self-care and self-medication. Because of inadequate and unhygienic conditions in the hospitals, these facilities may be thought of as places to die rather than get well. Medical facilities and services are very limited and do not meet Western standards. Thailand is easily accessible from Vientiane across the Friendship Bridge linking Laos to Nong Khai, Thailand. Those who are able may seek medical care in Thailand.

Ethnic/Race Specific or Endemic Diseases: Endemic diseases include chloroquine-resistant malaria, melioidosis, schistosomiasis (in southern Laos), and gnathostomiasis. Lao are at risk for dengue fever, iodine deficiency in the mountainous regions, cholera, pulmonary paragonimiasis (lung fluke), and poliomyelitis (which was still endemic in 1994). A majority of the population does not have access to potable water, increasing the risk for water-borne illnesses. Cholera outbreaks occurred in 1993 and 1994. More than 500,000 tons of unexploded ordnance is left over from the Vietnam War, causing approximately 120 casualties per year. Laos also has numerous mine fields that pose a hazard. Automobile accidents are also a health risk because of poorly maintained vehicles and roads. The World Health Organization's (WHO) estimated prevalence rate for HIV/AIDS in adults ages 15 to 49 years is 0.05%. The estimated number of children from birth to 15 years living with HIV/AIDS is less than 100. An estimated 130 adults and children died of AIDS in 1999, and about 280 children have lost their mother or both parents to AIDS since the beginning of the epidemic. The majority of cases are among heterosexuals, although it is estimated that only about one fifth of HIV cases are reported.

Health Team Relationships: In traditional families the oldest male makes health care decisions and may answer questions directed to a female patient. Doctors are considered authority figures and experts, therefore patients are told little about their conditions, medications, or diagnostic procedures. As a result, patients may give poor medical histories. Nurses are considered inferior to doctors, and their knowledge base is not equal to Western standards.

Families' Role in Hospital Care: Many family members may accompany the patient to the hospital and remain with the patient for the duration of the stay, providing physical care, equipment and supplies, and food.

Dominance Patterns: The basic family unit often involves three or four generations living together. Decision making is influenced by the astrological and lunar calendars. Women defer to men's decisions in most matters of the outside world; however, women frequently control the home and the community economy.

Eye Contact Practices: Looking directly and steadily into the eyes of someone who is respected or an elder is considered rude.

Touch Practices: A person's head is believed to be the seat of life. It is revered and is not touched. Only parents are permitted to touch the heads of their children. A female's breast is accepted dispassionately as a means of feeding infants, whereas a female's lower torso is considered extremely private. Women cover the area between the waist and knees, even in private. Females who sit with their legs crossed are considered offensive, and pointing the sole of the foot toward anyone is extremely rude. Hand-shaking has gained wide acceptance among men; however, it is not generally acceptable among women. Touching or kissing between brother and sister is not allowed. Waving the hand with the palm up is unacceptable.

Perceptions of Time: Emphasis is not placed on the urgency of getting a task done. Punctuality is reserved for important circumstances.

Pain Reactions: Pain may be severe before relief is requested. Many Buddhists believe that pain in this life may pave the way for a better reincarnation.

Birth Rites: Abandoned or relatives' children who are incorporated into the family may be inadvertently implied to be birth children. The husband may not be welcomed in the delivery room but may play a major role in traditional home births. The preferred delivery position is squatting. Some may consider vernix to be accumulated sperm. Circumcision is generally unknown. Newborns are not given compliments so that evil spirits will not capture them, so it is not unusual, when a Westerner compliments a baby, for the mother to say "No—ugly baby!" Traditionally the woman must remain inside the home for 1 month after delivery, but many need to return to work so this is not always possible. Traditional mothers may lie near or sit over a smoldering charcoal brazier for several days after delivery to help "dry up the womb." The newborn's age is considered to be 1 year at birth. The birth rate is 37.84 births per 1000 people. The last reported (WHO) maternal morality rate per 100,000 live births (1990) was 650, and the infant mortality rate was 89 per 1000 live births. The 1998 total fertility rate is 5.7 children born per woman. Life expectancy at birth is estimated to be 53 years.

Death Rites: Lao prefer quality of life over quantity of life because of the belief in reincarnation and the expectation of less suffering in the next life. Death at home is preferred, and cremation and burial are practiced. People who die in hospitals or from accidents are not cremated and are taken directly from the hospital or scene of the accident to a temple and buried quickly. After death the body is cleaned and dressed in good clothes, and the face is washed with coconut water. White flowers and candles may be put into the deceased person's hands. In some areas, jewels or money (in a wealthier family) and rice (in a poorer family) are put in the mouth of the deceased in the belief that these objects will help the soul when it encounters gods or devils.

Food Practices and Intolerances: Glutinous rice (sticky rice), a salad—*tam mahoun*—made of green papaya, and hot chilies are the main foods. *Lop* (raw or cooked meat pounded together with herbs and spices) is eaten at celebrations. *Lao-lao,* a form of locally prepared rice liquor, is particularly enjoyed by the men daily, as is *Mekong* whiskey. Soup made of rice and water and occasionally with small pieces of shellfish or meat (rice soup) is a popular food for the sick.

Infant Feeding Practices: Colostrum is considered poisonous and believed to cause diarrhea in an infant. Newborns are not allowed to breast-feed until the mother has a full milk supply, so rice paste or boiled sugar water is substituted during this time. For several days after birth (or weeks if it is the mother's first child), the mother eats large amounts of salt and fat. During this time she does not eat red meat, fruits, or vegetables, although she can eat small amounts of chicken.

Child Rearing Practices: A fat infant is considered a healthy one. Methods for calculating the age of an infant may vary by as much as 2 years. At approximately age 6, a strict upbringing begins, independence is discouraged, and parents demand obedience. The oldest child (whether a boy or girl) is responsible for the younger siblings if the parents become ill, are old, or die. Segregation of females from males is common. Literacy rates for males is 69% and for females is 44%, and 43% of the population is 14 years or younger. Laos has numerous cases of childhood malaria, a significant contributor to morbidity in children.

National Childhood Immunizations: BCG at birth; DTP at 6, 10, and 14 weeks; OPV at 6, 10, and 14 weeks; measles at 9 months; vitamin A at 1 to 4 years during third round of routine services; and TT for pregnant women and CBAW. The reported percentages of the target population vaccinated are as follows: BCG, 69; first dose of DTP, 83; third dose of DTP, 53; MCV, 42; Pol3, 57; TT2plus, 45; and vitamin A, 87.

Other Characteristics: The family name is written first and followed by the given name, and married women officially use their husband's last name. Given names are used almost exclusively. Family names are used only for formal occasions or on written documents.

BIBLIOGRAPHY

Anothay O, Pongvongsa T: Childhood malaria in the Lao People's Democratic Republic, *Bulltn WHO* 76(suppl 1):29, 1998.
D'Avanzo C: Bridging the cultural gap with southeast Asians, *MCN Am J Matern Child Nurs* 17:204, 1992.
Dance-David AB: Melioidosis, *Curr Opin Infect Dis* 15(2):127, 2002.
Kagen CN, Vance JC, Simpson M: Gnathostomiasis. Infestation in an Asian immigrant, *Arch Dermatol* 120(4):508, 1984.
Lawson LV: Culturally sensitive support for grieving parents, *MCN Am J Matern Child Nurs* 15:76, 1990.
Shadick KM: Development of a transcultural health education program for the Hmong, *Clin Nurse Spec* 7(2):48, 1993.
Yee B et al: Pulmonary paragonimiasis in Southeast Asians living in the central San Joaquin Valley, *West J Med* 156(4):423, 1992.
http://www.odci.gov/cia/publications/factbook/geos/la.html
http://travel.state/gov/laos.html

◆ LATVIA (REPUBLIC OF)

MAP PAGE (861)

Laima M. Karosas

Location: Latvia, one of the three Baltic states, regained its independence after the dissolution of the Soviet Union. The Baltic Sea is to the north, Estonia to the northeast, the Russian Federation and Belarus to the south, and Lithuania to the west. The eastern part of the country, a fertile lowland, has lakes and hills. The total land area of Latvia is 64,100 km^2 (24,749 square miles).

Major Languages	Ethnic Groups	Major Religions
Lettish	Latvian 52%	Lutheran
Russian	Russian 34%	Russian Orthodox
Lithuanian	Belarussian 5%	Roman Catholic
	Ukrainian 3%	
	Polish 2%	
	Other 4%	

Health Care Beliefs: Acute sick care; little emphasis on health promotion. Although health promotion and disease prevention is considered important, resources are first allocated to in-patient care. Preventative services are scarce, and health promotion and disease prevention programs, especially for women, have deteriorated during the past 10 years. Younger people take a more active role in health care, and recent public literature pieces have emphasized primary care, especially in regards to women's health. Free universal care is provided primarily in health care facilities rather than in community settings. However, payment in the form of gifts or money is expected for most treatments.

Predominant Sick Care Practices: Biomedical, holistic, traditional, and magical-religious. Folk healers are often consulted, and cupping is widely practiced. Latvia has a blend of Christian and pagan beliefs; for example, a pagan ritual may be accompanied by recitations of verses from the Bible. It is recognized that health care is at a crossroad in Latvia. The entire system of health care is being reorganized and consolidated from the previous Soviet political and health system, which emphasized hospitalization rather than primary care.

Ethnic/Race Specific or Endemic Diseases: Because of the poor quality of the industrial air, childhood asthma is a serious health risk. Hepatitis, tuberculosis, diphtheria, tick-borne encephalitis, endemic goiter, and nutritional deficits are significant health concerns. The World Health Organization's (WHO) estimated prevalence rate for HIV/AIDS in adults ages 15 to 49 years is 0.011%. The estimated number of children from birth to 15 years living with HIV/AIDS is less than 100.

Health Team Relationships: Before Latvia broke away from the Soviet bloc, the word *nursing* had no meaning, doctors directed all activities and were not questioned, and people could not differentiate between medicine and nursing. Patients still receive very few medical explanations, and "consent" is not a recognized concept. Bribes to doctors may allow people to obtain commodities that otherwise would not be available. Older people view health care professionals as either all-knowing or incompetent. Younger patients question health care providers and seek out better care if warranted, even if they have to go to a private clinic. Doctors and nurses are referred to by title.

Families' Role in Hospital Care: Caring for hospitalized family members is not a cultural phenomenon—it is imperative if a patient is to survive a hospital stay. Little food is provided by the hospital, and patients must obtain their medications elsewhere. During a lengthy hospital stay, patients go home on Saturdays to take a bath. Families provide linens and often clean hospital rooms themselves.

Dominance Patterns: Traditionally, men have a slightly more dominant role, but the women make most of the decisions. Husbands and wives both work, and women are responsible for the household, children, food shopping, and food preparation.

Eye Contact Practices: Direct eye contact is necessary when discussing serious matters.

Touch Practices: Touch is uncommon even within families. A handshake between males is common at the beginning and end of an interaction and between both sexes in professional situations.

Perceptions of Time: Latvians practice present-oriented crisis management in the health care setting. Past traditions, including how older adults have healed illnesses, are important. Little emphasis is placed on health promotion or prevention. Younger people are beginning to prepare for the future, whereas the older generation expects to be cared for by the young.

Pain Reactions: Patients who are terminally ill may not be provided with pain medications because of the scarcity of supplies. Bearing pain in silence is considered admirable.

Birth Rites: Almost all births occur in hospitals and include doctors and possibly a midwife, who may or may not be a nurse. Few fathers choose to be present during delivery and are not encouraged to coach labor. Courses for natural childbirth and prenatal and postpartum care are available. The semiseated position is common for delivery. Circumcision is not practiced.

Death Rites: If an illness is fatal, the family is told first, and they then decide whether the patient should be told. Traditionally, funerals are not sad times. Singing and laughing are common and after the funeral, family and friends have a large, happy party.

Food Practices and Intolerances: Traditionally, the preferred main meal has been lunch but because of modern-day working schedules, it is now the evening meal. Potatoes, seasonal vegetables, bread, meat, and soups are common. Great quantities of milk and other dairy products, tea, coffee, and alcohol are consumed. Meat is considered an essential part of the diet, especially for males.

Infant Feeding Practices: Breast-feeding is encouraged more than bottle-feeding, but many women state that they do not produce enough breast milk. Food is introduced at 4 to 5 months.

Child Rearing Practices: Children are cooperative and reared using disciplinary styles ranging from logical reasoning to authoritarian rule. Fathers may be very involved or detached. Both parents usually work, and many families are headed by single mothers. The grandmother often takes care of her grandchildren. Women are entitled to maternity leave at 32 weeks gestation and may continue until the child is 3 years old. Maternity leave wages are only a percentage of a woman's regular rate; therefore many women choose to return to work earlier

National Childhood Immunizations: BCG at birth; DPT at 3, 4?, 6, and 18 months; OPV at 18 months and at 7 and 14 years; hep B at birth and at 1 and 6 to 8 months; IPV at 3, 4?, and 6 months; MR at 15 months and 7 years; rubella at 15 months and 12 years; DT at 7 years; and Td at 14 years.

BIBLIOGRAPHY

Kalnins I: Pioneers in academia: higher education for nurses in Estonia, Latvia, and Lithuania, *Nurs Outlook* 43(2):84, 1995.

Kalnins I, Barkauskas VH, Seskevicius A: Baccalaureate nursing education development in two Baltic countries: outcomes 10 years after initiation, *Nurs Outlook* 49(3):142-7, 2001.

Kalnins ZGP: Nursing in Latvia from the perspective of oppressed theory, *J Transcultural Nurs* 3(1):11, 1992.

Nadisauskiene RJ, Padaiga Z: Changes in women's health in the Baltic republics of Lithuania, Latvia and Estonia during 1970-1997, *Int J Gynaecol Obstet* 70(1):199-206, 2000.

Priede-Kalnins Z: Latvia: nursing reborn, *Nurs Health Care* 16(3):148, 1995.

Priede-Kalnins Z: Oppression's influence on behavior: first hand impressions, *J Cult Diversity* 2(3):83, 1995.

Van Damme P: Hepatitis B: vaccination programmes in Europe-an update, *Vaccine* 19(17-19):2375-9, 2001.

♦ LEBANON (LEBANESE REPUBLIC)

MAP PAGE (864)

Salim M. Adib and Ismat Fayez Mikkey

Location: Lebanon is a parliamentarian republic on the eastern shore of the Mediterranean Sea. It is bordered by Syria to the north and east and by Israel to the south. Lebanon has a total land area of 10,452 km² (4000 square miles). The country is 215 km (134 miles) long, and from east to west the distance ranges from 25 to 90 km (16 to 56 miles). A long and narrow coastal plain runs parallel to the Mediterranean and is overshadowed by the Lebanon Mountains, which culminate at 3088 m (with the highest point in the Middle East). Another mountain range, the Anti-Lebanon Mountains, runs parallel to the Lebanon range and creates a natural border with neighboring Syria. Between the two mountain ranges is a fertile plateau, the Bekaa Valley.

Major Languages	Ethnic Groups	Major Religions
Arabic (official)	Arab 95%	Muslim 70%
French	Armenian 4%	Christian, other 30%
Armenian	Other 1%	
English		

Health Care Beliefs: Acute sick care; traditional. The Lebanese generally understand and accept the biological mechanisms of health and disease. However, if pressed, many still attribute disease at least partly to the "evil eye" of jealous acquaintances (the power of people to harm others merely by looking at them), exposure to cold air or water, or the wrong food combinations. In addition to modern drugs, the Lebanese still widely believe in the virtues of wild herbal concoctions from the mountains. Years of civil war and Israeli occupation (from 1975 to 2000) have resulted in massive destruction to the country's infrastructure, including its health care system. In accordance with the liberal *laissez-faire* philosophy of Lebanon, the country has no national health policy. Health is largely a private sector industry, and the reconstruction of the health care facilities has largely been conducted by private organizations. Obtaining health care is now very expensive for most people in Lebanon. The role of government is limited to operating a few small dispensaries and clinics. The government also attempts, at increasingly greater costs and with decreasing success, to provide the uninsured citizens from lower socioeconomic levels subsidized access to private health care. In 2000, more than 80% of the budget of the Ministry of Public Health was used to subsidize private hospitals for treatment of patients who could not afford health care expenses. The relative youth of the Lebanese public and their health awareness from better education have thus far prevented the country from facing unusual and uncontrollable public health problems. However, current neglect of environmental problems such as air, water, and marine pollution, in addition to the gradual aging of the population, may lead to some major health issues in the coming years.

Predominant Sick Care Practices: Biomedical and magical-religious. The majority of citizens live in major cities and are unlikely to consult traditional healers or wear amulets as a first option for treatment. Such people tend to seek health care professionals' help as their primary choice. However, people from rural areas who have less access to modern care may decide to use available traditional practices. Despite their large reliance on modern medicine, the Lebanese are superstitious and prefer to ensure additional "heavenly" support for their health problems. Couples struggling with infertility consult a doctor for medical advice and a religious person *(sheikh)* for amulets. Lebanese Christians (and many non-Christians) visit shrines of the Virgin Mary and other saints and make vows to offer alms or other gifts if they are healed.

Ethnic/Race Specific or Endemic Diseases: No particular diseases are reportable in Lebanon. Acute diarrheal diseases caused by contaminated food and water are common in the summer. Travelers need to be cautious when eating or drinking, especially the further they are from Beirut. The main causes of death in Lebanon are cardiovascular diseases and cancer, as they are almost everywhere except in the poorest nations, where infectious diseases are still the major killers. Regarding infectious diseases, leishmaniasis still persists at a low level, mostly in the rural northern region of Akkar bordering Syria. Brucellosis persists as an endemic disease in the Bekaa, where unpasteurized milk and dairy products are consumed directly after they are produced. Lebanon shares with other Mediterranean populations a higher prevalence of some genetic diseases including thalassemia and glucose-6-phosphate dehydrogenase (G6PD) deficiency. Lebanese have higher rates of familial Mediterranean fever than do people in other countries, and it is most often diagnosed in Armenian families. Approximately 6% of about 70,000 newborns per year have minor or major congenital problems. This prevalence is also higher than the worldwide level of 1% to 2%, most likely because of higher numbers of consanguineous marriages in the more traditional rural areas. HIV and AIDS are still rare, and it is estimated that fewer than 5000 have become infected since the beginning of the National AIDS Program in 1984. The World Health Organization's (WHO) estimated prevalence rate for HIV/AIDS in adults ages 15 to 49 is 0.09%.

Health Team Relationships: The health care system is still largely male dominated, and patient-doctor relationships are still marked by paternalism. Doctors are dominant in doctor-nurse relationships, and nurse-doctor interactions are very limited, occurring during rounds (in the morning and evening) or when nurses are calling a doctor to discuss a patient.

Families' Role in Hospital Care: During hospital admission, many of the close relatives accompany patients to mitigate their uncertainties and worries and occasionally answer questions for the patients. When visiting hospitalized friends, visitors usually bring chocolate or flowers. Close relatives who stay most of the day with a patient show their hospitality to visitors by serving them coffee or candy.

Dominance Patterns: The Arab countries are known as having male-dominated societies. Although the father is usually the head of the family and its breadwinner, most of today's mothers work. Even in rural areas, informal work of women—tending to the farm animals and maintaining crops—is very valued as men try to obtain formal employment, often away from home. Caring for children whose mothers are working is the responsibility of the child's grandmother; however, this practice is becoming rare as more and more couples move away to start nuclear families. Extended families are becoming the exception rather than the norm. Many urban couples rely on nurseries or on inexpensive domestic servants from Southeast Asia or East Africa to care for small children while both parents are busy earning a living. Women in Lebanon have equal rights, including the right to vote. Women currently have only three seats in the parliament (of 128 seats), but more women have begun competing in the open election process. The civil code for marriage and inheritance varies depending on the declared religious affiliation of the individual; therefore Lebanese citizens must be affiliated with a legal religious group. Men and women intermingle in daily life and are largely free to choose their spouses. Nevertheless, up to 20% of marriages are still consanguineous, mostly among first-degree cousins in the more rural parts of the country. All marriages in Lebanon must be performed by a religious minister; however, civil marriages of Lebanese citizens performed outside Lebanon are duly registered in the country, allowing couples from different religious backgrounds to marry without having either one of the spouses change their religion. Public demands for civil marriages to be performed in Lebanon have been increasing lately. Like all other Arab countries, Lebanon does not automatically grant Lebanese nationality to non-Lebanese men who marry Lebanese women, but it does for non-Lebanese women who marry Lebanese men. All modern behaviors and dress codes are acceptable and common in and around Beirut but may be increasingly less acceptable in areas further away. Modest dress is recommended in the traditional parts of the country and is particularly important when visiting mosques and other religious places. The ethnically and religiously diverse Lebanese people are generally friendly and hospitable.

Eye Contact Practices: People from the Middle East who are of the same gender are likely to stand quite close to each other (less than 18 inches apart). A wider distance is kept during male-female encounters, but this is less true in the more central areas of Lebanon.

Touch Practices: Although public displays of affection are not generally accepted, they do occur in Lebanon and are generally tolerated. Young couples may engage in intense displays of affection on campuses, on the beach, and in nightclubs—mostly in urban areas. Recently, some Muslims who are adopting more religiously conservative attitudes have been avoiding shaking hands with strangers of the opposite sex.

Perceptions of Time: In Lebanon, people are expected to arrive at their appointments on time, although the congested urban traffic may not always allow them to do so. Like all Arabs, the Lebanese like to begin their meetings with numerous social niceties. They serve tea or coffee and inquire about the health and family of others before getting down to business. Ignoring those social rules may occasionally be perceived as rude and inconsiderate.

Pain Reactions: Pain reactions in Lebanon cannot be specifically characterized, although men may be less vocal than women.

Birth Rites: The fertility rate in Lebanon is the second lowest in the Arab world (after that of Tunisia), with 2.8 children born per female of reproductive age. When a mother gives birth, her relatives, friends, and neighbors visit to congratulate her and give her gifts, which are usually baby items. Today, most births in Lebanon occur in hospitals, and the average period of hospital stay is about 3 to 4 days. Many families now offer visitors boxes of sugar-coated almonds to mark the "sweetness" of the event. Traditionally, the sweetness was emphasized by serving a special semolina pudding heaped with dry coconut and nuts *(moghli)*. Most males are circumcised because it is part of the culture and for cleanliness reasons. Most families prefer to circumcise their male infants during the first week of age, but others might postpone it for many years. Many Christians, who do not have to circumcise males for religious reasons (as Muslims do), still chose to do so. During the postpartum 40-day period, Muslim mothers are not allowed to perform religious rituals (pray, fast during Ramadan), and sexual intercourse is prohibited until she has no remaining postpartum vaginal discharge. For Christian families, baptism is a corollary to birth. The religious ceremony generally takes place between 3 months and 1 year of age and is attended by friends and family members. A dinner, which may be fairly lavish and elaborate, is usually offered after the baptism.

Death Rites: Donation of human organs is allowed under Lebanese law, and all dead bodies must be buried and cannot be cremated. Autopsy is permitted if ordered by a judge for legal reasons or recommended by doctors and allowed by the family members. Soon after the death of a Muslim, the body is washed and wrapped in a white cloth, taken by male relatives and friends to the mosque for prayer, and then buried without a coffin in the cemetery. Christians have no washing rituals. Prayers are recited at churches by both sexes, but only men are expected to go with the coffin to the burial grounds. Cemeteries are all administered by religious denominations; therefore all deceased Lebanese must be identified as part of a denomination to be buried. Loud expressions of sorrow and grief are acceptable from male and female relatives alike. Relatives of the deceased person go back to the person's home and accept condolences for 3 days. During these days, most people serve traditional sugar-free coffee as a sign of sadness for the deceased, but they occasionally serve snacks and soft drinks at meal times and during hot summers. Christians in Lebanon invite friends and relatives to a remembrance ceremony marking the fortieth day after death, after which it is acceptable to forgo the black ties and dresses of the grieving period. Some women, especially those in the mountain villages, may chose to wear black dresses for the rest of their lives to mark their status as widows.

Food Practices and Intolerances: The staple food in Lebanon is wheat, which is eaten in breads and as cracked, grilled wheat *(borghoul)* in various foods. The cuisine relies heavily on vegetables, grains, and lamb meat. Lebanese food has become famous in Lebanese restaurants started by the diaspora all over the world. Some well-known dishes include *hummus,* a dip consisting of mashed chickpeas and sesame butter with lemon, garlic, and olive oil; *fatoush*, a pita bread salad seasoned with lemony summac herbs and olive oil; and *tabbouleh,* a parsley-mint salad with *borghoul*. Lebanese cuisine has now become part of a larger Middle Eastern cuisine that is found with slight local variants throughout that part of the world. For a quick breakfast, many Lebanese buy oven-baked *manakish* pies covered with *zaatar* (a mix of oregano or thyme, sesame, and sumac) and olive oil. At a typical restaurant meal in Lebanon, the *mezza,* a large version of small vegetarian and meat-based dishes, is served first so that it can be slowly enjoyed with the local drink, *arak*. *Arak* is an alcoholic drink of distilled grapes with a hint of anise, which may remind some of the French *pastis* or Greek *ouzo*. The main course may consist of grilled skewered chicken and lamb or other more elaborate dishes. Desserts include Arabic sweets and the fresh fruits for which Lebanon is famous in the Middle East. Food is often scooped using pieces of pita bread. The *narghileh* (water pipe) may be smoked with or after meals by both sexes; it has been a tradition since the Ottoman nineteenth century. All types of specialized and ethnic restaurants are found in Beirut today. Lebanon has no food or alcohol restrictions whatsoever.

Infant Feeding Practices: The majority of women prefer to breast-feed their infants.

Child Rearing Practices: Lebanon has no specifically Lebanese child rearing practices. Practices vary widely by socioeconomic levels; children in rural areas have more outdoor freedom than those in urban areas, where parks and leisure spaces are almost nonexistent.

National Childhood Immunizations: DPT at 2, 3, 4, at 15 to 18 months and at 4 to 6 and 10 to 12 years; OPV at 2, 3, 4, and 15 to 18 months and at 4 to 6 and 10 to 12 years; hep B at birth and at 1 and 4 months; MMR at 9 to 10 and 15 to 18 months and at 5 to 6 years; and DT at 6 to 8 and 10 to 12 years. BCG is no longer included in the vaccination program, which is different from neighboring countries in which the disease is still endemic.

Other Characteristics: The population of Lebanon is estimated to be approximately 4 million, of which about 300,000 are Palestinian refugees primarily from the 1948 war. Lebanon is one of the most pluralistic countries of the Arab world. Its population, composed of a mixture of Christians and Muslims, has historically been a cultural bridge between East and West. The Christian Maronite *(Marooni)* and the Muslim Druze *(Durzi)* communities are groups that are primarily specific to Lebanon. These communities compose the historical mountain core from which the modern Republic of Lebanon has emerged. Lebanon has one of the best education systems in the Middle East, with a general literacy rate of more than 85%, one of the highest in the Arab world. Beirut and its surrounding coastal and mountain areas are sociologically cosmopolitan, where Arabic culture blends with Western influences, primarily French and American.

BIBLIOGRAPHY

Adib SM, Hamadeh GN: Attitudes regarding disclosure of serious illness in the Lebanese public, *J Med Ethics* 25:399–403, 1999.

Ammar W, Jokhadar A, Awar M: Health sector reform in Lebanon, *J Med Liban* 46(6):328, 1998.

Beydoun MA: Marital fertility in Lebanon: a study based on the population andhousing survey, *Soc Sci Med* 53(6):759, 2001.

Farhood LF: Testing a model of family stress and coping based on war and non-war stressors, family resources and coping among Lebanese families, *Arch Psychiatr Nurs* 13(4):192, 1999.

Hamadeh GN, Adib SM: Cancer truth disclosure by Lebanese doctors, *Soc Sci Med* 47(9):1289, 1998.

Hamadeh GN, Adib SM: Changes in attitudes regarding cancer disclosure among medical students at the American University of Beirut, *J Med Ethics* 27:354, 2001.

Kandela P: Lebanese medicine—still struggling against the odds, *Lancet* 355(9207):907, 2000.

Kabakian-Khasholian T et al: Women's experiences of medical care: satisfaction or passivity, *Soc Sci Med* 51(1):103, 2000.

Littlewood R: Social institutions and psychological explanations: Druze reincarnation as a therapeutic resource, *Br J Med Psychol* 74(pt 2):213, 2001.

Sidani YM, Gardner WL: Work values among Lebanese workers, *J Soc Psychol* 140(5):597, 2000.

◆ LESOTHO (KINGDOM OF)

MAP PAGE (863)

Location: Lesotho is landlocked and completely surrounded by South African territory. The country consists of high plateaus, hills, and mountains, and more than 80% of the country is 1800 m above sea level. The climate is temperate, with cool or cold, dry winters and hot, wet summers. In winter, snow often closes mountain passes, and temperatures often drop below freezing at night, even in the lowlands. The majority of the people live in rural areas, and some can be reached only on horseback or by airplane. The total land area is 30,350 km^2 (11,718 square miles), slightly smaller than Maryland, and the capital is Maseru. The total population is 2,143,141, and population pressures are forcing settlements in marginal areas, resulting in overgrazing and soil erosion. The gross domestic product per capita is $2400.

Major Languages	Ethnic Groups	Major Religions
English (official)	Sotho 99.7%	Christian 80%
Sesotho (official)	Other 0.3%	Indigenous beliefs 20%
Zulu		
Xhosa		

Health Care Beliefs: Acute sick care only, usually in the form of crisis care, with prevention a low priority. Although the government has attempted to promote primary health care, political unrest and social instability have done great damage to the health infrastructure. Lesotho has an urgent need for health promotion activities at all levels. Because of poor sanitary conditions, diarrheal diseases in infants and children are a major cause of morbidity and mortality, and efforts have been made to teach mothers how to perform oral rehydration therapy at home. This practice has had some limited success. Rural communities often have numerous individuals with undiagnosed HIV infection or AIDS and other sexually transmitted diseases, combined with very little knowledge of high-risk sexual behavior. For example, in one study, 11.6% of the women and 38% of the men had had sex during the previous several months with a person who was not their regular partner; none had used condoms. Studies of dam construction workers revealed noise-induced hearing loss in 92%, and 5.4% had developed pneumoconiosis from chemicals and dust. Health and safety are low priorities in this country because of the daily struggle for survival.

Predominant Sick Care Practices: Biomedical when available and traditional. People consider biomedical treatment to be effective. Hospitals are the highest level of care and located in urban areas; rural areas are serviced by health centers and frequently staffed by village health workers. When people are ill, they usually try to reach a hospital because they believe they will receive higher quality care, a practice that has overloaded urban hospitals. To address this the Ministry of Health developed advanced health centers that were meant to be an intermediate level between the two facilities. Although this has relieved some of the congestion in health centers, costs seem to be as high as they are in the hospital. In general, medical facilities are minimal, and many medications are unavailable. Lesotho has no reliable emergency or ambulances services. Good medical care can be obtained in Bloemfontein, South Africa, which is 90 miles west of Maseru. Magical-religious and traditional systems of care are also used in Lesotho with traditional healers and herbalists. Water extracts, primarily from boiling the roots of medicinal plants (usually found at high altitudes), are often effective for various complaints. For example, bulbine narcissifolia is used to heal wounds and as a mild purgative. Studies of medicinal plants used by healers and herbalists indicate that these plants have true healing qualities, such as moderate to very high antibacterial activity against gram-positive and gram-negative bacteria.

Ethnic/Race Specific or Endemic Diseases: Endemic diseases include schistosomiasis, typhoid, hepatitis A, and rabies. The people are at risk for acute respiratory tract infections, pneumonia, tuberculosis, and diarrhea (in children). In 1989, there was an outbreak of diphtheria in older children and adults in Lesotho; the younger people were most likely to die. Tap water is not reliably potable and is therefore a source of disease. Because of intertribal hostility and the widespread use of alcohol and cannabinoid drugs, violence-related injuries are very common and put a strain (in addition to HIV/AIDS) on the health care system. Lesotho also has numerous automobile-related deaths given the small size of the country. In the 1980s, Lesotho seemed to be somewhat protected from the HIV epidemic. The virus is, however, spreading rapidly to neighboring villages near construction projects, especially with the influx of migrant construction workers from other areas. The World Health Organization's (WHO) estimated prevalence rate for HIV/AIDS in adults ages 15 to 49 is very high: 23.57%. About 240,000 adults and children are living with HIV/AIDS. The estimated number of children from birth to 15 years living with HIV/AIDS is 8200. The estimated number of adults and children who died of AIDS in 1999 is 16,000, and the number of currently living children who lost either their mother or both parents to AIDS is 29,469.

Health Team Relationships: In the rural areas the village chief is the leader and helps people make health care changes and decisions. Primarily, hospital aids perform nursing care.

Families' Role in Hospital Care: The socioeconomic conditions make it imperative for relatives to participate in the care of their family members when they are in a hospital. Traditional birth attendants deliver many infants in rural areas, but many of them have little knowledge of aseptic technique and how to handle emergency situations. The maternal mortality rate was reported to be 610 deaths per 100,000 live births in 1990. The Ministry of Health has made efforts to provide midwifery education in the form of "Safe Motherhood" modules.

Dominance Patterns: As in many developing countries, women are not men's equals. They are considered minors culturally and depend on their husbands for economic survival. The cultural position of women in regard to alcoholic beverages facilitates a vicious cycle. They women usually brew and sell the alcohol, and they then often struggle with alcoholism themselves as they cope with drinking husbands. Although men can drink without censure, husbands can divorce their wives for drinking—a disastrous consequence for a woman. Unusual for African countries, literacy rates are higher for women (93%) than men (72%).

Infant Feeding Practices: Interviews with women in Lesotho indicate that although breast-feeding is central to the culture, exclusive breast-feeding is almost an unknown concept and rarely ever practiced. Complementary feedings are introduced very early in the infant's life, which reduces the amount of breast milk (and nutrition) they receive and gives them an irregular diet of milk and other protein-rich foods. Contemporary mothers also routinely give water to very young infants, often because nurses suggest it. Another major problem is that water is a potential reservoir for pathogens. Fewer than 5% of the people in many areas use latrines or know how to maintain a clean water supply. In one survey, mothers reported that about 18% of the children who were 5 or younger had recently had an episode of diarrheal illness. Apparently the pattern of early supplementation is a newer trend, because the grandmothers stated they breast-fed more than their daughters, although not exclusively; and only occasionally gave their infants a thin gruel. The grandmothers also correctly thought it was important to feed a child with diarrhea, which contrasts with more current beliefs about limiting food for those with diarrhea. The total fertility rate is 4.08 children born per woman, and the birth rate is 31.24 births per 1000 people. The infant mortality rate is 82.77 deaths per 1000 live births.

Child Rearing Practices: About 40% of the population is 14 years old or younger. Corporal punishment is common in schools, causing academic impairment, physical injuries, and psychological damage. Studies of rural children 15 years and younger show stunting, a sign of chronic under-nutrition, even within the first year of life, and the prevalence of iodine-deficiency goiter is 18%. Many of the health problems of children stem from a lack of resources in the home. Although statutes in the region state that a man must support his legitimate and illegitimate children, weaknesses in the law make it hard to enforce. Women are also unaware of the law or are afraid of being physically abused or receiving other forms of retribution if they address the issue. A network of women who study women's legal rights in Lesotho is attempting to enforce the laws more effectively because they believe that if the financial burden is shared by both parents, men will have a financial stake in controlling women's fertility.

National Childhood Immunizations: BCG at birth; DTP at 6, 10, and 14 weeks; OPV at birth and 6, 10, and 14 weeks; measles at 9 and 18 months; DT at 18 months; and TT for pregnant women, +4 weeks, +6 months, +1, +1 year. The reported percentages of the target population vaccinated are as follows: third dose of DTP, 69, and Pol3, 67.

Other Characteristics: Lesotho experienced significant civil unrest in 1998, but relative stability has returned. However, the deteriorating economic conditions threaten the health and safety of the population.

BIBLIOGRAPHY

Almroth S, Mohale M, Latham MC: Unnecessary water supplementation for babies: grandmothers blame clinics, *Acta Paediatr* 89(12):1408, 2000.

Aarmstrong A: Maintenance payments for child support in Southern Africa: using law to promote family planning, *Stud Family Plann* 23(4):217, 1992.

Colvin M et al: Health and safety in the Lesotho Highlands Dam and Tunnel Construction Program, *Int J Occup Environ Health* 4(4):231, 1998.

Colvin M, Sharp B: Sexually transmitted infections and HIV in a rural community in the Lesotho highlands, *Sex Transm Infec* 76(1):39, 2000.

Jooste PL et al: Nutritional status of rural children in the Lesotho highlands, *East Afr Med J* 74(11):680, 1997.

Kravitz JD et al: Quantitative bacterial examination of domestic water supplies in the Lesotho highlands: water quality, sanitation and village health, *Bull WHO* 77(10):829, 1999.

Mphi M: Female alcoholism problems in Lesotho, *Addiction* 89(8):945, 1994.

Monyooe LA: Perspective reports of corporal punishment by pupils in Lesotho schools, *Psychol Rep* 73(2):515, 1993.

Pepperall J et al: Hospital of health center? A comparison of the costs and quality of urban outpatient services in Maseru, Lesotho, *Int J Health Plann Mngmnt* 10(1):59, 1995.

Shale TL, Stirk WA, van-Staden J: Screening of medicinal plants sued in Lesotho for anti-bacterial and anti-inflammatory activity, *J Ethnopharm* 67(3):347, 1999.

Touchette P et al: An analysis of home-based oral rehydration therapy in the Kingdom of Lesotho, *Soc Sci Med* 39(3):425, 1994.

Quotsokoane-Lusunzi MA, Karuso P: Secondary metabolites from Basotho medicinal plants. I. Bulbine narcissifolia, *J Natural Prod* 64(10): 1368, 2001.

Touchette P et al.: An analysis of home-based oral rehydration therapy in the Kingdom of Lesotho, *Soc Sci Med* 39(3):425, 1994.

http://www.odci.gov/cia/publications/factbook/geos/lt.html

http://travel.state.gov/lesotho.html

◆ LIBERIA (REPUBLIC OF)

MAP PAGE (862)

Location: Liberia is located on the Atlantic coast of southwestern Africa, with Sierra Leone and Guinea to the north, Cote d'Ivoire to the east, and the Atlantic Ocean to the south and west. It is mostly flat, with rolling coastal plains rising to rolling plateau and low mountains. Much of the country is covered with dense tropical forests that experience a heavy annual rainfall. The climate is tropical—hot and humid, with dry winters that have hot days and cool or cold nights and wet, cloudy summers with frequent rain. The total land area is 111,370 km² (43,000 square miles), slightly larger than Tennessee. Monrovia is the capital. The total population is 3,225,837. Liberia is a developing country in which 70% of the population works in agriculture. The gross domestic product (GDP) per capita is $1100, and 80% of the population is below the poverty line.

Major Languages	Ethnic Groups	Major Religions
English (official)	African 95%	Indigenous 40%
African languages	Americo-Liberian 2.5%	Christian 40%
	Congo people 2.5%	Muslim 20%

Most of the population is made up of indigenous people including Kpelle, Bassa, Gio, Kru, Grebo, Mano, Krahn, Gola, Gbandi, Loma, Kissi, Vai, and Bella. About 2.5% are descendents of repatriated slaves known as Americo-Liberians, and 2.5% are descendents of immigrants from the Caribbean who had been slaves. African languages include more than 20 languages of the Niger-Congo group.

Health Care Beliefs: Acute sick care; ethno-medical beliefs predominate. Health promotion efforts are frequently unsuccessful because of the social and economic problems of the country. For example, efforts to promote the home use of a sugar and salt solution to prevent dehydration in children with diarrhea have been minimally effective. Traditional ethno-medical views tend to predominate. Notions of sorcery, witchcraft, or taboo violations are often expressed as the etiology of diseases such as sexually transmitted diseases. Mental illness is attributed to supernatural forces and thought to be best treated by traditional healers. People with epilepsy are shunned and discriminated against in educational environments, employment arenas, and marriage because the disease is considered highly contagious and shameful. Liberia has a high prevalence of epilepsy; parasitic infections, particularly neurocysticercosis, are important etiological factors.

Predominant Sick Care Practices: Traditional and biomedical when available. Hospitals and medical facilities are poorly equipped and incapable of providing even basic services. Medications are scarce and unavailable in most areas. Health care expenditures constitute a major part of domestic spending, particularly for those seeking Western health. Traditional healers handle many cases of serious diseases such as HIV and AIDS. Treatments usually comprise decoctions from the leaves and roots of medicinal herb plants. They are usually administered as teas but may also be given as enemas or vaginal implants during a 2- to 4-day period.

Ethnic/Race Specific or Endemic Diseases: Endemic diseases include falciparum malaria (which is hyperendemic), cholera, schistosomiasis, onchocerciasis *(sowda),* meningitis, neurocysticercosis, polio, Lassa fever, and hepatitis A and B. Liberians are also at risk for Shigella infection, typhoid fever, leprosy, yellow fever and severe malnutrition. Liberia has had cholera and Ebola virus outbreaks. Dust-laden harmattan winds blow in from the Sahara Desert from December to March, causing episodes of respiratory illness. Vehicular travel is hazardous and traffic accidents are a common cause of death and disability. Liberians also have high rates of sexually transmitted diseases. The World Health Organization's (WHO) estimated prevalence rate for HIV/AIDS in adults ages 15 to 49 is 2.8%. The estimated number of children from birth to 15 years living with HIV/AIDS is 2000. The estimated number of children and adults who have died since the beginning of the epidemic is 34,000, and 4500 died in 1999. Liberia currently has 20,337 living orphans. HIV transmission is primarily through sexual intercourse; a major co-factor is the presence of other sexually transmitted diseases.

Families' Role in Hospital Care: Tradition dictates that the family accompanies the patient to the hospital and takes care of cooking and laundry; however, centralized hospital services are the current trend.

Dominance Patterns: Transactions for major health care expenditures are usually handled by the men, using their own personal income and whatever belongs to the couple. Women are more likely to spend their personal income on treating the more minor health conditions affecting themselves and their children. Dominance differences exist among different villages and groups. For example, Kpelle wives have input into most financial decisions but defer to men on issues of Western health care and educational expenditures. Physical and sexual violence against women (estimated to be more than 50%) was documented during the civil war.

Birth Rites: The traditional midwife is valued and active in rural Liberia; however, maternal mortality is very high. The infant mortality rate is also high: 132.42 deaths per 1000 live births. Widespread premarital sex and lack of contraception results in illegal abortions, pregnancy-related school dropout, and the potential for sexually transmitted disease transmission, including HIV. The birth rate is 46.55 births per 1000 people, and the total fertility rate is 6.36 children born per woman. Life expectancy at birth is 49.96 for men and 52.91 for women.

Food Practices and Intolerances: Food shortages have been problematic because of continuing social upheaval.

Infant Feeding Practices: Some parents may strongly believe that Western medicine's pills or injections can cure severe malnutrition in children.

Child Rearing Practices: Female circumcision and excision is widespread among some groups. As many as a third of all children die before their fifth birthday. Targeted child survival programs are helping reduce these numbers. Literacy rates are 53.9% for males and 22.4% for females; these figures are gradually improving as a result of improving school systems.

National Childhood Immunizations: BCG at birth; DTP at 6, 10, and 14 weeks; OPV at birth and 6, 10, and 14 weeks; measles at 9 months; vitamin A at 9 months for infants and BCG, OPV0 or DTP1 for postpartum women; YFV 6 months and every 10 years; and TT every 14 years, +1, +6 months, +1, +1 year. The reported percentages of the target population vaccinated are as follows: BCG, 45; third dose of DTP, 48; MCV, 52; Pol3, 52; TT2 plus, 25; and vitamin A, 26.

Other Characteristics: A devastating civil war ended in 1997. Civil unrest continues, despite slow infrastructure restructuring. Thousands of displaced persons were reported in the cities in 2002, and many thousands have become refugees in the Republic of Guinea. Law and order is still considered very limited. Liberia is becoming a more common transshipment point for heroin from Southeast and Southwest Asia and cocaine from South America that is bound for European and U.S. markets.

BIBLIOGRAPHY

Becker SR, Thornton JN, Holder W: Infant and child mortality estimates in two counties of Liberia: 1984, *Int J Epidemiol* 22(suppl 1):42, 1993.

David S: Health expenditure and household budgets in rural Liberia, *Health Trans Rev* 3(1):57, 1993.

Gage AJ, Meekers D: Sexual activity before marriage in sub-Saharan Africa, *Soc Biol* 41(1-2):44, 1994.

Green EC: The anthropology of sexually transmitted disease in Liberia, *Soc Sci Med* 35(12):1457, 1992.

Long N: Meals distributed in Liberia, *Front Lines* 32(5):7, 1992.

Parr NJ: Pre-marital fertility in Liberia, *J Biosoc Sci* 27(1):1, 1995.

Rosemergy I, Robinson J: Suffer the little ones, *NZ Nurs J* 84(4):18, 1991.

Swiss S et al: Violence against women during the Liberian civil conflict, *JAMA* 279(8):625, 1998.

Wright J: Female genital mutilation: an overview, *J Adv Nurs* 24:251, 1996.

http://www.odci.gov/cia/publicaations/factbook/geos/li.html

http://travel.state.gov/liberia.html

◆ LIBYA (LIBYAN ARAB JAMAHIRIYA)

MAP PAGE (862)

Suher M. Aburawi

Location: Libya, located almost at the center of northern Africa, has a total land area of about 1,750,000 km² (675,500 square miles) (about the size of Alaska), with a northern coast of about 2000 km on the Mediterranean. The land spans more than 1600 km (994 miles) from east to west and north to south. Therefore climatic conditions vary from a mild Mediterranean climate along the coast to an extremely dry desert interior. The terrain is mainly low lying, with hilly regions in the northeast and northwest and the Tibesti Mountains in the south.

Major Languages	Ethnic Groups	Major Religions
Arabic (official)	Berber and Arab 97%	Sunni Muslim 97%
English	Other 3%	Other 3%

Approximately 3% of the population is made up of Greeks, Maltese, Italians, Egyptians, Pakistanis, Turks, Indians, and Tunisians, most of whom are expatriate workers. The Libyan population is about 5,000,000. Arab Berbers (or Berber Arabs) make up most of the population. (The ethnic distinction is unclear.) Historically, the original Berbers of northern Africa assimilated Romans, Greeks, Arabs, and Copts, and in modern history many population movements brought people from Crete and Turkey. It is hard today to distinguish whether a person has Arab or Berber ancestors, and it could be assumed that ethnic differences related to health conditions, practices, and attitudes are negligible. However, two small ethnic groups are distinct from the majority of the population—the

Tuareg, who live in the southwest and frequently move between Libya, Algeria, and Niger, and the Tabu tribes in Tibesti. Differences between the Tuareg or the Tabu and the rest of the population in terms of endemic diseases or susceptibility to diseases are not known. Arabic is spoken by almost everyone. Old Hamitic languages are also being used by a small percentage of the population in the northwest hilly region and among the Tuareg and Tabu tribes. English is widely used for activities relating to health care and technology (with drug prescriptions and medical records being written in English), and it is practically the second language in business, industry, and tourism. Almost 100% of the population, excluding expatriate workers, is Sunni Muslim.

Health Care Beliefs: Acute sick care; folk medicine. To Libyans, folk medicine is synonymous with herbal medicine. Herbal medicine is considered primary health care in mild cases of illness with generally known etiologies, especially for treatment of symptoms such as stomachaches, diarrhea, coughs, or spasms. The choice of herbs depends on previous evidence of success. In the rare cases in which medical practitioners fail to provide a cure, people seek out herbal medicine. Some reports indicate that diseases such as asthma, nephrolithiasis (kidney stones), some tumors, and hypertension are being effectively treated with herbs. Public awareness of psychotherapy has yet to emerge. Seeing a psychoanalyst is embarrassing and rare and is done with complete discretion. (The general mindset is that "only a crack would go to a shrink.") In the very rare cases when professional medical practitioners cannot provide a remedy, people may seek out supernatural treatments for psychological and physical ailments. Reading the Koran is generally believed to provide people with the strength to resist physical and psychological ailments and help in recovery; however, few would make that choice. Some, although very few, still use amulets for protection from malicious acts involving spirits or spells, but their use is kept secret from police for fear of prosecution. During private conversations, people mention hearsay reports about the successes and failures of amulets. Self-prescribing treatments for illness is common to either save time or money, and individuals in pharmacies may make suggestions as well. Antibiotics are practically sold as over-the-counter drugs, although all believe this should not be done.

Predominant Sick Care Practices: Biomedical and magical-religious. Free health care is provided by a state-run system of hospitals (some of which are specialized) and clinics. Hospitals usually include out-patient departments. Since 1990, Libya has had a proliferation of private clinics offering their services to those who can afford them. The advantages of these clinics are better nursing and hospitality arrangements. Many doctors and surgeons also have private practices. Though state health policies emphasize the advantages of primary health care, the general public tends to consult specialists when medical services are needed. Going to a pediatric or obstetric hospital for related services is the norm, regardless of the condition. The general public complains about the quality of health care services, although they have confidence in the doctors' skills. People usually complain about poor management, a lack of professional competence in nursing and paramedical staff, and a shortage of resources.

Ethnic/Race Specific or Endemic Diseases: Historically, the endemic disease list has included malaria, plague, cholera, measles, meningitis, diphtheria, tetanus, and polio. Reported cases of these diseases have been decreasing dramatically during the last 30 years, and the numbers of reported cases are not alarming. Currently, limited sporadic outbreaks of measles and cholera are usually expected. Emerging diseases such as HIV and AIDS and hepatitis B are priorities for health authorities. The World Health Organization's (WHO) estimated prevalence rate for HIV/AIDS in adults ages 15 to 49 years is 0.05%. WHO has no estimates for children from birth to 15 years living with HIV/AIDS.

Health Team Relationships: Medical doctors, who are skeptical about the skills of nursing staff, do not delegate power or responsibilities to them. The general public shares these convictions and attitudes, thus interns have the most direct contact with patients; otherwise, such contact is reduced. This phenomenon led to the introduction of university-level nursing education programs in the late 1990s; medical technology university education also was introduced in the early 1990s.

Families' Role in Hospital Care: Hospital food is nothing other than tasteless; hence for decades it has been the custom to bring food to in-patients. The previous lack of confidence in nursing staff made it essential for family members to stay with the patient for as long as needed. Despite occasionally limited resources, these practices are strongly resisted by the hospital management and health care staff members, and family members are only allowed to stay with a patient when the family's presence benefits the patient.

Dominance Patterns: Traditionally, the husband and father is responsible for earning the family's income, whereas the wife is responsible for household chores. Children are the mother's responsibility, although boys become the father's responsibility when they become teenagers. The father's dominance over children is more prevalent—a fact that is a detriment in child development and may be a seed for psychological disorders. This pattern has been changing during the past 25 years because of developments in education, increasing percentages of working women, and the proliferation of nuclear families. Although still important, male dominance (i.e., of the husband, father, or boss) is becoming more moderate.

Eye Contact Practices: Religious women are not expected to make direct eye contact with men who are not immediate family members. For the majority, eye contact is acceptable even between men and women, and it is permissible to make direct eye contact with seniors.

Touch Practices: Timidity is a virtue and a teaching of Islam. Most of the females' bodies and private parts of the males' bodies are not exposed to people of the opposite sex (other than parents, children, and some siblings) unless need or necessity dictates. Similar restrictions on touching apply to the whole body. Thus exposing or touching the body or parts of it does not hinder physical examinations or procedures of medical staff members. However, patients with diseases of the genitals prefer a doctor or a nurse of the same sex.

Perceptions of Time: The espoused theory of time is, "Time is as a sword. If you don't cut it, it cuts you." However, in practice the theory is quite different. Although almost everyone preaches that time is precious, an important percentage of time is consumed in social interactions. Those who are ill will not tolerate wasted time; they expect a prompt response to their symptoms. Although other professionals may have a fairly relaxed attitude about time, medical and health care professionals must value time.

Pain Reactions: A woman's voice is considered disgraceful if it is heard by strange men, hence women keep pain to themselves. For men, an expression of pain is a sign of weakness.

Birth Rites: The birth of an infant is usually celebrated. The birth of a boy—or of a girl who is born after a mother already has several boys—is more celebrated. Although Islam states that parents should be satisfied with God's gifts, whether boys or girls, parents become temporarily depressed after having a second or third female child in a row. Circumcision is a religious rite for Muslims and is performed on all males, usually during their first 5 years. Today, it is often performed at a hospital or clinic during the first week after birth because most births occur in hospitals. Female circumcision (clitoridectomy) is not performed.

Death Rites: Muslims bury a dead person as soon as possible, usually within 24 hours. Funeral rituals are short and attended by family, friends, and acquaintances. All who attend the funeral visit the family of the deceased person to offer condolences, usually within the 3 days after burial.

Food Practices and Intolerances: The diet primarily contains starchy components derived from wheat (e.g., couscous, pasta, bread, rice), whereas the main protein sources are lamb, chicken, camel, and beef. Conventional Libyan dishes are fatty because of the excess of animal fat and vegetable oils (i.e., olive, sunflower, and corn oils). With improving health and fitness awareness, the consumption of fish, vegetables and fruits is increasing, and the consumption of fats in general is decreasing. According to Islamic tradition, only specific meats can be eaten, and pork and carrion are forbidden. Most if not all Libyans fast from sunrise to sunset during the month of Ramadan, which occurs for 1 month every lunar year.

Infant Feeding Practices: Breast-feeding is common; about 91% of women breast-feed for 11 months, and no significant differences between urban and rural women have been noted. Most women who do not breast-feed have medical or physiological reasons.

Child Rearing Practices: The infant usually sleeps in a rocker in the parents' bedroom until the age of 12 to 18 months. Boys are separated from girls at about 10 years old. Libyan social rules require obedience to parents and respect for all older adults. Bad and good behaviors result in punishments or rewards. Punishments vary from mild physical reprimands to taking away allowances. Rewards are usually candy, toys, and other items depending on age of the child.

National Childhood Immunizations: BCG at birth and 6, 10, and 14 weeks; DTP at 6, 10, and 14 weeks and 18 months; OPV at birth, at 6, 10, and 14 weeks, and 18 months; hep B at birth, 6 weeks, and 8 months; measles at 8 and 18 months. Because the majority of births occur in hospitals, it is easy to remind parents of immunization requirements. The reported percentages of the target population vaccinated are more than 90% for most (BCG, 99%; first dose of DTP and polio, 98.2%; second dose of DTP and polio, 97.2%; third dose of DTP and polio, 95.7%; and measles, 92%). School admissions at ages of 6 and 12 require a medical check-up and a review of immunization status. The meningitis vaccination is given at age 6, and tetanus, polio, and PCG are given at 12 years. Hepatitis B has been administered at birth since 1989.

BIBLIOGRAPHY

Centers for Disease Control: *Malaria information for travelers to North Africa,* http://www.cdc.gov/travel/regionalmalaria/nafrica.htm.
Department of Health: *Development of health services in the years 1969–1988,* Department of Health, Sirte, Libya, 1989.
Department of Health: *Health in Libya,* Department of Health, Tripoli, Libya, 1980.
Health Information and Documentation Center: *Statistical bulletin,* Sirte, Libya, 1993.
League of Arab States: *Arab maternal and child health indicators,* League of Arab States, Cairo, Egypt, 1999.
PAPCHILD Project: *Libya maternal and child health survey—preliminary report,* Secretariat of Health and Social Affairs, Sirte, Libya, 1997.
Tripoli Health Department: *1989 annual report,* Tripoli Health Department, Tripoli, Libya, 1990.
World Health Organization: *Global epidemic detection and response,* Geneva, 2002, http://www.who.int/emc/surveill/index.html.
World Health Organization: *WHO report on global surveillance of epidemic-prone infectious diseases,* Geneva, 2000, WHO.

◆ LIECHTENSTEIN (PRINCIPALITY OF)

MAP PAGE (860)

Location: The tiny country of Liechtenstein is a democratically run constitutional monarchy located between Austria and Switzerland, with Austria to the north and east, and Switzerland to the south and west. It is mostly mountainous (because of the Alps), and the Rhine Valley comprises its western third. The climate is continental, with cold, cloudy winters with frequent snow and rain, and cool to moderately warm summers. The total land area is 160 km² (62 square miles), almost the size of Washington, DC. The capital is Valduz. The population is 32,528, and 71% is between the ages of 15 and 64 years. Unemployment rates are low in this prosperous country (1.9%), and the gross domestic product per capita was estimated to be $23,000 in 1998. The literacy rate is reported to be 100%.

Major Languages	Ethnic Groups	Major Religions
German (official)	Alemannic 88%	Roman Catholic 80%
Alemannic dialect	Italian, Turkish, other 12%	Protestant 7%
		Other 5%
		Unknown 8%

Health Care Beliefs: Active role; health promotion important. Liechtenstein has an ongoing commitment to a community health promotion project called *Mauren Aktiv,* which encourages exercise and better health habits and was implemented in the 1990s. This program has increased offerings of health promotion projects by 100%, and evaluations indicate that the program's success has been enhanced by volunteer activity and the support of health professionals.

Predominant Sick Care Practices: Biomedical. Good medical care is widely available in the country.

Ethnic/Race Specific or Endemic Diseases: Endemic diseases are cardiovascular diseases and alveolar and cystic Echinococcus infections. People are at risk for Borna disease, a rare central nervous system disorder caused by the Borna disease virus, and tick-borne encephalitis (TBE). The World Health Organization (WHO) has no estimated prevalence rates for HIV/AIDS in adults or children.

Birth Rites: The birth rate is 11.53 births per 1000 people, and the infant mortality rate is low at 4.99 deaths per 1000 live births. The total fertility rate is 1.5 children born per woman. Life expectancy at birth is 75.32 years for men and 82.6 years for women.

National Childhood Immunizations: No immunization data are available from WHO but because the country has excellent health services, adequate coverage is probably the norm.

Other Characteristics: Multilateral organizations involved in international guidelines for financial sector oversight have found gaps in Liechtenstein's financial services controls that make the country vulnerable to money laundering for illegal drug revenues.

BIBLIOGRAPHY

Batliner B: Evaluation of a community-oriented health promotion project "Mauren Aktiv," *Sozial Praventivmed* 43(5):262, 1998.

Caplazi P et al: Borna disease in Switzerland and in the principality of Liechtenstein, *Schweiz Arc Tierheilkd* 141(11):521, 1999.

Eckert J: Epidemiology of *Echinococcus multilocularis* and *E. granulosus* in central Europe, *Parassitologia* 39(4):337, 1997.

Krech T et al: Endangering of the Liechtenstein population by the early-summer meningoencephalitis virus, *Schweiz Med Wochensch* 122(34):1242, 1992.

http://www.odci/gov/cia/publications/factbook/geos/ls.html

http://travel.state.gov/switzerland_liechtenstein.html

◆ LITHUANIA (REPUBLIC OF)

MAP PAGE (861)

Laima M. Karosas

Location: Lithuania is located in eastern Europe on the eastern shore of the Baltic Sea. Latvia is to the north, Belarus to the east and southeast, Poland to the southwest, and the Russian Federation to the west. The land is characterized by gentle rolling hills, forests, lakes, and rivers. The total land area is 65,200 km² (25,174 square miles).

Major Languages	Ethnic Groups	Major Religions
Lithuanian (official)	Lithuanian 80%	Roman Catholic 89%
Russian	Russian 9%	Other 11%
Polish	Polish 7%	
	Belarussian 2%	
	Other 2%	

Health Care Beliefs: Acute sick care; some health promotion efforts. Although health promotion is considered important, resources are first allocated to in-patient care. Preventative services are scarce, and health promotion and disease prevention programs, especially for women, have deteriorated over the past 10 years. Younger people take a more active role in disease prevention and health promotion. Free universal care is provided, primarily in health care facilities rather than in community settings. However, payment is expected for most treatments.

Predominant Sick Care Practices: Biomedical, holistic, traditional, and magical-religious. The breakup of the Soviet Union, with its accompanying political, social, and economic alterations, also created major changes in the health care system of Lithuania. In the current process of changing from the Soviet system of hospital-based care to a primary care system that will better serve the needs of the population, resources are limited in all aspects of care. Health care providers receive low pay and often expect gifts of money or goods, limiting access to the best care. Older adults are more likely to consult folk healers but also seek help from the biomedical system if folk medicine fails to produce results. For protection or to overcome illness, some believe in the "evil eye" and in prayer.

Ethnic/Race Specific or Endemic Diseases: Lithuanians are at risk for phenylketonuria, thyroid disorders, and nutritional deficiencies. Endemic diseases include tuberculosis (the rate of which is consistently increasing), cardiac diseases, hepatitis, rabies, and influenza. Alcoholism is a growing problem. More than 75% of the rural population and 50% of urban dwellers drink to excess. Drinking alcohol is tolerated during working hours, including in health care facilities. The World Health Organization's (WHO) estimated prevalence rate for HIV/AIDS is 0.02%. The estimated number of children from birth to 15 years living with HIV/AIDS is less than 100.

Health Team Relationships: Nurses and doctors are predominantly female, and nurses follow doctors' orders. Nursing patterns reflect 50 years of Soviet influence. A significant percentage of people who are nurses did not select nursing as a career but were directed into it. Introductory social conversations are uncommon. Expression of feelings may not be encouraged by professional caregivers. Asking questions of a health care provider is considered a challenge to authority, therefore information may not be shared freely. Patients address the health care professionals by title rather than by name. Patients may offer gifts to health care providers to ensure quality care.

Families' Role in Hospital Care: Family members are expected to assist with bathing, feeding, comforting, and elimination needs.

Dominance Patterns: Traditionally, men assume a slightly more dominant role; however, the men and women share responsibility for decision making. Decisions are usually not made quickly and are debated at length. The woman is usually responsible for the household, children, food shopping, and food preparation.

Eye Contact Practices: Eye contact practices vary, and eye contact may shift during conversations. Direct eye contact is used when communicating serious matters; however, older adults may avoid direct eye contact when speaking to health care personnel. Direct eye contact can be considered a challenge to authority in some situations, such as those involving older male doctors.

Touch Practices: Touch is uncommon even within families. A handshake between males is common at the beginning and end of an interaction and for both sexes in professional situations.

Perceptions of Time: In the health care arena, Lithuanians focus on present-oriented crisis management. Past traditions, including how older adults healed illnesses, are important. Little emphasis is placed on health promotion or prevention. Individuals can still meet with a practitioner if they are late for an appointment at a public institution, but this may not be true for an appointment with a practitioner in private practice. Doctors are notoriously late and do not apologize for making patients wait for appointments or treatments. It is the duty of the patient to wait to be seen without complaint.

Pain Reactions: Pain tolerance is valued, although pain relief is both desired and requested. Verbal expressions of pain indicate a higher level of pain. During labor, women are encouraged to keep silent and be stoical. Because of short supplies, pain medications may be limited or unavailable in hospitals.

Birth Rites: Almost all births occur in hospitals and are attended by a doctor and possibly a midwife, who may or may not be a nurse. The father may choose to be present during delivery but is not permitted to coach labor. Courses for natural childbirth and prenatal and postpartum care are becoming more popular. The semiseated position is common for delivery. Circumcisions are not performed.

Death Rites: If an illness is fatal, the family is told first; they decide whether the patient should be told. A dying person is not left alone without family members. After death an open coffin permits others to view the body for up to 3 days. Burial occurs on the third afternoon after a church service. Cremation is not practiced. Grief may be expressed verbally, and crying in private is expected.

Food Practices and Intolerances: The preferred main meal is in the evening. Potatoes, seasonal vegetables, bread, meat, and soups are common. Great quantities of milk, other dairy products, tea, coffee, and alcohol are consumed.

Infant Feeding Practices: Breast-feeding is encouraged more than bottle-feeding. Many women state that although they want to breast-feed, they do not produce enough breast milk. Most women transfer to bottle-feeding between 3 and 30 days after the birth. Infants are not fed on demand during the first 2 weeks of life but instead are fed every 4 hours (which could contribute to the lack of milk production problem). Foods are introduced at 4 to 5 months.

Child Rearing Practices: Children are cooperative and reared using disciplinary styles ranging from logical reasoning to authoritarian rule. The grandmother may have a valued position in child rearing, especially in single-parent families or families in which both parents work. Sharing of possessions is verbally encouraged but may not be enforced. Some children may do chores at home or be taught to rely more on their parents. Women are entitled maternity leave at 32 weeks' gestation and are allowed to continue the leave until the child is 3 years old. Maternity leave wages are only a percentage of a woman's regular rate; therefore many choose to return to work earlier.

National Childhood Immunizations: BCG at birth, 11 months, and 6 to 7 years; DTP at 3, 4 to 5, 6, and 18 months; OPV at 6 to 7 and 12 years; hep B at birth and 1 and 6 months; IPV at 3, 4 to 5, and 18 months; MMR at 15 to 16 months and 12 years; Td at 6 to 7 and 15 to 16 years.

BIBLIOGRAPHY

The Baltic states: a reference book—Estonia, Latvia, and Lithuania, Tallinn, Riga, Vilnius, 1991, Encyclopedia.

Birutis AL: *Country nursing-midwifery profile: Lithuania.* Paper presented at the third meeting of the European Chief Governmental Nursing Officers, Bucharest, Romania 1993.

Birutis AL: The facts, needs and prospects; Lithuania. In *Nursing in the world,* Tokyo, 1992, International Nursing Foundation of Japan.

Birutis AL: *Guidelines for the development and reconstruction of nursing profession in Lithuania,* Amsterdam, 1992, The European Nursing Congress.

Birutis AL: *Nursing in Lithuania.* Paper presented at the second meeting of Selected Nursing Leaders, World Health Organization Regional Office for Europe, Copenhagen, 1993.

EUROHEALTH, World Health Organization Regional Office for Europe: *Lithuania: health sectors review report,* Copenhagen, 1991.

Kalnins I, Barkauskas VH, Seskevicius A: Baccalaureate nursing education development in two Baltic countries: outcomes 10 years after initiation, *Nurs Outlook* 49(3):142-147, 2001.

Kalnins I: Pioneers in academia: higher education for nurses in Estonia, Latvia, and Lithuania, *Nurs Outlook* 43(2):84, 1995.

Karosas L: Nursing in Lithuania as perceived by Lithuanian nurses, *Nurs Outlook* 43(4):153, 1995.

Karosas L: Nurse practitioner revisits Lithuania, *Npnews* 2(1):3, 1994.

Nadisauskiene RJ, Padaiga Z: Changes in women's health in the Baltic republics of Lithuania, Latvia and Estonia during 1970-1977, *Int J Gynaecol Obstet* 70(1):199-206, 2000.

Stuttle C: Midwifery in Lithuania, *Midwives Chron Nurs Notes* 107(1275):144, 1994.

Van Damme P: Hepatitis B: vaccination programmes in Europe—an update, *Vaccine* 19(17-19):2375-9, 2001.

Vasyliunas R: Where's home? *J Multicult Nurs Health* 1(3):30, 1995.

World Health Organization Regional Office for Europe: *Highlights on health in Lithuania,* Copenhagen, 1992.

◆ LUXEMBOURG (GRAND DUCHY OF)

MAP PAGE (860)

Alexandre R. Bisdorff

Location: Luxembourg is a small country in western Europe with a temperate climate. It has borders with France (to the south), Belgium (to the west), and Germany (to the east). The total land area is 2586 km² (998 square miles) with a population of 441,300, resulting in a relatively high population density of 170.6 inhabitants per square kilometer. Most people work in services and industry, and 2% work in agriculture. Every day a large part (46%) of the working population commutes from neighboring countries to work in Luxembourg. Luxembourg also has a very high percentage (37.3%) of foreigners living in the country. The most important foreign communities are (with percentages calculated as a part of the whole foreign community) as follows: Portuguese (35.4%), Italian (12.3%), French (12.2%), Belgian (9.2%), German (6.4%), British (3%), Dutch (2.4%), other European Union (6.1%), and other (12.9%). Luxembourg is a constitutional monarchy headed by the Grand Duke. The state is organized like a modern democracy, with a parliament voted for by general elections and based on the principle of separation of powers.

Major Languages	Ethnic Groups	Major Religions
Luxembourgish	Celtic base with	Roman Catholic 97%
French	French and	Protestant and
German	German blend	Jewish 3%

Luxembourg has three official languages: Luxembourgish, French, and German. The main spoken language is Luxembourgish *(Lëtzebuergesch),* a language with Germanic roots going back to the fourth century and specific to the region of Luxembourg and neighboring areas in Belgium, France, and Germany. *Lëtzebuergesch* has sufficiently differentiated itself from its parent language such that it is no longer readily understood by Germans. The most important language used for official and legal documents is French, whereas the main language used in the daily newspapers is German. This unusual situation of the simultaneous use of several languages has historical and geographical origins; the territory and population of the country is small and involved in permanent exchanges with its neighboring countries. Every Luxembourger who grew up in this country speaks at least Luxembourgish, French, and German. Immigration from other countries means that people can speak another mother tongue. English is taught in secondary schools.

Health Care Beliefs: Active participation; health promotion important. Preventative medicine is primarily organized by government bodies. For example, all school children are seen once a year by a doctor, who informs the parents of any problems. Vaccination programs are suggested by the Ministry of Health, and social security pays for most vaccines. A number of doctors working for the administration deal primarily with occupational medicine. Certain health promotion activities are actively encouraged, such as yearly mammography for women in middle age and yearly Pap tests for women of every age. Some private initiatives offer programs for back exercises and injury prevention. In general, the trust in scientific medicine is relatively high; however, many patients use alternative practices, particularly if they have chronic or progressive diseases or ill-defined symptoms. Care for mental illness is provided by general practitioners and psychiatrists. Mental and to some extend neurological diseases are still associated with a stigma. Fear associated with these diseases was much stronger during and after World War II because of the eugenics practiced by the Nazis who had occupied Luxembourg.

Predominant Sick Care Practices: Biomedical and alternative. Luxembourg has 1083 doctors: 361 general practitioners, 721 specialists, and 266 dentists. This corresponds to 2.5 doctors per 1000 inhabitants (not including dentists), and the country has 5.6 hospital beds per 1000 inhabitants. Most doctors have trained for at least a few years in neighboring European countries because Luxembourg has no medical school offering a complete medical education. All doctors working in Luxembourg must show that they have achieved the European Union standards of skills. Doctors work in hospitals, and most specialists in hospitals also have a practice in the community. The majority of medical services are offered locally, but patients may be referred abroad for rare or highly specialized services. It is mandatory that every doctor practicing in Luxembourg is automatically in the public social security system covering most of the population. Patients have free access to general and specialized practitioners and do not need a referral. Doctors and some other health professionals work as self-employed individuals and are paid on a fee-for-service basis. Tariffs are strictly regulated and the object of regular negotiations among doctors or other health professionals and the social security system. Generally, patients pay the doctor first and then receive a refund from social security. Magical or unfounded health practices are a marginal phenomenon, but some doctors offer alternative medicine, which is not covered by social security.

Ethnic/Race Specific or Endemic Diseases: The most common illnesses in Luxembourg, as in most developed countries, are cardiovascular diseases, cancer, hypertension, and diabetes mellitus. Orthopedic problems such as chronic backaches and hip and knee arthrosis are also common as well, as are disabilities resulting from dementia and stroke in older adults. Major differences in causes of disease of the various nationalities living in Luxembourg are unknown. The World Health Organization's (WHO) estimated prevalence rate for HIV/AIDS in adults ages 15 to 49 is 0.16%. WHO has no estimates for children from birth to 15. The incidence of HIV infection from 1990 to 2000 was 9 to 10 cases per year (about 2.5 cases per 100,000).

Health Team Relationships: The health system is doctor driven. Because of the free access to any doctor, patients have free choice in out-patient and in-patient settings except in emergencies. Therefore popular doctors have a big workload and fill hospital beds and surgical rooms. Hospitals have an interest in recruiting busy doctors of different specialties to ensure excellent services and to justify the pay for nurses and other personnel.

Families' Role in Hospital Care: The role of the families in hospital care is mainly to serve as a source of emotional support and help to make medical decisions regarding invasive tests and treatments for patients who are unable to do so. Families often bring food to their relatives, although it is unnecessary. Visitors for in-patients may arrive in the afternoon and stay overnight in special circumstances (e.g., when a patient is dying). One parent often stays overnight with children. The number of visitors may be limited when a patient is in intensive care or has an infectious disease.

Dominance Patterns: By law, men and women have equal rights and duties. Mothers tend to play a more important role in care of ill children because they stay with them at home or in the hospital. Currently most doctors are men, but the number of women entering medicine is growing, particularly in the areas of general medicine and pediatrics.

Eye Contact Practices: Eye contact is direct when people, including doctors and patients, talk to each other. A patient who avoids eye contact immediately causes the health professional to wonder whether the patient is extremely anxious, is shy, or has a mental disorder.

Touch Practices: Shaking hands is the normal way of greeting patients and their relatives before a medical consultation. Physical touching is quite acceptable during a physical examination. Touch practices do not vary between sexes, regardless of whether a male doctor is treating a female patient or vice versa.

Perceptions of Time: People value their cultural heritage because it is part of their identity. Most perceive that the ever-increasing European integration will result in many changes that will decrease national self-determination. On the whole, this is considered positive for the people. Patients like to take advantage of the latest achievements of scientific medicine and find it quite normal that the social security system will pay for such services, as it has during the last few decades. Many hope that scientific progress will result in better options for health care or cures for fatal diseases. On the other hand, some are concerned that future developments in molecular biology and embryology could lead to discrimination and abuse. Patients usually make appointments to see doctors, and doctors who are on a schedule may charge a small supplemental fee. Generally, patients have to wait before being seen, but waiting times of several hours are not the norm. Luxembourg has no significantly long waiting lists for specialists or elective surgeries such as cataract procedures or joint replacements.

Pain Reactions: The spectrum of pain reactions reflects the multicultural nature of Luxembourg. Luxembourgers behave much like other Northern

Europeans, tending to be stoical, but many patients with Mediterranean backgrounds are more expressive. Professionals need to consider cultural differences in the expression of suffering to make adequate assessments of Luxembourgers.

Birth Rites: Nearly all births occur in a hospital, and hospitals allow fathers to be present during childbirth. After birth the father registers the newborn and its name with the local authorities. Regardless of whether the couple is married, the child's surname is always the father's. Relatives bring flowers to the mother in the hospital, where she usually stays for several days as an in-patient before going home with the newborn. Every newborn is examined by a pediatrician, and some screening tests for common genetic diseases are performed. No differences in procedures or family rituals exist between male and female infants.

Death Rites: Death is not a topic most people consider very much during their lives. Only a few people carry or write "do not resuscitate" (DNR) statements. Most people die in hospitals or nursing homes and if a person's death is expected, family members often ask to stay with the patient. Most Luxembourgers declare being Roman Catholic, although only a small minority are actively practicing Catholics. However, religious celebrations of baptism, marriage, and funerals are very common. By law, doctors are allowed to take organs for transplantation from patients who are brain dead if no statement of refusal has been written by the person. In practice, most people have written such a statement, and close relatives are asked for their consent. It is usually unacceptable to overrule a family's wishes, and they often refuse to allow organ donations from deceased relatives. Luxembourg does not do regular autopsies; they are actually quite rare. Most autopsies are requested by attorneys for forensic reasons such as in cases of violent death or deaths with unknown causes or that occurred under suspicious circumstances.

Food Practices and Intolerances: Food in Luxembourg is comparable to food in most Western countries. Carefully preparing food and matching it with the correct wines is highly regarded and takes its inspiration from France. The many foreign communities, especially the French, Italian, and Belgian, also have enriched the local cuisine.

Infant Feeding Practices: Breast-feeding is encouraged for at least 6 weeks after birth because of scientific evidence of benefits. No attitudes are specific to the culture.

Child Rearing Practices: Most children have their own room and do not sleep in their parents' room after infancy. Many parents allow their children to come to their bed at night but try to stop the habit gently. Child rearing in Luxembourg is not particularly strict or authoritarian, and physical punishment is largely rejected. Ideally, children are supposed to grow up to become responsible adults, not submissive subjects. Most families are small, with one or two children. In many families, grandparents take over a part of the child rearing, allowing both parents to work. Some children become spoiled under these circumstances, and lines of authority can become unclear when too many adults are involved in their upbringing.

National Childhood Immunizations: Following are the official recommendations of the Ministry of Health of Luxembourg for childhood immunizations; the program is voluntary: BCG at 1 to 2 months; OPV at 2, 3, 4 to 6, at 11 to 12 months, at 5 to 7 and 12-15 years, and every 10 years; DTP at 2, 3, 4 to 6, and 11 to 12 months; MMR at 14 to 15 months and 5 to 7 years; hep B at 1, 2, 3, and 4 to 6 months; HIB at 2, 3, 4 to 6, and 11 to 12 months; meningitis C at 14 to 15 months; tetanus at 5 to 7 and 12 to 15 months and every 10 years.

BIBLIOGRAPHY

Autier P et al: The Luxembourg Mammography Programme: a breast cancer screening programme operating in a liberal health care system: 1992–1997, *Int J Cancer* 20:97(6):828–32, 2002.

Kuffer C: Towards quality in Luxembourg, *Nurs Standard* 9(2):7, 1994.

Lynch J et al: Income inequality, the psychosocial environment, and health: comparisons of wealthy nations, *Lancet* 21:358(9277):194–200, 2001.

Scheiden R et al: Cervical cancer screening in Luxembourg, *Eur J Cancer* 36(17):2240–3, 2000.

Service Central de la Statistique et des Etudes Economiques, Luxembourg: http://www.statec.lu

World Health Organization (June 2000): *Epidemiological fact sheets by country,* Geneva. Retrieved March 1, 2002, from http://www.unaids.org/hivaidsinfo/statistics/june00/fact_sheets/index.html

World Health Organization (2001): *WHO vaccine-preventable diseases: Monitoring system,* Geneva. Retrieved March 1, 2002, from http://www.who.int/vaccines/

◆ MACEDONIA (REPUBLIC OF)

MAP PAGE (860)

Velibor B. Tasic

Location: Macedonia (the former Yugoslav Republic) is a continental country located in the southeastern part of the Balkan Peninsula. It borders Yugoslavia on the north, Bulgaria on the east, Greece on the south, and Albania on the west. The total land area is 25,333 km^2 (9,781 square miles). Macedonia has lakes, many mountains, and rivers. It is a country rich in culture, tradition, and history. The ethnic majority are Macedonians, followed by people of Albanian descent. Ethnic minorities include Romas (Gypsies), Turks, Serbs, and Vlahos. The country is mainly agricultural. The total population was estimated to be 2,021,000 in 2000.

Major Languages	Ethnic Groups	Major Religions
Macedonian (Cyrillic alphabet)	Macedonian 65%	Eastern Orthodox Christian 67%
Albanian	Albanian 22%	Muslim 30%
Turkish	Turkish 4%	Other 3%
	Serb 2%	
	Roma (Gypsy) 3%	
	Other 4%	

Health Care Beliefs: Acute sick care; traditional. People in Macedonia want to learn about health, evidenced by the fact that in newspapers and television one of the most popular topics is health. Under the communist system the state was active in health promotion and disease prevention (e.g., had early recognition of breast and genital cancers). Unfortunately, people do not receive regular preventable check-ups; even health care workers are poor role models. For example, the majority of those at professional risk for infection with hepatitis B have not been vaccinated. Tuberculosis is still a significant problem, despite the fact that mobile stations are available to detect the disease early. Some efforts have been made to rehabilitate those with mental handicaps and integrate them into society after discharge from a hospital; however, many are prejudiced toward people with mental illness, and even families may not want them back. They are isolated during prolonged hospitalizations, and the treatment they have received is often inadequate. In rural communities, traditional practices are still carried out, especially with newborns. For example, coffee powder is put on an umbilical cord that will not stop bleeding. This folk practice has practical benefits because coffee is rich in vitamin K, which is important for the clotting process. On the other hand, this procedure may subject a newborn to infection. When an infant has jaundice, a traditional treatment is to make a small incision on the infant's forehead with a knife. It is believed that the wound releases the jaundice and cures the infant. Infants with jaundice are also dressed in yellow clothes so that their yellow skin is less noticeable. Infants wear amulets on their hands and fingers and special pieces of velvet on their eyes to protect them from the "evil eye," or the power of a person to harm others merely by looking at them. After delivery, infants are kept in the house for 6 weeks to allow the immune system to mature and protect the infant from infections. Pregnant women also are discouraged from going to the cemetery because evil spirits might take the infant from them; in some rural communities, only a mother-in-law can deliver a woman's baby. Umbilical cords are cut with razors, increasing infection and mortality risk for the newborn. When infants have complications, people attempt to transport the mother to the hospital before birth or immediately after. Too frequently infants come too late to the intensive care unit or die on their way to the hospital. In Europe, Macedonia has the second highest infant mortality rate. (Albania has the highest.) A new project by the World Bank has been established to decrease perinatal mortality. Macedonia has initiated a comprehensive program to prevent the high morbidity and mortality of newborns by using standard protocols. Surfactant also has become available in Macedonia and has been effective in reducing mortality of premature infants with respiratory distress syndrome.

Predominant Sick Care Practices: Alternative; magical-religious; bio-medical when available. Under the previous regime the health system was structured, and the medical field was held in high esteem. However, during the past decade, after the separation of the former Yugoslav Republic, significant transitional changes took place. Health insurance was previously almost free but now is tied to employment. Because many people are currently unemployed, few people can go to a doctor. Until recently, medications could be bought without a prescription in drugstores. Because access was easy, self-treatment was common and based on information from news, television, friends, or colleagues from the office. This practice led to abuse of drugs, particularly antibiotics, with resultant drug resistance (e.g., the resistance of *Escherichia coli* against co-trimoxazole is 48%). If initial self-treatment was unsuccessful, people then consulted a doctor. Scheduled doctors' visits are unusual in Macedonia, examinations are considered poor, and often little discretion between doctor and patient exists, especially in public facilities. Not surprisingly, people are unsatisfied with public health services and prefer to consult doctors working in private offices or hospitals if possible. If patients have their own health insurance, they pay a small amount to participate in the public health system. In the private system the entire amount must be paid and although not expensive by Western European standards, prices are high compared with average salaries of Macedonians. Rather than consulting a doctor, some consult with nonmedical staff members, or *paramedics,* who claim to cure people with herbs, bioenergy, or semimagical treatments. At times, the actions of these practitioners have serious consequences. A paramedic using herbs or special teas may forbid a person to use doctor-prescribed drugs. If a person has insulin-dependent diabetes, the cessation of insulin can lead to serious consequences such as diabetic ketoacidosis or coma and death. Circumcisions that are ritually performed in Muslim communities are frequently done without anesthesia by non-professionals, most of whom are religious leaders. In addition to causing great pain to the child, a frequent complication is meatal stenosis. A rare complication of this procedure—poststreptococcal glomerulonephritis—is a consequence of an infected circumcision wound. Treatment with bioenergy is especially popular, and all cities or villages have a bioenergy practitioner. Diseases treated with bioenergy include nocturnal enuresis, lumboishialgia (back pain as a consequence of spinal compression of the sciatic nerve), epilepsy, certain types of cancer, and many central nervous system diseases. Treatment with herbs or tea is popular for the flu, diarrhea, kidney stones, and menstrual problems. Macrobiotic diets are particularly popular among patients with cancer. Those with incurable diseases may undergo some very unpleasant procedures; for example, some believe that drinking blood from a turtle may help cure patients with leukemia.

Ethnic/Race Specific and Endemic Diseases: After World War II, many diseases such as malaria and syphilis were eradicated, and the incidence of rheumatic fever, acute poststreptococcal glomerulonephritis, and tuberculosis significantly decreased. The southern part of the country still has cases of hereditary Mediterranean anemia (thalassemia), a specific hematological disease affecting those of Macedonian ethnicity. Certain parts of the country still have cases of *kalaazar* (leishmaniasis). The worsening economy and low educational level have been instrumental in the increased incidence of tuberculosis, acute poststreptococcal glomerulonephritis, and rheumatic fever, particularly among Albanians. The prevalence of tuberculosis is 58.8 per 100,000 Albanians versus 32.9 per 100,000 in the general population. Iron-deficiency anemia is common among children, and occasionally, children develop kwashiorkor. During the summer, diarrhea is common and lately has been known to progress to toxicosis with bad outcomes, especially in malnourished children. Macedonia has had occasional epidemics of hepatitis A. Hepatitis B is a serious problem; the prevalence of carriers in the population has been estimated to be up to 8%, and vaccinations for hepatitis B are uncommon. Hepatitis C infection has become a serious problem, especially among patients on dialysis. The main causes of death are cardiovascular diseases (56%); malignant diseases (17%); symptoms, signs, and undefined situations (8%); respiratory diseases (4%); poisoning and trauma (4%); endocrine diseases (3%); digestive system diseases (3%); and others (5%). The World Health Organization's (WHO) estimated prevalence rate for HIV/AIDS in adults ages 15 to 49 years is 0.01%. The estimated number of children from birth to 15 years living with HIV/AIDS is less than 100. The first person with HIV was registered in 1987, and the first person with AIDS—a person with hemophilia who was infected by blood products from abroad—was registered in 1989. By December 31, 2001, the total number of officially registered HIV/AIDS cases since the beginning of the epidemic was 59. Of the 43 people who have developed AIDS since the beginning of the epidemic, 37 have died. These data do not represent the country's actual infection rates because no random testing has been done. It is impossible to determine which part of the country or which nationality has the highest incidence rate. Infection rates seem to be highest in people ages 30 to 39, followed by those who are 20 to 29. The average age of infection among those who use drugs is 19 to 29 years, and three cases of vertical transmission have been reported. The dominant mode of transmission is heterosexual, although figures may include males who are in homosexual or bisexual relationships. For cultural and religious reasons, as well as social, it is still very difficult for Macedonians of any nationality to speak openly about their sexual behavior.

Health Team Relationships: The new educational health care system is focusing on teamwork between the nurses and the doctors. A harmonious relationship exists for the most part, influenced by social and cultural environments. Patients generally respect medical staff members. An initiative has been developed to create special programs for the health care of children, particularly children with special problems—those for which communication among the general doctor, pediatrician, and parents is crucial. The system is moving toward greater integration of patient needs with needs of health care professionals and better overall communication among parties.

Families' Role in Hospital Care: The hospitals cannot provide the care for patients common in Western European countries. Food, drugs, accommodations, and hygiene are all inadequate, which is the reason relatives still accompany and care for hospitalized patients. Mothers of children younger than 3 years are allowed to stay in the hospital without charge. Older children are accompanied by a parent and if a bed is available, costs for the parent's stay are charged to the family. Food is usually brought to the hospital but does not always meet therapeutic recommendations; for example, if a family of a child who has acute glomerulonephritis brings fruit, drinks, or salted meals, the food could result in increased blood pressure and worsening of the child's health. During the transition into a new health care system, efforts toward open communication among patients, family, and staff members are being made, even among those in intensive care. The parents of critically ill children or infants who are in incubators or receiving mechanical ventilation assistance are allowed to touch the children skin to skin after thoroughly washing their hands.

Dominance Patterns: In the urban environment, differences between sexes are not as important. However, in some rural areas, women continue to be predestined to remain in the home, where cooking, cleaning, and the education of children have been traditionally and primarily women's tasks. Men's roles relate to making money for the family and doing more difficult physical labor.

Eye Contact Practices: Making direct eye contact signifies trust, and avoidance of eye contact is interpreted as shame or lying. Direct eye contact may be avoided when the authority of one individual intimidates the other.

Touch Practices: Youths have more freedom in expressing their feelings physically, and differences exist between those in rural and urban surroundings and those who are modern or conservative. The relationship between male doctors and female patients is delicate. In some rural areas, women still go to a doctor accompanied by their husbands or someone else, especially when a gynecological examination is performed. Some women, particularly women from Muslim areas, prefer to be examined by female doctors.

Perceptions of Time: Punctuality is not typical, and the majority of people are late, even to doctors' appointments, frequently causing chaos. Macedonians tend to live in the present, facing only daily social, economic, and political problems. They often think about the past with nostalgia. This is true particularly for young people who feel hopeless about future prospects for employment, living conditions, or travel. Unfortunately, many young people look to their future by emigrating to Canada or Australia.

Pain Reactions: Men are expected to be strong when in pain, whereas women are expected to cry and yell. Children are trained to cope with pain in early childhood. Children's rights are not fully recognized, and poor pain control and prescription of intramuscular injections in the hospital make many children permanently frightened of hospital care. People in general still strongly believe that injections have more power than drugs taken orally. Unfortunately, many painful procedures such as bronchoscopies and colonoscopies are performed without any medication or analgesic relief. The problem of pain has rarely been seriously considered, especially in the public system. In private practice, somewhat more attention is paid to the issue of pain.

Birth Rites: Macedonians are not actively involved in birth control methods. In 2000 the number of deliveries was 29,357, and the number of abortions was 10,129. Most women have three ultrasounds during pregnancy and deliver in hospitals with the assistance of professionals. Only 3.7% of deliveries are performed at home without professional help, which is usually provided by older women. In the past, newborn tetanus was very common because people would cut the umbilical cord with a razor or unclean scissors. Newborns are kept in the hospital for several days if they have no complications. Since 2000, some obstetric hospitals have started the United Nations Children's Fund (UNICEF) rooming-in program; newborns are kept with their mothers constantly unless mother or child has serious complications. Some families are happier when a boy is born, and his birth may be celebrated by shooting a gun. In some cases, the father does not even want to take his infant home when it is a girl. Elective cesarean sections are considered for infants who may have low Apgar scores, asphyxia, or unpredictable neurological outcomes. Traditional women still believe they should suffer the pain of delivery with little expression. Infant mortality is about 11.8 per 1000 newborns; 72.5% of deaths occur during the first 4 weeks of life and 27.5% within the first year. The most common causes of the infant mortality are prematurity and low birth weight (31.5%) and congenital malformations (16%).

Death Rites: Customs differ between Muslim and orthodox populations. For orthodox burials, candles are lit in the home, and family, relatives, and close friends spend the night with the body. The burial ceremony is conducted by a priest, the coffin is lowered into the ground, and people throw earth on it. After the funeral ceremony, participants are invited to have a meal at the home of the deceased person. It is still believed that the spirit of the person is present during the 40 days after the death. Because of this belief, on the fortieth day after death the family invites relatives and friends to a lunch to celebrate the presentation of the person to God. According to Muslim custom, men carry the coffin, and women follow behind separated from the men. If a death occurs in the hospital, Muslims forbid autopsy; the orthodox do not have such rules. According to Macedonian law, an autopsy must be performed if a death occurs within 24 hours of admission or when the cause of the death is unclear. Organ donations are not performed, so this issue has not been regulated. The only option for people with renal failure is kidney transplantation from a living relative.

Food Practices and Intolerances: Basic foods are bread, dairy products (e.g., yogurt, milk, cheese), and meat. Sheep and cows are raised in the mountains and villages, so meat and milk are inexpensive. Milk is generally given to infants rather than formula, which is expensive relative to the low incomes of most individuals. This practice leads to a higher incidence of rickets and sideropenic anemia. Many inexpensive products contain high carbohydrates and no proteins, predisposing people to malnutrition. The country is mainly agricultural and produces many vegetables and fruits, so theoretically the diet should be healthy. Traditionally, only women prepare meals, and on Friday families have a traditional bean dish. On Sunday, people have a traditional family lunch of baked meat, usually chicken, pork, or beef. The most typical Macedonian food is *ajvar*—mild paprika peppers, possibly with other vegetables. The peppers are baked, chopped into very small pieces, and fried in oil (possibly with tomato and other spices). Afterward the mixture is put into glass bottles or cans and sterilized (i.e., canned) for the winter. Muslims never consume pork or alcohol. Most individuals eat with knives, forks, and spoons, but some Muslim and Gypsy families still use their hands.

Infant Feeding Practices: Because of difficult social and economic conditions, children generally do not have the most nutritious diet possible. The dominant foods are carbohydrates and fats. Breast-feeding is favored by health professionals but not practiced or accepted by many modern mothers. UNICEF strongly promotes exclusive breast-feeding, emphasizing its advantages over artificial (formula) feeding. Various formulas are on the market, but they are expensive.

Child Rearing Practices: Macedonians still have very conservative views of family behavior. The father controls power and discipline, and the mother devotes her time to the education and care of the children. Parents expect children to be calm and obey rules. Children are not employed before they are 18 and therefore are economically dependent on their parents until that age.

National Childhood Immunizations: The following vaccine schedule is not posted on the WHO immunization Web site: TBC at 3 days and at 7 and 14 years; diphtheria at 4, 5 1/2, and 7 months and 2, 4, 7, and 14 years; tetanus at 4, 5 1/2, and 7 months and 2, 4, 7, 14, and 18 years; pertussis 4, 5 1/2, and 7 months and 2 and 4 years; polio at 4, 5 1/2, and 7 months and 2, 7, and 14 years; morbilli at 13 months and 7 years; parotitis at 13 months and 7 years; and rubella at 13 months and 7 and 14 years (for girls). The standard European schedule is accepted. Macedonia received a certificate from the international community through WHO 2 years ago for eradication of poliomyelitis. Infectious diseases are now very rare because of well-developed vaccination programs.

BIBLIOGRAPHY

Economist Intelligence Unit: *The former Yugoslav Republic of Macedonia: country profile,* 1997, Health Care Systems in Transition—Republic of Macedonia, Copenhagen, 2000, European Observatory on Health Care Systems.

Republic Institute for Health Protection: *Annual report 2000,* Macedonia.

Skopje Public Health Institute report for 2001: Center for Prevention and Treatment of Drug Abuse, Public Health Organization Psychiatric Clinic, 2001, Skopje.

Tasic V: Doctoral dissertation, University Sv.Kiril i Metodij, 1997, Skopje.

Tasic V, Polenakovic M: Poststreptococcal glomerulonephritis following circumcision, *Pediatr Nephrol* 15:274–275, 2000.

United Nations Children's Fund International Child Development Center: *Women in transition. Regional monitoring reports,* No 6, Florence, 1999, UNICEF.

World Bank: *The former Yugoslav Republic of Macedonia—health sector transition project,* Report No 15399–MK, 1996.

◆ MADAGASCAR (REPUBLIC OF)

MAP PAGE (863)

Katharine Quanbeck and Stanley D. Quanbeck

Location: Madagascar, the fourth largest island in the world, is situated in the Indian Ocean across the Mozambique Channel from southeastern Africa. The island contains a central plateau bordered on the east by an escarpment covered with rain forest; vestiges of the original virgin forest remain in a few areas. Lining the vast coast are regions varying from semiarid and grassy grazing lands, to spiny forests, to sharp cliffs, to white intermingled with black (titanium) sandy beaches connecting with the expanses of coral reefs. The total land area is 587,041 km^2 (226,597 square miles). Although Madagascar gained independence from France and became the Malagasy Republic in 1960, this "great red island" nation also has a history of its nationals attempting to unify Madagascar. The most recent census (1997) estimated the population of Madagascar to be 16 million. The literacy rate varies widely from 5% in the coastal regions to 90% in the highlands. Madagascar is the eleventh poorest country in the world, and an estimated 75% of the island population lives below the poverty line. In the past 40 years, Madagascar's population has doubled, and its forest area has greatly decreased.

Major Languages	Ethnic Groups	Major Religions
Malagasy	Malayo-Indonesian	Traditional (animist) 43%
French	Cotiers	Roman Catholic 25%
	Arab	Protestant 25%
	French	Muslim 7%
	Indian	
	Creole	
	Comoran	

The Malagasy language varies widely in vocabulary, syntax, and intonation from one region to another. In several waves of immigration, a vast variety of people came to be called *Madagascar.* Oral traditions indicate that some came from Egypt and Abyssinia, India, Malaysia or Borneo, and Sumatra or Polynesia. Some claim that the Malagasy language is closely tied to the Malayo-Polynesian group; others in Madagascar claim that they find equally strong Semitic (possibly Hebrew) and Chaldean similarities. Bantu words are also significant. Royalty clans throughout the island use the "respect language" when addressing or referring to honored persons. The language consists of specific words that are to be used only with clan elders. Certain specified parts of the body (e.g., head, ears, eyes, buttocks) can only be referred to with this language. When addressing an older adult, a person would not say *"your* eyes" *("ny masonao, Dadatoa Jaona"),* rather, "That with which you see, respected sir" *("ny fijerinao, Ro Andria or Nahoda").* Deoxyribonucleic acid (DNA) studies indicate that about a third of Madagascar's people contain blood similar to types found in the Far East, another third show similarities to Bantu-type DNA, and the remaining third seem to have a mix of Middle Eastern types (most likely Arab and Hebrew). French and English are well known by the limited percentage of the populace who has had an adequate education. In some clans, illiteracy is 95%; they consider most other Malagasy ethnic groups to be foreign *(vezaha),* and all languages other than the one they speak are considered French. Each clan has its own specific oral tradition about its ancestry, cultural practices, and institutions. Animists are practitioners of an ancestral cult that either follows shamans' directives given to traditional kings or queens, venerate ancestral spirits, or worship and obey spirits dwelling in a sacred tree or a boa constrictor. Syncretism also exists. Some have a high priest, and some a specific elder that holds the sacrificial knife.

Health Care Beliefs: Acute sick care; traditional. Since about 1975, mobile teams have worked with villagers, encouraging vaccinations and promoting nutrition, breast-feeding, disease recognition, maternal and child care, preventive practices, and sanitation and hygiene principles. In many areas, training of community health workers has been taking place since 1980 through hospitals, dispensaries, and primary health care centers in remote villages, even among illiterate populations, using a participatory approach and methods appropriate for adult learning.

Predominant Sick Care Practices: Magical-religious and biomedical when available. It is not uncommon for an ill person to first consult with a shaman or an herbalist or to receive treatment from them simultaneously with treatment from a doctor, nurse, or medical assistant using biomedical care. Depending on the healer, who can be a man or woman, the person may use sticks or pieces of wood and coins mixed with rum. Use of this concoction is coupled with "calling on a healer spirit" to possess the healer. If a female patient enters a hospital wearing a silver bracelet attached to her hair at the top of her head, it indicates she has an indwelling spirit (i.e., is possessed, or *tromba*). Spirit possession syndromes are widespread throughout the island, and the interplay between such syndromes and overt mental illness is being studied by Malagasy doctors. Community health workers (primarily women) also do monthly growth monitoring and nutritional counseling, teach use of hand-grinding mills, teach women about solar cooking, distribute food to underweight children, and distribute food during famines. They also visit from door-to-door in their villages to remind people about vaccination days, check on use of oral rehydration gruels for those with diarrhea, and remind those being treated for tuberculosis to show up for supervised daily medication administration or intermittent sputum checks. They also know who is being treated for leprosy. Early famine alert warnings usually come from these workers, who speak with appropriate outside officials. They are involved in cooperatives of kitchen gardens and sewing, supervising protection of the water supply, and repairing or requesting new water wells. Mass projects, such as mebendazole for intestinal parasite control, surveying sexually transmitted diseases, or cervical cancer prevention research, can only be carried out with the involvement of these workers, and they serve as examples of positive health practices. Even shamans and herbalists in such villages work in coordination with health workers, and it is not unusual for villagers to choose their shamans to be the people who are trained to be their health workers. If harmful, traditional practices are addressed by Malagasy trainers often through role-plays that are followed by questions and dialogue; otherwise, traditions are respected.

Ethnic/Race Specific or Endemic Diseases: Although Madagascar has some cases of chloroquine-resistant malaria, chloroquine still suppresses the symptoms in a very high percentage of cases and thus is still the drug of choice. Tuberculosis continues to be a major problem. The treatment is a multidrug therapy for 2 months, two drugs for 6 months, and three sputum checks to monitor progression. Infection with HIV is suspected and tested in a person found to be resistant to the tuberculosis regimen. Schistosomiasis (bilharzias—both *Schistosoma mansoni* and *S. haematobium*) is prevalent. Pigs are permitted to run loose in villages, creating the perfect environment for cysticercosis. A high prevalence of cysticercosis-based epilepsy exists. Training to reduce morbidity and mortality at the grassroots level for acute respiratory illnesses (ARIs) has only begun. Oral rehydration for the control of diarrhea has been taught for more than 20 years but has not yet reached all remote areas. Lack of clean sources of water, lack of education, and taboos against defecating in the same place more than once all contribute to the problem. Drives to encourage breast-feeding for the first 6 months still have not prevented malnutrition and stunted growth in all regions. In areas where flooding or drought with famine occurs frequently, stunting is endemic. It is common for the boy of fraternal twins to be favored, offered the breast milk first and more frequently, and given food supplements if not thriving. The female twin often displays signs of neglect and intestinal parasites—a constant problem, especially for infants and children across the entire eastern coastal rainforest region. Neither training in basic sanitation and hygiene nor community-based regular deworming programs have been effective in ridding the population of parasites, although better educated, wealthier individuals are more apt to periodically treat themselves with mebendazole. In addition to the previous endemic diseases, people in Madagascar are at risk for many others. In spite of the grave economic situation caused by political instability, poor management of resources, and social disintegration resulting from mining lifestyles, the rural Malagasy want help to improve their community health situation. Sexually trans-mitted diseases are pervasively present in all areas but the central highlands, where sex workers receive weekly check-ups and treatments and where sex before marriage is much less common than it is elsewhere. HIV and AIDS are rapidly increasing problems in sapphire-mining regions. Only in the past several years have any groups seriously begun intensive programs of testing and education. In some regions of the rain forest, filariasis leads to severe physical defects such as scrotal elephantiasis or hydroceles as large as basketballs; in other regions, it leads to disfiguring elephantiasis of the leg. Filariasis can also lead to chronic malaise and ill health, affecting both sexes throughout the eastern rainforest region. Attacking this disease would take World Health Organization (WHO) involvement, which is not currently occurring. If all villagers could have at least one bedding net with insecticide in their homes, it would affect the endemic properties of filariasis and malaria. The numbers of leprosy cases are decreasing, but the disease has not been eradicated in remote rural areas, especially areas with poverty, poor hygiene, and lack of sanitation. Goiter and cretinism have been a problem in certain regions far from the sea because of iodine deficiencies in soil and water. The government is making a concerted effort to provide iodized salt to these areas. Mental illness also is a significant problem. In seven indigenous care and treatment centers of the Malagasy Lutheran Church, 743 patients were diagnosed in 2001 as having either psychosis or neurosis. Life expectancy is 52 years for men and 57 years for women. The WHO's estimated prevalence rate for HIV/AIDS in adults ages 15 to 49 is 0.15%. The estimated number of children from birth to 15 years living with HIV/AIDS is 450. Initiatives exist emphasizing primary prevention that includes counseling and HIV testing, treatment of sexually transmitted diseases, and education through local and private media plus grassroots organizations such as schools, church groups, and community advocacy groups. Education methods include drama, peer groups, songs, and dancing, all of which are activities representing lifestyles and valued forms of communication that are meaningful to specific indigenous groups.

Health Team Relationships: Doctors are at the top of the echelon, especially in more modern biomedical treatment centers. In remote areas where no doctor will work, nurses and even untrained people are addressed as *radoko* (doctor) by villagers, and their care is sought, trusted, and followed. This is particularly true in regions with high illiteracy rates, especially if a nurse has developed rapport with villagers. Nearly half of Malagasy doctors are women, most of whom are from the central highlands groups. Whether doctors are dominant to paramedical practitioners depends mostly on the individual doctor's attitude. Still, doctors seem to be associated with an unspoken attitude of dominance and condescension that nurses, sociologists, and paramedical professionals often complain about. Doctors receive higher salaries because of their perceived social status and class.

Families' Role in Hospital Care: Illness generally involves the entire extended family. Family members assist relatives who are hospitalized by cooking for them in kitchens at adjacent or nearby hospital guest-housing quarters. On the other hand, in more modern hospitals in larger cities, food is cooked and brought to the patient by the hospital staff members. Although the country had a dearth of medication in the early 1980s, the situation has gradually improved, although dental care supplies and reagents for laboratories are still difficult to obtain. Emulation of traditional beliefs and practices reigns in Madagascar; elders in each clan rule—their word is law and followed exactly regardless of whether the elder is right or wrong. Such respect for clans also relates to care of ill and well family members. This practice can lead to the financial ruin of those who earn a respectable living and has led to the ruin of more than one self-supporting institution such as a hospital. This occurs when traditional practices dictate that the income in the hospital must be used for the functioning of families, institutions, or groups related to the hospital in any way.

Dominance Patterns: The extended family, or clan, is vitally important. Elders and ancestral spirits are respected and honored, as are traditional consecrated elders who perform sacrifices and high priests who guard the clan's worship place. Clans are primarily patriarchal, even though women do head some clans. In some clans, wives are the advisors of their husbands; in other clans a woman may be the leading elder, and it is not unusual for such a clan leader to be the judge for her clan's people. Royalty clans abide by the "great lady" concept. A son's ability to become king depends completely on his mother's identity. Royalty clans have also had queens, and one still reigns in northwestern Madagascar. Women usually hold the family's money. In this nation of wide contrasts, well-educated female leaders exist in every walk of life and in many regions. Anyone who earns a dependable salary can be expected to use it to care and provide for the entire extended family. Nuclear families do exist, but the emphasis is on the entire clan; often cousins are called "siblings" and nieces and nephews are called "children," therefore one person can have several "mothers."

Eye Contact Practices: Although in many clans, it is common to avoid eye contact with people in authority, it is uncommon in other clans. When children are being disciplined, they may have difficulty looking into the eyes of the adult who is speaking, even when they are requested to do so. As with many other customs, the issue of eye contact varies among various clans, even ones who are neighbors.

Touch Practices: Among some clans, young boys and girls and even husbands and wives may avoid physical contact in public. It is considered taboo for a couple for whom a marriage is being arranged or considered to be seen together in public. Therefore many believe that if a young man and woman are seen alone together, they will not marry. This practice is governed by family and clan values. Touch also affects traditional health care and healing methods used. Traditional healers called *mpitsapa* are believed by many to have the power to heal by stroking, lightly massaging, or touching. For instance, it is said that a broken bone can be healed by such a *mpitsapa* touching and manipulating the bone. In many clans, it is very common and acceptable for two female friends or two male friends to walk down the street holding hands. Preschool-age children in families often sleep packed together in one bed, and it seems that sitting close to each other with bodies touching is more comfortable than sitting apart. Handshaking is the most common form of greeting, but some groups kiss the cheek three times. Parents are affectionate with their children and even dote on them. Children tend to be raised to depend on their parents and each other rather than to think and act independently in their clan-oriented society. Extended family members assume major roles in child rearing. It is not unusual for a grandmother to demand to raise a grandchild.

Perceptions of Time: Punctuality traditionally holds no value for most clans. It is far more important to give adequate attention to politeness—to inquire about each family member and show respect by chatting—than it is to remember to reach an appointment on time. This mindset tends to be true even among those who know the vital importance of punctuality to Europeans. Variations in perceptions of time exist among clans. Some tend to focus on past traditions almost totally, some never consider the future—and tomorrow does not yet exist—and some live completely in the present. Educated individuals have trained themselves to function by acknowledging the future, and they are the best at planning, ordering medications ahead of time, training others to be in charge in the future, and writing reports so that future efforts and activities acknowledge past mistakes or successes. Many believe that the way an event occurred was preordained by God. Some also believe in astrology.

Pain Reactions: Pain is shown and expressed by many clans, although some train their children to be tough and repress discomfort, pain, and fear, regardless of whether they are boys or girls. If these children do express their pain, they are unworthy of their clan title (which begins "Of the family of..." or "Descendant of..."). These clans tend to express toughness bluntly and freely and readily use a method of relating called *mifampiziva*—a teasing, insulting pleasantry among people of specific clans who have established this special type of communication.

Birth Rites: Pregnancy is associated with various food taboos that vary from clan to clan. Taboos can involve eggs, chicken, or seafood, and the pregnant woman is watched by elders to ensure she is not endangering her fetus. In most clans, sons are much more celebrated than daughters, even though daughters can help the mother with home duties. In clans that value education, some grant equal opportunities to boys and girls. When finances become a problem, it is the sons who receive continuing education, not the daughters. For many Malagasy clans, educating their children is a top priority. In remote villages in some regions, the mother squats and gives birth under a tree, occasionally alone. She cuts the cord with a shell or other sharp object and is then expected to go back and work the fields. In other clans, it is customary for the mother to *mifana*—sit beside a fire bundled in a heavy blanket with the infant. She is fed a milky sauce of small fish so that she can produce breast milk. If a woman is admired, she may sit beside the fire for up to 6 months, growing fatter and fatter. In some clans, the women begin breast-feeding before cutting the umbilical cord so that she can pump any remaining nutrients out of the cord into the breast milk. Most remote rural clans insist that only women can assist a woman with childbirth. These women are usually trained birth attendants who may have received a certain amount of training in labor, childbirth, and handling complications. In some royalty clans, it is still forbidden for a king's numerous wives to be treated by a male health worker. Many rural villagers do not name their infants for several months or a year after birth because of the high infant mortality. The Malagasy Health Ministry encourages women giving birth to have assistance from professional midwives, have regular check-ups throughout the pregnancy, receive tetanus vaccines, and receive monthly chloroquine treatments. Regardless, in remote villages, which are 50 to 100 km from the nearest midwife, traditional practices prevail. In such villages, it is not unusual for a woman who has been in labor for a day or two and cannot deliver her infant to ride in a wooden-wheeled ox cart for 2 or 3 days to get to a surgical center. Distances are great, but the suffering is greater. It is a miracle when such a mother survives the delivery of a dead infant after so much time. This is not uncommon in remote areas. The average number of living children born to women ages 15 to 49 years is 6.6. Contraceptive use is 19.4%, and the percentage of mothers receiving prenatal care is 76.8%.

Death Rites: It is not unusual for a family or clan member to thank a doctor when a family member dies, saying, "You have done all you can, and we have done our best as well, to care for our loved one." Traditionally, many tend to place death in the hands of *Zanahary* or *Andriananahary*, their almighty and omnipotent creator god. Families ordinarily stay with those who are dying, touching or holding them. Organ donation would be taboo if it were possible, and autopsies are only rarely permitted. Many fear that a body part could be stolen; if a leg is surgically amputated, the body part must be buried in its own tomb. Among those who no longer follow traditional practices, a wake is held for one or a few nights, giving the family members the opportunity to travel from far away to attend the funeral. If the deceased person was Christian, a religious service is conducted by a pastor or priest before the burial. In clans who use large family tombs built above ground, the clan elder officiates at the family grave opening and even reviews the names of those buried in the tomb and on which shelf they are resting. He also then informs the family which remaining shelves belong to those who are the living—the shelves where they will eventually go to "lie with their fathers." Some bury the dead in caves or holes in or on top of a rocky mountain, and some bury the bodies under a large pile of rocks on a high place such as a hill or on the side of a highway. Occasionally, standing stones are incorporated strategically into the cement or rock wall surrounding the rock-filled grave. *Alo-alo*—carved, wooden markers similar to totem poles—mark the tops of many graves in addition to cow horns indicating the number of cows that were slaughtered for the funeral festivities. Christians are often buried in a Western-style grave with a tombstone or standing stone marker, but many are also buried among their fellow villagers, in a traditional rock and cement above-ground grave, although it is marked by a cross and scripture passage from the Bible. The whole clan is expected to contribute money, food (e.g., a cow), and labor to make the grave, a process that can last for several months or even a year or longer. These clans may erect temporary houses near the gravesite and live there while involved in grave construction. Standing stones pepper the countryside throughout a good proportion of the island, commemorating those who died elsewhere and possibly indicating the might or valor of the deceased. Among some clans in the central highlands who reopen the grave periodically, the corpse is taken around the ancestral village and given new grave cloths. This gesture shows respect for ancestors, respect that is similar to the total respect granted living elders in a clan. Before an elder dies, it is common for the person to designate the clan member who is to become the clan elder or leader, and it is not uncommon for a woman to be chosen. In many regions, the more important a person is, the more cattle are killed after the person's death and the longer the wake and the burial. For royalty, it is not uncommon to wait six 6 to 12 months or 2 years before the burial, and the spouse is expected to sit at the side of the corpse during the ceremony. For Christians, a wake of one to a few nights is common, as is walking to the grave site, carrying the coffin or body, and singing hymns. Formalin, which is used to preserve the body, is rarely available in rural communities, although it is much appreciated when it can be obtained. The common lamentation involves sharp cries, wailing, and weeping by women, which begins anew every time new visitors arrive to pay their respects. The sharp cries of lamentation are startling. In some clans the king may be buried in the trunk of the largest tree the clan is able to find; clansmen often have to go scores of kilometers to find it and then have to spend much money hiring a truck to carry it to the village. Dancing en route to the burial site is not uncommon and is accompanied by revelry and singing.

Food Practices and Intolerances: In the central highlands and wherever rice can be grown, rice is the staple food and is eaten with a topping *(laoka)* of meat, dried beans, lentils, and greens or other vegetables, and tomatoes. Cassava, sweet potato, other locally available greens, and watercress are also commonly combined with beans or meat and served as a topping. It is common for rice to be the basis of what is eaten; only a few spoonfuls of topping are included. Snacks vary, but a favorite is rice cakes *(mokary)*, which may be sweetened, *sambosse* (an Indian triangular-shaped snack), or a meatball or two. Although some clans eat absolutely nothing but rice, it is common for most to enjoy eating whatever fruit is in season as a snack or dessert or as the mainstay of the diet when it is in season. Elsewhere on the island, staples such as cassava, sweet potato, taro root, and corn are the only foods eaten. These staples might be combined with greens, soured milk *(habobo)*, lentils, or dried beans. Garbanzo beans are widely used to supplement breast milk if a child is malnourished or has stunted growth. The beans are cooked until they become a milky consistency and then spooned into the mouth of the malnourished infant; breast-feeding continues. The rice-eating Malagasy truly believe they cannot feel full and have not eaten a meal unless they have eaten rice. In fact, the verb meaning "to eat" is *mihinam-bary,* which translates as, "to eat rice." Those whose staple is not rice use a different verb—*sakafoi;* it involves the root word "food," thus *misakafo* means "eat food." Food is usually eaten with a large spoon. In the central highlands, a fork and knife may be used.

Infant Feeding Practices: In some clans, traditionally mothers spooned herbal teas into the mouths of their newborns while holding the infant's nostrils shut. Such clans believe colostrum is unhealthy, so this process continues until the "real milk" comes in. The Health Ministry is addressing this problem by emphasizing breast-feeding only for the first 6 months. Mothers who have become convinced of the benefits of breast-feeding have been known to brag about the fact that their infants are so healthy and have only been fed breast milk. Bottles are seldom used, although some children have had slow growth because of improper use of formula. Gruels are introduced by 6 months and consist of rice or two parts carbohydrate food, one part lentil or dried bean, and part peanut. The four-part gruel is especially used to feed children with stunted growth or who are malnourished. Mashed fruit is also used to supplement the gruel and breast milk after 6 months of age. Infants who do not have an appetite are fed a mixture made of egg yolk beaten into orange or tomato juice, a mixture that usually perks up appetite. Health workers teach those whose infants have diarrhea or are vomiting to continue breast-feeding and to offer liquid gruels as oral rehydration and electrolyte replacement mixtures. Family spacing programs and child survival efforts center on growth monitoring and nutritional counseling, with food supplementation when needed.

Child Rearing Practices: Children are loved and carried constantly by their parents, older siblings, and grandparents. Rural women carry infants on their backs, as do some urban and educated women. Urban parents have also been seen carrying an infant in a front pack. Traditionally, it was not uncommon for a child to be breast-fed for 2 years or more. The family is generally permissive, and discipline usually involves guidance, talking, urging, and distracting rather than outright confrontation or castigation. Toilet training is often begun at a young age—within the first few months after birth. The mother or another female is expected to take the child outside and sit on the ground night and day with her legs out in front of her so that she can cradle the infant on the anterior aspect of her ankles until the infant eliminates. The adult sleeping with the infant anticipates when the child has the urge to urinate. Mothers are often considered poor parents if their children urinate in their beds. Infants and young preschoolers are accustomed to being held, having attention, and being played with, so it seems rather natural for Malagasy infants to be content and quiet and willing to sit with an adult or older child, calmly gazing around. Praise is used liberally. Parents and grandparents, older siblings, aunts, and uncles are all involved in child rearing. Older children are encouraged to play outside and ignored as they sing in harmony, as loudly as they desire. In many clans, children are taught from a young age to be silent when older adults are talking and obey without question, as well as to show respect for their elders at all times. Many clans also teach children to stand when older adults enter the room and offer their seat to the most respected adult. People in Madagascar hope for many children, so for most, being infertile is a terrible burden. When asking how many children or grandchildren a family has, it is common for people to also ask how many of them are boys. People want to have children even though half their offspring may not survive infancy because of breast-feeding difficulties and diarrhea or survive the preschool years because of malnutrition and diseases. The percentage of children younger than 3 years with stunted growth is 48.3%. Poverty is one reason the extended family is so vitally important in the life of a child. After a drought or flood, families turn to their extended family and the community for help. A joy of parents is giving their children the opportunity to go school. Another joy is knowing that their children will care for them in their old age. In addition to poverty, health is affected by taboos and deadly regulations imposed by traditional restrictions of shamans, who may demand that children herd cattle or be prevented from studying even if the village has a school. Children who are allowed to begin school are often forced to quit after the fourth year either to take care of siblings, plant and harvest the fields, or in the worst-case scenario, travel to the nearby city to become a prostitute because the family is starving. All but one clan circumcises infants, and the event is often accompanied by feasting, merriment, and dancing. Some circumcise in the first year, but other clans wait until age 7 or 8 and then circumcise all the village boys of that age during one ceremony in the village's special house, near special water, and with special instruments. For some clans it is a duty or privilege of the maternal uncle to eat with a banana the foreskin of a child who has just been circumcised. In other clans, the foreskin is inserted in the muzzle of a shotgun and fired into the air as a symbol of future virility.

National Childhood Immunizations: BCG at birth; DPT at 6, 10, and 14 weeks; OPV at birth and 6, 10, and 14 weeks; measles at 9 months; vitamin A at 6 to 11 months; and TT for pregnant women at first contact, +4 weeks. The percentages of children ages 12 to 23 who received their vaccinations are as follows: BCG, 66; DPT and polio (three doses), 48.4%; polio (three doses), 47.7%; and measles, 46%.

BIBLIOGRAPHY

L'arche de noé dans l'Océan Indien, un thème d'origine de l'homme dans les contes malgaches et comoriens, *Etudes Océan Indien* 16, 1993.

Beaujard P: La violence dans les sociétés du sud-est de Madagascar, *Cahiers D'etudes Africaines* XXXV:2–3, 563–598, 1995.

Dahl OC: *Migration from Kalimantan to Madagascar,* Oslo, 1991, Norwegian University Press, The Institute for Comparative Research in Human Culture.

Dahl O: *Malagasy meanings—an interpretive approach to intercultural communication in Madagascar,* 1993, Stavanger, Norway.

Dewar RE, Wright HT: The culture history of Madagascar, *J World Prehistory* 7(4), 1993.

Fanony F, Gueunier N: Le mouvement de conversion à l'Islam et le role des confréries musulmanes dans le nord de Madagascar, Cheminements, *ASEMI* XI:1-4, 51-168, 1980.

Faublée J: Notes sur un clan du sud-est de Madagascar, *J Africanistes* 62(2), 1992.

Feeley-Harnik G: *A green estate—restoring independence in Madagascar,* Washington and London, 1991, Smithsonian Institute Press.

de Flacourt E: *Histoire de la grande isle Madagascar,* Paris, 1995, Editions Karthala, Paris.

Graeber D: Dancing with corpses reconsidered: an interpretation of famadihana (in Arivonimamo, Madagascar), *Am Ethnol* 22(2):258–278, 1995.

Gueunier N: La genèse de l'homme Blanc—récits d'origine du sud-ouest de Madagascar, *Etudes Océan Indien* 15:227–259, 1992.

Heurtebize G: *Mariage et deuil dans l'extrême-sud de Madagascar,* Paris, 1997. Museum of Art and Archeology, Antanarivo, Madagascar.

Lambek M: Taboo as cultural practice among Malagasy speakers, *Man (NS)* 27:245–266, 1988.

Larson PM: *Making ethnic tradition in a pre-colonial society: culture, gender, and protest in the early Merina kingdom, 1750–1822,* doctoral dissertation, 1992, University of Wisconsin—Madison, Madison, Wisconsin.

Lupo P: *Mélanges ancêtres et Christ—un siècle d'evangelisation dans le sud-ouest de Madagascar, 1897–1997,* Ambozontany—Fianarantsoa, Madagascar, 1997.

Luzzatto L, Notaro R: Protecting against bad air—perspectives: Malaria, *Science* 293, 2001.

Nurse GT, Weiner JS, Jenkins: *The peoples of Southern Africa and their affinities, 1985,* Oxford University Press.

Pearson MP: Tombs and monumentality in Southern Madagascar: preliminary results of the central Androy survey, *Antiquity* 66(253): 941–948, 1992.

Rajemisa-Raolison R: *Dictionnaire historique et géographique de Madagascar,* Madagascar, 1966, Fianarantsoa.

Rakibolana Malagasy: Madagascar, 1985 Fianarantsoa (Ambozontany).

Ralaimihoatra-Nicole G: *Et si la lune ne revenait pas? Madagascar—le secret des Vazimba,* Saint-Denis de la Réunion, 2001 Editions Grand Océan, St-Denis, Reunion (island).

Randriamihajanirina D: *FISAKANA—Tsa Hanim-boay…!* Antananarivo, Madagascar, 1999.

Sharp L: *The possessed and the dispossessed—spirits, identity, and power in a Madagscar migrant town,* Los Angeles, 1993, University of California, Berkeley.

Exorcists, psychiatrists, and the problems of possession in Northwest Madagascar, London, 1994, University of California Press.

Tishkoff S et al: Haplotype diversity and linkage disequilibrium at human G6PD: recent origin of alleles that confer malarial resistance, *Science* 293, 2001.

Tyson P: *The eighth continent—life, death, and discovery in the lost world of Madagascar,* New York, 2000, Harper Collins.

Underhill P et al: Maori origins, Y-chromosome haplotypes and implications for human history in the Pacific, *Human Mutation* 17:271–280, 2001.

◆ MALAWI (REPUBLIC OF)

MAP PAGE (863)

Chiwoza R. Bandawe

Location: Malawi is a small African country occupying a southern part of the East African Rift Valley. It has a total land area of 119,140 km^2 (45,988 square miles), of which 20% is water. It is landlocked and borders Mozambique, Tanzania, and Zambia. Its topography is varied, ranging from the Rift Valley floor at sea level to the majestic Mulanje Mountain at 3000 m. Malawi attained its independence from Britain in 1964 and was ruled by a one-party dictatorship until 1993, when internal and external pressure ushered in a multiparty system of government. Elections were held in 1994, and a new democratically elected government came into power. Malawi has a national population of 9.7 million people. It has been described as one of the poorest countries in the world, with a macro economy of US$70, and 60% of the population living below the absolute poverty line. The country is predominantly agricultural based, and 85% of the population lives in rural areas.

Major Languages	Ethnic Groups	Major Religions
English	Chewa	Christian 75%
Chichewa (national)	Nyanja	Islam 20%
Chitumbuka	Tumbuko	Other 5%
	Yao	
	Lomwe	
	Sena	
	Tonga	
	Ngoni	
	Ngonde	
	Asian	
	European	

English is the official language in government, parliament, the judiciary system, and secondary and tertiary education systems.

Health Care Beliefs: Acute sick care; traditional. Social psychologists who have studied Malawians argue that they are able to maintain two different belief systems about health and well-being without any sense of conflict or contradiction. In other words, Malawians understand the causes of diseases according to Western scientific explanations and traditional explanations, which involve mysticism and the role of spirits and ancestors in the cause of disease. Hence most people seek out traditional healers and Western-trained medical doctors. An increasing number are also turning to prayers with a strong Pentecostal Christian emphasis conducted by various religious men and women. People primarily attribute mental illness to traditional factors such as being bewitched.

Predominant Sick Care Practices: Biomedical and magical-religious. Primary health care is the major focus of the Malawi health services delivery system. It has been asserted that health education in Malawi cannot be carried out without consideration of other health programs. Health education is therefore "a support service which catalyses other components so that action is taken by individuals, families and communities... and behaviour change is the end product" (Bomba, 1990, p. 1). Currently the Malawi government's information, education, and communication activities are guided by health education strategies. It is believed that increased public awareness "facilitates involvement and participation, and promotes activities which will foster health and encourage people to want to be healthy, know how to stay healthy and do what they can individually or collectively to maintain health and seek help when needed" (Bomba, 1990, p. 4). Because of material and financial resource limitations, the government has had to focus on activities that directly affect vulnerable groups, especially women and children. The country has one national mental hospital, and common causes for admission include substance abuse and schizophrenia.

Ethnic/Race Specific or Endemic Diseases: Malaria is the major illness that affects Malawi. It is the leading cause of out-patient visits and in-patient admissions and the leading cause of death among children younger than 5 years. Other illnesses, in decreasing order of importance, include lower respiratory tract infections (such as tuberculosis), diarrheal diseases, and malnutrition. The country is recognizing the seriousness of the HIV and AIDS epidemic. The World Health Organization's (WHO) estimated prevalence rate for HIV/AIDS in adults ages 15 to 49 years is 15.96%. The estimated number of children from birth to 15 years living with HIV/AIDS is 40,000. Since the first cases of AIDS were diagnosed and reported in Malawi in 1985, HIV-related diseases have precipitated an epidemic of unprecedented proportions. A senior official from the National AIDS Control Programme (NACP) estimated that 70% to 80% of adult in-patients had AIDS-related illnesses in 2000. Between 1985 and June 1999, a cumulative total of more than 53,000 AIDS cases were officially reported to the NACP. However, because most cases are not reported, the NACP estimates that the actual figure for this period was more than 265,000. The incidence of HIV as recorded through Sentinel Surveillance sites has risen rapidly in the 1990s. Prevalence rates among pregnant women attending clinics in Blantyre rose from 3% in 1986 to 35% in 1996. Nationally, 16.4% of the population between the ages of 15 and 49 is infected with HIV. The NACP estimates that 46% of all new infections in 1998 were among young people ages 15 to 24 years and of those, 60% were female. Among people ages 15 to 19, HIV infection rates are five times higher among females. The cumulative AIDS cases between 1995 and 1998 show that more women are infected in the 15- to 29-year-old age group, whereas more men are infected in the 30 and older age group. NACP projections of HIV indicate that the number of Malawians living with HIV is likely to increase to more than a million during the next 10 years. The cumulative number of children who have lost either their mother or both parents to HIV/AIDS since the epidemic began is estimated to be 390,000. HIV/AIDS–related conditions now account for more than 40% of all hospital admissions and are likely to increase.

Health Team Relationships: Because of the low doctor-patient ratio (1 doctor for every 46,000 people), doctors are not the authoritative health care workers in most health settings. Clinical officers, medical officers, and nurses play the key roles. The mental health care system is virtually run by psychiatric nurses because Malawi has no psychiatrists. In the eyes of the community, medical personnel have a high social status in Malawi.

Families' Role in Hospital Care: The family plays a critical role in the health care of hospitalized patients. Usually the wife or the mother stays in the hospital with the patient. Because of this practice, most public hospitals have guardian shelters built near the hospitals. They are responsible for moment-to-moment care of patients in a health care sector that is severely understaffed.

Dominance Patterns: Men are usually dominant. Even in matrilineal societies, it is the uncle or brother on the maternal side who has the decision-making responsibilities.

Eye Contact Practices: Modesty is the rule.

Touch Practices: Physical touch among men is restricted to handshakes or holding hands. Hugs, even among close traditional family members, are very rare. Many men hold hands with each other as they walk down the road, and it has no sexual connotations whatsoever. Women are more expressive and often hug each other in public. Traditional men and women do not touch in public, and the sexes are kept separate. Some urban Malawian men and women who have been exposed to Western influences may hold hands.

Perceptions of Time: The Malawian bioethicist, Mfutso-Bengu, writes that people in traditional Malawi have a "natural time zone" that allows them to listen to their body. Time is the servant and not the master; the focus is therefore on relationships, not time. Malawians often spend a considerable amount of time greeting others and asking about their families rather than just getting down to business. Time in Malawi is not linear; it is cyclical and based on the seasons of the calendar year. Time is tied to events. Because the relatively low literacy rate of 48%, many rural women think of history in relation to particular events (e.g., a child's birth being "before the great drought").

Pain Reactions: It is not shameful to express physical pain. Men are expected not to express emotional pain, but it is acceptable for women to cry.

Birth Rites: The birth of an infant is a big event in Malawi. During the seventh month of pregnancy, women give the mother advice. The father is told to refrain from sexual intercourse from this time until 4 months after birth. Traditional birth attendants play an important role in the delivery of the child. The naming process of the infant is taken seriously. The infant is normally named after an ancestor who was highly regarded.

Death Rites: Death is never a private family affair; it is a community event. The whole community stops its activities and gives its full support to a bereaved family. An overnight vigil is held until the day of the burial. Men spend the time outside the house, whereas women remain inside the house and usually sing if the deceased person had any church affiliation. Burial takes place within 2 to 3 days. Death causes the community to feel fractured, and people participate in funeral rituals regardless of whether they personally knew the deceased person. For instance, if a close relative of a work colleague dies, the co-workers attend the funeral and give support to the grieving relatives. In Malawi a dead person is only considered physically dead; Malawians believe the spirit moves on to the spirit world. The grave is dug on the day of the funeral, and the ceremony usually takes place in the afternoon after everyone has eaten at the house, which is where the funeral takes place. People usually have an opportunity to view the body, and a religious ceremony follows. The funeral ceremony itself does not end until the coffin is lowered and the grave has been filled with soil. Women openly wail, and men put their hands on one side of their face. Organ donations are not really an issue because the health care facilities lack the technical resources for organ donation. Autopsies are acceptable when the family wants to establish the cause of death. Because the person's spirit is moving on to the next world, those conducting the autopsy have to assure the family that they will leave the body intact after the autopsy.

Food Practices and Intolerances: The basic foods in Malawi are corn, rice, cassava, groundnuts, dark-green leafy vegetables, sorghum, millet, fish, and fruit (which vary by season). The stable diet is *nsima,* a solidified crushed corn. Men and young children get first choice of the available food, and the most popular foods include beef and fried chicken. Malawians, especially when eating *nsima,* eat with their hands. Men and women in rural areas normally eat separately.

Infant Feeding Practices: Breast-feeding is almost universal. The period of weaning in rural Malawi is normally extended until about 9 months, when children are introduced to other foods.

Child Rearing Practices: Young children are tied to the back of their mother or another female relative and therefore have frequent and close contact with the mother. At night they usually sleep in the mother's bed or on the floor beside her bed. Child rearing in traditional Malawi settings is a communal responsibility. Children who are old enough move in to live with their peers. *Chinamwali* is the period of transition from childhood to adulthood. Children have a traditional "training school," during which time girls and boys separately go to an isolated location and are taught the ways of adulthood. This training involves songs and various rituals. Politeness and obedience are encouraged in girls, whereas boys are encouraged to be bold and take leadership positions.

National Childhood Immunizations: BCG at birth or during first clinic appointment; DTP at 6, 10, and 14 weeks; OPV at birth and 6, 10, and 14 weeks; measles at 9 months; vitamin A at 6 to 12 months; and TT at 15 to 45 years, +4 weeks, +6 months, +1, +1 year. The Malawi government runs the Malawi Expanded Program of Immunization. By age 12 months, a child should have received the complete schedule of vaccinations. The demographic and health survey for 2000 showed that 70% of children ages 12 to 23 months were fully vaccinated. Coverage for the first doses of polio and DTP was 96%. The dropout rate was 17% and 12% for polio and DPT vaccines, respectively. Approximately 3% of children ages 12 to 23 months had received no vaccinations. The mother's educational level is associated with compliance with childhood immunizations.

BIBLIOGRAPHY

Ager A et al: Perceptions of tropical health risks in Mponda, Malawi: attributions of cause, suggested means of risk reduction and preferred treatment, *Psychol Health* 12:23–31, 1996.

Bomba WG: Strengthening of IEC and social mobilization unit of Ministry of Health, Lilongwe, Malawi, 1990, Ministry of Health.

Chowa GC: The potential use of mass media in health education in Malawi, master's thesis, United Kingdom, 1995, University of Manchester.

Kaspin D: A Chewa cosmology of the body, *Am Ethnol* 23(3):561–578, 1996.

MacLachlan M, Carr SC: From dissonance to tolerance: towards managing health in tropical countries, *Psychol Dev Soc* 6:119–129, 1994.

MacLachlan M, Chimombo M, Mpemba N: AIDS education for youth through active learning: a school-based approach from Malawi, *Int J Edu Dev,* 17(1):41–50, 1997.

MacLachlan M, Nyirenda T, Nyando C: Attributions of admission to Zomba mental hospital: implications for the development of mental health services in Malawi, *Int J Soc Psych* 41(2):79–87, 1995.

Malawi Government and World Bank: *Malawi AIDS assessment study: volume I,* Lilongwe, Malawi, 1998, NACP.

Malawi Government and World Bank: *Malawi AIDS assessment study: volume II.* Lilongwe, Malawi, 1998, NACP.

Malawi National Statistical Office: *1998 population and housing census: report of preliminary results,* Zomba, Malawi, 1998, Malawi Government.

Mfutso-Bengu JM: *In the name of the rainbow: politics of reconciliation as a priority of social pastoral care in South Africa and Malawi,* Frankfurt am Main, 2001, Peter Lang.

Ministry of Health and Population: *Malawi national health plan: 1999-2004,* Lilongwe, Malawi, 1999, The Ministry.

National Statistical Office (Malawi) and ORC Macro: *Malawi demographic and health survey 2000.* Zomba, Malawi, and Calverton, Maryland, 2001, National Statistic Office.

Republic of Malawi: *Statement of development policies: 1987–1996,* Lilongwe, Malawi, 1986, Office of the President and Cabinet, Department of Economic Planning and Development.

Shaba B et al: Palliative versus curative beliefs regarding tropical epilepsy as a function of traditional and medical attributions, *Central Afr J Med* 39:165–167, 1993.

◆ MALAYSIA

MAP PAGE (867)

Abdul Manaf Hamid

Location: Malaysia has two separate land areas. Western Malaysia is the southern part of the Malay Peninsula, and eastern Malaysia includes Sabah and Sarawak on the island of Borneo. Malaysia is situated in southeastern Asia, surrounded by Thailand, Indonesia, Singapore, and Brunei Darussalam. The country is covered with tropical jungle and has a mountain range running from north to south surrounded by a very long coastal line. Malaysia has a total land area 329,758 km^2 (127,286 square miles), a population of 21 million, and a population density of 64 people per square kilometer.

Major Languages	Ethnic Groups	Major Religions
Malay (official)	Malay and other	Muslim (Malays)
Tamil	indigenous 59%	Buddhist (Chinese)
Mandarin	Chinese 32%	Hindu (Indians)
Hokkien	Indian 9%	Other

Malaysia is multiracial and multicultural. In addition to the major ethnic groups, it also has the tribal groups of Iban, Kadazan, Dusun, and Malanau. All ethnic groups are free to maintain their own cultures and traditions as long as they do not offend people of other cultures or religions. The national and most prevalent religion is Islam, although other religions are practiced freely.

Health Care Beliefs: Modern, traditional, and herbal; other complementary medicine. Although modern medicine is the most popular, all major ethnic groups have their traditional medicine practices. The Malay practice *bomoh,* the Chinese *sinseh,* and the Indians *ayuvedar.* Herbal medicine is now becoming more popular. In fact, some herbs are considered functional or healthy foods. Complementary medicine such as homeopathy and acupuncture are considered alternatives to modern medicine.

Predominant Sick Care Practices: Biomedical and traditional. The health care delivery system was geared toward achieving health for all by 2000. This was emphasized in all aspects of primary, secondary, and tertiary health care. The primary health care team plays a central role in prevention and early detection of diseases or health problems in the community. Health center staffs are led by doctors, but the main service activities such as antenatal and postnatal care, immunizations, child health care, family planning, health and nutritional education, and treatment of minor ailments are the responsibility of community nurses. Public health inspectors oversee other environmental health factors such as water supply, waste and sewage disposal, and sanitary latrines. Community clinics are available in every 5-km radius to ensure that everyone has access to health services.

Ethnic/Race Specific or Endemic Diseases: The epidemiology and endemicity of diseases seem to relate more to geographical location, stage of community development, and seasonal variations (e.g., rainy or dry season) than to ethnicity or tribal distribution. For example, dengue and dengue hemorrhagic fevers commonly occur in urban areas, whereas malaria is more common in rural areas, especially in the swampy coastal areas or jungle fringes. Seasonal variation in disease occurrence is mainly a result of changes in the breeding pattern of vectors. Vector-borne diseases peak in dry seasons, whereas water- and food-borne diseases increase after flooding. Cholera and typhoid outbreaks are related to water supply. Rural areas and poor urban areas are at high risk for water contamination. Noncommunicable diseases have a similar pattern. Cardiovascular disease is the major killer in Malaysia, and its prevalence is associated with lifestyle rather than ethnicity. A sedentary lifestyle, fat- and cholesterol-laden food, and cigarette smoking are all factors increasing Malaysians' risk for diseases typical of developed countries. Malaysia is in a period of transition and has the diseases of developed nations, such as cardiovascular diseases, diabetes mellitus, hypertension, and obesity, and diseases of developing countries, such as tuberculosis, sexually transmitted diseases, food- and water-borne diseases, and chronic energy deficiency. The World Health Organization's (WHO) estimated prevalence rate for HIV and AIDS in adults ages 15 to 49 is 0.42%. The estimated number of children from birth to 15 years living with HIV/AIDS is 550.

Families' Role in Hospital Care: Strong family ties exist. Community and family support in decision making concerning care of the sick, those with disabilities, and older adults is strong. Hospitalization or institutionalization is sought as a last resort. Visiting patients, bringing them food, and accompanying them in the ward are the norm. Family members take turns spending the night with their hospitalized relatives.

Dominance Patterns: The head of the family is usually a man, although the dominant figure may vary. For example, the grandfather may have more power than the rest of the family members, and the mother-in-law may have input in decision making. Gender issues do not affect dominance patterns of the family significantly. Taboos for menstruating women are quite common. The Malay previously referred to menstruation as "dirty," but now it is referred to as "a monthly affair." Because of modern lifestyles, women have more freedom.

Touch Practices: Medical examinations by the opposite sex are acceptable, although some patients prefer to be examined by doctors of the same sex. Eye contact and physical touching while taking a patient's history and performing a physical examination are normal. Exposure of private body parts such as women's breasts and genitalia is minimized. A chaper one may be required if a male doctor examines a female patient.

Perceptions of Time: Generally speaking, punctuality depends on the occasion. Malaysians are usually punctual for prayers, business appointments, and job interviews. On other occasions, especially those involving larger groups, such as wedding ceremonies, public speeches, meetings, and festive parties, being 30 minutes late is common. Being on time for personal appointments or dates depends on the individual. Although time perceptions change with time, currently many Malaysians other than city dwellers still move at a leisurely pace.

Pain Reactions: Pain tolerance and reactions seem to be related to ethnicity. Indians seem to have the lowest threshold of pain, followed by the Chinese and Malay; during labor, Indian women tend cry out the most. The Chinese immediately seek medical advice for pain or discomfort. Malays usually wait for a while and then consult traditional practitioners; modern practitioners are their last resort.

Birth Rites: Primigravida women, grand-multipara women, and women with medical problems must give birth in a hospital. Home or domiciliary deliveries are encouraged for mothers with uncomplicated second, third, or fourth pregnancies and are usually attended by trained personnel. Pregnant women with potential complications who go to community clinics or health centers are referred to district or general hospitals for further assistance. When the abdomen of a pregnant woman becomes obviously larger at the fifth or sixth month of gestation, the family throws a small party to announce the expected arrival of an additional family member. During pregnancy, it is believed that certain foods must be avoided; for example, pineapple and papayas are "sharp" and may cause abortion. Pumpkins and leafy vegetables produce flatulence and are also avoided. Food supplementation with vitamins or iron should be avoided because the Malay believe they may cause the infant to become too large and result in a difficult delivery. A pregnant mother is not allowed to participate in certain activities such as sewing or killing or injuring an animal because they are thought to deform the infant. Pregnant women must have their food cravings fulfilled, otherwise their infant may develop a mental problem or a "watery mouth." Eating fresh-water fish is encouraged because it helps heal wounds. Participation in household activities is encouraged to promote an easy delivery. During labor, traditional birth attendants and trained midwives are called to assist. The traditional birth attendant performs the necessary rituals, and the midwives assist in the birth, cutting the cord, bathing the infant, and taking care of the perineum. After childbirth the mother's autonomy and control are unquestioned, and she may eat and drink whatever she likes. She is encouraged to eat high-energy food such as chocolate and rice porridge and hot spices such as ginger and garlic to keep the body warm. Today's mothers are becoming conscious of their appearance, so the tradition of sleeping near a fire and wrapping the stomach with herbal mixtures has been abandoned because it can scald and blister the skin. Traditional massages are still performed to improve uterine contractions and involution. Birth attendants do the massage as midwives bathe the mother and infant daily for a week. On the seventh day after birth, a small party is organized to name the infant and is followed by another party on the seventh week (42 days) after birth to mark the end of the puerperium.

Death Rites: Death is thought of a journey into the next world. All of the family and community members gather to pay their last respects and bid farewell to the deceased person. Death rites differ according to religion. Muslim burials are carried out as soon as possible, preferably on the day of death. Other religions may have funerals a few days later. Cremation is not allowed for Muslims, although people of other religions may choose cremation. In a Muslim burial, the body is wrapped in a white cloth and buried without a coffin in the ground. Malaysian Muslims forbid organ donation after death, although giving blood or other parts of the body, such as skin, bone marrow, or kidneys, while a person is alive is acceptable. Autopsies are uncommon and only performed for forensic reasons; the body must be buried intact.

Food Practices and Intolerances: Staple foods for Malaysians are rice and bread, but the diet includes a large variety of foods. Rice and bread are eaten with meat, fish, poultry, and vegetables, and fruit is served as dessert. Foods restrictions primarily involve those who are fasting during Ramadan. Muslims do not consume pork, carrion, blood, or alcoholic beverages. Hindus do not eat beef, and Buddhists are often vegetarians. Traditional Malaysians sit on the floor and eat with their hands from an individual plate. Today, many eat at a table and use forks and spoons. The Chinese may use chop sticks.

Infant Feeding Practices: The majority of mothers breast-feed their infants. Mixed feeding (breast- and bottle-feeding) usually starts when mothers resume working. Breast-feeding usually lasts for 18 months, but exclusive breast-feeding may only last for 4 months. Solid foods are given to infants as young as 4 months of age. Mashed banana and rice porridge are common infant foods.

Child Rearing Practices: Children's likes and dislikes are generally considered; therefore mothers find it difficult to give medicine to a sick child or ask a child to go to school. Children sleep with parents for the first few years. Toilet training occurs later, usually after a child learns to talk. Disciplining children is usually the father's duty because he is considered a fierce and strict figure. Most parents expect their children to be obedient, and corporal punishment is acceptable. Male circumcision usually is performed between the ages of 6 to 15 years, although it can be done as young as at birth or as old as 20 years old. Female circumcisions are unusual, although some communities in Malaysia still practice it symbolically by making a small niche on the clitoris at birth.

National Childhood Immunizations: BCG at birth and 7 years if no scar; DTP at 3, 4, 5, and 18 months; OPV at 3, 4, 5, and 18 months and 7 years; hep B at birth and at 1 and 5 months; measles at 9 to 12 months; rubella at 12 years; DT at 7 years; and TT at 15 years and for pregnant women at 18 weeks gestation, +1 month. Other vaccines such as meningococcal and chickenpox vaccines are available on request.

Other Characteristics: Malaysians do not have a "family name." Their last name is the father's name, but they are always addressed by the first name. Women do not change their names after marriage.

BIBLIOGRAPHY

Annual report, Malaysia Ministry of Health, 1997.

Chen PC: Traditional and modern medicine in Malaysia, *Am J Chin Med* 7(3):259, 1979.

Lonergan S, Vansickle T: Relationship between water quality and human health: a case study of the Linggi

River Basin in Malaysia, *Soc Sci Med* 33(8):937, 1991.

◆ MALDIVES (REPUBLIC OF)

MAP PAGE (866)

Location: Formerly the Maldive Islands, the country is made up of atolls; it has more than 1200 small coral islands (about 220 of which are inhabited). No island's area is greater than 13 km^2 (5 square miles), and all areas are flat. Maldives is located in the Indian Ocean off of the southern tip of India. Inhabitants are primarily Islamic seafaring people, probably descendents of people from India and Sri Lanka. Before becoming a republic, Maldives was a sultanate. Most transportation involves a boat or sea plane. Maldives has two monsoon periods: the northeast *(ruvai)* from December through March and the southwest *(ulhangu)* from April to November. The temperature is approximately 82° F all year. The total area is 300 km² (116 square miles), about 1.7 times the size of Washington, DC, and Male is the capital. With a population of 310,764, the Maldives is one of the world's least developed countries, with a per capita gross domestic product (GDP) of $2000.

Major Languages	Ethnic Groups	Major Religions
Maldivian Divehi (official)	Sinhalese	Sunni Muslim (state religion) 100%
English	Dravidian	
Arabic	Arab	
Hindi	African	

Divehi is a dialect of Sinhala, and English is spoken primarily by government officials. No religions other than Muslim are permitted, and adherence to Islam is required for citizenship.

Health Care Beliefs: Acute sick care; traditional. Attitudes about health and hygiene-related concerns are very conservative, and the country has little focus on health promotion and disease prevention. Despite rapid population growth, family planning programs were not effective until the 1980s, when nongovernmental programs focused on improving overall health and included a focus on birth spacing and later age of marriage. The World Health Organization (WHO) monitored the use of various contraceptive methods for 4 years in the mid-1980s, but by the 1990s the government still had not taken action to reduce the number of children born per couple. Abortion is not legal. Because it is an Islamic culture, women are very modest about exposure of the body during physical examinations. Health care beliefs are influenced by traditional beliefs involving evil spirits called *jinnis* that can come from the land, sea, or sky. When modern medical methods cannot adequately explain reasons for illness, *jinnis* are often thought to be the cause, and people resort to using various charms and spells to combat them. Some observers have identified a magical-religious system parallel to Islam known as *fandita,* which provides a way for people to deal with actual or perceived problems.

Predominant Sick Care Practices: Magical-religious and limited biomedical when available. Medical facilities' resources are very limited, and some medications are not available. The capital has one private and one government-operated hospital. Efforts have been made to implement a primary care system to provide basic health care in areas outside of the capital.

Ethnic/Race Specific or Endemic Diseases: Endemic diseases include chloroquine-sensitive malaria, diarrheal diseases, and respiratory problems. Water-borne diseases (e.g., cholera, typhoid, gastroenteritis) are prevalent because of the lack of a potable water supply; the fresh-water table is shallow and easily contaminated by organic and human waste. Efforts have been made to address this problem in Male, but no sewage plans exist in the other islands. Like Tristan de Cunha and the Caroline Islands, Maldives has the highest prevalence for asthma in the world. People are at risk for polio, β-thalassemia, histoplasmosis, tuberculosis, eye infections, salmonella, leprosy, and filariasis. Since the 1970s, WHO has carried out numerous disease-eradication projects. The WHO's estimated prevalence rate for HIV/AIDS in adults ages 15 to 49 years is 0.05%. WHO has no estimates for children from birth to 15 years.

Dominance Patterns: Individual freedoms related to religion and workers' and women's rights are restricted. The legal system is based on Islamic law. A significant gap exists between the elite on Male (the traditional home of the sultans) and the populations of the other islands. Ruling families in Male control much of the government, business, and religion. Regional control over atolls is exerted by *atolu verin,* or atoll chiefs, and the *gazi,* or community religious leaders. About 80% of the households consist of a single nuclear family rather than an extended family, and the man is the head of the household. Descent is patrilineal. Women maintain their maiden names after marriage, and inheritance of property may be through both males and females. Muslim men may have as many as four wives; however, divorces are easy to obtain by men or women. In fact, Maldives has one of the highest divorce rates in the world. According to a recent census, almost 50% of women older than 30 had been married four or more times, and half the women had been married by age 15. The status of women is surprisingly high; the country has had four sultanas (female sultans). Women do not wear veils and are not strictly secluded except in mosques and during certain public gatherings.

Birth Rites: The infant mortality rate is high at 63.72 per 1000 live births (but is lower than the rate of 120 per 1000 in the 1970s). The total fertility rate is 5.5 children born per woman. Life expectancy rates at birth are 61.39 for men and 63.8 years for women.

Death Rites: Autopsies are uncommon because the body must be buried intact. Cremation is not permitted. For Muslim burials the body is wrapped in special pieces of cloth and buried without a coffin in the ground as soon as possible after death.

Food Practices and Intolerances: Only 10% of the land is arable. Food produced includes coconuts, taro, fish, and limited fruits and vegetables such as millet, corn, sweet potatoes, and watermelons. Fish and rice are staple foods; meat and chicken are consumed primarily on special occasions. National dishes include fish soup, fish curry, and fried fish. Alcohol is not generally available in this Muslim country, but a local brew *(raa)* is made from the crown of the palm trunk. A local nut *(arecanut)* is commonly chewed with cloves, lime, and betel leaf after dinner. Nutritional studies have reported marginal nutritional status and marginal malnutrition because of low intakes of fat, fruits, and vegetables (leading to low levels of beta-carotene, vitamin C, fiber, and folic acid). These deficiencies are of particular concern for children.

Child Rearing Practices: Unmarried adults usually remain with relatives rather than live on their own. About 45.63% of the population is 14 years or younger. Maldives has three types of schools: Koranic schools, Dhivehi-language schools, and English-language schools. Most students attend Koranic schools that charge a fee rather than the free government-sponsored schools. University education is unavailable. Literacy rates are high: 93.3% for males and 93% for females.

National Childhood Immunizations: BCG at birth to 3 years; DTP at 6, 12, and 18 weeks; OPV at birth and +1, +1, +1, +1 month; hep B at birth and at 1 to 2 and 2 to 3 months; measles at 9 months; vitamin A at 6 months to 14 years; and TT CBAW at 15 to 49 years ×5. Maldives has achieved high levels of immunization. The reported percentages of the target population vaccinated are as follows: BCG, 99; first dose of DTP, 98; third dose of DTP, 97; third dose of hep B, 45; MCV, 99; Pol3, 97; TT2 plus, 100; and vitamin A, 98.

Other Characteristics: Maldives has an active tourist trade and rapid economic growth that have resulted in modernization of the infrastructure and improved social indicators.

BIBLIOGRAPHY

Anonymous: Progress towards poliomyelitis eradication—Southeast Asia region, 1997-1998, *Morbid Mortal Wkly Rep* 48(11):230, 1999.

Golder AM et al: Dietary intake and nutritional status of women and pre-school children in the Republic of the Maldives, *Public Health Nutr* 4(3):773, 2001.

Turner KJ: Epidemiology of the allergic response, *Ciba Found Symp* 147:205–222: 1989.

Wolstenholme RJ: The disease spectrum in a Maldivian (Adduan) population, *Trans Roy Soc Trop Med Hygiene* 78(4):505, 1984.

www.cia.gov/cia/publications/factbook/geos/mv.html

http://memory.loc.gov/cgi-bin/query/r?frd/cstudy:@field(DOCID+mv0017″

http://www.lonelyplanet.com/destination/indian_subcontinent/maldives/culture.htm

http://travel.state.gov/maldives.html

◆ MALI (REPUBLIC OF)

MAP PAGE (862)

Kathleen Slobin

Location: Mali is a landlocked country in the Sudanic belt of West Africa and has a total land area of 1,204,021 km^2 (464,873 square miles), of which nearly 60% is desert. Its southern borders, which parallel the meandering Senegal and Niger Rivers, are fixed by the boundaries of

Guinea, the Ivory Coast, Burkina Faso, and Niger. Its northern border juts upward into the Sahara Desert, adjoining Mauritania to the northwest, Algeria to the northeast, and Senegal in the west at the Faléme River. Only 11% of Mali's total surface supports cultivation, resulting in a large variation in population density from 70 persons per square mile in the south to 5 persons per square mile in the north. The population distribution corresponds to Mali's three climate zones. The southern Sudanic zone receives 20 to 60 inches (508–1524 mm) of rainfall a year, the middle Sahelian zone receives 7 to 20 inches (179–508 mm), and the northern Sahara zone receives only minimal rain and has temperatures between 120° to 140° F (35°–45° C). The water and flood plains of the Senegal and Niger Rivers support transport, commerce, cultivation, animal husbandry, and fishing. They also serve as routes for cultural diffusion. The Republic of Mali was preceded by a progression of state societies, of which three were major kingdoms: the Sonike Empire of Ghana in the tenth century, the Mandigo Empire of Mali in the fourteenth century, and the Songhai Empire of Gao in the sixteenth century. French invasion and colonization of the area began in the late nineteenth century, resulting in the establishment of the French Sudan in 1920 after World War I. In 1958 the colony claimed independence as the Sudanese Republic and joined Senegal to form the Mali Federation. In 1960 the Federation split, and Sudan claimed its present name of Mali.

Major Languages	Ethnic Groups	Major Religions
French (official)	Mande (Bambara,	Muslim 90%
Local languages	Malinke, Sarakole) 50%	Indigenous beliefs 9%
	Peul (Fulani) 17%	Christian 1%
	Voltaic 12%	
	Songhai 6%	
	Tuareg/Moor 10%	
	Other 5%	

Mali is among the poorest of developing countries, with approximately 70% of its 11,008,518 people living in rural areas. Approximately 47.2% of the population is younger than 15 years of age, 49.73% are between 15 and 64, and 3.07% are 65 and older. Mali has many different ethnic groups who support a wide variety of living languages and dialects. About 10% of the population is nomadic, and some 80% are engaged in farming and fishing. The many ethnic groups, tradition-based and largely subsistence economies, and the wide range of urban to rural lifestyles make it difficult to generalize about cultural beliefs and practices. Voltaic groups include the peoples who speak Dogon, Senoufo, and Mossi. Although French is the language of government, other official languages include Bamankan (Bambara), Bomu, Bozo, Dogoso (Dogon), Fulfulde (Fulani), Hasanya, Mamara, Maninkakan (Malinke), Soninke, Sonoy, Syenara, Tamasheq, and Xaasongaxanno. Forty living languages are regularly used in Mali. Official estimates of religious affiliation do not adequately reflect the variation in beliefs and practices encountered in urban and rural areas. Many who proclaim themselves Muslim or Christian continue to integrate indigenous rituals, meanings, and practices into their relatively new faiths. What is most evident, especially among the villages in rural areas, are forms of syncretism in which authority, daily habits, and rituals surrounding birth and death bind the old and the new.

Health Care Beliefs: Acute sick care; traditional. Health care beliefs and practices reflect the evident ethnic and religious diversity that facilitates medical pluralism. The traditional view of illness is associated with a lack of balance between the physical and spiritual being. Today, even as urban and town dwellers accept the efficacy of biomedicine for some illnesses, they tend to retain their belief in indigenous medical practices, which involve the spiritual and emotional aspects of illness etiology. Although open to varying interpretations, indigenous classification systems identify illness as being in one of the following categories: illnesses of God, illnesses of the bush, illnesses of the ancestors, and sorcery. Illnesses of the bush are said to be caused by spirits or wind. Illnesses of the ancestors are punishments for breaking local customs or mores. Illnesses resulting from sorcery are caused by a person's enemies, people who use curses, poisons, or charms to harm others. Illnesses of God refer to simple, short-term sicknesses that follow a natural course. The illnesses in this category, such as malaria or influenza, are most readily adapted to the physical and mechanical framework of biomedicine

Predominant Sick Care Practices: Biomedical and magical-religious. In Bamako, as in other administrative centers and larger towns, publicly funded, biomedical clinics staffed by doctors, nurses, and nurse practitioners operate in proximity to Muslim religious healers and indigenous specialists. Treatment choices among urban and village residents depend more on the type and duration of illness than on the proximity of care. Typically, biomedical treatments are sought by individuals who have acute ailments such as fever, diarrhea, and stomach pain attributed to natural causes. Indigenous treatments are sought by those who have an illness that persists and becomes associated with sorcery or spirit possession. Within the indigenous sector of medicine, ill people or family members may consult *diviners* for an initial diagnosis and then consult healers who are known for their ability to treat the diagnosed illness. The healer in turn may prescribe a complex set of remedial measures that may include a combination of herbal medicine, prayers, amulets, sacrifices, or good deeds. In this sector, physical ailments are treated as culturally significant manifestations of disorder. Treatments, in turn, are activities that restore health and support the desired unfolding of events.

Ethnic/Race Specific or Endemic Diseases: Endemic diseases in Mali include chloroquine-resistant malaria, yellow fever, cholera, syphilis, leprosy, brucellosis, onchocerciasis, trypanosomiasis, and schistosomiasis. The

Centers for Disease Control recommends the following vaccines for travelers: hepatitis A and B, meningococcal meningitis, yellow fever, rabies (because of the risk of exposure through wild and domestic animals), typhoid, and booster doses for tetanus and diphtheria, measles, and polio. However, infant and child mortality rates in Mali continue to be high. The rate from 1992 to 1996 was 123 per 1000 live births for infants younger than 1 year and 238 per 1000 live births for children younger than 5 years. The immediate causes of death were malaria, respiratory and diarrheal infections, and malnutrition. The World Health Organization's (WHO) estimated prevalence rate for HIV/AIDS in adults ages 15 to 49 years is 2.03%. This percentage is the numerical equivalent of 100,000 adults and children. The estimated number of children from birth to 15 years living with HIV/AIDS is 5000. Of adults with HIV/AIDS infection, 53,000 are women. Since 1999, an estimated 9900 people have died of AIDS. The estimated number of children who have lost their mother or both parents since the beginning of the epidemic is 45,000.

Health Team Relationships: Health team relationships are organized hierarchically, with biomedical doctors maintaining diagnostic and treatment authority over nurses and other technical staff. Similarly, in maternity clinics where routine visits are conducted by a nurse with technical or lay staff, the nurse consults with a doctor but maintains authority over technical staff. In rural areas, these arrangements vary depending on the availability of trained personnel. Biomedical practitioners may consult or work with local healers if such an arrangement is thought to be in the best interest of the patient. Furthermore, biomedical personnel may train village birth attendants or other village health aids to act as clinic liaisons, provide simple medications, and administer prescribed injections. Finally, health and illness in Mali are family affairs, and the health team typically works to establish good relationships with members of a patient's family.

Families' Role in Hospital Care: In urban areas and especially in small towns, the family is the primary caregiver in the hospital. Family members typically provide meals, monitor the patient's condition, and attend to all of the patient's daily needs. The relationship between the doctor and the family is important and characterized by a certain interdependence maintained by communication and mutual respect. Forms of interaction between health care personnel and family members are not unlike those found between indigenous healers and their clients; therapeutic relationships are facilitated by responsive, open, and negotiated forms of communication.

Dominance Patterns: Dominance patterns vary across the many ethnic groups. Among settled agricultural groups (e.g., Bambara, Dogon), village life is typically ordered by extended families and sustained by a male hierarchy in which the oldest male is accorded the most respect. Among the nomadic groups, whose subsistence largely depends on animal husbandry (e.g., Fula [Fulani], Tuareg), male hierarchies are sustained in the smaller family groups. Traditionally, village and clan hierarchies are usually ordered in accordance with descending relationships of dominance from families of the chief, or royal family, to commoners, to persons of caste, who typically are artisans (e.g., blacksmiths, leather workers, musicians). Furthermore, dominance patterns are involved in the rather strict separation of male and female roles; males are responsible for major crop production, family economy, and decision making. Women are responsible for food preparation, providing water and cooking fuel, gardening, and child care. Marriage and family customs generally follow the patrilineal pattern, with wives becoming members of the husband's family household. Many groups also practice polygyny. Wives are subordinate to their husbands. Men have conjugal rights, paternity rights to the children, and control over their wives' labor; wives must request land and permission to work from their husband. Still, through their gardening and marketing skills, women may develop some financial independence. This pattern differs among nomadic groups (Fula and Tuareg), in which monogamy and nuclear family units tend to promote greater intimacy between husbands and wives. In 1995 the literacy rate, with "literate" defined as people 15 years and older who are able to read and write, was 31% for the total population, with 39% for males and 23% for females. The gender disparity in literacy correlates with 1996 reported differences in school attendance for boys (14.4%) and girls (7.3%).

Eye Contact Practices: Variations in eye contact in public tend to be dictated by gender relationships and positions of authority. Women lower their eyes and heads while talking to a man or a stranger; however, when women work in the marketing arena, work next to men in the fields, or make a request, their eye contact is more direct. In general, modesty and respect are the rule for men and women.

Touch Practices: Practices vary among ethnic groups. Generally, men and women do not shake hands. Young adolescent women and men may hold hands while walking down the street, but this is uncommon among adults. Certain groups, (e.g., Dogon), have various comportment taboos. For example, in certain Dogon villages, menstruating women are isolated, and all women of childbearing age remove their shoes on village pathways and may not enter the blacksmith's forge. These practices are more strictly observed in villages where either the chief or the majority of inhabitants observes indigenous religious practices.

Perceptions of Time: Perceptions of time among Malians are typically related to seasonal agricultural requirements. The temporal ebb and flow of the river flood planes are significant for nomadic groups. Among practicing Muslims, daily prayers break the day into five units. Furthermore, when recounting events or telling stories, time might be organized according to a birth, a death, or a national or religious holiday. In urban centers, use and perception of time is beginning to reflect European influence.

Pain Reactions: Malians tend to be stoical in their response to life's difficulties and pain. Women in the predominant ethnic groups rarely cry out during childbirth. Child rearing practices, which promote modesty, nobility, and shame as responses to self-promotion or self-display, prepare men and women to tolerate and bear adversity.

Birth Rites: Normally, the birth of a boy is preferred; however, girls are appreciated because they will later bear children and through marriage will strengthen the family. Because all the ethnic groups in Mali are patrilineal, children are said to belong to their father. In case of divorce the child stays with the mother until weaning or soon thereafter and then joins the father's household. Today, an estimated 23.7% of infants are born in a maternity clinic or with the aid of a skilled birth attendant. Among village and nomadic groups, women go through childbirth alone or with the help of their mother or mother-in-law. The birth of a child signals that a female is a true woman because she can bear children. Her next duties are to raise the child and continue to have more children. Generally, a newborn stays in the confines of the birth place, being nursed and protected by the mother. At about a week of age, the infant is baptized, given a name, and presented to the community. The total fertility rate is 6.81 children born per woman. Life expectancy is 47.02 years. Mali continues to have a high infant morality rate at 121.44 deaths per 1000 live births and a high maternal mortality rate of 577 per 100,000 live births. Approximately 23% of children younger than 3 years of age are seriously malnourished.

Death Rites: Because of the diversity of ethnic groups in Mali, rituals associated with death vary. Although Muslims typically wrap the body in cloth and bury it without a coffin in the ground within 24 hours, many continue to follow traditional indigenous practices. Both Muslim and traditional practices include periods of mourning when relatives and community members stop work and pay their respects to the bereaved family. Some groups, such as the Dogon, are known for the elaborate ritual practices associated with the death of significant members of the community. On an appointed day about a year after such a death, the young men dress in costumes and masks to represent spirits of the bush. They enter the village, and dance and escort the dead person's spirit out into the wilderness.

Food Practices and Intolerances: The diet varies enormously depending on economic status and primary form of subsistence. Many urban dwellers have adopted the full European diet with fish, meat, vegetables, and rice. Rural inhabitants typically eat millet porridge, couscous, or rice with either a vegetable or fish sauce. Seasonally available vegetables such as tomatoes, carrots, okra, and onions and fruits such as mangos are also eaten. Nomadic groups rely heavily on animal milk products, although they incorporate dietary grains purchased from or traded with local farmers. For holidays and celebrations, animals (goats or sheep) may be killed and roasted for the entire community. On such occasions, millet beer is produced by women and sold to the men who drink and enjoy the added revelry. Muslims do not eat pork.

Infant Feeding Practices: The majority of Malian women nurse their infants until age 2 years. About 90% of women nurse their infants until 9 months, when the rate drops to 80%; it drops to 72% at 15 months and 47% at 19 months. Approximately 17% are still nursing at 35 months. Typically, weaning occurs at approximately 2 years or when another child is born. Weaning is a critical and difficult time for children because mothers have few nutritious substitutes for breast milk. Typically, young children are given liquid millet porridge until they are able to adjust to a more adult diet. Although eggs, fish, and vegetables might be available seasonally or on certain occasions, they are typically not prepared for young children.

Child Rearing Practices: Although child rearing practices may vary from group to group, parents typically incorporate three major stages. During the first 3 years, children stay near their mother's side. Infants are wrapped on the mother's back and nursed on demand and learn the language and the rhythms of the household. At the second stage, from 7 to 8 years, the child plays freely among members of the extended family. Boys join their brothers and male cousins, and girls play with their sisters and begin to help their mother with daily chores. During the third stage, which lasts until puberty, children's behavior is seriously monitored to ensure the development of certain values (e.g., modesty, nobility, respect, diligence) prized by the group. At the end of this stage, boys are circumcised and girls, who are typically circumcised at a younger age, begin to menstruate.

National Childhood Immunizations: BCG at birth; DTP at 6, 10, and 14 weeks; OPV at birth and 6, 10, and 14 weeks; measles at 9 months; and yellow fever at 9 months. By 1999, 84% of children 12 to 23 months had received the BCG, 52% had received the third dose of DTP, 52% had received the Pol3, and 57% had received the MCV.

BIBLIOGRAPHY

Adams AM, Madhavan S, Dominique S: Women's social networks and child survival in Mali, *Soc Sci Med* 54:165–178, 2002.

Centers for Disease Control (2002): http://www.cdc.gov/travel/wafrica.htm

Central Intelligence Agency (2001): http://www.cia.gov/cia/publicaitons/factbook/geos/ml.html

Coppo P: *Médecine traditionnelle, psychiatrie et psychologies en Afrique,* Rome, 1988, Il Pensiero Scientifico Editore.

Demographic and Health Survey (1995): http://www.childinfo.org/cmr/Kh98/KH8AX1IM.pdf

Demographic and Health Survey: *Enquete demographique et de Santé, Mali 1996–1996,* Calverton, Md, 1996, Cellule de Planification et de Statistique do

Ministere do las Sante, Direction Nationale de la Statistique et de l'Informatique et Macro International.

Dieterlen G: Méchism de l'impureté chez les Dogon, *J Société Africanistes* 17:81–90, 1947.

Ethnologue (2002): *Languages of Mali,* http://www.ethnologue.com/show_country. asp?name=Mali

Feierman S: Struggles for control: the social roots of health and healing in modern Africa, *African Stud Rev* 28(2/3):73–147, 1985.

Griaule M: *Masque Dogon,* Paris, 1963, Institut D'Ethnologie.

Imperato PJ: *Historical dictionary of Mali,* ed 2, Metuchen, 1986, The Scarecrow Press.

Organization Mondiale de la Santé 2000: *Mali: Fiche épidémilogique sur le VIH/ SIDA et les infections sexuellement transmissible,* http://www.Who.int/emc/diseases/hiv.

Slobin K: Healing through the use of symbolic technologies among the Dogon of Mali, *High Plains Appl Anthropol* 16(2):136–143, 1996.

Slobin K: Repairing broken rules: care-seeking narratives for menstrual problems in rural Mali, *Med Anthropol Quart* 12(3):363–383, 1998.

Trimingham JS: *A history of Islam in West Africa,* London, 1962, Oxford University Press.

United Nations Children's Fund (2001): *UNICEF Global data base: skilled attendant at delivery,* http://www.childinfo.org/eddb/maternal/datavase2.htm.

United Nations Children's Fund: *Enfants et femmes au Mali.* Paris, 1989, L'UNICEF aux Editions, L'Harmattan

World Health Organization and United Nations Children's Fund (2001): *Review of national immunization coverage 1980–1999,* http://www.childinfo.org/eddb/immuni/ index.htm

Zahan D: 1970. *The religion, spirituality, and thought of traditional Africa,* Chicago, 1970, University of Chicago Press (Translated by K Erza and LM Marin).

◆ MALTA (REPUBLIC OF)

MAP PAGE (860)

Mark Muscat, Charles Savona Ventura, Brenda Murphy, and Maria Ellul

Location: The Maltese archipelago consists of three islands: Malta, Gozo, and Comino. It is located in the middle of the Mediterranean Sea 93 km (58 miles) south of Sicily and 288 km (179 miles) from the nearest point on the North African mainland. Together the islands have a total land area of 316 km² (122 square miles). The largest island of the group is Malta. Valletta, the capital, is the cultural, administrative, and commercial center of the Maltese islands. Topographically the islands consist of a series of low hills with characteristic terraced fields and several natural harbors. The climate is Mediterranean, with mild, rainy winters and hot, dry summers. The annual rainfall averages 578 mm, most of which falls from September through March.

Major Languages	Ethnic Groups	Major Religions
Maltese (official)	Maltese 100%	Roman Catholic (official) 91%
English (official)		Other 9%

The Maltese are descendents of ancient Carthaginians and Phoenicians, with strong Greco-Roman and Arab influences. European elements, namely Italian, Spanish, and French with traces of Anglo-Saxon origins, were assimilated. With a population of 382,525 in 2000 the country has one of the highest population densities (more than 1000 people per km^2) in the world. Five percent of the enumerated population in the 1995 census was born outside Malta; most of them were born in the United Kingdom, Australia, Canada, and the United States and are emigrants who returned. English and Maltese are the official languages, although Italian is widely spoken. Maltese has Semitic roots mixed with romance languages and is a good representation of the cultural heritage of the country

Health Care Beliefs: Active involvement; health promotion important. The population is becoming increasingly aware that prevention of disease is better than treating it, so more individuals are becoming health conscious and attempting to follow general guidelines of health promotion. Health promotion and education have become more established during the past 10 years. Consequently, the population is generally more aware of healthy lifestyles and their connection to prevention of common diseases such as diabetes, heart disease, and certain lifestyle-related cancers. A national health promotion agency financed by the health sector provides the impetus for most national campaigns for health education as well as related literature for public consumption. Mental illness is still feared, so those who are mentally ill or have disabilities are marginalized.

Predominant Sick Care Practices: Biomedical and religious. The Maltese are very health conscious when they feel unwell. Their first step is usually to consult their family doctor, although they frequently consult a specialist even for relatively minor disorders. In spite of their reliance on standard health services, their religious traditions often play a role, particularly among the older adults and very religious people or when they are facing a chronic or incurable disease. In these situations, the Maltese pray, participate in religious activities, and attend faith-healing services.

Ethnic/Race Specific or Endemic Disease: A major disease among Maltese is late-onset diabetes mellitus and its complications. It is a significant national health problem, with a prevalence of 10.3% in adults older than 35 years. Coronary heart disease and stroke are the major cause of morbidity and mortality. Cancers account for 25% of deaths, with lung, breast, and large bowel malignancies being the most common. Accidents are an important cause of death in those younger than 65 years. Communicable diseases of major public health significance include food-borne illnesses such as salmonellosis, *Campylobacter* infections, and recently, meningococcal disease. Murine and tick-borne typhus, leishmaniasis, and brucellosis are endemic to the islands. Certain genetic blood disorders such as thalassaemia typically found in the Mediterranean region are also found in Malta. The World Health Organization's (WHO) estimated prevalence rate for HIV/AIDS in adults ages 15 to 49 is 0.12%. This rate is considered low, and the major mode of transmission is through men who have sex with men. WHO has no estimates for children from birth to 15 years. So far, no local outbreaks of HIV infection have occurred among those who use intravenous drugs.

Health Team Relationships: Health services continue to be controlled by doctors, and they tend to assume a dominant position over other health care professionals. However, in the last 2 decades, the nursing profession has taken stock of its situation and established its importance, enabling self-management in the state health services. In spite of the apparent lack of harmony, working relationships between doctors and other health professionals are generally good. The renewed professional status of nurses is still unappreciated by clients. In contrast, doctors are often more respected, especially by the older generations.

Families' Role in Hospital Care: Generally, families pay close attention to their hospitalized relatives, regularly visiting them and bringing food. In spite of the close and caring family unit, sick and incapacitated older individuals are often left as in-patients in the hopes they will obtain early admission into the state's hospice for older adults.

Dominance Patterns: Malta has a typical patriarchal culture; however, it has significant Mediterranean cultural and social factors. For example, macho behaviors and attitudes can pervade especially all-male events. Mothers are often in control in the domestic arena, especially for education and child care issues. When family members are sick, the husband's mother plays an active role in caregiving and domestic organization. Legislative changes in family law and equal opportunities have been in place since the 1990s, and more skilled and professional women have been entering the workforce. However, male dominance still remains the norm on executive boards, in top management positions, and in the civil service. As in other Western countries, the paradigms and tensions of gender balance prevail.

Eye Contact Practices: It is considered polite to maintain eye contact during a conversation. The listener maintains the eye contact continuously, whereas the speaker may avert the eyes occasionally during the dialogue.

Touch Practices: The Maltese have basic Mediterranean attitudes, and both sexes are very expressive when speaking, using gestures and hand movements. Physical touching, particularly of arms and shoulders, is part of this expression. During greetings, a simple handshake is expected and may be accompanied by hand, arm, or shoulder clasping or an embrace, depending how well the individuals know each other. Kissing both cheeks is also common, especially between women and between women and men they know (e.g., family members, close friends).

Perceptions of Time: Because of their relaxed Mediterranean attitudes, the Maltese do not consider punctuality to be extremely important, regardless of social class. In general the Maltese feel the need to look toward the future. They tend to maintain traditions but at the same time adapt to change.

Pain Reactions: Attitudes and reactions to pain are generally Mediterranean, or overtly expressive.

Birth Rites: The majority of births occur in hospitals and involve standard medical practices. Although several Maltese folklore beliefs are related to childbirth, they are now basically extinct. However, doctors today are still asked questions associated with old beliefs passed on from previous generations. The infant mortality rate is 6.1 per 1000 live births. The birth rate has been steadily decreasing and is currently one of the lowest in the Mediterranean region, with a male to female ratio of 0.98.

Death Rites: Mourning involves demonstrative expressions of emotions by surviving family members and close friends. Nevertheless, attitudes are generally positive because of the strong belief in a Christian afterlife. Wearing black or dark clothing at the time of death and for a period thereafter is a mark of respect for the deceased person. Organ donations and autopsies have in the last 2 decades become more and more acceptable.

Food Practices and Intolerances: The Maltese diet is traditionally Mediterranean but has become more westernized in recent years. Convenience foods have gradually gained popularity in Maltese families, especially in two-income families, who usually have less time to prepare food with wholesome ingredients. However, in general, the public has become more aware of the importance of a low-fat, low-sugar, and no-salt diet, resulting in an increased consumption of low-fat milk products and whole-grain breads and cereals.

Infant Feeding Practices: Mothers predominantly bottle-feed, although during the last 7 years, breast-feeding has become more popular. However, rates are still low, with a current rate of 41% within 30 minutes of delivery. Even when mothers begin breast-feeding, they usually only do so for a short time. Maltese mothers are known to introduce weaning foods early in the infant's life, despite discouragement by health professionals. Many grandparents still think that a big baby is a healthy one.

Child Rearing Practices: Child rearing practices in Malta vary. Infants often sleep with their parents, but they generally have their own bed when they are older. The mother is usually the disciplinarian, although the father becomes involved when stronger disciplinary measures are needed. Children are expected to excel in education. Schooling is compulsory for all children ages 5 to 16 years and is provided free by the state. Approximately 33% of children attend church or private schools. People pay a voluntary contribution for church schools and a mandatory fee for private schools.

National Childhood Immunizations: BCG at 12 to 14 years; DTP at 2, 3, and 4 months, DT at 3 to 4 months; OPV at 2, 3, and 4 months and 3 to 4 and 16 years; hep B at 9 years; HIB at 2, 3, and 4 months; MMR at 15 months and 7 years; and Td at 15 to 19 years. In recent decades, the incidence of certain vaccine-preventable diseases in Malta has decreased significantly because of the availability of free, effective vaccines combined with improved living standards. Diphtheria, tetanus, and polio vaccines are required by law, and vaccinations against rubella are required by law for female children ages 10 to 13. Coverage rates are higher than 90% for diphtheria, tetanus, poliomyelitis, pertussis, and *Haemophilus influenzae* type B.

Other Characteristics: According to 2000 data, Malta scores high on the human development index, with a life expectancy of 74.32 years for men and 80.16 years for women. Malta depends heavily on imports because of their lack of any natural resources. The main income-generating industries are in the service and manufacturing arenas.

BIBLIOGRAPHY

Abela AM: *Gender issues and statistics,* Proceedings of a workshop of the Central Office of Statistics in collaboration with the Department for Women's Rights, Valletta, May 1998.

Abela AM: *Shifting family values in Malta: a western European perspective,* 1994, Media Centre, Institute for Research on the Signs of the Times (DISCERN).

Camilleri F: *Gender trends in Malta: a statistical profile,* Workers' Participation Development Centre, University of Malta, Commission for the Advancement of Women, 1996.

Department of Public Health: *Notifiable infectious diseases annual reports.*

Maltese Government: *The Maltese islands.* Retrieved February 1, 2002, from http://www.magnet.mt/info/location.html

National Immunisation Service: *Immunisation schedule.* Retrieved February 7, 2002, from http://health.gov.mt/immunisation

National Immunisation Service, Department of Primary Health Care: *Annual reports. The health of the Maltese nation.* Retrieved February 1, 2002, from http://www.health.gov.mt/indexnext.html

National Obstetric Information System, Department of Health Information, WHO-OBSQID Project: *Birth and delivery statistics from all birthing centres, annual summary report 2000.* Retrieved February 5, 2002, from http://www.health.gov.mt/indexnext.html

National Office of Statistics: *Demographic review 2000.* Retrieved February 1, 2002, from http://www.nso.gov.mt/cospubs/demography/2000/index 2000.htm Accessed 1 February 2002.

National Office of Statistics: *Shipping and aviation statistics 2000.* Retrieved February 1, 2002, from

http://www.nso.gov.mt/cospubs/shipping/2000/index2000.htm

Sultana RG, Baldacchino G, eds: *Maltese society: a sociological inquiry, Msida, Malta,* 1994, Mireva Publications.

World Health Organization: *WHO vaccine-preventable diseases: monitoring system,* Geneva, 2001. Retrieved March 1, 2002, from http://www.who.int/vaccines

World Health Organization: Epidemiological fact sheets by country, *Geneva, 2000.* *Retrieved March 1, 2002, from* http://www.unaids.org/hivaidsinfo/statistics/june00/ fact_sheets/index.html

◆ MAURITANIA (ISLAMIC REPUBLIC OF)

MAP PAGE (862)

Ould El Joud Dahada

Location: Covering 1,030,700 km² (397,850 square miles) Mauritania is one of the biggest countries in Africa, about three times the size of New Mexico. The country is divided into 13 regions called *wilaya* in Arabic; every *wilaya* is divided into departments or *moughataa*. The country is two thirds arid desert, and the climate is dry and hot. It is windy and dusty from February to May, and the rainy season is from June to October. The Atlantic coast is 754 km (467 miles) long and has a pleasant oceanic climate. The country is bordered in the south by Senegal (and the Senegal River separates the two countries), by Mali in the south and east, Algeria and the western Sahara in the north, and Atlantic Ocean to the west. The Capital is Nouakchott and contains a fourth of the total population.

Major Languages	Ethnic Groups	Major Religions
Arabic (official)	Mixed Maur/	Sunni Muslim 100%
Pular	Black 40%	
Soninké	Maur 30%	
Wolof	Black 30%	
French		

The population is estimated to be 2,548,157. Nouadhibou (the economic capital), Ziffa, and Zouerate are the largest cities after Nouakchott. The principal ethnic groups are Arabic, Toucouleur, Soninké, and Wolof. French is widely used in government and administrative offices.

Health Care Beliefs: Acute sick care, traditional, indigenous healers. The population has three kinds of care systems: modern medicine where it is geographically available; traditional medicine, which primarily involves herb plants, leaves, and roots; and *marabou* (traditional healers) who cure by using prayers, amulets, and other traditional methods. Pharmacy owners prescribe medications and treat illnesses, especially for those in the lower socioeconomic classes. Private clinics primarily exist in large cities but are inaccessible for the majority of the population. Self-medication with over-the-counter medications including antibiotics and other drugs is common.

Predominant Sick Care Practices: Magical-religious, alternative and biomedical when available. The Mauritanian health system is mainly based on primary health care, with essential services and medication comprising the first level of care. The second level (the hospital) in the *wilaya* is almost nonexistent. The tertiary level in the capital, Nouakchott, involves two general national hospitals: the Centre Hospitalier National and Cheikh Zayed Hospital. The area also has a specialized neuro-psychiatric hospital. Other medical institutions exist such as the School of Public Health, Institute for Medical Specialization, National Hygiene Center, National Transfusion Center, and National Orthopedic Center. Mauritania has no medical colleges.

Ethnic/Race Specific or Endemic Diseases: The compulsory reportable diseases are malaria (but only in the southeastern and central regions), pertussis, diphtheria, meningitis, typhoid fever, hepatitis B, cholera, and acute flaccid paralysis. Diseases preventable through immunization are diphtheria, neonatal tetanus, tetanus, measles, poliomyelitis, pertussis, tuberculosis, and hepatitis B. The World Health Organization's (WHO) estimated prevalence rate for HIV/AIDS in adults ages 15 to 49 years is 0.52%. The estimated number of children from birth to 15 years living with HIV/AIDS is 260. Since 1987, 6500 people have been infected with HIV, 1400 have died, and 1500 children have lost their mother or both parents because of HIV/AIDS. The people are regaining their awareness of and becoming more political engaged in the issue of HIV/AIDS.

Health Team relationships: Doctors and nurses are respected by the population.

Families' Role in Hospital Care: Having family and friends visit while hospitalized or ill at home is important. Although the presence of so many visitors occasionally interferes with the work of medical staff members, their assistance is needed because there are not enough staff members to look after every patient. The family assumes some respon-sibility for direct care. They also bring home-cooked meals to hospitalized patients and take turns staying with them 24 hours a day.

Dominance Patterns: The extended family includes uncles, aunts, cousins, nephews, and nieces. Tribal and ethnic life has a great influence on individuals and organizations. Respect for older adults is the norm. In general, family decisions are made by the men, but women are involved in the discussions. Women in Mauritania have the same rights as men and are very respected and free.

Eye Contact Practices: Direct eye contact is maintained during discussions and consultations.

Touch Practices: Among the Touchouleurs, Sonoinkés, and Wolofs, women and men greet each other by shaking hands. Arab men are not allowed to shake the hands of women or touch them and vice versa, if they are not "brothers." Between men and between women, greetings consist of shaking hands and embracing.

Perceptions of Time: Mauritanians are casual about punctuality and oriented to the present. Definitions of "early" and "late" are flexible.

Pain Reactions: Men tend to be stoical about pain. Women and children express pain more freely.

Birth Rites: Procreation is very important in this society, and the fertility rate is 6.3 children born per woman. Being infertile is considered a great tragedy, and usually the woman is assumed to be the problem. Pregnant women are respected by their husband and relatives, and they generally get everything they want because people believe that if they do not, their infant may be born with an abnormality. Husbands are not present during labor and birth, although the presence of a family member (who must be a woman) for natural births or cesarean sections is common. Male and female circumcisions are common. About 50% of all births occur at home, which contributes to the high maternal mortality rate (930 per 100,000 live births). Newborns are named on the seventh day after birth, and the event is celebrated by feasting. The mother has a rest period for 40 days after the birth and stays with her parents. Girls may have their ears pierced in the fist year of life. Working parents continue to collect their salaries, and working mothers usually have flexible hours and time to breast-feed. The life expectancy at birth for women is 54.8 and for men is 52.8 years. The infant mortality rate remains high at 74 per 1000 live births, and the maternal mortality rate is very high at 930 per 100,000 live births.

Death Rites: Death rites are governed by Islam. The body is wrapped in a shroud and buried as soon as possible. Before the burial, as many people as possible pray the "death prayer," and men recite from the holy Koran in the home. All groups have the same death, burial, and the cemetery rituals. Cremation is not allowed.

Food Practices and Intolerances: Food practices in Mauritania do not vary and are limited to dishes such as red meat, fish, rice and meat, rice and fish, and couscous and meat. Those in the middle and upper classes eat a great deal of red meat, particularly lamb and sheep. Camel is preferred by Arabs and beef by the Touchouleurs, Soninké, and Wolofs. The consumption of fruit, vegetables, and salads is increasing. Mauritanians do not regularly eat out or stay in hotels; they prefer to stay with parents or friends. Food restrictions are those dictated by the Muslim religion; for example, it is forbidden to eat pork or drink alcoholic beverages.

Infant Feeding Practices: Mothers generally breast-feed until their children are 2 years of age.

Child Rearing Practices: Children are treated affectionately, and kissing and holding children are signs of affection. School begins at 5 years with Koran school, and modern school follows at about 7 years of age. Children in the upper classes attend nurseries and preschools.

National Childhood Immunizations: BCG at birth; DTP at 6, 10, and 14 weeks; OPV at birth and 6, 10, and 14 weeks; measles at 9 months; and TT at 14 years.

BIBLIOGRAPHY

Office National de la Statistique: http://www.ons.mr

Organisation Mondiale de la Santé: http://www.oms.mr

Synthèse du profil pauvreté en Mauritanie 2000: Office National de la Statistique, October 2001.

World Health Organization and United Nations Children's Fund: *Revised 1990 estimates of maternal mortality: a new approach by WHO and UNICEF,* 1996, WHO.

◆ MAURITIUS (REPUBLIC OF)

MAP PAGE (863)

Geeta Oodit

Location: Mauritius is a small volcanic island in the Indian Ocean surrounded by coral reefs; it is 855 km (531 miles) off the east coast of Madagascar. Its nearest neighbor is Reunion to the southwest. The total land area is 1869 km^2 (718 square miles), almost 11 times the size of Washington, DC. Approximately 49% of the land is arable, and 22% is covered by forests and woodland. Mauritius is a developing country with a multiethnic population. It has a high population density—about 611 people per square kilometer.

Major Languages	Ethnic Groups	Major Religions
English (official)	Indo-Mauritian 68%	Hindu 52%
French	Creole 27%	Christian (mostly
Creole	Sino-Mauritian 3%	Roman Catholic) 28%
Hindi	Franco-Mauritian 2%	Muslim 17%
Urdu		Other or none 3%
Bhoipuri		
Hakka		

Health Care Beliefs: Active involvement; health promotion efforts increasing. Prevention and health promotion are practiced in Mauritius. People fear mental illness, and people with mental disorders are marginalized. Mauritians do not believe that diseases can be cured with heated coins or cups. They do practice acupuncture, and people often take herbs as a primary relief measure. Reiki has recently become a popular means for curing such symptoms as stress, insomnia, and hypertension. From 1987 to 1988, smoking prevalence decreased 23% in men and 61% in women, likely because of increases in the cigarette tax, health promotion programs, and a concerted effort to decrease cigarette advertising. Measures also have been taken to improve the cardiovascular health of

Mauritians (e.g., encouraging them to use soybean oil instead of coconut oil for frying). These steps have improved lipid levels and decreased disease risk. Most of the people believe in God, and some consider sickness to be God's will.

Predominant Sick Care Practices: Biomedical, traditional and religious. Most consult doctors; however, some consult traditional healers. It is estimated that approximately 94 species of plants are used in traditional medicine on the island. Health care services are free in public hospitals for everyone and are of good quality. Mauritians in low-income groups particularly benefit from these services, which are accessible to all. Mauritius has five main hospitals throughout the island, and all are well equipped; it also has some private hospitals. Private companies offer health insurance, but few Mauritians are able to afford it. For primary health care, the people first go to a community health center managed by a doctor and nurses; one is usually within a 1-mile radius.

Ethnic/Race Specific or Endemic Diseases: Mauritians are at very high risk for hepatitis A and less risk for hepatitis B and sickle cell anemia. Patients with sexually transmitted disease and prison inmates have a high incidence of infection with hepatitis C virus (46.2% and 43.8%, respectively). They are also at risk for cryptosporidiosis and malaria. Bronchial asthma is an increasing problem and seems to be largely attributable to house dust mites, which are considered to be the most serious allergen on the island. Mauritians are also at risk for epidemic dropsy from oil contaminated with argemone seed and for glucose-6-phosphate dehydrogenase (G6PD) deficiency. Schistosomiasis is endemic in the districts of Pamplemousses, Port Louic, and Grand Port. β-Thalassemia is prevalent because of the gene flow from India to Mauritius. Type II diabetes is endemic, with high prevalence rates in all ethnic groups and a high incidence of diabetic retinopathy. Mortality from coronary heart disease is among the highest in the world. Insulin resistance syndrome has been reported in a high proportion of Mauritians with premature heart disease. The seroprevalence of cytomegalovirus infection is very high in those who donate blood: 94% of males and 100% of females. Mortality from stroke is very high (like in eastern Europe and the former Soviet Union countries): 268 per 100,000 men and 138 per 100,000 women. Industrialization in the last 10 years has been accompanied by a 30% increase in breast cancer incidence. Life expectancy at birth is 72 years. The World Health Organization's (WHO) estimated prevalence rate for HIV/AIDS is 0.08%. WHO has no estimates for children from birth to 15 years. As of October 2001, 269 cases of HIV/AIDS had been reported (173 males and 96 females) in Mauritius. In 1998, 8% of sex workers were found to be infected.

Health Team Relationships: Relationships are doctor driven. Doctors are respected by patients and other members of the health care team.

Doctors and nurses in the service sector have a good working relationship. Nurses provide basic care and counseling and all participate in a 3-year nursing course. In addition, the Institute of Health provides refresher courses every 2 years.

Families' Role in Hospital Care: Families do not stay in hospitals overnight. However, they do visit patients, and some relatives bring food in the morning and afternoon even though food is provided by the hospital. Because health care is free, patients do not pay unless they are treated in a private hospital or clinic, which provide more personalized care and service. In these situations, families pay the bill, which includes drug costs. Families play a key role in providing care and taking responsibility for the relative. Responsibility for care of older family members is shared by the children.

Dominance Patterns: Mauritius is a patriarchal society. Men dominate the home and social sphere. Literacy rates are 87% for men and 79% for women. Women's status has been evolving, and women are playing a large role in the development of the country and the family. Because of the free education, boys and girls go to secondary schools and universities. Girls perform better than boys in the arts and even in the sciences. Women have high aspirations and delay marriage, mostly by choice. Gender inequality still exists, especially among those in the poorer and lower classes.

Eye Contact Practices: In general, direct eye contact is acceptable and expected.

Touch Practices: Mauritian culture is characterized by kissing, but shaking hands is common when people do not know each other well. If people are close, then embracing is perfectly acceptable. Doctors and nurses are allowed to touch patients for examination purposes; however, when a male doctor is examining a female patient, a female nurse always assists him.

Perceptions of Time: In general, Mauritians are conscientious about being on time for appointments.

Pain Reactions: Different individuals react differently according to their sociocultural backgrounds. Mauritians of Asian origin seem to be very sensitive to pain, whereas those of African descent seem to be more capable of enduring pain. For example, when people of Indian/Asian origin receive a Norplant or Minilap insert, they seem to feel much pain, whereas those of African descent (i.e., Creoles) seem to tolerate the pain better.

Birth Rites: Mauritius is a multicultural society. Each ethnic group has particular rites and rituals that are performed to celebrate the birth of a child. Indo-Mauritians participate in community bathing on the sixth and twelfth days after birth to celebrate. The mother bathes in water that has been boiled with different kinds of herbal leaves. (A priest is normally consulted regarding the appropriate timing of this bath.) Special food (seven varieties of greens) is cooked, and special spices are incorporated that cleanse the body and soul. Cumin seeds are boiled, and the mother drinks the resulting water. Mauritians' preference for boys, which was very common in the past, is gradually disappearing. The maternal mortality rate is 120 per 100,000 live births, and the fertility rate is 1.9 children born per woman. The infant mortality rate is 15 per 1000 live births. Studies indicate that congenital cytomegalovirus infection is highly likely to be associated with mental retardation and deafness of Mauritian children. The incidence of breast-feeding has decreased from 86% to 72% since 1985. According to surveys, only 16% of infants from 3 months and younger are exclusively breast-fed. About 29% of infants between the ages of 6 and 9 months are given breast milk and complementary foods and liquids. Only 12% of infants from 12 to 15 months receive at least some breast milk along with complementary foods. Therefore many women limit breast-feeding and begin supplementing breast milk when the infant is very young.

Death Rites: A funeral is a social event, so families and friends gather for a 1-night vigil under a tent erected for the event. Black coffee is served, and neighbors provide support, informal counseling, and food for the bereaved family. Burial and cremation (for Hindus) tend to be dignified, although it is acceptable for relatives to cry. The government provides some monetary allowances for funerals. Death is accepted as an inevitable event. Autopsies are acceptable, although organ donations are not popular among Mauritians.

Food Practices and Intolerances: Basic foods are rice, *chappati* (flat bread), grains, vegetables, and either seafood or meat. Different communities have different eating habits. The food of Indo-Mauritians tends to be spicy, and curries served with *chappati* are popular. They also often prepare Chinese and Indian food as well. Creoles rely more on dishes that are not vegetable-based (e.g., beef, pork, seafood) and tend to eat more tinned meat and fish. Muslims eat more beef and less lamb. Mauritians are quite health conscious and on weekdays, they often consume more soup, bread, and pasta and eat more rice on the weekend. Asians in villages often eat with their hands, but this practice is changing. At weddings, food is served in a banana leaf and eaten with the hands. Many people in urban areas eat with a fork, knife, and spoon. Recent efforts promoting the substitution of palm oil with soybean oil for frying have been effective in some parts of the population, reducing the lipid levels of those groups.

Infant Feeding Practices: Fewer women are breast-feeding, regardless of their ethnic origin. Many women try to breast-feed for at least up to 3 months, but working women may find this more difficult, and many women are joining the labor market.

Child Rearing Practices: Child rearing involves a mixture of leniency and discipline, and spanking is allowed. Parents are very loving and enjoy parenting, but at the same time they are pressured to raise their children in a disciplined way. Usually the mother is responsibility for raising the children. Children normally sleep with both parents until they are 5 or 6 years old. Both parents are responsible for disciplining children.

National Childhood Immunizations: BCG at birth; DTP at 3, 4, and 5 months; OPV at 3, 4, and 5 months; measles at 9 months; and DT at 2 and 5 years.

BIBLIOGRAPHY

Chandrasekharan N, Sundram K: Fall in cholesterol after changes in composition of cooking oil in Mauritius, *Brit Med J* 314(7079):516, 1997.

Cox HS et al: Decreasing prevalence of cigarette smoking in the middle income country of Mauritius: questionnaire survey, *Brit Med J* 321(7257):345, 2000.

Gorakshakar AC et al: β-Thalassemia gene flow from India to Mauritius, *Am J Hematol* 65(3):263, 2000.

Grummer-Strawn LM et al: Infant feeding patterns on Mauritius Island, 1991, *Soc Sci Med* 43(12):1697, 1996.

Khittoo G et al: Mutation analysis of a Mauritian hereditary breast cancer family reveals the *BRCA* 26503delTT mutation previously found to recur in different ethnic populations, *Human Heredity* 52(1):55, 2001.

Manraj M et al: Genetic and environmental nature of the insulin resistance syndrome in Indo-Mauritian subjects with premature coronary heart disease: contribution of α3-adrenoreceptor gene polymorphism and β-blockers on triglyceride and HDL concentrations, *Diabetologia* 44(1):115, 2001.

Pultoo A et al: Detection of cytomegalovirus in urine of hearing-impaired and mentally retarded children by PCR and cell culture, *J Comm Dis* 32(2):101, 2000.

Sarti C et al: International trends in mortality from stroke, 1968 to 1994, *Stroke* 31(7):1588, 2000.

Schwarz TF et al: Hepatitis C and arboviral antibodies in the island populations of Mauritius and Rodrigues, *J Med Virol* 44(4):379, 1994.

◆ MEXICO (UNITED MEXICAN STATES)

MAP PAGE (857)

Eric Dumonteil and M. Rubí Gamboa Léon

Location: Located between the United States and Central America, central Mexico is a high plateau with mountain chains on the east and west and oceanfront lowlands. The total land area is 1,972,550 km² (761,603 square miles). The coastline is 9,329 km (5,798 miles). The United States is to the north, the Gulf of Mexico to the east, Belize and Guatemala to the south, and the Pacific Ocean to the west.

Major Languages	Ethnic Groups	Major Religions
Spanish 99%	Mestizo 60%	Catholic 89%
Nahuatl 2%	Native American 30%	Protestant 6%
Maya 1%	White 9%	Other 5%
Other 4%		

Health Care Beliefs: Passive role; acute sick care only. Common beliefs include *mal de ojo* ("evil eye"), *empacho* (problems caused by a bolus of food stuck to the stomach wall or blocking the intestine), *caida de mollera* (a fallen fontanel), *susto* (the result of a frightening or traumatic emotional experience), and *mal puesto* (a hex or illness imposed by another). Health is believed to be a matter of chance or God's will. Diseases are believed to be influenced by "hot" and "cold" imbalances. "Cold" illnesses are caused by the invasion of the body from the exterior and are generally incapacitating (resulting in alterations of motor and sensory functions, pain, and immobility). "Hot" illnesses are believed to be generated from within the body and result in irritation (e.g., skin rash, fever, cough). Theories about causes of illness include contagions, excessive work, cold or "air" exposure, food contamination, punishment from God, bewitchment, or transgression of moral and social rules. Spiritual diseases may be cured through *limpias* (cleansing of the soul) or *leída de la suerte* (reading of the destiny). Prayer and the use of religious relics, rosaries, and crucifix may also be used, in addition to various amulets. Being a healthy male is part of appearing macho, meaning that men seek health care less frequently than women. Thus males are perceived as being healthier than females or children. The severity of a patient's illness may be determined partly by pain or the appearance of blood. Some consider stomachaches and headaches to be illnesses.

Predominant Sick Care Practices: May include biomedical, magical-religious, traditional, and self-medication practice—all focusing on cure of acute illness rather than prevention and based on Western, pre-Hispanic, African, and Catholic elements. Mexico has approximately 30,000 *parteras* (traditional midwives) and 10,000 *curanderos* (healers) treating 15 to 20 million patients in Mexico. People of all socioeconomic and educational levels use biomedical and folk health systems, sometimes simultaneously. Additional folk healers include *yerberos* (herbalists) and *sobadors* (masseuses). Homeopathic and other alternative medical practices, as well as practices with oriental influences such as naturopathy and spiritism, are becoming more popular. Because the cultural context of medical and folk practices are fundamentally completely different, the two systems have historically been perceived as conflicting, and traditional healers have been marginalized within the health system. However, recent years have involved a move toward greater integration of both health practices (although it has been only partially successful), and several attempts at legislating traditional folk medicine (through registration, licenses, and training) have been made in some states. Some biomedical practitioners are also beginning to accept and use traditional medicine. Biomedical practice is divided into private medicine (primarily for upper-class patients), public medicine (administered by the Secretaria de Salubridad y Asistencia), and socialized medicine (represented by the Instituto de Seguridad y Servicios Sociales de los Trabajadores del Estado and the Instituto Mexicano del Seguro Social) The sale of drugs—other than narcotics, barbiturates, and other addictive drugs—is uncontrolled; pharmacists can be consulted, and self-medication is widely common.

Ethnic/Race Specific or Endemic Diseases: Endemic diseases include chloroquine-sensitive malaria, leishmaniasis, Chagas' disease, with no or little risk in urban areas. Mexicans are at risk for gastroenteritis and intestinal infectious diseases, obesity, diabetes, tuberculosis, dengue fever, high hemoglobin and hematocrit levels, and alcoholism. The World Health Organization's (WHO) estimated prevalence rate for HIV/AIDS in adults ages 15 to 49 is 0.29%. The estimated number of children from birth to 15 years living with HIV/AIDS is 2400. In Mexico, HIV/AIDS principally affects men (with a male/female ratio of 6:1).

Health Team Relationships: The health care system is doctor driven, with a strict and vertical organization of power and duties. Practitioners may believe that patients have no right to question them. The practitioner is considered an outsider, which affects the power relationships with the patients. On the other hand, the *curandero,* or folk healer, is a member of the nuclear or extended family network and able to create a special relationship with the patient, who is considered in a more integral context. The government has attempted to incorporate traditional healers into the system. Family interdependence takes precedence over independence, so self-care is not an important concept. Personal matters are discussed and handled within the family. Valued behaviors by health care practitioners include being informal and friendly, including family members in interactions, giving careful and concrete explanations, sharing experiences, taking time to listen, and inquiring about the patient's health. Health care practitioners of the same sex as their patients are preferred, and people have greater confidence in older practitioners.

Families' Role in Hospital Care: Family members are expected to be involved in care, and frequently accompany hospitalized patients. The male head of household should be consulted before health care decisions are made and should be included in any counseling sessions. The mother is not allowed to give consent for her child's treatment, and family decisions supersede decisions made by health care providers. Female health care providers and family members other than a person's spouse may not give care at home if that care involves touching adult male genitalia.

Dominance Patterns: The family structure is patriarchal; however, gender roles are becoming more democratic. The mother is in charge of running the household and decides when health care will be sought, behavior that has been encouraged by the health system because it presents health as a domestic problem. Mothers also play an important role in self-medication. Deference is given to elders, fathers, and grandfathers. The collective needs of the family, whether extended or nuclear, take precedence over those of the individual. Some ethnic groups in the state of Oaxaca have a matriarchal structure (Tecas).

Eye Contact Practices: In rural or periurban areas, sustained direct eye contact is rude, immodest, and even dangerous for some. Problems from a person with *mal de ojo* ("the evil eye") can result from excessive admiration. Women and children are thought to be more susceptible to *mal de ojo;* therefore children may avoid direct eye contact with others.

Touch Practices: Touch is used often. Touching people while complimenting them neutralizes the power of the evil eye. Closeness and physical contact are valued in familiar situations. However, excessive embracing, especially between men or between fathers and sons, may be badly perceived. People with rural origins are more reserved and less demonstrative.

Perceptions of Time: The tendency is to focus on the present and be relatively unconcerned about the future. The concept of time is relaxed. *Mañana* may or may not mean "tomorrow."

Pain Reactions: Emotional self-restraint and stoical inhibition of strong feelings and emotional expression are common, as is an impressive tolerance to pain. In rural areas, medical care is not sought unless an illness is severe. Expressions of pain may be a self-help relief mechanism. Pain relief might be refused as a means for atonement. During labor women loudly repeat *"Aye, yie, yie"* requires long, slow breaths, thus it is becoming a culturally and medically appropriate method of pain relief.

Birth Rites: Practices associated with pregnancy may include sleeping flat on the back to protect the infant, keeping active to ensure a small infant and an easy delivery, avoiding cold air, and continuing sexual intercourse to lubricate the birth canal. Folk practices include satisfying *antojos,* or food cravings that can cause an infant to have a characteristic mark such as a strawberry spot if they are not satisfied, and *cuarentena,* a 40-day relaxation period during when the mother rests, stays warm, avoids bathing and exercise, and eats special foods that promote warmth. It is inappropriate for a husband to be with his wife during birth; he is not expected to see his wife or child until both have been cleaned and dressed. A woman's mother, sister, or both may be present during delivery. Approximately 55% of infants are born in hospitals, where the number of cesarean sections have increased in the past years (and now account for 30% of all births). Traditional deliveries are also popular, and 45% of both urban and rural mothers deliver with the assistance of *parteras.* Women in the culture have great confidence in *parteras* because they are from the same socioeconomic class and have the same cultural values as the mothers. A coin or marble that has been wiped with alcohol may be strapped firmly to an infant's navel to make it attractive.

Death Rites: Small children may be shielded from dying and death rituals. Family members take turns staying continuously with the dying person in the hospital. Grief can be quite expressive; for example, *el ataque* consists of hyperkinetic and a seizure type of behavior pattern that releases emotions. Death rituals include overnight mourning at the funeral home before burial. For many, the funeral is a day of music, dancing, and rejoicing, especially after the death of a child. All Souls' Day is a major celebration of the day that souls travel home to the living and are remembered.

Food Practices and Intolerances: Lactose intolerance is common. Prenatal vitamins are thought to be a hot food and are not supposed to be taken during pregnancy. Dietary staples such as rice, corn, and beans provide complete proteins. Tortillas (corn flour), beans, and chilies (hot peppers) are the main diet of many poor families, and malnutrition is still very common. Poor food and water hygiene are a source of major gastroenteritis and intestinal infectious diseases. Pineapples, pumpkins, peanuts, sweet potatoes, squashes, avocados, papayas, and mangos are native to Mexico.

Infant Feeding Practices: Colostrum may be thought of as bad milk, therefore bottle-feeding may be used until the breasts fill with "normal" milk. Breast-feeding is common during the first 4 months.

Child Rearing Practices: Birth control methods other than the rhythm method are not popular in the Catholic population. Mexicans tend to overprotect newborns. Children are expected to strictly respect and obey their parents and elders, and the older adults often help with child rearing. Older brothers may discipline younger siblings. Families are more protective of girls, so boys are granted greater overall freedoms.

National Childhood Immunizations: The national immunization protocol was changed in 1999: BCG at birth and 6 years; pentavalent vaccine (DTP+HB+HIV) at 2, 4, and 6 months and at 2 and 4 years; OPV at 2, 4, and 6 months; measles at 9 months and 6 years; and DTP booster at 2 and 4 years.

Other Characteristics: It is believed that a high fever may be broken by using warm blankets and hot drinks. Intravenous solutions *(sueros)* are also available and may be infused at home by family members or folk healers. The first surname is the father's, and the second is the mother's. A married woman adds "de" before the husband's surname. Human beings are measured with the palm open and held vertical to the ground at the correct height. The fifteenth birthday is an important social event for girls. In many rural areas, people strongly believe in the relationship between the body and social or cosmic equilibriums.

BIBLIOGRAPHY

Alvarez-Gordillo GC et al: Percepciones y prácticas relacionadas con la tuberculosis y la adherencia al tratamiento en Chiapas, México, *Salud Publ Mex* 42(6):520, 2000.

Avila-Curiel A et al: La desnutrición infantil en el medio rural Mexicano, *Salud Publica Mex* 40:150, 1998.

Castaneda Camey X et al: Traditional birth attendants in Mexico: advantages and inadequacies of care for normal deliveries, *Soc Sci Med* 43(2):199, 1996.

Flores M et al: Consumo de energía y nutrimentos en mujeres Mexicanas en edad reproductiva, *Salud Publica Mex* 40:161, 1998.

Gomez DO: La regulación de la práctica médica en México, *Rev Invest Clin* 51(4):245, 1999.

Gonzalez-Perez GJ et al: Caesarean sections in Mexico: are there too many? *Health Policy Plan* 16(1):62, 2001.

Jones ME, Bond ML: The Mexican health care system: implications for nurses in the United States, *J Multicult Nurs Health* 2(2):12, 1996.

Nigenda G et al: La práctica de la medicina tradicional en América Latina y el caribe: el dilema entre regulación y tolerancia, *Salud Publ Mex* 43(1):41, 2001.

Santos-Preciado JI: Nuevo esquema de vacunación en México, *Salud Publ Mex* 41(1):1, 1999.

Taddei-Bringas GA et al: Aceptación y uso de herbolaria en medicina familiar, *Salud Publ Mex* 41(3):216, 1999.

http://www.unaids.org/hivaidsinfo/statistics/june00/fact_sheets/index.html
http://www.who.int/vaccines/

◆ MOLDOVA (REPUBLIC OF)

MAP PAGE (861)

Valentina Teosa

Location: Moldova is located in southeast Europe and occupies a territory of 33,700 km² (13,008 square miles). In the north, east, and south it is bordered by the Ukraine and in the west the Prut River separates Moldova from Romania. Moldova has a population of approximately 4.3 million. The landscape is extremely varied, ranging from the hills of central and northern Moldova to the Dniester steppelands and the South Moldovan plain, or the Budzhak Steppe. Moldova's chief asset is its black soil, which covers 80% of the territory. Forests cover more than 9%.

Major Languages	Ethnic Groups	Major Religions
Moldovan (official)	Moldavan 58%	Eastern Orthodox 98%
Russian	Romanian 7%	Jewish 2%

According to most linguists, the Moldovan language is practically the same as Romanian, therefore it is often referred to as *Moldovan/Romanian*. As a heritage from Soviet times Russian is commonly used. Two languages are spoken in the country—Moldovan/Romanian and Russian. Moldova has always been a multiethnic state. About 35% of the population is made up of various minorities: 13.8% Ukrainian, 13% Russian, 3.5% Gagauz, 2% Bulgarian, and 1.5% Jewish. Much smaller in number are people from the following national groups: Belorussian, Polish, German, and Roma (Gypsy). The Gagauz population is historically of Turkish origin and has Orthodox beliefs.

Health Care Beliefs: Acute sick care; traditional. The society's level of knowledge about health and disease has increased overall. It is understood that good health involves good nutrition and physical exercise. It is unlikely that anyone now believes that a person can be healed by such practices as rubbing heated coins over a diseased area; however, traditional beliefs fly in the face of current medical knowledge. For example, girls and women are actively discouraged from sitting directly on cement or stone because they believe that their reproductive systems will be damaged by the cold radiating out of those materials. In addition, a vinegar compress is still considered an effective treatment for fevers. The hard economic conditions during the last few years have been particularly difficult for those with mental illness; they were previously marginalized and are now neglected by the society.

Predominant Sick Care Practices: Biomedical and religious. The network of clinics, polyclinics, dispensaries, hospitals, maternity homes, and children's dispensaries is spread widely across Moldova. The new architecture of health care at the regional level includes regional hospitals that provide complex care, district hospitals, outpatient clinics, and rural preventive outpatient clinics. Medical treatment is generally free, but the country has many private medical centers where patients pay for their treatment. Private clinics have to be licensed and adhere to professional codes, as do public facilities. Doctors are most often consulted when people are in pain. People who simply do not feel well consult a family doctor at the clinic; if they feel too sick to leave the house, they send for the doctor. The doctor asks the patients about the symptoms of their illness, does a comprehensive examination, and perhaps gives an injection to relieve pain. Alternate healers are not generally consulted, and wearing amulets for prevention of illness is not a common practice. Praying for health is very common, although people also consult a doctor.

Ethnic/Race Specific or Endemic Diseases: Tuberculosis is a significant problem, with an incidence rate of 72 cases per 100,000 people. The people of Moldova, particularly rural laborers, are at high risk for chronic respiratory diseases of nontuberculous etiology. The sexually transmitted disease incidence is 208 cases per 100,000 people. Moldova has high hepatitis B endemicity and high rates of acute perinatal infections with the virus. Infants must be consistently vaccinated against hepatitis B. In addition, Moldova has a fairly high incidence of hepatitis C and D infection among children and pregnant women. The hepatitis C virus is also considered endemic in the dialysis centers in Moldova. Malaria imported from Azerbaijan is closely monitored by health officials. From 1994 to 1996 a diphtheria epidemic occurred after the disease had been almost nonexistent for 20 years. Fortunately, it was controlled by mass immunization campaigns. The World Health Organization (WHO) does not report HIV/AIDS prevalence estimates for Moldova, but locally available statistics provide a fairly accurate picture of the current situation. The first cases of HIV infection were recorded in 1987. From 1987 to 1995, only solitary cases were detected but since 1997, HIV/AIDS has been considered endemic. By October 2001, 1436 Moldavian citizens were infected with HIV/AIDS, and 25 have died. Individuals from 15 to 40 years of age account for 94% of all cases. In the first years of the epidemic the usual mode of transmission was sexual contact. In December 1995 the first case of infection contracted through injectable drug use was noted. Since 1996, HIV/AIDS has been highly prevalent among those addicted to drugs, and in 2001, 83% of all those infected were using injectable drugs. Of those in the total population who are infected, 74.15% are men and 25.85% are women. Predictions of future incidence of HIV infection are not favorable because of the increasing number of those addicted to drugs and the tremendous increase of HIV/AIDS in women who are commercial sex workers and have been spreading the disease to their clients. During the last several years the following patterns have been observed: decreases in the average age of those infected, an increase in the percentage of infected women, and an overall increase of the number of AIDS cases.

Health Team Relationships: The doctor is considered to be the chief of the health care team and plays the dominant role in decision making. Nurses are expected to take care of patients and perform tasks such as giving injections or changing surgical dressings. Working relationships between nurses and doctors are usually good.

Families' Role in Hospital Care: Relatives or friends buy everything necessary for the treatment of a hospitalized family member, and in some hospitals this includes medications. Visits with patients take place according to the timetable of each particular institution. Only close relatives can visit maternity wards. It is acceptable for patients to spend the weekend with the family and then return to the hospital.

Dominance Patterns: There are strong negative attitudes toward women in rural communities, where patriarchal traditions still dominate. Since time immemorial, the role of women has been to take care of the family, cook, and raise the children. During the last 2 decades, women's involvement in professional, scientific, and political life has increased. In 2000, 9% of the parliament consisted of women; in 2002, it increased to 13.3% and for the first time a woman became the speaker of the parliament.

Eye Contact Practices: It is customary to maintain direct eye contact with people while talking. During conversations with friends, not looking into another person's eyes indicates a lack of respect or sincerity. Traditionally, it is prohibited for people outside the family to look directly at an infant's face until the baptism ceremony because of fear of the "evil eye" (i.e., the power of a person to harm others simply by looking at them). Direct eye contact with those in a higher social class is acceptable.

Touch Practices: Touch is considered acceptable in the health care field, and some women have male gynecologists. People of rural origin are more reserved and less demonstrative in their attitudes and emotions. Traditional people shake hands when meeting each other. On arrival and departure, kissing acquaintances is normal. Gestures are common during interpersonal communications.

Perceptions of Time: People strive to make their plans, visits, and appointments at a particular time; thus punctuality is an important issue. However, in rural communities, punctuality and the concept of being on time for an appointment are relative because of more relaxed attitudes in the provinces toward time. Moldavian culture tends to focus on previous times and traditions. Youth are more liberal and tend to think more of the present and future.

Pain Reactions: Women in particular tend to react to pain very emotionally, and anesthetic drugs are frequently used. Pain reactions are individual and usually judged by such parameters as facial grimaces, body position, stature, and limited movement. In rural areas, people often avoid seeking medical care unless their pain is severe.

Birth Rites: Pregnancy is considered a very delicate period for a woman's health, so the family takes great care to offer pregnant women the best quality and largest quantity of food they can. Women are typically cared for by professionals during and after delivery. Most infants, other than those being born in emergency situations, are delivered in hospitals. Until recent years, fathers and other family members were not allowed to assist in the birth. Today, the father is often present in the delivery room. The birth of a child is a time for family feasting and visits to the newborn. Mothers generally bathe babies every day in the first month after birth, and breast-feeding mothers restrict foods likely to distress the baby. Moldovans tend to celebrate the birth of a son or a daughter equally, although some fathers are especially happy when a son is born. Because the majority of Moldavans are Orthodox, the birth of a child is strongly associated with the baptism ceremony, which is a religious and a family occasion. Until the baptism ceremony, infants are protected from the "evil eye" by limited contact with strangers. Parents usually decide on the infant's name according to family tradition and the calendar of religious holidays. The infant mortality rate is approximately 20 per 1000 live births.

Death Rites: The family expresses grief through crying and wailing at the moment a person dies. Family members and close friends dress in black and official suits. Depending on the religious background and traditions of the person who died, a priest might be summoned to conduct the burial service. The family offers meals out of respect to the deceased on the burial day and the ninth and fortieth day after the death. Family members continue to go to the cemetery and bring flowers to the tomb, especially on sacred days or special anniversaries. Organ donations and autopsies are acceptable with the family's approval. Moldova has no tradition of cremation. Bodies are buried in graves, usually according to the rites of the Eastern Orthodox religion.

Food Practices and Intolerances: Moldovans have few food intolerances. The majority of people eat three times a day. Because most people now work during the day, during the last 10 years most people have preferred that the largest meal be in the evening rather than at lunch. Most prefer to eat at home. Before the Christmas and Easter holidays, dietary restrictions for religious reasons are common. The national cuisine is noted for its abundance of fruit and vegetables. Typical Moldavian food includes vegetables (tomatoes, cucumbers, onions) with special Moldovan cheese, soups such as zama and ciorba, and national meals, which are *mamaliga* and *sarmale*. In rural communities, Moldovans are hurt if a guest refuses an offered glass of wine because the people have a long-standing tradition of winemaking. Meat and meat products are preferred for dinner. Meals are usually eaten at a table with a spoon, knife, and fork.

Infant Feeding Practices: It is considered traditionally important and is socially expected for women to breast-feed their babies, and most do so for at least 4 months. Differences in feeding newborns and infants primarily depend on whether the mother lives in an urban or a rural area and whether she is employed. Village women breast-feed more often and longer, and women concerned about returning to work breast-feed much less frequently and for shorter periods.

Child Rearing Practices: In some families, fathers play the dominant role and children are brought up in relatively conservative surroundings. In families with only one parent and in multigenerational families, the grandparents usually participate freely in the child rearing process. Children usually sleep in their own beds. It is common for children to attend kindergarten, particularly if their mothers are working. In rural communities, children may be punished severely and be involved in housekeeping and agricultural work from an early age.

National Childhood Immunizations: BCG at birth and at 6 to 7 and 14 to 15 years; DTP at 3, 4 1/2, 6, and 22 to 24 months; OPV at 3, 4 1/2, 6, and 22 to 24 months and 6 to 7 years; hep B at birth and 1 and 6 months; measles at 12 months; mumps at 12 months; DT at 6 to 7 years; and Td at 14 to 15, 20, 25, 30, and 35 years. Vaccination coverage is reported to be 98%. As a result the morbidity associated with hepatitis B in newborns is five times lower.

Other Characteristics: As a result of the well-known political and socioeconomic changes that took place in the country during the last decade, the Republic of Moldova is currently experiencing a significant socioeconomic crisis. The country has a high incidence of poverty, an exhausted health care infrastructure, and a deteriorating reproductive potential and gene pool. The country has also experienced a total decline in the volume of personal goods and services and consumption. Levels of consumption in 2000 compared with 1990 are lower. The level of consumption of fish and fish products decreased 3.4 times, fruit and berries 3.3 times, sugar and confectionery products 4.9 times, meat and meat products 2.7 times, and milk and dairy products 2.5 times. This decline may have eventual negative long-term consequences for the health of the population. The sharp decline in living standards has negatively affected the population structure as well. From 1990 to 2000 the population of the Republic of Moldova decreased, primarily because of migration outflow. Fewer children have been born since 1990 but the rate is beginning to stabilize, and females from 15 to 19 years have increased birth rates. Although stabilization of the birth rate is considered good, the increased rate is associated with young (often single) women and having negative social consequences. It leads to the potential deterioration of health in young mothers and children, creates obstacles in raising the educational and professional level of young people, increases the number of individuals needing social assistance, and reduces the well being of young families. The decline in living standards and the current crisis in the public health system has led to an increase in the mortality rate. In addition, because of alcohol and tobacco use, murders, and suicides, men have a life expectancy of 63.7 years compared with 71% for women.

BIBLIOGRAPHY

Bejan-Volc I: *Femeile în comunit˘ile rurale: tendin˘e 'i afirm˘ri,* Chissinau, Moldova, 2000.

Iuri-Apostol E: *Eutanasia—o problem' a deontologiei medicale. Materialele conferin˘ei ˘tiin˘ifice anuale a colaboratorilor 'i studen˘ilor,* Chissinau, Moldova, 1997.

Moldova National Study: *Gender, poverty and employment,* ILO Program, Chissinau,, Moldova, 2001.

Moldova National Study: *HIV/AIDS situation and social-economical sphere,* ILO Program, Chissinau,, Moldova, 2001.

National human development report, 1999–2000, Republic of Moldova, UNDP Moldova, 2000, 2001.

Report status of women in the Republic of Moldova, UNDP Moldova, 1999.

Republica Moldova: *Pia˘a muncii ˘i dezvoltarea social'. L-ul anuar economic i social,* Chissinau, Moldova, 2000.

Situa'ia mamei ˘i a copilului în Republica Moldova. Realit˘i ˆi tendin'e, Raport National, Chissinau, Moldova, 1997.

◆ MONACO (PRINCIPALITY OF)

MAP PAGE (860)
Location: Monaco is a tiny 1 km² (0.6 square miles) hilly wedge of coastal land on the French Mediterranean.

Major Languages	Ethnic Groups	Major Religions
French (official)	French 47%	Catholic 95%
English	Monegasque 16%	Other 5%
Italian	Italian 16%	
Monegasque	Other 21%	

Ethnic/Race Specific or Endemic Diseases: The World Health Organization (WHO) has no reported prevalence statistics for HIV/AIDS for Monaco.

National Childhood Immunizations: There are no reported immunization schedules for Monaco but WHO reports that in 1999, 100% of the population was vaccinated for BCG, the third dose of DTP, the third dose of hep B, the third dose of HIB, MCV, and Pol3.

◆ MONGOLIA

MAP PAGE (865)

Laurie Elit

Location: Mongolia is a landlocked country north of China and south of Russia. Mountains in the northwest, vast deserts in the south, and steppes of grass-covered plains in the central and eastern regions make up the 1,500,000 km^2 (579,000 square miles) of the country. It is divided into 20 *aimags* (with a population of 12,232 to 117,024 per *aimag*) and two large cities. (Ulaan Baatar has a population of 673,664, and Darkhan has a population 90,433.) In 1999, 2,400,000 people inhabited the country. Half of the people are nomadic and depend on camels, cattle (including yaks), horses, sheep, and goats for their livelihood.

Major Languages	Ethnic Groups	Major Religions
Mongolian (90%)	Mongol 90%	Tibetan Buddhist and
Russian	Kazak 4%	Shamanism 95%
	Chinese 2%	Muslim 4%
	Russian 2%	Christian and other 1%
	Other 2%	

Different ethnic groups speak with slight dialects or accents (i.e., Buryat), but the different groups have no problems understanding each other. Since 1944, the Russian Cyrillic alphabet has been used to write the language. The most common second language is Russian, and all medical training is still in Russian. Literacy is 90%.

Health Care Beliefs: Acute sick care; traditional. Most Mongolians do not fully understand the health care principles of preservation of health and disease prevention. Before 1921, health practices were based exclusively on Buddhist-Tibetan traditions, with lamas as the main health practitioners.

Commonly the lama is asked to say a prayer on behalf of the sick patient or advise him on a course of sutras or prayers.

Predominant Sick Care Practices: Ethnomedical, biomedical and magical-religious. The country is increasing its use of traditional medicines, including certain foods (wolf), acupuncture, and cupping (application of heated cups to the affected body part). Some of the traditional beliefs about healing are that drinking mother's urine cures many diseases, walking in cold water causes tonsillitis, applying a freshly cut dog ear to an affected area heals burns, putting a newborn puppy on the liver area cures liver cancer, fermented mare's milk is good for gut disease, and vitamin injections cure many illnesses. Currently, health care is available for those with health care insurance. The national health insurance program is based on the principle of cost sharing: the employee or self-employed individual pays a basic fee for the program, and the government pays the rest of the cost. However, many individuals are unable to participate in the insurance program because they do not have the cash to make direct payments. Children receive health care provided they are registered in their home district, even when parents are unable to afford insurance.

Ethnic/Race Specific or Endemic Diseases: Mongolia has a high maternal mortality rate and high mortality rate among young men. The incidence of some communicable diseases is high (i.e., diarrhea and respiratory illness in young children, viral hepatitis, tuberculosis, brucellosis, and sexually transmitted diseases). Brucellosis usually affects nomads because of their consumption of unboiled milk and homemade cheeses and handling of freshly killed meat or cow dung (used for building fires). Bubonic (black) plague is seasonal; the plague infects marmots, squirrels, and rats and is transmitted to humans by flea bites. The increase in cardiovascular disease causes 4600 deaths annually. In addition, 30% of the population older than 40 has hypertension, and rheumatic fever and rheumatic heart disease are significant medical and health problems. The rate of cancer is increasing, with the leading causes of cancer in 1997 being liver, stomach, cervix, and lung. Alcoholism rates and tobacco use are high. Currently, the incidence of HIV/AIDS is low. The World Health Organization's (WHO) estimated prevalence rate for HIV/AIDS in adults ages 15 to 49 is 0.01%. WHO has no estimates for children from birth to 15 years. A 1997 Memorandum of Understanding was created between the United Nations Country Team and the Government on HIV/AIDS and other sexually transmitted diseases; all Mongolians stipulate that individuals who are abroad for more than 3 months must be screened when they return to the country.

Health Team Relationships: Mongolian medicine is a mixture of Western technology, Oriental practice, and folk treatment. During the communist era, the health care system was a clone of the model set up in the former

Soviet Union. The country had a nationwide network of government facilities, with service delivery, human resources, and infrastructure being centrally planned. Mongolia had community-based *feldschers* (health care workers) and doctors supported by a hierarchy of hospitals and mobile emergency teams. Physician assistants (including midwives) staffed approximately 1200 medical stations *(somon)* in the rural areas, and doctors staffed 29. The country had 12 *sum* hospitals with consulting rooms, an in-patient ward, and a delivery room, and three *aimag* (general hospitals). This system led to a high degree of specialization among doctors (pediatrics: 21%, obstetrics: 6%, public health: 6%, preventative diseases: 6%, and oncology: 0.5%). These specialty units also resulted in a great deal of compartmentalization in that doctor interactions stayed within their specialties. Although rural areas had few doctors, cities had a high number of doctor per person; for example, 49% of doctors are concentrated in the capital city Ulaan Baatar. Since 1993 the government has restructured health services through the implementation of a development program supported by funds from the Asian Development Bank. The program design was based on a dialogue among stakeholders who determined needs, with the goals of continuous improvements in access and availability of health care and better delivery of services. A major goal was to redistribute resources from the hospital sector to primary care and prevention. Currently, Mongolia has 84 family group practices with 334 doctors servicing 17% of the population. These doctors have moved from hospital-based clinics to clinics in their target population areas, and performance contracts specify the level of essential services, such as emergency coverage, to be given. From a personnel perspective, 65% of doctors are women. Unlike North America and western Europe, the social and economic status of the doctor is low; however, doctors have traditionally run the health care system. Nursing exists as a profession in Mongolia, but doctors do not trust nursing assessments of patients. The quality of nursing care is being addressed by developing nursing care standards, and education in management issues. The health team does not tell patients when they are dying. In addition, details of operations are not explained to the patients. These practices are thought to protect the patients. For example, a woman who is having a hysterectomy could be divorced by her husband because she is no longer able to have children.

Families' Role in Hospital Care: Family members are expected to be supportive during illness, providing personal comfort and food for the patient. Families provide basic care for hospitalized relatives; they bring meals, clean the sheets, and deliver medications. However, families are not allowed in hospital rooms in major city hospitals or in consulting rooms. Patients must go down to a reception area or have another patient go to the reception area to get supplies from the family. If a patient needs help getting to the bathroom or eating, they depend on their roommates.

Dominance Patterns: Mongolians have a profound respect for elders, and the social fabric of the country revolves around the family unit. Women have traditionally enjoyed a position of respect and relative equality, but each gender has its own role. Women are primarily responsible for the sheep, animals that are important for daily sustenance. Men are primarily responsible for horses, which are considered animals of prestige, war, and sport. Women remain subordinate to men; however, attitudes are more flexible when the men are away for military or other duties. Women are torn between the desire to have children, which is considered a civic duty, and the desire for higher level jobs requiring commitment of time and energy. In the 1979 census, 34.9% of employed women worked in agriculture (a decreasing trend), 14% worked in industry, and 11.5% worked in education and art. Women have more of the lower paying jobs, and only a token number have higher professional and administrative positions, even though girls are three times more likely than boys to receive a higher education. To remedy this situation, Mongolia joined the Convention to Eliminate All Types of Gender Discrimination in 1981. However, a 1999 survey indicated that about 33% of Mongolian women were subjects of some form of domestic violence; 10% stated they had been battered by their husbands or another male living in the home. UNIFEM (United Nations) and the Mongolian government signed a memorandum of understanding in September 1999 that focused on policies to ensure the economic security of Mongolian women, improve the situation of rural women, increase the representation of women at management and decision-making levels, eliminate all forms of violence against women, and ensure increased access of women to information and technology.

Eye Contact: In urban areas, it is considered polite to make eye contact when talking. In the rural areas, herders are reluctant to make eye contact with those in authority, and if a woman makes eye contact with a man, it is considered flirting.

Touch: Mongolians live communally with four or more people in each room and have a very small circle of personal space. It is normal for friends of all ages and of the same sex to walk arm-in-arm or hand-in-hand. Men slap the backs of other men, and it is usual to greet one another with a handshake. Mongolians do not use outward signs of affection such as hugging or kissing, and adults never touch another adult's head.

Perception of Time: Immense travel distances and unreliable transportation mean that it is normal to be flexible about appointment times. Appointments can sometimes be delayed by a day, or they may happen spontaneously. Most people live in the present, so planning can be an issue. Young people, especially in urban areas, are thinking more about the future.

Pain Reactions: Older people and people from rural areas are very stoical. This is partly a result of the limited availability of narcotics for postoperative or palliative pain. Acupuncture and herbs are often used to relieve pain, and hot mineral baths in volcanic springs are used for muscle and joint pains.

Birth Rites: During the communist regime (1920 to 1990), child bearing was promoted as a woman's patriotic obligation, and material incentives were given to promote large families. The state mandated maternity leaves of 120 days with pay. The state also gave a family allowance that provided subsidies at the level of an industrial wage for families with more than 4 children younger than 16 years of age, bestowed the second-class Order of Maternal Glory and subsidies for five to eight children, and bestowed the first-class Order of Maternal Glory and subsidies for more than 8 children, in addition to a 2-week, all-expenses paid vacation at a spa. This incentive program resulted in large families, with 22.8% of families having 5 to 6 members, 16.1% of families with 7 to 8 members, and 11.8% of families with more than 8 members. Families also were exempt from certain taxes. Paralleling Mongolia's economic transition period, maternal mortality that was 120 per 100,000 live births in 1990 increased to 157 per 100,000 live births in 1998. The change for the worse was a result of the closing of maternal rest homes and the poorer quality of emergency medical care in geographically isolated areas. In the last 5 years the quality and quantity of antenatal care has increased; 90% of pregnant women now receive some antenatal care, and 94% of deliveries take place in hospitals. Soon after delivery, a particular type of mushroom is eaten that helps increase uterine contractions (i.e., is a folk medicine method used to decrease postpartum bleeding). As Mongolian women embrace modern medicine, they remain rooted in past traditions. For example, a popular antenatal belief is that two pregnant women should not give each other the traditional Mongolian greeting in which the younger woman supports the arms of the older women because it may cause the infants to switch their sex. The leading cause of maternal morbidity is anemia associated with poor nutrition. Women are released from domestic work for 36 days after delivery, and they are not allowed to bathe in cold water because it is believed to lead to arthritis or edema. Although husbands or older mothers provide physical and psychological care for the new mother, other people are expected to stay away for a month. Mongolians have traditions about which gifts to bring and how to present the gifts since bringing the wrong gift or presenting it incorrectly could dry up the mother's milk or make her breasts sore. A newborn is not named for at least a week, and some names are chosen to confuse the spirits; for example, the name *Enbish* means "not this one" and is a plea to the spirits to leave the infant alone. When an infant is sick, parents may change the child's name to confuse the spirits so that the child is left un-harmed. Likewise, boys may be dressed as girls. Traditionally, children do not have their hair cut until they are 3 to 5 years old.

Death Rites: It is taboo to talk about death. During the dying process, patients are usually in the home and depend on the care of family because Mongolia does not have a home nursing system. Families decide who is allowed to be present. In acknowledgment of the insufficient care for the dying in Mongolia, a palliative care society and center has been formed. All people (other than Kazak Muslims) who die in the hospital automatically have an autopsy. The main religion in Mongolia is Buddhism. In keeping with the religion, most bodies are buried in the traditional fashion with a lama, family, and friends present. The ceremony is long, with all attendees staying at the graveside until the ground is covered and the cement slab is poured over the site.

Food Practices: The Mongolian diet in rural areas is based on meat and dairy products. Tea is flavored with milk and salt. *Airag* (fermented mare's milk) is the Mongolian national drink and tastes like bubbly buttermilk. Yogurt, milk, cheese, and fermented milk are easily obtained from the milk of horses, goats, yaks, camels, and cows. Boiled mutton in flour is a favorite dish, and it is considered a great honor to be given a sheep's tail. Other meat dishes include beef, horse, and camel. All parts of the animal are eaten. With the exception of potatoes and onions, fresh vegetables and fruits must be imported and therefore are rare in the countryside. Only 30% of households can or dry foods for later consumption. Mongolians consume significant amounts of alcohol, but it has a seasonal nature. Consumption increases during the milking season, when homemade milk vodka distilled from fermented milk can be produced quickly and cheaply on a daily basis. Food is served on a large platter. In rural areas the food is usually first served to the husband and fathers, and in urban settings the women serve the children first. It is polite to accept food with the right hand, with the left hand supporting the right hand at the elbow. Knives are rare, so most people eat with a spoon and fork. Drinks such as *airag* are consumed from a shared bowl.

Infant Feeding Practices: Most infants are breast-fed. It is common to use fat from a boiled sheep's tail as a comforter. At 4 months, 75% of infants are exclusively breast-fed, but only 21% are by 6 months. Approximately 30% of children are weaned on *bantam,* a porridge of wheat flour and meat mixed in boiling water, 20% on rice porridge with sugar and butter, and 19% on *zutan,* a porridge of wheat flour only. The 1992 Mongolian Child Nutrition Survey showed that the main nutrition problems in children are protein energy malnutrition, iodine deficiency, vitamin D and A deficiencies, and iron deficiency anemia. Of children younger than 5, only 35% consumed meat three or more times per week. As a result, 33% of children younger than 5 years of age have rickets, and 42% have anemia. Attitudes and knowledge about infant feeding were explored by the Nutritional Research Center and World Vision Mongolia. When women were asked what they thought caused bowed legs, 36% said they were related to diet, 19% said they were because a child had not been breast-fed, 17% believed they were caused by horseback riding, and 15% said they were related to sunshine. These responses demonstrate that a combination of traditional and biomedical beliefs still influence attitudes toward health and the causes of illness.

Child Rearing: The extended family lives in a *ger,* which is a one-room circular tent. Beds are placed around the periphery around a central wood or dung-burning stove. While parents work, grandparents, relatives, and young "elder siblings" care for younger children. During the absence of parental caretakers, statistics indicate that children are at high risk for injury and death. Child rearing is strict, and fathers are usually responsible for disciple. Smacking children on the bottom is common and accepted.

National Childhood Immunization: BCG at birth and at 8 and 15 years; DTP at 2, 3, and 4 months and 2 years; OPV at birth, at 2, 3, and 4 months, and at 2 and 8 years; hep B at birth and 2 and 8 months; measles at 8 months and 1 and 3 years; DT at 2 and 8 years.

ACKNOWLEDGEMENTS: This chapter could not have been written without the help of numerous people: R. Cosstick (of the United Nations Children's Fund); Dr. Erdenejargal, B. Irhig of the Joint Christian Services, R. Reimer of the Peace Corps; R. Salmela of the World Health Organization; and G. Venning of Volunteer Services Overseas.

BIBLIOGRAPHY

Batjargal J et al: *Care practices for young children in Mongolia,* 2000, Ministry of Health Mongolia and United Nations Children's Fund.

Bolormaa D: Mongolia's national drug policy, *World Health* 2:28, 1995.

Brill MT: *Enchantment of the world. Mongolia,* Chicago, 1992, Children's Press Chicago.

Davidson I: The wealth of Khan, *American Way,* 1991.

DeGlopper DR: *The society and its environment in Mongolia—a country study,* Federal Research Division, Library of Congress, 1991, Washington, DC.

Foggin PM et al: Health status and risk factors of seminomadic pastoralists in Mongolia: a geographic approach, *Soc Sci Med* 44(11):1623–1647, 1997.

Grennway P, Storey R, Lafitte G: *Mongolia,* Melbourne, 1997, Lonely Planet.

Johnstone P: *Operation world,* 1993, Grand Rapids, Mich, Zondervan Publishing House.

Kachondham Y et al: Child health and nutritional status in Ulaanbaatar, Mongolia: a preliminary assessment, *Asia Pac J Public Health* 6(4):226–232, 1992.

Kotilaninen H: Rehabilitation of the hospital infrastructure in a developing country, *World Hosp Health Serv* 37(2):25–28, 34-35, Ulaanbaatar, 2001.

Neupert RF: Early-age mortality, socio-economic development and the health system in Mongolia, *Health Transit Rev* 5(1):35-57

Nutrition Research Center and World Vision Mongolia: *Micronutrient status, coverage and knowledge, attitudes and practices in children under five and pregnant and lactating women in Bulgan, Tov and Ulaanbaatar, Mongolia,* July 2001.

O'Rourke M, Hindle D: Mongolia's system-wide health reforms: lessons for other developing countries, *Aust Health Rev* 24(2):152–60, 2001.

Salmela R: Personal communication, 2000.

United Nations Systems in Mongolia: *1999 annual report,* http://www.unmongolia.mn/ who/index.html

World Health Organization: *WHO vaccine-preventable diseases: monitoring system,*
    Geneva, 2001. Retrieved March 1, 2002, from http://www.who.int/vaccines/"
World Health Organization: *Epidemiological fact sheets by country,* Geneva, 2000.
    Retrieved March 1, 2002, from http://www.unaids.org/hivaidsinfo/statistics/
    june00/fact_sheets/index.html
http://www.un-mongolia.mn/publications/mou-aids.htm

◆ MOROCCO (KINGDOM OF)

MAP PAGE (862)

Location: Morocco is located on the northwestern coast of Africa just
south of Spain, across the Strait of Gibraltar. The North Atlantic Ocean is
to the west and northwest, the Mediterranean Sea to the northeast, Algeria
to the east and southeast, and the western Sahara to the southwest. The
total land area is 446,550 km^2 (172,368 square miles) slightly larger than
California. Rabat is the capital. The Atlantic coast has fertile plains, whereas
the Mediterranean coast is mountainous and subject to earthquakes. The
climate is Mediterranean but becomes more extreme in the interior.
Morocco is a developing country, and about 19% live below the poverty
line. The total population is 30,645,305, with a GDP per capita of $3500.

Major Languages	Ethnic Groups	Major Religions
Arabic (official)	Arab Berber 99.1%	Muslim 98.7%
Berber dialects	Non-Moroccan 0.7%	Christian 1.1%
French	Jewish 0.2%	Jewish 0.2%

French is spoken in government, diplomacy, business, and postprimary
education settings.

Health Beliefs: Acute sick care; traditional. Moroccans believe that those
with the "evil eye" (the power to harm others merely by looking at them)
can affect the health and well-being of individuals.

Predominant Sick Care Practices: Biomedical and magical-religious.
Adequate medical care is available, especially in Casablanca and Rabat.
However, not all facilities meet high-quality standards, and it is not
always possible to attain specialized care or treatment. Medical facilities
are adequate for situations that are not emergencies. Ambulance service
is seldom available for medical emergencies. Hope, optimism, and the
positive advantages of treatment should be stressed. Recent research
indicates that women may prefer to give birth outside of health institutions
primarily because of concerns regarding quality of care, rather than ethnic
or traditional preferences.

Ethnic/Race Specific or Endemic Diseases: Endemic diseases include hydatid
cystic disease, tuberculosis, trachoma (southern Morocco), leishmaniasis,
and hepatitis A. Moroccans are at risk for hepatitis E, Q fever, myco-
toxicoses, malaria (in certain regions), typhoid fever, schistosomiasis,

and ascaridiosis. A major health issue is that water supplies are frequently contaminated by raw sewage; there also is silting of reservoirs and oil pollution of coastal waters. The World Health Organization's (WHO) estimated prevalence rate for HIV/AIDS in adults ages 15 to 49 is 0.03%. WHO has no estimates for children from birth to 15 years.

Families' Role in Hospital Care: Family members or close friends accompany the patient and expect to participate in care or take on a vigilant, supervisory role.

Dominance Patterns: Men and women have contrasting social roles, and the father has the authority in the family. According to the constitution, all citizens are equal, but non-Muslims and women face discrimination in traditional practices and the law. Spousal violence is common. A wife who has been abused has the right to complain to the police, but she would do so only if she were prepared to bring criminal charges against the husband. Physical abuse is legal grounds for divorce, but divorce is granted only if the woman has two witnesses to the actual abuse who will support her in court. Medical certificates of injury do not suffice in the legal system. If the court rules against the woman, she is returned to the husband's home. Few women dare to report abuse. If a man murders his wife, the sentence is generally light. The criminal code provides severe punishments for men convicted of rape or sexual assault of a woman or girl other than their wives. The women bear the burden of proving their innocence, however, and because of the stigma attached to loss of virginity before marriage, most assaults are not reported. Victims' families may offer men who have raped women the opportunity to marry their victims to preserve family honor. Women seeking divorce have few practical alternatives. They may offer their husband money to agree to the divorce (a *khol'a* divorce). The husband must agree and is allowed to specify how much will be paid, with no limit. The *Moudouwana,* a code based on Islamic law, states that women can inherit only half as much as male heirs. When women do inherit property, male relatives may pressure them to relinquish their part. Some well-educated women pursue careers in medicine, law, and education but few make it into the upper echelons of their professions. Literacy rates are 41% for males and 67% for females.

Touch Practices: It not unusual for men to walk hand-in-hand in public.

Pain Reactions: In hospital settings, pain relief is expected, so pain medications may be persistently requested because of the belief that an ill person must conserve energy for recovery. Outside of hospital settings, pain is usually expressed privately to family members or close relatives and friends. During labor and childbirth, it is expected that women will be vocal about pain.

Birth Rites: About 35% of the population is between infancy and 14 years of age. The total fertility rate is 3.05 children born per woman. The birth rate is 24.16 births per 1000 people. The infant mortality rate is 48.11 deaths per 1000 live births, and life expectancy at birth is 67.2 years for men and 71.76 years for women.

Death Rites: Muslim beliefs may or may not discourage organ donations or transplants, but Muslim doctors usually recommend transfusions to save lives. Autopsies are uncommon because the body must be buried intact. Cremation is not permitted. For Muslim burials, the body is wrapped in special pieces of white cloth and buried without a coffin in the ground as soon as possible after death.

Food Practices and Intolerances: Pork, carrion, alcohol, and blood consumption are forbidden for Muslims. The national dish is couscous— finely ground semolina that is usually accompanied by lamb and vegetables. Sweet mint tea is the drink of choice. Although Morocco is a Muslim country, it has no general ban on alcohol. Ramadan fasting is practiced, with exemptions for the sick and children.

National Childhood Immunizations: BCG at birth; DTP at 6, 10, and 14 weeks; OPV at birth and 6, 10, and 14 weeks; hep B at birth and 6 weeks and 9 months; measles at 9 months; vitamin A at 9, 15, and 21 months. The reported percentage of target population vaccinated: BCG, 99; first dose DTP, 97; third dose of DTP, 95; third dose of hep B, 43; MCV, 93; Pol3, 95; TT2plus, 90; and vitamin A, 40.

Other Characteristics: Morocco is an illegal producer of hashish; trafficking is increasing for domestic and international drug markets. Shipments of hashish are mostly directed to western Europe. Morocco is a transit point for cocaine from South America destined for Western Europe.

BIBLIOGRAPHY

Andrews MM, Boyle JS: *Transcultural concepts in nursing care,* ed 2, Philadelphia, 1995, Lippincott.
Obermeyer CM: Pluralism and pragmatism: knowledge and practice of birth in Morocco, *Med Anthropol Quart* 14(2):180, 2000.
Storti C: *The art of crossing cultures,* Yarmouth, Me, 1990, Intercultural Press.
http://state.gov/www/global/human_rights/1999_hrp_report/morocco.html
http://travel.state.gov/morocco.html
http://voyage.dfait-maeci.gc.ca/destinations/report_e.asp?country=Morocco
http://www.odci.gov/cia/publications/factbook/geos/mo.html

◆ MOZAMBIQUE (REPUBLIC OF)

MAP PAGE (863)

Location: Mozambique stretches along the southeastern coast of Africa, bordering the Mozambique Channel, between South Africa and Tanzania. The country has uplands in the center, high plateaus in the northwest, mountains in the west, and coastal lowlands that cover nearly half of the country. The total land area is 801,590 km^2 (309,413 square miles), slightly less than twice the size of California, and the capital is Maputo. The climate is tropical to subtropical, and cyclones are common. The population is 19,371,057, with 44% working in agriculture. The country has experienced civil war, severe drought, crop failure, and famine. Major migration has occurred to urban and coastal areas, resulting in pollution of surface and coastal waters. In 1994, Mozambique was ranked one of the poorest countries in the world. The economy grew at an annual 10% rate from 1997 to 1999, one of the highest growth rates in the world, but slowed in 2000 because of devastating floods from tropical cyclone, Gloria. The gross domestic product (GDP) per capita in 2000 was estimated to be $1000, and the unemployment rate is high at 21%. Approximately 70% of the population lives below the poverty line.

Major Languages	Ethnic Groups	Major Religions
Portuguese (official)	Indigenous tribal groups	Indigenous beliefs
Indigenous dialects	(Shangaan, Chokwe,	50%
	Manyika, Sena, Makua,	Christian 30%
	and others) 99%	Muslim 20%
	Europeans, Euro-Africans,	
	Indians 1%	

Health Care Beliefs: Acute sick care; passive role. It is widely believed that herbs, amulets, and charms can influence health and illness. The people also strongly believe in the existence of an invisible, internal "snake" (called *nyoka* by Tsonga and Shona speakers), described as a power or force that lives in the stomach but can move throughout the upper part of the body. This belief may be related to sorcery or witchcraft but also may be symbolic of the need to respect the body and protect it from impurities. Prevention efforts are urgently needed to counteract general lack of health care knowledge and traditional beliefs regarding illness etiologies. For example, studies in cholera-prevalent areas indicate that people do not associate the disease with consumption of unclean water or contamination of water supplies caused by a lack of latrines or toilets.

Predominant Sick Care Practices: Magical-religious, traditional and biomedical where available. Health care is nationalized and includes a policy of primary health care. However, medical facilities are rudimentary and not up to Western standards, and many medications are not available. Maputo's Sommerschield Clinic provides some general, non-emergency services. Traditional healers, as well as diviner mediums known as *impandes,* have a strong role in the belief system of the people and a role in treatment of illness. Traditional healers *(curandeiros)* often use a combination of herbal and magical medicine and are a comfortable traditional choice for many people. Individuals may seek out traditional healers because of inadequate financial resources to pay for biomedical treatments, but the choice also affected by cultural comfort. Because of the extreme scarcity of doctors in Mozambique and as part of a culturally appropriate strategy, the government is actively seeking the assistance of traditional healers. Healers have been recruited through national associations of traditional healers, of which there are several in southern Africa. Healers are considered to be trusted advisors by the people and can relate to the culture in areas where educational efforts may be considered taboo. For example, healers are involved in HIV/AIDS prevention programs and receive instructions about transmission and condom use that they then bring back to the villages.

Ethnic/Race Specific or Endemic Diseases: Endemic diseases include cholera, schistosomiasis, helminth infections, chloroquine-resistant malaria, endomyocardial fibrosis, hepatitis A and B, and bilharzias. People are at risk for Newcastle disease virus, hepatocellular carcinoma (whose high rates seem to be associated with hepatitis A and B prevalence), poliomyelitis, rabies, tuberculosis, meningococcal meningitis, typhoid fever, diphtheria, tetanus, and dietary cyanide exposure from eating cassava. After the severe floods in 2000, Mozambique had outbreaks of cholera and malaria in the refugee camps. A recent study in Maputo city suggested that the leading causes of death are perinatal disorders, malaria, diarrheal disease, tuberculosis, lower respiratory tract infections, road traffic accidents, anemia, cerebrovascular disease, homicides, and bacterial meningitis. HIV/AIDS is a major source of morbidity and mortality in Mozambique. The World Health Organization's (WHO) estimated prevalence rate for HIV/AIDS in adults ages 15 to 49 is 13.22%. The estimated number of children from birth to 15 years living with HIV/AIDS is 52,000. Currently 1.2 million people in the country have HIV/AIDS. The death rate from AIDS in 1999 was estimated to be 98,000, and 310,000 children have lost either their mother or both parents to AIDS since the beginning of the epidemic. In 1998, 17% of women at an antenatal clinic tested positive for HIV, and 20% of those younger than 20 years of age tested positive. Among female patients at a sexually transmitted disease (STD) clinic in Maputo, HIV prevalence increased from 5% in 1993 to 8% in 1997. Outside of Maputo, HIV prevalence in male patients at an STD clinic was 37% in 1998; prevalence was 26% in 1997 among female patients at an STD clinic.

Health Team Relationships: Governmental efforts to employ traditional healers in conjunction with standard medical care have been successful. The doctor shortage has placed the responsibility of maternity care on personnel such as traditional birth attendants, midwives, and technicians. Surgical technicians have been trained to do cesarean sections, hysterectomies, and other surgical procedures. Nurse midwives are trained to perform screenings for syphilis—a major cause of poor pregnancy outcomes—and the data indicate that this approach has already decreased perinatal mortality by about 20%. This demonstrates what the WHO has long known—that increasing the education of midwives in developing countries can significantly decrease maternal mortality. Studies of 6-month pediatric nurse training programs at provincial hospitals also demonstrate that additional education results in significant decreases in deaths of hospitalized children.

Dominance Patterns: Mothers usually spend the little they earn on daily food and health care for the family, and they often must request more money for these expenses from their spouses. Not surprisingly, the mothers who are able to earn more have more bargaining power in the family. Although men have the dominant role in many families, some ethnic groups are matrilineal, such as the Macua in northern Mozambique. In a matrilineal kinship system the husband and his family cannot mistreat or reject the wife, which gives her considerable protection against abuse. However, when women are infertile, they are excluded from certain social activities and traditional ceremonies, creating a very difficult situation for the woman. Studies show that a lack of bargaining power affects women's ability to negotiate sex, and results in adolescent pregnancies and illnesses from STDs. It has been demonstrated that middle-class women have fewer sexual partners, use condoms more often, challenge gender norms, and are generally more assertive toward men than working-class women, who may depend on their partners for material support. Literacy rates are 58.4% for males and only 27% for women. It is well known that increasing educational levels of women usually means better health for their families because they know more about factors affecting health and disease.

Birth Rites: The majority of infants are born at home in the presence of a traditional birth attendant or relative. Rural infants who are born at home may be delivered onto the ground and left untouched until the placenta is delivered. It is considered very important to have numerous children; the total fertility rate is 4.82 children born per woman, and the birth rate is 37.2 births per 1000 people. However, couples are encouraged to space births. Given the status of health care and prevalent diseases in Mozambique, pregnancy poses serious mortality risks for women and their children. Women frequently seek contraceptive methods such as herbs, charms, or amulets from indigenous healers, although oral contraceptives, intrauterine devices, and injectable drugs are available from family planning clinics run by the government. The Macua in northern Mozambique who are seeking treatment for infertility visit traditional healers much more frequently than modern hospitals; their beliefs about the causes of infertility are traditionally rather than biomedically based. Because of these beliefs, almost all commit adultery in the hope of conceiving. The estimate for maternal mortality was very high in 1990 (the last reported statistic from UNAIDS/WHO) at 1500 deaths per 100,000 live births. The maternal mortality rate in this region is about 100 times higher than that of developed countries, and the rate may be even higher because of serious underreporting. Estimates do not include the approximately 60% of people who do not go to health facilities. Adolescent maternal mortality is associated with malaria, pregnancy-induced hypertension, puerperal sepsis, and septic abortion; 75% of these deaths are deemed avoidable. The infant mortality rate is high at 139.2 deaths per 1000 live births, and infant deaths are frequently associated with maternal malaria and syphilis. The life expectancy at birth is very low by any standard: 37.25 years for men and 35.62 years for women.

Food Practices and Intolerances: Sorghum and beans are common foods, and oil is used to cook food over open fires. Meat is an expensive commodity.

Infant Feeding Practices: Breast-feeding until the infant is 18 months old is encouraged. One out of four babies dies before the age of 5 years. About 42.72% of the population is 14 years or younger.

National Childhood Immunizations: BCG at birth; DPT at 2, 3, 4 months; OPV at birth and 2, 3, and 4 months; measles at 9 months; and TT for pregnant women ×2. The reported percentages of the target population vaccinated are as follows: BCG, 99; first dose of DTP, 99; third dose of DTP, 88; MCV, 97; Pol3, 87; and TT2 plus, 61.

Other Characteristics: Mozambique is a southern African transit point for South Asian hashish, South Asian heroin, and South American cocaine that are likely destined for European and South African markets. Mozambique is a producer of cannabis (for local consumption) and methaqualone (for export to South Africa).

BIBLIOGRAPHY

Agadjanian V: Women's choice between indigenous and Western contraception in urban Mozambique, *Women Health* 28(2):1, 1998.

Bique-Osman N et al: An intervention study to reduce adverse pregnancy outcomes as a result of syphilis in Mozambique, *Sex Trans Infect* 76(3):203, 2000.

Da Luz-Vaz M, Bergstrom S: Mozambique—delegation of responsibility in the area of maternal care, *Int J Gynaecol Obstet* 38(suppl):37, 1992.

Dgedge M et al: The burden of disease in Maputo City, Mozambique: registered and autopsied deaths in 1994, *Bulltn WHO* 79(6):546, 2001.

Fleming J: Mozambican healers join government in fight against AIDS, *J Int Assoc Physic AIDS Care* 1(2):32, 1995.

Gerrits T: Social and cultural aspects of infertility in Mozambique, *Patient Educ Couns* 31(1):39, 1997.

Granja AC et al: Adolescent maternal mortality in Mozambique, *J Adolesc Health* 28(4):303, 2001.

Green EC, Zokwe B, Dupree JD: The experience of an AIDS prevention program focused on South African traditional healers, *Soc Sci Med* 40(4):503, 1995.

Green EC: Purity, pollution and the invisible snake in southern Africa, *Med Anthropol* 17(1):83, 1996.

Machel JZ: Unsafe sexual behaviour among schoolgirls in Mozambique: a matter of gender and class, *Reprod Health Matters* 9(17):82, 2001.

Nsungu M, Jonga M: Does a direct cholera threat necessarily improve the knowledge, attitude and practices on the disease? *Cent Afr J Med* 42(5):125, 1996.

O'Heir JM: Midwifery education for safe motherhood, *Midwifery* 13(3):115, 1997.

Pfeiffer J, Gloyd S, Ramirez-Li L: Intrahousehold resource allocation and child growth in Mozambique: an ethnographic case-control study, *Soc Sci Med* 53(1):83, 1982.

Pisacane A: Reduction of child hospital mortality in Mozambique through a nurse training program, *Ann Trop Paediatr* 5(1):7, 1985.

Songane FF, Bergstron S: Quality of registration of maternal deaths in Mozambique: a community-based study in rural and urban areas, *Soc Sci Med* 54(1):23, 2002.

http://www.odci.gov/cia/publications/factbook/geos/mz.html

http://travel.state.gov/mozambique.html

◆ MYANMAR (UNION OF BURMA)

MAP PAGE (867)

Soe Soe and Myint Aye Mu

Location: Myanmar occupies the northwestern portion of the Indochinese peninsula and has a total land area of 671,000 km^2 (259,006 square miles) about the size of France and England combined or the state of Texas. It shares borders with China, India, Thailand, Laos, and Bangladesh. Myanmar consists of a narrow mountain range, a plateau, a flat, fertile delta, and a long coastline stretching from the Bangladesh border in the northwest to the Malay Peninsula and Thai territory in the southeast. Burma became Myanmar in 1989 because the name *Burma* implies only Burman, which is just one of the many ethnic groups in the country. On the other hand, *Myan* means "fast," and *Mar* means "healthy." Myanmar has a population of 48 million.

Major Languages	Ethnic Groups	Major Religions
Burmese (official)	Burman 65%	Theravada Buddhist 87%
English	Shan 10%	Christian 5%
	Karen 7%	Muslim 4%
	Rakhine 4%	Animist 3%
	Chin <4%	Hindu 1%
	Kachin <4%	
	Mon <4%	
	Kayah <4%	

All major ethnic groups have their own language and script. English is the second language at school. In addition to the previously mentioned groups, Myanmar has more than 100 minor ethnic groups.

Health Care Beliefs: Acute sick care; traditional; increasing interest in health promotion. According to Buddhism, health is the most important gift in life. Thus people in Myanmar greet each other by saying "How are you?" instead of "Good day." The people pay close attention to their diet by choosing the proper amount of the correct foods. Certain sayings attest to the importance of food, such as "foods are nutrients as well as medicines"; "a suitable amount is medicinal, but overdose is dangerous"; and "a bad step or a mouthful of bad food can be fatal." Nutrients are categorized as "cold" or "hot" and further subdivided into six categories according to taste: salty, bitter, sweet, sour, spicy, and *phan,* a combination of slightly bitter and sour. Special news articles on good and bad food appear each month in popular journals, explaining which foods are cold and hot and which tastes promote good health. Most people of the older generation prepare foods and eat them according to these articles. Food taboos are common. For example, lactating mothers are not allowed to eat red meat because they believe it will cause "wind colic" in infants. Depression is rare because of the comfort and support provided by family members, and fortune tellers are believed to have tricks that can cancel bad luck. Religion also plays a part in Myanmar life because bad luck is believed to be the consequence of bad behavior in previous lives. It is therefore rare for a person to sue for malpractice because anything that goes wrong is thought to be deserved. In the same way, suicide is uncommon because Buddhists believe that it will be repeated in the person's next 500 lives. Blood donation is encouraged, because people believe that whatever is given is returned in some way. For example, those who do not give to the poor could end up living in poverty. People emphasize natural products for inner health and outer appearance. Women use a special scented plant known as *thanakha* (the botanical term for which is *Limonia acidissma linn*) as a cosmetic. It is ground with water over a specially prepared stone called a *kyauk-pyin*. The semiliquid product (a homogeneous paste) obtained from the bark is used for the face, and the inner part (containing sediment) is used for the rest of the body. *Thanakha* has a very pleasant odor, soothing effect, and protects the skin from sunburn; thus women put a thick layer on their cheeks, forehead, and nose when going out in the sun. Modern women prefer to use cosmetics for a day in the city but *thanakha* in the evening. Plant products are used to shampoo the hair, after which coconut oil is applied. Most women prefer to keep their hair long, often to their ankles, because long, black, thick hair is regarded as one of the five characteristics of a beautiful lady.

Predominant Sick Care Practices: Biomedical and traditional practices. Traditional practices consist of remedies from plants, massages with or without plant extracts, and acupuncture involving pointed instruments made of several metals. Biomedical treatment is preferred for severe illness and by urban dwellers. Minor forms of diabetes, hypertension, skin disease, hair loss, and symptoms such as nausea, giddiness, dysmenorrhea, constipation, indigestion, and colic are treated with the traditional medications that are common in almost every house. For example, a minor form of diabetes is treated with an indigenous medicine made of bitter gourd, and muscle pain and fatigue are treated by massage. Acupuncture is reserved for chronic pain. Traditional acupuncture in Myanmar (which is often done by untrained personnel) is gradually being replaced by Chinese acupuncture. Public biomedical and traditional health care services are provided by dispensaries and hospitals for free. A referral from a dispensary is needed for admission to a biomedical hospital. In private clinics and hospitals, patients can make an appointment directly with a specialist, and family members can visit or stay with the patient at any time. Therefore private services are preferred but must be paid for in cash because social health insurance does not cover them. Myanmar also has free dispensaries and hospitals where doctors and nurses provide voluntary services, as well as special clinics and hospitals for Buddhist monks and nuns.

Ethnic/Race Specific or Endemic Diseases: The population has a genetic risk for hemoglobin E disease, thalassemia, and to a lesser extent glucose-6-phosphate deficiency (G6PD). Nutritional goiters are common in those living in the mountain ranges and delta areas. Malaria is endemic in the forested mountains and border areas, and chloroquine-resistant malaria is found at the border of Thailand. As in other developing countries, the people are at risk for infectious diseases such as acute respiratory tract infections; diarrhea; hepatitis A, B, C, and E; polio; tetanus; diphtheria; intestinal worms; plague; dengue; rabies; and typhoid. Snake bites from vipers during rice harvesting season cause high mortality because of the superstition that wearing boots in the rice field annoys the spiritual guardians of the field. Blood donations are systematically screened for hepatitis B and HIV. Postpartum and neonatal beriberi is common in some isolated and remote villages because of a lack of proper food during pregnancy and lactation. Liver cancer is very common in males, second only to lung cancer. It occurs at relatively early ages (35 to 50), with the youngest recorded case in a 29-year-old man. The high liver cancer rate may be related to the high hepatitis B carrier rate and the prevalence of aflatoxin in street food such as ground nuts and chili, which men eat more often. The incidence of uterine fibroids is high in single women, and more than 70% of women must have them surgically removed after age 40. Breast and cervical cancer are the most common cancers in single and married multiparous women, respectively. The World Health Organization's (WHO) estimated prevalence rate for HIV/AIDS in adults ages 15 to 49 years is 1.99%. The estimated number of children from birth to 15 years living with HIV/AIDS is 14,000.

Health Team Relationships: Health care is doctor-driven, with active participation of the patient and all family members. Myanmar has three medical institutes; two are in Yangon, the capital city situated in lower Myanmar, and one is in Mandalay, the former capital in upper Myanmar. About 600 medical doctors graduate yearly. Entrance to professional institutes such as medical institutes depends on grades obtained on high school final examinations. The highest scorers go to the medical institutes because Buddhists believe saving lives is the most noble work possible. The medical course lasts 7 years and includes a final 1-year internship in a teaching hospital. After internship, 2 years of service in township hospitals equipped with specialists are needed before attending post-graduate courses. Postgraduate master's degrees, and more recently, doctoral degrees for specialties, are granted after 2 and 5 years, respectively. The institute of dental medicine and school for health assistant training are in Yangon. Health assistants are allowed to measure blood pressures and inject vaccines and medications. In remote villages at the grassroots level, dispensaries are run by health assistants. Myanmar has two institutes for general nursing care, one in Yangon and one in Mandalay. The nursing course lasts 3 years. Nurse training for midwifery is offered in all seven divisional hospitals and lasts 6 months. A person who has both trainings is called a "double certificate holder." The four grades of technicians have different levels of responsibility and expertise. The country has four initiatives for endemic diseases: malaria, leprosy, tuberculosis, and trachoma. School health teams are present in each township and composed of medical doctors, dental surgeons, and nurses. They visit schools in the township and perform general medical check-ups of teachers and students, vaccinations, health education, and inspection of the food sellers. Health education includes personal hygiene, environmental sanitation, the life cycle of fecal-orally transmitted diseases and vector-borne diseases. Sex is not discussed among friends, relatives, or family members, and sex education is not introduced because sex is regarded as wrong and prohibited before marriage. Attitudes toward virginity are strict, and out-of-wedlock pregnancy is unacceptable. Kissing or embracing between a couple in public is regarded as shameful. Even a friendly kiss or holding a woman's hand without her permission is regarded as an insult and could be punishable with 5 years of prison. Friendly kisses to young girls younger than 5 years are allowed, but after age 5, kisses or body contact are prohibited, even by family members of the opposite sex. Extramarital sex is prohibited: monogamy and loyalty to one's marriage partner is stressed. Prostitution is illegal. Arranged marriages by parents are becoming less popular; however, approval of the prospective spouse by the parents is common because children display great loyalty and gratitude towards them. It is considered indecent for a woman to expose her body, so when being examined she must be covered with a thin sheet of cloth. If the doctor is a man, another woman must be present during the examination. Health education is promoted on television each evening and includes topics such as nutrition and common illnesses such as influenza and diarrhea. Sex education is provided by health personnel only to adults at special meetings. Homosexual men can be found in Yangon, Mandalay, and in other big cities. They wear women's clothes and speak like women. They speak a special language among themselves and usually earn their living as a person with the ability to contact spirits (*natgadaw*) or as hairdressers. Homosexual women are very rare, and they dress like men.

Workers' clinics and hospitals are present in each township for those engaged in either governmental or private industry, and they also can go to public dispensaries and hospitals. Social welfare personnel are present in public and workers' hospitals, providing help for those who cannot afford medications, transportation to hospitals, or rehabilitation. The Ministry of Health has five main departments: the Department of Health, Department of Health Sciences, Department of Health Planning, Department of Traditional Medicine, and Department of Medical Research. The Myanmar pharmaceutical industry under the Ministry of Industry in Yangon produces essential medications and monovalent and polyvalent antiviper and anticobra snake venoms.

Families' Role in Hospital Care: Families stay with the patient in the hospital, perform basic care, and provide meals and clean linen. If essential medicines are not available in the hospital, the family must purchase them. Both fathers and mothers discuss the health of their children and participate in decision making: it is usually the mother, however, who takes care of the children.

Dominance Patterns: Women have the same rights as their male counterparts in health decisions, but have more dominance regarding the economy of the house. They are often teased that they are the "home ministers." However, it is believed that a lady cannot become a God, and is not allowed to go to a place higher than the God statues or monks.

Eye Contact Practices: Direct eye contact between friends is the norm. Direct eye contact is considered polite and necessary especially when greeting a person. Regardless of age, a confidential connection between health care personnel and patients necessitates eye contact.

Touch Practices: Hugs and kisses for young children from family members, friends, or health personnel are common, but touch among adults, especially between opposite sexes, is not. Regardless of age or gender, touching is considered natural by health care professionals, especially to comfort and assure patients. The frequency of touching in nursing care situations increases with very sick patients, older patients, and when needed to relax and comfort patients.

Perceptions of Time: Punctuality is not stressed, and excuses are usually accepted for lateness if it is not a life-and-death situation. People are reluctant to say "no" to requests, even though the request may involve something that is difficult to accomplish in time.

Pain Reactions: Women are freely allowed to express pain; men are expected to bear it with less of an overt reaction.

Birth Rites: Women in urban areas practice family planning, and contraceptive pills and injections are preferred to condoms. Hospital stays are 24 hours for multiparous women and 5 days for first-time mothers because of their episiotomies. In villages, women prefer to give birth at home either with traditional birth attendants or midwives. The puerperium is 45 days after the delivery, during which time women do no work. The focus is on involution of the uterus, regaining abdominal muscle, and encouraging the free flow of breast milk. The mother eats rice, vegetable soups with fish or chicken, and baked, dried fish. In some villages, chicken is not consumed because some think it causes an allergic reaction. Traditionally, the mother and infant avoid exposure to the smell of frying foods. A name is chosen after consulting an expert who uses the time and date of the infant's birth to select a name that should bring good health, success, and prosperity. A family name is not compulsory, and it is also not required for a woman to change her family name after marriage. Only the children are required take the father's name. The formal name-giving ceremony usually takes place when the child is about 6 months old. Before this event, parents give the child a nickname that is often chosen before birth.

Death Rites: People prefer a quality life to a long one because Buddhists believe in reincarnation and less suffering in the next life. Those who are dying are helped to recall past good deeds, which enables them to achieve a fit mental state. Patients prefer to die at home among family members. Autopsies are permitted, and cremation is preferred—usually on the third day after death. On the seventh day after death, the family has a ceremony to announce to the person's spirit that it is free to go. Relatives, friends, and neighbors support the family and accompany them at the funeral and ceremony. Some people donate their eyes and bodies after death for corneal transplants and human anatomy education.

Food Practices and Intolerances: In villages, breakfast is rather heavy and consists of sticky rice with fried beans or baked dried fish with green tea. In the city, it is usually rice noodle soup with fish or wheat noodle soup with chicken, as well as tea with milk and sugar. White rice with curry made of fish, meat, or shrimp, and vegetable soup and salads with fish sauce are eaten at lunch and dinner. Traditional curry contains oil, onions, garlic, and ginger. For cooking, groundnut oil and more recently sunflower oil are used. Sesame oil is used for salads. People tend to prefer fresh-water fish, shrimp, and crab rather than food from the sea. The most commonly eaten meat is chicken. In some parts of the country, people do not eat pork because they say that their spiritual bodyguards would not like it, and some do not eat beef because they use working cows in the fields and thus owe a debt of gratitude to them. In between the three meals, snacks can be sticky rice cakes, pickled tea-leaf salad, appetizers, or nuts. In essence, people eat throughout the day. During ceremonies guests are served food and drinks. Alcohol prepared from fermented rice and fermented palm juice is consumed by the men but never by the women.

Infant Feeding Practices: Most infants are breast-fed; however, breast-feeding may be delayed for several days because people believe that colostrum is bad for infants. Women know that certain foods and medications can pass through the breast milk, so nursing mothers are aware of foods that can be harmful. However, if her infant is constipated, the mother drinks tamarind juice so that it can be transferred to the child. A semiliquid rice mixture is introduced when the child is 1 month old, and vegetables and fruits are gradually added at about the third month. A special pillow for the infant made of broken rice grains is made so that it can adapt to the infant's head and prevent flattening of the back of the head or one side of the skull.

National Childhood Immunizations: BCG at 6 weeks; DTP at 6, 10, and 14 weeks; OPV at 6, 10, and 14 weeks; measles at 9 months; and TT at first antenatal contact, +1 month.

BIBLIOGRAPHY

Aung Than B et al: Thalassaemia-hemoglobin E disease and thalassaemia major, *Trop Geogr Med* 23:25–29, 1971.

Aung Than B, Hla P, Khin KN: The incidence of alpha-thalassaemia trait III, *Trop Geogr Med* 23:23–25, 1971.

Aung Than B, Hla P: Haemoglobinopathies in Burma. I. The incidence of hemoglobin E, *Trop Geogr Med* 23:15–19, 1971.

Fawcett B: Midwifery training in Burma, *Nurs Times* 86(30):30, 1990.

Myint-Oo M, Tin-Shwe, Marlar-Than, O'Sullivan WJ: Genetic red cell disorders and severity of falciparum malaria in Myanmar *Bulltn WHO*: 73:659–665, 1995.

National health plan, 1996-2001: Forum on health sector development, Planning Document Series-3, The Government of the Union of Myanmar.

Shein H et al: Knowledge, attitude and practice against malaria in a rural Myanmar village, *Southeast Asian J Trop Med Pub Hlth* 29:546–549, 1989.

Soe S, Than-Than, Khin-Ei-Han: The nephrotoxic action of Russell's viper venom. *Toxicon* 28:461–467, 1990.

Soe S et al: Comparative study between molecular hybridization and electron microscope for the detection of hepatitis E virus, *Southeast Asian J Trop Med Pub Hlth* 24:477–479, 1993.

Soe S et al: Hepatitis B surface markers in hepatocellular carcinoma. *Myanmar Hlth Sci Res J* 8:12–14, 1996.

Soe S et al: The peripheral lymphocyte mitogenic responses of apparently healthy Myanmar blood donors, *Myanmar Hlth Sci Res J* 7:14–16, 1995.

Soe S et al: Phytohemagglutinin (PHA) induced peripheral lymphocyte blastogenic response in cancer patients, *Myanmar Hlth Sci Res J* 8:125–129, 1996.

Soe S et al: Renal histopathology following Russell's viper (*Vipera Russelli*) bite, *Southeast Asian J Trop Med Pub Hlth* 24:193–197.

Soe S et al: Some characteristics of hospitalized HIV seropositive patients in Myanmar, *Southeast Asian J Trop Med Pub Hlth* 24:18-22, 1993.

Tun-Lin W, Thu MM, Than SM, Mya MM: Hyperendemic malaria in a forested hilly Myanmar village, *J Am Mosq Contr Assoc* 11:401-407, 1995.

http://www.cia.gov/cia/publications/factbook/geos/bm.html#Intro

http://www.lonelyplanet.com/destinations/south_east_asia/myanmar/http://www.myanmar.com/ACOCI/CULTURE/beauty.html

◆ NAMIBIA (REPUBLIC OF)

MAP PAGE (863)

Jörg Klewer

Location: Namibia is located on the southwestern corner of Africa and covers a total land area of 834,295 km² (317,827 square miles). Namibia has been an independent democracy since 1990. It is divided into 13 districts, and the capital, Windhoek (190,000 citizens), is centrally located. The estimated population is about 1.8 million, with an annual population growth of 3.1%. Namibia shares long borders with Angola in the north and Botswana in the east. The Caprivi Zipfel, a small corridor from the northeastern edge of Namibia, touches Zambia and Zimbabwe. Its natural boundaries are the Kunene, Kavango, and Zambezi river systems in the north and the Orange River in the south. Topographically, Namibia can be divided into four distinct regions: the Namib and Kalahari Deserts, the Central Plateau, and the northern savannah grasslands.

Major Languages	Ethnic Groups	Major Religions
Afrikaans (common)	Black 88%	Christian 80% to 90%
German	White 6%	Indigenous 10%
English (official)	Mixed 6% to 20%	
Indigenous		

Namibians are a heterogeneous mixture of many cultures. The oldest inhabitants are the San, also called "Bushmen," now only living in the Kalahari Desert. Thousands of Bushmen served during the independence war in the South African army because they are very skilled in picking up trails and surviving in the desert. After Namibia became independent, many of them moved to South Africa because they were disliked by the new Namibian government. The second oldest inhabitants are the Damara. This former nomadic population lives in the northwestern part of Namibia, the Damaraland. The Nama in southern Namibia, near Keetmanshoop, have an old culture and migrated into Namibia from the south. They have a great natural talent for music. More than 70% of the Namibian population are Bantu ethnicities: Owambo, Herero, Kavango, Caprivi, and Tswana. The majority are the Owambo (650,000), living as farmers in the northern parts of the country (Owamboland). Eight Owambo sub-tribes live in Namibia; the largest is the Kwanyama. The most striking feature of the traditional Owambo social system is their practice of matrilineal descent. The Herero are a pastoral cattle-breeding population living in the eastern part of Namibia (Hereroland). The Herero women wear Victorian-style dresses adapted from the wives of Rhinish missionaries. The Himba women (a tribe of Herero descent) in the Kaokoveld (northwest Namibia) rub their bodies with a mixture of red ochre and fat. They wear traditional body ornaments and garments. Their hairstyles correspond to their age, sex, and social status. The Kavango are traditionally farmers and live at the banks of the Okavango River in northeastern Namibia. They create very skillful carvings. Their eastern neighbors are the Caprivi, living in the Caprivi Zipfel, primarily near Katima Mulilo. The Tswana are cattle-breeding people who originated in Botswana and migrated into Namibia in the middle of the nineteenth century. They live now in the southeastern parts of Namibia around Gobabis. A small group is the Basters. They are descendents of white South African farmers who married native women in the Cape area. In the middle of the nineteenth century, they migrated to central Namibia and live now around Rehoboth, not far from Windhoek. Approximately 80,000 people of European descent live in Namibia and are primarily descendants of the German colonialists (approximately 20,000; Namibia was a German colony from 1884 to 1918) and of Afrikaan-speaking South Africans. These South Africans moved to Namibia after World War I. More than eleven languages are indigenous to Namibia. People commonly speak two or three languages, and more than 50% of the population speaks Oshiwambo. Indigenous languages are included in school at the primary level. At the secondary level, English is the medium of instruction. European languages spoken are German, Portuguese, Spanish, and French. Traditional beliefs are more common in the San and Himba populations and primarily comprise holy fires and spiritual contacts to ancient tribal chiefs. Some Islamic and Jewish communities do exist.

Health Care Beliefs: Acute sick care, traditional, increasing emphasis on prevention. Because of the shortage of medical doctors, Namibian nurses have taken over many duties. The country is covered by a network of more than 280 primary health care clinics, where one to five nurses provide vaccinations, screening examinations, and health education (about water safety, breast-feeding, tuberculosis awareness, prevention of HIV/AIDS). For patients with minor illnesses (e.g., headache, sore throat, small wounds), primary health care clinics also offer medical treatment. Patients with major diseases are sent to the hospital, occasionally by an ambulance (if one is available). Furthermore, indicators for health statistics are collected and analyzed by primary health care nurses. Mobile nursing teams assist these nurses, and the teams go to outreach points in the rural area using off-road vehicles. They provide health education, vaccinations, and medical treatment to the population. As a result, the incidence of many preventable infectious diseases has decreased significantly. Poster campaigns were also launched by the government and international organizations to promote breast-feeding, use of malaria nets, use of condoms to prevent HIV and other sexually transmitted diseases, tuberculosis awareness, and awareness of land mines (that were left over from the war for independence). After 1990 the government initiated a program to build water holes and wells not more than 2 km (1.25 miles) away from human settlements to ensure a safe water supply for all Namibians. Simultaneously, programs were initiated to build latrines outside traditional houses and collect garbage for dumping or burning. Mental illness is feared. People in the rural area often consider mental illnesses to be magical—conditions caused by witches or ghosts. Patients with mental illnesses are first brought by their family to traditional healers or witches to get rid of the spell. The individual "treatment" depends on the specialty of the witch or traditional healer. If a patient does not improve after traditional treatments, the family usually brings the patient to a primary health care clinic or directly to a hospital.

Predominant Sick Care Practices: Predominantly government-operated (public) health care system based on Western (biomedical) medicine. Also, some alternative and magical-religious therapies. The health system is comparable to the South African health care system. The regional and district hospitals are well equipped with medications and technical equipment and offer the services of medical doctors in out-patient and in-patient departments. Health care (including medications) is nearly free; only a small fee must be paid. Therefore people mainly go to public health care facilities. In addition, private practices and pharmacies do exist in urban areas (mainly in central and southern Namibia), but these practices are only available to patients who can afford private health insurance. Traditional healers are widespread in the northern regions. Different types of traditional healers exist—those practicing traditional massage techniques, especially on patients with musculoskeletal problems; those using herbal mixtures; and those who treat by making several parallel short incisions (1 to 2 cm) in the skin on the painful part of the body. Occasionally these traditional healers create amulets to prevent the wearer from contracting specific diseases. People in the northern regions tend to visit traditional healers and go to the public health facilities. In some cases, patients who are admitted to the public hospital get unofficial treatments from traditional healers, which can conflict with Western-based medical therapies. Health care authorities fight against these practices. One major problem with herbal mixtures of traditional healers is that most of the healers' experience was lost during the war of independence. Herbal mixtures are created that often contain toxic herbs, leading to severe intoxication and renal failure. Some of these traditional healers occasionally claim that they have found a way cure AIDS and sell the useless mixtures at high prices. Because of this practice, no policies have been developed to integrate traditional healers into the health care system. In addition, people in the northern regions believe in witches and witchcraft. These witches normally live in villages in the rural area. They are normally contacted by people who believe they are bewitched, seek treatment for witchcraft, or want to put a spell on a person. Some people believe that these witches are able to take the shapes of snakes, spiders, or black bulls so that they can go to other villages.

Ethnic/Race Specific or Endemic Diseases: The current major health problems in Namibia are HIV/AIDS, sexually transmitted diseases, viral hepatitis, tuberculosis, and malaria. Tuberculosis and HIV (often in combination) are a countrywide tragedy. Additional health problems, especially in the northern parts of Namibia, are tropical malaria, schistosomiasis, endemic plague, vitamin deficiencies and malnutrition, leprosy, rabies, complication from snake bites and scorpion stings, and diarrhea. Because of the open fires in traditional houses, respiratory tract infections and burns are common among children. In urban areas, traffic accidents, violence (primarily stab wounds), and alcohol abuse are health problems. Injuries from bomb blasts and exploding land mines are still a problem in northern Namibia, often affecting children who find the explosives. In northern Namibia, especially in the Kavango territory, an acquired form of immune thrombocytopenia called *onyalai* exists, and about 660 cases of *onyalai* are counted each year. The disease is mainly found in Namibia, with lower incidence in the surrounding countries. The clinical hallmarks are hemorrhagic bullae on the mucosa of the oronasopharynx, and hemorrhage from ruptured bullae; epistaxis or gastro-intestinal bleeding is severe and may cause shock and death. Chronic thrombocytopenia often ensues, and recurrent episodes of clinical bleeding are common. The causative agents are mycotoxins from contaminated millet, sorghum, or maize. The average life expectancy in Namibia is approximately 63 for females and 59 for males. Because of the HIV/AIDS epidemic, a decrease in statistical life expectancy is expected. Namibia is one of the countries most heavily affected by the epidemic. The World Health Organization's (WHO) estimated prevalence rate for HIV/AIDS in adults ages 15 to 49 years was 19.54% at the end of 1999. The estimated number of children from birth to 15 years living with HIV/AIDS is 6600. Until the end of 2000 the total number of people with HIV was officially 83,000 cases, but about 15,000 new HIV cases were registered in 2000. Women account for 56% of all reported new infections, and anonymous surveys among pregnant women revealed the highest prevalence of HIV in the urban areas of Katima Mulilo (33%), Windhoek (31%), Oshakati (28%), and Walvis Bay (28%). HIV prevalence is also high in rural sites close to main roads, such as Onandjokwe (23%), Swakopmund (23%), and Keetmanshoop (17%). In a few rural sites such as Gobabis, Rehoboth, and Opuwo, the HIV prevalence is still less than 10%. The median age of death from AIDS is 34 for women and 38 for men. More than 12,000 deaths from AIDS have been reported since the beginning of the epidemic. The number of deaths from all causes in adults accounts for 51% of all reported deaths, but many of these deaths are directly attributable to AIDS. The increasing number of deaths from tuberculosis, pneumonia, and diarrhea in this age group suggests that HIV is the underlying cause in many of these cases. The number of free condoms distributed increased from 8.7 million in 1998 to 11.2 million in 2000, and this trend holds some promise for decreasing the transmission AIDS.

Health Team Relationships: Generally, medical doctors command significant power in relationship to nurses and patients. When patients seek health care, they usually prefer to be examined and treated by a doctor. Patients prefer to be seen by a white doctor rather than a black one because they think that white doctors receive better training. Only Cuban doctors (of which there are several in the public health care system) are disliked, because Cuban doctors have been involved in serious medical malpractice cases during previous years. Cooperation between medical doctors and nurses is usually good. It seems that nurses trained in Windhoek have better skills and are more motivated than nurses trained in Oshakati, where training is more conservative. Therefore highly motivated younger nurses try to find jobs in hospitals in the south. Most patients going to primary health care clinics or hospital out-patient departments expect a prescription of oral medication or injections to address their underlying health concerns. To fulfill these expectations, patients with no therapeutic need for medications get some multivitamin tablets to prevent disappointed patients from receiving unnecessary treatment at the hands of traditional healers.

Families' Role in Hospital Care: Namibian hospitals provide full-service care, including a hospital bed, meals, and nursing care. In pediatric wards the mothers often stay with their children and assist the nurses in the daily care of their children. Family members are allowed to stay with patients in the wards only during visiting hours. The rest of the day, family members stay outside the hospital. Despite regular meals of good quality, family members are usually allowed to bring in soft drinks and home-cooked meals.

Dominance Patterns: In Namibia, women and men have equal rights, but Namibian families are traditionally dominated by a male patriarch. The wife has to serve and cook for her husband, maintain the house, work in the fields, and bear enough healthy children. Officially, only monogamy is allowed, but in the rural area of northern Namibia, polygamous relationships can be found; this practice is legitimized by traditional weddings, and each wife has her own cooking facilities. Changes in family patterns are not common. Other male family members take over the patriarch's role if he dies or has a severe illness. In urban communities such as Windhoek, these traditional roles are less fixed. Women have professional jobs and are in political positions.

Eye Contact Practices: Eye contact is normally not avoided, even when people in superior positions are present.

Touch Practices: Physical touching by traditional hugging or handshaking is common. Greeting a friend or relative is normally accompanied by ritualized handshaking. Physical touching is accepted during medical examinations. Members of the opposite sex holding hands in public are becoming more common in urban areas but are still uncommon in rural areas.

Perceptions of Time: In general, punctuality is not a major issue in Namibia, and appointments and other commitments may not be kept in a timely fashion. This is usually a result of the lack of personal and public watches, especially in rural areas. People who do not have a watch estimate the daily time by looking at the direction and intensity of the sun or the appearance and shape of the moon. The small plastic bags used to hand out prescribed medications are covered with sun and moon symbols, symbolizing the times when the patients should take the medication. Events that occurred several weeks before, such as the last menstrual period of pregnant women, are often described in terms such as "when the full moon was over the big tree." Accordingly, health professionals need some knowledge about the lunar year and regional features. Each Namibian culture has its own history, which has been influenced by colonialism and the war of independence. However, the situation in Namibia has improved in past decades, and the country has become a young multicultural democracy. People tend to combine living in the present and reaching for future goals (such as good health and work for all Namibians) because Namibia is still progressing.

Pain Reactions: Traditionally, it is expected that men should be stoical, but it is acceptable for women to express their pain. Males and females, even in rural areas, express physical pain through body movements, screaming, crying, and occasionally hysteria. These reactions can complicate some medical procedures. Extensive and loud expressions of emotional pain are much more common from females. Some males express grief over the loss of a loved person by cutting their hair.

Birth Rites: Pregnancy and labor, even when difficult, are regarded as natural processes. In traditional rural communities, pregnant woman continue their daily life activities including working on the farm until they are close to delivery. The primary health care system includes antenatal clinics that provide regular physical examinations, health education, and free iron, folic acid, and vitamin A supplements. Pregnant women definitely appreciate these antenatal clinics. Some women wear amulets or other magical ornaments to influence pregnancy, although it is not very common. At the estimated time of delivery, pregnant women go to the birthing facilities at the hospitals. They may come alone, or their relatives may bring them. Normally, the women stay alone in the hospital with other pregnant women until they are close to labor. In general, husbands do not enter delivery rooms. Maternity wards are well equipped and managed by qualified nurses and midwives, and women are closely observed before and after delivery. In cases of complicated births, a gynecologist or surgeon is usually available to perform a cesarean section. Analgesia is not routinely used for normal births. The number of home births is decreasing, but they still occur. After a home birth, mother and infant go to the postnatal clinic or hospital for follow-up care. Labor pain is tolerated in various ways. Multiparous women and women who accept pregnancy and birth as a natural process are not expressive about the associated pain. They arrive at the hospital, deliver the infant, are happy if the child is healthy, and leave the hospital after a few days. Primigravida women and young women may react more to pain by crying and screaming in the delivery room. The birth of a newborn is a happy event for the whole family and is usually celebrated with relatives and neighbors. Parents are proud of their newborns, and girls and boys are both celebrated. Sons can help the father tend the cattle and increase the size of the clan, and girls can work on the farm and receive a bride prize before marriage.

Death Rites: Deaths are considered natural and are marked by celebrations. The initial reaction to the death of a relative or friend is shock and denial, followed by a period of mourning and acceptance. Because of the number of fatalities caused by the war and now being caused by the AIDS epidemic, people have developed a fatalistic perception of death, resulting in a reduced emotional response and stoical reactions. Consequently, abridged burial ceremonies are becoming more common because most families are faced with the death of several members. The bodies are buried in a cemetery, especially if the person was a Christian. Traditionally, bodies were buried in the cattle pasture to remove all traces of the burial through the footprints of the cattle. Occasionally the family destroyed the traditional house and moved somewhere else to avoid any contact with the deceased and the associated ghost. Even though most of the Namibians are Christians, the traditional beliefs in witchcraft as a cause of death are still present, although officially denied. No one discusses organ donation in Namibia because no transplant surgery unit exists in the country. Because of a shortage of pathologists, autopsies are not performed routinely. Occasionally surgeons perform requested autopsies, but the procedures are often superficial and only related to a specific question. Forensic autopsies are normally accepted.

Food Practices and Intolerances: Meat is the staple food—either game (e.g., kudu, antelope, ostrich) or domesticated animals (e.g., cattle, goats, chicken). Agriculture is only widespread in northern Namibia. Meat is normally served grilled or dried; well-spiced dried meat of beef or game is called *biltong*. Cows are expensive; therefore people prefer to eat goat or chicken. Meat is eaten with potatoes (boiled or fried), corn, rice, or porridge made from pumpkins. Near the coast, fish is alternated with meat and is either grilled naturally or salted and grilled. In northern Namibia, *omahango (mahango),* a kind of millet, is the basic vegetable. *Omahangu* plants grow up to 3 m and are cultivated on every small farm. In poor families, porridge made from *omahangu* flour is served each day, usually without meat but occasionally with eggs. To enrich their food and obtain some protein, people in northern Namibia collect special large caterpillars from the trees and serve them fried, salted, or both. During the rainy season from November to April, fish and frogs living in the rivers are harvested, dried in the sun, and used to enrich soups and porridges. All traditional meals are normally served in earthenware or wooden vessels or on plates made of palm tree leaves or wood. All meals are traditionally eaten with the fingers, even meat that has been chopped with knives. Spoons are usually used for soups. In northern Namibia, fruits such as guava, bananas, and different palm tree fruits are cultivated and highly appreciated. In Namibian towns, all kinds of fruit and vegetables are available because they are imported from South Africa, Zambia, or Angola, but they are expensive and unaffordable for ordinary Namibians. *Omahangu* flour is also used to brew *otombo*, a traditional beer made of *omahango* flour and brown sugar. *Otombo* is easy to brew in open bowls and tastes sweet but intoxicates people and is a major public health problem in Northern Namibia, leading to domestic violence, alcoholism, and unemployment. In the past, traditional liquor was distilled from palm tree sap, but it led to extermination of palm trees and its production is now prohibited by law. Because of endemic goiter, all salt in Namibia for human and animal consumption must be iodized. Women generally do all kitchen chores, and traditionally a good wife is one who can prepare various dishes for her husband. In restaurants, especially for tourists, the dishes are normally prepared in a European fashion. Because of the colonial history of Namibia, traditional dishes are not usually served.

Infant Feeding Practices: Since the country's independence, the Namibian Ministry of Health and Social Service has promoted breast-feeding for at least 6 months after birth. Breast-feeding is natural, satisfies all infant needs, and is the cheapest way to feed children, so primary health care facilities educate pregnant women about its advantages. The problem of HIV infection from breast-feeding is recognized, and women who are infected with HIV can get formulas from health facilities for free. Unfortunately, infant formula is not always available, so these mothers are forced to continue breast-feeding. International companies have also begun to advertise and sell industrial milk products and infant formulas in Namibia. These advertisements suggest that artificial food is healthier than breast-feeding, and young parents are tempted to buy it even when they cannot afford it. Because of the high cost of infant formula, mothers dilute it—often with contaminated or inadequately boiled water, causing malnutrition and diarrheal disease. An additional problem is the increasing amount of soft drinks given to small infants. They are more expensive than traditional food and fruits and lead to malnutrition (kwashiorkor) and dental caries.

Child Rearing Practices: Children are reared by their parents and any relatives who live nearby, and young children generally with their mother, who teaches them how to behave and the difference between right and wrong. Because of the lack of jobs, numerous Namibian men work in southern Namibia, especially in Windhoek, Swakopmund, Walvis Bay, and Oranjemund. Therefore many children grow up without their fathers and see them once or twice a year. Respect for older adults is traditionally a very important value to instill in children, and it is typically enforced by beating them. Occasionally older children, usually girls, or grandparents look after younger siblings or children of relatives or neighbors. Normally small children stay with their parents in one traditional house, and when they grow older they sleep in the children's house on the traditional farm. Urbanized Namibian families live in modern houses, and children sleep in separate rooms. When children grow up, boys stay with male relatives and learn how to tend cattle and other livestock owned by the family. They may also be educated in tracing game and hunting. Girls remain with their mother and other female relatives and learn how to get wood and water, maintain the house, and work in the fields. At 6 to 7 years of age, they are sent to school, so working in the fields or tending animals is reduced to afternoon hours and weekends. This causes sometimes conflicts, especially when parents do not understand the importance of education. An emerging problem is the escalating number of children who have lost their mother or both parents to AIDS; many children grow up with their grandparents or relatives. Although orphanages exist, they cannot cope with the increasing number of orphans. The first National Orphans and Vulnerable Children Conference was held May 2001 to develop a program to address this problem.

National Childhood Immunizations: BCG at birth; DPT at 2, 3, 4, and 11 months; OPV at birth, 6, 10, and 14 weeks, 10 to 15 years, and every 10 years; MMR at 9 to 12 months and 2 to 5 years; and Td at 5 and +5 to 10 years. Vaccinations against meningitis are only administered during outbreaks, and MMR is combined with an oral dose of vitamin A solution when possible. Immunizations are offered for free on a daily basis at most health facilities, and national immunization days are regularly organized. Vaccinations are documented in individual health passports, but they are often lost or destroyed by mice or the tropical climate; children with unknown or unclear immunization records receive full immunizations. In 2000, WHO declared Namibia free of neonatal tetanus.

BIBLIOGRAPHY

Biellik RJ et al: Polio outbreaks in Namibia, 1993-1995: lessons learned, *J Infect Dis* 175(suppl 1):30-36, 1997.

Forster N: *Brief review of the year 2001,* Republic of Namibia, 2002.

Government of Namibia: http://www.grnnet.gov.na

Joint United Nations Programme on HIV/AIDS: *Namibia—epidemiological fact sheet, 2000 update,* Geneva, 2000.

Ministry of Health and Social Service: http://www.healthforall.net/grnmhss

Ministry of Health and Social Services: *Epidemiological report on HIV/AIDS for the year 2000,* Republic of Namibia, Ministry of Health and Social Services, 2001.

Ministry of Health and Social Services: *Report of the 2000 HIV sentinel sero survey,* Republic of Namibia, Ministry of Health and Social Services, 2001.

The Namibian: http://www.namibian.com.na

◆ NAURU (REPUBLIC OF)

MAP PAGE (856)

John Dixon

Location: Nauru is a small, oval-shaped coral atoll situated in the southwestern portion of the Pacific Ocean—just below the equator and halfway between Australia and Hawaii. It has a total land area of 21 km^2 (8.1 square miles), about one-tenth the size of Washington, DC. Its unique, barren terrain of jagged limestone pinnacles on the central plateau is the product of 90 years of continuous phosphate strip mining. Only its very narrow fertile coastal belt is inhabitable. Nauru has a tropical climate tempered by cool sea breezes, although it is subject to high humidity (averaging 70% to 80%) and heavy but erratic rainfall averaging 6 to 8 inches (15 to 20 centimeters) per year. Nauru was settled approximately 3000 years ago by intrepid seafaring Polynesian and Melanesian explorers. Nauruans thus originated from a mixture of people from Polynesia, Micronesia, and Melanesia, although they have predominantly Polynesian characteristics. Little is known of traditional Nauruan culture, which was based on a fishing and hunting lifestyle, although it is known that the ancestors believed in a female deity—*Eijebon*—and a spirit land—an island called *Buitani*.

Major Languages	Ethnic Groups	Major Religions
Nauruan	Nauruan 58%	Protestant 67%
English	Other Pacific Islander 26%	Roman Catholic 33%
	Chinese 8%	
	European 8%	

The indigenous spoken language is Nauruan, a distinct Pacific Island language, although the use of spoken and written English is virtually universal. Chinese pidgin English is also spoken. Until the end of the eighteenth century the 12 tribes that made up island society lived in isolation and generally peacefully as a kingdom. This changed forever when the Nauru was discovered in 1789. Soon after, the introduction of firearms, alcohol, foreign germs, and colonial exploitation began destroying the island, its people, and their traditional culture. The Germans began a Nauruan cultural deterioration when they banned traditional island dancing and eventually other cultural practices after they annexed Nauru as part of the Marshal Islands Protectorate under the 1887 Anglo-German Convention. The cultural legacy of 50 years of Australian hegemony is the Nauruans' addiction to Australian Rule's Football, their love of Foster's lager, and other Australian sociocultural and sporting icons. Nauru thus supports a hybrid culture in which Christian and contemporary Western customs coexist with traditional customs. Nauru's hybrid culture has produced a people with a distinctive set of values. They have a good spirit, which has enabled them to stand up to more than 2 centuries or more of fractious British, American, and German seafarers; three colonial empires; and the military might of Japan. They are hospitable, honest, jovial, and unassertive. They place high value on friendliness, kindliness, and compassion. They prefer to work together, help each other, and treat everyone the same. They see much merit in harmony and justice.

Health Care Beliefs: Acute sick care; some health promotion. Sickness prevention and health promotion campaigns are undertaken by the government occasionally. With the assistance of the World Health Organization (WHO) in the mid-1990s, the capacity for implementing health promotion programs, in collaboration with nongovernmental organizations, communities, schools, and youth groups, was improved. Tobacco control and substance abuse prevention policies have also been developed; however, there is a general lack of media-generated health information because of the paucity of local media. It is a popularly held belief that physical bulk signifies prosperity and prestige.

Predominant Sick Care Practices: Biomedical and traditional. The sick seek care from two well-equipped public hospitals, which in 2001 employed all the 14 doctors and 59 nurses in Nauru. Traditional healers still practice their craft. The Nauruan government is now looking to Cuba to augment its supply of trained and experienced health and medical personnel. These hospitals provide adequate care for routine treatments. Because sophisticated medical services are quite restricted, the government pays for Nauruans to receive specialist treatment when required overseas, notably in Australia and New Zealand. In the mid-1990s, 265 patients were referred for such treatment. About 9% of the national budget is spent on health care.

Ethnic/Race Specific or Endemic Diseases: In 1962, James Neel, an American geneticist, presented a now widely accepted theory that Nauruans, along with other Micronesians, have a "thrifty gene" that enables them to store surplus sugar as fat, which predisposes them to life-threatening illnesses such as diabetes, heart disease, and strokes—known collectively as the *New World syndrome*. The population's general health is not good and life expectancy is low given the relatively high living standards. Very few people live beyond 65 years of age. The·leading causes of morbidity (by hospital admissions) in the mid-1990s per 10,000 people were respiratory infections (100.94); accidents, poising, and violence (55.66); diarrheal diseases (46.23); skin and musculoskeletal infections (36.79); and stomach, duodenum, and large bowel diseases (35.85). The leading causes of institutional mortality in the mid-1990s per 10,000 people were cardiovascular disease and hypertension (23.69), respiratory tract infections and pneumonia (19.11), malignant neoplasms (16.98), stillbirths (12.26), and end-stage renal failure (in those with diabetes, 10.38). Alcohol consumption is a serious social problem with health implications. It leads to physical assaults and dangerous driving, making traffic accidents a cause of many deaths. Drinking, particularly *kava,* a bitter-tasting beverage made from the root of a pepper shrub, is an important part of social and ceremonial life. Smoking is a widespread practice, and more than half the population smokes. Nauru's per capita tobacco consumption one of the highest in the world, especially among women. The country also has a high incidence of obesity. Most Nauruans, who are physically large like anyone of Polynesian stock, are classified as class 1 obese (70% of men and 56% of women). Diabetes affects 40% to 45% of the population (41% of men ages 30 to 64 and 42% of women ages 30 to 64). Among those older than 65 years of age, the prevalence rate could be as high as 55%. Type 2 diabetes (non–insulin-dependent diabetes) is found in children. Nauruans have a high incidence of hypertension, heart disease, and cancer. Lymphatic filariasis remains endemic, and dengue fever is a serious risk. AIDS and HIV are not prevalent, and no cases have ever been reported. Homosexuality remains illegal; an active prevention strategy is in place that involves Health Ministry officials, the various religious denominations, and civil society.

Health Team Relationships: Doctors dominate the health care delivery system.

Families' Role in Hospital Care: Nauruans expect to do no more than visit hospitalized sick relatives during the designated visiting hours. Indeed, all medical and dental services are free for Nauruans and all government employees and their family.

Dominance Patterns: Despite their traditionally matrilineal society and their tradition of worshipping a female deity, women have a subordinate role in Nauruan society. Although Nauruan law gives them the same freedoms and protections as men, societal pressures limit their opportunity to exercise those rights fully. Limits are placed on their job opportunities. Anecdotal evidence suggests that alcohol abuse leads to spasmodic physical abuse against women and, although less frequently, against children. Such abuse is treated as a serious communal matter. Nauruans do not respond well to aggressive and argumentative people; diplomacy and tact are preferable to confrontation. A friendly, unassertive, co-operative approach is most likely to achieve successful interactions. The sexes have similar literacy rates: 93% for males and 96% for females.

Eye Contact Practices: Making direct eye contact is a sign of respect and caring.

Touch Practices: Physical touching is a manifestation of the Nauruans' friendliness, kindness, and compassion.

Perceptions of Time: Nauruans abide by "Pacific time," in which the past, present, and future are brought into accord by ensuring that whatever can be put off until tomorrow will be—with no guilt. Punctuality requires a degree of anticipation that is inconsistent with climatic and cultural imperatives.

Pain Reactions: Pain is to be endured stoically and silently by men but not necessarily by women.

Birth Rites: Nauruan women give birth in hospitals for free. The maternal mortality rate in the mid-1990s was 0. Births of all children are celebrated. The birth rate is 27.22 births per 1000 people, and the fertility rate is 3.61 children born per woman. The infant mortality rate is 10.71 deaths per 1000 live births, and general life expectancy is 57.7 years for men and 64.88 years for women.

Death Rites: Christian beliefs about death are common. Autopsies are acceptable, but organ donations are irrelevant because organ transplant operations cannot be performed.

Food Practices and Intolerances: Because of environmental degradation, the supply of fresh food and water is limited on Nauru. Only a small amount of fresh food is available; it is primarily fish (tainted with cadmium), which is eaten raw, especially by children, but is occasionally chicken, beef, pork, or a few locally grown fruits or vegetables. The islander diet is dominated by processed, imported foods—grisly turkey tails, mutton flaps, ice cream, and candy have become status symbols that are associated with affluence. The readily available junk food has become a staple part of the diet. Nauru has periodic droughts and limited natural freshwater resources. Roof storage tanks collect rain water, but the people must depend on a single, aging desalination plant and supplements of imported water.

Infant Feeding Practices: Nauruan mothers prefer to breast-feed their babies if possible, but no data have been collected.

Child Rearing Practices: Nauruan mothers have the dominant child caring and rearing responsibilities, although traditionally they were communal (tribal) responsibilities.

National Childhood Immunizations: BCG at 1 month and at 5 and 16 years; DTP at 1, 2, 3, and 18 months; OPV at 2, 4, 6, and 18 to 24 months; hep B birth and 1, 5, and 6 years; and MMR at 12 to 15 months. The percentages of 1-year-old children who have been immunized with the various vaccinations are as follows: measles, 100; BCG, 78; third dose of DPT, 50; and the third dose of polio, 36%.

Other Characteristics: Environmental degradation has turned the majority (90%) of central Nauru into a wasteland and threatens the limited remaining land resources; it is simply ignored by many Nauruans. They accept that the phosphate mines are just "up there," or "topside"; in other words, out of sight, out of mind. They accept that the source of their wealth—phosphate—has destroyed their land and is killing them. Ecological rehabilitation is a government priority, but little has been done, likely because of the projected cost: $230 million over 20 years. Nauru also faces other environmental threats that are a product of its location.

The greenhouse effect and risk of global warming could cause sea levels to flood the habitable coastal land area. Nauru also lies downwind of the French nuclear test sites in the Pacific. Since 1888, Nauru has been exploited by the Germans, British, Australians, New Zealanders, Japanese, and more recently the Nauruans themselves. Its people, culture, forest, soil, and ultimately sub-soil have been stripped or shipped away at the whim of colonial powers. The mining of 1000 years of bird droppings has been lucrative; however the valuable but finite phosphate reserves are virtually exhausted. Nauru's legacy is a standard of living that is among the best in the Third World, with a gross national product (GNP) per capita in excess of $7000. This certainly makes Nauruans the "poor little rich kids" of the Pacific Islands; they pay no taxes, live in government-subsidized housing, and get free health care and education. They have a penchant for a sedentary lifestyle, simple but well-equipped traditional houses, and luxury cars. They also have a very uncertain economic future, generally poor health, and an unenviable natural environment. However, in recent years they have been willing to support this lifestyle not only by accepting refugees seeking asylum in Australia for a payment but also by accepting dubious Russian bank deposits in its offshore banking operations—for a fee.

BIBLIOGRAPHY

Dowse GK, Zimmet PZ, Collins VR: Insulin levels and the natural history of glucose intolerance in Nauruans, *Diabetics* 45:1367-1372, 1996.

Hodge AM et al: Mortality in Micronesian Nauruans and Melanesian and Indian Fijians is not associated with obesity, *Am J Epidemiol* 143(5):442–455, 1996.

Humphrey ARG et al: Diabetics and nontraumatic lower extremity amputations: incidence, risk factors, and prevention—a 12-year follow-up study in Nauru, *Diabetes Care* 19(7):710–714, 1996.

Kovats RS, Bouna MJ, Haines A: *El Niño and health (WHO/SDE/PHE/99.4),* Geneva, 1999, World Health Organization.

McDonald CN, Gowdy JM: *Paradise for sale: a parable of nature,* Berkeley, Calif, 2000, University of California Press.

Petit-Skinner S: *The Nauruans: nature and supernature in an island of the central Pacific,* ed 2, San Francisco, 1981, MacDuff.

Silver K et al: Molecular scanning for mutations in the beta3-adrenergic receptor gene in Nauruans with obesity and non–insulin-dependent diabetes mellitus, *J Clin Endocrinol Metab* 81(11):4155–4158, 1996.

World Health Organization: *Press release* (WHO/46, 12 June), Geneva, 1997, World Health Organization.

World Health Organization: *World health report 2000,* Geneva, 2000, World Health Organization.

www.atlapedia.com/online/countries/anuru.html
www.cdc.gov/tobacco/who/nauru.html
www.cia.gov/publications/factbook/geos/nr.html
www.commonwealthfoundation.com
www.earth.nwu.edu/people/emile/nauru.html
www.ethnologue.com/show_country.asp?name=Nauru
www.hellopacific.com/news

www.news.bbc.co.uk/hi/english/world/asia-pacific
www.state.gov
www.tbc.gov.bc.ca/cwgames/country/nauru/nauru.html
www.time.com/time/pacific/magazine.
www.un.org/ga/aids/statements/docs
http://www.who.org

◆ NEPAL (KINGDOM OF)

MAP PAGE (866)

Narbada Thapa

Location: Nepal is a landlocked country in southern Asia with a diverse, multilingual, multireligious, and multiethnic population of 23.2 million. It is situated between China in the north and India in the south, east, and west. The total land area is 140,800 km^2 (53,363 square miles). Two thirds of the country is covered by hills and mountains, including Mount Everest, the highest peak in the world (8848 m). More than 90% of the population lives in rural areas and depends on agriculture. Because of the difficult terrain, transport and communication are sparse or nonexistent in most of areas. Tourism, especially trekking and mountaineering, have recently increased overall prosperity, but the gross national product (GNP) per capita is still very low at $1100 per year. Geography and altitude influence the types of health problems and the availability of health care. Nepal has more than 60 caste, or ethnic, groups, who speak more than 40 languages. Ethnic groups can be classified into two broad categories: the Indo-Aryans, or Indo-Nepalese, and the Tibeto-Mongoloids, or Tibeto-Nepalese.

Major Languages	Ethic Groups	Major Religions
Nepali	Chhetri 16%	Hindu 85%
Maithali	Brahmin 14%	Buddhist 8%
Bhoipuri	Magar 7%	Muslim, Christian 7%
Tharu	Tharu 7%	
Tamang	Newar 6%	
Newari	Tamang 5%	
Others (more than 35 languages)	Others (more than 50 caste, or ethnic, groups) 45%	

Tibeto-Mongoloids, which include Sherpas, Tamang, Rai, Limbu, Magars, and Kirantis, primarily live in the northeastern part of the country. The bulk of the Hill and Terai (low land) groups include Indo-Aryans such as the Chhetri, Brahmin, Tharus, and Danuars.

Health Care Beliefs: Acute sick care; traditional. Particularly in rural Nepal, illness is believed to be caused by purposeful intervention of an agent such as a supernatural being (e.g., deity, a god), an inhuman entity (e.g., ghost, ancestor, evil spirit), or a human being (e.g., witch, sorcerer). Sick people are literally thought of as victims—the objects of aggression or punishment directed specifically against them or their family. The treatment of disease depends on the belief of the cause. For example, people who believe that the cause of the disease is naturalistic in origin seek biomedical or ayurvedic treatments from various sources such as a pharmacist, grocer, hospital, clinic, or health care provider or rely on home remedies such as herbal preparations. Likewise, people who believe that the cause of their disease is the wrath of a god, the influence of an evil spirit, sorcery, or breech of a taboo, seek treatment involving witchcraft and magic, pray, and perform rituals to please the god or deity and priest, and use charms and amulets. Spiritual practices include praying, singing hymns, cupping, and rubbing or burning the skin with a heated spoon. Beliefs in the effects of "hot" and "cold: foods are also common. Mental illness is thought to be the result of sins in the past life.

Predominant Sick Care Practices: Biomedical, magical-religious, and traditional practices. Health care treatments include indigenous, Western, and ayurvedic medicine. More than 70% of the people use traditional methods of treatment (involving faith or spiritual healers, priests, and home remedies) before seeking biomedical treatment. Ayurvedic medicine and natural therapies have become popular in recent years.

Ethnic/Race Specific or Endemic Diseases: Chloroquine-resistant malaria, and kalazar are endemic in Nepal, with no risk in urban and hilly regions. The patterns of diseases vary according to geographical setting and socio-economic conditions rather than ethnicity or race. Nepalese are at risk for cholera, Japanese encephalitis, leprosy, diarrhea, nutritional deficiencies, pneumonia, tuberculosis, and hepatitis. Common causes of death among children are respiratory tract infections, diarrhea, and malnutrition. The World Health Organization's (WHO) estimated prevalence rate for HIV/AIDS in adults ages 15 to 49 is 0.29%. The estimated number of children from birth to 15 years living with HIV/AIDS is less than 930. Men in the younger age groups are most affected. Life expectancy is 58 years.

Health Team Relationships: The majority of doctors are men, and nurses are primarily women. People and patients pay more respect to doctors than nurses. Although nurses are highly qualified, the doctors' dominance over nurses exists in hospital settings. Paramedics and community health workers are also important providers of health services on the community level. Generally, attitudes toward all health providers are positive. In most settings, people are reluctant to receive care from a person of the opposite sex.

Families' Role in Hospital Care: In Nepal, people live together in extended family units. If one member gets ill, other members of the family take care of the person. Families stay with hospitalized relatives, helping them eat and perform hygiene tasks, as well as providing psychological support. They also purchase medications, take specimens to the lab if necessary, pay hospital bills, and do anything else that is necessary. Providing care for ill family members is considered an act of love and respect and is done out of a sense of responsibility.

Dominance Patterns: The family unit is important, but gender inequities exist in the society. Because Nepal has a patriarchal society, young women move to the home of their in-laws after marriage, where they immediately assume the responsibility for many chores and are low on the family hierarchy. Men are more powerful and the decision makers in most families except in the Tibeto-Mongoloid ethnic group. In certain special situations such as the selection of a daughter-in-law, pregnancy, childbirth, and care of newborns, mothers-in-law and older women are most influential. Sons are responsible for looking after their parents in their old age.

Eye Contact Practices: Looking into a person's eyes during a conversation, especially of a senior citizen or woman, is considered disrespectful and impolite. It is believed that some individuals have the ability to cast a spell on another by just looking at their faces, foreheads, palms, or body in general. When individuals cast this "evil eye," the subject faces misfortune and will become ill. A witch can injure others by the power of her eyes; she may destroy others with a curse or make them ill. Witches are generally believed to be female.

Touch Practices: Men are not allowed to touch women unless they have a specific reason for doing so. Only a mother, sister, daughter, or wife can be touched by a male family member. The head is considered the place of God and is not to be touched by another unless necessary. Older adults can touch a younger person's head to extend good wishes. Spiritual healers touch the forehead or other parts of the body of an ill person during the process of diagnosis and treatment, a practice that is considered acceptable. Handshaking is uncommon between men and women. Dress tends to be traditional, and a woman who immodestly exposes her body is culturally unacceptable.

Perceptions of Time: Traditionally, punctuality is not considered to be very important. More recently, perceptions have been changing, and punctuality is becoming more important and appreciated. Time is very important during rituals such as birth, death, and marriage, when timing is strictly followed according to a priest's calculations. Nepalese people live between the past and present and are trying to establish a better future.

Pain Reactions: People generally have a high tolerance for pain and discomfort. Men and rural people are more stoical than people from urban areas. Women from rural areas do not express pain, even during childbirth. People remain quiet and even smile while experiencing pain, which causes health practitioners to underestimate the severity of the problem and delay treatment.

Birth Rites: Pregnancy is considered a natural process, so no special attention is given to most pregnant women. To ward off evil spirits and ensure a safe pregnancy and birth, a pregnant woman wears a protective band around her neck. During his wife's pregnancy, a husband is not allowed to slaughter an animal, and a pregnant woman does not eat spicy food. Pregnancy before marriage is unacceptable and is a very sensitive issue. Because there are legal and social considerations relative to the decision to abort a baby, many women get abortions from un-trained persons or quack healers, and these women frequently become septic. Unsuccessful attempts to abort the baby illegally may compel women to have the baby and then try to kill the newborn or discard it. More than 80% of deliveries take place at home and are attended by untrained people, such as a mother-in-law, another relative, or a traditional birth attendant. In rural areas, many women give birth alone in animal sheds. Males, unmarried girls, and children are not allowed to be in an area where childbirth is taking place. The period of childbirth and menstruation is considered a "polluted period" for the women, so no one is allowed to touch them because of issues related to the deities and gods. People believe that if a deity or god becomes angry, the mother and infant may develop health problems. Therefore the mother stays isolated for 7 to 11 days after birth in a separate room that is kept warm and draft free. The mother and newborn sit in the sun each day and have oil massages with hot mustard oil that is often cooked with *Trigonella fonnum (methi)*, a spice believed to have healing powers. Male and female infants are given equal care. Special foods given to the mother include meat, rice, mustard oil, cumin, soup with trachysperous ammi *(jwano),* a spice believed to increase the mother's milk production sugar candy, and butter. *Methi* and *jwano* are also used in curries. Women reduce their salt intake for 6 to 10 days because salt is believed to cause swelling and infections in the mother. Green spinach, pumpkins, and apple consumption is also restricted for 2 to 3 months after delivery because they are considered "cold" food that can cause diarrhea in children as they drink their mother's milk. Food restrictions are not as strict among the Tibeto-Mongoloid ethnic group.

Death Rites: Death is considered as the natural process of life, and people believe God decides the timing of birth and death for all living beings. Most older people try to do good deeds to ensure a place in heaven or increase their wealth and decrease their suffering in the next life. Death at home is preferred to death in a hospital. After death the body is washed and wrapped with a new, special cotton cloth. If the dead person is a married woman, she is dressed as a new bride. Relatives and friends express their grief; they are present when death is expected and after the death as well. Autopsies are uncommon unless the death has unusual characteristics that require investigation. In most cases the body is cremated immediately after death. The son and wife of the dead person stay isolated for 13 days and eat plain food they cook themselves. Salt, meat and meat products, vegetables, beans and grains, and spices are restricted. Rituals are performed 13 days, 45 days, 3 months, 6 months, and every year after the death to keep the dead person's soul at peace. The family offers meals and household goods through a priest out of respect to the dead person. The mourning ceremony is different in Sherpa and Lama ethnic groups. Some express grief through singing sad songs. Organ donation is considered a holy work. For example, donation of the eyes after death is believed to reduce the sins of the person, allowing entrance into heaven.

Food Practices and Intolerances: The staple foods are rice, chapatti, corn, dal (lentils), beans, green vegetables, meat, and fish. People eat three times a day—lunch, Tiffin, and dinner—and consume meat or fish once or twice a week. Traditionally, people eat with their hands. Elders and male members of the family eat first, and the daughter-in-law eats last. In mountain areas, potatoes and barley are staple foods.

Infant Feeding Practices: Women breast-feed exclusively for 3 to 6 months and then introduce supplementary foods. Nearly all mothers breast-feed their babies. Weaning foods are introduced at the age of 5 months to daughters and the age of 6 months to sons. After a weaning ceremony the child is allowed to eat normal adult foods. Cow's milk is commonly used. More than 50% of the children in Nepal are malnourished.

Child Rearing Practices: Child rearing is undertaken primarily by the grandmothers and elder siblings. Sons are preferred. Infants up to 6 months old are massaged in oil, often mustard oil, and placed in the sun several times a day. The oil, which is absorbed by the body, is believed to make the child strong and prevent air from going into the body. This practice is based on the belief that cool air passing through the body of the mother and newborn could make them sick with diseases thought to be caused by coldness, such as pneumonia, diarrhea, abdominal pain and distension, dysentery, and edema. To keep the shape of the infant's head round, a pillow made of mustard seed is made and molded to the infant's head. Because of limited access to health services and lack of awareness, most women do not use maternal and pediatric health clinics, resulting in maternal mortality rates of 1500 women per 100,000 live births and an infant mortality rate of 79 per 1000 live births. Discipline and obedience are encouraged. Children go to school at the age of 3 to 5 years, but education for girls has a low priority. The adult literacy rates for males and females are 41% and 14%, respectively.

National Childhood Immunizations: BCG at birth or at first contact; DTP at 6, 10, and 14 weeks; OPV at 6, 10, and 14 weeks; measles at 9 months (up to 36 months); and TT CBAW at 15 years. The Expanded Program of Immunization (EPI) is one of the priority programs of the

Nepalese government. The immediate objectives of the EPI programs were to eliminate or reduce neonatal tetanus and measles and to eradicate poliomyelitis by 2000. Although these objectives have not been met, the last reported morbidity rates were 0.0002% for neonatal tetanus, 0.031% for measles, and 0.0001% for polio. According to 1998 and 1999, reports, the coverage level for BCG and measles vaccine is higher than 90% and 80%, respectively, whereas the coverage rate for the third dose of DPT and third dose of OPV is approximately 76%. However, because of the difficult geographical considerations, coverage is still not uniform within the country, with some districts achieving 100% coverage and others staying far behind.

BIBLIOGRAPHY

Gautam M: Malnutrition in Nepal: a review, *J Nep Med Assoc* 34:141–151, 1996.

Department of Health Services: *Annual report 1998/1999,* Kathmandu, Nepal, Department of Health Services, Ministry of Health.

Desjarlais RR: Poetic transformations of Yolmo "sadness," *Cult Med Psychiatry* 15(4):387, 1991.

Jones CM: The meaning of being an elder in Nepal, *Nurs Sci Q* 5(4):171, 1992.

Mahat G, Phiri M: Promoting assertive behaviours in traditional societies, *Int Nurs Rev* 38(5):153, 1991.

Ogilvie L: Nursing in Nepal, *Can Nurse* 91(6):25, 1995.

Sharma A, Ross J: Nepal: integrating traditional and modern health services in the remote area of Bashkharka, 27(4):343, 1990.

World Health Organization (June 2000): *Epidemiological fact sheets by country,* Geneva. Retrieved March 1, 2002, from http://www.unaids.org/hivaidsinfo/statistics/june00/fact_sheets/index.html

World Health Organization. (2001): *WHO vaccine-preventable diseases: monitoring system,* Geneva. Retrieved March 1, 2002, from http://www.who.int/vaccines/

◆ NETHERLANDS (KINGDOM OF THE)

MAP PAGE (860)

Frits van Merode

Location: The Netherlands is situated in the northwestern part of Europe at the North Sea. Because of the warm gulf, the climate is mild. Most of the country is flat, and a substantial part is gained from the sea and protected by dikes: 60% of the Dutch live below sea level. The country has the typical characteristics of a coast country, especially the western part, which is also known as *Holland*. It has large ports (including Rotterdam, the largest port in the world) and an elaborate infrastructure into the continent (especially Germany). Schiphol is the third largest airport of western Europe. The Netherlands is one of the smallest countries in the world with a total land area of 37,330 km² (14,413 square miles), but it ranks in the world's top 10 in export volume and top 20 for gross national product (GNP). In the past, the Netherlands had colonies:

Indonesia, New Guinea, Surinam (Dutch Guyana), and the six Caribbean Islands, of which Curacao is the largest, located north of Venezuela. The Caribbean Islands are independent in their domestic affairs but belong to the Kingdom of the Netherlands. The Netherlands has large groups originating from these former colonies.

Major Languages	Ethnic Groups	Major Religions
Dutch (official)	Dutch 96%	Roman Catholic 34%
Frisian	Moroccan, Turk, other 4%	Protestant 25%
		Muslim 3%
		Other 2%

Dutch is the official language and spoken by almost everyone; most speak English as a second language. Protestants live primarily in the northern and western part of the Netherlands; Catholics live in the south. Primarily, immigrants from northern Africa (especially Morocco) and Turkey adhere to Islam. A large part of the Dutch population does not actively practice religion.

Health Care Beliefs: Active role; prevention important. Prevention is one of the cornerstones of Dutch health care. All municipalities have a legal obligation to have a policy for prevention and hygiene. Often the tasks resulting from this obligation are outsourced to a municipal or regional community health service (Gemeentelijke Gezondheidsdienst or GGD). Aside from the numerous national prevention programs (e.g., eating practices, smoking cessation, hygiene) health is largely considered an individual responsibility. Individuals also are becoming increasingly assertive about what they want from health care providers, an attitude that is not always appreciated by providers because they feel that they are being thrust into negotiation situations.

Predominant Sick Care Practices: Biomedical and limited alternative practices. Sick care practices predominantly involve standard medicine. A small proportion (6.4%) of the population seeks help from homeopathic and alternative medical practitioners. Some private insurance companies reimburse these nonstandard practices up to a certain amount of Euros. The Dutch health care system is a gate-keeping system; a distinction is made between general care and specialist care. General practitioners and dentists provide general care. Only with a referral from a general practitioner can patients generally access medical specialists, who almost always have their practices in hospitals. Costs of health care were 33,043,000,000 Euro (roughly equivalent to $US) in 2000, which is 8.2% GNP. Costs for nursing and care are 24% of total health care expenditures, and 25% of these costs relate to psychological disorders, primarily dementia. About 75% of nursing and care costs are spent for women, whereas their share in total health care costs is only 59%, a result of their higher life expectancy: 80.6 years for women versus 75.5 for men. Overall estimates of the health condition of the Dutch population are as follows: very good, 25.9%; good, 54.5%; reasonable, 11.6%; sometimes good, sometimes bad, 5.8%; bad, 2.3%.

Ethnic/Race Specific or Endemic Diseases: Infectious diseases and accidents, back and neck problems, and contact eczema have the highest incidence. The main causes of death are coronary heart diseases and stroke (more than 10,000 deaths per year). Illness prevalence (more than 1,000,000 cases per year) is the highest for anxiety and hearing disorders and back and neck complaints. The World Health Organization's (WHO) estimated prevalence rate for HIV/AIDS in adults ages 15 to 49 is 0.19%. The estimated number of children from birth to 15 years living with HIV/AIDS is 100. The incidence of AIDS is less then 500 cases per year.

Health Team Relationships: The doctor has a dominant position in Dutch health care. Nurses have been becoming more important as process managers, a change that was especially taking place in 1990s. In addition, during the 1990s, hospitals changed their organizational structures in a way that integrated doctors more into hospital management. Most hospitals have implemented a structure that resembles a divisional organization, in which each division has a doctor as the medical manager. The position of nurses has become more central in the health care system through the introduction of specialized nursing (e.g., diabetes nursing, asthma nursing). In most hospitals, nurses work in teams involving a mixture of patient-centered and task-oriented nursing.

Families' Role in Hospital Care: Families do not play a role in hospital care. However, some hospitals are experimenting with training the families of patients to assume certain care roles after discharging the patient. The goal of hospitals is to shorten the length of stays, therefore the role of families in providing care outside the hospital is becoming more important. This "informal" care is an important part of nursing and care for patients. This development is stimulated by a nursing shortage and the increase in demand for care as the Dutch population grows older.

Dominance Patterns: Men and women are relatively equal in the Netherlands.

Eye Contact Practices: During conversations, direct eye contact is essential.

Touch Practices: Some touching is acceptable, but most people are conservative about touching others.

Perceptions of Time: Punctuality is highly valued, and it is expected that a person should never be late, even 5 minutes, for an appointment. Even for informal visits (e.g., with friends), it is customary to make an appointment. Even if a person has an invitation to "drop by," it is expected that the person will confirm the appointment at least several hours before the visit. It is important to arrive exactly on time because it is also considered impolite to arrive too early (even a few minutes).

Pain Reactions: The reaction of individuals toward pain is moderate—neither stoical nor expressive. Some pain is considered natural; for example, during childbirth, analgesics are neither expected nor required. However, the term "unbearable" pain is used in discussions about euthanasia.

Birth Rites: Many consider a home birth with the assistance of midwives to be supreme; therefore it is encouraged. However, because of a shortage of midwives, the demand for home births is greater than the number of midwives. Many cities have "open birth centers" with delivery rooms that can be rented. These centers do not have to be connected to a hospital. The father is expected to support the mother during the delivery. It is becoming quite usual for couples who are not married but are living together to have a child. Of the total of 206,619 babies, 155,080 were born to married couples. The age at which women have their first child is increasing (26.4 years in 1950 versus 29.1 years in 2000), although this trend seems to have reached a plateau. The mean age of mothers having a child is 30.7 years. The fertility rate is 1.7 children per woman, and overall fertility rates are decreasing.

Death Rites: Euthanasia is allowed under strict conditions. The person must have a medical problem, the euthanasia must be conducted by a doctor, peer consultation must be involved, and a report must be submitted by the practicing doctor that can be checked by the ministry of justice. It is expected that close family remain with dying relatives. The Netherlands has a national organ donation register of all Dutch people that indicates whether they are willing to have their organs donated to another person or for scientific study (which are two different categories). However, the immediate family must also give permission to use the organs in many situations. It is difficult for doctors and nurses to talk with families about organ donation immediately after they have lost a loved one, so they country still has a significant shortage of donor organs.

Food Practices and Intolerances: Breakfast often consists of a combination of yogurt products, bread, coffee or tea, cereal, cheese, and juice. People have sandwiches for lunch. The main meal is in the early evening. Potatoes, rice, or pasta with meat or meatballs is the main meal (which is eaten in the evening, at about 5 or 6 PM). Young people are adapting to the American way of eating, with no strict times for meals and more frequent consumption of snack or fast foods, a particular problem for children in secondary school. A fork, knife, and spoon are used for most meals. It is unacceptable to use the hands for other than small sandwiches, small cakes, and biscuits.

Infant Feeding Practices: Breast-feeding is becoming more popular.

Child Rearing Practices: Children begin school when they are 4 years old. They do not sleep with their parents. Children are taught to be assertive. Parents are neither too permissive nor too strict.

National Childhood Immunizations: DtaP at 2, 3, 4, and 11 months; IPV at 2, 3, 4, and 11 months and 4 years; MMR at 14 months and 9 years; DT at 4 and 9 years; HIB at 2, 3, 4, and 11 months.

BIBLIOGRAPHY

Centraal Bureau voor de Statistiek: http://statline.cbs.nl/StatWeb
http://www.rivm.nl/nationaalkompas/data/gezondheidstoestand
http://www.xpat.nl/chapter.html

◆ NEW ZEALAND/AOTEAROA

MAP PAGE (856)

Lynne S. Giddings

Location: Located in the South Pacific, Aotearoa/New Zealand is approximately 2012 km (1200 miles) east of Australia. New Zealand consists primarily of two islands: North Island and South Island, which are separated by Cook Strait. Climatic conditions range from semitropical in the north to cool temperate in the south, with glaciers in the southwest. New Zealand has volcanic activity (e.g., volcanoes, hot springs, mud pools), predominantly in the North Island. A mountainous chain stretches along the spine of the North and South Islands, and abundant pastoral plains support the mainly agricultural economy. Geographical isolation has created a natural biological border so that many worldwide diseases (malaria and most tropical diseases) are not present. New Zealand has no snakes or dangerous carnivores except for a mildly poisonous native spider—the katipo. The population of Aotearoa/New Zealand in the year 2000 was 3,830,000.

Major Languages	Ethnic Groups	Major Religions
English (official)	European 75%	Christian 81%
Maori (official)	Maori 15%	Hindu, Confucian 1%
	Pacific Islander 5%	Other 18%
	Asian 4%	
	Other 1%	

Maori, the *tangata whenua* ("people of the land") of New Zealand, were the first people to settle in the land. In 1840 a treaty was established, Te Tiriti O Waitangi, with the British royalty. This founding document forms the bicultural basis for the government's approach to issues concerning health. Numerous waves of immigration have come to New Zealand since 1840, including Scots, English, Irish, Chinese, Dutch, Pasifika, and recently, Asian immigrants and refugees from around the world. Sports are an important focus for cultural identity. Popular sports include water sports (e.g., swimming, canoeing, rowing, yachting), mountaineering, skiing, netball, squash, cricket, and rugby.

Health Care Beliefs: Active role; holistic; health promotion important. Although the health care system is primarily based on the biomedical model, alternative therapies and holistic practices are popular and include acupuncture, osteopathy, homeopathy, naturopathy, and indigenous (Maori) herbal remedies.

Predominant Sick Care Beliefs: Biomedical and traditional. Health care is largely government funded and hospital based. However, private and voluntary organizations are working in the community to provide specialized assistance such as the Plunket Society (family, mother, and baby care), Women's Refuge and Saftinet (domestic violence), Cancer Society, Intellectually Handicapped Society (IHC), and other specialist medical and disability support groups. Since the 1970s, deinstitutionalization has transformed mental health services. Care and treatment of mental illness is largely community based, and the range of services includes supported accommodation, individual community support, cultural services, medical and multidisciplinary treatments, and 24-hour crisis services. Antidiscrimination programs and the political work of the consumer movement supplement the community focus.

Ethnic/Race Specific or Endemic Diseases: The major causes of death (with rates per million of mean population in 1996) are malignant neoplasms, 2063; ischemic heart disease, 1833; and cerebrovascular disease, 735. The Maori and Pasifika populations have an increased incidence of diabetes (three to five times higher than the norm), asthma (one and a half times higher), heart disease, and smoking-related diseases. Smoking causes at least 22% of all cancer deaths in New Zealand and is the single greatest preventable cause of early death among Maori and non-Maori New Zealanders. It is estimated that 20% to 25% of the overall population smokes. However, approximately 45% of Maori men smoke, 57% of Maori women smoke, and 12% of young Maori (ages 10 to 15 years) smoke regularly. The World Health Organization's (WHO) estimated prevalence rate for HIV/AIDS in adults ages 15 to 49 is 0.06%. The estimated number of children from birth to 15 years living with HIV/AIDS is less than 100.

Health Team Relationships: The medical profession dominates the health care system, and people are successfully challenging the patriarchal structure. The system includes indigenous health services (often *marae-,* or tribal-based *iwi* buildings and land, which have a strong spiritual and cultural dimension), independent midwives (the preferred childbirth practitioner), consumer advocates (addressing patient rights and mental health issues), and independent nurse practitioners (with prescribing rights).

Families' Role in Hospital Care: Family involvement in the care of a hospitalized relative is encouraged and supported. Visiting hours are extended, and special arrangements can be made for family and significant others to stay overnight with a patient. *Whanau* (family) rooms are available in most hospitals, providing accommodations and acknowledging the special needs of patients and their extended families.

Dominance Patterns: Social and community issues such as domestic violence, older adult, child, and sexual abuse have become a focus of concern for government and other agencies since the early 1990s. However, reliable population-based rates of family violence are not yet available. Since the emancipation of women in 1893, gender inequality has been a contentious issue. Inequalities between genders still exist in relation to salaries, promotions, and child rearing practices. Although women are represented at the highest level in New Zealand (e.g., prime minister, governor general, chief justice), gender inequalities continue to affect all levels within society. For example, currently the average wages for women in public service can be as much as $41,000 less than the wages of their male colleagues. These gender differences are compounded by various forms of prejudice, including racism and heterosexism.

Eye Contact Practices: Some groups maintain eye contact (e.g., Europeans), whereas others (e.g., Maori, Pasifika) consider it polite to avert their gaze.

Touch Practices: It is difficult to generalize cultural interpersonal practices in New Zealand because of the effects of European colonization and cultural mixing over time. However, a diverse range of practices exist, ranging from reserved English and European practices with limited touching and a focus on the nuclear family, to Maori *marae*-based living, with its more open expressions of intimacy and focus on the extended family *(kwhanau* and *hapu)*.

Perceptions of Time: Modern European perceptions of time predominate.

Pain Reactions: Pain reactions vary according to gender and cultural characteristics. Some groups can be stereotyped as more stoical (e.g., Pasifikas and males).

Birth Rites: Childbirth and child rearing practices vary depending on cultural identity. Traditionally (and increasingly since the early twentieth century), childbirth has taken place in hospitals and is monitored by doctors and obstetricians. More recently, women have been choosing home births under the guidance of midwives. For people who identify themselves as Maori, the connection with the land, or *whenua,* is strong. For many Maori an infant's connection to the land is confirmed through the burial of the placenta, which is also called *whenua,* soon after birth.

Death Rites: Death rites vary widely and depend on cultural and religious practices. Many families of European origin leave the body at a funeral home, and burial or cremation follows a religious or secular service. More recently, because of the influence of Maori funeral practices, New Zealand European (Pakeha) families are asking for their loved ones to be returned home so that family and friends can mourn together until a burial or cremation. Maori funeral practices involve a *tangi* or *tangihanga* mourning that is held on the *marae* for 3 days and 3 nights. This period is a time of farewell speeches, tears, and mourning as extended family members and friends attend to the body before burial.

Food Practices and Intolerances: Availability of nourishing food (e.g., seafood *[kaimoana]*, lamb, beef, a wide variety of vegetables and fruit including kiwi), and a high incidence of physical activity (with two out of every three people being active during their leisure time) contribute to a generally healthy population. However, abundant dairy and meat products have also contributed to high rates of heart disease, diabetes, and the increasing incidence of obesity. Fast food, a recent phenomenon, is exacerbating this situation.

Infant Feeding Practices: In New Zealand, Plunket nurse records suggest that breast-feeding rates were about 80% in 1938 but then decreased until 1968, when they were only about 41%. From 1974 to until today, the trend has been increasing. In 1992, 80% to 90% of women were breast-feeding when discharged from the hospital after birth, and 40% to 60% were still breast-feeding at 4 months, statistics similar to those in other Western countries.

National Childhood Immunizations: DTaP at 6 weeks and 3, 5, and 15 months; OPV at 6 weeks, 3 and 5 months and 4 and 11 years; hep B at 6 weeks and at 3 and 5 months; HIB at 6 weeks and at 3 and 15 months; MMR at 15 months and 4 and 11 years; and Td at 11 years and then every 10 years. Of the 145 countries listed in the United Nations Children's Fund (UNICEF) report The State of the World's Children 1998, 74 had higher immunization rates than New Zealand for DTP at age 1 year.

ACKNOWLEDGEMENTS: I acknowledge the help of librarians, Donna Jarvis and Andrew South, Akoranga Library, AUT, Auckland, New Zealand.

BIBLIOGRAPHY

Bateman New Zealand encyclopedia, ed 5, Auckland, New Zealand, 2000, Bateman.
Cancer Society of New Zealand: Retrieved February 18, 2002, from http://www.cancernz.org.nz/
Coney S: *Standing in the sunshine: a history of New Zealand women since they won the vote,* Auckland, New Zealand, 1993, Viking.
Davis P, Ashton T: *Health and public policy in New Zealand,* Auckland, New Zealand, 2001, Oxford University Press.
Davis P, Dew K: *Health and society in Aotearoa New Zealand,* Auckland, New Zealand, 1999, Oxford University Press.
Domestic Violence Centre (New Zealand): http://www.dvc.org.nz/stats.htm
Intellectually Handicapped Society: http://www.ihc.org.nz/about/index.asp
Lange R: *May the people live: a history of Maori health development 1900–1920,* Auckland, New Zealand, 1999, Auckland University Press.
Maori to English translation: http://www.classysisters.co.nz/Maori-dictionary.html
Mental Health Commission: http://www.mhc.govt.nz
Ministry of Health: http://www.moh.govt.nz
Ministry of Health: *Family violence: guidelines for health sector providers to develop practice protocols,* Wellington, New Zealand, 1998.
Ministry of Health: *Our health, our future: hauora pakari, koiora roa: the health of New Zealanders 1999,* Wellington, New Zealand, 1999.

Plunket Society: http://www.plunket.org.nz

Sports Commission of New Zealand: http://www.hillarysport.org.nz

Statistics New Zealand (includes New Zealand Yearbook): http://www.stats.govt.nz

Statistics New Zealand: *New Zealand official yearbook 2000,* Wellington, New Zealand, 2000.

Treaty of Waitangi, http://www.govt.nz/aboutnz/treaty.php3

United Nations Children's Fund Report: *State of the world's children 1998.* Retrieved February 18, 2002, from http://www.unicef.org/sowc98/refs.htm

World Health Organization (June 2000): *Epidemiological fact sheets by country,* Geneva. Retrieved March 1, 2002, from http://www.unaids.org/hivaidsinfo/statistics/june00/fact_sheets/index.html

World Health Organization (2001): *WHO vaccine-preventable diseases: monitoring system,* Geneva. Retrieved March 1, 2002, from http://www.who.int/vaccines/

◆ NICARAGUA (REPUBLIC OF)

MAP PAGE (857)

Mary Ruth Horner and Bonnie J. Brownlee

Location: Nicaragua is located in the middle of Central America, bordered on the north by Honduras and on the south by Costa Rica. The Caribbean Sea lies to the east and the Pacific Ocean to the west. Nicaragua is divided topographically into three regions—the Pacific, the central, and the Atlantic. The total land area of Nicaragua is 129,494 km² (49,998 square miles), and the population is concentrated in the Pacific region (approximately 62%), the location of the capital, Managua. The central region has approximately 33% of the country's population and the Atlantic region, which makes up approximately 50% of the area, has the remaining 6% of the population. The population in 2001 was 4,918,393.

Major Languages	Ethnic Groups	Major Religions
Spanish (national)	Mestizo 69%	Roman Catholic 95%
	White 17%	Protestant 5%
	Black 9%	
	Amerindian 5%	

The indigenous and Creole populations (mainly in the Atlantic region) speak Miskito (or other indigenous languages), Creole English, or both.

Health Care Beliefs: Acute sick care; passive role. Overall, Nicaraguans are not involved in health promotion in terms of prevention. The preventive services that do exist for women concentrate on the reproductive stage of life, and the services offered focus on family planning, prenatal care, childbirth, the puerperium, and timely detection of cervical and breast cancer (offered in urban areas). Immunization rates for children are impressive: 100% for measles, 97% for DPT, and 94% for polio. For adolescents, prevention of drug addiction and of unwanted pregnancies or pregnancy at a young age is stressed. Nevertheless, most seek health care for treatment of current symptoms. Mental illness is understood, yet treatment through the public health system is generally inadequate because health resources and training concentrate more on other types of illness. The people have no widely practiced traditional rituals for curing illness; however, prayer is a very common among the majority Catholic population.

Predominant Sick Care Practices: Biomedical and traditional. Western health care is provided through the national public health system, various social security plans for workers (who comprise 5% of the population), nongovernmental or church-sponsored programs, and the private sector. Although private sector providers are increasing, the Ministry of Health continues to be the main provider of services for the Nicaraguan population as a whole. The Ministry of Health's health center is the most common source of out-patient care, accounting for three fourths of all services provided. Although community-level health posts exist, they are used very little because of lack of personnel and insufficient drugs. Nicaragua's indigenous population and its Anglo-speaking groups on the Atlantic Coast are more likely to seek health care from indigenous healers, especially for illnesses that are believed to be mental or spiritual in nature. Herbs and other locally grown plants are used for their medicinal qualities. Nevertheless, the trend is toward Western practices. For example, immunization of infants is widely accepted and has contributed to great reductions in infant and childhood mortality.

Ethnic/Race Specific or Endemic Diseases: Although the Nicaraguan population is racially and ethnically diverse, poverty determines who has special health needs. Approximately 44% of the entire population lives below the international poverty line, as does 60% of the rural population. The health burden for rural families is exacerbated by distance from health services. Approximately 25% of the rural population lives more than a 2 hour-walk from a health center. Rural families are therefore more likely to become ill but less likely to seek medical attention. Life expectancy in rural areas is 56 years, compared with 66 for the overall population. Health statistics for Nicaragua are beginning to reflect a very curious situation; causes of death of infants and children younger than 5 years are common diseases of poverty (e.g., acute diarrheal disease, respiratory infections), whereas the major causes of death in adults are diseases of the rich, such as cancer, hypertension, diabetes, and cardio-vascular problems. Only two thirds of the population has access to safe drinking water, a situation that increases the high incidence of diarrheal diseases. Ironically, although suitable drinking water is scarce for many, the population as a whole also contracts two water-related diseases carried by mosquitoes—malaria and dengue fever. Chloroquine resistance, migration, increased rainfall, and a shortage of resources (e.g., to rebuild the country after Hurricane Mitch) all contribute to the increased rates of mosquito-borne illness. One group with significant health risks is agricultural workers who work on large farms where pesticide use is heavy. The vast majority of chemical products used in Nicaragua are pesticides, and their fairly uncontrolled use in agriculture makes acute pesticide poisoning the major health problem among agricultural workers. The World Health Organization's (WHO) estimated prevalence rate for HIV/AIDS is 0.2%. The estimated number of children from birth to 15 years living with HIV/AIDS is <100.

Health Team Relationships: The Ministry of Health oversees Nicaragua's health services. In recent years the Ministry of Health has decentralized operations, delegating functions to integrated local health care systems (Sistema Lôcal de Atencion or SILAIS). In addition, a private health care system (consisting of seven hospitals, 200 out-patient clinics, and other laboratories and pharmacies) serves a small portion (perhaps 7%) of the population. In terms of health team relationships, doctors generally control the operations of hospitals and clinics. Likewise, medical doctors and nurses generally have good working relationships. Patients tend to prefer speaking directly with doctors about their ailments. In rural areas, doctors often have a revered status among patients.

Families' Role in Hospital Care: Practices vary. Hospitals in Managua generally restrict family visits and the types of items visitors bring to patients. In other areas, particularly rural areas, policies are more lenient, and it is not uncommon for family members to bring food and other supplies. In some maternity wards, female family members are permitted to stay with the new mother.

Dominance Patterns: Some argue that Nicaragua has a patriarchal society, whereas others think that it is matriarchal. Certainly, the Sandinista revolution drew women into public life in new ways and spawned a women's movement in the country resulting in gender equality that was ensured in the national constitution. Still, many of the traditional values and customs are still being practiced. Traditional values include the notion that a woman's place is in the home and her role is to raise her children. Traditionally, men have had the freedom to have extramarital affairs and leave the home chores to their women. Also traditionally, women have been the caregivers.

Eye Contact Practices: Eye contact is not avoided. Flirting is common.

Touch Practices: Touching is acceptable. People often kiss on the cheek when they are being introduced to a stranger. Men may touch each other (with a hand on the shoulder) while talking. Women may hold hands. Nicaraguans, even those who work together, often shake hands when they greeting each other.

Perceptions of Time: Punctuality is not a major issue. People operate on *tiempo nica*, meaning they come to events whenever they decide to, which is usually not at the posted time. Meetings tend not to start on time. Nicaraguans live in the present. Although many yearn for what they recall as "the better times" (often the era preceding the current one) and hope for better times in the future, they certainly operate in the present.

Pain Reactions: Nicaraguans tend to react to pain quietly. At times of death, family and friends gather for wakes and may cry together.

Birth Rites: On average, every Nicaraguan woman gives birth to five children, and 25% of women begin having children while they are still adolescents. Nicaraguan families are following a worldwide trend toward having their children in a health facility, especially hospitals in urban areas; if the birth takes place at home, they are likely to have a trained person in attendance. Only 20% of births take place without a trained attendant, and nearly 50% take place in a health care institution. Practices at birth are governed by standard protocols of the clinic or hospital; specific ethnic or religious practices are allowed as long as they do no harm to the mother or child. For the most part, mothers are allowed to eat what they like before, during, and after the birth. Newborns are normally breast-fed within an hour after birth. However, mothers must be constantly convinced that it is more beneficial to give the newborn the nutrient-rich colostrum than to wait several days for regular breast milk. Although Nicaragua's macho culture still slightly favors the birth of a son, this preference does not seem to affect parents' decisions about educating their daughters—national literacy rates are equal for women and men.

Death Rites: Family members are present at death. Death rites are predominantly governed by Catholic religious ceremonies. In some rural areas, newborn infants are not named until at least a week after birth because of the fear that the infant may die. Similarly, registration of newborns may also be delayed to prevent unnecessary effort (e.g., a trip to the health center) and fees in case the infant dies soon after birth. Organ donation is acceptable but not generally possible because the technology is not available. Autopsies are rare. However, a "verbal autopsy" is a method often used by health organizations trying to understand the causes of maternal death and developing strategies to lower the rate. When a woman dies before, during, or after childbirth, the verbal autopsy consists of a series of structured interviews with people who were familiar with the situation and have insight into the specific circumstances surrounding the woman's death.

Food Practices and Intolerances: Basic staples of the diet are rice, beans, corn tortillas, and chicken. Black coffee sweetened with sugar is the most popular beverage, and children begin consuming it at a young age. Rural families consider animals such as pigs, goats, cows, and chickens to be assets. Thus they are more likely to sell them or use them for bartering than to consume them. The general diet of poor families is based on carbohydrates such as rice, potato, cassava, and other root vegetables (e.g., *quequisque*.) Fresh fruit and vegetables are abundant and low priced when they are in season, and many rural families grow their own. The two greatest barriers to a good diet are income (regardless of food available in the market) and education. (Low educational levels are associated with poor diets, even when nutritious foods are available and affordable.) The need for mothers to work outside the home and commute for long distances has been leading to more reliance on ready-made foods. Families of all income brackets commonly consume processed foods such as noodles, Magi soup, bread, cookies, and crackers. Wealthier families also consume imported soft drinks, snack foods, and gourmet items. Western-style utensils are used throughout the country, but Chinese use chop sticks.

Infant Feeding Practices: Nicaraguan mothers understand the importance of breast-feeding and almost without exception, their infants begin their lives nurtured by breast milk. However, the duration of breast-feeding is not ideal. Only one third of mothers breast-feed exclusively for the first 3 months, and the international recommendation is that exclusive breast-feeding should continue for at least 4 months. Many mothers erroneously believe that because of the country's warm climate, the infant needs additional fluids, so they provide water, juice, teas, thin gruels, or even infant formula in addition to breast milk. By the time the infants are 4 months old, approximately 50% are already receiving cereal-based gruels in addition to breast milk. In many cases, mothers who would normally continue to breast-feed exclusively must return to work; therefore babies are often fed poor substitutes while the mother is away. The diets for children are often lacking in sufficient fruits and vegetables, especially those rich in vitamin A. Because many of these foods are not expensive and readily available in the market, the main barrier to a diverse nutritious diet is lack of understanding. Children need to be encouraged to eat green and orange vegetables, and Nicaraguan mothers of all income brackets are generally not motivated and do not take the time (if they are working mothers) to do so. The high prevalence of chronic undernutrition in Nicaraguan children is most often a combination of food shortage (either because of low production or low purchasing power), repeated illness, and poor feeding practices.

Child Rearing Practices: Children are very valued in Nicaragua, and child rearing practices tend to be permissive. Infants generally sleep with their parents. Children are raised in large families, and many members of the extended family take an active part in raising them and providing support to the parents. Grandparents are especially valued in this regard. Children in poor families, who constitute the majority of the Nicaraguan population, are expected to help with household chores at a young age. When not in school, these children are also likely to work in the informal labor market, either with their parents or independently. This is true in rural families and urban families alike.

National Childhood Immunizations: BCG at birth; DTP at 12 months; OPV at 2, 4, 6, and 12 months and 2 to 4 years; DTPHH at 2, 4, and 6 months; MMR a +1 year; and DT at 6 to 9 and 10 to 14 years, +15, +15, +15 years.

BIBLIOGRAPHY

Country study handbook for Nicaragua: Retrieved March 14, 2002, from http://lcweb2.loc.gov/frd/cs/nitoc.html

David A et al: Letter from Central America: availability of HIV care in Central America, *JAMA* 286(7):853-860, 2001.

Kodrich K: *Tradition and change in the Nicaraguan press: newspapers and journalists in a new democratic era,* Lanham, Md, 2002, United Press of America.

Pan American Health Organization information on Nicaragua: http://paho.org
http://centralamerica.com/nicaragua/info/general.html
http://web5.infotrac-college.com/wadsworth/session/932/128/20799256/3!xrn_1_0_A77336906
http://www.lanoticia.com.ni
http://www.laprensa.com.ni
http://library.thinkquest.org/17749/health.html
http://wwsw.nuevodiario.ni

◆ NIGER (REPUBLIC OF)

MAP PAGE (862)

Location: Located in the interior of northern Africa, Niger is dominated by the Sahara Desert and the *Sahel* (the "shore" of the desert). Algeria and Libya are to the north, Chad is to the east, Nigeria is to the south, Benin and Burkina Faso are to the southwest, and Mali is to the west. The total land area is 1,267,000 km^2 (489,189 square miles), slightly less than twice the size of Texas. The country experiences periods of famine and drought. Four fifths of the land is uninhabitable desert, and much of the population lives in the narrow fertile belt south of the Niger River. The total population is 123,337,822. The gross domestic product (GDP) per capita is $200. Literacy rates are low: 21% for males and 7% for females. Larger cities do not always have electricity and running water.

Major Languages	Ethnic Groups	Major Religions
French (official)	Hausa 56%	Muslim 80%
Hausa	Djerma 22%	Indigenous beliefs,
Djerma	Fula 9%	Christian 20%
	Tuareg 8%	
	Beri-Beri (Kanouri) 4%	
	Arab, Toubou,	
	Gourmantche 1%	
	Approximately 1200	
	French expatriates	

Health Care Beliefs: Acute sick care; passive. Niger has linguistic taboos against speaking words related to sexuality, even for midwives. Muslims pray five times a day, and religion is an integral part of their beliefs about illness etiologies: "God gives life and health, and God knows why sickness is necessary."

Predominant Sick Care Practices: Traditional, holistic and biomedical when available. Primary health care and medical practices are based on an ancient, complex, and traditional set of practices that include herbs, Islamic treatments of religious prayers, recitation of verses, and appeals to different spirits. Although the government has a system of primary health care services, surveys indicate that it is frequently not used enough because of the high costs of medications (29%), service charges (19%), easy access to traditional healers (39%), and difficulty of getting transport to a health care facility (30%). Respondents also complain about the unfriendly attitudes of health care workers (3.6%) and wasting time at the facility (7.8%). Direct-user charges and indirect insurance payments recently implemented in government health care facilities were accompanied by an increased quality of services. The increase in quality was thought to outweigh the cost disadvantages.

Ethnic/Race Specific or Endemic Diseases: Endemic diseases include malaria, hepatitis A and B, schistosomiasis, dracunculiasis, and meningococcal infections. People are at risk for leprosy, tuberculosis, enteric fever, yellow fever, and cholera. The World Health Organization's (WHO) estimated prevalence rate for HIV/AIDS in adults ages 15 to 49 is 1.35%. The estimated number of children from birth to 15 years living with HIV/AIDS is 3300. The number of children who have lost their mother or both parents to AIDS since the beginning of the epidemic is 31,000. During 1999, 6500 adults and children died of AIDS. Life expectancy at birth is 49 years in Niger.

Health Team Relationships: Because of a belief that mentioning an illness can cause it to occur, patients may describe illnesses in broad and general terms, especially when children are involved. The socioeconomic status of women prevents them from receiving proper treatment when they are diagnosed with serious illness such as AIDS, which results in abortions, transmission of the disease to infants, and crushing debts.

Dominance Patterns: Polygamy is practiced. The wife is responsible for all activities related to raising children and maintaining the household. Study findings indicate that educated wives need the support of educated husbands to limit family size. Women in the Souloulou region are cloistered in their homes and cannot leave without the permission of their husbands or until they are of a certain age. When outside of the home, they must cover their heads and bodies. A length of cloth called a *zane* is wrapped around the waist and tied to the side. A shirt is worn on top, and another length of cloth is tied over the head. Homes often comprise multiple families.

Pain Reactions: A comprehensive plan for cancer pain has not yet been formulated in the West Africa subregion. It is reported that 70% to 90% of patients report severe pain. Oral preparations of strong opioids are generally unavailable, and few can understand the concept of taking medications at certain prescribed intervals.

Birth Rites: Research has demonstrated a high prevalence (50%) of food and nonfood pica in pregnant women (with nonfood pica being significantly higher). The maternal mortality rate is very high: 1200 per 100,000 live births. It is said that women occasionally refuse to push during labor because they fear it will result in more pain after birth. Shouting or crying during birth is not allowed. The placenta is buried in or near the house, with the maternal side facing the sky. Traditional first-time mothers give birth in their parents' house, where they are isolated in a room with their mother or a traditional birth attendant and deliver in the squatting position. A 40-day period of rest is observed after the birth. Niger has the highest child mortality in the world according to United Nations Children's Fund (UNICEF) figures. The infant mortality rate is 112 per 1000 live births. The total fertility rate is 6.8 children per woman.

Death Rites: Muslim doctors may recommend transfusions to save lives, but organ donations and transplants are occasionally unacceptable. Autopsies are uncommon because the deceased must be buried intact, and cremation is not permitted. For Muslim burials the body is wrapped in special pieces of white cloth and buried without a coffin in the ground as soon as possible after death (often within 24 hours). Deaths (like births) are celebrated by most inhabitants in villages. Life is considered a gift from God, and "only God knows why misfortune and death, especially premature death, is necessary."

Infant Feeding Practices: Because of the belief that breast-feeding weakens the mother, infants are quickly weaned if the mother discovers she is pregnant again. A popular weaning food is millet flour and water *(hura).*

Child Rearing Practices: Children are sent to live with grandparents or an older female for an unspecified period if their mother must work in the fields or becomes pregnant again or if the children become ill. The surrogate parent assumes all responsibility (except financial) for the child. Female circumcision and excision is widespread within some groups.

National Childhood Immunizations: BCG at birth; DTP at 8, 12, and 16 weeks; OPV at birth and 8, 12, and 16 weeks; measles at 9 months; vitamin A at 6 months; YFV at 9 months; and TT at first contact, +4 weeks, +6 months, +1, +1 year. The reported percentages of the target population vaccinated are as follows: BCG, 44; first dose of DTP, 41; third dose of DTP, 25; MCV, 25; Pol3, 36; and TT2 plus, 31.

BIBLIOGRAPHY

Amadou M: The sun rose more than twice on Amina, *Safe Motherhood* 18(2):11, 1995.

Chawla M, Ellis RP: The impact of financing and quality changes on health care demand in Niger, *Health Pol Plann* 15(1):76, 2000.

Chmielarczyk V: Transcultural nursing: providing culturally congruent care to the Hausa of northwest Africa, *J Transcultural Nurs* 3(1):15, 1991.

Jaffre Y, Prual A: Midwives in Niger: an uncomfortable position between social behaviours and health care constraints, *Soc Sci Med* 38(8):1069, 1994.

Katung PY: Socio-economic factors responsible for poor utilization of the primary health care services in a rural community in Niger, *Niger J Med* 10(1):28, 2001.

Prual A et al: The quality of risk factor screening during antenatal consultations in Niger, *Health Pol Plann* 15(1):11, 2000.

Soyannwo A, Amonour-Boadu SD: Management of cancer pain—a survey of current practice in West Africa, *Nigerian Postgrad Med J* 8(4):175, 2001.

Uchudi JM: Spouses' socioeconomic characteristics and fertility differences in sub-Saharan Africa: does the spouse's education matter? *J Biosoc Sci* 33(4):481, 2001.

Wright J: Female genital mutilation: an overview, *J Adv Nurs* 24:251, 1996.

◆ NIGERIA (FEDERAL REPUBLIC OF)

MAP PAGE (862)

Adebowale A. Adeyemo

Location: Nigeria is Africa's most populous nation, with an estimated 124 million people. It is located in West Africa, bordered on the west by the Republic of Benin, on the north by the Republic of Niger, and on the east by the Republic of Cameroon. The country occupies a land area of 923,768 km^2 (356,667 square miles), and the vegetation ranges from mangrove forest on the coast to desert in the far north. The country is divided into three natural geographical zones (north, west, and east) by two rivers: the River Niger (which runs from west to east) and the River Benue (which runs from east to west). Both rivers meet at a confluence just south of the geographical center of the country and run southward into the sea. Population growth has been quite rapid, from 55.7 million in the 1963 national census to 88.5 million in the 1991 census. The population of Nigeria is predominantly rural, with about 41% living in urban areas. Major urban centers include Lagos, Ibadan, Kano, Onitsha, Kaduna, and Port-Harcourt. The population is quite young, with 47% younger than 18 years of age. Children younger than the age of 5 comprise about 20% of the population, and women of child-bearing age comprise another 20%.

Major Languages	Ethnic Groups	Major Religions
English (official)	Hausa, Fulani 20%	Muslim 50%
Hausa	Yoruba 21%	Christian 40%
Yoruba	Ibo 18%	Indigenous beliefs 10%
Ibo	Ijaw, Kanuri, Ibibio,	
Fulani	Tiv 10%	
	Other groups 31%	

Nigeria has one of the most ethnically diverse populations in the world, with more than 380 distinct ethnic groups. The major groups include the Edo, Efik, Fulani, Hausa, Igbo, Ijaw, Kanuri, Tiv, Urhobo, and Yoruba. The three largest ethnic groups are the Hausa-Fulani in the north, the Yoruba in the west, and the Igbo in the east. However, as noted, many other ethnic groups exist, and Nigeria has entire states in which none of the three largest ethnic groups comprise a majority or even a significant minority. Administratively, Nigeria consists of 36 states and a Federal Capital territory. They are further divided into 774 local government areas (LGAs). Nigeria came into being as a nation-state in 1914 when the British colonial administration merged the North and South Protectorates and the colony of Lagos into one administrative unit. The nation became independent in 1960 and a republic in 1963. For most of Nigeria's history since independence, it has been under military rule. Nigeria returned to democratic rule in May 1999 under a presidential system of three tiers of government: federal, state, and local. The federal government comprises an executive arm (led by the president), a bicameral legislative arm (with the senate and house of representatives), and a judiciary arm. Each state has its own governor and house of assembly, and each local government has a chairman and council.

Health Care Beliefs: Active participation; health promotion important. Prevention and health promotion are widely practiced. In traditional society, these often involve either general health promotion issues (such as personal cleanliness, good nutrition, and environmental hygiene) or specific taboos (such as the belief that pregnant women should not walk in the hot sun or their fetus could have congenital malformations). Today, immunization of children and pregnant women, exclusive breast-feeding, and growth monitoring of children are practiced with varying degrees of success. Mental illness is widely feared and carries considerable social stigma. It is usually blamed on spiritual causes such as evil spirits, demons, ghosts, the gods, or human agents of such spirits (such as wizards and witches). Because of this belief, it is probable that indigenous healers treat more patients with mental illnesses, although an increasing proportion is treated in modern hospitals. Indigenous treatment of mental illness often involves the patients living with the healers in their compound. Divinations are carried out to ascertain the source of the illness, after which treatment with herbal preparations is often accompanied by rituals and sacrifices. Patients go home when it is believed that they are again in their "right mind." The social stigma that mental illness confers is considerable and applies to the whole family. Because mental illness is believed to be potentially hereditary, members of families with individuals who are mentally ill often find it difficult to find spouses because others do not want to risk having affected children, thereby stigmatizing their own extended families. Religion and indigenous medicine are closely interwoven. Illness is believed to be caused by four sources: natural, supernatural, mystical, and hereditary. A wide variety of treatment methods may be used including herbal preparations that are drunk, inhaled, rubbed into scarification marks, or used as an enema; divination aids (such as stones and bells); and rituals and sacrifices.

Predominant Sick Care Practices: Traditional, biomedical and magical-religious. Nigeria has a three-tiered health care system comprising primary, secondary, and tertiary care. The primary care system is meant to be the first point of contact for an ill person (in addition to providing such services as immunization and health education and promotion). Secondary health care mainly comprises general hospitals with radiology and surgery, and they are intended to treat sick people that cannot be treated at the primary care level. Tertiary health care comprises the specialist and university teaching hospitals that provide the most sophisticated care available, mainly through referrals from the lower levels of health care. In addition to these levels, some patent medicine vendors, or "chemists," officially sell nonprescription, over-the-counter drugs and often serve as major sources of health care delivery. In reality, health care in Nigeria is pluralistic, with people using official and unofficial sources of health care delivery. Unofficial sources include indigenous healers, diviners, fortune tellers, herbalists, bone setters, and traditional birth attendants or midwives. These categories are not exclusive, and a particular healer may assume two or more of these roles. Some indigenous health practitioners are specialists in specific areas such as mental illness or circumcision. Indigenous healers have considerable status and are increasingly organized, having fairs and sponsoring television advertising. More recently, people have turned to religious or spiritual sources, usually in the Christian Pentecostal churches, where the belief in miraculous healing for all who have faith is a basic tenet. Many people often seek health care from multiple sources.

Ethnic/Race Specific or Endemic Diseases: The illnesses that affect the country the most are infectious. Among children, malaria, respiratory tract infections, diarrhea, vaccine-preventable diseases (especially measles and tetanus), and malnutrition are major causes of illness and death. Sickle cell anemia is the single most common serious hereditary disorder, affecting about 3% of all newborns. Burkitt's lymphoma and leukemia are the most common cancers among children. Among adults, aside from malaria and other infections, hypertension is likely the most common noncommunicable disease, affecting up to 14% of adults. In addition, pregnancy-related complications related to infection and bleeding cause considerable morbidity among women, whereas accidental injuries are a major problem for men. The most common cancers are cervical and breast among women and prostate and liver among men. The World Health Organization's (WHO) estimated prevalence rate for HIV/AIDS in adults ages 15 to 49 is 5.06%. The sentinel site seropositivity rate for the year 2000 was 5.8%. The estimated number of children from birth to 15 years living with HIV/AIDS is 120,000. Sentinel survey estimates for seropositivity in pregnant women in antenatal care were 5.4% in 1999. The number of reported AIDS cases in 1999 was 18,490 (an increase from 2829 in 1995). However, the numbers vary considerably by region. For example, the north central zone of the country had twice the prevalence of the southwest zone (7.1% compared with 3.5%).

Health Team Relationships: The health team is led by a doctor. The doctors and nurses often have a good working relationship, although it varies from place to place and is often worse in the larger hospitals. Patients' attitudes toward doctors and nurses are usually positive, although many complain that they do not spend enough time with them. This attitude is hardly surprising considering the heavy caseload that doctors and nurses routinely carry, which greatly limits the amount of attention any one patient can have. Medical practice is still more paternalistic than it is in Europe and America.

Families' Role in Hospital Care: Families play a major role in hospital care. They often accompany patients to clinics and emergency facilities, especially on their first visit. Families are often expected to stay with admitted patients, not necessarily on the ward but somewhere on the hospital premises. Because hospital fees are unaffordable for most and no health insurance exists, families contribute funds to pay for hospital bills. Hospital policies about bringing food to the patients vary from extremely permissive to extremely strict; the larger tertiary centers tend to be stricter.

Dominance Patterns: The culture is male dominated. Even in a few communities with matrilineal lines of inheritance, the men still dominate. This is true even during times of illness, when decisions about seeking health care and treatment are usually made by the household head. Indeed, some people may have to wait for days to obtain care because they are waiting for the head of the household to return home and grant permission to go to a hospital. However, in female-headed households these traditional patterns are no longer followed.

Eye Contact Practices: Eye contact is common and not avoided because of status or gender. However, age is greatly respected, so younger people may avoid direct eye contact with an older adult. In some places, no one (with a few exceptions) is expected to make direct eye contact with a traditional ruler.

Touch Practices: Physical touching is acceptable, but public displays of affection are unusual. Children touch each other during play and hold hands, which is normal. Men may shake or touch hands but are unlikely to walk down the street holding hands. Women may hug one another, especially after a long separation.

Perceptions of Time: Time is flexible, and people do not often get to appointments on time. This is considered normal for social occasions; a person may say an event starts at 10 for 10:30 AM, meaning the occasion will actually start at 10:30. For official or business appointments, punctuality is important, although it may be impossible to be on time because of the poor infrastructure (poor roads, poor transportation systems, bad phone network). The culture throughout Nigeria values past traditions, and these are invoked in discussions of almost all issues. However, there is a dynamic tension between looking backward to tradition and looking forward to "modernization."

Pain Reactions: Pain reactions vary considerably from place to place. For example, the Fulani (in the north) and the Igbo (in the east) are generally perceived to be stoical, whereas the Yoruba (in the west) are usually very expressive. However, men are expected to tolerate pain more easily and be more stoical in the face of severe pain than women. Children are allowed to express pain but are often admonished to learn to be more tolerant of it.

Birth Rites: Birth rites vary considerably from place to place. In many instances the mother is confined indoors for a varying period of time after birth, often for 40 days. During this period, she has hot baths once or twice a day, breast-feeds the infant, and does little else. Relatives usually help to perform the usual household chores, and the children's grand-mothers (if alive) are expected to help the mother take care of them. A naming ceremony usually takes place on the seventh or eighth day of life; with some ethnic groups, this may be as late as 3 months. Depending on the context of the birth, a son may be celebrated more than a daughter, but it is probably more accurate to say the birth of the first-born son is celebrated more than other births. With urbanization and changes in life-style, many of these customs are breaking down. For example, few women are still completely confined for 40 days after a birth before resuming their normal activities. The total fertility rate is more than 6 children per woman. The mortality of children younger than 5 was more than 100 per 1000 in the 1990s—192 per 1000 in 1990 and 147 per 1000 in 1995. Maternal mortality was estimated to be 800 per 100,000 live births in 1995. More than a third (36%) of children younger than 5 were underweight in 1990. Thus social indicators show that Nigeria is a country with low gross domestic product, high external debt burden, high child and maternal mortality, and high fertility.

Death Rites: In most Nigerian cultures, death means the person assumes another existence and becomes one of the ancestors who watch over the living and can be consulted in times of difficulty. Some Nigerians believe in reincarnation, often in two very different contexts. In one context a child born shortly after the death of a grandparent of the same sex is often considered to be the reincarnation of the deceased relative and therefore may be named after the person. In the second, some dead children are believed to reincarnate and be born again to the same woman, only to die again at about the same age. Although death is universally mourned, the death of an older person (who is thought to have lived a long and full life) is often celebrated with elaborate ceremonies. If death occurs at home, family members may be present, and they usually take responsibility for preparing the corpse for burial. Among Muslim families, burial usually takes place the same day (before sunset), and autopsy and organ donation are generally prohibited. However, many non-Muslims also prohibit autopsies because they are considered mutilation of the corpse. Some also believe that whatever information is obtained during an autopsy is not of any practical use because it does not bring the dead person back to life.

Food Practices and Intolerances: Food practices vary, but staple foods include roots and tubers (e.g., yams, cassava, cocoyam), grains and cereals (e.g., millet, guinea corn, maize, rice), and legumes. Palm and peanut oils are often used when cooking soups and stews that contain tomatoes, peppers, or other vegetables and meat or fish. Chickens and goats are often kept in villages. The items available may vary. For example, in the north where cattle are kept, milk is available and more likely to be consumed than it is in the south. In coastal areas seafood (e.g., crabs, shrimps, other shellfish) is a significant part of the diet. Traditionally, food is eaten with the fingers, but in urban areas and among the more educated, the use of cutlery (i.e., a knife, fork, and spoon) is more common. It is believed that some foods, such as pounded yams, are best eaten with the fingers, regardless of the time and place.

Infant Feeding Practices: Breast-feeding is universal, and it is a major social issue if a woman does not breast-feed her child at all. Even if the mother dies during delivery, a wet nurse may be used if the child lives. However, water or herbal preparations may also be given to the infant in addition to breast milk. Women traditionally breast-feed for at least 2 years; this period is only shortened by a new pregnancy, which would be considered shameful because Nigerians often consider it taboo for breast-feeding women to have sexual intercourse. They also consider it taboo for a pregnant woman to breast-feed, so a woman who gets pregnant must stop breast-feeding. Weaning and introduction of food takes place at approximately 4 to 6 months, and by the second year of life, most children are eating from the family pot.

Child Rearing Practices: Child rearing practices vary from place to place, but overall is more strict than permissive. Children are expected to be well disciplined, show good manners, be quiet, and be respectful and obedient to adults. Child rearing is considered a task for the whole family, including the parents, grandparents, uncles, and aunts, although bad behavior is usually blamed on the mother. Older children (especially girls) help care for the younger ones. Children learn household and other chores as they grow older. Boys may be spared from performing any household chores in traditional societies.

National Childhood Immunizations: BCG at birth; DTP at 6, 10, and 14 weeks; OPV at 6, 10, and 14 weeks; measles at 9 months; vitamin A at

9 months; and TT CBAW at first contact, +4 weeks, +6 months, +1, and +1 year.

Other Characteristics: The country has abundant natural resources. Major agricultural products include cocoa, rubber, groundnuts, palm oil, cotton, cassava, yams, corn, millet, and rice. Mineral resources include petroleum, coal, tin, columbite, and gold. However, petroleum has been the mainstay of foreign exchange earnings for Nigeria in the last 3 decades. Indeed, Nigeria is the sixth largest producer of crude oil in the world and earns several billion U.S. dollars annually from sales of crude oil alone. However, these earnings have not translated to a healthy national economy because of decades of mismanagement and corruption under dictatorial government by successive military regimes. Thus at the end of 1999, the GDP was only $310. Economic hardships during the 1990s meant that social sector spending was far less than required. The health and education sectors in particular were deprived of much needed support and funding. It is only with the advent of democratic governance at the end of the decade that the social sector began receiving increased attention.

BIBLIOGRAPHY

Federal Office of Statistics, Macro International: *Nigeria demographic and health survey, 1990,* Federal Government of Nigeria. {1992}

Iwu MM: *African ethnomedicine,* Nsukka, Nigeria 1982, University Publishing Series.

Jegede AS. Culture-bound terminology in the interpretation of illness in the Yoruba community in Nigeria, *J Contemp Health* 4:74–75, 1996.

Jegede AS: *African culture and health,* Lagos, Nigeria, 1998, Stirling-Horden Publishers Limited.

Madauci I, Isa Y, Daura B: *Hausa customs,* Zaria, Nigeria, 1968, Northern Nigeria Publishing Company Limited.

National Population Commission, Macro International: *Nigeria demographic and health survey 2000,* Federal Government of Nigeria.

Odebiyi AI: Food taboos in Nigeria and child health: the views of traditional healers in Ile-Ife, *Soc Sci Med* 28:985–996, 1989.

Obisesan KA et al: The family planning aspects of the practice of traditional healers in Ibadan, Nigeria, *West Afr J Med* 16:184-190, 1997.

Okunribido OO et al: Cultural perceptions of diarrhea and illness management choices among Yoruba mothers in Oyo State, Nigeria, *Int Quart Comm Health Ed* 17:309–318, 1997.

Olupona JK, Falola T, eds: *Religion and society in Nigeria: historical and sociological perspective,* Ibadan, Nigeria, 1991, Spectrum Books Limited.

Omoradion FI: The sociocultural context of health behaviour among Esan communities, Edo State, Nigeria, *Health Trans Rev* 3:131–150, 1993.

Omotade OO et al: Perceptions and first line home treatment of diarrhoeal diseases in Ona Ara Local Government Area of Oyo State, *Niger J Paediatr* 21(suppl):80–87, 1994.

Social Sciences and Reproductive Health Research Network: *Male responsibility in reproductive health: the construction of manhood in Nigeria,* Ibadan, Nigeria, 1999, Social Sciences and Reproductive Health Research Network.

◆ NORWAY (KINGDOM OF)

MAP PAGE (860)

Bodil Ellefsen

Location: Norway occupies the western part of the Scandinavian peninsula in northwestern Europe and extends approximately 483 km (300 miles) above the Arctic Circle. It consists of 385,155 km² (148,693 square miles), including Svalbard and Jan Mayen. The coastline, including fjords, is 21,192 km. More than two thirds of the country is uninhabitable because of glaciers, mountains, moors, and rivers. Inhabitants per square kilometer were estimated to be 30 in 2001, and the population is 4,504,000. Approximately 21% of the population is younger than 16 years of age, 65% are between 16 and 66 years of age, and 14% are 67 years of age and older. Life expectancy for an individual born in 1999 was 75.6 for men and 81.1 for women. Norway is a constitutional monarchy.

Major Languages	Ethnic Groups	Major Religions
Norwegian (official)	Norwegian 99%	Evangelical Lutheran
Lapp- and Finnish-	Lappish 1%	(state church) 86%
speaking		Roman Catholic, other
minorities		Protestant 3%
		Other 1%
		Unknown or none 10%

Health Care Beliefs: Active participation; health promotion important. Norwegians are actively involved in health care, and illness prevention and health promotion are practiced and valued. Health promotion is emphasized, particularly in prenatal and child care (of children from 18 years of age and younger), and pregnant women, children, and adolescents receive regular physical examinations to ensure wellness. Being clean, resting, exercising, eating healthy food, and taking cod liver oil are believed to improve health, so these practices are followed by a large percentage of the population. People tend to consider their health good even if they have one or more diseases. Although mental illness has been socially stigmatized in Norway, this problem is slowly decreasing as people become more accepting of counseling and drug therapies for various mental health complaints.

Predominant Sick Care Practices: Biomedical, with some alternative practices. The biomedical model dominates the health care system, and Norwegians consult doctors for health care. A primary care practitioner plan was introduced in 2001, and all citizens are being encouraged to choose a general practitioner, who refers them to specialists as necessary. Alternative health care practices such as acupuncture, homeopathy, chiropractic, and naturopathy may be sought for some health care problems. Use of homeopathic medicine and holistic approaches such as acupuncture are increasing in Norway. The country has a nationalized health and social care service that is financed through indirect taxation. Those using the system pay a minimum fee for doctor visits, tests, and prescription medication. A hospital stay is entirely covered without fee. Older adults and those with disabilities account for 45% of all expenditures in health and social care. The basic tenets of the system are equity, equality, and solidarity for all residents.

Ethnic/Race Specific or Endemic Diseases: Heart and circulatory diseases, malignant neoplasms, and diseases of the respiratory system account for 95% of all deaths. Although lifestyle-related heart and cardiovascular diseases are decreasing, cancer, musculoskeletal ailments, and respiratory diseases are increasing and are the most common causes of long-term sick leave and disablement. Immigrants to Norway from eight countries in the Middle East, Asia, and South America have had an impact on the health care system because they experience more anxiety, depression, and diabetes than Norwegians. For example, only 1% of Norwegians between the ages of 45 and 66 have diabetes, compared with 9% of immigrants. This statistic is 19% among immigrants from Pakistan, which has increased the need for adequate screening of these populations. The World Health Organization's (WHO) estimated prevalence rate for HIV/AIDS in adults ages 15 to 49 is 0.07%. The estimated number of children from birth to 15 years who are living with HIV/AIDS is less than 100. HIV testing is systematically done for blood donations, pregnant women, and patients with sexually transmitted diseases. By the end of 2000, 2194 HIV cases had been reported. Among cases reported from 1997 to 2000, 68% were heterosexuals, 25% were homosexual men, and 7% were using injectable drugs. Since the beginning of the epidemic, 534 individuals have died of AIDS.

Health Team Relationships: Depending on the setting, health care may be both doctor and nurse driven. In the formal sense the doctor has more power and influence during the admission, treatment, and discharge of patients. However, doctors and nurses often collaborate and discuss patients and tests, medications, and further exploration of health problems. Working relationships are usually good, but questions about leadership roles in various situations that occur in hospital wards and units create occasional tension in the working relationship. Patients are generally open and direct in their relationship with nurses, whereas they tend to adopt a more formal and detached attitude toward doctors. New patient rights legislation that was passed in 1999 was developed to provide better health services to patients and increase their confidence in the system. Patients are granted essential health assistance from specialists, the right to a medical examination within 30 days, the right to a second opinion, and the right to choose their hospital. Norwegians want to be given options and have a role in decision making. Although the new patient rights legislation does not always function optimally, it makes it easier for patients to influence their treatments, participate more actively, be provided with information, and access their medical records on request. The new law also has rules for handling patient complaints, provisions for patient representatives, and provisions that govern special rights for children.

Families' Role in Hospital Care: Norway is divided into five health regions. Hospital services are organized so that each of the five areas has three types of hospitals: district, central, and regional. The district hospitals are small and designed to meet the requirements of the local community with respect to internal medicine, surgery, obstetrics, x-ray, and laboratory. Central hospitals are larger, with more than 200 beds. They provide a much broader range of services and are intended to meet the needs of areas beyond the local one. Regional hospitals cover much wider areas and have highly specialized functions and services. The nursing and medical staffs provide all care in hospitals. Visiting hours are fairly liberal, and young children are allowed to visit. The rights of children in hospitals are protected by regulations based on Norwegian legislation, which addresses teaching, housing of parents (with one allowed to remain at all times), and the economic rights of parents. Children are usually placed in rooms with other children, parents often stay overnight, and friends and siblings are allowed and encouraged to visit. Provisions are made for children to continue their education when they are ill for long periods.

Dominance Patterns: Norwegians have a passion for equality in society and in the relationship between the sexes. However, the female partner continues to do most of the domestic work in families. Norwegians usually take time to make a decision, and matters tend to be debated at length. Families usually share the decision-making responsibilities, child rearing, and other household duties to some degree. When a partner is ill, the other partner assumes household duties as necessary and cares for the ill partner. However, as a general rule, women have the primary responsibility for caring for sick relatives. Treatment of men and women is considered to be fairly equal in the workplace, but discrimination still occurs; women may receive lower wages than men for the same job, or men may receive preferential treatment during hiring.

Eye Contact Practices: Direct eye contact if usually preferable and acceptable.

Touch Practices: The Norwegian culture accepts touching, especially in familiar settings, and younger people are the mostly likely to have the most contact. Although touching between individuals of the same or opposite sex is accepted, it is considered more acceptable for women to touch other women than for men to touch other men.

Perceptions of Time: Norwegians are both present and future oriented, although many people have the attitude that if things are going well today, they do not have to worry about tomorrow. People tend to be punctual, with a 5- to 10-minute deviation. Being more than 10 minutes late is considered inconsiderate.

Pain Reactions: Individuals are traditionally expected to react with stoicism to pain, and extremely emotional expressions of discomfort are not the norm. However, health professionals provide pain relief as necessary, monitor pain in hospitalized patients, and encourage attitudes promoting the admission of pain and expectations of pain relief.

Birth Rites: The infant mortality rate in Norway is among the lowest in the world. Many mothers attend prenatal birth preparation courses, and natural childbirth is common. Most births take place in hospitals, and the father is encouraged to be in the delivery room to support the mother. After delivery the infant is placed on the mother's abdomen for bonding, and rooming-in is common (i.e., having the infant stay in the hospital room with the mother at all times). To allow the new mother to rest, infants may be taken to the nursery at night if the mother desires.

Death Rites: The majority of Norwegians die in health care institutions rather than at home. The closest family members are usually with the dying person, because they believe that no one should die alone. A religious ceremony accompanies most cremations or burials, and family and friends are present to comfort the family of the deceased. Organ donations and autopsies are considered acceptable.

Food Practices and Intolerances: Breakfast may consist of a combination of yogurt products, bread, coffee or tea, cereal, cheese, salami, and juice, and people generally have a sandwich for lunch. The main meal is eaten in the early evening. Potatoes with meat or meatballs and boiled or fried fish are traditional food staples. Rice, spaghetti, and pizza are becoming more popular, especially among young people. Great quantities of milk are also consumed. When the main meal is eaten at midday or early afternoon, another light meal is eaten between 8 and 10 PM. A fork, knife, and spoon are used for most meals, and it is unacceptable to use the hands unless eating small sandwiches, small cakes, or biscuits.

Infant Feeding Practices: Breast-feeding is encouraged and common. In 1999, 92% of Norwegian mothers were breast-feeding 1 month after the birth of the infant; 80% were breast-feeding 6 months after birth.

Child Rearing Practices: Child rearing practices are quite permissive, although when discipline is necessary, it is shared by both parents. Children are allowed to participate in decision making and generally have a great deal of autonomy. Children do not begin school until they are 6 years of age.

National Childhood Immunizations: BCG at 13 to 15 years; DPT at 3, 5, and 11 to 12 months; HIB at 3, 5, 11 to 12 months; DT at 11 to 12 years; polio at 6 years; MMR at 15 months and 12 to 13 years.

BIBLIOGRAPHY

Blom S, Ramm J: Ikke flere syke, men når de først blir syke, *Samfunnsspeilet* 3:6–15, 1998.

Haukelien H: *Vocation and bureaucracy,* master's thesis, Oslo, 2000, University of Oslo.

Hydle I: *Anthropological perspective on medicine, insurance and the law,* Oslo, 1997, Tano-Aschehoug.

Ministry of Health and Social Affairs: *The health and social affairs sector in Norway,* Oslo, 2001.

Nortvedt L, Kase BF: Children's rights in Norwegian hospitals—are children and parents satisfied? *Tidsskr Nor Laegeforen* 4(120):469–471, 2001.

Official Statistics of Norway: *Annual report 2001,* Oslo, Norway.

Ramm J: We do not complain until it is needed, *Samfunnsspeilet* 2:14–21, 1997.

Tønjum L: When women give up breastfeeding, *Tidsskriftet Sykepleien* 89(8):48–51, 2001.

Vikan ST: An uneven process towards equality, *Samfunnsspeilet* 4:13–25, 2001.

◆ OMAN (SULTANATE OF)

MAP PAGE (864)

Euan M. Scrimgeour

Location: The Sultanate of Oman is located on the southeast corner of the Arabian Peninsula. It is a primarily hot and dry country with a narrow coastal plain, and a wide arid plateau, which is largely desert. It is mountainous to the north and south. Most of the deep valleys in the north have adequate water resources and are fertile, with numerous, isolated small villages. The district of Salalah on the south coast is the only part of the Arabian Peninsula affected by the Indian summer monsoon (from June to August), when it is relatively cool and rainy (with daytime temperatures of 28° C and nighttime temperatures of 22° C). Frankincense trees thrive in this region.

Major Languages	Ethnic Groups	Major Religions
Omani	*Omani*	*Omani*
(1.5 million):	*(1.5 million):*	*(1.5 million):*
Arabic	Omani Arab 75%	Ibadi, Sunni,
Swahili	East African	Shiaa Muslim 75%
Baluchi (Urdu)	Omani Arab 15%	Other 25%
Persian	Baluchi 9%	*Expatriates (0.6 million):*
Expatriates	Lawati 1%	Christian, Hindu,
(0.6 million):	*Expatriates*	Other 75%
Malayalam	*(0.6 million):*	Muslim 25%
English	Indian 70%	
	Other 30%	

The Ibadi language derives from an early, fundamentalist sect of Islam. The majority of Omanis speak Arabic, but English is widely spoken by all ethnic groups living in Oman. Isolated from the rest of Oman by deserts, the hill people of southern Dhofar Province have a seminomadic, tribal lifestyle and speak a distinct Arab language, Jabali. Many Dhofari women (and many rural Omani women) still wear masks covering their nose, cheeks, and mouth. Oman previously had a coastal enclave, Gwadar, Baluchistan, on the coast of Pakistan (until 1958), and large numbers of Baluchis have settled in Oman. Until 1964, Oman administered Zanzibar; after its independence, many hundreds of thousands of Swahili-speaking, ethnic Omani Arabs migrated to Oman. Today, many of the latter group occupy important roles in many professions (e.g., banking, commerce, oil production, and medicine). The majority (70%) of Indian expatriates working in Oman are from Kerala, speak Malayalam, and are Christian. Fewer Pakistani, Sri Lankan, Filipino, and various European nationalities are employed in Oman. Although Omanis are very devout and pray 5 times a day, they permit non-Muslims to practice their own religions. Until 30 years ago, Oman was one of the most isolated and backward countries in the Middle East, with only 5 km of surfaced road. In 1970 the youthful, progressive Sultan Qaboos bin Said assumed control from his aging father and with the help of primarily British foreign advisers, he immediately began to modernize his country. Today, Oman is one of the most advanced and progressive countries in the region, although it retains much of its traditional customs and way of life. With a large, youthful population, a large proportion of which is being educated at secondary-school levels, Oman has decreed that Omanization is to be strongly promoted in every occupation. Thus within the past 5 or 10 years, numerous expatriates (e.g., Indians, Pakistanis) who have unskilled or semiskilled labor jobs (e.g., drivers, gardeners, cleaners) have been replaced by Omanis. The policy has now been extended to shop keepers and businessmen and is having more of an impact on white-collar workers, teachers, and even academic staff.

Health Care Beliefs: Active participation with emphasis on health promotion. Omanis believe that ill health is an inevitable part of life, not divine retribution. The overriding characteristic of all patients and their families is acceptance of Allah's will. Disease prevention is strongly promoted by the Ministry of Health.

Predominant Sick Care Practices: Biomedical and traditional. Oman has an excellent health care system, with countrywide primary health care clinics and modern regional hospitals. Muscat, the capital, has two well-equipped and staffed tertiary referral hospitals. In the past, patients traditionally consulted village healers for herbal remedies and skin cautery over affected areas. Many Omanis continue to seek this treatment before (and even after) receiving modern medical care. Many Indians working in Oman seek traditional ayurdevic medical treatment. When a patient is admitted to a hospital, the family provides strong support. As a rule, very elderly, incapacitated patients are cared for in their own homes, in accordance with religious teaching. Long-term geriatric hospitals are not available. Blood transfusions are routinely available. Patients do not accept amputations easily because they believe the body should be intact at the time of death.

Ethnic/Race Specific or Endemic Diseases: Health care is essentially free for Omanis, but all expatriates and their employers must pay for treatment. Adult Omanis have a high prevalence of diabetes mellitus, hypertension, and atherosclerotic arterial disease (causing strokes and myocardial infarction). Obesity is comparatively unusual. Among children, acute respiratory tract infections and gastroenteritis are common. Some infectious diseases such as diphtheria, poliomyelitis, and probably leprosy, have been eradicated. Malaria is now rare (so prophylaxis for visitors is unnecessary), and tuberculosis, brucellosis (which is largely restricted to the Salalah region), and sexually transmitted disease incidences are decreasing. A single focus of schistosomiasis persists in permanent lakes and streams in the Salalah district. The World Health Organization's (WHO) prevalence rate for HIV/AIDS in adults ages 15 to 49 is 0.11%. WHO has no estimates for children from birth to 15 years. HIV is primarily contracted by heterosexual contact, and non-Omanis who are found to be infected are repatriated.

Health Team Relationships: When the first modern hospitals were built in the 1970s, they were staffed almost entirely by foreign doctors and nurses. A few senior doctors were Omanis from Zanzibar who had graduated in the United Kingdom. The first graduates from the medical school of the Sultan Qaboos University graduated in 1989 have gradually filled junior posts and now more frequently, consultant posts. Nurses have been largely recruited from the Philippines, India, and Malaysia, with Europeans, and some foreign-trained Omanis occupying senior posts. Omanis are now being trained locally as nurses. The medical teams are doctor driven, but the team spirit is strong, and nurses are held in very high esteem. Patients and their families are invariably pleasant and grateful for medical care, and medical litigation is almost unknown.

Families' Role in Hospital Care: Relatives almost always accompany a patient to hospital, using their own transportation rather than ambulances, which are generally reserved for emergencies. A family member stays with patients if they are seriously ill. Families do not help patients with personal care or eating tasks (unless the patients are small children). Families do have a role in decision making about invasive procedures (e.g., lumbar puncture) or surgical operations. A patient's illness must be explained in detail to the family. At times a senior family member forbids an operation even when a patient agrees to it. It is not uncommon in these situations for the family to remove the patient from the hospital against medical advice and seek an opinion in another hospital or even overseas, often in India or Jordan.

Dominance Patterns: Oman is essentially a male-dominated society, particularly in rural areas of the country. In urban, more Westernized families, men and women are more equal. Arranged marriages are customary, but today they are usually conducted only with the agreement of both marrying partners.

Eye Contact Practices: Women tend to avoid eye contact with men they do not know and in general, eye contact is indirect between strangers. Men usually avoid looking directly at women, especially if the women are alone. However, when women wear the traditional face mask (which covers the nose and mouth but leaves most of the face uncovered), they tend to have more confidence in eye contact with strangers.

Touch Practices: Handshaking is restricted between individuals of the opposite sex. Males do not shake hands with women, although women may shake each other's hands. Males may greet good male friends or relatives with an embrace and a kiss on both cheeks.

Perceptions of Time: In traditional desert tribal life and in early times in coastal towns, Omanis had a relaxed attitude when conducting their affairs. Time was not dictated by the clock and was marked by the timing of the five daily prayers, which changed during the lunar cycle. As a result, patience was an attribute that was encouraged and valued. Today, Omanis have adjusted well to the rapid pace of modern life and the need to be punctual and conscientious in their work commitments. As a rule, Omanis are punctual for appointments.

Pain Reactions: Most patients are relatively stoical in response to pain. They rely implicitly on Allah and are prepared to withstand considerable discomfort and pain without complaint. However, the administration of analgesics, including opiates, is routine when required.

Birth Rites: The majority of women go to antenatal clinics. About 40% of infants in rural areas are born in hospitals, and almost 90% of infants in urban areas are born in hospitals. Abortion is not permitted except in exceptional medical situations. During birth the mother or mother-in-law of the woman in labor must be present. The birth of a son is usually greeted with extra enthusiasm, and all boys are circumcised. The infant mortality rate is 17.6 per 1000 live births. Birth spacing, with a gap of 2 years between births, is the basis of the national policy to limit family size. About 44% of the population is younger than 15 years, and the life expectancy for men and women is 70 and 74 years, respectively.

Death Rites: When a Muslim dies, the body is washed, wrapped in special cloth, and buried without a coffin in the ground. When a patient dies in hospital, the family removes the body immediately for a private burial. Autopsy is almost invariably refused. Both cadaver and living donor organ transplantations (e.g., renal, bone marrow) are carried out in Oman.

Food Practices and Intolerances: Pork is forbidden for Muslims, and all meat must be halal (dispatched with Islamic rites). During the holy month of Ramadan, Muslims fast during daylight hours. Unless given special permission, patients are not permitted to swallow any medication that contains nutrients or fluid or receive injections. Food is eaten only with the right hand. Muslims are not permitted to drink alcohol; however, alcohol is available in larger hotels and in licensed restaurants for expatriates (who are also permitted to have alcohol at home). Narcotic addiction is uncommon in Oman.

Infant Feeding Practices: Almost every infant is breast-fed in Oman, a practice strongly promoted by the Ministry of Health. As a result, gastro-enteritis in infants is unusual. However, the occasional HIV-positive mother will be advised to bottle-feed her infant (as opposed to the policy in developing countries, where the risk of fatal gastroenteritis exceeds the risk of contracting AIDS). Weaning starts at 6 to 8 months, and most mothers stop breast-feeding at 2 years.

Child Rearing Practices: Both parents help raise the children, frequently with the help of grandparents or other relatives. Discipline tends to be quite permissive but when it is required, both parents are involved. Spanking and other forms of physical punishment are generally discouraged.

National Childhood Immunizations: BCG at birth; DTP at 6 weeks and 3, 5, and 18 months; OPV at birth, 6 weeks, 3, 5, 7, and 18 months, and 6 to 7 and 17 to 18 years; hep B at birth, 6 weeks and 7 months; measles at 12 months; MMR at 18 months; DT at 6 to 7 years, Td at 12 to 13 years; TT at 17 to 18 years, then every 10 years or CBAW ×5. (In addition, 200,000 units of vitamin A are given at 7 and 12 months.) The national coverage rates for BCG, HBV, DPT, and OPV exceed 98%.

Other Characteristics: Omanis are renowned for their friendly and tolerant attitude toward foreigners. Almost all wear traditional dress: embroidered caps or turbans and white robes, or *dishdasha.* for men, and head scarves and the black *abeiya* (ankle-length cloak) for women. As noted, many rural women still wear the Omani face mask. Permission must always be obtained before photographing any Omani, including a child; as a rule, women do not agree to be photographed. Foreign women are expected to dress modestly but are not required to wear a head covering. All forms of communication including magazines, films, television, and videos are strictly censored, and any material deemed morally offensive is banned.

BIBLIOGRAPHY

Robison G: *Oman: Arab gulf states,* Melbourne, 1993, Lonely Planet Publications.
Scrimgeour EM, Mehta FL, Suleiman AJM: Infectious and tropical diseases in Oman: an epidemiological review, *Am J Trop Med Hyg* 61:920–925, 1999.
Thesiger W: *Arabian sands,* London, 1991, Penguin Books.
Vine P: *The heritage of Oman,* London, 1995, Immel Publishing.

◆ PAKISTAN (ISLAMIC REPUBLIC OF)

MAP PAGE (866)

Shehzad Parviz

Location: Located in South Asia, Pakistan borders India in the east, China in the northeast, and Iran in the southwest; Afghanistan abuts its western and northern edges. The Arabian Sea is Pakistan's southern border and has 1064 km (661 miles) of coastline. Pakistan's Hindu Kush and Himalayan Mountains contain the second highest peak in the world. Pakistan has desert lands in the east and areas of alluvial plains along the Indus River. The total land area of Pakistan is 796,095 km^2 (307,361 square miles), nearly four times the size of the United Kingdom. Approximately 37% of the population lives in urban areas, and the rest live in rural areas.

Major Languages	Ethnic Groups	Major Religions
Punjabi	Punjabi 66%	Sunni Muslim 77%
Sindhi	Sindhi 13%	Shi'a Muslim 20%
Pashtu	Pashtun 9%	Other 3%
Balochi	Balochi, other 12%	
Urdu (national language)		
English (official language), other		

Health Care Beliefs: Acute sick care; traditional. People believe that health and sickness are provided by God. Sickness may be attributed to some evil deed done in the past or sorcery. Those who are mentally ill are considered by some to be possessed by an evil spirit, or *gin.* Mental illness is considered a stigma; therefore those who are affected may not seek psychiatric care. Doctors and family members avoid telling patients about a grave diagnosis such as cancer because they may get very depressed. If someone gets ill, is cured, or has a child, it is very common for them to give money, *sadiqa,* to the poor or needy to obtain good wishes and inhibit evil spirits. Some may sacrifice goat or sheep and distribute the meat to the poor. Women may believe that reproductive tract infections are caused by "melting bones," consuming foods with that are "hot," poor personal hygiene, and procedures such as dilatation and curettage. They do not generally perceive sexually transmitted diseases as the cause of reproductive problems. Many would not clean wounds from a dog bite at all, and only a few would apply an antiseptic or water; instead, many would instead use red chilies, calcium carbonate, herbal medicine, or ground tobacco or would perform a ritual. Injections and intravenous fluids are considered more effective than oral medication. It is common for doctors to overprescribe antimicrobials, vitamins, minerals, and injections.

Predominant Sick Care Practices: Allopathic, homeopathic, and indigenous methods. All three methods are used concurrently by some. Pakistan has many modern private hospitals, and government hospitals provide free or subsidized care. People prefer to go to private hospitals or doctors if they can afford to. Among those who are sick, about two thirds in urban areas and one third in rural areas consult private doctors; less than one sixth use the government health facilities.

Ethnic/Race Specific or Endemic Diseases: Endemic diseases include chloroquine-resistant malaria (including urban areas), tuberculosis, acute respiratory tract infections, bacillary dysentery, typhoid fever, amoebiasis, and rabies. Diarrhea is the chief cause of death among children. Almost two thirds of children younger than age 5 have mild to moderate protein-energy malnutrition. The World Health Organization's (WHO) estimated prevalence rate for HIV/AIDS in adults ages 15 to 49 is 0.10%. The estimated number of children from birth to 15 years living with HIV/AIDS is 1600. The estimated number of adults and children who died of AIDS in 1999 is 6500. The estimated number of children younger than 15 years who have lost their mothers or both parents to AIDS since the beginning of the epidemic is 7900.

Health Team Relationships: Criticizing a person of higher status or rank is unacceptable. Men traditionally fill positions of authority; therefore female health care workers are under the authority of male doctors and hospital administrators. Nursing is perceived as a menial occupation, and nurses are not trained to make decisions or to be change agents. Traditional practitioners are called *hakims*.

Families' Role in Hospital Care: Hospitals supply meals, but they are usually of substandard quality. In government hospitals, patients who do not have needed medicines must buy them from an outside pharmacy or simply not take them. Female wards in hospitals are separated from male wards, and men cannot stay overnight.

Dominance Patterns: Women are governed by different laws than men. Women are expected to be obedient to men and are discouraged from making decisions. In some places, it is preferable that women stay in their homes and go out only if they are completely physically covered and unrecognizable. Women do have access to higher education. Most medical schools have more women than men, although most opt not to practice after graduation because of family obligations. Women feel they have limited control over their lives, exemplified by young marriages, high expectations that newlywed women conceive, and poor access to contraceptives. Women frequently express a strong preference for sons, primarily for economic reasons, reflecting women's subordinate position in society and the low economic value placed on women's work. Most women wear a soft cloth *(dupatta)* around the neck or over the head; they almost always wear traditional clothes. However, men are allowed to wear Western clothes. Mortality statistics are higher for women than men, possibly because men receive preferential treatment. The adult illiteracy rate in

2000 for those older than 15 years is 69% for females versus 40% for males.

Eye Contact Practices: A peripheral gaze or no eye contact may be preferred during male-female interactions. The eyes remain down as a sign of obedience during interactions with older adults or persons in a superior position.

Touch Practices: Male and female health care professionals are both reluctant to physically expose a patient, even during an examination. Male and female patients are reluctant to expose body parts to health care professionals of the opposite sex. Members of the opposite sex do not shake hands or embrace another person unless the person is a close family member. Women embrace and kiss on the cheek when greeting other women; men shake hands and embrace.

Birth Rites: The maternal and infant mortality rates are high; approximately one fourth of births are attended by trained health personnel. (Traditional birth attendants are called *dai*.) A *tawiz*, which is an amulet containing Koranic verses, is placed around the neck or shoulder of the infant. After 1 month of age, the infant's head is shaved because birth hair is considered unclean. The head shaving is accompanied by a family function known as *haqiqa,* during which a goat or sheep is sacrificed.

Death Rites: Muslim beliefs about organ donations or transplants vary, but the procedures are very uncommon. In contrast, Muslims believe it is acceptable to use blood transfusions to save lives. All family members congregate when a relative is dying. Death is usually ascribed to a fate determined by God. A holy Imam does not have to be present at death; however, a Muslim should recite the following Declaration of the Faith or help the patient recite it: "There is no God but God, and Muhammad is his messenger." When the person dies, others recite the following: "We all belong to Allah, and we shall return to him." According to Islamic tradition the family members must wash the body before the funeral. Autopsies are uncommon because the body must be buried intact. Cremations are not permitted. For Muslim burial, the body is wrapped in special pieces of cloth and buried without a coffin in the ground.

Food Practices and Intolerances: Pakistanis have three meals a day—breakfast, lunch, and dinner—and food practices vary. Pashtuns and Balochis are meat lovers but also eat a special kind of bread called *tandoori roti* that is made in a furnace. The Punjabi staple diet consists of lentils, rice, and bread known as *chapatti*. Food tends to be spicy, and the diet is high in fat. Spicy chicken is very popular. Milk tea is consumed every day at work and during the evening. *Kahwa,* a yellow tea without milk, is preferred in the morning during winter. Consumption of alcohol, pork, carrion, and blood is forbidden to Muslims. Ramadan fasting is practiced by all except for those who are sick or traveling. The mean daily intake of calories and micronutrients is lower for rural than urban children.

Infant Feeding Practices: Breast-feeding is recommended by the Islamic faith, and women may breast-feed for up to 2 years. The popularity of breast-feeding is declining. More than half of the women who breast-feed do so for more than 1 year. Two thirds of mothers do not give their infants colostrum. The majority of women are providing supplemental bottle-feedings by 5 months. The most common reason for starting bottle-feeding is worries about insufficient breast milk. Mothers who are illiterate, poor, or have had girls may stop breast-feeding sooner.

Child Rearing Practices: Some associate dehydration and malnutrition, and even marasmus, and inevitable death with spirits and close contact with "unclean" women—in other words, women who are menstruating or did not take a ritual bath after sexual intercourse. The most traditional Pakistanis may wrap their infants in cow dung to give them the strength and warmth needed for growth. Some mothers do not associate a lack of growth with lack of food. A sick child is a reflection of the mother's carelessness and social disgrace; therefore the family of the sick child may be ostracized. The duration of breast-feeding is decreasing. The high fat content in the buffalo milk that is fed to some infants makes it hard to digest. Each Muslim boy and girl is taught to read the holy book, the Koran, at a young age and to read it completely at least once. Boys receive preferential treatment in educational settings and child rearing. Although education for women is increasing, the family considers a girl's marriage to be more important than a career.

National Childhood Immunizations: BCG at birth; DTP at 6, 10, and 14 weeks; OPV at birth and 6, 10, and 14 weeks; measles at 9 months; and TT at first contact and 4 weeks after first dose.

Other Characteristics: People with medical emergencies in cities with ambulances usually do not use them. This practice is not only a result of poor accessibility but also a result of cultural barriers and an inability to recognize the danger signs of true emergencies.

BIBLIOGRAPHY

Ahmad WI: Patients' choice of general practitioner: intolerance of patients' fluency in English and the ethnicity and sex of the doctor, *J R Coll Gen Pract* 39(321):153, 1989.

Bhatti LI, Fikree FF: Health-seeking behavior of Karachi women with reproductive tract infections, *Soc Sci Med* 54(1):105–117, 2002.

David S, Lobo ML: Childhood diarrhea and malnutrition in Pakistan: part I: incidence and prevalence, *J Pediatr Nurs* 10(2):131, 1995.

David S, Lobo ML: Childhood diarrhea and malnutrition in Pakistan: part II: treatment and managements, *J Pediatr Nurs* 10(3):204, 1995.

David S, Lobo ML: Childhood diarrhea and malnutrition in Pakistan: part III: social policy issues, *J Pediatr Nurs* 10(4):273, 1995.

Galanti GA: *Caring for patients from different cultures,* ed 2, Philadelphia, 1997, University of Pennsylvania Press.

Hakeem R, Thomas J, Badruddin SH: Rural-urban differences in food and nutrient intake of Pakistani children, *J Pak Med Assoc* 49(12):288–294, 1999.

Haq MB: Lady health visitors: public health nursing education in Pakistan, *J Cult Diversity Health* 1(2):36, 1994.

Harnar R et al: Health and nursing services in Pakistan: problems and challenges for nurse leaders, *Nurs Adm Q* 16(2):52, 1992.

Hezekiah J: The pioneers of rural Pakistan: the lady health visitors, *Health Care Women Int* 14(6):493, 1993.

Kamal IT: The traditional birth attendant, *World Health,* Sept-Oct, p 6, 1992.

Karim MS: Disease pattern, health services utilization and cost of treatment in Pakistan, *J Pak Med Assoc* 43(8):159–164, 1993.

Kulsoom U, Saeed A: Breast feeding practices and beliefs about weaning among mothers of infants aged 0-12 months, *J Pak Med Assoc* 47(2):54–60, 1997.

http://www.ncbi.nlm.nih.gov:80/entrez/query.fcgi?cmd=Retrieve&db=PubMed&list _uids=9798028&dopt=Abstract Postexposure treatment of rabies in Pakistan, *Clin Infect Dis* 27(4):751–756, 1998.

Raftery KA: Emergency medicine in southern Pakistan, *Ann Emerg Med* 27(1):79, 1996.

Raglow GJ, Luby SP, Nabi N: Therapeutic injections in Pakistan: from the patients' perspective, *Trop Med Int Health* 6(1):69–75, 2001.

Razzak JA, Cone DC, Rehmani R: Emergency medical services and cultural determinants of an emergency in Karachi, Pakistan, *Prehosp Emerg Care* 5(3):312–316, 2001.

Sbaih LC: Women in the "developing world" and their perceptions of health: an area for examination by the nurse from the "developed world," *J Adv Nurs* 18:1524, 1993.

Weisfeld GE: Sociobiological patterns of Arab culture, *Ethnol Sociobiol* 11:23, 1990.

Winkvist A, Akhtar HZ: God should give daughters to rich families only: attitudes towards childbearing among low-income women in Punjab, Pakistan, *Soc Sci Med* 51(1):73-81, 2000.

Zindani N: Pakistani nurses vision for change, *Int Nurs Rev* 43(3):85, 1996.

◆ PALAU (REPUBLIC OF)

MAP PAGE (856)

Location: Palau is an archipelago of more than 200 islands in a chain about 560 kilometers (400 miles) long; located in the western Pacific Ocean southeast of the Philippines.

Major Languages	Ethnic Groups	Major Religions
English (official all 16 states)	Composite of	Christian 67%
Palauan (official in 13 states)	Polynesian,	Modekngei
Sonsorolese, Angaur, Japanese,	Malayan, and	(indigenous
Tobi (in one state each)	Melanesian	beliefs) 34%

Ethnic/Race Specific or Endemic Diseases: The World Health Organization (WHO) has no reported prevalence statistics for HIV/AIDS for Palau.

National Childhood Immunizations: DTP at 2, 4, 6, and 15 months and 4 years; OPV at 2, 4, and 6 months and 4 years; hep B at birth and at 2 and 6 months; HIB at 2, 4, 6, and 15 months; and MMR 12 and 15 months.

◆ PANAMA (REPUBLIC OF)

MAP PAGE (857)

Claude Vergès de López

Location: The Republic of Panama is situated between the Caribbean Sea on the north, the Republic of Colombia on the east, the Pacific Ocean on the south, and the Republic of Costa Rica on the west. The total land area is 75,517 km² (29,157 square miles). From east to west the country is divided by a chain of mountains, the Cordillera Central, with elevations of more than 3000 m, and from north to south by the Panama Canal, which is 80 km long and stretches from the Caribbean Sea to the Pacific Ocean. Panama City, the capital of the Republic, has 708,438 inhabitants and is on the Pacific Coast of the Panama Canal. Colon is on the Atlantic coast (Caribbean Sea), with 174,059 inhabitants. The country is politically divided into nine provinces and five Amerindian territories. The climate is tropical, with temperatures between 25° C and 32° C, and 77% humidity. Panama has two seasons: a dry season that lasts from December to April and a rainy season that lasts from May to December.

Major Languages	Ethnic Groups	Major Religions
Spanish (official)	Mestizo 70%	Roman Catholic
English	Amerindian, mixed	(official) 85%
	(West Indian) 14%	Protestant 15%
	White 10%	
	Amerindian 6%	

Spanish is the most disseminated language, but in Panama City and Colon, almost 25% of the inhabitants speak English. The Amerindian population is bilingual (speaking Spanish and indigenous languages). Primary school is obligatory, and illiteracy (close to 12% in 2000) is primarily restricted to Amerindians (with exception of the Kunas) and very poor people. The number of Protestant churches has increased, and some Amerindians and Afropanamanians practice their own indigenous religions. Witchcraft practitioners and those who perform magic rituals are disseminated among the population. The total population is about 2,839,177, consisting mainly of Hispano-Amerindians and Afropanamanians. The Amerindian population is 10% of the total population and consists of six groups: Kuna (21.6%) in the San Blas Islands and Darien, Embera and Wounaan (7.9%) in Darien (the Colombian frontier), Ngöbe-Buglé (65.5%) in the three western provinces, and the Bokotas, Teribes, and

Bri Bri (less than 3%) in Bocas del Toro (the Costa Rican frontier). Minority ethnic groups consist of Chinese, Jews, and Hindustanis. About one third of Panamanians are younger than 15 years old.

Health Care Beliefs: Acute sick care; increasing efforts in area of disease prevention. The Ministry of Health and some doctors' associations are very active in the promotion of healthy lifestyles, and prevention is a part of medical services. Coverage of the development program for children younger than a year old has been almost 94% since 1992. Inhabitants of urban areas are open to prevention campaigns; lifestyle problems are generally related to poverty. In rural areas the concepts of prevention are less understood, although prevention of childhood diseases and hygienic delivery of infants are becoming increasingly accepted (79% in 1999). Other programs, such as reproductive and sexual health, birth control, and cancer prevention for women meet some resistance. Men do not frequently attend health programs before the age of 50. Amerindians generally do not attend for economic or cultural reasons (beliefs and languages barriers of language) and because of what they consider to be the dominating attitude of doctors and nurses. Some of the Embera and Wounaan groups believe that illness can be drawn out with heated coins, but this belief is disappearing with migration from the countryside and the extension of services by the Ministry of Health. Mental illness is generally feared but accepted, probably because of the influence of African and Amerindian beliefs. People with mental illness who are not dangerous live with their relatives. The members of the upper class are the least accepting of those with mental illness.

Predominant Sick Care Practices: Biomedical and traditional. Western health care is offered through the national public health system, an employment-linked prepaid health and retirement plan called *Seguro Social,* and through a high, fee-for-service private urban sector. Medical services of the Ministry of Health cover the entire country, with 60 hospitals, 215 health centers and polyclinic centers, and 520 health subcenters. Five public and three private highly specialized hospitals are located in Panama City. Panama has 3475 doctors, 788 dentists, and 3185 nurses. Doctors receive their degree in Panama but do their specialty rotations in Mexico, Brazil, the United States, or Europe. Panama has 519 inhabitants per doctor in urban areas and 2402 per doctor in rural areas. The government pays 80% to 100% of hospital costs, depending on the family's income. Amerindians have their own healers, but they also use Western medical services, primarily after a community member has had a positive experience with the Western health service. New generations of those attending school are also more open to modern medicine. Relationships between healers and doctors often conflict, primarily because of the rejection of indigenous beliefs among doctors. Self-medication, excluding antibiotics, is common. Herbs and other locally grown plants are widely used for their medicinal qualities and are sold in the open markets.

Ethnic/Race Specific or Endemic Diseases: The ten principal causes of death in the country since 1995 (with little variations between the first and the second one) have been cancer (primarily prostate and gastric cancer among men and cervical cancer among women), all forms of violence (automobile accidents, aggression, and suicide), ischemic heart disease, cerebrovascular diseases, diabetes mellitus, chronic pulmonary illnesses, HIV/AIDS, other heart illnesses, prenatal illnesses, and pneumonia. In 2000, the life expectancy was 76 for women and 72 for men. The total mortality rate was 5 per 1000, and infant mortality was 20 per 1000 live births. The number of children per woman (fertility rate) was 2.5. Afropanamanians are usually affected with sickle cell disease, though a decrease in rates has resulted from obligatory screenings at 1 year and other health promotion programs that have been in place since 1986. Diabetes and cardiovascular diseases particularly affect Afropanamanian women older than 40. Amerindian communities have all the diseases common among the poor: respiratory tract infections, diarrhea, and other infectious diseases at younger than 5 years with high mortality rates; complications of pregnancy and high maternal mortality among women; and tuberculosis in both sexes. Life expectancy is almost 15 years less than the median life expectancy of Panamanians. The World Health Organization's (WHO) estimated prevalence rate for HIV/AIDS in adults ages 15 to 49 is 1.54%. The estimated number of children from birth to 15 years living with HIV/AIDS is 670. The first case of AIDS was diagnosed in 1984, and the numbers of those infected are rapidly increasing; females are at particular risk for infection. From 1988 to 2000, estimates of women infected have increased from one sixth to one third of the population. Blood transfusions are controlled by the Ministry of Health, and AIDS transmission through transfusions account for 5% of cases. Transmission is primarily heterosexual (84%) because of resistance of men to using condoms and multiple sexual partners.

Health Team Relationships: Health team relationships depend on many different factors—the type of service provided (with hospitals being more hierarchical than health centers), the style of the head of the team, the number of years of close work, and the academic preparation and professional experience of each member of the team. Generally, health teams with a majority of doctors have good relationships. The term *doctor* is used to express respect or affection, and nurses are addressed by *miss*. In public practice as in private, attitudes toward doctors and nurses are generally trusting. People are generally unassertive toward doctors and, although to a lesser degree, toward nurses. If they do not trust a doctor or nurse at one health service, they go to another health service. In the last several years a more challenging attitude has been observed, and the media has had discussions about cases of medical malpractice. Individuals who feel they have received poor treatment have the right to a "people's defender" (a lawyer named by the government for defense of the human rights).

Families' Role in Hospital Care: Since 1980, families have been staying with their hospitalized children in the Child Hospital of Panama to take care of them, but food from the outside is prohibited. The hospital has special facilities for mothers from rural areas, and every parent can have access to the library to read about their children's illness. In other hospitals, families stay only when patients have special needs, but they can bring the patients food and in some situations, medications. Ngobe families and a special rural group of Hispano-Amerindian people, with strong Spanish traditions, move near the hospital when a family member is ill to care for the person until recovery or death.

Dominance Patterns: Men dominate Panamanian culture, but work for legal equity between men and women has been in process since 1995. Health maintenance and care of the ill are the responsibilities of women, who take care of every member of the family. Women have access to all sorts of services and can choose what they prefer for themselves or for family members. In the median and upper classes, male dominance is apparent only if the costs of services are too high or during very important decision making. In the lower classes, control of the economic resources of the family is in the hands of men, and they make the decisions regarding women's sexual and reproductive health.

Eye Contact Practices: Eye contact is generally maintained in most but two situations, the most important one involving eye contact with a newborn. Mothers, worried about women with the "evil eye" (i.e., the power to harm the newborn through her gaze), try to avoid interacting with these women until they can arrange a witch ceremony to combat the curse. The other situation involves interactions with Ngobe people, who think that pregnant women should avoid eye contact with men, although this belief does not tend to be as relevant during interactions with health practitioners.

Touch Practices: Physical touching is acceptable, but men prefer that only male doctors examine them for sexually related diseases. Women say that they prefer female doctors for sexually related examinations, although they often change their minds after having a respectable and positive experience with a male doctor. It is always best to examine patients of the opposite sex in the presence of a nurse or other doctor, particularly if the examination involves the genitalia. Use of touch is used to make personal or social contact in urban areas. Men greet each other by shaking hands or an embrace, and kissing one cheek is common between women, or men and women, as an initial greeting. In rural or indigenous areas, touch is used only between members of the same family.

Perceptions of Time: Punctuality is an issue for people who interact with public or private health services. People may arrive nearly 2 hours before appointments, but the doctors may consider being behind schedule as a sign that they are successful. Panamanian culture is very reality based, and people tend to live in the present. The focus on the past is limited to older adults and academics, and a focus on the future is often associated with those in politics or who are wealthy.

Pain Reactions: Reactions to pain depend on culture and education. Stoicism seems to characterize Amerindian and rural people, whereas those with high levels of education may cry calmly and discreetly. Very expressive reactions are the norm among Afropanamanian or Hispanopanamanian people, and shouting, screaming, and gesticulating are not uncommon.

Birth Rites: In urban areas, 99.7% of deliveries involve professional assistance, whereas in rural areas the coverage is 80% and is 54% in Amerindian territories. Maternal mortality rates are reported to be between 0.5 (urban) and 0.8 (rural) per 1000 live births. The poor coverage of Amerindian territories can be attributed to their long distance from any health care center, language barriers, the high cost of transportation, preferences for delivery in a vertical position (assisted by the husband or mother), and the traditional practice of burying the placenta. The Ministry of Health has an active program of family planning in its centers, including contraceptives and intrauterine devices at minimal cost; the coverage of women ages 20 to 40 years was almost 61% in 1998. This program is facing opposition by the Catholic church and men, particularly in poor and rural communities.

Death Rites: Death is perceived as a significant loss, even when the person was older. All family members are usually present at a relative's death, and the death ceremony (which is familiar and religious) is a social event in the community. When a person is dying in the hospital, staff members allow the family to visit, and the parents can stay with the person until the priest or the pastor arrives. Rural and Amerindian people prefer to take deceased family members home themselves because of transportation costs and to perform their own ceremonies. Organ donations and autopsies are not usually acceptable; acceptance depends on the educational level of the family, and the decision of whether to allow the procedure to be performed is made by all adult members.

Food Practices and Intolerances: The basic diet and preferred foods are related to the social and economic status of families, as well as their ethnic background. In the upper classes, families adopt the typical Western diet or the cultural diet of the ethnic group to which they belong (e.g., Jewish, Italian, Jamaican). Hispanopanamanian families commonly eat rice with meat and beans. Ngobe families eat rice with beans and occasionally chicken, but from July to September, they eat only once a day. Panamanians' favorite foods are traditional ones, but people enjoy soft drinks such as Coke and Pepsi. They usually use a fork, knife, and spoon, and it is unusual to eat with hands.

Infant Feeding Practices: Breast-feeding is considered a common cultural practice among Amerindian and rural families and a healthy choice in urban areas. The Ministry of Health promotes breast-feeding through the health services, and bottle-feeding is prohibited in maternity hospitals. In rural areas infants are breast fed until they are a year old and occasionally until they are 2 years. In urban areas, the ability to breast-feed often depends on the working needs of the mother. The Work Code allows 3 months for breast-feeding and then 1 hour of work time until the infant is 6 months old. Mothers follow the recommendations of doctors and nurses about the gradual introduction of solid foods as their infants grow and develop during the first year. In the Amerindian population, infants between 8 months and a year (who have their first teeth) eat what the family is eating.

Child Rearing Practices: Child rearing practices are very permissive, although parents and grandparents may spank children when they consider it necessary. Generally the father is the head of the family, but discipline is the responsibility of both parents. Until 1 to 2 years, children sleep with their parents or (if they are in the upper class) with a "nana." They then sleep with their brothers or sisters or alone. In very poor families, houses have only one room, so these separations are impossible.

National Childhood Immunizations: BCG at birth; DTP at 4 to 6 years; DTPHH at 2, 4, 6, and 15 months; OPV at birth, 2, 4, and 6 months, and 4 to 6 years; measles at 9 months; MMR at 15 months and 11 to 12 years; *Haemophilus influenzae* B and yellow fever at 1 and 10 years in high-risk areas; DT CBAW ×3; and hepatitis A and B in the first year of age. The National Program of Immunizations is supported by PHO-WHO.

Other Characteristics: Panama is considered a median economic country with great disparities among families' incomes and an important urban middle class

BIBLIOGRAPHY

Biesanz J, Biesanz, M: The people of Panama, 1977, Greenwood Press, New York.
Contraloría de la República de Panamá, Dirección de Estadística y Censo: *Panamá en Cifras*, 2001, Panama.
Heckadon S: *Panama en sus usos y costumbres*, Biblioteca de la Cultura Panameña, tomo 4, Panama, 1994, Editorial Universitaria.
Ministerio de Salud: *Memorias*, Panama, 1999.
Pan American Health Organization: *Health in the Americas*, pp 432–441, Scientific Pub No 569, 1998, Washington, DC.
Pan American Health Organization: *Health Statistics from the Americas*, Scientific Pub No 567, 1998, Washington, DC.
Rudolf G: *Panama's poor—victims, agents and historymakers*, 1999, University Press of Florida, Tampa.

◆ PAPUA NEW GUINEA (INDEPENDENT STATE OF)

MAP PAGE (856)

Major Franklin H.G. Bridgewater

Location: Papua New Guinea is in the South Pacific and comprises the mainland and approximately 600 offshore islands, with a total land area of 461,690 km² (178,259 square miles). The mainland constitutes the eastern portion of the island of New Guinea, and Irian Jaya, a province of Indonesia, comprises the western portion. From the border with Indonesia, Papua New Guinea reaches east. The island of New Guinea has one of the largest unspoiled rain forests in the world. Papua New Guinea's mainland is thickly forested, with dense jungle and relatively unexplored mountains. The climate is temperate in the highlands of the mainland (4° C [39° F] to 32° C [90° F]) and tropical in the coastal lowlands and islands. A predictable daily weather pattern for the highlands is early fog, a pleasant morning, afternoon rain, and a cool or cold night. The coastal and island areas are hot and humid with temperatures ranging between 20° C (68° F) and 32° C (90° F) and have a wet season with varying intensity.

Major Languages	Ethnic Groups	Major Religions
Pidgin English	Papuan 95%	Indigenous beliefs
English (official)	Other (Negrito,	(animist, pantheist)
Motu	Micronesian,	34%
Other	Melanesian,	Roman Catholic 22%
	Polynesian) 5%	Lutheran 16%
		Other Christian 28%

As a result of isolation caused by the rugged terrain, an extremely large number of diverse tribes and language groups evolved. More than 700 different languages and dialects have been recorded. Pidgin English developed as a common means of communication. It primarily derives from English but incorporates elements of German, Malay, Motu (a language of the Port Moresby area), and other local words; it has a limited vocabulary. Although English is the official language, it is spoken by only 1% to 2% of the population. Some have advocated for a division of the population into two major groups, Papuan and Melanesian. Others suggest smaller groupings such as Papuans (from the south of the mainland), Highlanders, New Guineans (from the north of the mainland), and Islanders. The latter suggestion is more in line with the country. This variability in culture and physical characteristics makes it impossible to produce cultural statements that apply to all of Papua New Guinea. Perhaps the most consistent tenet is the importance of land and the manner in which it is held.

Health Care Beliefs: Traditional; both active and passive involvement. The people have a widespread belief that evil spirits are a reality and inhabit some jungle and forested areas. Illness may be attributed to personal actions that have offended these spirits or the work of a sorcerer acting at the behest of a hostile individual. Basically, the people have no precise differentiation between mental and physical illness. Some people simply accept an illness—and that any investigations into its cause will "*kamap nating,* or "come-up with nothing." Most health promotion is carried out at the village level by direct personal contact or in small groups with the use of basic illustrative posters. Some additional teaching occurs at hospital clinics and in schools.

Predominant Sick Care Practices: Biomedical and magical-religious. In the towns and larger centers, most people accept modern health care practices. However, even those who are avowed Christians may follow traditional practices to treat illness, which involve animist and pantheist practices. In some cultures, particular individuals assume a healer's role and may receive payment, whereas in others, relatives may accept this responsibility. Certain leaves and botanical preparations are thought to have curative qualities. Placating the aggrieved spirits is common to promote healing. Traditions vary from region to region, and some from the Lufa, Daru, Kwikila, Samarai, and Rigo subprovinces have been documented.

Ethnic/Race Specific or Endemic Disease: Malaria is endemic in the lowlands and coastal areas, and chloroquine-resistant forms may be encountered. Effective chemical prophylaxis and appropriate clothing are essential to avoid contracting the disease. People are also at risk for tuberculosis and leprosy. In addition, pig-bel (enteritis necroticans), a severe form of gastroenteritis, is encountered in the highlands and caused by a specific bacterium. It is associated with the pig feasts, which are an important cultural feature of the region. A person with pig-bel may need surgery, but immunizations against the organism are now common in the highlands. Anemia affects all age groups and is associated with chronic malaria and worm infestation. Kuru, a spongiform encephalopathy, affected the Kuku Kuku, a small group in the Fore area. Its relationship to the local practice of cannibalism has been investigated; the disease stopped appearing in the youngest age group in 1964, and then progressively ceased affecting older age groups thereafter. Kuru, like bovine spongiform encephalopathy (BSE, or "mad cow disease") in Europe, may have been transmitted to humans through the food chain. Sexually transmitted diseases are common, particularly in urban areas. The World Health Organization's (WHO) estimated prevalence rate for HIV/AIDS in adults ages 15 to 49 years is 0.22%. The estimated number of children from birth to 15 years living with HIV/AIDS is 220.

Health Team Relationships: Government aid posts are staffed by people trained in first aid and basic hygiene and are scattered throughout the country. Subprovincial and provincial centers have more advanced health care and education because of the hospitals and more highly trained personnel, but access to these facilities may be limited by weather, transportation, and finances. Health care relationships between members of the opposite sex are definitely reserved. AusAID, the Australian Government's overseas aid program, has significantly supported the Papua New Guinea government with providing health care in numerous areas. The provision of aid by personnel on military deployments highlights certain features. Although overtly beneficial, such aid creates dependence and may denigrate local workers, invite abuse of the system by local practitioners, create an undesirable secondary economy, and develop unrealistic expectations. Civilian health care workers should consider these aspects when considering such units currently in Papua New Guinea.

Families' Role in Hospital Care: Almost all parents and families actively provide care for their hospitalized children and family members. Families consider it a duty and an obligation to provide companionship and care, including provision of food and firewood. These practices have economic and social implications. Hospital budgets are constrained, so additional food is needed for patients. Extra help is always needed and may be used for performing basic nursing tasks. Some may have unjustified concerns that care provided by an outsider (someone other than a tribal member, or *wantok* ["one-talk"]—a person who speaks the same language), may be prejudiced in some way and provide substandard or even harmful care or treatment.

Dominance Patterns: Male dominance and individuality are important to some. Condom use to prevent the spread of HIV/AIDS is a challenge for health care professionals because it is important to obtain the husband's approval for use of contraceptives. Polygamy is practiced in some areas. In rural areas, women are responsible for growing and preparing food and tending children and animals. Pigs are highly valued, so piglets are breast-fed if necessary. Girls may be married by the age of 14 years.

Touch Practices: The sight of young men and women holding hands with members of the same sex is common and simply indicates valued companionship. Grooming a friend in various ways, such as combing hair or removing lice, may occupy a considerable amount of time. Children, particularly if they are White, may be patted or stroked incessantly by young and old and male and female indigenous Papua New Guineans.

Time Perception: Generally, little effort is made to adhere to a strict schedule, and events are often allowed to happen at their own rate. A request to rigidly follow a set program may lead to intense frustration and create animosity.

Birth Rites: Approximately two thirds of women receive some antenatal care. Most births are supervised only by a local tribal midwife or older female family member. A delivery that becomes complicated usually eventually enters the health care system but often at a late stage, a practice that is associated with high infant mortality. Almost all infants are breast-fed. In remote areas dominated by traditional practices, infants with physical anomalies may be left to die, unattended and unfed. When infant mortality was higher, children were not named until their first birthday.

Death Rites: Death rites, including various forms of burial, vary enormously between regions. Women in some cultural groups are expected to express grief; however, men are not. Traditionally, when Highlander women experience the death of a husband, they amputate a finger just above the first knuckle as a sign of their sorrow. These wounds often heal well. Illness and death can be the provocative event that begins a "pay-back" for previous misdeeds. Those held responsible for the death are required to recompense the aggrieved party in some way. Such "pay-backs" may initiate a conflict that continues for a long period. An extreme example occurred in the Highlands in 1972. An islander doctor and the driver of a vehicle involved in an accident in which a child was killed stopped to give help and were immediately stoned to death by local villagers. Historically, amputated body parts have been valued and buried. It is assumed that the deceased will be buried in the same plot and be able to use the appendages again in the next life. Organ donations are not performed in this community, but if they were available they would likely conflict with traditional beliefs.

Food Practices and Intolerances: Sweet potatoes *(kaukau)* are eaten as the staple food in the highlands, and sago palm (*saksak,* which is almost pure starch) is eaten in the lowlands. Taro, bananas, and greens are common. Dietary iodine deficiency was a cause of endemic goiter in the highlands. The widespread use of iodine supplementation by injection provided the initial solution to this problem. Pig feasts are a highlight and may be used to celebrate significant social occasions. The consumption of large amounts of poorly cooked, contaminated pork that has been passed for several days from person to person and area to area as a gift (according to tradition) is responsible for the previously mentioned outbreaks of pig-bel. People know certain plants can cause them to become intoxicated and that alcoholic beverages can be produced in numerous ways (*hom-bru,* or "home-brew"). Intoxication can be a serious, socially disruptive problem and result in public brawls and domestic violence. More and more automobile accident fatalities are being associated with alcohol—approximately 20% in 1979. Alcohol consumption is associated with a large and growing health problem in contemporary Papua New Guinea. Perhaps the most common recreational drug is betel nut *(buai).* It is chewed with mustard and lime, producing characteristic red saliva. Some have proposed an association between this habit and oral cancer.

Infant Feeding Practices: Breast-feeding may continue until a child is 4 or 5 years old and may help prevent pregnancy. In the past, when breast-feeding was replaced by bottle-feeding, it was frequently associated with an infant's failure to thrive because of an inadequate understanding about formula preparation and hygiene. Legislation was introduced, and prescriptions are now required for infant formula.

Child Rearing Practices: Significant differences in child rearing are apparent among various groups, and changes are occurring throughout the country. Previously, during tribal fighting in some areas, warriors were banned from having conjugal relationships. The lack of tribal fighting has made this restriction obsolete, resulting in an increase in young siblings within a family grouping. Discipline for young children is generally verbal, but they may receive an occasional slap. At a young age, girls assume responsibility for sibling care. Boys have a longer period without such responsibilities. Parents often encourage secondary education for their sons but not their daughters. The parents may be concerned about their daughter's safety in an area other than her home or believe that females simply do not need such an education. The practice of demanding a "bride price" is still common and creates significant difficulties.

National Childhood Immunizations: BCG at birth; DTP at 1, 3, and 4 months; OPV at birth and 1, 2, and 3 months; hep B at birth and at 2 and 3 months; measles at 6 and 9 months; TT at first and second contact and next pregnancy; and pig-bel at 1, 2, 3, and 4 months and during the first and last year of community schooling.

BIBLIOGRAPHY

Alto WA, Albu RE, Irabo G: An alternative to unattended delivery: a training programme for village midwives in Papua New Guinea, *Soc Sci Med* 32(5):613, 1991.

Avue B, Freeman P: Some factors affecting acceptance of family planning in Manus, *PNG Med J* 34(4):270, 1991.

Biddulph J: Child health in Papua New Guinea: a 30 year personal perspective, *Med J Aust* 154(7):439, 1991.

Bridgewater FHG: Poisoning with angel's trumpets, *PNG Med J* 11:26–28, 1969.

Bridgewater FHG et al: Provision of emergency surgical care in a unique geopolitical setting, *ANZ J Surg* 71,606–609, 2001

Burton-Bradley BG, ed: A history of medicine in Papua New Guinea vignettes of an earlier period, Kingsgrove, Australia, 1990, Australian Medical Publishing Company.

Hetzel BS: From Papua New Guinea to the United Nations: the prevention of mental defect due to iodine deficiency, *Aust J Public Health* 9(3):231, 1995.

Neuhaus S, Bridgewater FHG, Kilcullen D: Military medical ethics: issues for 21st century operations, *Aus Defence Force J* 151:49–58, 2001.

Reade MC: Medical assistance to civilians during peacekeeping operations: wielding the double-edged sword, *Med J Aust* 173: 586–589, 2000

Reuben R: Women and malaria: special risks and appropriate control strategy, *Soc Sci Med* 37(4):473, 1993.

Sharaz J: Motherhood in Papua New Guinea, *Midwives* 107(1299):102, 1996.

Spear SF et al: Nurses as a key PHC link in Papua New Guinea, *Int Nurs Rev* 37(l):207, 1990

http://www.ausaid.gov.au/country/papua.cfm

http://coombs.anu.edu.au/SpecialProj/PNG/Index.htm

◆ PARAGUAY (REPUBLIC OF)

MAP PAGE (859)

Richard G. Bribiescas

Location: Paraguay is a landlocked South American nation with a total land area of 406,752 km^2 (157,006 square miles), about the size of California. Brazil and Bolivia border the country to the north, and Argentina and Uruguay border it to the east and south. The eastern departments are characterized by subtropical woodland, whereas the Chaco region to the north is sparsely populated and consists primarily of dry scrubland.

Major Languages	Ethnic Groups	Major Religions
Spanish (official)	Mestizo (mixed Spanish and	Roman Catholic 90%
Guarani (official)	Indian) 95%	Protestant 5%
	Whites, Amerindians 5%	Other or none 5%

Paraguay is one of the few Latin American nations to adopt an indigenous language as an official language. Spanish is taught in school and is the predominant language in urban areas, whereas Guarani is the language of choice in rural communities. The population in 2002 was 5.5 million, and most of the population lives near the two major cities of Asuncion and Cuidad del Este. Although most communities consist of individuals of mixed Amerindian and European descent, isolated communities of Amerindians with limited European influence live in the eastern departments of Canindeyú and Alto Paraná and the northern regions of the Gran Chaco. Major indigenous groups include the Ache, Ayoreo, Chiripa, Guarani, Lengua, and Maká. Approximately 5% of the population consists of Protestants, including several Mennonite colonies.

Health Care Beliefs: Acute sick care; traditional; Western-based. Health care beliefs are very diverse and reflect the differences among the various Paraguayan communities. People in many communities, especially those in the rural areas, either believe in some aspects of or practice *yuyos* (pronounced "YOO yohs"), a form of herbal and spiritual home medicine. The practice derives from indigenous medical beliefs, mainly from the Guarani, Maká, and Chiripa peoples. The use of *yuyos* is quite complex and involves not only the use of an herb for the particular ailment but also interactions with spiritual aspects of the herb.

Predominant Sick Care Practices: Biomedical and indigenous. Sick care practices vary widely among communities and are driven primarily by socioeconomic status. Although much of the population is familiar with or practices *yuyos,* traditional Western-based medicine is widely accepted and desired by those who can afford it. Indigenous healers and *yuyos* are especially prevalent among the Ayoreo peoples of the Chaco and the Guarani, Chiripa, and Maká communities in eastern and central Paraguay. Among nonindigenous Paraguayans, the use of *yuyos* is more prevalent in rural areas, although it may simply be a result of lack of access to contemporary Western medical resources.

Ethnic/Race Specific or Endemic Diseases: Chagas' disease is the most endemic vector-borne disease in Paraguay. The prevalence of *Trypanosoma cruzi* infection in all of Paraguay is 11.6%, although 5.7% (1995) and 4.1% (1996) seropositive results for *T. cruzi* antibodies were noted in blood transfusion tests. Surveys of indigenous populations in the Chaco region indicate that up to 80% of the people are seropositive for *T. cruzi,* which emphasizes the broad range of variation in Paraguayan society to risk of exposure and infection. A 1995 survey of 5042 pregnant women in the departments of Paraguarí and Cordillera revealed a 15% prevalence rate of *T. cruzi* infections. Approximately 1000 cases of cutaneous leishmaniasis infection are reported each year, although lack of reporting is a serious concern. Most cases (85%) occurred in the departments of Canendiyú, Alto Paraná, and San Pedro. Most of these cases involved the development of new agricultural land; men older than 20 were the most affected by this disease. Malaria is a constant problem, especially in rural areas such as the departments of Alto Paraná, Caaguazú, and Canindiyú, which account for 90% of 1000 cases of malaria caused by *Plasmodium vivax*. However, the infection rate has stabilized and did not increase from 1996 to 1999. Since the 1988 and 1989 outbreak of dengue fever (serotype 1) that infected more than 40,000 Paraguayans, no new cases have been reported, although the primary vector, *Aedes aegypti,* is still common. Tuberculosis is a major health issue, especially in rural and indigenous communities. In 1992 and 1993 the annual incidence rate for tuberculosis was 43.3 per 100,000. In 1994 it was 38.4, in 1995 it was 36.1, and in 1996 it was 37.2; 95% of cases were pulmonary. The Maka and Chamacoco communities have the highest rates of tuberculosis infection—10 times higher than the rest of the Paraguayan population. In addition, 80% of indigenous households are infested with *Triatoma infestans*, the vector of Chagas' disease. Asthma is common in South America, although in an extensive survey, Paraguay had the lowest incidence of asthma mortality in South America. Interestingly, Paraguay reported that more asthma deaths occurred in the home (88%) than in other Latin American nations, suggesting significant underreporting of this disease. Among older adults (65 and older) the primary causes of death are cardiovascular disease (28%), malignant neoplasms (13%), diabetes (6%), pneumonia and influenza (4%), and hypertension (3%). Although data are incomplete, the 1992 census reported that 5335 individuals in the capital of Asunción had some form of physical disability, whereas the National Institute for the Protection of Exceptional People in 1995 reported 22,000 people with disabilities. Accidents and violence have become an increasing concern in rural and urban areas. Drug trafficking and armed assaults are becoming more common. Automobile accidents are more frequent and severe because of the opening of new asphalt roads, the growing number of large vehicles such as logging trucks on the road, and poor traffic control. In 1995, 58% (130) of highway deaths involved individuals between the ages of 15 and 24, and 24% were between 25 and 44; 80% of those killed were male. The World Health Organization's (WHO) estimated prevalence rate for HIV/AIDS in adults ages 15 to 49 years is 0.11%. The estimated number of children from birth to 15 years living with HIV/AIDS is less than 100. A total of 253 cases of AIDS were reported in Paraguay between 1986 and December 1996, resulting in a fatality rate of 57%. The age group most affected by AIDS is individuals who are 30 to 34 years. Males are more likely to be infected than females, although the rate for females has been increasing; the majority of infections (66%) are thought to have resulted from sexual contact. Although initial cases primarily involved homosexual men, heterosexual men are becoming infected more frequently. In addition to sexual contact, 12% of infections are thought to involve intravenous drug use, 3.8% are from blood transfusions, and 2.9% are through perinatal transmission. Current information suggests that individuals between the ages of 20 and 24 years have the highest risk, and 0.2% of blood donations test positive for HIV. A cross-sectional sampling between March 1994 and September 1998 of individuals with HIV-1 infection in Peru, Ecuador, Uruguay, and Paraguay revealed that genotype B was found in 98.3% (228 of 232) of the individuals tested. Moreover, genotype F was found for the first time in Paraguay. Life expectancy at birth for males is 68 years and for females is 72 years.

Health Team Relationships: Paraguay has 5.1 doctors per 10,000 people, so the issue of doctor-nurse relationships is somewhat irrelevant in most areas. However, the doctor predominantly controls the relationship. Although nurses offer some basic care, doctors dictate the strategy of treatment.

Families' Role in Hospital Care: Family care and attention in hospitals is crucial, especially in rural areas. Food and basic necessities such as sheets, blankets, and pillows are often unavailable and are provided by the family or in some cases by relief workers such as religious missionaries. In urban hospitals, it is more likely for these basic necessities to be provided—but only after the family or patient has demonstrated the ability to pay for services.

Dominance Patterns: Men in Amerindian and non-Amerindian communities have a dominant role in social and political matters. Nonetheless, women's influence in social and familial situations varies among cultures. For example, in indigenous communities such as the Ache, women play a significant role in political and social matters and are likely to play a central role in guiding their family's health care practices.

Eye Contact Practices: Paraguayans have no social taboos against direct eye contact, although younger women may be more reluctant to maintain eye contact with an unknown male.

Touch Practices: Shaking hands is a common form of greeting in Paraguay, especially between males. Females do not usually shake hands, although it is not uncommon to do so. Some indigenous groups do not shake hands within others in their community but understand that it is the norm among Paraguayans of European decent.

Perceptions of Time: Most communities, rural and urban, understand the importance of punctuality, although practical factors, such as the availability of transportation, child care, or the freedom to leave a job, may make some seem chronically tardy. The tradition of the afternoon siesta, which involves returning home for a meal and a rest between approximately 3 and 6 PM, can affect the ability to set appointment times, especially in urban areas where commuter traffic is a constant problem.

Pain Reactions: Pain reactions are not especially stoical or expressive compared with those of Americans.

Birth Rites: According to the Pan American Health Organization (PAHO), 36% of deliveries are performed by trained medical personnel. In 1995, 40% of births that occurred in a Ministry of Health facility were attended by doctors, 40% by nurses or midwives, 16% by traditional birth attendants, and the remaining 4% by others, including family members. Birthing practices vary widely among communities, especially among indigenous groups. For example, an Ache father is never present during a birth; instead he may be out hunting or getting food for his wife and new infant. Newborns are given an Ache name based on a special aspect of the mother's diet during her pregnancy. For example, the name *Chachugi* may be given if the mother ate an unusual amount of wild boar *(chachu)* meat. Similar customs are evident in other tribes as well. According to the Paraguay Demographic and Health Survey of 1990, 38.7% of rural women practiced some form of birth control, compared with 56.8% among urban dwellers. Education level was positively associated with contraceptive use. Among rural women using contraceptives, *yuyos* was the most common form of birth control (used by 88% of women). Older women, those who already have children, and rural women are most likely to use *yuyos* compared with women who have more education and live in urban areas. Although *yuyos* practices are widely known and accepted, their contraceptive efficacy has not been clinically demonstrated. The desire to stop having children was positively associated with the number of children a mother already had. Among those with no children,

2.3% wanted to prevent pregnancy; additional related statistics follow: 1 child, 10.1%; 2 children, 33.6%; 3 children, 52.2%; 4 children, 56.2%; 5 children, 64.2%; 6 or more children, 70.8%. Of those using modern birth control, the most common methods were oral contraceptives, intra-uterine devices, and sterilization of the female. Among those not using any birth control, the most common reason was a desire to become pregnant, followed by a dislike of using contraceptives, a fear of side effects, a lack of sexual activity, and older age. Infant mortality among indigenous groups in Paraguay is quite high, ranging from 64 deaths per 1000 live births among the Maká to 185 per 1000 in the Chamacoco community. The infant mortality rate for Paraguay overall is 27 per 1000 live births, and the mortality rate of children younger than 5 years is 47 per 1000 live births. The maternal mortality rate is 123 per 100,000 live births; 35% of births involve trained personnel.

Death Rites: Most death rites follow the traditional practices of Roman Catholicism. Family members are often present and play an active role in funeral planning. Autopsies are uncommon, so families should be approached with sensitivity and care when an autopsy is necessary. Although the official doctrine of the Catholic church understands the need for autopsies in certain situations, Paraguayan Catholics have not had much exposure to these changes and may be fearful about an autopsy of a loved one. Similarly, organ transplantation is relatively new to Paraguay, although cardiac and renal transplants are becoming more common. Latin America as a whole accounts for 12% of global renal transplants. Nonetheless, the availability of transplants in Paraguay is extremely limited and restricted to the most modern urban hospitals. Death rites of indigenous groups vary widely. For example, the body of a deceased Ache may be bound at the wrists and ankles with twine from vines and buried in a fetal position in a simple grave with many of their possessions such as knives, glasses, cups, and clothing.

Food Practices and Intolerances: Manioc *(mandioca),* a starchy root, is usually eaten at most meals. It is typically served peeled and boiled, although it may be fried or made into flour to make traditional Paraguayan bagel-like breads known as *chipa*. Meats such as roasted chicken, boiled beef, and pork are also common fare. In general, traditional Paraguayan food is not heavily spiced. Use of eating implements such as forks, knives, and spoons is expected and common in all but the poorest communities, who cannot afford them. Dried and ground leaves of the *yerba* mate plant are used extensively to make warm tea known as *mate* ("MAH the") or cold tea known as or *te tade* ("teh dah DEH"). *Mate* with sugar and other spices added is known as *cocido*. *Mate* is usually consumed socially throughout the day in the company of several friends, acquaintances, or family members. *Mate* is drunk from a communal cup known as a *bombea* ("bom BEEAH") and a filtered straw, the *wompa* ("wohm PAH"). The cup is passed from person to person. When people decide they have had enough, they simply say "gracias" when the *wompa* is offered to them again. *Mate* has a slight stimulant affect, similar to but distinct from caffeine. Although some have proposed that *mate* has beneficial health effects, some studies have linked *mate* consumption with esophageal cancer, although the heat of the drink and not its ingredients seems to be the most risky aspect.

Infant Feeding Practices: According to the 1990 Demographic and Health Survey conducted by the Paraguay Center of Population Studies, the mean duration of breast-feeding was 11 months, although data on variations were unavailable. Breast-feeding is a common practice in rural and urban settings. No customs that would seem unusual to Westerners are practiced. Virtually all Ache infants are weaned by approximately 3 years.

Child Rearing Practices: In urban areas, children are raised in typical Western fashion. Depending on socioeconomic status, mothers breast-feed discretely in public; poorer mothers often nurse a child in public to keep a job such as selling *chipas* or *mate* on the street. In rural regions, breast-feeding is discrete and not uncommon.

National Childhood Immunizations: BCG at birth; DTP at 2, 4, 6, and 18 months and 4 years; OPV at 2, 4, 6, and 18 months and 4 years; TT/dT CBAW ×5; DTPHH at 2, 4, and 6 months; measles at 12 months; MMR at 1 and 4 years; and YFV younger than 1 year along endemic borders. The Pan American Health Organization reports the following immunization coverage percentages for children younger than 1 year: DPT, 82%; third dose of OPV, 82%; BCG, 87%; and measles, 60%.

Other Characteristics: When arriving at a person's home, it is rude to knock on the door. The common practice is to clap the hands loudly two or three times. Approximately 39% of the population (59% urban, 7% rural) has access to drinking water services, with "access" being defined as being within 200 m of a water source; 32% (22% urban, 44% rural) has access to sanitation services. Urban systems include basic latrines and septic tanks, whereas rural facilities include mostly latrines. The percentage of the population living in poverty as reported by the PAHO is 21.8%.

BIBLIOGRAPHY

Bull SS, Melian M: Contraception and culture: the use of *yuyos* in Paraguay, *Health Care Women Int* 19:49–60, 1998.

Castellsague X et al: Influence of mate drinking, hot beverages and diet on esophageal cancer risk in South America, *Int J Cancer* 88:658–664, 2000.

Hill K, Hurtado M: Ache life history: the ecology and demography of a foraging people, New York, 1996, Adline de Gruyter Press.

Krayacich de Oddone N et al: Paraguayan pharmacies and the sale of pseudo-abortifacients, *J Biosoc Sci* 23:201–209, 1991.

Mazzuchi N et al: Latin American registry of dialysis and renal transplantation: 1993 annual dialysis data report, *Nephrol Dial Transpl* 12:2521–2527, 1997.

Neffen H et al: Asthma mortality in Latin America, *J Invest Allergol Clin Immunol* 7:249–253, 1997.

Pan American Health Organization (1999): *Paraguay: basic country health profiles, summaries 1999*. Retrieved February 11, 2002, from http://www.paho.org/English/SHA/prflpar.htm

Patterson MC: A medical survey of a South American Indian tribe in the Paraguayan Chaco, *Trop Doctor* 10:124–128, 1980.

Population Council Paraguay: Results from the demographic and health survey, *Stud Fam Plann* 23:137–141, 1992.

Russell KL et al: Emerging genetic diversity of HIV-1 in South America, *AIDS* 14:1785–1791, 2000.

Santiago-Delpin EA, Garcia VD: Organ transplantation in Latin America, *Clin Transpl* pp 115–122, 2000.

Schmeda-Hirschmann G: Magic and medicinal plants of the Ayoreos of the Chaco Boreal (Paraguay), *J Ethnopharmacol* 39:105–111, 1993.

Simancas LC, Zuniga MRG: Population policies and reproductive health in Paraguay, *Cadernos de Saúde Pública* 14:105–114, 1998.

U.S. State Department (2002): *Background note: Paraguay*. Retrieved February 3, 2002, from http://www.state.gov/r/pa/bgn/1841.htm

World Health Organization: Guiding principles on human organ transplantation, *Lancet* 337:1470–1471, 1991.

◆ PERU (REPUBLIC OF)

MAP PAGE (859)

Haq Nawaz and Devon Graham

Location: Peru is located on the western coast of South America and is the continent's third largest country in land area (after Brazil and Argentina) and fourth largest in population (after Brazil, Argentina and Colombia). It covers a total land area of 1,285,222 km^2 (496,225 square miles) (roughly three times the size of California). The country is divided into three broad geographical regions—the Pacific Coast, the Andes Mountains, and the Amazon lowlands—and 23 departamentos (provinces). The capital, Lima, on the central Pacific coast, is the most populous city in Peru. The rugged Andes Mountains run the length of the country. The eastern third is covered by largely intact Amazon rain forest. The major rivers in the eastern part of the country include the Napo (flowing from Ecuador into Peru), the Ucayali (which includes the headwaters of the Amazon River), and the Marañon, which joins with the Ucayali to form the Amazon River itself. The climate varies by the region. Coastal areas are arid and mild, the Andes are temperate to frigid, and the Amazon lowlands are typically warm and humid.

Major Languages	Ethnic Groups	Major Religions
Spanish (official)	Amerindian 45%	Roman Catholic 90%
Quechua (official)	Mestizo (European,	Other 10%
Aymara	Amerindian) 37%	
Other native	White 15%	
languages	Other (Japanese,	
	Chinese, Black) 3%	

The population was estimated to be 25.7 million in 2000, with a majority (70%) residing in urban areas. The population is concentrated in larger urban centers on the Pacific coast, with the lowest population density in the Amazon lowlands. The capital, Lima, has an estimated population of 8.27 million—approximately one third of the total population. White and Mestizo populations are concentrated along the coast and in urban areas in the highlands. Pure Amerindian populations are found primarily in the Andean highlands (particularly in the south), on the eastern slopes of the Andes, and in the Amazon lowlands. Spanish is the principal language of government, commerce, and education. Quechua and Aymara are widely spoken among the Amerindian population of the highlands, whereas various languages of the Quechua language family are spoken among scattered tribes in the Amazon lowlands. Peru has two primary social classes, a rich upper class (predominantly of Spanish and European background) and a poor lower class (primarily Amerindian and Mestizo), as well as a small but increasing middle class. The official religion is Roman Catholic, although Protestant and other sects are increasing rapidly in many areas. Catholicism in the highlands has been heavily influenced by Amerindian beliefs dating from the Inca Empire. In the Amazon lowlands, rural people often meld Catholicism with traditional animist beliefs.

Health Care Beliefs: Acute sick care; traditional. In urban areas, most people have a basic understanding of disease and its etiology. In remote and the poorest urban areas (with high proportions of immigrants from rural areas), many people have a limited education, and folklore and native concepts of disease are prevalent. Many consider illness to be a direct result of witchcraft, whereas others may believe it to be caused by "hot" and "cold" imbalances. In one study in which mothers in Lima were interviewed about their beliefs about children's diarrhea, most mothers thought that diarrhea was caused by ingesting "cold" food, with consequent invasion of the body by "cold" elements. Milk was withheld as a treatment. Similarly, a survey conducted by the authors revealed that only 34% of the people in some Amazon villages believe that mosquitoes cause malaria. Approximately 47% of people in the survey reported using alternative health care, and approximately 73% strongly believed that alternative health care was effective.

Predominant Sick Care Practices: Biomedical, alternative and magical-religious. The predominant sick care models are biomedical and magico-religious, with the latter being most prevalent in areas with proportionately high numbers of Amerindians. Many medications are available without a prescription, and pharmacists may prescribe medications to people who discuss their various symptoms. Modern medicine may be combined or supplanted by traditional medical practices. Many communities have *curanderos*, *shamans,* or *brujos* who are consulted in cases of illness or misfortune. *Curanderos* can be men or women and function primarily as herbalists, using a wide range of plant species to treat an equally wide range of medical conditions. Many rural people maintain small medicinal plant gardens for home treatment of common conditions, and most rural people (and many urban ones) are familiar with the medicinal uses of various plants. *Shamans* (exclusively men) combine herbal medicine with magico-spiritual beliefs and practices and are consulted for particularly serious cases and for cases in which evil spirits or influences may be involved. *Shamans* practice what would be considered in western European culture to be white magic. In contrast, *brujos* (warlocks) and *brujas* (witches) practice black magic and are consulted for the purposes of casting harmful spells or curses on perceived enemies. *Brujos* and *brujas* are rarely publicly acknowledged and maintain a low profile. *Curanderos* and *shamans* are well known and respected. In urban areas, holistic and New Age medical practices are becoming more common. Peru has several systems of health care. Branches of the military and police each have their own independent hospital or clinic system to attend to their employees and their families. The EsSalud hospital system is the social security and insurance health system in the country, with participants (or their employers) making monthly payments into the system. Numerous private hospitals and clinics cater primarily to the middle and upper classes. However, the majority of the population is served by the public health system operated by the Peruvian Ministry of Health. This was previously a fee-based system, although students who were enrolled in school were entitled to free medical care. In January 2002 a new system of medical care was instituted for Peruvians with no other medical coverage. To access this system, participants must register with the public health system, which requires a background check to ensure that they do not have any other health coverage. After a satisfactory check, medications and most procedures are free. Public hospitals are located in larger urban centers, and areas outside of these cities have a network of small hospitals (with one or two doctors) or health posts (*puestos de salud*—operated by a doctor or nurse). Most communities have a health promoter *(promotor de salud),* an unpaid member of the community who receives some medical and public health training. The health promoter is responsible for such tasks as assisting professional medical personnel during vaccination campaigns, promoting sanitary practices in the community, and reporting any contagious disease outbreaks. In theory, health promoters receive a basic medical kit for use by the community. Many people, particularly those in rural areas, are reluctant to go to clinics or hospitals when they are ill. Rural people (other than school children) rarely benefit from any form of health coverage and consequently must pay for consultations and medications. Although cost is one deterrent, clinics and hospitals are difficult to access for many rural people, and many hours or even days of travel away. Mental illness, schizophrenia, and epilepsy are not common. Peru has institutions in some larger cities for those with mental illness, but in smaller urban centers and rural areas, those thought to have a mental illness are either cared for by family members or are homeless, living in the street, subsisting from charity. The same is true of children born with birth defects or Down syndrome. Such conditions may be thought of as the result of a curse or actions of evil spirits. Most medications, including antibiotics, are available without a prescription at pharmacies. Narcotics are available by prescription. Many available medications are produced nationally or in neighboring Colombia, and prices are relatively low. However, people from the lower economic classes may still find that medications are unaffordable.

Ethnic/Race Specific or Endemic Diseases: Malaria and dengue fever are prevalent, and tuberculosis is a major public health problem. Like most underdeveloped countries, diseases linked to poor hygiene and infections are common and include yellow fever, diphtheria, salmonella, and typhoid fever. Incidence of malaria varies with terrain and local environment and is higher in the tropical northern coast and lowland Amazon jungle. The prevalence of cholera is higher in rural and jungle areas of the country. The indigenous population in rural areas is at a disadvantage and has higher rates of infectious diseases. Indigenous rural people lack many amenities such as safe drinking water that are available to the urban population, which partially explains the differences in health. For example, the maternal mortality rate in urban areas is 185 per 100,000 live births, whereas in rural areas it is as high as 448 per 100,000 per live births. The World Health Organization's (WHO) estimated prevalence rate for HIV/AIDS in adults ages 15 to 49 is 0.35%. The estimated number of children from birth to 15 years living with HIV/AIDS is 640. According to the Pan American Health Organization (PAHO), as of 2001 Peru had a total of 10,539 cases of AIDS and 4342 deaths attributed to AIDS. The total number of new AIDS cases has remained steady at approximately 1000 cases per year. However, underreporting and incorrect diagnosis are significant problems. The number of new cases of AIDS is approximately three times higher in men than women; however, this gap is narrowing. For instance, in 1997 the ratio of male to female cases was 4.7, while in 1999 the ratio narrowed to 3.3. Approximately 3% of all cases are infants who are infected at the time of birth. Major modes of transmission are heterosexual (47%) and homosexual or bisexual contact (48%).

Health Team Relationships: Peruvians are conscious of their status and title. Most people (other than close friends and family) with an advanced degree or position are addressed by their title or position as a sign of respect and recognition. The term *doctor* is used (with or without the surname) when addressing medical doctors. Likewise, *enfermera* and *technico* are used to address nurses and lab technicians. The health care system has a clear hierarchy of responsibility and authority.

Families' Role in Hospital Care: In most cases the family is involved in the care of hospitalized family members. Although larger hospitals provide food, smaller clinics and hospitals may not have this capability, so family members are consequently responsible for providing food for patients. One or more family members often stay with patients for part of the day, although they may stay all day and night with relatives who have critical or terminal conditions. Families are generally involved in decisions concerning medical procedures, and the extended family may come together to raise money to pay for expensive treatments. Patients and families are generally deferential to medical personnel, and prevention of or interference with medical examinations and procedures is rare.

Dominance Patterns: Families are male-dominated, although women may play a strong role in maintaining family finances and determining activities. Older, more established families are the most likely to have a strong male leader. Young couples often live with the wife's family until they establish a household of their own. Likewise, aging parents generally live with the family of one of their children. The extended family may include godparents and godchildren. Godparents are expected to be involved in important aspects of the lives of godchildren (e.g., higher education, marriage, illness) and are usually friends (or relatives) of the family. Naturally, godparents of higher economic standing are desirable. Children are given the surnames of their fathers' and mothers' families, with the mothers' surname coming last. The second surname is often not used in daily life but is given on all documents and used for formal occasions. Women are very active in all levels of politics and even in small, remote communities, they may be elected to positions such as village chief. Women are also becoming more involved in business, education, and medicine, and near parity has been achieved in medical school admissions. Women are poorly represented in the military, although Peru was the first South American country to train women military pilots.

Eye Contact Practices: Direct eye contact is common within and between sexes and among social classes.

Touch Practices: Men and women typically greet female acquaintances by touching cheeks on one or both sides of the face; lip contact with the other person's cheek is common but not necessary. Men greet other men with a handshake, and men and women also use a handshake for greeting women with whom they are not familiar. Greetings in a professional relationship generally include a handshake. Amerindians of the Peruvian highlands are generally more reserved in social settings than urban people or Amerindians of the Amazon lowlands. Touching during conversations is common.

Perceptions of Time: Among rural people, time is relative to other events, rather than being a discrete entity. Rural people are very aware of what day it is, and what important events occur on which days (thanks to the medium of radio, and to the elementary schools that are present in all but the smallest communities), but there is little urgency (or, in most cases, need) to initiate or complete tasks by certain times or dates. Urban people are necessarily more time conscious. Punctuality is expected of employees of lower status, but not necessarily for higher-ranking individuals. One measure of social standing and/or importance of position is how long people will wait for you.

Pain Reactions: Pain may be expressed vocally and through facial expressions. However, rural people, whether adults or children, are often stoical. Often the health care provider may have to ask direct questions about whether a patient has pain. Men seem to be expected to bear pain better than women, and women seem to be more vocal about their pain. Many people, particularly those in rural areas, may avoid visiting hospitals or clinics until medical conditions are aggravated or severe. People may be observed carrying out daily tasks despite having medical conditions that are quite painful.

Birth Rites: Births usually occur at home, particularly among the lower classes. A midwife generally assists the expectant mother, and female relatives may help as well. Fathers are not usually present for labor and delivery. Hospital deliveries are increasingly common in urban areas and among the upper classes. Male circumcisions are not routine. Infants are baptized soon after birth (if they are Catholic), although in some remote areas a priest only visits once a year; he baptizes all the infants born since his last visit and gives a Mass for those who have died. In rural areas, parents take little or no time off from their normal schedule after a birth, although female members of the extended family typically assist new mothers. In urban areas, working women continue to work well into their pregnancies and generally take some time off after delivery. Births of boys and girls are celebrated. Family sizes are smallest in urban areas and highest in the rural Amazon lowlands, in which 10 or more children per family is not uncommon. Government programs encourage family planning through various methods, including extending breast-feeding, the rhythm method, condom use (which is also promoted for preventing HIV transmission), intrauterine devices, vasectomies, and tubal ligations. Tubal ligations are common among rural women but are generally only performed after a woman has had 5 to 8 children. Few men obtain vasectomies, and condom use is not widespread except among younger educated people in urban areas. Tubal ligations and vasectomies are free in government hospitals. The infant mortality rate has been decreasing steadily and was 39 deaths per 1000 live births in 2000. As the infant mortality has decreased, the life expectancy has slowly but steadily increased from 53.6 years in 1970 to 69 years in 2002. Communicable diseases, respiratory tract infections, and intestinal infectious diseases are the most common cause of death in infants.

Death Rites: Death rites are class dependent but always involve an outward show of grief and respect for the deceased. In smaller communities, most community members join the funeral procession and interment rituals. In the highlands and Pacific coastal areas of Peru, cemeteries are a conspicuous feature of many communities. Elaborate tombstones and mausoleums are common, even for relatively poor families. Family plots are the norm, and graves are visited at least annually to place flowers and religious items and clean the plots or mausoleums. In the Amazon lowlands the dead are buried in simple graves in small cemeteries located away from villages because of fears about ghosts. Graves are marked with a simple wooden cross and periodically cleared of encroaching vegetation. Coffins are used in urban areas and among the higher social classes, with elaborate coffins being used by upper classes. Poor families may rent coffins for processional purposes. In rural areas, poorer people may simply wrap the body in a blanket or sheet. Burial is usually the day after death, and relatives have a wake, or *vela* ("candle"), for the person the night before the funeral. In urban areas, it is common for poorer families to have a procession with one or two musicians and family members carrying religious images and a collection box. Donations from passersby and area businesses are used to defray funeral expenses. Embalming and cremations are rare and practiced only by some of the upper class. Autopsies and organ donation occur only in the larger urban centers. Most of the country does not have the technical ability or facilities for organ donations. Autopsies may be performed in larger hospitals after familial permission. Peruvians have no taboos about autopsies, and they are not considered mutilation of the dead.

Food Practices and Intolerances: Rural people often eat two meals per day, one at midmorning and another meal in the late afternoon or early evening. Meals at different times of the day are often very similar. Urban people typically eat three meals, including a light breakfast and more substantial midday or evening meal. Most meals are prepared and eaten at home, although those in the urban middle and upper classes eat out regularly. Utensils are used for most foods, but it is common to use the hands to consume fruit, fish (i.e., to remove bones), and various other food items. Rural people working away from home may take a prepared lunch wrapped in a large leaf, and the meal is typically eaten with the fingers. Washing hands before eating is uncommon for rural people unless their hands are heavily soiled. Diet varies considerably among regions. On the coast, large amounts of fish and seafood are consumed, and various irrigated crops are widely available, including vegetables and grains and starches such as rice, corn, and potatoes. Processed and "fast" foods are widely available in urban areas. In the mountainous highlands, dietary staples are corn, potatoes (many varieties), and indigenous grains such as quinoa and kiwicha. Meat protein in the mountains comes in part from *cuy* (guinea-pig) and llama. In mountain and coastal regions, better recognized domesticated animals (e.g., cattle, pigs, sheep, chickens, turkeys) are also raised, and some dairy industry is active. In the Amazon lowlands, fish is consumed at most meals, and fish allergies are common. Basic starches include manioc *(yuca)* and plantains *(plátano)*, and some rice and corn are also cultivated. Few vegetables are cultivated or consumed, and almost no dairy products are consumed in other than larger urban areas. Native and introduced fruit trees of many species are commonly planted around homes and villages, and children often consume fruit. A wide variety of wild game is also eaten in the Amazon lowlands, including monkey, *peccary* (wild pig), deer, *paca* (a large nocturnal rodent), and wild birds. Snakes are considered inedible. Chickens, ducks, and pigs are commonly raised domestic animals in the Amazon, whereas cattle and water buffalo are rare. Indigenous alcoholic beverages are prepared and consumed in all parts of the country. In the coastal area and highlands, the common alcoholic beverage is *chicha*, prepared from fermented germinated corn kernels. In the Amazon lowlands, *masatto* is prepared from cooked and chewed manioc root. *Aguardiente*, or firewater, distilled from sugar cane juice, is widely available in the Pacific and Amazon lowlands. Children in rural areas often drink lightly fermented *chicha* or *masatto*. Alcoholism is a problem among the poorer classes and occurs in rural and urban areas. Smoking of processed or crude tobacco is widespread but because of economic factors, most people do not smoke large quantities daily or on a regular basis. In the highlands, it is common to chew coca leaves for their mild stimulant effects to combat fatigue and the effects of altitude, and use of the coca leaf is not considered drug abuse. In the Amazon lowlands, consumption of the *ayahuasca* hallucinogenic drink (prepared from *Banisteropsis* vines, *Psychotria* leaves, and other plant additives) for medical, magical, and spiritual purposes is likewise an accepted practice. Peru has an increasing problem in larger urban areas with abuse of hard drugs (cocaine, heroine, various designer drugs).

Infant Feeding Practices: The government promotes breast-feeding as the best option nutritionally for infants, which also serves as a natural contraceptive measure. Breast-feeding in public is accepted and common in rural areas, although less so in urban centers. Infant formula is available only in urban areas, and most rural people do not have access to it or cannot afford it. In urban areas, middle-class families often feed their children formula to indicate their superior social status. The period of exclusive breast-feeding is usually very short, and supplementation with solids and other foods begins at a relatively young age. Approximately 40% of children younger than 3 months receive food to supplement breast-feeding, and only 32% at age 4 to 6 months are exclusively breast-fed. By age 9 months, approximately 6% are breast-feeding exclusively. Growing children often share the food eaten at home, and obesity in infants or children is considered a sign of health. Chronic malnutrition is prevalent (up to 40% of young rural children) and is attributable to inadequate food intake, poor food preparation, presence of intestinal parasites, and frequent illnesses. Children of mothers with no formal education fare the worst; 50% are either undernourished or malnourished.

Child Rearing Practices: Children are treated affectionately and are rarely alone. Physical discipline is rare, and children are expected to help with household chores at a young age, particularly in rural areas. By the age of 8 to 10 years, boys are assisting their fathers with clearing fields, fishing, and care of domestic animals, and girls are helping with cooking, caring for younger siblings, and other domestic chores. Older sisters routinely care for younger siblings, and all members of extended families (and even entire villages) are involved in child rearing. Parents are not overly protective, and children regularly play unsupervised on streets and in empty lots in urban areas. In the Amazon lowlands, children play in canoes and in the water and learn to swim at a young age. It is common to see toddlers in canoes being paddled around by slightly older siblings. Grandparents typically live with the family of one of their children and help to keep an eye on grandchildren. Upper-class families often hire a nursemaid or nanny to care for children. Middle- and upper-class children are generally enrolled in private or parochial schools, whereas other children receive a public school education. Peruvian law dictates that all children attend 6 years of school, but many children in rural areas and from poorer families often miss school because no school is nearby or they need to help support the family. The normal school day is half a day (either morning or afternoon/evening), and the school year is from April to December. January to March is harvest time in many parts of the country, and children are needed to help with the crops. Children who are homeless (because either both parents have died or their families are too poor to support them) can be found in the larger cities. These children support themselves by begging or doing odd jobs for spare change. The government encourages these children to attend school, but enforcement is difficult. Girls often marry or live with a man from the age of 16 and older, whereas men are typically a few years older. Young couples frequently live with the wife's family and thus continue to help care for younger relatives. Eventually the young couple builds or obtains a house of their own. Except among the middle and upper classes, children do not have private rooms; they share a single room with their siblings or parents. In rural areas, sleeping arrangements are often a mattress or mat on the floor. In areas with malaria, government programs provide each family with a large mosquito net under which most family members sleep. In urban areas, most people use standard beds. In rural and urban areas, people are becoming more aware of the problem of sexual abuse of children, and public campaigns to raise awareness of and prevent sexual abuse have been initiated in recent years.

National Childhood Immunizations: BCG at birth; DTP at 2, 3, and 4 months; OPV at birth and 2, 3, and 4 months; hep B at birth and 2 months; HIB at 2, 3, and 4 months (in endemic areas); measles at 12 months; vitamin A at 6 to 11 and 12 to 23 months; and YFV at 9 months in endemic areas. Average rates of childhood vaccination are generally higher than 90%. Hepatitis B vaccinations are administered only in areas of the country in which hepatitis B is endemic (e.g., Rio Pastaza, Rio Napo area), areas where coverage is almost 100%. Childhood immunizations have been free from their initiation, as is treatment for numerous medical conditions that are considered public health threats, such as malaria, yellow fever, dengue, cholera, and tuberculosis. Government health programs emphasizing malaria and dengue prevention, AIDS prevention, family planning, prevention of infant diarrhea, cholera, and other health-related problems are prominent in urban areas.

Other Characteristics: Peru is considered to be a developing country. The per capita gross domestic product (GDP) in 2000 was $2101 per year. According to government statistics, by December 2001 the unemployment rate had increased to 9% in urban areas; however, the actual rates are thought to be substantially higher. Failed economic reforms between 1960 and 1990 pushed the country into a deep recession. With recent economic stability and the elimination of previous terrorist and drug-production activities, the country's considerable tourism potential is being increasingly exploited. The government is the single largest employer in the country.

BIBLIOGRAPHY

Central Intelligence Agency: *Peru: The world factbook.* Retrieved February 7, 2002, from http://www.odci.gov/cia/publications/factbook/geos/pe.html

Economic Commission for Latin America and Caribbean, Economic Development: *Economic survey of Latin America and the Caribbean 1999–2000,* LC/G.2102-P/I, December 2000.

Economic Commission for Latin America and Caribbean, Economic Development Division: *Preliminary overview of the economies of Latin America and the Caribbean 2000,* LLC/G.2123-P/I, December 2000.

Encuesta Permanente de Empleo en Lima Metropolitana: *Inform de empleo,* No. 1, Lima, Peru, Instituto Nacional de Estada e Informatice, 2002.

Escobar GJ, Salazar E, Chuy M: Beliefs regarding the etiology and treatment of infantile diarrhea in Lima, Peru, *Soc Sci Med* 17(17):1257–1269, 1983.

Library of Congress, Federal Research Division: *Peru—a country study. Country studies. Area handbook series.* Retrieved February 7, 2002 from http://lcweb2.loc.gov/frd/cs/petoc.html

Nawaz H et al: Health risk behaviors and health perceptions in the Peruvian Amazon, *Am J Trop Med Hyg* 65(3):252–256, 2001.

Pan American Health Organization: *Biannual report. Regional program on AIDS and STIs,* December 2001, World Health Organization AIDS Surveillance in the Americas, Division of Disease Prevention and Control; World Health Organization, PAHO, and UNAIDS Working Group on Global HIV/AIDS and STI Surveillance.

Pan American Health Organization: *Biannual report. Regional program on AIDS and STIs,* May 2000, World Health Organization AIDS Surveillance in the Americas, Division of Disease Prevention and Control; World Health Organization, PAHO, and UNAIDS Working Group on Global HIV/AIDS and STI Surveillance.

Pan American Health Organization: *Country immunization profile. Peru,* Washington, DC, March 2001, PAHO, Pan American Sanitary Bureau, Regional Office of the World Health Organization.

Pan American Health Organization: *Health in the Americas*, Scientific Pub No 5691998, 1998, Pan American Sanitary Bureau, Regional Office of the World Health Organization.

Peruvian Ministry of Health: Personal communication, February 2002.

U.S. Department of State, Bureau of Western Hemisphere Affairs (April 2001): *Peru, background notes.* Retrieved February 7, 2002, from http://www.state.gov/r/pa/bgn/2056.htm

World Bank Group: *Peru at a glance, 2000 data*. Retrieved February 7, 2002, from http://www.worldbank.org/data/

◆ PHILIPPINES (REPUBLIC OF)

MAP PAGE (867)

Lorraine Antolin D'Avanzo (Consultant: Nelly P. Alamo)

Location: An archipelago approximately 500 miles off the southeast coast of Asia, the Philippines consists of approximately 7000 volcanic islands, of which 880 are inhabited. The larger islands—Luzon in the north, Visayas in the central region, and Mindanao in the south—are crossed with mountain ranges. Only approximately 7% of the islands are larger than 1 square miles. Its boundaries are the Luzon Strait to the north, Philippine Sea to the east, Celebes Sea to the south, Sulu Sea to the southwest, and the South China Sea to the west. Luzon and Mindanao account for 66% of the land area.

Major Languages	Ethnic Groups	Major Religions
Pilipino (i.e., Tagalog, official)	Christian Malay 91%	Roman Catholic 83%
English (official)	Muslim Malay (Moro) 4%	Protestant 9%
Other	Chinese 2%	Muslim 5%
	Other (upland tribal) 3%	Buddhist, other 3%

Eleven languages and 87 dialects are indigenous in the archipelago. Dialects such as Tagalog, Cebuano, Ilocano, Hiligaynon, Bicolano, Waray-Waray, Pampangan, and Pangasian are still the native languages for much of the population. The Philippines has been named one of the most disaster-prone areas on earth, with floods, earthquakes, volcanic eruptions, typhoons, tsunamis, land slides, ferry accidents, and Muslim insurgents all being significant problems. After centuries of intermarriage, Filipinos have become a blend of Chinese, Malay, Spanish (Mestizos), Negrito, and American. Although church and state have been officially separated since the 1990s, the Roman Catholic Church's influence on the government is reflected in the prohibition of divorce and the lack of resources allocated to family planning.

Health Care Beliefs: Crisis health care; passive role. Mental illness is highly stigmatized and is usually believed to be rooted in witchcraft or demonic possession; for example, people with the "evil eye" can curse another person with their eyes or mouth. If orthodox medical therapies are unsuccessful, an illness may be attributed to forces of nature, dwarfs, spells, sins, or past misdeeds.

Predominant Sick Care Practices: Biomedical, magical-religious and traditional. Modern medicine is based on the germ theory and involves scientifically educated practitioners. The traditional system is based on taboos set by supernatural forces. Those in urbanized areas tend to consult professional providers. Magico-religious forms of care are most common in remote areas, and home remedies are often used. A sense of fatalism stems from beliefs that ghosts and spirits control life and death. Usurping the powers of the gods is believed to have a cause-and-effect relationship to subsequent misfortunes. In general, many individuals alternate between the two systems, using a combination of home remedies, professional providers, and traditional healers. Poverty has made mainstream health care unaffordable for most of the rural population (with approximately 41% living below poverty line) and is used as a last resort. Alternative therapies such as herbal, unapproved medications, consultation with an *albularyo* or a *hilot* (village healer), faith healing and prayer are the norm outside of major cities. *Albylaryos,* or *medicos,* lack formal education of any kind and are the primary dispensers of health care. *Hilots* are midwives and chiropractic and massage practitioners; it is believed that individuals born by breech delivery are destined to become *hilots*. Because fees are thought to decrease their powers, *albylaryos* and *hilots* are paid with goods or services. The health care system is considered adequate in urban areas and minimal in rural areas, similar to the situation in other Southeast Asian countries. Improvements in public and private sector health programs are attempting to fill in the gaps in health care delivery. Some employees receive medical and dental benefits from their employers. Private insurance is available for those who can afford it, and may people choose private-pay systems. Some government-sponsored hospitals charge very minimal fees for their services, and public assistance programs are a safety net for the poor.

Ethnic/Race Specific or Endemic Diseases: Endemic diseases include chloroquine-sensitive and chloroquine-resistant malaria (although not in urban areas) and tuberculosis. Vitamin A deficiency is a common cause of childhood blindness, and the country has dengue hemorrhagic fever outbreaks every 2 to 3 years. Significant morbidity from noninfectious diseases is attributed to diarrhea, bronchitis, bronchiolitis, pneumonias, influenza, hypertension, heart disease, chickenpox, and typhoid and paratyphoid fever. Infectious diseases continue to be the leading cause of morbidity and mortality, with approximately 75 Filipinos dying of tuberculosis every day. The Philippines has the worst tuberculosis problem in the

Western Pacific, with an estimated 30 million people infected (32% of the population). Of the 69 provinces, 66 have endemic malaria and in rural areas, infection rates are 40% to 60%. The leading causes of mortality in descending order are heart disease, vascular system diseases, pneumonia, accidents, cancer, tuberculosis (all forms), chronic obstructive pulmonary disease (COPD) and other respiratory diseases, diabetes mellitus, and nephritis and nephritic syndrome. The World Health Organization's (WHO) estimated prevalence of HIV/AIDS in adults ages 15 to 49 years is 0.07%. The estimated number of children from birth to 15 years living with HIV/AIDS is 1300. Most HIV infections are transmitted through heterosexual activity. Although prevalence is low, an active sex industry and a considerable population of those who use intravenous drugs has prompted a national prevention and control program for HIV/AIDS and other sexually transmitted diseases.

Health Team Relationships: Authority is respected and it is believed that a professional's time is valuable; therefore a health problem must be serious or it is not mentioned. Nurses may carry out a doctor's order rather than question it. In the same way, rather than give a "no" answer to a question, patients may remain silent or respond with a hesitant "yes." An influential group member often makes group decisions. An intermediary may be used for confrontational situations. In the late 1980s and early 1990s, approximately 500,000 migrants maintained a Philippine residence but worked abroad. Nurses and doctors have migrated to the United States for training and work experience. Many have remained in the United States and have become permanent residents. The Philippines has approximately 33,000 health professionals, including 9500 doctors. Approximately 1700 hospitals with 85,000 beds are concentrated in urban areas.

Families' Role in Hospital Care: Loyalty is a social imperative, so children may feel an obligation to parents who are ill and spend hours giving care. Because loyalty to the immediate family comes first, patients can expect full care from family members, and often several members of the family help each other care for loved ones. Because of the close family bonds, care is also traditionally provided for more distant extended family members as well. Traditional values are clung to, particularly in rural areas. The family is central to Filipinos' identity, and kinship ties are central to friendships and relationships.

Dominance Patterns: The interests of the family are considered before any individual needs. Obligatory tasks of caring for the family unit are played out, strengthening the unit structure. For example, the oldest child is educated through the family's efforts; therefore the child is expected to continue to "sacrifice" for the next sibling and so on. Protection against outsiders, dependency, harmony, and reciprocity of obligation are group values. Women in the Philippines have always enjoyed greater equality with men than in most other parts of Southeast Asia, with unquestioned rights to legal equality and inheritance. Literacy rates for women are higher than for men, and it is common for women to be appointed to important positions in business and government. However, although women are eligible for high-level positions, in reality they are frequently held by men. Women traditionally control the family finances yet are generally submissive to men and have tolerated a double standard of sexual conduct (although this is changing). Restricted divorce laws are considered by some to be an infringement on women's liberty and by others to be a protection against abandonment and loss of support. In rural areas, wives usually stay at home to take care of the children. When the children are grown, the wife then helps the husband earn their livelihood.

Eye Contact Practices: Some fear eye contact; however, if it is established, it is important to return and to maintain the eye contact.

Touch Practices: Touch is considered a friendly gesture and more encouraged between friends who are the same sex. It is not unusual to see girls walking together arm-in-arm. In some parts of the country, it is believed that an "evil eye" curse that has been placed on a child can be neutralized by putting a bit of saliva on the finger and making the sign of the cross on the child's forehead while giving a compliment.

Perceptions of Time: Filipinos have a relaxed sense of time. Time generally moves ahead slowly, and they have the attitude that "We'll get there when we get there." Being an hour late for appointments is considered perfectly acceptable. Life is lived from day to day.

Pain Reactions: Pain is endured for as long as possible. High thresholds of pain are expected, especially if a cure is financially out of reach. People also may seem stoical if they believe pain is the will of God and that God will give them the strength to bear it.

Birth Rites: Filipino women are modest. They often delay or neglect receiving prenatal care and Pap tests to avoid being examined by male doctors. Millions of poor Filipino women have little or no access to adequate family planning or reproductive health care. Approximately 20 million women are in their childbearing years, and their greatest health risks are related to pregnancy and childbirth. Department of Health studies indicate that more Filipino mothers die from pregnancy and childbirth than from any other cause because of hemorrhaging, hypertension, and abortive outcomes. The high fertility rate (3.42 children born per woman) has grave consequences for social welfare, economic growth, and the environment. USAID is targeting poor Filipinas to reduce the birth rates (which is currently 27.37 births per 1000 people). It is believed daily bathing and shampooing during pregnancy results in a clean baby and that sexual intercourse may harm the woman and the infant. In the past, women were encouraged to stay in bed for a week or more after birth, and bathing or showering were prohibited. These practices are now obsolete. Restricted activities, rather than total bed rest, are now the norm. In rural areas, new mothers take a special bath with warm water and herbal leaves at some point after birth. After the bath, regardless of the room temperature, the new mother wears warm clothing and keeps covered with blankets if necessary to keep warm.

Death Rites: Patients are frequently not told about a poor prognosis because relatives prefer not to add to the person's suffering. Family members who die are kept for 1 week in the family home for bereavement. Religious ceremonies are held nightly, and family and friends have a feast on the ninth day after the burial. The Organ Donation Act of 1991 promotes transplantation of organs in the Philippines.

Food Practices and Intolerances: Rice is the staple food. Preferred foods are a mixture of fish, vegetables, and native fruits. Malnutrition is a continuing problem. In the late 1980s, reports indicated that 3% of preschoolers had third-degree malnutrition, and 18% had second-degree malnutrition. Targeted food assistance for preschoolers and lactating mothers is believed to have improved these numbers. In the late 1980s, consumption of milk tripled and fats and oils nearly doubled, changes that are believed to be contributing to increases in cardiovascular diseases.

Infant Feeding Practices: Breast-feeding is common until 2 years of age, although the percentage of breast-fed babies has decreased in the past 2 decades. Infants are usually fed on demand. Timed or scheduled feedings are unusual. Mothers who are not employed usually feed their babies on demand. Even infants who are breast-fed, begin receiving solid foods when they have teeth or even as young as 4 months. Infants are fed with mashed cooked rice and fruits such as bananas.

Child Rearing Practices: Infants are not usually separated from their mothers and until they are toddlers sleep with their parents in cribs in the parents' room. Disposable diapers are used by those who can afford them. Washable diapers are usually used for infants until they are 1 year. Infants are toilet trained at a young age without diapers, and they learn quickly not to urinate on themselves. Children stay with parents until they are married, regardless of their age. Parents have the responsibility to send their children to school, which is the reason older children are obligated to help their parents or younger siblings.

National Childhood Immunizations: BCG at birth; DPT at 6, 10, and 14 weeks; OPV at 6, 10, and 14 weeks; hep B at 6, 10, and 14 weeks; measles at 9 months; and TT at first contact during pregnancy, +4 weeks, +6 months, +1, +1 year. The estimated percentages of the population vaccinated are as follows: BCG, 81%; first dose of DTP, 80%; third dose of DTP, 79%; hep B, 3%; Pol3, 75%; and MCV, 80%.

Other Characteristics: Filipinos are hospitable people, and a person can stop by for a visit without any previous notice. Visitors can expect a meal during their unexpected visit. Filipinos are also quite sensitive emotionally and tend to value shared rather than private possessions or property. A bond between two people may be formed on the basis of *utang na loob.* For example, it is assumed that when a gift is given, it will be repaid; some debts (such as obligations to parents) can never be fully repaid, so the obligation lasts for generations. Gifts may result in long-term dependencies in which the giver and the debtor feel free to request other favors over time. As Filipino society becomes more modernized and urban, the predominantly rural concept of *utang na loob* is becoming less important. The guerilla group Abu Sayyaf has created inner turmoil in the republic through kidnappings and other terrorist activities in its pursuit of an independent Islamic state. The Philippines exports locally grown marijuana and hashish to East Asia, the United States, and other Western countries and is a transit point for crystal methamphetamine and heroin.

BIBLIOGRAPHY

AIDS and infectious diseases. Retrieved February 16, 2002, from http://www. usaid-ph.gov/aids%20&%20id_usaid.htm

Althen GL, Jaime J: *Assumptions and values in Philippine, American and other cultures, class materials,* Portland, Ore, 1991, Summer Institute of Intercultural Communication.

Chernack C: Speak up ... Dula Pacquaio, *NJ Nurse* 25(6):3, 1995.

Davis CF: Culturally responsive nursing management in an international health care setting. In Brown BJ, ed: On the scene, *Nurs Adm Q* 16(2):36, 1992.

Luyas G: How Filipino mothers care for their young children, *UT Nurse* 5(1):7, 1991.

Philippines: The role and staus of the Filipina. Retrieved February 16, 2002, from http://memory.loc.gov/cgi-bin/query/r?frd/cstudy@field

Population, health and nutrition. Retrieved February 16, 2002. http://www. usaid-ph.gov/health_usaid.htm

Rowell M: Eradication of vitamin A deficiency with 5 cents and a vegetable garden, *J Ophthalmic Nurs Tech* 12(5):217, 1993.

Spector RE: *Cultural diversity in health & illness,* ed 4, Stamford, Conn, 1996, Appleton & Lange.

Stuart G: *Albularyos and hilots*. Retrieved March 1, 2002 from http://www. stuartxchange.com/Albularyo.html

Williamson NE: Breastfeeding trends and the breastfeeding promotion program in the Philippines, *Int J Gynaecol Obstet* 30(suppl 1):35, 1990.

Wilson S: The Filipino elder: implications for nursing practice, *J Gerontol Nurs* 20(8):31, 1994.

World Health Organization (June 2000): *Epidemiological fact sheets by country,* Geneva. Retrieved March 1, 2002, from http://www.unaids.org/hivaidsinfo/statistics/ june00/fact_sheets/index.html

World Health Organization (2001): *WHO vaccine-preventable diseases: monitoring system,* Geneva. Retrieved March 1, 2002, from http://www.who.int/ vaccines/

◆ POLAND (REPUBLIC OF)

MAP PAGE (860)

Irena Wrońska and Danuta Zarzycka

Location: Poland is a north central European country with an opening to the Baltic Sea. Most of the country consists of broad plains, except for the Carpathian Mountains to the north and the Oder and Neisse Rivers to the west. Poland borders Russia, Lithuania, Belarus, and Ukraine on the east; Slovakia and the Czech Republic on the south, and Germany on the west. The total land area is 322,577 km² (124,547 square miles), and the capital is Warsaw. The total population is 38,609,400. The older the age group, the higher the percentage of women; the percentage of women age 65 and older is 62.2%, whereas the percentage of men is only 37.8%.

Major Languages	Ethnic Groups	Major Religions
Polish	Polish 98%	Roman Catholic 95%
	German, Ukrainian,	Russian Orthodox,
	Belarussian 2%	Protestant, other 5%

Poland also has smaller numbers of Lithuanians, Jews, Gypsies, and Muslims.

Health Care Beliefs: Active role; prevention important. The majority of Poles believe that health is the most important human value; therefore an increasing number of people are taking care of their own health by such steps as daily physical exercise, low-fat diets, and more involvement in sports during holidays. This healthy way of living is promoted by the mass media, such as television and newspapers. In the last few years the attitudes toward those with mental illness have changed. The quality of care for people with mental disorders has improved, and people with less serious mental impairments are being integrated into the work force. Because society's level of knowledge about health and disease has increased, few people believe in traditional treatments such as healing with heated coins. Nevertheless, cupping is still considered useful and is used as a home remedy for influenza.

Predominant Sick Care Practices: Primarily biomedical with some traditional. Poland has a public health care system with free basic and specialist care for everyone. It also has private diagnostic and therapeutic units run by professional doctors. Alternative healing in the form of bioenergy therapy, acupressure, and massage are popular, as is spiritual healing. It is estimated that millions of people use these therapies. According to surveys, most people (95% of respondents) who consult folk medicine practitioners also say they simultaneously consult practitioners in the public health care system. Wearing amulets to prevent illness is no longer common practice, whereas praying for better health is typical because most Poles are Christians.

Ethnic/Race Specific or Endemic Diseases: The highest mortality rates are from diseases of the circulatory, respiratory, and digestive systems and cancer. A major endemic health problem is iodine deficiency in regions far from the ocean, causing goiter and the risk of retardation, hypothyroidism, and cretinism. Other endemic diseases include toxoplasmosis in the eastern Lublin region bordering Ukraine, Lyme borreliosis, *Mycoplasma pneumoniae,* human alveolar echinococcosis, tick-borne encephalitis in the northeastern part of the country, and *Trichinella* infections in animals, which is transferred to humans as they eat the meat. Hepatitis A is classified as a risk. The World Health Organization's (WHO) estimated prevalence rate for HIV/AIDS in adults ages 15 to 49 is 0.06%. WHO has no estimates for children from birth to 15 years. From 1985 to 1998, 5298 HIV cases were reported. Estimates from the Ministry of Health and Social Welfare reveal that as many as 20,000 people were infected, 70% of whom were 20 to 45 year olds. HIV is being found in people of younger ages, and the incidence in women is increasing. The mode of transmission is primarily heterosexual. Many Poles continue to have the misconception that HIV is only a problem of people who are addicted to drugs and that people who are not are not at risk.

Health Team Relationships: Doctors are dominant in the health care system, as is true in other European countries. In some situations, the dominance takes the form of autocratic, superior-subordinate relationships, but in others, the dominance of doctors is considered natural by nurses because of doctors' superior knowledge and level of responsibility. However, nurses are not submissive; they foster the partnership relationships necessary for care of patients. Patient-doctor interactions tend to be more formal, whereas patient-nurse relationships are more informal, natural, and un-ceremonious.

Families' Role in Hospital Care: In the last few years the contact between patients and their families has improved because Polish hospitals have removed the strict visitation rules. In many hospitals, families are allowed to visit their relatives just after the morning doctors' rounds, and visits in the afternoon are now common. The meals served in hospitals are usually sufficient, but families may bring snacks, mineral water, and juice to patients.

Dominance Patterns: The matter of who dominates male-female relationships involves Polish history and tradition. For ages, women have played an important role in the family life of Poles, and men have respected their role. Men, on the other hand, provided for the entire family and played an important role in professional, scientific, and political life. These relationships began to change in the second half of the nineteenth century, as they did in many countries, when women began to claim their rights to study and to work. The twentieth century was the time of women's emancipation, as they increased their active participation in professional and political life. Today, many women have important, even dominant, roles in Poland. Men and women in Poland are generally considered partners and tend to cooperate.

Eye Contact Practices: Differences in eye contact are relative to timing and circumstances. Most people avoid extended periods of direct eye contact when standing close to someone. Male-female eye contact follows the pattern of most Western societies, where direct eye contact usually means attentiveness, interest, and attention.

Touch Practices: Touch is socially acceptable within limits of propriety and depends on age and gender, the range and character of the relationship, and the situation in which it occurs. Touching between members of the same sex is generally more socially acceptable than it is between members of the opposite sex. Doctors and nurses have historically used touch to communicate empathy. Shaking hands is common during greetings and during Roman Catholic religious services means "peace be with you."

Perceptions of Time: People consider punctuality to be important, although the importance varies depending on location. Rural people tend to be more relaxed about time, whereas people living in large cities who have professional jobs are more bound to strict time schedules. Tradition is valued, which is reflected in the preserved cultural objects, historical buildings, and other monuments of national identity. A distinctive characteristic of Poles is their hospitality and enjoyment of traditional celebrations, especially religious feasts such as Christmas and Easter. Differences in orientation to the present, future, or past reflect a person's age and life experience. Young people primarily live in the present and future, which is natural. Older adults, as is true in most cultures, tend to focus on past memories because thoughts of the future may conjure images of loss of independence and death.

Pain Reactions: Poles usually have high levels of pain tolerance, and differences can be attributed to gender, educational level, and past and current experiences of pain (i.e., frequency, duration, cause, intensity). Pain is monitored as a vital sign and assessed by evaluating facial expressions, body position, and movement. Poles usually use modern medicine for pain relief, and all citizens, regardless of their formal rights, are entitled to free pain relief.

Birth Rites: Most children are born in hospitals, and fathers are often present in the delivery rooms. In most Polish families the birth of a child evolves into a family festivity involving visits to the newborn and gifts. Mothers avoid certain foods when they are breast-feeding (e.g., beans, peas, cabbage) but consume vegetable and fruit juices in the postpartum period. Boys and girls are equally valued, although fathers are especially happy when a son is born. Because most Poles are Roman Catholic, the baptism ceremony is an important event. The average life expectancy is 69.8 years for men and 78 years for women.

Death Rites: The traditions in many regions of Poland determine patterns of behavior for those who are dying and those who are providing companionships for the dying. Those who are dying must be reconciled with their enemies and God. They bid farewell to friends and family members, reveal inheritances, and fulfill life obligations. Until recently, most people died at home, but today most die in hospitals because Poles are more concerned about prolonging life whenever possible. A "good death" is thought to be a painless death that occurs during sleep or suddenly at an older age and one that does not involve equipment artificially sustaining life. Those in the process of dying are in the presence of their family and friends. Most people support the transplantation of human organs from cadavers. Bodies are buried in the ground, usually according to the rites of Roman Catholicism. Poland has no tradition of cremation.

Food Practices and Intolerances: Poles consume large amounts of animal fats and sugars, although recent trends show this is decreasing. The Polish diet, except among those who live near the Baltic Sea, is lacking in iodine because of the low iodine content of soil and water. The use of iodized kitchen salt is actively promoted. Consumption of vegetables, fruits, milk, and milk products is low, and Poles tend to prefer white flour products. Eating habits include irregular meal schedules, no breakfast, heavy dinners, and hasty meal consumption. Typical foods include potatoes, soups, sauerkraut stew, sausage, and *piernik* (cake with honey). Poles are fond of spices such as horseradish, garlic, and mushrooms. About 90% of meals are eaten at home with a spoon, knife, and fork.

Infant Feeding Practices: After World War II, bottle-fed infants were the norm, but during the 1990s breast-feeding increased. About 50% of women breast-feed their children for 6 weeks, and most continue for 14 weeks. Better educated and rural women are more likely to breast-feed and to do so for longer periods. Breast-feeding is a commonly accepted and socially expected behavior, evidenced by the associations for the support of breast-feeding and the national promotion programs. Goat milk is often used as an alternative to breast milk.

Child Rearing Practices: Various birth planning methods are used; abortion is only allowed in exceptional situations. Children are usually brought up in nuclear families in which decisions about upbringing are made by both parents. In multigeneration families the grandmother plays an important role in caring for the children. Crèche, nursery school, and others are popular, and parents rely on these places for their children to learn negotiation, proper behaviors, and necessary educational tasks. As in all Western countries, upbringing and education of children and youth is considerably influenced by the mass media, primarily television and the Internet.

National Childhood Immunizations: BCG at birth, 12 months, and 7, 12, and 18 years; DTP at 2, 3 to 4, 5, and 16 to 18 months; OPV at 2, 3 to 4, 5, and 16 to 18 months and at 6 years; hep B at birth and at 1 and 6 months; measles at 13 to 14 months and 7 years; DT at 6 years; and Td at 14 and 19 years. Poland has high immunization rates—98.8% children age 2 years in 1999: tuberculosis, 95.8%; DTP, 97.7%; pertussis, 97.5%; measles, 94.5%; polio, 97.6% of 2 year olds; hep B, 98.9% of 2 year olds; and rubella, 97.4%.

BIBLIOGRAPHY

Andrews MM, Boyle JS: *Transcultural concepts in nursing care,* ed 2, Philadelphia, 1995, Lippincott.

Blunt E: Emergency nursing in Poland, *J Emerg Nurs* 19(6):22A, 1993.

Cook LJ: Notes from work in Poland with a perinatal education program, *Neonatal Net* 5:61, 1992.

Grajcarek A: *AIDS. How to reduce the risk of HIV infection in nursing practice,* Warsaw, 1999, NIPiP.

Kawczyńska-Butrym Z: Family context of health and illness, Warsaw, 1995, CEM.

Kawczyńska-Butrym Z: *Nursing family. Theory and practice,* Warsaw 1997, CEM.

Latalski M: *Public health,* 1999, AM, Lublin.

Lenartowicz H: Polish nursing in action, *Nurs Adm Q* 16(2):64, 1992.

Nelson F: Citizen Ambassador Program of People to People International's hospice delegation to Russia and Poland, *Am J Hospice Palliat Care* 12(4):6, 1995.

Piatkowski W: Non-medical health care in Poland in the twentieth century, Warsaw, 1988, CEM.

Reid J: A trip to Poland examines their midwifery, *KY Nurse* 42(4):15, 1994.

Rocznik S: *Republic of Poland year-book,* Warsaw, 2000, GUS.

Roemer MI: Recent health system development in Poland and Hungary, *J Comm Health* 19(3):153, 1994.

Sekula W: *Food consumption in Poland during 1950-1996 calculated by energy and nourishing component,* Warsaw, 1997, Borgis.

Spector RE: *Cultural diversity in health and illness,* ed 4, Stamford, Conn, 1996, Appleton & Lange.

Wronska I, Lidbrink M: Letter from Poland, *Nurs Times* 92(3):221, 1996.

Walden–Ga?uszko K, Majkowicz M, Trzebiatowska I: The idea of "good death" at medical staff, *Psychooncology* 1:39-43, 1997.

◆ PORTUGAL (PORTUGESE REPUBLIC)

MAP PAGE (860)

Rosa Ribeiro Costa, Rui Moreno, and Ricardo Matos

Location: Portugal is located in the southwestern part of Europe in the Iberian Peninsula and has a total land area of 90,000 km^2 (34,749 square miles). It is mountainous in the north and flat in the south and is crossed by three major rivers that originate in Spain. Portugal also has two small archipelagos of volcanic origin: the Azores and the Madeira. The winters are usually cold and wet, and the summers hot and dry.

Major Language	**Ethnic Groups**	**Major Religions**
Portuguese	Homogeneous Mediterranean stock on mainland, and in Azores On the Madeira Islands also African (less than 100,000)	Roman Catholic 96% Protestant 1% Other 3%

Ethnically, Portugal is quite homogenous as is most of the Mediterranean. The presence of ethnic minorities has increased in recent years, with immigrants from Africa, India, and China. Politically, Portugal has been a republic since 1905, a democracy since 1974, and a member of the European Union since 1985. Portugal has experienced a major decrease in religious practices in the last few years, particularly in the cities.

Health Care Beliefs: Traditional and Western; active role. The rural areas have a significant amount of tradition-based medicine. Religion-based limitations on health care, such as the prohibition of donated blood or blood products, are rare.

Predominant Sick Care Practices: Biomedical. Nurses are more concerned with other aspects and dimensions of care.

Ethnic/Race Specific or Endemic Diseases: The only disease specific to Portugal is Joseph disease. However, cardiovascular disease and diabetes incidence is increasing. The World Health Organization's (WHO) estimated prevalence rate for HIV/AIDS in adults ages 15 to 49 years is 0.74%. The estimated number of children from birth to 15 years living with HIV/AIDS is 500.

Health Team Relationships: Nurses and medical doctors work together in a hierarchical relationship; doctors are dominant. Doctors and nurses also have separate tasks during care, with doctors attempting to cure and nurses attempting to provide daily care. Formally, the relationships are good, and communication tends to be less hierarchical and more cooperative.

Families' Role in Hospital Care: Formally, the involvement of the family is very limited, although their role is expanding to include participation in decision making and provision of care. This change in family roles is particularly affecting the specialties of oncology and pediatrics.

Dominance Patterns: The family structure is patriarchal; however, a strong movement toward more democratic gender roles is taking place and is affecting young couples particularly in the major cities. The mother is traditionally in charge of running the household and deciding when health care practitioners should be consulted. Deference is given to older adults, fathers, and grandfathers, especially in the more traditional areas of the country.

Eye Contact Practices: Direct eye contact is an important part of communication in Portugal. It is generally believed that looking others directly in the eyes is a sign of honesty.

Touch Practices: The Portuguese consider touch to be socially acceptable. In health care, touch is frequently used to as a form of nonverbal communication, especially to reassure patients.

Perceptions of Time: The Portuguese tend to live in the present, but they consider past traditions and habits to be important as well.

Pain Reactions: Except in small rural areas, public expressions of pain are unusual.

Birth Rites: Most births (97.8%) occur in hospitals with doctors in attendance. In rural areas, midwives still have a major role in delivering babies. Portugal has no established, organized system with medical and nursing support for home birth. Birth control is used by most of the population.

Death Rites: Widows are expected to remain unmarried for at least 1 year and to wear black clothing for the rest of their lives unless they marry again. Bodies are buried. Cremation is not accepted by the general population and is uncommon in major cities.

Food Practices and Intolerances: Most Portuguese have a Mediterranean diet that is high in fish, vegetables, fruit, and olive oil. Fast food is becoming more common in major cities and among young people. The consumption of alcohol is higher in rural areas and is increasing among young people in the major cities. In the last few years, red wine, which is believed to have cardiovascular benefits, is being replaced by beer and imported spirits.

Infant Feeding Practices: Most infants are breast-fed during the first 3 months after birth. At approximately the fourth month after birth, mothers progressively introduce soup, meat, and vegetables and then add fish at approximately the eighth month. Between 1 and 2 years, all foods are introduced to children.

Child Rearing Practices: Children are expected to strictly respect and obey their parents and older adults, and the older adults often help with child rearing. Families are usually more protective of girls.

National Childhood Immunizations: BCG at birth and at 5 to 6 and 11 to 12 years; DTP at 2, 4, 6, and 18 to 24 months; OPV at 2, 4, and 6 months and 5 to 6 years; hep B at birth and 10 to 13 years; HIB as of 2000; MMR at 15 months and 11 to 12 years; and DT at 5 to 6 years.

BIBLIOGRAPHY

Barreto A et al: *A situação social em Portugal, 1960-1999,* Lisbon, 1999, Instituto de Ciências Sociais da Universidade de Lisboa.

Boavida J, Borges L: Community involvement in early intervention: a Portuguese perspective, *Infants Young Child* 7:42, 1994.

Cobb AK: The role of the lay midwife in childbirth in rural Portugal, *West J Nurs Res* 17:353, 1995.

http://www.dgsaude.pt/
http://www.ics.ul.pt/
http://www.ine.pt/
http://www.min-saude.pt/
http://www.unaids.org/

◆ QATAR (STATE OF)

MAP PAGE (864)

Nigel J. Shanks

Location: Qatar is a peninsula that only appeared 4000 years ago and is situated halfway along the west coast of the Arabian Gulf. Together with numerous islands and reefs, the country covers a total land area of 11,437 km² (4416 square miles), with 700 km of coastline. The topography of Qatar consists of flat, rocky surfaces at or below sea level. However, the Jebel Dukhan in the west have some spectacular limestone outcrops and sand dunes that reach a height of 60 m near the inland sea. Qatar has a moderate desert climate with long, hot, humid summers (and temperatures ranging from 25° C to 55° C) and short, mild winters with some rainfall (i.e., an average of 70 mm annually). The sovereign state of Qatar became independent on September 3, 1971, and is one of the Gulf Cooperative Council (GCC) states in addition to Saudi Arabia, Kuwait, Oman, the United Arab Emirates, and Bahrain.

Major Languages	Ethnic Groups	Major Religions
Arabic (official)	Arab 40%	Sunni Muslim 95%
English	Pakistani 18%	Other 5%
Hindi	East Indian 18%	
Urdu	Iranian 10%	
	Other 14%	

The people of Qatar are the descendents of ancient Arabians who migrated from the Arabian hinterland. The Qataris have strong historical and family ties to the other gulf Arab states because of the migratory nature and freedom of movement of the Bedouin tribes. Qatar also has families of Persian origin. Most (60%) of the inhabitants of Qatar live in the capital of Doha, but large numbers of people also live in the towns and villages of Wakrah, Dukhan, Umm Said, Al Khor, and Madinat Shamal. (The population distribution is 88% urban and 12% rural.) Twenty-five percent of the population is Qatari, and the remainder is foreign nationals with residency status, the vast majority of whom are Arab, Pakistani, Indian, and Iranian. All official documents must be completed in Arabic, but English is widely spoken, particularly in business and health care arenas. Qatar is an Islamic state, and most have orthodox beliefs. Islamic law *(Shari'a)* is the main form of legislation.

Health Care Beliefs: Active role; Western and traditional. Belief in traditional or Koranic healing practices persists in Qatar, albeit in conjunction with conventional medicine. Traditional practices range from the recitation of healing verses from the Koran to anointing patients with special oils, to cauterizing certain body parts (thus many older Qataris have cautery scars). The traditional approach is dying out. Recently, numerous complementary medical clinics (e.g., chiropractic, massage, reflexology) have been established in Doha.

Predominant Sick Care Practices: Biomedical, alternative and religious. Health care is available to residents and visitors at government health centers. For a small fee, residents can purchase an annually renewable health card and register at the nearest primary health care center. Treatment and prescriptions are heavily subsidized. All health care provision is under the auspices of the Ministry of Health, which is charged with providing health services in all fields of specialization and establishing and organizing hospitals, health centers, and quarantines. The Hamad Medical Corporation manages the main governmental hospitals. The Hamad Hospital is the main hospital in Doha and offers a full range of medical specialties. In addition to government hospitals, Qatar has private hospitals and clinics. Qatar Petroleum, the state oil and gas company, and its subsidiaries are also mandated to provide primary health care for their employees and dependants, principally in the industrial areas. However, the vast majority of health care services are in the public health care system.

Ethnic/Race Specific or Endemic Diseases: Infectious diseases are less of a concern primarily because of the extensive immunization programs that are in place. Obesity and diabetes mellitus are becoming more common, as are hypertension and heart disease. These changes are thought to be partly a result of changes in dietary habits. The traditional diet of rice, fish, and small amounts of red meat has changed to one that is higher in animal fat and sugar because of the advent of a plethora of Western fast-food outlets and importation of preserved foods. Asthma is also very common. Injuries from automobile accidents are a major problem as well; seat belt legislation was introduced in February 2002. Non-Qatari residents are required to be screened and test negative for hepatitis (B and C), tuberculosis, and HIV infection before obtaining full residency status. The World Health Organization's (WHO) estimated prevalence rate for HIV/AIDS in adults ages 15 to 49 is 0.09%. WHO has no estimates for children from birth to 15 years. Qatar has a limited amount of natural fresh water, so the people are becoming more dependent on desalination facilities.

Health Team Relationships: Relationships among different health care professionals tend to be collaborative. The roles of doctors and nurses are clearly defined in the hospitals. The health team has a true hierarchy, with the doctor at the top and the nurse at the bottom. The nurse is not allowed to do anything unless instructed to do so—not even change dressings after operations.

Families' Role in Hospital Care: Families and patients have a right to and expect a high level of health care. Patients generally have at least one relative stay with them during their hospital stay. Families may be very demanding of health care professionals to ensure that the patient receives care and attention. Gifts of sweets and chocolates are common and may lead to conflicts with dietary restrictions. Families also expect to be allowed to spend as much time, whenever they like, visiting a patient. These frequent visits can lead to conflicts between hospital routines and family desires.

Dominance Patterns: Qatar has a patriarchal culture, and the family has the top priority. Polygamy is common among men, who are largely regarded as providers and protectors. Families tend to be large and extended because polygamous relationships tend to be complex. Tribal ties are still strong. Important decisions relating to family life are always made by the father. When a boy reaches 7 years, he is entrusted to the care of his father, who accompanies him everywhere; thus the bonds between father and son are strong. Women are playing an increasingly important role in society, and many work in professions such as teaching and medicine. Women always cover their head with a scarf, generally wear a veil, and are usually accompanied by a male relative when they go out to shop. Recently, women have experienced great liberalization and enhanced personal freedom. The traditional restrictive practices are no longer the norm as they are in Saudi Arabia.

Eye Contact Practices: Men maintain eye contact with other men during conversation. Eye contact between men and women is brief and limited.

Touch Practices: Touching between men and women is discouraged. Kissing, shaking hands, and holding hands is quite acceptable among males.

Perceptions of Time: Qataris live for today and do not to dwell on the past. They tend not to think of the future because it is ordained by Allah.

Pain Reactions: Reactions to pain are varied and can be stoical or vocal. It is more acceptable for women to express pain. Medical practitioners are reluctant to provide adequate pain medications. For example, intravenous opiates for severe pain are rarely given to those with traumatic injuries. Qatar has no hospice movement, and pain relief is generally inadequate.

Birth Rites: Large families are encouraged through the provision of state benefits for each child and a desire to increase the population. The estimated birth rate in 2001 was 15.91 births per 1000 people. The population growth rate estimate for 2001 was 3.18%. Qataris generally prefer to have boys, particularly as their first-born child. The infant mortality rate was estimated in 2001 to be 21.44 deaths per 1000 live births. After birth, Qatari women tend to stay with their mothers (the infant's grandmother) for up to 40 days to recover, allowing the grandmother to care for the infant.

Death Rites: Death or a poor prognosis is generally only discussed with male members of the family. Islamic regulations *(Fatwah)* state life support can be discontinued when certain conditions are met and that organ donations are acceptable. However, family desires are the ultimate deciding factor. When a death has occurred, male members of the family are not expected to show their grief, whereas women can be very vocal. Religious beliefs dictate that the soul moves on to a better place after death, which can be a great comfort to the family members. Autopsies are uncommon because of the religious mandate that the body must be buried intact. Interment is carried out usually within 1 day after death, and the body is buried wrapped in special shrouds without a coffin in the ground. Cremations are not permitted. Deaths are frequently announced in national newspapers. Condolences are received by family members, with separate venues for males and females. Organ transplantations are acceptable.

Food Practices and Intolerances: The traditional diet in Qatar is fish and rice, with a small amount of red meat. However, all types of ethnic and international foods are available in Qatar. Food is good and cheap, and multinational fast-food chains are found all over the country. Numerous large hotels have world-class restaurants and are licensed to serve alcohol. Pork, blood, and carrion consumption is forbidden for Muslims, so these foods are not imported into the country. Fasting during the holy month of Ramadan is mandatory for all adults other than children and those who are sick, although it is common for those who are hospitalized to fast between sunrise and sunset. Eating, drinking, and smoking in public during Ramadan is forbidden. It is acceptable to eat with the fingers, but only the right hand can be used because the left is considered unclean.

Infant Feeding Practices: Breast-feeding is the usual practice for women in Qatar and may continue for 1 year, depending on the mother's health and quantity of milk.

Child Rearing Practices: Child rearing tends to be permissive, and discipline is usually inconsistent. Infants often sleep with mothers until they are 1 or 2 years of age. Child rearing is often the responsibility of older female siblings or domestic servants. Education is provided from the primary to the university level by the state. It is free, and the state provides textbooks, paper, transportation, sports clothes, and equipment at all levels. Qatar has much invested in and pays significant attention to sports. Participation of young people is encouraged. More emphasis is placed on male activities, especially soccer, and males and females are segregated during sport and fitness activities. However, females are taking a more active role in fitness pursuits than they have in the past.

National Childhood Immunizations: BCG at birth; OPV at 2, 4, 6, and 18 months and 4 to 6 years; hep B at birth and at 2 and 6 months; DTPHIB at 2, 4, 6, and 18 months and 4 to 6 years; measles at 9 months; MMR at 15 months; and DT 4 years.

Other Characteristics: Restrictions for those who are not nationals are not as severe as they in some other Arab countries. For example, females are allowed to drive and go out alone. Female Qataris are allowed to vote and hold high office. Alcohol is available from a syndicate for expatriates with a liquor license, and it also is served in some hotels in Doha. The recent discovery and development of large natural gas reserves have given Qatar a substantial income, and it currently has the fastest growing economy in the world and the largest per capita income.

BIBLIOGRAPHY

Al-Madfa H, Abdel-Moati MA, al-Gimaly FH: Pinctada radiata (pearl oyster): a bioindicator for metal pollution monitoring in the Qatari waters (Arabian Gulf), *Bull Environ Contam Toxicol* 60(2):245, 1998.

Al-Shahiri MZ, Kinchin-White J: Continuous quality improvement. A proposal for Arabian Gulf Medical Associations, *Saudi Med J* 21(1):135, 2000.

Chaikhouni A et al: Coronary angiography in Qatar: the first ten years, *Angiology* 49(8):625, 1998.

Gehani AA et al: Myocardial infarction with normal coronary angiography compared with severe coronary artery disease without myocardial infarction: the crucial role of smoking, *J Cardiovasc Risk* 8(1):1, 2001.

Helmi I, Hussein A, Ahmed AH: Abdominal trauma due to road traffic accidents in Qatar, *Injury* 32(2):105, 2001.

McGivern SA: Patient satisfaction with quality of care in a hospital system in Qatar, *J Healthc Qual* 21(1):28, 1999.

Shanks NJ, Papworth G: Environmental factors and heat stroke, *Occup Med* 51(1):45, 2001.

World Health Organization (June 2000): *Epidemiological fact sheets by country,* Geneva. Retrieved March 1, 2002, from http://www.unaids.org/hivaidsinfo/statistics/june00/fact_sheets/index.html

World Health Organization (2001): *WHO vaccine-preventable diseases: monitoring system,* Geneva. Retrieved March 1, 2002, from http://www.who.int/vaccines/

◆ ROMANIA

MAP PAGE (860)

Mary G. Schaal and Adriana Vilan

Location: Romania is in southeastern Europe, bordering the Black Sea, Hungary, Moldova, Yugoslavia, Bulgaria, and Ukraine. The total land area is 237,500 km^2 (91,699 square miles), and the capital is Bucharest. The highest peak of the Carpathian Mountains is 2544 m (8346 feet). The climate is temperate, with cold, cloudy winters and frequent snow and fog and sunny summers with frequent showers and thunderstorms. The population in 2000 was 22,435,205.

Major Languages	Ethnic Groups	Major Religions
Romanian (official)	Romanian 84%	Romanian Orthodox 70%
Hungarian	Hungarian 7%	Roman Catholic 6%
German	Serb, Croat, Russian,	(including 3% Uniate)
	Turkish, Roma	Protestant, Muslim,
	(Gypsy), 8%	Jewish 6%
	German, Ukrainian 1%	Unaffiliated 18%

Romanian is a Romance language derived primarily from Latin. Minority languages include Hungarian, German, Turkish, Serbo-Croatian, and Romani (the language of the Roma, or Gypsy, population). English and French are taught in many schools and are the most common second languages spoken in Romania. The adult literacy rate in Romania is 100%. Before 1989 the educational system heavily emphasized practical and technical studies. However, in recent years, management, business, and social sciences have become more popular.

Health Care Beliefs: Passive role; acute sick care, but health promotion considered important. Health promotion practices encourage prenatal and child care in particular. The health care system addresses acute problems and tertiary care; however, rehabilitation is not emphasized. Health education in Romania improved significantly in the last century. During the communist regime, people were given lectures in health care and medical treatment. Courses were organized to teach older people and women about symptoms of frequent diseases and ways to cure them. These efforts have improved the health care knowledge of the general population. In the rural areas, older people may use herbs in tea, lotions, or potions to treat illness, but it is not the predominant practice. A few people in the country are known as healers by the power of God, and they use their hands (bioenergy), herbs, and prayers to cure various diseases. Most healers are deeply religious and encourage people to have faith in God. They are usually consulted by people with terminal illnesses. Some older Gypsy women called ghicitoare (fortune tellers) serve as healers, although Gypsies use traditional medical services as well.

Predominant Sick Care Practices: Biomedical; coexisting holistic, folk, and Western medical practices. Health promotion and illness prevention do not predominate; the focus in on care for those who are ill. Romanians prefer medical treatment for their diseases, even in rural and remote areas of the country. Generally they respect the word of the doctor, who is highly respected and trusted. Although medical technology is not updated, Romania has hospitals and centers where people can receive health care, especially in the major cities. Romanians are beginning to consider regular check-ups for disease prevention. National health care services are paid by employers and the employees through salary deductions. In addition, private services are available for those who can afford them. Hospitalization is usually free, but often the patients must pay for medications. The house doctor can prescribe a limited amount of medication for free. A wider range of facilities and services is available for children and older adults.

Ethnic/Race Specific or Endemic Diseases: Industrial pollution influences health. Cardiovascular diseases, hypertension, viral hepatitis, and cancer are major adult problems, whereas malnutrition among those with HIV/AIDS or respiratory illnesses are more common among children than adults. The World Health Organization's (WHO) estimated prevalence rate for HIV/AIDS in adults ages 15 to 49 is 0.02%. The estimated number of children from birth to 15 years living with HIV/AIDS is 5000. Young people feel free to talk about homosexuality, and they discuss sexual practices and homosexuality to prevent HIV infection. Older people consider homosexuality a private issue and do not talk about it. Only since the 1989 revolution has the government acknowledged the existence of AIDS. Government officials and doctors frequently deny that HIV/AIDS is of any significance.

Health Team Relationships: The doctor is the primary authority in hospital settings, and nurses are subordinate. Nurses are given more respect if they are the only health care professionals in the setting. Doctors and nurses practice primarily in the hospitals, all of which are public. Some new and well-equipped private clinics are being established in Romania, and the best doctors practice in them after their work in the public arena. Doctors are licensed for practice, and their practice is guided by a professional code with strict guidelines for professional and patient relationships. Recently social workers and psychologists have been included on the medical teams of hospitals. Nursing education is provided by scoala postliceala sanitara (post high schools) and takes 3 years. Schools can be public or private. More recently, the nursing college in the University of Medicine and Pharmacy opened and different specialties are taught. National examinations are held after graduation for licensing and specialization (e.g., pediatrics, psychiatry, gynecology, surgery, public health).

Families' Role in Hospital Care: Families rally around people who are sick and play an important role in their care. Family members are expected to stay with patients, provide food, and assist with basic hygiene tasks, although the nurses and cleaning women help as well. It is expected for friends to visit those hospitalized patients.

Dominance Patterns: The principle of gender equality is new in Romanian society and has not yet been embraced by a significant percentage of the population. Women do not have an important role in decision-making processes, although Romania has many well-educated and professionally trained women. Women's nongovernmental organizations play an important role in increasing public awareness about the role of women in political and social life.

Eye Contact Practices: Direct, sustained eye contact is the norm. It is customary to maintain eye contact with other people while talking. Avoiding eye contact during conversations with friends portrays a lack of respect or insincerity.

Touch Practices: Two kisses on the check for greetings and farewells are common. Touch is an important part of nonverbal communication.

Perceptions of Time: Time schedules are followed more precisely in urban areas than they are in rural regions. Punctuality has not traditionally been a very important value, although perceptions have been changing, especially in the last 10 years, and punctuality is becoming more important and appreciated. Romanians try to focus on a better future, although it is hard for them to ignore the difficulties of the present and forget the sacrifices of the past. Romanians live primarily between the past and the present as they try to establish a future-oriented view.

Pain Reactions: Romanians typically have a high tolerance for pain and discomfort. Some are communicative about their pain, and others are stoical. Some prefer injections for pain relief. Women are not expected to cry out in pain during labor; loud verbal expressions in response to pain are considered shameful.

Birth Rites: Romanian women deliver their infants in a hospital. The delivery procedures are typical of Western practices, with the woman lying down and her legs elevated on leg rests. The pain of delivery is not usually eased with localized anesthesia. Pregnancy is considered a very delicate period in a woman's health, and the family takes great care to offer her the best quality and quantity of food they can. Women are typically cared for by professionals during and after their delivery. Women are treated for the different infections they are likely to contract because of imperfect sanitation conditions at maternity hospitals. Women do not stay long at the hospital and usually go home after the first or the second day after the delivery unless they have problems requiring special treatment. New mothers rely on an older woman, often the mother or mother-in-law, to care for her during the first 2 weeks at home. Mothers are encouraged to breast-feed and eat food that increases milk production. The family tries to ensure that the mother is emotionally stable because they believe that erratic emotions can spoil milk production. Infants must be named within the first 2 weeks and registered in the family register of city population. Visitors, friends, and family are expected to come and visit the family of the newborn and bring gifts, clothes, or money, to help the family. The mother's family of origin customarily buys the main clothes and crib for the infant. Parents usually decide on the name of the infants, but occasionally grandparents name them after themselves or with other names they prefer. This naming tradition is more common in rural areas, where the traditional family predominates. Mothers who have a job during their pregnancy get a 1-year leave. The employer pays 50% of her salary during this period. Many women take a shorter leave, especially those who work in the private sector because they do not want to lose their full salary. Abortion and contraceptives are legal.

Death Rites: Relatives and friends expend considerable effort to be present when a person is near death. The family starts expressing their grief through crying and wailing at the moment that the person dies. Family members and closer friends of the deceased person dress in black and official suits. Family members expect visits from all relatives, friends, and neighbors. The body is buried within 48 hours after the death. If the dead person was a young woman, she is dressed in a white bridal dress. If a young man dies, he is dressed in a bridegroom suit. Depending on the religious background of the person, a priest may conduct the burial service. The whole family and the closer relatives are in mourning for at least 40 days after the death. Autopsies are not routinely performed. Most people die at home and are embalmed and prepared for viewing in the home. If a person is ill and dies in a hospital, the embalming and preparation of the body occurs in the hospital. In either situation the body is dressed in nice clothes that are provided by the family; it lies in state in the home, usually in the living room. Often a few personal effects of the deceased person are placed in the coffin, such as jewelry, shaving implements, watches, glasses, writing implements, and cigarettes, and these items are eventually buried with the deceased. The family offers meals as a sign of respect to the dead person; these meals are offered on the day of the burial, on the fortieth day after burial, on the 6-month anniversary of the death, and on the 1-year anniversary of the death. The meal marking the 1-year anniversary ends the period of mourning. Few families continue to offer meals for very close family members after a year. Family members do continue to go to the cemetery and take flowers to the tomb, especially on sacred days, special anniversaries, birthdays, or special days for each family.

Food Practices or Intolerances: The majority of people eat three times a day. Traditionally, the largest meal is lunch (after 12 pm). Supper in the evening includes meat and vegetables, rice, pasta, or beans, and the meat and vegetables are well cooked. During the last 10 years, with the transition in the economy, people began working for the entire day and thus prefer the largest meal in the evening. Popular Romanian foods include mititei (seasoned grilled meat balls) and mamaliga (a cornmeal porridge served in many different ways). Wine and a plum brandy called tuica are popular beverages among Romanians, and placinta (turnovers) are a typical dessert.

Infant Feeding Practices: Breast-feeding is typical; most women recognize that it is healthy. However, women do not breast-feed in public. If breast-feeding is impossible for medical reasons or the mother simply chooses not to breast-feed, formula is available.

Child Rearing Practices: Child rearing is not specifically strict or permissive. Some children are extremely obedient, and some are not. Parents try to educate their children in a traditional way, but often children respond more to peer influence and ignore traditional values. Children are economically dependent on their parents; young adults often live with or receive financial support from their parents because of limited financial resources and increasing rates of unemployment. Many children have different caretakers. Grandparents are considered appropriate and very trustworthy caretakers, so they may supervise children when parents work. Despite their age, grandparents take excellent care of their grandchildren by telling them stories, playing with them, and accompanying them to and from school. Parents are very invested in the education of their children. Even when in difficult situations, they still try to sacrifice so that their children can be educated. Education in Romania is free and compulsory for children between the ages of 7 and 14, and most children choose to stay in school after age 14. The education of girls is considered much more important so that they will not be subject to family slavery. At the same time, fears about safety have hindered the education of some young women. Unfortunately, social disruption during the transition period (i.e., the postcommunist era) has made education more difficult because some village schools were destroyed, and many teachers left for more profitable occupations. Children who are likely to receive an inadequate education include Gypsies, children of illegal migrants to the cities, and children without families. Unfortunately, drug abuse is a growing problem of the youth in Romania because of the easy access to drugs and their doubts about the future.

National Childhood Immunizations: BCG at birth and 14 years; DTP at 2, 4, 6, 12, and 30 to 35 months; OPV at 2, 4, 6, and 12 months and 9 years; hep B at birth, 2 and 6 months, and 9 years; measles at 9 to 11 months and 7 years; and DT at 7 and 14 years.

BIBLIOGRAPHY

Buchanan J: Ceausescu's legacy, *Nurs Times* 86(7):16, 1990.
Campbell NN, Harbonne DJ, Norwich R: Medicine in Romania, *Br Med J* 300(6726):699, 1990.
Cassidy MD: Romania: haemodialysis, handicap and a sense of humor, *Lancet* 337(8737):353, 1991.
Dickman S: AIDS in children adds to Romania's troubles, *Nature* 343:579, 1990.
Ember L: Pollution chokes East-bloc nations, *Chem Engin News* 68(16):7, 1990.
Freedman DC: Gender identity and dance style, *East Eur Q* 23(4):419, 1990.
Houston S: Birth, abortion, family planning and child care in Romania, *Prof Care Mother Child* 3(2):41, 1993.

Lakey CK: Romania: a nursing journey, *Nurs Health Care* 16(3):144, 1995.

Lakey CK et al: Health care and nursing in Romania, *J Adv Nurs* 23(5):1045, 1996.

Lass A: The wedding of the dead, *Am Anthropol* 92(3):784, 1990.

Life after Ceausescu, *Economist* 314(7636):39, 1990.

Lutz S: Nurses begin Romanian mission, *Mod Healthcare* 21(34):13, 1990.

Lutz S: US execs find Romanian health system "depraved," *Mod Healthcare* 20(37):2, 1990.

Nolan P, Nolan M: Child of hardship, *Nurs Times* 87(12):16, 1991.

Rawlinson JW: Developing mental health nursing education in Romania, *Nurse Ed Today* 13(3):225, 1993.

Rudin C et al: HIV-1, hepatitis (A, B, and C) and measles in Romanian children, *Lancet* 336(8730):1592, 1990.

◆ RUSSIA (RUSSIAN FEDERATION)

MAP PAGE (861)

Gennadij G. Knyazev and Helen Slobodskaya

Location: Massive disintegration of the former Soviet Union's Communist Party and territory occurred in 1992. Declarations of independence by the republics of Latvia, Estonia, and Lithuania were followed rapidly by declarations of other republics. Russia extends from the western Black and Baltic Seas to the Pacific Ocean, and has a total land area of 17,075,200 km² (6,592,745 square miles). Its vast areas of plains and plateaus are punctuated by low mountain ranges. The climate varies from arctic severity during the winter to subtropical heat during the summer.

Major Languages	Ethnic Groups	Major Religions
Russian	Russian 81%	Russian Orthodox
Other	Tatar 4%	Muslim
	Ukrainian 3%	Other
	Chuvash, Bashkir, Belarusian, Moldavian 4%	
	Other 8%	

Most emigrants from the former Soviet Union speak Russian, and it is uncommon to overhear Ukrainian, Belarussian, Uzbek, or Armenian in Russian cities. On the other hand, in several republics inside of Russia, local languages may dominate, especially in rural areas, namely Bashkortostan, Tatarstan, Chechnya, Evenkia, the Jewish Autonomic Republic, the Republic of Tuva, Buryatia, the Chuvash Republic, the Kabardino-Balkarian Republic, Mari El, Sakha, and Udmurt.

Health Care Beliefs: Acute sick care; passive role; increasing efforts towards prevention. Medical information and advice about healthy food and the need for exercise frequently appears in the mass media, although some of it is of dubious quality. Cigarette advertisements (which are very common on city streets) always include the Health Ministry's declaration that smoking is unhealthy. Oriental traditional medicine such as Chinese medicine is popular. In Soviet times, schizophrenia was the primary diagnosed mental disorder, and the same is true today. Psychotherapy is an emerging field of uncertain quality. It is becoming popular among the wealthy, but most patients have illnesses of a psychosomatic nature. Fear of mental illness is widespread, not only because of prejudice and fear of being ridiculed but also because of the punitive characteristics of psychiatry in the former Soviet Union. Superstitions about magical healing properties of some drugs or objects are widespread.

Predominant Sick Care Practices: Official biomedical, alternative and magical-religious. Most people, especially those in the cities, go to out-patient clinics that are generally free. Drugs such as analgesics are not free. These clinics provide only a limited number of services, and the quality is generally not very good. Numerous private clinics have emerged recently in which services are better but are very expensive. Even in the state clinics, serious surgical operations are not free. They are very expensive and unaffordable for a considerable part of the population. Indigenous healers are rare in cities but still popular in rural areas, especially in the northern territories, where *shamans* practice among aboriginal people. Many charlatans have recently appeared in cities. They pretend to have extrasensory powers or to be magicians with the ability to heal; their advertisements are common in the mass media.

Ethnic/Race Specific or Endemic Diseases: For many years, opisthorchiasis foci have existed in the northern Ob River region and in the Kama and Vyatka Rivers basins. Natural foci of tick-borne encephalitis exist in Siberia, the Far East, and the Ural region of Russia. Tuberculosis incidence is increasing. Hepatitis delta virus genotypes I and II cocirculate in the endemic area of Yakutia. In Siberia, the prevalence of hepatitis B virus infection is about 10 times higher than it is in Japan. Biliary pathology in the far northern population is related to ethnic and geographical factors. Viliuisk encephalomyelitis seems to be endemic among the native populations of Yakutia. More cases of hemorrhagic fever with renal syndrome, tick-borne encephalitis, Crimean hemorrhagic fever, and West Nile fever (with a high proportion in urban populations) are being registered annually. An increase in the epizootic activity of the natural foci of plague is noted despite the absence of morbidity among humans. The outbreaks of tularemia are linked not only with the increased activity of natural foci but also with reduced immunization coverage in endemic regions. The main causes of death are cardiovascular diseases (58%), malignant tumors (18%), and traumas and poisoning (13%), and according to autopsy findings, alcohol-associated lesions of different organs (9%). Eastern Europe is experiencing higher rates of HIV/AIDS, and Russia is among the countries with the most alarming rate increases despite its relatively low reported prevalence rate. The World Health Organization's (WHO) estimated prevalence rate for HIV/AIDS in adults ages 15 to 49 is 0.018%. The estimated number of children from birth to 15 years living with HIV/AIDS is 1800. According to official statistics, as of September 2000, approximately 56,978 cases had been reported, including 951 children; AIDS was diagnosed in 409 cases (of which 129 were children). The regions with the highest number of HIV cases were Moscow (9861 cases), Irkutsk (7139 cases), and Kaliningrad (2865 cases).

Health Team Relationships: Doctors dominate. Patients' attitudes toward doctors and nurses are dubious.

Families' Role in Hospital Care: Family members generally do not stay with patients in the hospital. The exceptions are mothers of hospitalized infants and relatives of those who are seriously ill and whose care cannot be provided by the hospital. However, even if family members do not stay, they usually come as often as possible to help the patients and bring them food.

Dominance Patterns: Men dominate politics and business, but numerous women are health care professionals and school teachers. In the family the father traditionally dominates, although this pattern is changing. More than 20% of households in 1995 were headed by single-parent women, and this number is increasing.

Eye Contact Practices: Eye contact is not avoided, and gender differences are not great.

Touch Practices: Touch practices vary, but physical touching is not generally common. Three kisses on the cheek for greetings and farewells is now an exotic practice in Russia. Kisses on the cheek are still common among Orthodox believers greeting each other during the religious holidays, especially during Easter, the main Orthodox holy day. Generally, only men shake hands.

Perceptions of Time: Punctuality is not terribly important. Some people are punctual, but being late to appointments or breaking promises is common and generally not a problem. Traditions have changed several times in Russia during the last century and are still changing today. After the dissolution of the former Soviet Union, some older Russian traditions were revived. The older adults mainly focus on past traditions (i.e., traditions from Soviet times); middle-age and young people tend to look to the future.

Pain Reactions: Expressions of pain are acceptable for women and children, but men are expected to be stoical.

Birth Rites: The majority of births occur in maternity hospitals with the assistance of a midwife who is under the supervision of a doctor. After birth the woman is placed in a ward with others, and the newborn goes to the nursery with other newborns. Newborns are examined by a pediatrician and if no complications are involved, the mother and the infant stay in the hospital about 5 days and go home under the observation of the child clinic. New changes in obstetric care include wards where the mother and infant can stay together, shorter stays, and provisions for fathers to be present in the delivery room. Parents usually adhere to child care suggestions given by the clinic, including daily bathing and special recommended foods. The sex of the newborn makes no difference to modern Russian parents; any preferences are individual.

Death Rites: The death of a family member is usually considered a tragedy. As a rule, all family members, colleagues, and friends try to attend the funeral. Organ donations and autopsies are acceptable.

Food Practices and Intolerances: Meat or fish with potato garnish is the prevalent dish. Bread and sausage, eggs, and milk products are usual for breakfast. A type of ravioli and boiled buckwheat are among the favorite Russian foods. Cabbage, sauerkraut, carrots, and beets are staple vegetables in winter, whereas in the summer, apples, local berries, cucumbers, tomatoes, and salads are added to the diet. Recently, a vast range of fruits and vegetables have become available, but most of them are too expensive to be widely purchased; bananas and oranges are the most popular. It is unacceptable to eat with the hands or implements other than a fork, knife, and spoon. According to government regulations, alcoholic beverages (including beer) can only be sold to adults (those older than 18). Alcohol consumption and binge drinking have been increasing in the last years.

Infant Feeding Practices: Breast-feeding is the usual practice, especially during the first 6 months, but bottle-feeding is increasingly popular. Infant feeding in most areas is not culture specific and tends to be based on the recommendations of the child health clinics.

Child Rearing Practices: Permissiveness predominates, and children do no usually have strict rules. The mother is responsible for most of the discipline. Sleeping with parents is not common. Children are generally loved, and parents are often overly concerned about a child's success in school. Children are not expected to be quiet and obedient and are not discouraged from pursuing independent activities or confrontations. Traditional gender roles usually apply, especially for boys.

National Childhood Immunizations: BCG at birth and 6 to 7 years; DTP at 3, 4, 5, and 18 months; OPV at 3, 4, 5, 18, and 24 months and 6 to 7 years; mumps at 12 to 15 months and 5 to 6 years; D at 11 to 12 years; Td at 5 to 6 and 15 to 16 years.

BIBLIOGRAPHY

Avtsyn, A. P., A. A. Zhavoronkov, et al. (1994). [New data on the epidemiology and morphology of Viliuisk encephalomyelitis]. *Arkh Patol* 56(4): 39–44.

Ivaniushina, V., N. Radjef, et al. (2001). Hepatitis delta virus genotypes I and II cocirculate in an endemic area of Yakutia, Russia. *J Gen Virol* 82(Pt 11): 2709–18.

Kalichman, S. C., J. A. Kelly, et al. (2000). The emerging AIDS crisis in Russia: review of enabling factors and prevention needs. *Int J STD AIDS* 11(2): 71–5.

Khazova, T. G. and V. K. Iastrebov (2001). [Combined focus of tick-borne encephalitis, tick-borne rickettsiosis and tularemia in the habitat of Haemaphysalis concinna in south central Siberia]. *Zh Mikrobiol Epidemiol Immunobiol*(1): 78–80.

Korenberg, E. I., L. Y. Gorban, et al. (2001). Risk for human tick-borne encephalitis, borrelioses, and double infection in the pre-Ural region of Russia. *Emerg Infect Dis* 7(3): 459–62.

Kotel'nikov, G. A. and S. N. Malkov (1991). [The opisthorchiasis situation in the Kama-Vyatka river basin]. *Med Parazitol (Mosk)*(2): 9–10.

Krasnov, V. A. and G. S. Murashkina (1998). [Tuberculosis epidemiology-epizoology relationship in West Siberia]. *Probl Tuberk*(5): 8–11.

Malyutina, S., M. Bobak, et al. (2001). Alcohol consumption and binge drinking in Novosibirsk, Russia, 1985-95. *Addiction* 96(7): 987–95.

Ohba, K., M. Mizokami, et al. (1999). Seroprevalence of hepatitis B virus, hepatitis C virus and GB virus-C infections in Siberia. *Epidemiol Infect* 122(1): 139–43.

Onishchenko, G. G. (2001). [Infectious diseases in natural reservoirs: epidemic situation and morbidity in the Russian Federation and prophylactic measures]. *Zh Mikrobiol Epidemiol Immunobiol*(3): 22–8.

Rybinsky EM (1996) Childhood in Russia: reality and problems. Moscow: Russion Child Foundation Research Institute of Childhood (In Russian).

Takashima, I., D. Hayasaka, et al. (2001). Epidemiology of tick-borne encephalitis (TBE) and phylogenetic analysis of TBE viruses in Japan and Far Eastern Russia. *Jpn J Infect Dis* 54(1): 1–11.

Tsukanov, V. V. (1997). [The prevalence and structure of biliary tract diseases in the rural population of northern regions of Siberia]. *Ter Arkh* 69(2): 30–2.

Vinokurov, II, K. P. Samsonova, et al. (1993). [Characteristics of epidemiology and clinical course of pulmonary tuberculosis in inhabitants of Northern Russia]. *Probl Tuberk*(2): 19–20.

Zairat'iants, O. V. (2001). [Analysis of fatal outcomes according to the Moscow pathology service data (1996-2000)]. *Arkh Patol* 63(4): 9–13.

Zhuravlev, S. E., O. K. Galaktionov, et al. (1989). [Helminthiases among the population of northwestern Siberia. 1. Opisthorchiasis and mixed invasion in the native inhabitants of the Ob River basin and their clinical course]. *Med Parazitol (Mosk)*(5):54–7.

◆ RWANDA (RWANDESE REPUBLIC)

MAP PAGE (863)

Kizito Bishikwabo Nsarhaza and Michel Carael

Location: Rwanda is located in central Africa to the east of the Democratic Republic of Congo. It has a rugged landscape with high mountains and deep valleys. The principal geographical feature is the Virunga Mountains, which run north of Lake Kivu and include Rwanda's loftiest point, Volcan Karisimbi. Rwanda has twelve prefectures. In addition to the capital city,

Kigali, other major towns include Butare, Gisenyi, and Ruhengeri. The country covers a total land area of 26,338 km^2 (10,169 square miles), with a population that was estimated to be 7.6 million in 1994. With a density of 280 persons per square kilometer, Rwanda is one of the most densely populated countries in the world, and its population has a high annual growth rate that was estimated to be 3.6 in the 1990s because of a high fertility level and low contraceptive use. Approximately 5% to 10% of the population is living in urban areas.

Major Languages	Ethnic Groups	Major Religions
Kinyarwanda (official)	Hutu 80%	Christian 75%
French (official)	Tutsi 19%	Indigenous and
English (official)	Twa (pygmy) 1%	others 25%

Kinyarwanda (a Bantu language), French, and English are official languages, but Swahili is widely spoken. Most Christians are Roman Catholic. A small number of Tutsi are Muslim. Since its independence, ethnic violence has led to large-scale massacres and the creation of perhaps as many as 3 million refugees. Hutu and Tutsi leaders, at the national as well as local levels, have exploited intergroup tensions and violence in the neighboring state to justify their methods of political monopoly (dictatorship), physical exclusion (provoking refugee flows), and physical elimination (genocide).

Health Care Beliefs: Prevention; health promotion; passive role common. Rwanda has a national program for prevention of HIV/AIDS, with strong information, education, and communication components. The country was committed to achieving "health for all by the year 2000." Therefore primary health care through health promotion is an important aspect of the health programs and interventions.

Predominant Sick Care Practices: Biomedical, traditional and magical-religious. Rwanda has a wide range of health care practices. The population consults doctors or traditional healers depending on numerous factors: the practitioners' location (urban or rural), financial aspects (cost of treatment), cultural habits, and type of sickness. People practicing traditional religion wear amulets. They believe that the power inherent in the amulets will improve their living conditions and maintain their health. In the last decade, mental illness has become an important aspect of health promotion. Diagnostic symptoms of depression and posttraumatic stress disorder are locally described as being the results of the genocide. The "mental trauma syndrome" includes posttraumatic stress disorder symptoms and some depression and local symptoms. Rwanda also has a "grief syndrome" that includes other depression and local symptoms. The significance of mental illness and psychological disorders in the Rwandan population is widely understood by the international community as a consequence of the mass ethnic killings in 1994. Many health development programs have been put in place to reduce the psychosocial impact of that crisis. The centerpiece of the mental health system of Rwanda is the neuropsychiatric Hospital of Ndera, which plays a key role in decentralization of mental services and their integration with primary health care services. Effort has been made to integrate traditional medicine into the modern health system. For example, the Centre Universitaire de Recherche sur la Pharmacopée et la Medecine Populaire, which is affiliated with the Université Nationale du Rwanda, has set up a clinic for popular medicine. Often, healers prepare medications at the healing site, using fluids to treat health, love, and illness issues.

Ethnic/Race Specific or Endemic Diseases: Endemic diseases are not associated with any particular minority group, and biological differences among ethnic groups have not been identified. Major illnesses affecting the country are yellow fever, cholera, shigellosis, malaria, malnutrition, and tuberculosis. Among older patients, infections (which affect 38% of the patients) and liver cirrhosis (which affects 32%) are the most common problems. Hospitalized older adults occupy 18% of available beds in the medical department. Their disease pattern is different from that of younger patients, placing heavier demands on medical resources. Malaria and upper intestinal inflammation are less common in older adults, but liver cirrhosis, primary hepatocellular cancer, pneumonia, prostatic cancer, cardiovascular pathology, chronic renal pathology, and chronic lung disease tend to be more prevalent. Because of the 1994 crisis, Rwanda has a high prevalence of mental health problems, which requires psychosocial programs for large refugee populations that aim to strengthen community structures and supporting groups instead of focusing on individuals. The World Health Organization's (WHO) estimated prevalence rate for HIV/AIDS in adults ages 15 to 49 is 11.21%. Prevalence figures are as high as 19% in pregnant women attending urban antenatal clinics. The estimated number of children from birth to 15 years living with HIV/AIDS is 22,000. The number of children who have lost their mother or both parents to AIDS is estimated to be more than 172,000. The trend of the HIV epidemic in the country is alarming, particularly in rural areas. The latest epidemiological data collected after the genocide show evidence that in some rural setting, the incidence of HIV/AIDS increased tenfold from 1994 to 1998. The situation in the urban area has remained unchanged but is still very high. Women are more frequently infected than men, and the highest rates are among commercial sex workers. The overall child mortality rate is estimated to be 203 per 1000 people, one of the highest in Africa. The response to the HIV epidemic is getting more organized, and political commitment has increased. Among institutional arrangements to fight the epidemic, Rwanda has set up the National Commission on HIV/AIDS to ensure a coordinated multisectorial response to the epidemic. The National HIV/AIDS Control Program has been strengthened, and the country has developed a national strategic plan that involves all development sectors.

Health Team Relationships: Although health team relationships are doctor driven, the dominance of doctors does not impede good working relationships. Patients' attitudes toward doctors and nurses are characterized by submission. When accessible, health professionals are expected to have the knowledge and ability to cure illnesses. Patients' lack of information makes them dependent on health professionals, especially patients in rural settings or who are uneducated.

Families' Role in Hospital Care: Community and family ties are very strong in Rwanda. Families assist their hospitalized relatives; they tend to stay with patients and bring them food. This sign of solidarity has been accentuated by the exacerbated conflict among ethnic groups. Patients prefer to eat food brought by relatives than hospital food.

Dominance Patterns: An absolute patriarchal authority is common in Rwanda. Children, even when married, are completely dependent on their parents; the parent's support contributes to their overall wellness. In turn, respect, veneration, and assistance to parents is the norm. In general, Rwandan culture is male dominated. Men and women have separate conjugal roles (e.g., wife doing housework, husband doing gardening) and joint conjugal roles (e.g., wife and husband disciplining children). Some decisions and their implementation can involve extended families or community members (e.g., taking care of elderly, those with disabilities, and orphans). This practice is more common in rural areas than in urban settings. Families are helping cushion the psychological impact of the 1994 genocide. Women have an important role in cooking and taking care of older family members, children, and ill family members. In these areas, male dominance is limited or nonexistent. A woman never challenges her husband in public. However, women's remarks and even criticisms are encouraged in private and close family settings.

Eye Contact Practices: Eye contact is usually avoided as a sign of respect, not only between members of the opposite sex but also among generations. A youth never looks directly into the eyes of an older adult and usually bows when talking to the father. These practices are also expected from women during interactions with their husband.

Perceptions of Time: Rwandans and Western people have cultural perceptions of time. It is uncommon to get to appointments on time. In agricultural settings, seasons are the main reference for time, and moments are often defined in terms of events. This practice is based on the past-oriented focus of Rwandan culture. People are very patient; they tend to consider it normal for people to be late to appointments and forgive them easily. However, educated people tend to be less patient and are more easily irritated by a lack of punctuality. This leads to a dual perception of punctuality in the culture. During official activities, people make efforts to be prompt. During unofficial activities, time has little meaning; for example, discussions may be extended with little regard for their length.

Pain Reactions: Stoicism is encouraged in Rwandan culture because expressions of pain are considered a sign of weakness. Calmness and serenity are praised, but the calmness is not passive. People are encouraged to stay calm and stoical when facing adversity and to concentrate their energy on preparing a response.

Birth Rites: For life to be worthwhile and meaningful, it is believed to be essential to have children. Childbirth traditionally takes place in a banana plantation, where women are assisted by female relatives. Today, numerous women give birth in maternity hospitals, and they are often accompanied by their daughters or another female relative. Men do not traditionally witness childbirth because it is considered a secret activity in which only women participate. After delivery, traditional woman are not expected to do any work in the household and are considered impure until they are ready for sexual intercourse with the father of the infant (usually a week or more after delivery). If birth occurs after a divorce, the wife still must have sexual intercourse with the father of the infant. During this period the husband takes care of the children and household duties. Rwanda has numerous other postpartum sexual rites. The mean birthweight (with twins excluded) was estimated to be 3160 g in 1997 but decreased to 3043 g in 2000, and the prevalence of low birthweight was 12.5%. Cesarean sections are done in approximately 26% of hospital deliveries—a cesarean rate of 1.1% in the population. The maternal mortality rate in hospitals has been estimated to be 600 per 100,000 live births between 1997 and 2000. Efforts are being made to educate at-risk women to give birth in health centers, and early referrals of women to the hospital are being reinforced.

Death Rites: The body is exposed for viewing for a limited number of days (not more than 3), and people visit the family. All family members are expected to attend the bereavement ritual. Men are separated from the women, and each group grieves in specific ways.

Food Practices and Intolerances: Basic food in Rwanda is composed of cassava, beans, potatoes, and cassava leaves, and beans are the favorite food. Rwandans have a wide range of ways to cook beans; they are often combined with other foods such as corn or meat. Rwandans have no reported food intolerances, but cultural practices limit people's consumption of certain foods. For example, lamb is not a common food, and women are not allowed to eat certain parts of chickens. Some foods are thought to have magical powers to facilitate pregnancy or the delivery of an infant. On average, rural inhabitants eat two meals per day, and the main meal is eaten in the evening. Main meals differ according to altitude. In zones with a tropical climate, the diet comprises four main foods: beans, sweet potatoes, cassava, and bananas, with the first two providing 50% of the total energy supply. At high altitudes the main foods are pulses (beans), cereals (maize), and potatoes, and protein intakes are very low, resulting in protein malnutrition that affects 5% to 6% of children. Vitamin A deficiency is also prevalent. The prevalence of undernutrition in unstable areas such as refugee camps has been estimated to be 19.5% in men and 13.1% in women and is even higher in those older than 60. The production of semen is thought to be favored by a healthy diet and beverages such as sorghum porridge, or *igikoma*, sorghum beer *(ikigage)*, and milk *(amata)*. Healers say that beverages higher in alcoholic content than sorghum beer, such as banana beer *(urwaga),* manufactured beer, and whisky, dehydrate the body and delay ejaculation. It is the usual practice to eat with the hands. Only a few people, especially families that have adopted Western culture, use a knife and spoon and eat from individual rather than collective plates.

Infant Feeding Practices: Maternal milk *(amashereka)* is generally used; breast-feeding is common in Rwanda. The average duration is 16 months, but it can last more than 3 years. Rwanda has no postpartum sexual taboos limiting breast-feeding as do other Great Lakes cultures. Breast-feeding is suspended when the mother is sick or in the case of a subsequent pregnancy because these situations are believed to provoke diarrhea in a breast-feeding infant. Bottles are occasionally used and powdered milk is sold at the market, but the powder is generally unaffordable for poor people. Bottles are considered a necessity for women who have jobs as servants taking care of children. Children are not fed with solid food until they start crawling.

Child Rearing Practices: Child discipline is a role of all the men in the community (e.g., fathers, uncles, grandfathers), although final decisions rest with the parents. However, because children spend most of their time with their mothers, the mother's influence is profound. Child rearing is permissive during the breast-feeding period. Children sleep with the parents until they start eating solid food and are treated tenderly. Children are expected to be respectful to their parents all of their lives. Finger sucking is discouraged, occasionally by putting hot spices on fingers. Children usually stay with their mothers while they do household chores (e.g., cultivation, fetch water, prepare meals) and accompany them to social activities such as wedding ceremonies. Later, they are regularly sent to spend time with their relatives. Sharing, strict respect, generosity, the importance of giving gifts, and a sense of community are taught to children, and children are taught to admit their errors (e.g., when they break household articles).

National Childhood Immunizations: BCG at birth; DTP at 6, 10, and 14 weeks and 15 1/2 months; OPV at birth, at 6, 10, and 14 weeks, and at 15 1/2 months; measles at 9 months; vitamin A at 6 to 11, and 12 to 59 months; and TT at first contact, +4 weeks, +1, +1, +1 year.

BIBLIOGRAPHY

Rwanda. In *Columbia Encyclopedia*. Retrieved February 5, 2002, from http://www.bartleby.com/65/rw/Rwanda.html

Cammaer G: *Le temps conçu et le temps vecu. Un problème de communication interculturelle,* Tervuren, Belgique, 1992, Annales des Sciences Humaines, Musée Royal de l'Afrique Centrale.

Caraël M, Msellati P, Bartos A: *Etude de faisabilité,* Alaitement et VIH au Rwanda, Unpublished manuscript, 1983.

De Jong JP et al: The prevalence of mental health problems in Rwandan and Burundese refugee camps, *Acta Psychiatr Scand* 102(3):171, 2000.

Ilinigumugabo A: *L'espacement des naissances au Rwanda: niveaux, causes et consequences,* 1989, Institut de Démographie, Louvain la Neuve.

Meheus A et al: *Santé et maladie au Rwanda,* Brussels, 1982, Administration Generale de la Cooperation au Développement.

Mets TF: The disease pattern of elderly medical patients in Rwanda, central Africa, *J Trop Med Hyg* 96(5):291–300, 1993.

Pieterse S, Manandhar M, Ismail S: The nutritional status of older Rwandan refugees, *Public Health Nutr* 1(4):259–264, 1998.

Rahlenbeck S, Hakizimana C: Deliveries at a district hospital in Rwanda, 1997—2000, *Int J Gynaecol Obstet* 76(3):325–328, 2002.

Taylor C: The concept of flow in Rwandan popular medicine, *Soc Sci Med* 27(12), 1988.

United Nations Joint Programme on HIV/AIDS 2000: *Rwanda. Epidemiological fact sheet on HIV/AIDS and sexually transmitted diseases, 2000 update,* UNAIDS, February 2002, http://www.unaids.org/hivaidsinfo/statistics/fact_sheets/pdfs/Rwanda_en.pdf

Yourassowsky V, Van der Borght K: *A nutritional survey in the Republic of Rwanda,* Annales des Sciences Humaines, No 87, Musée Royale de l'Afrique Centrale, Tervuren, Belgique, 1975.

◆ SAINT KITTS AND NEVIS (FEDERATION OF SAINT KITTS AND NEVIS)

MAP PAGE (858)

Location: St. Kitts and Nevis are two volcanic islands with mountainous interiors that are located in the eastern Caribbean Sea among the northern Leeward Islands. The islands are about 72 km (45 miles) northwest of Antigua. The climate is tropical, tempered by sea breezes, and has little seasonal variation. The population is primarily rural and concentrated along the coast. The total land area is 261 km^2 (104 square miles); St. Kitts is 168 km^2 (65 square miles), and Nevis is 93 km^2 (36 square miles). The total area is equivalent to approximately 1.5 times the size of Washington, DC. St. Kitts and Nevis are a constitutional monarchy, and Queen Elizabeth II as the head of state. The capital is Basseterre. The population of both islands is about 38,726, and 61% of the total population is between the ages of 15 and 64 years.

Major Languages	Ethnic Groups	Major Religions
English	Black African descent 99%	Anglican
	British, Portuguese,	Other Protestant sects
	Lebanese 1%	Roman Catholic

Ethnic/Race Specific or Endemic Diseases: Hepatitis A and B are endemic. Islanders are at risk for dengue fever, salmonellosis, and babesiosis, and they have a high incidence of diabetes mellitus. The World Health Organization (WHO) has no estimated prevalence rates for HIV/AIDS in adults or children.

National Childhood Immunizations: BCG at birth or 5 years; DTP at 2, 4, 6, and 18 months; OPV at 3, 4, 6, and 18 months and at 12 and 17 years; hep B at birth and at 1 and 6 months; MMR at 12 to 15 months and 5 years; DT at 12 and 17 years; and TT at first contact, +4 weeks, +1 year. The reported percentages of the target population vaccinated in 200 were as follows: BCG, 100; first dose of DTP, 99; third dose of DTP, 99; third dose of hep B, 100; third dose of HIB, 12; MCV, 100; and Pol3, 99.

Other Characteristics: The life expectancy in St. Kitts and Nevis is 73.97 for women and 68.22 for men. The birth rate is 18.78 births per 1000 people. The total fertility rate is 2.41 children born per woman, and the infant mortality rate is 16.28 deaths per 1000 live births. The per capita gross domestic product is $7000. The islands are a transshipment point for South American drugs destined for the United States and Europe.

BIBLIOGRAPHY

http://www.odci.gov/cia/publications/factbook/geos/sc.html

◆ SAINT LUCIA

MAP PAGE (858)

Location: St. Lucia is one of the Windward Islands of the southeastern Caribbean between Martinique to the north and St. Vincent to the southwest. It is a volcanic island, and mountains run from north to south. St. Lucians are primarily descendants of Black African slaves. The island has a tropical climate. The total land area is 619 km^2 (238 square miles), and the population is just more than 147,000. The population is about evenly divided between rural and urban areas. Castries, the capital, contains about one third of the population. Despite a high emigration rate, the population is growing rapidly at 1.6% a year. St. Lucia has a Westminster-style parliamentary democracy, and the head of state is Queen Elizabeth II.

Major Languages	Ethnic Groups	Major Religions
English	Black African descent	Roman Catholic 90%
French patois	90%	Protestant 7%
(widely spoken)	Mixed African/	Anglican 3%
	European 6%	
	East Indian 3%	
	European 1%	

Ethnic/Race Specific or Endemic Diseases: Hepatitis A, pertussis, and mumps are endemic. The islanders are at risk for schistosomiasis and dengue fever. The World Health Organization (WHO) has no estimated prevalence rates for HIV/AIDS in adults or children.

National Childhood Immunizations: BCG at 3 months; DTP at 3, 4 1/2, 6, and 18 months; OPV at 3, 4 1/2, 6, and 18 months and 5 years; measles at 2 years; MMR at 12 months; and DT at 5 years. It is estimated that 75% of 1- and 2-year-olds must be immunized to eliminate endemic mumps virus transmission on the island. Vaccination coverage of 80% of 2-year-olds is needed to eliminate endemic pertussis. The reported percentages of the target population vaccinated in 2000 were as follows: BCG, 91%; first dose of DTP, 76%; third dose of DTP, 70%; and Pol3, 70%.

Other Characteristics: The life expectancy in St. Lucia is 74 years for women and 66 years for men. The infant mortality rate is 21 per 1000 people. The per capita gross domestic product (GDP) is $3866.

BIBLIOGRAPHY

http://www.state.gov/www/background_notes/stlucia_398_bgn.html

◆ SAINT VINCENT AND THE GRENADINES

MAP PAGE (858)

Location: St. Vincent and the Grenadine islands are among the Windward Islands of the southeastern Caribbean Sea. The large island of St. Vincent has forested mountains and the Soufriere volcano, which became active in 1979 and is a constant threat. The Grenadines are a chain of about 500 smaller islands. St. Vincent and the Grenadines is located about 34 km (21 miles) southwest of St. Lucia and 100 miles (160 km) west of Barbados and is north of Trinidad and Tobago. It is a parliamentary democracy, and the chief of state is Queen Elizabeth II. The total land area is 389 km² (150 square miles), about twice the size of Washington, DC. Kingstown is the capital. The population is about 115,982, and 64.04% of the population is between 15 and 64 years. The people are primarily descendants of Black African slaves. The climate is tropical—hot and humid with little seasonal variations.

Major Languages	Ethnic Groups	Major Religions
English	Primarily Black	Anglican 47%
French patois	African descent 66%	Methodist 28%
	Mixed 19%	Roman Catholic 13%
	East Indian 6%	Seventh-Day
	Carib Amerindian 2%	Adventist, Hindu,
	Other 7%	other Protestant 12%

Ethnic/Race Specific or Endemic Diseases: Hepatitis A is endemic. The islanders are at risk for schistosomiasis and dengue fever. The Black population, primarily of West African ancestry, are known to have a high prevalence of essential hypertension and high rates of end-organ damage. The World Health Organization (WHO) has no estimated prevalence rates for HIV/AIDS in children or adults.

National Childhood Immunizations: BCG at birth; DTP at 3, $4\frac{1}{2}$, 6, and 18 months; OPV at 3, $4\frac{1}{2}$, 6, and 18 months and $4\frac{1}{2}$ years; hep B at first contact, +2 more doses; MMR at 1 and $4\frac{1}{2}$ years; DT at $4\frac{1}{2}$ years; and TT for pregnant women, +6 weeks, +5 years. The reported percentages of the population who were vaccinated in 2000 are as follows: BCG, 99; first dose of DTP, 91; third dose of DTP, 99; MCV, 96; and Pol3, 100.

Other Characteristics: The life expectancy in St. Vincent and the Grenadines is 74.34 for women and 70.83 for men. The birth rate is 17.91 births per 1000 people. The infant mortality rate is 16.61 deaths per 1000 live births, and the total fertility rate is 2.06 children born per woman. The per capita gross domestic product (GDP) is low at $2800. Pollution of coastal waters and shorelines by pleasure yachts and other effluents have caused severe pollution in some areas, making swimming unhealthy. The islands are a transshipment point for South American drugs destined for the United States and Europe.

BIBLIOGRAPHY

Kotanko P et al: Essential hypertension in African Caribbeans associated with a variant of the α2-adrenoceptor, *Hypertension* 30(4):773, 1997.
http://www.odci.gov/cia/publications/factbook/geos/vc.html

◆ SAMOA (INDEPENDENT STATE OF)

MAP PAGE (856)

Stephen McGarvey

Location: Samoa is an independent nation formerly known as Western Samoa and is located in the Pacific Ocean. It consists of four inhabited islands, with the majority of the population residing on the islands of 'Upolu, the site of the capital Apia, and Savai'i. The total land area is

2849 km^2 (1100 square miles), of which Savai'i is 660 square miles (1709 km^2), and 'Upolu is 440 square miles (1140 km^2). The 1991 census revealed a total population of 161,298, of which approximately 34,000 resided in the Apia urban area. About 41% of the population was younger than 15 years.

Major Languages	Ethnic Groups	Major Religions
Samoan (official)	Samoan 92%	Christian 99.7%
English	Euronesian 7%	Other or none 0.3%
	European 1%	

English is widely used. The Euronesian population is a mixture of Europeans and Polynesians.

Health Care Beliefs: Acute sick care; passive role. The Samoan population is almost universally Christian, and people's health beliefs often attribute poor health to divine will. Patients have very little knowledge about obesity, diabetes, and hypertension. The health care system is attempting to inform and empower patients and provide continuing professional education for providers about the biology, sociobehavioral, and cultural factors that influence patient-provider partnerships in managing chronic diseases.

Predominant Sick Care Practices: Biomedical and traditional. The majority of the population seeks acute and chronic care for illnesses at the government hospital in Apia, four other district hospitals, and several health centers. A growing private sector also provides medical services. Many individuals consult traditional healers, although it is very hard to estimate the number of people using such services. The Samoan government's health care system is in the midst of a major review and modernization of curative, emergency, and preventive services. The changing patterns of morbidity from childhood infectious diseases to adult noncommunicable diseases such as diabetes and hypertension have been recognized, and are leading to a reemphasis on preventive medical services and public health primary and secondary prevention activities.

Ethnic/Race Specific or Endemic Diseases: One of the difficult issues facing Samoa and many developing nations is the emergence of adult noncommunicable diseases such as diabetes and hypertension. Modernizing Samoans have a high prevalence of these conditions because of their high proportion of overweight adults. Management of the diseases linked to obesity such as diabetes and hypertension requires cooperation and knowledge sharing between patients and health care providers. Despite the decrease in childhood infection rates, filariasis remains problematic, although the health department has preventive teams that visit villages and focus on vector control and treating infected individuals. Tuberculosis cases decreased from 94 in 1991 to 51 in 1996. The World Health Organization (WHO) has no estimated prevalence rates for HIV/AIDS for adults or children in Samoa. Recent data on HIV indicate four cases were diagnosed in 1996. Life expectancy at birth is 63.5 years for men and 65.6 years for women.

Families' Role in Hospital Care: Families of some hospitalized patients are involved in their direct care, which includes provision of food.

Pain Reactions: Research among Samoan migrants in California has suggested a tendency toward stoicism in the face of pain, although this has not been studied in the Samoan archipelago.

Food Practices and Intolerances: The basic Samoan diet includes taro, a root crop, bananas, coconuts, breadfruit, fresh fish, canned fish, and canned beef. Imported food such as rice, flour, and convenience foods have become more prevalent in Samoa, especially in the Apia area.

Infant Feeding Practices: Many women breast-feed, and the weaning period varies significantly. The 1991 infant mortality rate according to the census was 19.8 per 1000 live births.

Child Rearing Practices: Child rearing is indulgent and lenient during infancy and early childhood. Mothers provide the primary care, but other females, especially older siblings and other relatives, participate as well. As children become older, they are expected to learn to be obedient to parents, older siblings, and older village members. Some have described a socialization pattern involving suppression of strong emotions because it can disrupt the small villages; this may be especially true for females. The mortality rate for children younger than 5 years according to the 1991 census was 27 per 1000 live births.

National Childhood Immunizations: BCG at birth; DTP at 6, 10, and 14 weeks; OPV at 6, 10, and 14 weeks; hep B at birth and at 6 and 10 weeks; measles at 9 months and 5 years; DT at 5 years; and TT antenatal 7 and 9 months and 6 weeks postpartum. Data from 1992 to 1994 indicated that more than 92% of children received vaccinations against diphtheria, tetanus, pertussis, polio, measles, and hepatitis B.

BIBLIOGRAPHY

Annual report 1993 and 1994, Apia, Samoa, 1996, Department of Health, Government of Samoa, Government Printing Office.

Baker PT, Hanna JM, Baker TS: *The changing Samoans, behavior and health in transition,* New York, 1986, Oxford University Press.

Collins VR et al: Increasing prevalence of NIDDM in the Pacific Island population of Western Samoa over a 13-year period, *Diabetes Care* 17(1):288-296, 1994.

Galanis DJ et al: Dietary intake of modernizing Samoans: implications for risk of cardiovascular disease, *J Am Dietetic Assoc* 99:184-190, 1999.

Gerber ER: Rage and obligation: Samoan emotion in conflict. In White G, Kirkpatrick J, eds: *Person, self, and experience: exploring Pacific ethnopsychologies,* Berkeley, 1985, University of California Press.

Health sector strategic plan 1998-2003: partnerships in health, Apia, Samoa, 1998, Government of Samoa, Government Printing Office.

Howard A: Polynesia and Micronesia in psychiatric perspective, *Transcul Psych Res Rev* 16:123–145, 1979.

MacPherson C: Samoan medical belief and practice, Auckland, New Zealand, 1990, Auckland University Press.

O'Meara T: *Samoan planters: tradition and economic development in Polynesia,* Fort Worth, Tex, 1990, Holt, Rinehart, & Winston.

McGarvey ST: Obesity in Samoans and a perspective on its etiology in Polynesians, *Am J Clin Nutr* 53:1586S–1594S, 1991.

Report of the Census of Population and Housing 1991, Apia, Samoa, 1993, Government of Samoa, Government Printing Office.

◆ SAN MARINO (REPUBLIC OF)

MAP PAGE (860)

Location: San Marino is the smallest state in Europe after the Holy See and Monaco. It claims to be the oldest republic in the world, founded in the year 301. This small independent republic is landlocked in southern Europe and is an enclave in central Italy. It has a strong, independent history. Its location in the Apennine Mountains gives it a rugged terrain. The total land area is 61.2 km^2 (23.6 square miles), which is less than half the size of Washington, DC. The climate is Mediterranean, with mild to cool winters and warm, sunny summers. The total population is about 27,336, and 68% of the population is between the ages of 15 and 64.

Major Language	Ethnic Groups	Major Religions
Italian	Italo-Sammarinese 99%	Roman Catholic 99%
	Other 1%	Other 1%

Predominant Sick Care Practices: Biomedical. San Marino has a national health service and is making serious attempts to promote health education interventions through general practitioners.

Ethnic/Race Specific or Endemic Diseases: Hepatitis A, C, and E; cardiovascular disease; diabetes mellitus; and cutaneous leishmaniasis are endemic, as are intestinal parasites in children. San Marino has a high incidence of gastric cancer, accounting for 9% of all deaths and 335 of all cancer deaths. The age-adjusted death rate from gastric cancer is the highest in the world. In recent years, the incidence of respiratory tract and colorectal cancer has also increased. The World Health Organization (WHO) has no estimated prevalence rates for HIV/AIDS in children or adults.

National Childhood Immunizations: Although the immunization schedule for San Marino has not been published, the WHO reported percentages of the population vaccinated in 1999 are as follows: third dose of DTP, 99; third dose of hep B, 97; third dose of HIB, 95; and MCV, 100.

Other Characteristics: The life expectancy in San Marino is 85.1 for women and 77.68 for men. The birth rate is 10.76 births per 1000 people. Infant mortality rates are 6.21 deaths per 1000 live births. The total fertility rate is 1.3 children born per woman. The per capita gross domestic product is very high at $32,000.

BIBLIOGRAPHY

Conti EM et al: Cancer mortality in the Republic of San Marino, *Int J Epidemiol* 15(3):420, 1986.

Mamon J, Paccagnella B: Patient counseling by general practitioners: Republic of San Marino's experience, *Health Educ Q* 18(1):135, 1991.

http://www.odci.gov/cia/publications/factbook/geos/sm.html

◆ SÃO TOMÉ AND PRÍNCIPE (DEMOCRATIC REPUBLIC OF)

MAP PAGE (863)

Location: The smallest country in Africa, this country comprises small, mountainous, volcanic islands that straddle the equator. They are located 240 km (150 miles) off Gabon on the west coast of Africa in the Gulf of Guinea. The two main islands are São Tomé, which has dense, mountainous jungles, and Príncipe, which has jagged mountains. Smaller islands—Caroco, Pedras, and Tinhosas—are close to Príncipe, and Rolas is close to São Tomé. The total land area is 1001 km² (386 square miles), more than five times the size of Washington, DC. The capital is São Tomé. This republic is a developing nation. It attained independence from Portugal in 1975, but democratic reforms were not instituted until the late 1980s. Príncipe has had self-government since April 1995. The population is 165,034, and 48% is between the ages of 15 and 64 years. Most people are engaged in subsistence agriculture and fishing. The climate is tropical and humid, and the islands are beset with soil erosion and exhaustion.

Major Language	Ethnic Groups	Major Religions
Portuguese (official)	Mestico	Christian (Roman
	Angolares (descendents	Catholic, Evangelical
	of Angolan slaves)	Protestant, Seventh-
	Forros (descendents	Day Adventist) 80%
	of freed slaves)	Indigenous beliefs 20%
	Servicais (contract	
	laborers from	
	Angola, Mozambique,	
	and Cape Verde) and	
	their children (Tongas)	
	Europeans (primarily	
	Portuguese)	

Predominant Sick Care Practices: Biomedical where available and traditional. Medical facilities on São Tomé and Príncipe are extremely limited. The country only has one hospital—on the island of São Tomé—and several clinics. The level of medical care is extremely low. Medications are unavailable, and only minor medical needs can be addressed.

Ethnic/Race Specific or Endemic Diseases: Yellow fever, schistosomiasis, nonfilarial elephantiasis, and filariasis are endemic. Malaria is mesoendemic. People are at risk for toxoplasmosis, human parvovirus, intestinal helminthiasis, and injuries from automobile accidents because the roads are poorly maintained and the country has no street lights anywhere other than the capital. The World Health Organization (WHO) has no estimated prevalence rates for HIV/AIDS in children or adults.

National Childhood Immunizations: BCG at birth; DTP at 6, 10, and 14 weeks; OPV at birth and 6, 10, and 14 weeks; measles at 9 months; vitamin A at 9 to 59 months; yellow fever at 12 months; and TT CBAW. The reported percentages of the population vaccinated in 2000 are as follows: BCG, 81; third dose of DTP, 82; MCV, 69; Pol3, 87; and TT2 plus, 75.

Other Characteristics: The life expectancy in São Tomé and Príncipe is 67.07 for women and 64.15 for men. The birth rate is 42.74 births per 1000 people. The infant mortality rate is very high, with 48.96 deaths per 1000 live births. The total fertility rate is 6.02 children born per woman. The per capita gross domestic product (GDP) is very low at $1100. Fecal pollution throughout the territory causes unhygienic conditions and is considered dangerously unhealthy.

BIBLIOGRAPHY

Pampiglione S, Visconti S, Pezzino G: Human intestinal parasites in Subsaharan Africa II. Sao Tome and Principe, *Parassitologia* 29(1):15, 1987.
http://www.odci.gov/cia/publications/factbook/geis/tp.html
http://travek,stat,giv/saotome_principe.html

◆ SAUDI ARABIA (KINGDOM OF)

MAP PAGE (864)

Nigel J. Shanks

Location: The Kingdom of Saudi Arabia (1,960,582 km² or 758,981 square miles) occupies most of the Arabian Peninsula and has 2,640 km of coastline. The Red Sea and the Gulf of Aqaba are on the west, and the Persian Gulf is on the east. A mountain range spans the length of the western coastline, and east of the mountains is a massive plateau—the *Rub Al Khali* (the Empty Quarter)—which contains the world's largest sand desert. Saudi Arabia borders Iraq (for 814 km), Jordan (for 728 km),

Kuwait (for 222 km), Oman (for 676 km), Qatar (for 60 km), the United Arab Emirates (for 457 km), and Yemen (for 1458 km). Saudi Arabia has a harsh, dry desert climate, with great temperature extremes. Natural hazards include severe sand storms, electrical storms, and flash flooding.

Major Languages	Ethnic Groups	Major Religions
Arabic (official)	Arab 90%	Muslim (official) 99%
	Afro-Asian 10%	Other 1%

The Saudi family, who is allied with the Wahabis (a fiercely fundamental Islamic sect), united the warring tribes of the Arabian Peninsula through numerous military campaigns and territory acquisitions. Abdul Aziz Ibn Saud was proclaimed King of the Hejaz in 1926 in the Great Mosque of Mecca, entrusting the Saudi dynasty with the keeping of Islam's holy places. Today, the king of Saudi Arabia is called the *Custodian of the Two Holy Mosques*. The total population of 22,757,092 includes 5,360,526 nonnational expatriate workers, the vast majority of whom come from Egypt, Pakistan, India, and the Philippines. Ninety percent of the national population is ethnic Arabs who are descendant of the indigenous tribes and still today maintain strong tribal affiliations. Most of the population lives in and near the larger cities, with a small number of nomadic Bedouin tribes. The tenets of the kingdom are enshrined in Sharia law, and the public practice of other religions is forbidden. The vast majority of the population (85%) is Sunni Muslim, but 15% (mainly on the east coast) are Shiite Muslims. With two of the most sacred sites in Islam (Mecca and Medina) within its borders, Saudi Arabia considers itself the birthplace and heart of Islam.

Health Care Beliefs: Acute sick care, traditional, passive role. In Islam, people believe that "there is no disease that Allah has created except that He also has created its remedy, except for one ailment, namely old age." Even though advanced medical care is available, some Saudis (particularly those in nomadic tribes) still favor traditional Koranic medicine. According to a common traditional view, illness is not necessarily related to human behavior but is caused by spiritual agents such as *jinn,* the "evil eye" (the power of a person to harm others merely by looking at them), or the will of Allah. Prevention and treatment of disease are therefore based on appealing to the spiritual agent responsible, using methods such as prayer to Allah, votive offerings, or amulets to ward off the evil eye. Local practitioners specialize in various treatments, such as exorcism for mental illness, setting broken bones, herbal remedies for many ailments, and cauterization. However, consultations with these local, untrained healers are decreasing as access to more effective health care and health education becomes more available. Many believe that intrusive procedures such as injections and intravenous fluids are more effective than noninvasive treatments. Nomadic tribes and people in remote areas may only seek treatment when they are in the terminal stages of an illness.

Predominant Sick Care Practices: Biomedical, alternative and magical-religious. Health care is free to all Saudi citizens. Modern, state-of-the-art health care is available in the major cities (Riyadh, Dharan, and Jeddah) in the main hospitals affiliated with the Ministry of Defense and Aviation, national guard, and universities. These facilities are flagship hospitals, very well equipped with modern technological equipment, and offer a high standard of care. Some private hospital facilities are available, but the quality of health care varies. Saudi Arabia has numerous public hospitals and primary health care centers throughout the country, but they tend to be less well equipped than flagship hospitals, poorly staffed, and unsanitary. Islamic beliefs and culture pervade all aspects of health care, and Koranic traditional medicine is still practiced, particularly among people in remote locations in Saudi Arabia, although the practices are diminishing with the development of more modern health care facilities.

Ethnic/Race Specific or Endemic Diseases: Hepatitis is endemic throughout the Arabian peninsula, and 80% of the indigenous population has positive markers for hepatitis B infection. Chloroquine-sensitive malaria is a problem in the Tihama southern coastal plain, especially in Jizan, Asir, and Al Qunfudhah; however, measures are being taken to eliminate breeding grounds for mosquitoes by spraying with insecticide. Bilharzia (schistosomiasis) is a continuing but minor problem in Jizan, Al-Bahah, Asir, Najran, Medina, Al-Jawf, Hail, and Taif. Eliminating infestations of the bilharzia parasite and preventing reinfestation are a continuing challenge. Poliomyelitis has largely been controlled through vaccination. Cases of leishmaniasis have occurred in almost every province with the expansion of agricultural lands, which provide breeding grounds for disease-carrying sand flies. Trachoma is considered one of the main causes of blindness in the Kingdom, despite programs to combat the disease. Asthma is exceedingly common and tends to be seasonal, developing when the pollen count from certain grasses is high. Obesity and heart disease are endemic because of Western changes in dietary and lifestyle habits. Diabetes mellitus is very common and usually non-insulin dependent, and its clinical symptoms are different than they are in the West. For example, patients can tolerate extremely high blood sugar levels (more than 10 times normal) and have minimal symptoms. However, the long-term consequences of the disease (e.g., peripheral vascular problems, retinopathy, renal and heart disease) are the same. Poor dental hygiene is common and results in dental caries; the adverse sequelae of frequent consumption of carbonated soft drinks are obvious. Morbidity and mortality caused by major trauma from automobile accidents is high, despite public health campaigns promoting seat belts and defensive and safe driving practices. Although consanguineous marriages are discouraged, they are common, which results in many congenital abnormalities (some of which are very rare and confined to Saudi Arabia). Sickle cell trait is particularly common, and sickle cell crises are common in the accident and emergency departments. The World Health Organization's (WHO) estimated prevalence rate for HIV/AIDS in adults ages 15 to 49 is 0.01%. WHO has no estimates for children from birth to 15 years.

Health Team Relationships: Most doctors in Saudi Arabia are now Saudi nationals and tend to be well respected by their patients. Doctors are the dominant force in the health team. The majority of nurses are expatriate workers, mostly from the Philippines. Nursing is not a respected profession in Saudi Arabia, and nurses are thought of as servants. However, efforts are being made to rectify this situation through the establishment of schools of nursing within the kingdom to train Saudi nationals in the science of nursing.

Families' Role in Hospital Care: Most patients have an attendant or sitter with them for the duration of their stay in hospitals to ensure optimum care and attention. Sitters may be a family member but is usually a servant. Family members are often very demanding because they want to ensure that patients receive proper care and attention. Gifts of sweets and chocolates are common, and families expect to be able to visit for as long as and when they desire. These frequent visits can conflict with dietary restrictions and hospital routines.

Dominance Patterns: Saudi Arabia has a patriarchal culture. All important decisions are made by the oldest male family member. The Saudi mother is revered, and most sons seek their mothers' opinion on family issues. Women are primarily confined to the home to run the household, and they are not expected to play a prominent role in the family—this is generally perceived as a protective measure. However, younger Saudi females are now acquiring positions in teaching and medicine in increasing numbers. Women are usually not allowed to give consent for medical procedures; husbands or brothers give consent for them. In emergency situations a woman can give consent if her signature is witnessed by two men who are Saudi nationals. Polygamy is allowed for men but is quite uncommon.

Eye Contact Practices: Eye contact among men is expected during conversation and is a sign of honesty and integrity. Eye contact between men and women is discouraged, and if it occurs it is expected to be brief. Women can only make direct eye contact with other women and family members.

Touch Practices: Touching between men and women is forbidden except among family members. It is acceptable and quite common for men to kiss one another on the cheek and hold hands in public. Greetings and handshaking among men may be prolonged.

Pain Reactions: Reactions to pain are as for any nationality, rather than specific to Saudi culture. However, Bedouins tend to be more stoical than city dwellers. Pain is expressed verbally and nonverbally and with emotion. Pain-relieving medications are demanded frequently and must be provided immediately.

Perceptions of Time: *Inshallah,* or "as Allah wills," is the norm in Saudi Arabia. *Inshallah* can mean anything from "immediately" to "never." The concept may be used as a euphemism for "no." Time has little meaning in any situation other than business, and social rituals continue while appointments go by unheeded. It is common for people to arrive for hospital appointments late or on the wrong day.

Birth Rites: Large families are the norm and are encouraged by family pressure and state child benefits. The estimated birth rate in 2001 was 37.34 births per 1000 population, with a population growth rate of 3.27%. The overwhelming preference is for male children, particularly for the firstborn. Women can be divorced by their husbands if they do not bear sons. Childlessness is pitied, and infertility is considered a condition that must be rectified. Husbands and other male members of the family may be present at the birth, but at births in hospitals, they are rarely present. Most Saudi women prefer a doctor for the birth rather than a midwife. Celebrations and congratulations are effusive but are delayed for up to 3 months after birth. Saudi women are considered unclean after birth and may be sequestered in their home, or more commonly, in their mother's home, for up to 40 days. The 2001 infant mortality rate was estimated to be 51.25 per 1000 live births.

Death Rites: It is believed that only Allah knows the true prognosis for a patient, so confronting a patient with a grave prognosis shatters hope and can create mistrust. Islamic regulations *(Fatwah)* state that life support can be discontinued when certain conditions are met. Transplants are performed, and transplantation of human organs is completely acceptable; however, the desires of the family are considered the most important factor. Death is usually only discussed with male family members. After death the body must be washed ceremonially (possibly by a family member), after which no non-Muslim is allowed to touch the body. Interment is usually carried out within 1 day after death, and the body is buried in the ground wrapped in a shroud without a coffin. Cremations are not allowed. Autopsies are very rare because the body must be buried intact. When a family member dies, male family members are expected to repress any outward signs of grief. Women are frequently very vocal in their grief, wailing and ululating. Men and women receive condolences in separate venues for up to 3 days after death.

Food Practices and Intolerances: The traditional Saudi diet is rice, chicken, fish, and a small amount of red meat. Dates and *laban* (buttermilk) are common snacks. All types of ethnic, international, and fast foods are available in towns and cities across Saudi Arabia. The standard and variety of cuisine is among the best in the world. It is acceptable to eat with the fingers of the right hand, particularly at communal feasts. Pork, blood, carrion, and alcohol consumption is forbidden, so they are not imported into the country. Fasting between sunset and sundown is mandatory during the holy month of Ramadan for all people other than pregnant women, breast-feeding women, children, and those who are ill. However, some hospitalized patients fast even though they are ill. Eating, drinking, and smoking are forbidden in public places during Ramadan.

Infant Feeding Practices: Breast-feeding is the preferred method of infant feeding. It is acceptable in public and may continue for 18 months to 2 years. However, many mothers actually employ "wet nurses," and thereafter the care of the children is transferred to either an older female sibling or a maid. Infants who are not breast-fed are generally fed with premixed formulas or dried Nido milk.

Child Rearing Practices: Child rearing tends to be permissive. Discipline is inconsistent and is largely the responsibility of the female members of the family. Care is often the responsibility of older female siblings or servants. Families are generally large, and several families live in the same housing compound. Children are not taught how to play, and today they spend many hours watching television, creating widespread childhood obesity and exercise-shy children. Education is free for all Saudi citizens, but boys and girls are segregated and educated separately. Boys are raised in the female section of the household until they are 10 years of age, then they are transferred to the male part of the household; parenting is largely the responsibility of the father from this point on. Discipline is strict and firmly enforced. Females are considered adults by the age of 12 or at puberty. Although it has been outlawed, female circumcision still occurs on occasion among Saudi nationals, and it remains fairly common among Sudanese expatriate workers' families.

National Childhood Immunizations: BCG at birth; DPT at 6 weeks, 3, 5, and 18 months, and 4 to 6 years; polio at 6 weeks, 3, 5, and 18 months, and at 4 to 6 years; measles at 6 months and 12 months; and hep B at birth, 6 weeks, and 6 months. Child allowances are paid only after proof of completion of childhood vaccinations.

BIBLIOGRAPHY

al-Nasser AN, Bamgboye EA, Alburno MK: A retrospective study of factors affecting breast feeding practices in a rural community of Saudi Arabia, *East Afr Med J* 68(3):174, 1991.
al-Shammari SA: Help-seeking behavior of adults with health problems in Saudi Arabia, *Fam Pract Res J* 12(1):75, 1992.
Anderson R: Saudi Arabian culture, *Nurs Adm Q* 16(2):20, 1992.
Ballas E: Health meanings of Saudi women, *J Adv Nurs* 21(5):853, 1995.
Davis CF: Culturally responsive nursing management in an international health care setting, *Nurs Adm Q* 16(2):36, 1992.
El Hazmi A et al: Diabetes mellitus and impaired glucose tolerance in Saudi Arabia, *Ann Saudi Med* 16(4):381, 1996.

Reece D: Covering and communication: the symbolism of dress among Muslim women, *Howard J Comm* 7(1):35, 1996.

Sebai ZA, Bella H: Laying the foundations of good health care, *World Health Forum* 11(4):385, 1990.

World Health Organization (June 2000): *Epidemiological fact sheets by country,* Geneva. Retrieved March 1, 2002, from http://www.unaids.org/hivaidsinfo/statistics/june00/fact_sheets/index.html

World Health Organization (2001): *WHO vaccine-preventable diseases: monitoring system,* Geneva. Retrieved March 1, 2002, from http://www.who.int/vaccines/

◆ SENEGAL (REPUBLIC OF)

MAP PAGE (862)

Location: Senegal is on the northwestern coast of Africa on the Atlantic coast. Mauritania is to the north, Mali is to the east, and Guinea and Guinea-Bissau are to the south. Senegal circles The Gambia on three sides. It is a developing country comprising primarily a rural population that lives by subsistence farming. The capital is Dakar. The country has one of the best transportation systems in Africa. Much of Senegal is low, rolling plains, with foothills in the southeast. Senegal has wet and dry seasons; the dry season is dominated by the harmattan wind. The total land area is 196,190 km^2 (75,749 square miles), slightly smaller than South Dakota. The population is 10,284,929, and the per capita gross domestic product is $1600.

Major Languages	Ethnic Groups	Major Religions
French (official)	Wolof 43%	Muslim 92%
Wolof	Pular 24%	Indigenous beliefs 6%
Pulaar	Serer 15%	Christian 2%
Jola	Jola 4%	
Mandinka	Mandinka, Soninke,	
	European, Lebanese 4%	

Health Care Beliefs: Acute sick care; passive role. USAID/Senegal has sponsored mass media interventions, targeted information campaigns, and research to help slow the spread of HIV/AIDS. Use of condoms and family planning are central to these approaches. Other programs are being conducted, such as child survival programs (which are nutritionally focused) and promotion of oral rehydration therapy for treatment of diarrheal disease in children.

Predominant Sick Care Practices: Traditional and biomedical where available. Major and minor illnesses can be treated in several hospitals or clinics in Dakar. Senegal has good office-based psychiatry services but no inpatient facility. Public hospitals do not meet American standards, but private clinics are considered to be at the level of small European hospitals and approaching American community hospital standards. Outside of Dakar, facilities are limited.

Ethnic/Race Specific or Endemic Diseases: Endemic diseases include West Nile virus; bilharziasis; goiter (which is regional); hepatitis A, B and C; schistosomiasis (that is resistant to or tolerant of praziquantel); and intestinal parasites (amebiasis). Chloroquine-resistant malaria is mesoendemic, particularly during the rainy season, and trachoma is highly endemic. People are at risk for yellow fever, onchocerciasis (which is regional), chanchroid, tuberculosis, measles, borreliosis, cholera, typhoid fever, and meningitis. Senegal recently had an outbreak of Chikungunya disease and a recent cessation in the transmission of dracunculiasis. Vitamin A deficiency is a major cause of childhood blindness. The World Health Organization's (WHO) estimated prevalence rate for HIV/AIDS in adults ages 15 to 49 is 1.77%. The estimated number of people living with HIV/AIDS is 79,000. Approximately 7800 adults and children died of AIDS in 1999. The estimated number of children who have lost their mother or both parents to AIDS and who were alive and younger 15 at the end of 1999 is 29,023. Life expectancy at birth is 60.94 for men and 64.22 for women.

Dominance Patterns: Customs relative to family life and women are consistent with Islamic culture. Literacy rates are 43% for males and 23.2% for females.

Birth Rites: The birth rate is 37.46 births per 1000 people, and the infant mortality rate is 56.75 deaths per 1000 live births. The total fertility rate is 5.12 children born per woman. USAID estimated the contraceptive prevalence rate to be 7% in 1997.

Death Rites: Muslim doctors may recommend transfusions to save lives. Autopsies are uncommon because the body must be buried intact. For Muslim burials the body is wrapped in special pieces of cloth and buried without a coffin in the ground as soon as possible after death. Cremations are not permitted.

Food Practices and Intolerances: Pork, carrion, blood, and alcohol consumption are forbidden. Food tends to be spicy. Ramadan fasting is practiced, with exemptions for the sick and certain other individuals.

Child Rearing Practices: Approximately 44% of the population is 14 years of age or younger. Female circumcision and excision is widespread in some groups. By the end of 2000, about 10,000 Senegalese (the majority of whom were women and children) were refugees, including about 5000 in Guinea-Bissau and 5000 in The Gambia. Approximately 5000 were internally displaced because of armed conflicts between separatists and the Senegalese military in southern Senegal's Casamance province. Land mines in Casamance province have made 80% of the farmland unusable and have resulted in approximately 500 deaths since 1977.

National Childhood Immunizations: BCG at birth; DTP at 6, 10, and 14 weeks; OPV at birth and 6, 10, and 14 weeks; measles at 9 months; YFV at 9 months; and TT for pregnant women ×2. The reported percentages of the target population vaccinated are as follows: BCG, 89; first dose of DTP, 79; third dose of DTP, 52; MCV, 48; Pol3, 49; TT2plus, 45; and YFV, 34.

Other Characteristics: Children younger than age 5 who migrate from rural to urban areas have higher mortality rates, but this problem is being addressed by the child survival programs that have been initiated. The country has other deep-seated problems, such as chronic unemployment, juvenile delinquency, and drug addiction. Senegal is a transshipment point for Southwest and Southeast Asian heroin being transported to Europe and North America. It is also an illegal cultivator of cannabis. As of April 2002, rebel groups were still active in southwestern Senegal.

BIBLIOGRAPHY

Brockerhoff M: Rural-to-urban migration and child survival in Senegal, *Demography* 27(4):601, 1990.
Rowell M: Eradication of vitamin A deficiency with 5 cents and a vegetable garden, *J Ophthalmic Nurs Tech* 12(5):217, 1993.
Wright J: Female genital mutilation: an overview, *J Adv Nurs* 24:251, 1996.
http://www.odci.gov/cia/publications/factbook/geos/sg.html
http://travel.state.gov/senegal.html

◆ SEYCHELLES (REPUBLIC OF)

MAP PAGE (863)

Conrad Shamlaye

Location: A group of 115 islands scattered in the western Indian Ocean east of Kenya and northeast of Madagascar form the Seychelles. The population of 80,000 is found primarily on the three main granitic islands of Mahé, Praslin, and La Digue. The total land area is 455 km^2 (176 square miles). Many of the islands are uninhabited coral atolls. The islands were all uninhabited until the latter part of the eighteenth century, when they were colonized by French settlers and African slaves. Later, as the islands transferred to British rule, the population grew with European settlers, liberated African slaves from the Eastern coast of Africa, and Indian and Chinese immigrants. French and African cultural influences remain strong.

Major Languages	Ethnic Groups	Major Religions
Seselwa (Creole; official)	Seychellois 100%	Roman Catholic 90%
English (official)		Anglican 8%
French (official)		Other, none 2%

Creole is the common language and is spoken by everyone. Although the population is predominantly of African origin, numerous marriages have taken place among members of different ethnic groups. The Seychellois are proud of their unique national identity, and ethnic origin is considered irrelevant. In addition to the larger religious groups, Seychelles has small communities of Bahai's, Muslims, and Hindus. Seychelles is classified as a middle-income country, with an economy that is based primarily on tourism and fishing. The Seychellois population is culturally homogeneous, with high levels of literacy and good health indicators. The Seychellois nation is open to international influences because most professionals train outside the country, most people travel frequently, contact with tourists is frequent, and people have universal access to radio, television, and telephone (and now the Internet).

Health Care Beliefs: Both active and passive roles; health promotion important. As a result of health education and promotion efforts during the past 3 decades and a high level of education and excellent literacy rate, the concepts of illness and disease are generally based on scientific facts. However, some older people believe that illnesses may arise from evil intentions of others. Wearing of amulets is no longer common, but a long-practiced tradition involving herbal home remedies for minor ailments and general health improvements still exists. Consulting herbalists, usually in addition to rather than instead of doctors, is not unusual. The people have a growing interest in legalizing and regulating herbalists to promote potentially useful natural therapies and discard ineffective traditional magical practices. However, herbalism is associated with witchcraft so in the past, practitioners were consulted frequently for help with harming others or protection from evil. No particular stigmas are attached to illnesses such as epilepsy or mental disorders. In fact, Sechellois are becoming increasingly aware of the rights and needs of those with disabilities, older adults, and other potentially vulnerable groups.

Predominant Sick Care Practices: Biomedical, traditional and alternative. During times of illness, people readily turn to doctors and the orthodox health system. Because of the policy of decentralizing health care services, community health centers are found throughout the primary populated islands, and many people use the services. Health care is free for all citizens in the predominantly government-funded modern health care system of health centers, which are staffed by multidisciplinary professional teams, and a central referral hospital offering the primary specialist services. The Seychelles has several individual private medical and dental practitioners and a growing number of complementary health practitioners.

Ethnic/Race Specific or Endemic Diseases: Changes in lifestyle resulting from increases in social and economic status have resulted in an epidemiological transition; cardiovascular diseases now account for more than one third of all deaths. Cancers are the second most common cause of death. Childhood infectious diseases have essentially been eradicated by preventive health programs, including immunizations, and general social and economic improvement. Health awareness is high among the population, and no particular ethnic or cultural differences in use of health care services exists. People are becoming aware that men need to be the focus of specific preventive programs targeting cardiovascular diseases and excessive alcohol consumption. The World Health Organization (WHO) has no estimated prevalence rates for HIV/AIDS for the Seychelles. However, the WHO reports that although prevalence is low to moderate, it is steadily rising. From December 1998 to December 1999 the number of known HIV cases rose from 56 to 67.

Health Team Relationships: The majority of doctors are non-nationals (e.g., Indians, Cubans, Africans, Europeans) on 2-year contracts. Difficulties in communication occasionally arise because the doctors do not speak Creole and must use nurses or nursing assistants as interpreters. Most patients expect to have a conversation with their doctors and a thorough consultation and complain if they think that the doctors have not adequately examined them. Community health teams are usually led by a nurse manager who is well accepted by the community; in hospitals, doctors and nurses share leadership roles. Emphasis is on professional team building, and health practitioners often interact with social service workers, schools, and community organizations. Health professionals are expected to be aware of and responsive to the needs of patients and their families. Doctors and nurses make house calls to care for individuals and get to know the social setting.

Families' Role in Hospital Care: The Seychellois are quite dependent on service providers (e.g., health care, social services, housing) and tend to expect quick referrals to specialists and hospitals. As a result, the trend toward hospital-based care and use of laboratory and radiological diagnostic facilities is increasing. Waiting lists for surgeries are generally weeks long. Family members are not encouraged to remain with patients overnight unless the patients are young children or have terminal illnesses. As a rule, family members do not help care for patients in the hospital, and all meals are provided.

Dominance Patterns: Seychellois society is fairly matriarchal. Women head many households and succeed in housing, feeding, clothing, and bringing up their children with little help from the children's fathers. Many children are given their mother's surname rather than their father's. However, although it is becoming more common for men to share the household duties, many employed women still fatalistically accept that their partners, even those who are unemployed, will not help with child care or domestic chores.

Eye Contact Practices: Patients expect to make eye contact with service providers of both genders.

Touch Practices: Generally, touch during physical examination is acceptable, although a nurse is required to be present when a doctor performs an intimate examination.

Perceptions of Time: The Seychellois are time conscious, expecting to be seen on time and to have health services provided courteously and efficiently. Patients frequently arrive well before their appointment time and complain if they have to wait too long.

Pain Reactions: Patients are generally quite stoical about pain and begin moving quite rapidly after surgery. However, they often feel that they are unable to resume work for long periods after surgery. This is also true even when they are diagnosed with illnesses such as high blood pressure and diabetes that should not cause extended disability.

Birth Rites: Almost all births occur in the hospital, and home births are considered unacceptable. More fathers are attending births. The Seychellois have no particular birth rites or preferences for a particular gender. Other practices, such as not eating eggs during pregnancy and not washing the hair for several weeks after delivery, are dying out. Three of four infants are born to unmarried women. Women tend to take on most of the responsibilities for child rearing, and the father is frequently absent from the household. The total fertility rate is now just at the replacement level, and children are highly valued. Child rearing practices are generally permissive.

Death Rites: Extended families are still common, although pressure for the government to provide residence and care for aging adults is growing. Dying at home is becoming less common as hospitalization and institutional care increase. Families strongly believe that patients must be visited by a priest before their death. The Seychellois have no particular death rites. Church funerals are attended not only by immediate family and friends but also by distant relatives and acquaintances. Postmortem medical examinations are generally acceptable if the relatives are approached with sensitivity about the topic. Organ donations are not performed, and no legal provisions address the procedure.

Food Practices and Intolerances: The Seychellois diet, as are many other aspects of the culture, is in a state of transition. The diet is still high in fish, which is usually highly spiced and eaten with rice and vegetables. Root crops such as cassava and sweet potato are also consumed, although perhaps less than they were previously. Eggs, fresh and processed meat, pasta, and potatoes are becoming more common parts of the diet, and fast-food outlets are becoming more common as well. People normally eat with a fork and spoon. The consumption of carbonated soft drinks is alarmingly high, especially among children.

Infant Feeding Practices: Breast-feeding rates are high during the first few weeks but decrease rapidly after the completion of maternity leave (which is 12 weeks). Some women believe that when they resume sexual relations after birth, they should stop breast-feeding because the sperm can enter the breast milk and harm the infant.

Child Rearing Practices: Beating of children (especially boys) is common, especially by fathers and stepfathers. However, corporal punishment is no longer permitted in schools. Parents and teachers frequently shout at children. Girls are generally expected to do more housework than boys, although boys are often given outdoor jobs such as sweeping the courtyard, feeding the dogs, and throwing out the trash.

National Childhood Immunizations: BCG at birth and 6 years; DTP at 3, 4, 5, and 18 months; OPV at 3, 4, 5, and 18 months and at 6 and 15 years; hep B at 3, 4, and 9 months; MMR at 15 months; YFV at 12 months; DT at 6 years; and TT at 15 years and every 10 years.

BIBLIOGRAPHY

National Youth Study Committee: *Reports of the National Youth Study,* 1998, Victoria, Seychelles.

Government of Seychelles (Management Information Systems Division): *Annual statistical abstracts,* MISD, Victoria, Seychelles, 2000.

Government of Seychelles (Ministry of Health): *National Policy for the Prevention and Control of HIV/AIDS and STIs,* November 2001.

Perdrix J et al. Patterns of alcohol consumption in the Seychelles Islands, *Alcohol Alcoholism* 34:773–785, 1999.

Shamlaye C et al: The Seychelles Child Development Study on neurodevelopmental outcomes in children following in utero exposure to methylmercury from a maternal fish diet: background and demographics, *Neurotoxicology* 16(4):597–612, 1995.

Shamlaye H: Report on the study of women discharged from the Victoria Hospital gynaecology ward with a diagnosis of abortion or threatened abortion between November 1993 and December 1997, *Singapore J Obstet Gynaecol* 29:8–19, 1998

◆ SIERRA LEONE (REPUBLIC OF)

MAP PAGE (862)

Durodami Radcliffe Lisk

Location: Sierra Leone is located on the western side of the African continent, bordered on the north and east by Guinea and on the southeast by Liberia. The remaining third of its border is formed by the Atlantic Ocean, with a heavily indented coastline of mangrove swamps and beautiful sandy beaches. The total land area is 71,740 km^2 (27,699 square miles). The country is just emerging from 10 years of civil war.

Major Languages	Ethnic Groups	Major Religions
Mende	Mende 30%	Muslim 60%
Temne	Temne 30%	Indigenous beliefs 30%
Krio (English based)	Kono, Limba, Krio 39%	Christian 10%
Limba	Creole, European, Lebanese, Asian 1%	

Health Care Beliefs: Acute sick care; traditional; passive role. People have little or no scientific concept of disease causation, and illnesses are blamed on enemies, witchcraft, or displeased ancestors. Charms are often worn to keep evil spirits away. Disease prevention is rarely practiced. Patients tend to prefer injections rather than tablets, and rectal suppositories are frequently unacceptable. Health promotion programs are usually based on focused group discussions complemented by traditional dancing and role playing, mainly involving women. Mental illnesses are regarded with suspicion and kept secret and are not considered to be in the domain of Western medicine. Practitioners with special spiritual powers are consulted to exorcise the devil causing the illness.

Predominant Sick Care Practices: Biomedical; traditional; magical-religious. Sick care practices depend on availability of services: 90% of the urban and 20% of the rural population have access to health care. Predominant practices in rural areas involve traditional healers and herbalists. Traditional birth attendants are trained in basic aseptic techniques and safe practices. Extensive, itchy skin rashes are believed to be caused by evil spells, so patients expect to be scrubbed vigorously and shown desquamated skin debris as evidence of removal of the offending cause. Even in urban areas, Western medicine is often abandoned in favor of traditional methods if the illness is prolonged or complicated.

Ethnic/Race Specific or Endemic Diseases: Malaria is holoendemic in Sierra Leone, accounting for significant morbidity and mortality, especially among children. Most infections are chloroquine-sensitive, but the prevalence of resistant infections is increasing. Onchocerciasis is endemic in the north, and schistosomiasis is endemic in the east of the country. Hypertension is common in urban areas, with a prevalence of about 25% in the capital Freetown and 14% in rural communities. Blood pressure is positively related to body mass and age. Diabetes is virtually nonexistent in rural villages. Ten years of civil war have created a large internally displaced population (approximately 30% of the population), which is susceptible to malnutrition, tuberculosis, HIV/AIDS, and diarrheal diseases. The World Health Organization's (WHO) estimated prevalence rate for HIV/AIDS in adults ages 15 to 49 years is 2.99%. The estimated number of children from birth to 15 years living with HIV/AIDS is 3300. However, this statistic may be an underestimate because very few community-based prevalence rates of HIV infection have been done as a result of the civil war. Low rates were recorded in the early 1990s, but they have sharply increased in the past several years because of war conditions. Rates are higher among those in the fighting forces and displaced populations.

Health Team Relationships: The doctor is head of the health team in health planning and the hospital. However, district clinics are administered by community health officers, who are high school graduates with 3 years of paramedical training from a college. In urban areas, doctors' clinics are complemented by practices run by *dispensers,* who are essentially nurse practitioners with a nursing background and 3 years of training in pharmaceuticals and basic clinical skills. Nurses play supporting roles in hospitals and clinics. Patients tend to be subservient to their healers and readily accept their decisions.

Families' Role in Hospital Care: Families and friends provide much support for those who are ill, particularly during hospitalizations. They provide food and medications, help with hygiene tasks, and provide moral support. Family members stay with the patients most of the day and frequently spend the night, often sleeping on the floor.

Dominance Patterns: Sierra Leone has a male-dominated society. Traditionally, men have been the primary breadwinners, but this is changing, especially in urban settings. Women are still expected to fulfill traditional duties such as looking after the home and children and in rural areas, working on the farms. However, women have attained prominent positions such as Supreme Court judge, chief medical officer, commissioner of income tax, and university professor. Politics is firmly in the male domain, and very few women have made inroads into this arena.

Eye Contact Practices: Direct eye contact is considered rude or defiant, particularly when children or subordinates are being cautioned or reprimanded because they are expected to look down. Eye contact among equals is common and expected.

Touch Practices: Touching is common and in many instances may be considered intimate by Western standards. Handshaking is part of the greeting process. Touching of the arms, backs, or even thighs is common during conversation and has no sexual connotations. Men often hold hands with other men, and women readily embrace each other. Patients are unsatisfied if their doctors do not touch or examine them.

Perceptions of Time: Punctuality is not taken seriously. The phrase "Black man time" is lightheartedly used to mean "later than scheduled." Clinic appointments are impractical, and patients are served on a first-come, first-served basis. Sierra Leoneans live in the past, remembering the time when the country was known as the "Athens of West Africa" and had the first high school, university, railway, and television network in the subregion. Ten years of civil war have destroyed most of the country's infrastructure and left many despondent and pessimistic about the future.

Pain Reactions: Sierra Leoneans have a high pain tolerance, although it may vary according to tribe. For example, Fullah women are known to give birth with no assistance and in silence; they get up and begin moving about within a matter of hours after birth. Otherwise, pain is occasionally expressed through dramatic facial and vocal expressions.

Birth Rites: About 70% of all deliveries take place in the home. Traditional birth attendants deliver most of the infants born in villages, but in the towns obstetric services are available. In most cases mothers lie on their backs, but in some instances they squat. Babies are bathed almost immediately after birth. The buttocks of girls and limbs of boys and girls are "molded" to ensure a perfect figure when they grow up. In some cultures, people bury the placenta or a piece of the umbilical cord and plant a fruit tree at the spot of burial, thereby relating the birth to the universe. The tree becomes known as the child's tree; fruits from the tree are sold, and the money used to buy things for the child. The naming ceremony is on the seventh day after birth for girls and the ninth day for boys. During the naming ceremony an older female family member takes the infant out of the house for the first time. Piercing of girls' ears and circumcision of boys take place soon after birth.

Death Rites: Death rites are an important part of Sierra Leonean custom. The Muslim and Christian communities have some differences in their funeral ceremonies. In some cases the family begins preparing for death long before a patient dies. Families have been known to withdraw financial support for medication once it is clear that a patient is going to die and start saving instead for the funeral. When the patient dies, family members will congregate at the home of the deceased and openly grieve. For Muslims, burial takes place the same day. The body is laid in a room in the house, and prayers are said for several hours. Men and women tend to segregate in different rooms, and women usually do not attend the burial ceremony. Christians spread funeral activities out over several days or even weeks. Family and friends visit the deceased person's home daily to say prayers and commiserate with close family members. The night before the funeral is the wake, when prayers are recited and religious songs are sung. Tributes are delivered well into the early hours of the morning. Food and drinks, including alcohol, are served. On the day of the funeral, the family has a "laying out" ceremony. The body is laid out in the house or a public place for a final public viewing. It is then taken to the church for the funeral service before interment. After the burial, family and friends return to the house for refreshments. Further commemorations take place on the seventh and fortieth days after death and on the first, fifth, and tenth anniversaries. During these occasions, black-eyed peas are cooked, some of which are on a table with a glass of water for the dead person. Autopsies are uncommon because of family reluctance to grant permission. Often an order from the coroner is required.

Food Practices and Intolerances: The staple food is rice, which is eaten every day. In rural areas in particular, tuberous plants such as yams, cassava, and sweet potatoes are included. Fermented cassava cooked into a thick paste called *foofoo* is also popular. Several varieties of green leaves are cooked with palm oil mixed with onions, pepper, meat, or fish as a sauce (*palava* sauce) for rice and *foofoo*. Traditionally, one main meal is eaten each day either in the morning or evening. Food is cooked by the women after they return from the farm or market. More westernized sections of society have three meals each day. Food is eaten either with a spoon or a hand. Forks and knives are used by the elite. Fruits are plentiful and eaten when in season. Food taboos are common during pregnancy and involve primarily protein-rich foods–especially chicken and eggs. Pregnant women are also discouraged from eating pepper and ginger because they may cause the infant to be haughty or have a bad temper. Some groups believe that fish causes worms in children, and children are also discouraged from drinking coconut milk because it is believed that it will make them stupid.

Infant Feeding Practices: In some tribes in Sierra Leone, colostrum is discarded, but prolonged breast-feeding is the norm. Bottle-feeding is actively discouraged. Mothers start introducing foods at 4 to 6 months but continue to breast-feed for up to 2 years. A government program to manufacture and distribute a weaning food *(Bennimix)* based on locally grown, protein-rich beniseed has been very successful. Breast-feeding also is used as a means of contraception and for child spacing. In addition, some nursing mothers move away from their husbands and stay with their mothers for several months after delivery. Forced feeding of infants is practiced by many groups and occasionally leads to death by aspiration.

Child Rearing Practices: Children's upbringing is strict and authoritarian, and although discipline is enforced by both parents it is usually by the mother. Relatives and any older members of the community also enforce discipline. Children do not talk back to parents or adults. Corporal punishment is common in school and in the home. Children are expected to help with domestic chores and develop housekeeping skills at an early age. Girls must learn to cook and look after younger siblings. In poorer communities, children, even those who attend school, are expected to contribute to the household income by helping to sell wares. Female circumcision is widespread but primarily limited to the clitoris; this is part of a more detailed initiation process involving tutorials in child rearing and other domestic practices. This takes place around puberty. Boys are circumcised at a young age, usually during the first year after birth. Uncircumcised boys are ridiculed by their peers. The education arena has no gender discrimination. Most primary schools are coeducational, but the older and more traditional secondary schools are segregated by sex. Children grow up with great respect and reverence for their parents, characteristics that are maintained throughout life as they care and support for their aging parents in later years.

National Childhood Immunization: BCG at birth; DTP at 6, 10, and 14 weeks; OPV at 6, 10, and 14 weeks; measles at 9 months; and TT for pregnant women and CBAW. The Expanded Program on Immunization has been in existence since 1978 and by 1993 achieved a full immunization rate of 62.7% in 1-year-olds against tuberculosis, measles, DTP, and polio. The civil war disrupted the program because of its inaccessibility to most of the country because of hostilities. After the recent end of the war a survey carried out in September 2001 revealed a rate of only 25.7% for fully immunized infants. This ranged from 74% for BCG to 36.7% for measles. In the same survey, only 17% of mothers completed the three doses of TT required to prevent neonatal tetanus in their infants.

ACKNOWLEDGMENTS: Belmont Williams, former chief medical officer of the Ministry of Health in Sierra Leone, made an important contribution toward this article.

BIBLIOGRAPHY

Bangura A, Lisk DR: Tobacco and cannabis smoking in secondary school children in Bo, Sierra Leone, *West Afr J Med* 14:157–160, 1995.

Ceesay M et al: The prevalence of diabetes in rural and urban populations in Southern Sierra Leone, *Trop Med Int Health* 2(3):272–277, 1997.

Central Statistics Office, Government of Sierra Leone: *National coverage evaluation survey,* December 2001.

Central Statistics Office, Government of Sierra Leone: *Sierra Leone in figures 1998,* http://www.sierra-leone.org

Lisk DR: Control of hypertension in Sierra Leone, *World Health Forum* 17:294–295, 1996.

Lisk DR, Gooding EC: Doctors' knowledge, attitude, and practice in the management of hypertension in a developing country, *Ethnicity Dis* vol 10, 2000.

Lisk DR, McEwen EK: The significance and trend of hypertension related deaths in urban Sierra Leonean Africans, *J Hum Hypertens* 10:215–218, 1996.

Lisk DR, Pabs-Garnon E: Pregnancy associated hypertension in urban Sierra Leonean Africans, *Ethnicity Dis* vol 10, 2000.

Lisk DR, Williams DEM, Slattery J: Blood pressure and hypertension in rural and urban Sierra Leoneans, *Ethnicity Dis* 9:254–253, 1999.

Palmer L, Lisk DR: Who prescribe better, doctors or dispensers? *World Health Forum* 18:352-354, 1997.

Williams B: *The health services in Sierra Leone,* 1981, Ministry of Health, Sierra Leone.

Williams B: *The traditional birth attendant—training and utilization,* 1979, Ministry of Health, Sierra Leone.

Williams DEM, Lisk DR: A high prevalence of hypertension in rural Sierra Leoneans, *West Afr J Med* 17:85–90, 1998.

◆ SINGAPORE (REPUBLIC OF)

MAP PAGE (867)

Consultants: Noriah Khamid Caron and Paul Zakowich

Location: A small island nation off the southeast coast of Malaysia, Singapore is one of the most densely populated areas in the world, with a total land area of only 659.9 km² (254.7 square miles), and a population of approximately 4 million. It is a leading economic power with one of the world's largest ports. Its boundaries are the Johor Straight to the north, the Pacific Ocean to the east, the Straight of Malacca to the southwest (separating Singapore from Sumatra), and the Indian Ocean to the west. Singapore has a lowland central plateau with a few hills and has hot, humid, tropical, and rainy weather with two distinct monsoon seasons. The gross domestic product (GDP) per capita is higher than many of the leading nations of Europe, and its economic power has contributed to high standards in health, education (with a 94% literacy rate), and housing. Most people live in the city of Singapore on the main island.

Major Languages	Ethnic Groups	Major Religions
Chinese (official)	Chinese 77%	Chinese: mainly
Malay (official)	Malay 14%	Buddhist, Atheist,
Tamil (official)	Indian 8%	and Christian
	Others 1%	Malays: mainly Muslim
		Minority Religions:
		Christian, Hindu,
		Sikh, Tao,
		Confucian

Health Care Beliefs: Passive role; fatalistic belief that life and death are beyond their control. Muslims have beliefs based on the four pillars of Islam: fasting, *fitrah,* pilgrimage to Mecca, and prayer five times a day. Muslims fear mental illness but believe in health promotion. The government health services actively promote preventive medicine, and since 1992 has had a program dedicated to prevention: the National Health Lifestyle Campaign.

Predominant Sick Care Practices: Biomedical; traditional; magical-religious. Muslims use holy water, pray, and go to Mecca. Hindus use amulets to ward off illness. Singapore has a dual system of health care delivery: a public system managed by the government and a private system of general practitioners and private hospitals. Eighty percent of primary care services are provided by doctors in private practice. Eighty percent of hospital care is provided by the public sector. The system stresses personal responsibility, and employees must contribute 6% to 8% of their monthly salary to a tax-deductible individual account. Self-employed individuals are also required to contribute. An endowment fund serves as a safety net for those who are poor. Although only 11% of the population is older than 60 years of age, this percentage will increase to 27% by the 2030, which will undoubtedly increase the overall costs of the system.

Ethnic/Race Specific or Endemic Disease: High-level medical services, safe water, and sanitation have increased overall health indicators for

Singaporeans. Endemic diseases include hepatitis B, typhus, melioidosis, and dengue hemorrhagic fever. Antimicrobial drug resistance is a significant problem. Singaporeans are at risk for hand, foot, and mouth disease and dengue fever. Leading causes of morbidity are the noncommunicable diseases—cancer, coronary heart disease, stroke, diabetes, hypertension, and injuries. Cancer and cardiovascular diseases account for approximately 62% of the total causes of death. The World Health Organization's (WHO) estimated prevalence rate for HIV/AIDS is 0.19%. The estimated number of children from birth to 15 years living with HIV/AIDS is less than 40.

Health Team Relationships: Singapore has approximately 5154 doctors, with one doctor per 730 people. Slightly less than half (48%) of the doctors are in the private sector. Singapore has 1 nurse per 244 people and a total of approximately 15,947 nurses; approximately 55% work in the public sector. Doctors have good relationships with nurses, and patients' attitudes toward doctors and nurses are also good. In general, doctors are held in high esteem and expected to know the cause of an illness just from a quick examination that does not involve a thorough history or physical examination. Patients also expect to receive several medications (e.g., vitamins, antibiotics) after each visit and feel cheated if they do not. They also expect to feel well soon after the visit, usually by the next day. Because of conflicts with this Western attitude, doctors must take time to explain medical practice so that patients will accept advice and comply with treatments. A large segment of primary medical care is also provided by Chinese doctors *(sinseh),* who treat with traditional herbs.

Families' Role in Hospital Care: Parents may stay overnight with their hospitalized children, and it is common to bring food to the hospital.

Dominance Patterns: Males are dominant. Parents may defer to the oldest son or daughter as they become older and unable to handle their affairs without assistance.

Touch Practices: The head is considered sacred, and it is offensive to pat a child on the head or hit another person in the head. Reaching over a patient's head to pass something to another person is rude, involving one of the pillars of Islam called *fitrah*. Malay custom does not allow touching between men and women, particularly in public.

Perceptions of Time: Malays are generally on time; other ethnic groups' attitudes toward time vary.

Pain Reactions: The Chinese tend to be more stoical about pain than other groups. Indians and Malays seem to have lower pain thresholds.

Birth Rites: Malays celebrate a son more than a daughter because he can protect the mother. Most Malay mothers breast-feed their infants, occasionally until they are 3 years old. Infant and maternal mortality rates are estimated to be 2.5 deaths per 1000 live births and 1.7 deaths per 10,000 live births, respectively.

Death Rites: The 1992 Medical Therapy, Education, and Research Act allows donation of organs and tissues from deceased persons for transplantation. Organ donation is encouraged by the government and well accepted by the Chinese; however, Malay Muslims are generally against the practice. Autopsies are done primarily for forensic rather than medical reasons.

Food Practices and Intolerances: In general, Malays eat at home, and the Chinese eat out. Favorite foods include seafood, sweet potato fritters, banana fritters, curry puffs, and all kinds of sweets. Malays and Indians use their hands to eat except in public, when they use forks.

Infant Feeding Practices: Infant feeding practices vary, but the government is encouraging breast-feeding.

Child Rearing Practices: Strict child rearing is the rule, and both parents are responsible for discipline. Young children usually sleep with their parents.

National Childhood Immunizations: BCG at birth and 6, 12, and 16 years if not immune; DTP at 3, 4, 5, and 18 months; OPV at 3, 4, 5, and 18 months and at 7 and 12 years; hep B at birth and 1, 5, and 12 months if mother is infected; MMR at 15 months and 12 years; and DT at 7 and 12 years. The Ministry of Health reports high levels of immunization coverage: 97% for tuberculosis, 91% for DTP, 90% for polio, 89% for hep B, and 89% for measles, mumps, and rubella.

Other Characteristics: Some friction exists among the various ethnic groups. However, the government actively promotes community cohesion and a sense of being a Singaporean first and foremost.

BIBLIOGRAPHY

Fong NP, Basir H, Seow A: Awareness and acceptance of hepatitis B vaccination in Clementi, Singapore, *Ann Acad Med Singapore* 19(6):788, 1990.
Ministry of Health Singapore (2001): *Fact sheets.* Retrieved December 16, 2001, from http://www.gov.sg/moh/faq/mfd/MFD-faq11.html
Ministry of Health Singapore (2001): *Principal causes of death 2000.* Retrieved December 16, 2001, from http://www.moh.gov.sg/hfacts/hfacts-gen-pcd.html
Straughan PT, Seow A: Barriers to mammography among Chinese women in Singapore: a focus group approach, *Health Educ Res* 10(4):431, 1995.
Wong ML et al: Influence of lifestyle behaviours on obesity among Chinese adolescents in Singapore, *Health Educ J* 54(2):198, 1995.
World Health Organization (June 2000): *Epidemiological fact sheets by country,* Geneva. Retrieved March 1, 2002, from http://www.unaids.org/hivaidsinfo/statistics/june00/fact_sheets/index.html
World Health Organization (2001): *WHO vaccine-preventable diseases: monitoring system,* Geneva. Retrieved March 1, 2002, from http://www.who.int/vaccines/

◆ SLOVAK REPUBLIC

MAP PAGE (860)

Ing. Slavka Barlakova

Location: The Slovak Republic (Slovakia) is an interior country situated in east central Europe. It was formerly part of Czechoslovakia. Slovakia's topography is characterized by fertile lowlands, hills, and snow-capped mountains (the High Tatras). The Danube is the primary river that flows through the country. The total land area of Slovakia is 49,035 km^2 (18,932 square miles).

Major Languages	Ethnic Groups	Major Religions
Slovak	Slovak 85%	Roman Catholic 70%
Hungarian	Hungarian 10%	Evangelical 7%
	Romany 2%	Greek Catholic 4%
	Czech 1%	Calvinistic 2%
	Ruthenian, Ukrainian,	Non-denominational or
	Russian, German,	atheist 17%
	Polish, other 2%	

Health Care Beliefs: Active role; health promotion encouraged. Slovaks are actively involved in health promotion. Exercise, a healthy diet, and rest are believed to promote and protect health. By law, children 18 years and younger visit doctors regularly, and regular examinations during pregnancy are obligatory. Fear of mental illness is slowly decreasing, and it is no longer acceptable to virtually imprison individuals with mental illness so that they cannot participate in public life. People today try to integrate those with mental illness into society if possible. Slovakia has special "protected shops" in which individuals with relatively minor disabilities can work safely.

Predominant Sick Care Practices: State system—primarily biomedical with some alternative therapies. The status of doctors in the society is very honored, and medical knowledge is at a high level. Health care systems are provided in hospitals and ambulatory care sites; primary, secondary, and tertiary care is available. Primary care is provided by three types of doctors: general practitioners for adults, children, and young people; gynecologists; and internal medicine practitioners. Maternity and infant care is free, and people recognize that this should be an important present focus for the health care system. When people are ill, they generally seek out doctors first, but some also consult natural healers, particularly if the recommended medical treatment is unsuccessful. Alternative therapies such as acupuncture, homeopathy, and natural healing are also well accepted.

Ethnic/Race Specific or Endemic Diseases: The major causes of deaths for adults are heart and circulatory diseases (55% of deaths), malignant neoplasms (22%), respiratory diseases (7%), injuries and poisoning

(7%), and gastrointestinal tract diseases (4%). Increases in cancer and cardiovascular diseases such as hypertension are believed to be caused by various factors, including chronic stress, frustration, and apathy in the population. Oxidative stress is also blamed because of people's high consumption of nicotine and alcohol and low intake of antioxidants. Children primarily have respiratory and gastrointestinal diseases and urinary infections. The majority of children die from injuries, followed by neoplasms and congenital abnormalities. Perinatal mortality is very low at 6.7%. The World Health Organization's (WHO) estimated prevalence rate for HIV/AIDS in adults ages 15 to 49 years is 0.005. The estimated number of children from birth to 15 years living with HIV/AIDS is less than 100. These rates are among the best in Europe. HIV tests are obligatory for those giving blood and during pregnancy, and they can be requested for free as well. Homosexual transmission of HIV has decreased slightly, but heterosexual transmission and transmission among those who are addicted to intravenous drugs is increasing. The official number of people who are HIV positive is 153, but detailed data are not available to the public. An educated guess by health care professionals in the Slovak Republic is that approximately 250 to 300 individuals are infected.

Health Team Relationships: The health team is doctor driven. Nurses are expected to take care of health maintenance tasks such as giving injections and prescribed medications and fulfilling treatment tasks. Under Slovak law, nurses have little power and are not allowed to make independent decisions, unlike many Western nurses. The working relationship between doctors and nurses is usually good, but tensions inevitably arise because medicine is such a demanding occupation.

Families' Role in Hospital Care: The medical and nursing staff members provide all hospital care. Visiting hours are quite liberal, and some wards allow small children to visit. The rights of children in hospitals are protected by Slovak law, which addresses issues such as teaching, housing of parents, information communication, and the economic rights of parents. Parents are allowed to stay with children in the hospital, and friends and relatives are allowed to visit.

Dominance Patterns: Men were previously in control of all decision making, but this has changed in the family and society. However, in Slovak society, men still have higher salaries and better jobs. In the home, women still do most of the domestic work, care for the children, and are the primary caregivers for sick relatives. Women are becoming increasingly more career oriented and more likely to expect that household and other obligations should be shared.

Eye Contact Practices: Long-lasting, direct eye contact is unacceptable and often regarded as hostile during interactions with strangers. It is customary to make direct eye contact during conversations with well-known individuals.

Touch Practices: Touching is acceptable, and it is common to give a person a hug in the street or shake hands when meeting a friend or acquaintance. Men are less expressive with other men than women are with other women.

Perceptions of Time: Punctuality is valued, but being 5 minutes late is usually not a concern. People live in the present and future, but because of the country's history of war and conflict, they often have concerns about what the future holds.

Pain Reactions: People react to pain very differently, and range from being stoical to being very expressive. However, even Slovaks with severe injuries tend to stay relatively calm, and health professionals expect patients to endure pain without unnecessary outward expressions of emotion. Crying out loud during labor and delivery is acceptable.

Birth Rites: Many mothers, especially those from middle-class backgrounds, attend prenatal birth preparation courses. Most infants are born in hospitals, and when conditions are appropriate the father is admitted to the delivery room. The mother has a choice of delivery options such as a natural birth with no anesthesia or birth with epidural anesthesia. Most women give birth in the conventional back-lying position, but hospitals are attempting to accommodate a range of other birth positions such as standing or births underwater. After the birth the infant is examined by a pediatrician, cleaned, shown to the parents, and taken to the nursery. Some hospitals allow the infant to stay in the mother's room ("rooming-in") on the second or third day if the birth had no complications and the mother requests it. Many hospitals do not have enough space, and staff members are often unwilling to conform to new methods. Therefore most mothers and babies are separated except for during feedings, which take place six times a day. This procedure is gradually changing as the positive benefits of rooming in are becoming more evident. Mothers and infants usually leave the hospital on the fifth day after birth; they leave on the ninth day if a cesarean section was performed.

Death Rites: Most people die in health care institutions, and the closest family members usually stay with the dying person. In cities, funeral providers have all-inclusive services, including cleaning and dressing the body, a coffin, and a ceremony accompanying cremation or burial in the ground. In the countryside, it is still common to display the body in an open coffin at home, particularly if the person was a Roman Catholic. This practice allows friends and relatives to have a last personal visit in the home, after which they accompany the coffin in the hearse on the person's journey to the cemetery. Organ donations and autopsies are acceptable.

Food Practices and Intolerances: Most people eat three times a day and consume approximately the same amount at lunch and dinner. Breakfast usually consists of a combination of bread, butter, jam, yogurt, salami, cheese, and tea, milk, or coffee. Traditional food staples are potatoes, rice, and pasta, combined with pork, beef, and poultry (that is stewed or roasted). Vegetables and fruit (including tropical fruits) are available most of the year. The most consumed foods are carrots, peas, cabbage, tomatoes, pepper, corn, cauliflower, kohlrabi, apples, pears, strawberries, raspberries, plums, pears, apricots, bananas, oranges, and lemons. A typical traditional meal is gnocchi with *brynza* (sheep cheese) and bacon topping and potato pancakes with sauerkraut. Forks, knives, and spoons are used for most meals. Pizza, hot dogs, and sandwiches with various fillings are the favorite among young people, in particular.

Infant Feeding Practices: Breast-feeding is typical, and women are encouraged to breast-feed as long as possible but at least 3 to 4 months. Because mothers understand that breast milk is the best and the only natural food for babies, Slovakia has several women's clubs providing breast-feeding support. These groups are led primarily by doctors and mothers with experience. Although breast-feeding in public is frowned on, it is not unusual to see a 20-month-old child being breast-fed. If breast-feeding is impossible for medical reasons, formula is available. In Slovak culture the image of a woman breast-feeding her infant is considered a pure and wonderful expression of womanhood.

Child Rearing Practices: Child rearing practices are quite permissive and loving. However, children are expected to obey rules and have good manners. Parents usually supervise their children, try to support them mentally and financially, and help them when they are ready to become independent. Both the parents are responsible for discipline. Physical punishment is unacceptable, but an occasional smack on the bottom is considered a part of raising a child. Small children often sleep in a room with their parents. The maternity leave by law is 3 years, and many mothers stay at home with their babies for the entire 3 years. Fathers and mothers are both allowed to be on maternity leave during the 3 years. According to the law, employers cannot eliminate the job of a person who is on maternity leave or refuse to allow the person to return to work after the leave.

National Childhood Immunizations: BCG at birth; DTP at 2, 3, 9, and 24 months; OPV at 2, 4, 14, and 16 months and 11 to 12 years; hep B at 2, 3, and 9 months; HIB at 2, 3, and 9 months; MMR at 14 months and 11 to 12 years; and DT at 5 to 6 years. Vaccinations are free and required.

BIBLIOGRAPHY

Demé M: *Slovakia 1995 (synoptic report on situation in society),* Zdravotníctvo, str.139–149.

Ginter E: Composition of nourishment and average of life in different parts of Europe, Ekológia & Zivot, ?, 3, str. 15–17, 1996.

Michalkova DM et al: Incidence and prevalence of childhood diabetes in Slovakia, *Diabetes Care* 18(3):315, 1995.

Rubens D, Gyurkovics B, Hornacek K: The cultural production of bioterapia: psychic healing and the natural medicine movement in Slovakia, *Soc Sci Med* 41(9):1261, 1995.

The National Report of the Slovak Republic on Population and Development, 1999, Bratislava, Slovakia (21 -st OZ VZ UN, New York, 30.6–2.7. 1999).

The Statistic Office of the Slovak Republic: *Report on health conditions of population,* Bratislava, Slovakia, 1996.

The Statistics Office of the Slovak Republic: *Slovak census 2001*, Bratislava, Slovakia, 2001.

The statistics yearbook of the government office of the Slovak Republic, Bratislava, 2000.

World Health Organization (June 2000): *Epidemiological fact sheets by country,* Geneva. Retrieved March 1, 2002, from http://www.unaids.org/hivaidsinfo/statistics/june00/fact_sheets/index.html

World Health Organization (2001): *WHO vaccine-preventable diseases: monitoring system,* Geneva. Retrieved March 1, 2002, from http://www.who.int/vaccines/

◆ SLOVENIA (REPUBLIC OF)

MAP PAGE (860)

Marija Bohinc and Miro Gradisar

Location: Slovenia is in the southeastern part of Europe. It was a part of Yugoslavia until June 1991, when it declared independence. Slovenia is 230 km from Vienna, Austria; 240 km from Budapest, Hungary; and 460 km from Milan, Italy. Slovenia is a green place in the heart of Europe. It is largely mountainous, and forests cover almost half of the land. The landscape is very diverse, with mountains, hills, villages, spas, and the sea. The total land area is 20,256 km^2 (7820 square miles), and the population is 2 million.

Major Languages	Ethnic Groups	Major Religions
Slovenian (official)	Slovene 88%	Roman Catholic 71%
English	Croat 7%	Lutheran 1%
German	Serb 2%	Muslim 1%
Italian	Italian, Hungarian 1%	Other 27%
	Other 2%	

In addition to Slovenian, which is the major language, most of the population also speaks Serbo-Croatian.

Health Care Beliefs: Active role; health promotion important. In 1994, researchers investigated the hierarchy of values for Slovenian people. Health and family were assessed as most important. Thereafter a special national program was developed for promotion of health, healthy lifestyles, and prevention and early detection of diseases of preschool children, students, women, and older adults. The program affects health care centers, nurseries, schools, and communities. The health promotion initiative is organized to promote healthy nutrition, exercise, smoking cessation, and lower rates of alcohol and drug consumption. An important role of primary health care is to improve people's tolerance for and acceptance of those with mental disorders and promote their integration into the community. Care for those who are homeless and unemployed is the domain of other health promotion programs and self-help groups. People with minor disabilities can live, study, and work in the community.

Predominant Sick Care Practice: Biomedical and alternative therapies. The state system is organized according to the World Health Organization's (WHO) Goals for Health in the Twenty-first century. It focuses on an active approach and individual responsibility for health. Doctors are trusted and appreciated for their knowledge, but patients are more demanding relative about being included in decision making because they are informed about their rights. In the past, doctors had more of a paternal role. Medical knowledge, expertise, technology, and practice are excellent in Slovenia. Primary health care takes place in health care centers. Secondary care is provided by general hospitals and outpatient clinics, and tertiary care is provided by clinics and institutes. The vast majority of people are insured, so they have access to health care centers and emergency wards. Maternal infant care, preventive programs for scholars, and a portion of care for older adults are free. When people are ill, the first step they take is to visit a doctor in a health care center; 80% of the population solicits care at the primary level. Private health care is also developing in numerous different areas and involves various practitioners such as general doctors, private community nurses, and dentists. Community nurses are respected, valued, and an asset to the system. In addition to biomedical care, the use of alternative therapies is common, especially when standard medical treatment is not successful. Homeopathy, bioenergy, acupuncture, and natural healing methods are alternative treatment options.

Ethnic/Race Specific or Endemic Diseases: The major causes of death are cardiovascular diseases, cancer, injuries, poisoning, and gastrointestinal diseases. Increases in the incidence of cancer, cardiovascular disease, hypertension, high cholesterol, and diabetes are attributed to unhealthy lifestyles, excessive alcohol consumption, smoking, poor nutrition, and stress. Children primarily have respiratory, gastrointestinal, and urinary diseases. Prenatal mortality is very low and comparable to rates of Scandinavian countries. The World Health Organization's (WHO) estimated prevalence rate for HIV/AIDS in adults ages 15 to 49 is 0.02%. The estimated number of children from birth to 15 years living with HIV/AIDS is less than 100. By the end of 1999 the total number of people infected with HIV in Slovenia was 155 (46% of whom were homosexual men, 22% of whom were heterosexuals, and 8% of which were people who used intravenous drugs). HIV tests are obligatory for those who are giving blood, and they can be requested for free. Special programs address prevention of sexually transmitted diseases, and they are increasing their focus on heterosexuals and those who are addicted to intravenous drugs.

Health Team Relationships: The leader of the health team is the doctor, and the leader of the nursing team is the registered nurse. Slovenian nurses are becoming more independent and autonomous. Efforts to increase the academic level of nursing to the Bachelor of Science degree level are strong, and professional development is significant. Nurses can make independent decisions, and legislation for nursing practice is in process in parliament. It is expected that the relationship between doctors and nurses will be more synergistic in the future—more of a partnership and collaboration. However, current relationships are generally quite good between the professions.

Families Role in Hospital Care: Visiting hours in hospitals are very flexible and liberal. Relatives can visit an ill person almost any time (within the regulations of the hospitals) and beyond scheduled visiting hours if they have the permission of the doctor responsible for the patient. The rights of patients are in accordance with the 1994 Declaration of the Rights of Patients in Amsterdam and with health care laws of the country. All patients receive a brochure outlining their health care rights.

Dominance Patterns: In most cases, men have the highest positions. They receive better salaries and have access to better jobs. Most women are employed, and many of them are pursuing careers. They have as much education as men and as times are changing, more are moving into high-level and important managerial and leadership positions in all areas of public life. In the home, women still have the major responsibility for cooking, housekeeping, and taking care of children and sick relatives. In younger families the division of work is more balanced, and couples usually do not live with their parents.

Eye Contact Practice: Long-lasting, direct eye contact is not always acceptable. It is more common during conversational situations among people who know each other well.

Touch Practice: Touching is acceptable among friends or relatives. When meeting others, it is common to shake hands.

Perception of Time: Being on time is becoming more important. Popular proverbs say "to be on time is a nice habit" and "time is golden." It is very common, especially for older people, to be at least 5 or more minutes late for appointments. Younger people are more oriented to the future, and are prepared to change jobs more frequently than people did in the past.

Pain Reactions: People react very differently to pain. Reactions range from calm to serious, anxious, fearful, and powerless. It is not unusual for individuals to cry out and express their feelings.

Birth Rites: Many mothers and fathers, especially from the upper and middle classes, attend prenatal birth preparation courses for parents. Most infants are born in hospitals with excellent facilities, and fathers are allowed to be present during the delivery. Mothers can choose to have no drugs or to have a delivery with epidural anesthesia. Most women give birth in the conventional back-lying position, but hospitals are attempting to accommodate other options such as underwater births or births in the standing position. After the birth the infant is examined by a pediatrician, cleaned, and shown to the parents. Most hospitals promote rooming-in (keeping the infant and mother together in the same room) from the first day. Alternately, the infant may be kept in the nursery if the mother desires. Some hospitals are specifically considered "baby-friendly hospitals." Mothers and infants usually stay in the hospital until the third day after birth. Mothers who have had cesarean births leave with their infants on the seventh day after birth. Breast-feeding is promoted. According to the law, maternity leave is 1 year, and it can be extended if the infant was born prematurely. Both parents are allowed to take a maternity leave, which is a paid leave, and the employer cannot refuse to take the parents back when the leave is over.

Death Rites: Forty-six percent of people die in hospitals. The rest die in nursing homes, in their own homes, or at the homes of family members who are caring for the person. In cities, funeral facilities provide all services, including cleaning and dressing the body, coffin selection, and cremation or burial with an accompanying service or a ceremony. In the countryside, it is common to display the body in a place other than the home, often in a special hall in the village. Relatives and friends come to say good-bye, bring flowers, light candles, and pray for the dead person. The priest usually leads the funeral if the person was Roman Catholic. Organ donations and autopsies are acceptable with the previous permission of the deceased person or accountable persons.

Food Practice and Intolerances: People with more education tend to have healthier nutritional patterns. They eat more black bread, fish, and chicken and less pork and beef compared with those who have only an elementary school education. Women tend to have healthier habits than men. For example, according to population studies, women are more likely to have breakfast (although only 50% of the population has breakfast every day). Breakfast usually consists of the bread, milk, coffee, jam, honey, yogurt, cheese, eggs, margarine or butter, and tea. Traditional foods in Slovenia include vegetable soups, potatoes, rice, pasta with meat, and salads. Vegetables and all kinds of fruit are available and fresh throughout the year. The most consumed are apples, oranges, lemons, bananas, pears, plums, apricots, strawberries, green salads, cabbage, tomatoes, corn, cauliflower, kohlrabi, and beans. The typical Slovenian Sunday meal is beef soup, cooked beef with roasted potatoes, green salad, and fruit. Forks, knives, and spoons are used for most meals. Fast food is also becoming very popular, especially among young people, who eat all types of pizzas, hot dogs, and sandwiches.

Infant Feeding Practices: Breast-feeding is valued and considered a good investment in the health of the child. Women are educated to breast-feed for as long as possible but at least for 3 or 4 months. If breast-feeding is not possible for medical reasons, it is possible to use formula that can be prepared at home. In health care centers on the primary level of the national health care system, each community has a dispensary for infants and preschool children. Slovenia has prevention and health promotion programs for disease prevention, immunizations, and counseling, which are supervised by pediatricians, registered nurses, and community nurses in the home.

Child Rearing Practices: Child rearing practices are caring, loving, and permissive. Physical punishment is not allowed. Parents attempt to take good care of their children and support them financially, emotionally, and socially. They help children become independent so that they can finish secondary school and college or begin working and become independent. Most children have separate rooms for sleeping.

National Childhood Immunizations: BCG at birth, DTP at 3, 4 to 5, 6, and 18 months; DTP at 3, 4 to 5, 6, and 18 months; OPV at 3, 4 to 5, 6, and 18 months, and at 5 to 6 and 14 to 15 years; hep B at birth and 5 to 6 years; HIB at 3, 4 to 5, 6, and 12 months; MMR at 12 to 15 months and 5 to 6 years; and DT at 14 to 15 years. Vaccinations are free. Parents can refuse to have their children vaccinated, but they must then take responsibility for the health of their children.

REFERENCES

Bohinc M: Propositions for health educational work for children and the education of pedagogical workers, *Zdrav Var* 30(6,7):129–192, 1991.

European Parliament: Resolution on the status of non-conventional medicine. Session document A4 0075/97, pp 1–4, May 29, 1997, Copenhagen, WHO.

Filej B: The health center as a typical institution of primary health care in Slovenia, *European Nurse* 2(2):141–143, 1997.

Health Statistical Report Review: *Slovenia 2001, Zdrav Var* , 2001 (special issue). www.si.gov.si/ivz

Komadina D: Care for positive health, *Zdrav Var* 27(6,7,8):201–210, 1998.

Krasevec E, ed: *Promotion of health of socially disadvantaged groups in Slovenia,* pp 227-248, Institute of Public Health of the Republic of Slovenia, Slovene Foundation, Ljubljana, Slovenia, 1996.

National Program of Health Care of Republic Slovenia: *The health for all to 2004,* Official Report for Republic Slovenia, No 49, pp 6650–6678, 2002: 6.

Nurses Association of Slovenia: Ljubljana, Slovenia, 2000, www.zveza-dmszts.si

Obersnel Kveder D: Reproductive and sexual attitudes, *Zdrav Var* 36(1,2):4–6, 1997.

Strojin T: *The introduction of the health care law,* Official publication Republic of Slovenia, Ljubljana, Slovenia, 1998.

Tos N: *Slovenian public opinion. The attitudes of health, health care and health care insurance,* 1994, Institute of Social Science, University of Ljubljana, Ljubljana, Slovenia.

http://www.unaids.org/hivaidsinfo/

http://www.who.int/vaccines/

◆ SOLOMON ISLANDS

MAP PAGE (856)

Location: The Solomon Islands are an archipelago in the South Pacific Ocean to the east of Papua New Guinea and about 1200 miles northeast of Australia. Approximately 90% of the people are Melanesian, and 120 indigenous languages are spoken. The country achieved independence in 1978. The total land area is 28,450 km² (10,985 square miles), slightly smaller than Maryland. The land consists of forested mountains and low atolls, with 10 large and rugged volcanic islands and four groups of smaller islands. The climate is tropical monsoon, with few extremes of temperature or weather. However, the islands are vulnerable to volcanoes, typhoons, earthquakes, and tidal waves. The total population is 480,442, and the population is primarily rural. The capital is Honiara.

Major Languages	Ethnic Groups	Major Religions
Melanesian pidgin	Melanesian 93%	Anglican 34%
English	Polynesian 4%	Roman Catholic 19%
	Micronesian,	Other Protestant 43%
	European,	Traditional beliefs 4%
	Chinese 3%	

Pidgin is spoken throughout most of the country, and English is spoken by 1% to 2% of the population.

Health Care Beliefs: Active role; health promotion encouraged. Modern medical care is sought for most illness and injuries; however, traditional healers are also active and prescribe various herbs and other traditional medications. The islands have targeted prevention activities aimed at addressing the more serious problems faced by the residents. For example, it is generally agreed that accident prevention programs are needed to reduce injuries from coconut palm trees. Numerous children fall from the trees, and numerous others are injured from falling fruit. The government has implemented policies for prevention of malaria that focuses on early diagnosis and treatment at a health service, reduction of vector-human contact through use of insecticide-impregnated bed nets, and provision of chemoprophylaxis for pregnant women. However, protection against mosquitoes was found to be poor in the evening, which is when mosquitoes are most active. Selective primary care activity mobile unit teams may visit villages once or twice a year to seek out those who have malaria and provide chloroquine and primaquine treatments. Almost half of the gonorrhea infections are penicillin resistant, so the country has national guidelines for prevention and treatment for this and other sexually transmitted diseases. Regardless, public health clinics do not seem to adhere to the guidelines. Studies show that clinics do not properly collect data, serological testing for syphilis is low (28%), only 50% of the clinics have personnel that understand the national guidelines, and contact tracing is only performed 25% of the time. A high male/female notification ratio (3.6:1) for gonorrhea has been detected. Overall attention to public health fundamentals regarding prevention and treatment are not optimal.

Predominant Sick Care Practices: Biomedical and traditional. Villagers have stated that for serious illnesses such as malaria, antimalarial drugs are better than traditional medications or healers. Malaria poses a great risk to Solomon Islanders, and studies indicate that chloroquine resistance is about 25%. Hospitals and pharmacies are only found in population centers and mission facilities. The nearest reliable medical facilities are in New Zealand or Australia.

Ethnic/Race Specific or Endemic Diseases: Chloroquine-resistant falciparum malaria is hyperendemic. Other endemic diseases include human T-lymphotropic virus type 1 (HTLV-1), hepatitis A and B, penicillin-resistant gonorrhea (with a 45% rate of resistance), and vitamin A deficiency. Solomon Islanders are at risk for yaws; cholera; hepatitis A, C, and G; helminthic infections; diarrheal diseases; typhoid fever; infections from ritual scarification; and injuries from automobile accidents and coconut palm trees. Biotoxin poisoning from tropical fish and shellfish can occur.

Health Team Relationships: To improve educational opportunities for nurses, the Ministry of Health has implemented five post-basic nursing certificate courses for health workers using distance education modules. This program is proving to be highly successful for increasing skills and knowledge in these more remote areas of the world.

Birth Rites: Rapid population growth in the Solomon Islands is a private and public concern. The country has an extreme shortage of arable land, limited spots in schools, and health services that cannot keep up with the increasing demands of more people. Although people want smaller families, meager health resources and medical infrastructure, culture, and religion are hampering efforts to provide family planning services. The birth rate is 34.05 births per 1000 people.

Food Intolerances and Practices: The overall prevalence of malnutrition in children is about 28%. Malnourished children have been found to be at higher risk for malarial treatment failure. Vitamin A deficiency is common and a major cause of morbidity, mortality, and blindness (xerophthalmia) in children.

Child Rearing Practices: Approximately 44% of the population is 14 years of age or younger.

National Childhood Immunizations: BCG at birth and when beginning school; DTP at 2, 4, and 6 months; OPV at 2, 4, and 6 months; hep B at birth and 2 and 4 months; measles at 9 months; and vitamin A for underweight infants and children. The reported percentages of the target population vaccinated in 1999 were as follows: BCG, 99; third dose of DTP, 86; MCV, 96; and Pol3, 84.

Other Characteristics: Ritual scarification—the traditional practice of making incisions in the skin to create a pattern of scars—is still a culturally meaningful practice for Solomon Islanders.

BIBLIOGRAPHY

Furusyo N et al: Markedly high seroprevalence of hepatitis B virus infection in comparison to hepatitis C virus and human lymphotropic virus type-1 infections in selected Solomon Islands populations, *Am J Trop Med Hyg* 61(1):85, 1999.

Hess FI et al: Anti-malarial drug resistance, malnutrition and socioeconomic status, *Trop Med Int Health* 2(8):721, 1997.

Ishii A et al: Chemotherapeutic malaria control as a selective primary care activity in the Solomon Islands, *Parassitologia* 41(1–3):383, 1999.

Kenyon M et al: The community in the classroom: designing a distance education community health course for nurses in the Solomon Islands, *Pacific Health Dialog* 7(2):76, 2000.

Lucas RE: A survey to gather sexually transmitted disease epidemiological and management data in the Solomon Islands, *Tropical Doctor* 30(2):97, 2000.

Mammen L, Norton SA: Facial scarification and tattooing on Santa Catalina Island (Solomon Islands), *Cutis* 60(4):197, 1997.

Mulford JS, Oberli H, Tovosia S: Coconut palm-related injuries in the Pacific Islands, *Austr NZ J Surg* 71(1):32, 2001.

Rowling D et al: Family planning: personal and political perspectives from Choiseul Province, Solomon Islands, *Austr J Public Health* 19(6):616, 1995.

Schaumberg DA et al: Vitamin A deficiency in the South Pacific, *Public Health* 109(5):311, 1995.

http://www.cia.gov/cia/publications/factbook/geos/bp.html
http://www.healthfax.org.au/pacific.htm
http://travel.stat.gov/solomon_islands.html

◆ SOMALIA

MAP PAGE (862)

Helen D. Rodd

Location: Somalia is situated in Eastern Africa and has a strategic location on the Horn of Africa. It shares boundaries with Djibouti, Ethiopia, and Kenya, and its extensive 3000-km coastline borders the Gulf of Aden and the Indian Ocean. It is approximately the size of Texas (637,567 km^2 or 246,165 square miles), and the terrain is mostly flat with a more mountainous region in the north.

Major Languages	Ethnic Groups	Major Religions
Somali	Somali 85%	Sunni Muslim 97%
Arabic	Bantu groups 5%	Other 3%
English	Arab, other 10%	
Italian		

Somalia has 18 administrative regions and the capital city, Mogadishu, is located in the south. Since the late 1980s, Somalia has been ravaged by civil war, factional fighting, droughts, and famine. It is now undoubtedly one of the world's poorest and least developed countries. Accurate population statistics are difficult to obtain because many Somalis are nomadic, and many have fled the country. However, the population is estimated to be approximately 7 million, with an additional million refugees living in neighboring countries. Thousands of asylum seekers have resettled in Europe or the United States. The Somali language did not adopt a uniform orthography until 1973, and it is estimated that only 24% of the adult population is literate (36% of males and 14% of females).

Health Care Beliefs: Passive role; active sick care; traditional. Numerous illnesses are attributed to the presence of angry spirits within an individual. To appease these spirits, people may hold healing ceremonies, which may last 1 or 2 days and involve eating special foods, reading the Koran, and burning incense. Mental health problems are generally not acknowledged. An individual is either considered "well" or "mad," and Somalis have little understanding of mental illness. Unfortunately, psychological problems attributed to posttraumatic stress disorder and chewing *khat* (a leaf with hallucinogenic properties) are becoming more prevalent.

Predominant Sick Care Practices: Magical-religious; herbal; biomedical where available. Traditional medicine is widely practiced throughout rural and urban Somalia. Common practices include applying heated sticks to the skin ("fire burning") and blood letting. People often remove primary canine tooth buds (*ilko-dacowo,* or "fox teeth") from infants because it is believed that these teeth are the cause of many childhood ailments. The use of herbs and natural remedies provides a valuable adjunct to traditional medical practices. Most Somalis have had some experience with Western medicine, although they invariably only seek curative, not preventive, treatments. Numerous humanitarian and nongovernmental organizations are currently active in Somalia and work under the framework of the voluntary coordinating body, the Somalia Aid Coordination Body (SACB). These groups are striving to implement primary health care programs but are continually threatened by the highly unstable situation in Somalia.

Ethnic/Race Specific or Endemic Diseases: Somalia has one of the highest incidences of tuberculosis in the world, and cholera is endemic in most areas. The major causes of death in childhood are respiratory infections, malaria, and diarrhea-related sequelae. Sporadic outbreaks of measles also contribute to the high infant mortality. HIV/AIDS statistics are not yet available for all of Somalia. However, some baseline data obtained for northwest Somalia found the prevalence of AIDS to be less than 1%. Although HIV/AIDS prevalence rates remain considerably lower than those of neighboring African countries, some are concerned that Somalia is at risk for a serious epidemic in the future. Efforts to raise AIDS awareness are therefore in progress.

Health Team Relationships: Health care professionals in primary and secondary care settings are held in high regard. Nurses and auxiliary staff play an important role in service provision, particularly in rural areas. However, service provision in the main hospitals is predominantly headed by doctors. Numerous overseas agencies are involved in providing medical training within the local communities. The United Nations Children's Fund (UNICEF) in particular has a major role in designing and implementing new health policies.

Families' Role in Hospital Care: The family must assume a significant role in caring for a relative during a hospital admission. A patient depends entirely on relatives to provide their food while they are in the hospital.

Dominance Patterns: Women have a high status in the Somali family structure. The wife and mother is the head of the family unit and plays a major role in child rearing and keeping the family accounts. It is common for people to live with their extended family or jointly with another family; however, as in many Islamic cultures, men and women are separated in most other aspects of life.

Eye Contact Practices: Direct eye contact is considered extremely rude and is avoided by traditional Somalis.

Touch Practices: Physical contact between men and women is unacceptable unless it is among family members.

Perceptions of Time: Punctuality is not very important in Somali life. It is expected that individuals may be too early or, more commonly, too late for an appointment.

Pain Reactions: It is difficult to generalize about Somali pain thresholds and reactions to pain. However, the Somali do not like to show any sign of weakness, which is particularly evident during childbirth, when women are extremely stoical.

Birth Rites: Somali culture is extremely supportive of expectant or new mothers. After childbirth, new mothers remain at home and are cared for by female relatives and friends for 40 days (a period known as *afatanbah*). During this time, numerous special customs are observed. The mother is given special food and wears earrings made from string passed through a clove of garlic. The newborn infant is welcomed into the community, and neonatal care includes warm water baths, sesame oil massages, and passive stretching of the infant's limbs. An herb called *malmal* is usually applied to the umbilicus for the first 7 days of life. In addition, the baby wears a bracelet made from *malmal* to ward off evil spirits. At the end of the 40 days, a celebratory family gathering is held at a friend or relative's house to mark the first time the mother and infant have left their home since the birth. All boys and girls are circumcised. Boys are usually circumcised before 5 years, and the procedure is performed by a traditional doctor or hospital nurse or doctor. The most common form of female circumcision is infibulation, and a female member of the family usually performs the procedure on infants or young girls. During child-birth the mother's genital infibulation is opened and after birth is usually reinstated. Most women consider circumcision to be expected and desirable. The current fertility rate is 7.11 children born per woman, but the infant mortality rate is very high at 123.97 deaths per 1000 live births. The average life expectancy is 44.99 years for men and 48.25 years for women, and the overall population growth rate is estimated to be 3.48%.

Death Rites: When a person is about to die, relatives and friends gather to read special passages from the Koran and pray. After death, a male or female sheik attends the corpse, which is washed, perfumed, and wrapped in white cloth. The body is then taken to a mosque or directly to a grave prepared by the next of kin, where additional prayers are recited. The body is finally laid to rest facing Mecca. Somali believe that after death, a person's soul passes into *Barzakh*—the transition between the two worlds—until the day of judgment, when the soul and body will be reunited.

Food Practices and Intolerances: The food that Somali Muslims are allowed to eat (*halal* food) includes fish, grain, fruits, and vegetables. Conversely, *haram* food is forbidden and includes anything from an animal that eats another animal and is therefore unclean (e.g., a pig). Furthermore, even animals that are considered clean must be killed in a certain way to be *halal*. During Ramadan (an important religious festival during the ninth month of the lunar calendar), people pray, fast, and refrain from drinking during daylight hours. Rice is the staple component of the Somali diet and is usually mixed with meat (and called *isku-dhexkaris*). Vegetables are more commonly available in southern Somalia, whereas the nomadic northern Somali consume more milk and meat. However, extreme food shortages throughout Somalia continue to adversely affect the nutritional status of the population, and malnutrition is a chronic problem in all areas.

Infant Feeding Practices: Children are commonly breast-fed until they are 2 years of age, but supplementation with animal milk (usually with a cup, not a bottle) is common in early infancy. At the age of 6 months, the child receives a mixture of rice and cow's milk before the introduction of solid foods.

Child Rearing: Children usually sleep with their parents until the age of 2 years. Toilet training begins at a young age, as diapers are not usually used. The infant is regularly held over a small basin on the mother's lap.

National Childhood Immunizations: BCG at birth; DTP at 6, 10, and 14 weeks; measles at 9 months; TT CBAW at first contact, +1 month, +6 months, +1 year, + 1 year. However, data from UNICEF have indicated that childhood immunizations are not reaching all children in Somalia. In 1998, it was estimated that only small percentages of 1-year-olds were fully immunized against tuberculosis (57% immunized), DTP (24%), measles (47%), or poliomyelitis (24%).

BIBLIOGRAPHY

Arbesman M, Kahler L, Buck GM: Assessment of the impact of female circumcision on the gynecological, genitourinary and obstetrical health problems of women from Somalia: literature review and case series, *Women Health* 20:27, 1993.

Griffiths P et al: A transcultural pattern of drug use: qat (khat) in the UK, *J Psych* 170:281, 1997.

Harborview Medical Centre (1996): *Ethnic medicine guide,* http://www.ethnomed.org/ethnomed/cultures/Somali.html

Rodd HD, Davidson LE: "Ilko-Dacowo": canine enucleation and dental sequelae in Somali children, *Int J Paed Dentistry* 10:290, 2000.

United Nations Children's Fund (2000): *Somalia basic datasheet,* http://www.unicef.org/somalia/factfig/basic.html

United States Government Central Intelligence Agency (2001): *The world factbook—Somalia,* http://www.odci.gov/cia/publications/factbook/index.html

World Health Organization (2001): *WHO vaccine-preventable diseases: monitoring system,* Geneva. Retrieved March 1, 2002, from http://www.who.int/vaccines/

◆ SOUTH AFRICA (REPUBLIC OF)

MAP PAGE (863)

Hester Klopper

Location: The Republic of South Africa occupies the southernmost part of the African continent and has a total land area of 1,219,090 km² (470,691 square miles). It has common boundaries with the republics of Zimbabwe, Botswana, Namibia, and Mozambique and the kingdoms of Swaziland and Lesotho. To the west, south, and east, South Africa borders on the Atlantic and southern Indian Oceans and has a lengthy coastline of about 3000 km. The landscape is characterized by bush, veld, deserts, and forests on the majestic mountains peaks and wide, unspoiled beaches and coastal wetlands. South Africa is divided into nine provinces.

Major Languages	Ethnic Groups	Major Religions
English	African 77%	Christian 80%
Afrikaans	White 11%	Jewish, Muslim, Hindu,
IsiZulu	Colored 9%	other 20%
IsiXhosa	Indian, Asian 3%	
Sepedi		

According to the last published census results (1998), South Africa has a population of 40.58 million. Today, the country probably has approximately 45 million. The South African population consists of the

Nguni people (who comprise two thirds of the population), the Sotho-Tswana people (who include southern, northern, and western Sotho), the Tsonga, the Venda, Afrikaners, English, colored, Indians, and immigrants from the rest of Africa, Europe, and Asia. A few members of the Khoi and the San also remain. South Africa's constitution mentions eleven official languages, namely English, Afrikaans, IsiZulu, Sepedi, IsiNdebele, IsiXhosa, Sesotho, Setwana, SiSwati, Tshivenda, and Xitsonga. The 1998 census revealed the following use of languages: English, 8.6%; Afrikaans, 14.4%; IsiZulu, 22.9%; IsiXhosa, 17.9%; and Sepedi, 9.2%. Freedom of worship is guaranteed by the constitution, and the official policy is not to interfere with religious practices.

Health Care Beliefs: Passive and active roles; traditional; alternative; folk. The health care beliefs of South Africans are an integral part of the complex phenomenon of medical pluralism—the coexistence of different ways of perceiving, explaining, and treating illness. In South Africa, two broad groups of health care delivery can be identified: the system comprising allopathic, modern, and Western medicine and the complementary system comprising traditional, alternative, and folk medicine. Notwithstanding the fact that the allopathic medical system is dominant, South Africans strongly support traditional healers. Traditional healers tend to share the same sociocultural values as their communities, including beliefs about the origins, significance, and treatment of ill health. In the traditional (rural) societies, ill health and other forms of misfortune are often blamed on social causes, bad relationships, witchcraft, or supernatural causes (e.g., gods, ancestors). Traditional healers play a significant role in these societies. The healer focuses on the indigenous supernatural paradigm, historical legitimacy, sacred roles, tribal interest, and holistic treatment. It is important to note that natural and supernatural explanations of disease are often compatible. This can be illustrated by a story told by a social anthropology professor to a good friend who was a qualified nursing professional. The nurse's mother had become ill. It was evident that the nurse thought the origin of the illness could be witchcraft. The professor found it surprising that someone with scientific training would still believe in witches. "I know that the illness is a viral infection," said the nurse, " but I also need to know who sent the virus" (Boonzaaier, 1998). Mental disorders in particular are often considered by the African community to be supernatural and influenced by the ancestors.

Predominant Sick Care Practices: Biomedical and magical-religious. Western medicine has the official status supportive of the biomedical model. However, the various African cultures use traditional tribal medicine. Almost 50% of the African people consult a traditional healer before practitioners of Western medicine, or they consult them concurrently. As a result, many people receive a mixture of both forms of treatments. Treatments used by traditional healers may include ashes, amulets, and holy water. Since 1994 the government has made a concerted effort to unite the two existing systems of health care delivery. Health care is financed through two systems—the private and public health sectors. The private health sector is a crucial part of the current health care system. The total health care expenditure in South Africa is approximately 13% of the gross national product (GNP), and the private sector consumes nearly half of this amount. Despite these statistics the private sector provides care (which is primarily curative) to only 20% of the population. Private health care delivery is heavily concentrated in the densely populated wealthier urban areas and contributes little to alleviate the desperate shortages of resources in rural areas. Patients attending private health services need to pay for the service either as private patients in cash or through their medical plan. By April 1999, 168 private medical plans were registered in terms provided by the Medical Schemes Act, 1967 (act 72 of 1967). The Medical Schemes Act, 1998, was established on February 1, 1999. The intention of the act is to make affordable health care more accessible. The ANC Health Plan intends to ensure health services for all South Africans, primarily through the achievements of equitable social and economic development. The funding of health care, especially for the poor, will continue to come from general tax revenues. Free health care is provided in the public sector for children younger than 6, pregnant or nursing mothers, older adults, people with disabilities, and certain people who are chronically ill. Preventive and health-promotion activities, school health services, antenatal and delivery services, contraception, nutritional support, curative care for public health problems, and community-based care are also provided free in the public sector.

Ethnic/Race Specific or Endemic Diseases: The most common communicable diseases in South Africa are tuberculosis, malaria, measles, and sexually transmitted diseases. Malaria is endemic in the low-altitude areas of Northern Province, Mpumalanga, and northeastern KwaZulu-Natal. The highest risk area is a strip of about 100 km along the Zimbabwe, Mozambique, and Swaziland border. The disease should therefore be considered a regional, not a country-specific, problem. The malaria risk areas are divided into high-, intermediate-, and low-risk areas. In 1998, 26,440 cases and 198 deaths were reported, with the highest number of cases (14,575) occurring in KwaZulu-Natal. Tuberculosis has been a problem in South Africa for more than 200 years. The spread of the disease has been exacerbated by the unique pattern of mining, industrialization, urbanization, and politics. The epidemic is increasing by 20% per year, an increase resulting from the increasing poverty and the decreasing social status of the population. A complicating factor is the issue that tuberculosis is often not cured after the first attempt at treatment. HIV/AIDS are also complicating the disease; 40% to 50% of tuberculosis cases are associated with HIV infection. Cancer, cardio-vascular diseases, and strokes are thought of as diseases of the White man. (It has been reported that the incidence of myocardial infarctions in the Indian population is continuously increasing.) Approximately 1500 new HIV infections occur each day in South Africa. The mining industry has been the most affected, with a rate of HIV infection that is 7% to 17% higher than other groups. According to the 1998 ninth HIV National Survey, nearly 4 million South Africans are infected with HIV. The survey was based on 15,301 blood samples screened for HIV antibodies, which showed that an estimated 22% of women attending antenatal clinics nationally are infected. The survey also indicated that the prevalence of HIV in teenage girls between the ages of 15 and 19 years had risen from 12% in 1997 to 21% in 1998. The World Health Organization's (WHO) estimated prevalence rate for HIV/AIDS in adults ages 15 to 49 years is 19.94%. The estimated number of children from birth to 15 years living with HIV/AIDS is 95,000.

Health Team Relationships: Health personnel are considered the cornerstone for the realization of the Department of Health's vision. The main objectives are to integrate staff members, relocate them between urban and underserved areas, and reorient and retrain them. General practitioners play an important role in providing health care services. With the government's focus on primary health care, nursing professionals are playing a more important role because they are the frontline service providers. Other members of the health team include pharmacists and members of the allied health disciplines, such as physical and occupational therapists. Nursing professionals and doctors work as close teams in all disciplines of health care delivery.

Families' Role in Hospital Care: All hospitals—state and private—allow visitors during visiting hours. Family members are encouraged to assist when possible with the care of the patient, and many stay overnight to care for sick children. Because of financial constraints in state hospitals, families are more likely to provide bedding and food for hospitalized patients.

Dominance Patterns: A dichotomy exists relative to dominance patterns in South Africa. In most African households the father is the head of the family, or the patriarch, and usually the primary decision maker. In the Western (mostly White) households, men and women tend to have more equal relationships, and both help make decisions. Most of the women of South Africa contribute to its economic growth.

Eye Contact Practices: In most of the African cultures, it is an insult to make direct eye contact with superiors. A downward gaze is a sign of respect. In the other cultures, it is common to make direct eye contact. Guests and friends are usually greeted with a handshake, but family members are greeted with kisses.

Touch Practices: Touch practices also differ from culture to culture. In most African cultures, touching is common practice. In the more Western cultures, touching among family members (but not with others) is common. Hugs and kisses for children are very common. Nursing professionals often make physical contact with their patients to show they care; however, the doctor's role is such that limited physical contact occurs.

Perceptions of Time: Punctuality is not highly valued in South Africa; people operate according to what is often referred to as "Africa time." This lack of timeliness often causes friction in the business world. Health care practitioners simply expect patients to be late. Many primary health care nurses and doctors meet with patients who do not have an appointment. Patients simply show up, get in line, and wait their turn. When patients obtain a sick note from a doctor, they are not penalized for taking a day off from work.

Pain Reactions: Pain is primarily handled with respect, and patients are given the opportunity to discuss and describe their pain experiences. Analgesics are the primary treatment for pain relief, but lately more people have been using alternative therapies such as reflexology, aromatherapy, massage, and psychotherapy. In some hospitals, pain assessment forms are used to ensure effective pain management.

Birth Rites: The African and Western cultures in South Africa have major differences in birth rituals. Most infants of rural African women are born at home with the assistance of an older woman (often referred to as a *midwife,* although she has no formal training), and pain is not eased with any medication. The infants of women of the Western cultures are born primarily in a hospital with the assistance of a trained midwife. If the patient chooses one of the luxurious private hospitals for birth, they are able to have a medical doctor who is very often (in at least 70% of the cases) an obstetrician. Of the patients choosing private hospitals, 50% of their infants are born by cesarean section, often at the request of a mother who wants a planned delivery. After birth in the hospital, rooming-in is common (i.e., keeping the infant and mother together in the same room). Kangaroo care is used, and breast-feeding is usually the feeding method of choice.

Death Rites: In the Western cultures, most sick people die in a hospital setting, and family members are usually very involved in the patient's care. The funeral or cremation usually takes place within 4 to 7 days after the death. Occasionally a memorial service is held for the deceased in addition to the funeral or cremation service. The death is announced in newspapers, usually before the burial ceremony. In the African cultures the body is dressed in clothing provided by the family. The body lies in state in the house of a family member, usually in the living room. Family and friends of the deceased come and visit during a 2- or 3-day period. The visitation is followed by a service that precedes the burial. It is customary for all family and friends of the deceased to attend the funeral service and pay their last respects. After the service and burial ceremony, family and friends join in celebrating that the deceased is saved. It is not uncommon to slaughter a cow, 3 sheep, and 20 chickens for a funeral because most relatives or friends of the deceased person and the person's family participate in the celebration.

Food Practices and Intolerances: People from the urbanized communities usually eat three times a day, and may have the main course either at lunch or in the evening. The South African diet includes a wide variety of vegetables, fruits, fish, and meat such as chicken, beef, sheep, and pork. Because the diet is high in red meat, White males have a high incidence of high cholesterol and heart disease. The urban population also eats too many refined grains and breads. The rural South African's staple food is unrefined corn with seasonal vegetables, if they are available. Fifty-five to 60% of all South Africans are overweight, primarily because of the wrong diet or from overeating.

Infant Feeding Practices: Breast-feeding is the standard practice in South Africa, and most women are aware of its benefits. If for any reason a mother cannot or chooses not to breast-feed, formula is available. For White women, breast-feeding is a private affair. However, African women feed on demand, even in public.

Child Rearing Practices: Child rearing practices in South Africa have tended to be very strict; children are seen and not heard. Child rearing is the primary responsibility of the parents, but the task is shared by teachers at school. With the change of the school curriculum ("Curriculum 2005"), children are now taught to express their opinions freely and to think critically. South Africa strongly supports the United Nations Convention on the Rights of the Child by banning corporal punishment in schools. The common family structure of South Africa consists of a father and mother, but single-parent families are also relatively common. Because many African mothers work in the cities, their children are often left in the care of grandparents in rural areas. The grandparents take on the responsibility of raising the children, and the mother or father visits their children approximately every 3 months, depending on the travel distance. Working mothers are now granted 4 months of paid maternity leave, and fathers receive 5 working days of paternity leave.

National Childhood Immunizations: BCG at birth; DTP at 6, 10, and 14 weeks and 18 months; OPV at birth, 6, 10, and 14 weeks, 18 months, and 5 years; hep B at 6, 10, and 14 weeks; measles at 9 and 18 months; DT at 5 years; MMR at 15 months (optional); and TT CBAW.

BIBLIOGRAPHY

ANC: *A national health plan for South Africa,* Pretoria, South Africa, 1994, State Printers.

Boonzaaier E: Understanding disease: are 'first-world' and 'third-world' patients fundamentally different? *SA Family Practice,* Nov 1988.

Center for Health Policy: A national health service and the future of the private sector—the case for a national health insurance, 1991, JHB, University of the Witwatersrand.

Dennill K et al: *Aspects of primary health care,* Johannesburg, South Africa, 1995, Halfway House: Southern Book Publishers.

Dreyer M, Hattingh S, Lock M: *Community health nursing,* Johannesburg, South Africa, 1993, Halfway House: Southern Book Publishers.

Gilbert L, Selikow T, Walker L: *Society, health and disease. An introductory reader for health professionals,* 1996, JHB: Ravan Press (Pty) Ltd.

Government Communication and Information System: *South Africa yearbook, 2000/2001,* Pretoria, South Africa.

◆ SPAIN (KINGDOM OF)

MAP PAGE (860)

Henrietta Bernal

Location: Spain occupies most of the Iberian Peninsula in southwestern Europe. The total land area is 504,750 km^2 (194,884 square miles). Spain is bordered by the Atlantic Ocean on the west and the Mediterranean Sea on the south; Africa is only 16 km (10 miles) away. The Pyrenees Mountains in the northeast separate Spain from France. The Spanish people include groups that are originally from other parts of Europe and from the Mediterranean.

Major Languages	Ethnic Groups	Major Religions
Castilian Spanish	Spanish 73%	Roman Catholic 99%
Catalan	Catalan 16%	Other 1%
Galician	Galician 8%	
Basque	Basque other 3%	

Health Care Beliefs: Active role; minimal use of folk remedies; health promotion important. Some folk remedies might be practiced in the more extreme rural areas, but they tend to be those related to "grandmother's" cures for colds or headaches. In the early part of the century, such practices as cupping and folk remedies for warts were common, but these have mostly given way to modern medicine, with doctors and pharmacists playing a key role.

Predominant Sick Care Practices: Biomedical primarily. Spain is a modern western European country that is part of the European Common Market and NATO. The health care system is centralized and socialized and provides equal access to all. In general the citizens adhere to a Western medical model belief system and are more likely to use the modern medical system than alternative approaches. This is particularly true in urban areas.

Ethnic/Race Specific or Endemic Diseases: Spain has a very low infant mortality rate, a low birth rate, and is fifth in the world in length of life expectancy. The disease profile of Spain mirrors that of any developed country. Heart disease is the major cause of death, and HIV/AIDS, and substance abuse are increasing problems. The country is undergoing an immigration crisis as thousands of North Africans, Central Americans, and Eastern Europeans immigrate to Spain for a better life. The immigration is changing infectious diseases rates and places a great burden on the public health system. The World Health Organization's (WHO) estimated prevalence rate for HIV/AIDS in adults ages 15 to 49 is 0.58%. The estimated number of children from birth to 15 years living with HIV/AIDS is less than 100.

Health Team Relationships: People in higher socioeconomic groups ask about and expect to be fully informed about their problems and treatments. Children do not remain in bed in a hospital unless it is necessary. The nurse is transitioning from a dependent to a more collaborative role, but nurses and doctors still have specific tasks distinguishing their respective roles. In selected areas, nurse practitioners practice without supervision from a doctor. Friendliness, patience, efficacy, and professionalism are the qualities in the nurse that are the most highly valued by patients. Communication between nurses and patients is usually better than it is between patients and doctors.

Families Role in Hospital Care: Hospitals encourage the patient and family to collaborate in care. Some children continue their schooling while in the hospital. In most instances, families are expected to stay with relatives who are in the hospital and provide much of their personal care. Family members take turns staying with the patients, who are seldom left alone. As dual-career households increase, families are finding it harder to care for the growing population of older adults. Women have been brought to Spain from Central and South America to care for older adults because their children are working. Although families are hiring this extra assistance, placing a loved one in a nursing home is still very difficult for them.

Dominance Patterns: Spain has a very ethnically diverse society. Not only are there differences between Basques and Catalans, but rural and urban differences exist in food, music, and traditions. During the last 40 years, Spain has undergone great political, social, and economic changes, which have influenced the role of women. According to the Spanish constitution, women have equal rights; they are represented in all areas of employment and hold many elected offices. As a result the relationship between men and women parallels that of the rest of Europe. Although rural areas may still have traces of the more traditional male-dominant pattern, the younger generation of women is experiencing more equality with men.

Eye Contact: Direct eye contact is common among those in the younger generations.

Touch Practices: Touch practices vary greatly from region to region and within regions. Northerners tend to be less demonstrative and effusive. In general, compared with Americans, Spaniards tend to touch more.

Perceptions of Time: Although Spaniards have a reputation for having a casual attitude about time, the exigencies of modern society have made punctuality more important. Banks, stores, factories, and other establishments open on time, and public transportation tends to be reliable. Although all of this is true, the Spanish have a casual attitude about being on time for personal visits, dates, or other similar appointments.

Pain Reactions: Spaniards display a full range of pain reactions. Some are very stoical and do not admit they are in pain unless it is extreme, whereas some are extremely vocal. Hospice care is emerging in Spain as people begin to realize that patients need proper and adequate pain control.

Birth Rites: The birth rate is decreasing, and the age at which women are first becoming pregnant is increasing. Births usually take place in the hospital, and fathers may witness a delivery if there are no complications. The contraceptive methods used, in decreasing order of popularity, are condoms, birth control pills, intrauterine devices, diaphragms, and biological rhythm (which is used by religious couples who do not approve of other contraceptive methods).

Death Rites: The family has a wake for the deceased person for 24 hours, and some prefer to have a mass before the burial. The body is buried or cremated according to the person's previously stated desires. In some rural areas, only the men go to the cemetery, and the women stay in the church and pray the rosary; however, this practice is becoming uncommon.

Food Practices and Intolerances: Spanish food is not spiced liberally, but olive oil is an important ingredient. Breakfast is light, and the main meal is eaten during the afternoon siesta period. An early evening snack is eaten, and a multiple-course dinner is eaten late in the evening.

Child Rearing Practices: In the past, infant care was primarily the job of the women, but today the responsibility is beginning to be shared by the father. Education about sex role differences begins early. Students must pass a competitive qualifying examination to enter their desired field of education.

National Childhood Immunizations: DTP at 2, 4, 6, 15 to 18 months, and 5 to 6 years; OPV at 2, 4, 6, and 15 to 18 months and at 5 to 6 years; MMR at 15 to 18 months and 3 to 6 years; and Td at 14 to 16 years.

Other Characteristics: Spaniards have been called the "night owls of Europe" because they like to stay up late, partly because of the great weather in many parts of the country and partly because they like to have a good time. This characteristic is, of course, particularly true of young people. Although Spain has religious freedom, the Roman Catholic church has played a major role in the social life of Spain. Religious festivals are common throughout the country, and offer an opportunity for major and minor celebrations throughout the year. Children celebrate the feast of the three kings on January 5, a festival that includes gift exchanges. Television plays a major role in daily life and has been criticized because it is believed responsible for a decrease in book sales and reading.

BIBLIOGRAPHY

Beunza I et al: Diversity and commonality in international nursing, *Int Nurs Rev* 41(2):47, 1994.

Calvet IC et al: The role of the nurse from a user's point of view, *Enfermeria Clin* 5(2):61, 1995.

Cubel PML et al: A study of the demand for self care in the medical department of the Son Dureta Hospital in Palma de Mallorca, Spain, *Enfermeria Clin* 4(6):260, 1994.

Elsden C, Yarritu C: Development of nursing services in the Basque Autonomous Region, Spain, *Nurs Adm Q* 16(2):68, 1992.

Mondragón D: Health status and nursing's contribution in Catalonia, *Nurs Health Care* 14(10):520, 1993.

Moroan PL et al: The qualities of the nurse from the point of view of the patient, *Enfermeria Clin* 4(2):68, 1994.

Rendon DC et al: The living experience of aging in community-dwelling elders in Valencia, Spain: a phenomenological study, *Nurs Sci Q* 8(4):152, 1995.

Sims J: Nursing in Spain: times of change, *Nurs Times* 21(86):30, 1990.

◆ SRI LANKA (DEMOCRATIC SOCIALIST REPUBLIC OF)

MAP PAGE (866)

K.A.L.A. Karuppuarachchi

Location: Sri Lanka is a beautiful tropical island just off the southeastern tip of the Indian subcontinent. It has a total land area of approximately 62,705 km² (24,204 square miles). The central hilly area has mountains and plains and a mean temperature ranging from 14° C to 24° C, whereas the low-country plains and coastal areas have a mean temperature ranging from 26° C to 28° C. Sri Lanka has traditionally been an agricultural country, and Ceylon tea, which is grown in the central hills, is world famous for its taste. Other than tea and rubber exports, Sri Lanka's other major sources of income are tourism, the garment industry, and foreign remittances (employment especially in the Middle East).

Major Languages	Ethnic Groups	Major Religions
Sinhala	Sinhalese 74%	Buddhist 70%
Tamil	Tamil 18%	Hindu 15%
	Moor 7%	Christian 8%
	Burgher, Malay, Veddah 1%	Muslim 7%

The estimated population in 2000 was 19.4 million, with a population growth rate of 1.7%. The district of the capital city of Colombo has the highest population density. Sri Lanka has nine provinces and just more than half of the population is concentrated in the western, central, and southern provinces. The majority of the people are Sinhalese. The other significant ethnic groups include the Tamils, Moors, and Burghers. The Sinhalese speak Sinhala, whereas the Tamils and most Moors speak Tamil. The school children are encouraged to learn Sinhala and Tamil. Importance is also placed on English because knowledge of English is highly beneficial for social mobility and employment. The literacy rate in 1994 was 92.5% for males and 87.9% for females. Buddhism is practiced by most Sinhalese, Hinduism by most Tamils, Islam by the Moors, and Christianity by some Sinhalese, Tamils, and Burghers.

Health Care Beliefs: Active and passive roles; traditional. The majority believe that ill health has physical origins. However, some people, particularly those in rural areas, attribute it to supernatural or astrological influences. *Bodhi poojas*—pouring water on the *bo* tree, which is considered sacred— and visiting fortune tellers are also common.

Predominant Sick Care Practices: Biomedical; alternative; magical-religious. Western medicine is freely accessible to the people through the state health sector and has replaced traditional and indigenous practices. However, some people with chronic, debilitating, or mental illnesses rely on indigenous magico-religious rituals such as wearing enchanted threads or amulets, applying oils, and performing *thovil* (an exorcism ceremony). Trained and untrained ayurvedic practitioners have learned the art from their predecessors. Homeopathy and acupuncture are also practiced.

Ethnic/Race Specific or Endemic Diseases: Malaria is endemic in certain provinces. Other health problems include Japanese encephalitis, dengue hemorrhagic fever, and leptospirosis. Diarrheal diseases, filariasis, tuberculosis, and leprosy are also concerns. The morbidity and mortality associated with snake bites are also significant. Prevention of rabies is another important task. It is compulsory to report many of the communicable diseases, and the country supports public health programs for control. Alcohol-, tobacco-, and cannabis-related disorders are emerging health care problems. The suicide and deliberate self-injury rates have been alarming in the last few years. The World Health Organization's (WHO) estimated prevalence rate for HIV/AIDS in adults ages 15 to 49 is 0.07%. The estimated number of children from birth to 15 years living with HIV/AIDS is 200. HIV was first reported in Sri Lanka in 1987. By the end of December 2000, 358 cases had been reported, and 119 patients had been diagnosed with AIDS. Approximately 1.6 males get AIDS for every 1 female.

Health Team Relationships: Doctors are highly regarded, and traditionally most health care services have revolved around them. However, a multi-disciplinary approach to health care is becoming more popular in all areas including mental health, although it is primarily hindered by the lack of trained personnel.

Families' Role in Hospital Care: The extended family is usually involved in the care of hospitalized relatives. They take turns staying with the patients, and clean and feed them. They are also involved in decision making and long-term care if the patient has a chronic illness. The involvement of the family is helpful, especially for patients with mental illnesses because community care for these individuals is not well developed. However, rapid urbanization and disintegration of existing family networks is altering the traditional involvement.

Dominance Patterns: Men are usually dominant, especially in rural areas. However, women play a central role in the home. They are respected and revered by the children and are the primary caretakers of the home. Women traditionally wear *saree*. The work force has a considerable number of women in every sector, and women are in some managerial positions as well. Children usually have the father's surname.

Eye Contact Practices: Direct eye contact is common, regardless of sex.

Touch Practices: Touching is common among friends of the same sex who are talking. When greeting one another, Sri Lankans place their palms together in front of their chest, as if praying, and say *ayubowan,* or "long life." However, greetings in professional situations may be limited to a handshake.

Perceptions of Time: Punctuality is emphasized from childhood, and most ceremonies are performed at specific times designated as *naketh,* which are usually determined by astrologers. However, many Sri Lankans are relaxed about time during most other activities. They are proud to talk about Sri Lanka's previous prosperity and history.

Pain Reactions: Pain is expressed verbally by most.

Birth Rites: Most births occur in hospitals. The time of the birth is considered important, and horoscopes are developed based on it. Many believe the time of birth determines various aspects of the future, including education, employment, and marriage. Birth is a celebratory time for family and friends, and the mother and child are cared for by family members, especially by the grandmothers. The mother is fed a broth prepared with rice and chilies. Children of both sexes are equally valued, although certain families may prefer boys.

Death Rites: Family members are present at the time of a family member's death. Those who are dying are helped to recall their past good deeds to help them be in a sound state of mind at the time of death, which facilitates a better rebirth. When grieving, many Sri Lankans weep. Buddhists have priests chant *pirith,* or religious songs. Funerals vary according to religious rituals and rites. The family and friends attend the burial or cremation ceremony. Some families have burial plots in their ancestral lands, but the majority of people bury their family members in public cemeteries. The body is carried in a wooden casket, and some Sri Lankans play a special drum rhythm during the funeral procession. The funeral procession walks on white cloth or sand that has been placed on the ground. Flower wreaths are common. The community leaders and family pay a tribute to the dead person at the ceremony. On the seventh day and various intervals after the death, the priests are offered food in the belief that it will help the person during rebirth. Autopsies are generally acceptable, and Buddhism encourages organ donations.

Food Practices and Intolerances: Rice is the staple food and is eaten with curries of vegetables, fish, or meat. The food is spicy and hot, and coconut milk is used liberally in the curries. *Kiribath,* or milk rice, is a traditional specialty made with coconut milk and cooked for celebrations such as those for the new year. Most Sri Lankans eat with their right hand.

Infant Feeding Practices: Breast-feeding is popular, and most are aware of its benefits. Mothers may breast-feed their children for 2 to 5 years.

Child Rearing Practices: Children are raised in extended families that display tendencies towards overinvolvement and overprotection. Children have a religious upbringing and learn traditional values. Parents, older adults, and teachers are respected and occasionally honored with betel leaves.

National Childhood Immunizations: BCG at birth to 4 weeks; DTP at 2, 4, 6, and 18 months; OPV at 2, 4, 6, and 18 months and 5 years; measles at 9 months; measles-rubella at 3 years, rubella at 10 to 15 years (for those who did not receive it previously) and 15 to 44 years; DT at 5 years; adult tetanus-diphtheria at 10 to 15 years; and TT for first pregnancy ×2 and for subsequent pregnancies ×1 (up to fourth pregnancy).

BIBLIOGRAPHY

Department of Health Services: *Annual health bulletin,* Sri Lanka, 2000.
Kuruppuarachchi KALA, Rajakaruna RR: Psychiatry in Sri Lanka, *Psychiatric Bulletin* 23:686-688, 1999.
Ministry of Health, Epidemiological Unit: *Immunization schedule,* Sri Lanka, 2001.
World Health Organization (June 2000): *Epidemiological fact sheets by country,* Geneva. Retrieved March 1, 2002, from http://www.unaids.org/hivaidsinfo/statistics/june00/fact_sheets/index.html
World Health Organization (2001): *WHO vaccine-preventable diseases: monitoring system,* Geneva. Retrieved March 1, 2002, from http://www.who.int/vaccines
World Health Organization, Regional Office for Southeast Asia Suicide Prevention: *Emerging from darkness,* 2001.

◆ SUDAN (REPUBLIC OF THE)

MAP PAGE (862)

Ahmed M. EL Hassan and Muntaser Eltayeb Ibrahim

Location: Sudan lies in the northeastern part of Africa and is bordered on the west by Chad and Central African Republic; on the south by Congo,

Uganda, and Kenya; on the east by Ethiopia and Eritrea, and on the north by Libya and Egypt. Sudan, which is 1 million miles^2, is the largest country in Africa. The total land area is 2,505,810 km^2 (967,495 square miles). According to the 1993 census the total population was 25.6 million, of whom 78% is rural or nomadic. The urban growth rate is 4.6%, whereas the rural growth rate is 2.4%, a reflection of the high numbers of people migrating from rural to urban areas.

Major Languages	Ethnic Groups	Major Religions
Arabic	Black 52%	Sunni Muslim 70%
English	Arab 39%	Indigenous beliefs 25%
Tribal dialects	Beja 6%	Christian 5%
	Other 3%	

More than 100 languages are spoken in the Sudan. These languages can be categorized as three of the four of Greenberg's African language families: the Afro-Asiatic, the Niger-Kordofanian, and the Nilo-Saharan. These languages are disappearing and being replaced by Arabic, the language of trade and government. Other commonly spoken languages are Dinka, Nuer, Triggering, and Fur.

Health Care Beliefs: Traditional; active role; health promotion important. The Federal Ministry of Health and the television stations in the country sponsor health-promotion activities. In Khartoum state, *Omdurman,* a popular health-promotion television program is run by a senior doctor, and is broadcast live every week. It addresses major health problems and encourages dialogue among members of the public. The program invites senior doctors to participate in the discussion. Last year the program was chosen as the best Sudanese television show. The Federal Ministry sponsors a health education program and a museum in the capital of Khartoum that deals primarily with prevention of the major diseases in the country. Health centers have health promotion and prevention units, particularly for maternity and child health and nutrition. Some societies have been established for health promotion as well, such as the Friends of Diabetics Society and the Breast Cancer Society, which is sponsored by the Women's Initiative Group, a nongovernmental organization. The objective of the cancer group is to train women to perform breast self-examinations for early breast cancer detection. The groups also help the poorer patients with finances. Breast cancer is the most common type of cancer among Sudanese females. Mental illness is feared, and many believe it is the result of demonic possession. Most people, particularly those in remote villages and slums of large towns and cities, consult a holy man, or *Faki,* before a doctor. In a recent study by the department of clinical psychology at the University of Khartoum, a surprising number of educated people revealed that they had consulted *Fakis*. It was also revealed that the number of traditional healers in the country far outnumber the psychiatrists and psychologists. The treatment of patients with mental illness can be appalling. They are kept in solitary confinement, are given only bread and water, and may be beaten in an attempt to drive out the demons or evil spirits thought to possess the body. Some patients even develop scurvy. These individuals are eventually brought to the hospital because the scurvy prevents the beating wounds from healing. The previously mentioned study also revealed that traditional healers and psychiatrists collaborate by referring patients to one another. Traditional healers are not only consulted for psychiatric problems but also for organic diseases. Another form of traditional treatment is *zar,* which is commonly practiced in urban and rural areas in the northern part of the country and Ethiopia, where it probably originated. *Zar* is the name of a demon, or *jinni,* that is believed to cause many changes in a person's physical and psychological health and general welfare; for example, it can cause a person to become ill, a pregnancy or a birth, or a death. These invisible beings are believed to number 88 and be divided into two equal groups. Forty-four are controlled by a chief called *Warrar,* and the other 44 are controlled by another chief called *Mama*. In the Sudan, the Zar Mama is more influential; he is often mentioned and called on during the chants of the *Zar* ceremonies. During these ceremonies, the targeted patient goes into a trance under the influence of chants, burning incense, and the sound of drums. The songs are thought to appease the *jinni* or demon possessing the patient. During these trances and dances, the patient is free to indulge in activities that are normally taboo in everyday life; for example, women are allowed to smoke and drink. The patient may express suppressed needs, which may be therapeutic. The influence of the anima and the animus are obvious during these ceremonies. A woman may be dressed in a man's attire symbolizing certain idolized figures. Probably because of the influence of White men during British colonization of the country, patients dress in European attire and smoke a pipe. The resulting figure is known as a *khawaga,* a term used for any White man. Another figure that may be seen is the *Arabi,* or Arab. Those under the influence of the *Arabi* dress in the fashion of the Beja tribes (the Fuzzy Wuzzy of Kipling) of eastern Sudan. In contrast, men may dress as women during the ceremonies.

Predominant Sick Care Practices: Biomedical and magical-religious. Treatment-seeking behaviors vary from one part of the country to another. In remote rural areas, where the health services are poor or unavailable, patients still use traditional healers. Treatments given by traditional healers vary according to the type of disease but often include herbal medicines, scarification, and cauterization. In Muslim communities, patients are treated with recitations from the Koran. These verses are read over the affected body part, and the healer usually spits over the body part as well. This practice is common for treating headaches. Verses from the Koran may be written on a piece of wood. The writings are washed with water that is given to the patient to drink or rub on the affected area. Occasionally the verses are written on paper that is burned; the smoke is inhaled. The smoke practice is common when a disease is believed to be caused by someone with the "evil eye" (i.e., the power to harm other merely by looking at them) or possession by a *jinni*. Sorcery is practiced in Muslim and non-Muslim communities. The *faki,* or holy man, in the Muslim communities and other sorcerers in non-Muslim areas are called on to reverse the effects of witchcraft. Verses from the Koran and mysterious symbols are worn on amulets as protection against the evil eye. In paganism, belief in evil spirits and sorcery is common. For example, in the Nuba Mountains the *kujur* performs certain rituals to rid the patient of evil spirits. Roots of certain plants are often used to treat snake and scorpion bites in many rural parts of the country. Some roots are used as protective amulets. In urban areas, where modern medical facilities are available and people are more educated, patients usually consult a doctor. In the past, medical care was free. In the last 10 years, a fee-for-service system has been established. The poorer patients often cannot afford the cost of tests and treatment, so many more are seeking traditional treatments.

Ethnic/Race Specific or Endemic Diseases: Sudan has approximately 570 tribes that have been categorized into 56 ethnic groups on the basis of linguistic, cultural, and other ethnological characteristics. Malaria, tuberculosis, leprosy, cutaneous and visceral leishmaniasis, and schistosomiasis are the major endemic diseases in the country. The degree of endemicity varies, a fact that may be related to genetic or environmental factors. Some diseases are reported to be ethnically related, one of which is kala-azar. Evidence in an endemic focus shows that under similar exposure conditions, individuals from the tribes of southern Sudan and the Nuba Mountains are more susceptible to *kala-azar* than individuals from tribes of the northern Sudan. Sickle cell anemia is more common in the Messeyria tribes of Kordofan. The Beja tribes of the Red Sea hills are particularly susceptible to tuberculosis. In northern Sudan, diseases of affluence such as heart disease and diabetes are becoming important health problems. The World Health Organization's (WHO) estimated prevalence rate for HIV/AIDS in adults ages 15 to 49 years is 0.99%. WHO has no estimates for children. According to the AIDS Program of the Federal Ministry of Health, Sudan had 3512 confirmed cases by the end of 2000. This is probably an underestimation. It is estimated that approximately 400,000 people were actually infected by the end of 2000.

Health Team Relationships: Overall, doctors are dominant. In rural areas the midwife is highly respected and quite influential. Doctors and their assistants are highly regarded by the community. A commonly used name for a doctor is *Hakeem* (Arabic for "the wise").

Families' Role in Hospital Care: Family and friends play an important role in supporting patients in the hospital and at home. They stay with hospitalized relatives and bring them food. Mothers can stay with sick children in the ward. Among the Masalit tribes of western Sudan, those with a disease such as leprosy, which carries a stigma in many communities, are accepted and cared for by the family. They stay in a separate hut in the family's housing compound. Their clothes are washed by relatives, and their meals are prepared for them. In areas where leprosy is rare, the stigma is stronger. Many patients leave their families and are never heard from again.

Dominance Patterns: Generally speaking, men are dominant. However, with the recent increase in women's education, greater economic independence and emancipation of women have been evident in urban areas. Relationships between men and women are changing significantly, a change that is reflected in the enhanced role of women in the social and economic fields. Women won voting rights in the early 1960s, and many women now have senior positions in public and private sectors.

Eye Contact Practices: In certain situations, direct eye contact is prohibited. For example, conservative women do not have direct eye contact with unknown men, or with holy men.

Touch Practices: The handshake is a common greeting. In some Muslim factions, women are not allowed to shake hands with any men other than their husbands and first-degree relatives.

Perceptions of Time: Perceptions of time vary between rural and urban areas. In areas of traditional agriculture, the timing of events is related to the cycles of agricultural activities (e.g., harvest time, the rainy season, the flooding of the Nile). In urban areas, perceptions of time are similar to those in modern industrial societies, although the Sudanese are not known for being punctual. Today, during the current difficult chapter in the history of the nation, people often reminisce about the "good old days."

Pain Reactions: People in rural areas have a high pain tolerance. The younger generation, particularly in urban societies, has less of a tolerance.

Birth Rites: In rural areas traditional birth attendants assist with births. In the larger towns and cities, trained midwives are available. After birth the mother is confined to the house for approximately 40 days. In northern Sudan, she is taken with the infant to the Nile River, where part of the child's body is washed with water. This traditional relic remains from the time when the population in this area was Christian. This tradition might also have been practiced in the ancient kingdoms of Nubia. During the 40 days the woman cannot be visited by anyone who has seen a dead body or been to a cemetery. In rural areas the confined women wears a *mashahara,* which is a collection of beads and figures of humans and various animals. The *mashahara* is believed to ward off the evil eye and spirits. Immediately after birth a male relative recites in the infant's ear verses that are usually used for the call for prayers. Every newborn Muslim is named Mohamed or Fatima (after the prophet Mohamed and his daughter) at birth depending on the sex. On the seventh day after birth the infant is given a permanent name and a ram is sacrificed for the occasion. Boys are preferred. Among the Nilotic tribe of the Dinka of southern Sudan, where clans are traced through the male lineage, it is important for men to marry and produce a male child to maintain the lineage link. If no son is born, they face oblivion after death. If a boy dies, a brother or a close relative chooses a wife in the name of the dead boy; any children born are considered the dead boy's children. The birth of a girl is celebrated because she brings her family wealth when she marries, but she does not continue the family's lineage. Dinka women stay in their mother's house for the birth of their children, remaining in the hut for 5 days. Their mothers care for them and cut the umbilical cord. The placenta is placed in a skin and washed and is later buried by both women outside the house. The father sacrifices a bull or sheep, and the blood is spilled outside the hut. The grandmother dips her finger in the blood and smears it on the infant's forehead, neck, and chest; some is smeared on the mother as well. Some foods are taboo during pregnancy and while nursing. These foods include antelope, buffalo, and certain types of fish. If these rules are broken, it is believed that the child will die. Children are usually named after their ancestors. Nuba women give birth in their house. The umbilical cord is cut with a fragment of millet stalk, and the placenta is buried inside the hut. Traditionally the first-born male is named Kuku, the second Kafi, the third Tia, and the fourth with the female name Tutu. The first-born female is named Kaka, the second Toto, the third Kash, and the fourth Kiki.

Death Rites: In the hot climate of the Sudan the body is buried as quickly as possible to prevent decomposition. Women wail and lament, mentioning the virtues of the deceased. Muslims wash the body with water in a ritual dictated by the teachings of Islam. The body is then dabbed with perfumes and wrapped in new white cloth before it is finally buried after a short prayer. Inside the grave the body is laid on its right side with the face toward Mecca. Only men are allowed to attend the burial. The women follow the funeral procession for about 50 m. They wail and may throw sand on their uncovered heads, a sign of intense mourning. Mourning continues for 3 days, during which time the relatives of the deceased have visits from friends and relatives who are offering their condolences. The Dinka—the main Nilotic tribe of southern Sudan—dig a grave outside the hut and the body is buried in a fetal position with skins placed over and beneath it. If the deceased was a chief the four gravediggers remain near the grave for 8 days. A cow that produced milk consumed by the chief is killed, and the mourners eat it while they remain at the grave. Mourners do not drink milk. A bullock is sacrificed 4 days and 6 days after the death of the father and a brother, respectively. The animal is killed by repeated stabbing in the heart, and the males eat the meat. The sacrifice is repeated at intervals of months or years to propitiate the spirit of the deceased, or the spirit may cause the living to become ill. No one would touch the corpse of a mother's brother or the blood of his sacrifice because it is believed to cause the skin of the face to fall off as if it has burned. Among the Nuba of Kordufan, the family graves are shaped like a funnel. A 6- to 8-foot long shaft expands in its lower part into a space that is 3 feet high and 8 feet long. A couple of men are lowered in the grave to receive the body. Hoes, broken spears, and knives are buried with the corpse. In some clans, as many as 10 living sheep are buried with the body to appease the spirit of the departed. The spirit of the deceased is believed to stay in the grave with the body and leave occasionally to visit the village and appear to relatives in dreams. After the burial an animal is sacrificed and eaten by the blood relatives of the deceased. Husbands and wives do not eat the flesh of animals sacrificed for their spouse. The information on birth and death rites in the Dinka and Nuba is based on the publications of Seligman in the 1930s. It is likely that these rituals are still practiced by the tribes in their homelands. Those who have been displaced and no longer live in their tribal areas seem to have abandoned these practices and are following Christian or Islamic practices depending on their faith.

Food Practices and Intolerances: The Sudanese diet consists of vegetables, meat, regular bread, thin bread *(kissra),* and porridge made from sorghum, millet, or wheat. People living near the Nile and its tributaries or on the shores of the Red Sea eat fish. Meat is now becoming expensive, and poor people may not have meat except during festivities such as the Eid Eladha festival, when Muslims are required to sacrifice an animal, usually a sheep. Even the poor save money to celebrate this annual event. A popular dish affordable for many consists of beans with sesame oil that is eaten with wheat bread. The dish is usually eaten for breakfast and as an evening meal. *Aseeda,* a type of thick porridge made from sorghum or millet, is eaten with milk or stewed meat and vegetables. In some tribes, certain items of food are taboo. For example, the Beja tribes of eastern Sudan do not eat fish or eggs. Most eat with their hands.

Infant Feeding Practices: Most women breast-feed for 2 years according to the teachings of Islam. Nursing is supplemented by bottle-feeding if the mother feels she does not have enough milk. In urban communities, bottle-feeding is becoming fashionable and is increasing.

Child Rearing Practices: Child rearing is strict, and the father is responsible for most discipline. Children sleep with their parents.

National Childhood Immunizations: BCG at birth and first contact; DTP at 6, 10, and 14 weeks; OPV at 6, 10, and 14 weeks; measles at 9 months; vitamin A at 6 months; TT at first contact for CBAW, week 14 of gestations, +4 to 6 weeks. Vaccination coverage is reported to be high.

BIBLIOGRAPHY

Beasley A: Breastfeeding studies: culture, biomedicine, and methodology, *J Hum Lact* 7(1):7, 1991.

Eltom A et al: Thyroid function in the newborn in relation to maternal thyroid status during labour in a mild iodine deficiency endemic area in Sudan, *Clin Endocrinol* 55:485, 2001.

Meheus A, Antal GM: The endemic treponemas: not yet eradicated, *World Health Stat Q* 45(2–3):228, 1992.

Seligman CG, Seligman BZ: *Pagan tribes of the Nilotic Sudan*, London, 1932, Routledge & Kegan Paul.

Taha TET: Family planning practice in Central Sudan, *Soc Sci Med* 37(5):685, 1993.

Wright J: Female genital mutilation: an overview, *J Adv Nurs* 24:251, 1996.

ZijlIstra EE, el-Hassan AM: Leishmaniasis in Sudan: visceral leishmaniasis, *Trans R Soc Trop Med Hyg* 95(suppl 1):27, 2001.

◆ SURINAME (REPUBLIC OF)

MAP PAGE (859)

Carol Vlassoff and Dawn Bichel

Location: The Republic of Suriname is situated on the northeast coast of South America and is bordered by Guyana on the west, French Guiana on the east, Brazil on the south, and the Atlantic Ocean on the north. The country has a total land area of 163,820 km² (63,250 square miles) and consists of narrow coastal plain with swamps, rolling hills, and tropical rainforest. The population in 1980 was estimated to be 425,000 people. (A new census was planned for 2002.) The capital city is Paramaribo, distinguished by its fine (although deteriorating) wooden architecture dating from the Dutch period. The interior of Suriname covers about 85% of the total land area. Much of the interior is untouched and sparsely populated, consisting of dense flora and fauna. About 90% of the population lives in or around Paramaribo or in the coastal towns. The remainder is primarily Carib and Arawak Indians and Bush Blacks who are descendants of slaves who escaped in the seventeenth century; locally, they are called Maroons, and they are widely scattered throughout the interior.

Major Languages	Ethnic Groups	Major Religions
Dutch (official)	Hindustani (East	Hindu 27%
English	Indian) 37%	Protestant 25% (primarily
Sranan Tongo	Creole (Black,	Moravian)
(Surinamese)	mixed) 31%	Roman Catholic 23%
Hindustani	Javanese 15%	Muslim 20%
Javanese	Maroon 10%	Other or none 5%
	Amerindian 3%	
	Chinese 2%	
	European, other 2%	

Dutch is the national language, and Sranan Tongo (Surinamese) is also widely spoken. Suriname has been influenced by many cultures, yet little racial tension exists among the different groups. Surinamese of all backgrounds pride themselves on their ability to get along with one another.

Health Care Beliefs: Traditional; somewhat active role with increasing prevention activities. Governmental and nongovernmental organizations, development assistance agencies, and international organizations support the formal health care sector in Suriname, especially its health promotion aspects. For example, several organizations are involved in various aspects of prevention, care, and treatment of HIV/AIDS. An interreligious health committee promotes health through community leaders and provides information in a culturally sensitive way. A television series from South Africa called "Soul Buddyz" for children aged 8 to 12 has been introduced to address important health and social issues. Local nongovernmental organizations and development agencies also promote and host health days to increase awareness on topics such as water and sanitation, safe motherhood, and mental health. People in Suriname do not usually talk about mental illnesses because of the stigma surrounding mental health problems. Many think that illnesses such as epilepsy come from a spirit or person with the "evil eye" (the ability to harm others merely by looking at them). People with such illnesses do not usually consult a psychologist; they go to a traditional healer. It is common for families to hide away relatives who are mentally ill because they bring shame to the family. In the past, mental health institutions were unwelcoming, and very few people went to them for help. Paramaribo has one psychiatric institution that, despite limited resources, has established programs to encourage those with mental illness to visit the institution for in- and out-patient care. In 2001 a day care center was opened by the psychiatric center. Illnesses of older adults such as Alzheimer's are more accepted than illnesses of the young, because the illnesses of older people can be attributed to old age rather than evil spirits. Beliefs about mystical origins of disease are starting to change as a result of health promotion and public education.

Predominant Sick Care Practices: Biomedical, traditional healing and magical-religious. Medical services are provided through public and private hospitals in the two major cities, Paramaribo and Nieuw Nickerie. Primary health care is delivered through polyclinics of the Regional Health Services in the coastal area (including the urban areas), and through the Medical Mission in the hinterland. Although both are nongovernmental organizations, they now obtain most of the funding for their activities from the Surinamese government. Suriname has four types of health insurance: free care for the poor and near poor, which is financed through the Ministry of Social Affairs; subsidized health insurance for government workers that is provided through the State Health Insurance Foundation; free care for the approximately 40,000 people in the interior, which is administered through the Medical Mission; and privately financed health care for about 70,000 people who use either out-of-pocket funds or private (individual) and company (collective) insurance policies. Between 8% and 18% of the population pays for its own medical care. In general, most urban Surinamese try to use home remedies for illnesses not requiring immediate attention, but eventually they go to a doctor if their treatments do not work. Some people who do not have a health card and do not want to pay for treatment consult traditional healers because they do not charge as much for services and medications and will take delayed payments or payment in kind. Others consult traditional healers when they have a disease that they think either cannot be cured by a doctor or has been induced by black magic or an evil spirit. For example, some parents of children with malnutrition and diarrhea consult traditional healers, who wash the children with assorted herbs to cleanse them of evil spirits. People with chronic diseases such as hypertension and diabetes often consult a traditional healer because doctors do not prescribe medications that can cure them immediately. Mental illness and relationship problems are other common reasons for consulting a traditional healer because these situations are also thought to be caused by curses or evil spirits. Care from a doctor is not always accessible in rural areas, an additional reason some consult a traditional healer or bush doctor. Traditional healing, with its culture-specific rituals for certain ailments, is common among all ethnic groups. Many Amerindians and Maroons seek health care only from traditional healers. Hindustanis consult *pandits* (priests) and Maroons consult bush doctors for problems thought to be related to behavioral issues in their lives. Occasionally people consult medical doctors and traditional healers to determine which treatment works best for their problem. This use of two health systems is a serious problem in Suriname because the combination of medications can interact dangerously in the body, causing some to collapse and lose consciousness. Doctors have difficulty diagnosing and treating these patients because they are not aware of other remedies already tried. Prayers and amulets such as bracelets, belly necklaces, and stones are also commonly used by some groups to ward off illness. Some wear their amulets wrapped in cloth for no one to see, and some mothers put bluing agent behind the ears of their infants to ward off the "evil eye." Some also use amulets and prayer before they consult a doctor to protect themselves from the doctor. Many people strategically place amulets and ornaments in their homes to ward off evil.

Ethnic/Race Specific or Endemic Diseases: The top ten causes of death in decreasing order of importance are cardiovascular disease, cerebrovascular disease, accidents and injuries, cancer, gastrointestinal disorders, perinatal conditions, diabetes, acute respiratory tract infections, urogenital disorders, and HIV/AIDS. A national health information system is currently under development, but data on endemic diseases by ethnicity are limited. Because malaria occurs in the interior, the Maroons are mainly affected by this severe and recurring illness. Data collected on dengue for the year

2000 indicate that highest rates were among the Hindus (44%) and Creoles (18%). In the year 2000 malnutrition was most common among the Maroons (48%) and Creoles (25%). Data from 1995 to 1999 for leptospirosis indicate that Hindus (54%) and Creoles (18%) were most affected. Cardiovascular disease is the main cause of death for Surinamese adults older than 40 years of age. To determine the prevalence of cardiovascular risk factors within different ethnic groups, a nationwide epidemiological study was initiated in January 2000 by the Foundation for the Advancement of Scientific Research in Suriname. Preliminary results of the survey show that the prevalence of hypertension was significantly higher among Creoles (37.7%) and people of mixed origin (34.6%) compared with those of Asian origin (East Indian, 31%, Javanese, 27%). The prevalence of diabetes was slightly higher among the Hindustanis (13.4%) compared with the Javanese (11.7%), Creole (10.8%), and mixed group (10%), but this difference was not statistically significant. The prevalence of individuals without hypertension or diabetes was lowest in the Creole group (56.6%) and highest in the Javanese (64.5%). The combination of risk factors for hypertension and diabetes was less common among the Javanese (3.3%) compared with the mixed group (5.9), Creoles (5.4), and Hindustanis (5.1%). Two times more individuals of Asian origin had serum cholesterol levels greater than 6 mmol/L than did the other ethnic groups (East Indian, 18.6%, Javanese 19.3%, mixed 13.5% and Creole 10.8%). More than 70% of participants did not participate in regular physical activity. People with lower incomes and less education are more at risk for disease. The World Health Organization's (WHO) estimated prevalence rate for HIV/AIDS in adults ages 15 to 49 is 1.26%. The estimated number of children from birth to 15 years living with HIV/AIDS is 110. In Suriname, approximately 11% of new HIV infections in the first quarter of 2001 occurred in people less than 20 years of age, but statistics on AIDS deaths are not available. Given that the risks in Suriname are similar to those in the Caribbean as a whole (young initiation of sexual activity, young women having sex with older men), prevention is urgently needed to prevent the rapid spread of HIV/AIDS and other sexually transmitted diseases among adolescents.

Health Team Relationships: The health care system in Suriname is doctor driven, and doctors have a higher social status than nurses. However, doctors and nurses generally have good relationships. Patients consider the doctors to be responsible for diagnosis and treatment and therefore to have a more important role than nurses. The public considers the doctor to be an authority figure and the nurse to be a liaison between doctors and patients. As they do elsewhere, nurses would like to receive more recognition for their work. Rural health facilities rely more on nurses than urban facilities; they are more accepted and thought to play an important role in health care. Doctors visit the villages once a month and provide guidance to nurses when needed, but it is the nurses and health assistants who diagnose and treat patients.

Families' Role in Hospital Care: Families and friends of hospitalized patients can visit twice a day and are not allowed to stay overnight. Most family members bring food when a patient requests it. Although not required, family members frequently bring clean towels, sheets, and pillows because of the low standards of cleanliness in some hospitals.

Dominance Patterns: Men are generally dominant. They are often in higher and more powerful positions. Many women stay at home and care for their children while the men earn money for the family; women are expected to be subservient to men. Men are more dominant in public life than in the home, but attitudes and roles are changing as women, particularly of the younger generation, obtain more education and higher positions in the workforce and society. The head of the family is usually a man, especially in Hindustani and Asian groups. The Creole households are often headed by women, who provide for their own children and make all the decisions pertaining to the family. The Creole hierarchy's origins derive from Suriname's history of slavery. The men were forced to leave their families to work on plantations, leaving behind the women to make all decisions for the family. In the interior among the Maroons, a matrilineal structure exists in which decisions are made by the mother's brother, the mother's mother's brother (uncle), and so on. In the interior, most village leaders are men. They make all the decisions for their families and their village, and they often have more than one wife. Some men also live and work in more than one village and have more than one family in each village, which again leaves women alone with the children.

Eye Contact Practices: People usually make direct eye contact during conversations with acquaintances. Eye contact with strangers is usually avoided.

Touch Practices: Physical touching is acceptable but not common in public except during greetings. Professionals greet each other with a handshake. Friends of the opposite sex and female friends often greet each other with three kisses alternating on each cheek, and male friends greet each other with a handshake or pat on the back. Occasionally women friends hold hands; this has no sexual connotations whatsoever. Homosexuality is uncommon and not openly discussed or expressed.

Perceptions of Time: Punctuality is not a priority, and many people joke about their tardiness and attribute it to being on "Suriname time." Tardiness is sometimes blamed on the limited infrastructure, poor roads, and heavy traffic, but most Surinamese are tardy because they are expected to be. However, the importance of punctuality is increasing, especially for business meetings and other important appointments. For example, it is important to be on time for appointments at private medical practices or the appointment may have to be rescheduled. Traditionally, the people of Suriname have lived in the past, especially the older generation. The younger generation focuses more on the future but still has many traditional beliefs. Rural areas also seem to be more traditional than populated coastal areas. Some live in the present, such as those in poverty who are trying to survive one day at a time. Doctors find that living day to day is not just a social issue, it is a health issue because it is hard to convince those living in the present to take medications for future health, especially those with chronic diseases. Doctors have to relate medical issues to life today, being careful not to make patients worry about the future. The younger generation is changing as their education increases, and they are becoming more aware of modern health issues. For example, a doctor who wants to treat an older man for a chronic disease may ask the man to bring a child along to help explain the reasons for taking the medication.

Pain Reactions: Pain reactions vary among individuals and cultures. Doctors say that the Javanese have a high threshold for pain. If a Javanese person is crying from pain, doctors know that the situation is very serious.

Birth Rites: About 95% of women in the coastal area go to a hospital to give birth. A pregnant woman is the responsibility of an obstetrician or family practitioner, but the midwife delivers the infant. Pregnant patients consult a family doctor during pregnancy and at 36 weeks have additional consultations at the hospital with a midwife, doctor, or both. Midwives employed by the hospital must have a degree in nursing. Some women do not consult doctors and prefer to have midwives during pregnancy; some even give birth at home. Doctors deliver an infant during a medical emergency such as a cesarean, but midwives make all the decisions during the birthing process. If complications develop, the midwife calls for surgical assistance and tells the doctor what to do. A family member is allowed to be present during the delivery, and anesthetics are not used unless complications arise during the birth process. The mother and infant usually spend 3 days in the hospital if no complications develop. Usually the infant stays in a nursery and is brought to the mother for feeding for a half an hour each time. Visitors can see the infant through the window of the nursery. Very few hospitals let the infant stay in the same room as the mother. Working women are entitled to a 12-week maternity leave: 6 weeks before and 6 weeks after birth. Most pregnant women in rural areas are monitored and delivered by a health assistant; however, a health assistant is not always available, in which case traditional midwives deliver the babies. Some mothers who live in the interior prefer going to a traditional midwife, but problems often arise. If a problem occurs the patient is airlifted to a Medical Mission hospital, and if additional problems develop, she is transported to a hospital in Paramaribo. Women have many rituals after the birth of a child. Many tie their stomachs with string or bandages to help reduce its size. Some take herbal baths or steams to heal wounds and tighten the vagina, practices that are both common within the Maroon and Creole cultures. A thick stout of beer is also commonly consumed to cleanse the system. Many women do not leave the house until a month after birth (to protect the infant from the evil eye) unless they have to see a doctor. If they do, they protect the infant with amulets and bluing agent behind the ears. Traditional Islamic Surinamese never travel with small children at midnight because it is believed that the infants are most vulnerable to the spirits at this time. The Hindustani and Chinese celebrate the births of boys much more than girls because the boys will eventually have an income and pass down the family name for generations. When a girl is born, the family feels it has just lost a worker because she will eventually leave them to live with her husband's family. In addition, when a girl marries, a dowry must be provided to the husband. Although abortion is illegal, it is tolerated and performed by qualified doctors in Paramaribo. Despite overall decreases in fertility in recent years, the percentage of babies born to adolescent girls is increasing. Contraceptive use, although relatively high (40% to 50%) among women ages 15 to 44, is only 23% for married or in-union girls ages 15 to 19. An estimated 60% of first-time pregnancies among girls ages 15 to 19 are unplanned, and an estimated 8000 to 10,000 pregnancies end in abortion yearly.

Death Rites: Death is a time of respectful rituals, which vary by ethnic group and religion. Most deaths occur at home, and a doctor is called to confirm the death. The body is then taken to a mortuary to be prepared for subsequent rituals. Family, friends, and colleagues usually attend the ceremonies. Various ethnic groups are Christians, including Creoles, Hindustanis, and Javanese. Family and friends visit the mourners every night before the day of the funeral, which is usually within 2 to 3 days after the death. They bring food, sing, and pray to show support. The funeral takes place either at the home of the deceased or at a chapel, where a procession usually accompanies the coffin to the burial site. Christians may cremate the body. After the funeral, people visit and support the family of the deceased person for up to 7 days. Family members stay in mourning for about 8 weeks, sometimes longer. Mourning during the 8 weeks involves wearing dark clothes in the early stages and progressing to light-colored clothes near the end of the mourning period. White is worn on the day of the funeral. Christians must be baptized to be buried at the cemetery. During many Creole funerals, pallbearers dance and sing with the coffin, especially if the deceased person liked to sing, dance, and celebrate. In Creole ceremonies the preacher also knocks on the coffin and talks to the deceased person and then opens and closes the casket as a sign of respect, for the coffin is the person's last home. It is also common for Creoles to scream and cry aloud at the burial. In the Muslim culture, which includes many ethnicities, the bodies are buried within 24 hours after death, and the funeral starts at 3 PM the day after the death. Family and friends pay their respects and view the body at the home of the deceased the day of the funeral, before the ceremony. After prayers, a procession led by a *kaum* (preacher) goes to the burial site. At the burial, people kneel in prayer, and each family member takes a turn throwing dirt on the coffin. After the burial, family members return to the home for a traditional meal prepared by the women and blessed by the *kaum*. Ceremonies of mourning are held on the seventh, fortieth, one hundredth, and one thousandth day after the funeral. Family and friends visit the home of the mourners to pray and provide support. Muslims bury the deceased; they do not cremate. The Hindu death ceremony takes place as soon as possible after death, usually the same day. Ceremonies are held at home with prayers led by a *pandit* (preacher) and may last for several days. After the funeral the body is cremated and the ashes are thrown into the river by family members. The mourning period can last from several months to years and is signified by wearing dark clothes. Immediate male family members cut their hair very short just after hearing about the death of the loved one. The Maroon death ceremony involves praying to ancestors and sitting together in prayer before burial of the dead. The funeral can take place any time from a few days to a few months after death, and even longer if the deceased was the tribal chief. Ceremonies take place in the village, and a procession goes to the cemetery. Women, children, Whites, and men in Western clothes are not allowed to go the cemetery. The wives are not permitted to be present at the funeral of a deceased husband, and they must go into a mourning involving many restrictions such as isolation. The Maroons believe in reincarnation and that the soul stays with the body after death. It is only after a period of mourning that the soul can move to the world of the dead. Mourning must be observed by the spouse of the deceased and other close family members. Ceremonies of mourning occur on the eighth day and sixth week after the funeral. Mourning for a chief ends 1 year after the funeral. Various rituals mark the end of mourning, such as shaving of the widow's head. The mourning process is important to Maroons because they believe they must be ritually separated from the dead or they may become ill. Ceremonial practices differ according to traditional beliefs and Christian influence among the various Maroon groups, leading to numerous discussions during death rituals, and it is said that "there is no burial that goes without argument." The Amerindians also have traditional celebrations of death. When a person in the Awarak tribe dies, water is thrown around the body, and family members sit around the body until the day of the funeral. In the Carib tribe a ceremony takes place immediately after death, and people gather at the home of the deceased to prepare the body and commemorate the deceased with prayer, song, and dance. The body is suspended in a hammock and is lowered into a coffin for burial the following day. In the past, Caribs buried their dead in the vicinity of their homes, but this changed because of the influence of missionaries, who established cemeteries. Ceremonies of mourning follow on the eighth day and 1 year after the funeral and are accompanied by drumming and dancing. Family members of the deceased cut their hair short at the end of the mourning period. In Suriname, organ donations and autopsies are uncommon because it is difficult to get permission from families. People do not like to tamper with the dead; they want them to rest in peace. However, bodies and organs can be donated to the medical department at the academic hospital for student doctor training.

Food Practices and Intolerances: The Surinamese diet is as rich and varied as the ethnic makeup of the country. Rice is the main staple and is of very high quality. Cassava, sweet potatoes, plantains, and hot red peppers are also commonly used in Surinamese dishes. Well known Hindustani dishes are *roti*, a wheat-based flat bread served with curried vegetables and meat; *somosa,* fried pastry filled with vegetables and spicy potatoes; and *phulawri*, fried chick pea balls. Among the common Javanese dishes are *petjil*, vegetables served with spicy peanut sauce; *bami*, fried noodles; and *saoto* soup, chicken broth with bean sprouts, fried potatoes, noodles, peppers, and spices. Popular Creole dishes include *pom*, a puree of spiced tayer root and meat; *pastei*, pastry filled with meat and vegetables; and *moskie alesie*, rice mixed with meat, fish, white beans, vegetables, peppers, and spices. *Cassava bread* is a common dish among the Maroons and Amerindians. *Pinda alesie*, rice with peanuts, is also a popular Maroon dish. A popular Amerindian dish is *pepperwater,* which is a soup of fish and peppers. *Saw paw*, vegetables and meat steamed in sweet bread, is a popular dish among the Chinese. The enormous selection of tropical fruits in Suriname, which includes bananas, mangos, papayas, apples, grapefruit, tangerines, tangelos, watermelon, star fruit, custard apple, cashews, and palm nuts, are seasonal and can be expensive, yet they are well liked by everyone. Surinamese typically eat three meals a day. Most use a fork and spoon, but it is also quite common to eat with hands, especially among the Javanese, Hindustani, Maroons, and Amerindians. Knives are rarely used. Religious beliefs and traditional ceremonies play an important role in diet. Most Hindus do not eat beef or pork; they prefer vegetarian food and only eat meat such as chicken or fish, two to three times a week. Most Muslims do not eat pork and are forbidden to drink alcohol. Certain types of food and dishes are ceremony specific. For example, on the day of a funeral, Hindustanis do not eat meat, and they serve a sweet dish called *persade*. Hindustanis prepare 13 different types of vegetables before noon on the day of the ceremony, and all family members of the deceased must consume all 13 types. On the night before a funeral, Creoles eat sweet dishes of *sukrerkyi* and *asogri*. Porridge is blessed and generous amounts are served at Javanese birth ceremonies.

Infant Feeding Practices: Women in Suriname usually breast-feed during the first weeks after birth. However, they typically do not exclusively breast-feed for more than 1 to 2 months, at which time they begin to bottle feed as well. It is usually working women who combine formula and breast-feeding. Formula is available for those who cannot breast-feed, but it is expensive. Most women who do not work breast-feed for financial reasons. In the last few years, more mothers have become aware of breast-feeding as a healthy practice through educational campaigns promoting safe motherhood. Most women breast-feed (although not exclusively) for about a year, but it is common for members of some ethnic groups to breast-feed for 3 or 4 years regardless of whether they still have milk; they breast-feed to comfort their children.

Child Rearing Practices: Child rearing practices vary from family to family, and some are stricter than others. Both parents discipline the children. In female-headed households, the mother is responsible for the discipline. For the most part, children are expected to be quiet and obedient and are punished if they are not. Some children sleep with their parents for comfort or because no other bed is available. Occasionally in poorer households with many children, the youngest sleeps with the parents, and the others sleep on the floor.

National Childhood Immunizations: DPT at 3, 4, and 5 months and 1 to 5 years; OPV at 3, 4, and 5 months and 1 to 5 years; MMR at 1 year; DT at 4 years, +1 month; and TT for pregnant women, +1. The National Immunization Program has made great strides over the years; routine vaccinations are maintained at a reasonably high level. Immunization services are available at health posts only on scheduled days of the month because of a lack of functional cold-chain equipment at all facilities, poor accessibility in remote interior areas, and lack of qualified staff members. As a result, missed opportunities for vaccination are common. In addition, vaccinations are delayed until a sufficient number of children need them. The national immunization program has plans to develop and seek funding for the introduction of a pentavalent vaccine—one injection to immunize against five diseases.

Other Characteristics: Although Suriname ranks seventeenth in the World Bank's list of the world's richest countries, more than 60% of its population lives below the poverty line: 52% of the urban, 61% of the rural, and 91% of the interior population. As a result of the war and instability of the last 2 decades, Suriname is faced with a range of socioeconomic problems. The health sector has a shrinking financial base, insufficient investment in and poor maintenance of facilities and equipment, and too few drugs and reagents. In addition, many trained public health professionals, medical specialists, and registered nurses are leaving. Other problems include a shortage of qualified teachers, classrooms, and teaching materials; low wages, especially in the public sector; and increasing poverty among single-parent families, the majority of which are headed by women. Child labor, malnutrition, sexual abuse, and youth prostitution are reported to be increasing, although comprehensive data are lacking.

BIBLIOGRAPHY

Bakker WJ: *Health conditions in Suriname,* (Dr. Carol Vlassof) Paramaribo, Suriname, 1996, unpublished manuscript.

Duumi G et al: *Afdeling Cultuur Studies/Minov,* 1992, Paramaribo, Suriname.

Epidemiology data 1995-1999, 2000, Paramaribo, Suriname, Bureau of Public Health, Department of Epidemiology.

Epidemiology data 2000–2001, 2001, Paramaribo, Suriname, Bureau of Public Health, Department of Epidemiology.

Evaluation of the Immunization Programme of Suriname, Paramaribo, Suriname, 2001, Caribbean Epidemiology Center, unpublished manuscript.

Health in the Americas, 2002 edition, Washington, DC, July 2001, Pan American Health Organization.

The Maroni River Caribs of Suriname, 1971, Koninklijke Van Gorcum.

Pan American Health Organization and World Health Organization RGD Global Restructuring Project: *Progress Report XI,* July 1-Dec 31, 1999.

Sarafian I: *HIV/AIDS and out-of-school youth in Suriname: a focus group study,* 2001, unpublished manuscript.

Statistical Yearbook, Paramaribo, Suriname, 2000, Algemen Buro voor de Statistiek, Paramaribo.

Terborg J: Sexual behaviour and sexually transmitted diseases among Saramaka and Ndjuka Maroons in the hinterland of Suriname, Paramaribo, Suriname, 2000, Primary Health Care and Pro Health.

van Eer MY et al: *Ethnic differences in cardiovascular risk factors in Suriname,* Paramaribo, Suriname, 2000, unpublished manuscript.

World Health Organization (June 2000): *Epidemiological fact sheets by country,* Geneva. Retrieved March 1, 2002, from http://www.unaids.org/hivaidsinfo/statistics/june00/fact_sheets/index.html

World Health Organization (2001): *WHO vaccine-preventable diseases: monitoring system,* Geneva. Retrieved March 1, 2002, from http://www.who.int/vaccines/ http://www.cia.gov/cia/publications/factbook/geos/ns.html

◆ SWAZILAND (KINGDOM OF)

MAP PAGE (863)

Emma Dube and Nomsa Mary Gule

Location: Swaziland is located in southern Africa, with South Africa to the north, southeast, and west and Mozambique to the east. It is a land-locked, mountainous country that is slightly smaller than New Jersey. The climate is temperate. The total land area is 17,360 km^2 (6703 square miles) and has a population of 1,083,289.

Major Languages	Ethnic Groups	Major Religions
Siswati	Swazi 90%	Christian 60%
English	Zulu 2%	Indigenous beliefs 40%
	European 3%	
	Other 5%	

Health Care Beliefs: Indigenous; passive role. Disease prevention and health promotion are actively encouraged by nongovernmental organizations and various government health institutions, especially because of the high prevalence of HIV/AIDS in the country. People fear anyone who has a mental illness. Swaziland has numerous indigenous healers, including *sangomas, inyangas,* faith healers, throat scratchers, and traditional birth attendants, all of whom attribute illness primarily to supernatural forces, violations of indigenous rules, the environment, or the influence of the ancestors.

Predominant Sick Care Practices: Traditional, magical-religious and biomedical if available. Because most people attribute their illnesses to supernatural forces, they first consult indigenous healers. If healers cannot provide a cure, they then resort to doctors and nurses. If they still do not improve, they resort to prayer. One practice involves heating the tip of a cow's horn or neck of a bottle over an incision to draw out impurities from the body. Another involves inducing vomiting and diarrhea or taking steam baths to rid the body of toxins.

Ethnic/Race Specific or Endemic Diseases: Diseases endemic to the country are tuberculosis, kwashiorkor, infantile diarrhea, and dysentery. The country has had recent outbreaks of cholera, which are being contained; the country also had malaria outbreaks in the Lowveld during the summer months. Schistosomiasis, enteric fever, and advanced periodontal disease are prevalent. The incidence of leprosy is decreasing rapidly. The World Health Organization's (WHO) estimated prevalence rate for HIV/AIDS in adults ages 15 to 49 is 25.25%. The estimated number of children from birth to 15 years living with HIV/AIDS is 3800. One in three people between the ages of 15 and 49 years is infected with HIV.

Health Team Relationships: The health team tends to be doctor driven in hospitals and nurse driven in community clinics. Doctors and nurses have good working relationships. Most patients understand the different roles of doctors, nurses, and nurses' aids and are cooperative when dealing with members of the health system.

Families' Role in Hospital Care: The families' roles in hospitals are vital because of the serious shortage of nurses and doctors. Families often stay in the hospital to care for relatives, and they also bring food.

Dominance Patterns: Men dominate this culture, although when people are ill, women have a more prominent role in making decisions about health care.

Eye Contact Practices: Women and men avoid direct eye contact, as do people speaking with others of a higher status.

Touch Practices: Physical touching between men and women is unacceptable.

Perceptions of Time: Life has a relaxed pace compared with developed countries, and punctuality is often not important, particularly in rural areas. People who are late are operating on "African time." The country values past traditions and celebrates them with public holidays and ceremonies, so the Swazis have a very strong national identity. Many of the celebrations are in honor of the king.

Pain Reactions: People believe that pain and sickness are private and should be hidden from the general public.

Birth Rites: A pregnant woman does not linger in a doorway because she believes it could make her birth difficult. Some believe a child will be born lazy if a pregnant woman lies down for any great length of time during the day. A pregnant woman does not expose her stomach to anyone. During pregnancy, the mother tends to avoid eating liver and eggs because it is believed they can cause a child to be born without hair. Untrained traditional birth attendants assist in approximately 20% of deliveries. When a child is born, some traditionalists do not bathe their children in water and only use an herbal solution because it will protect the child from evil. The mother eats large amounts of boiled chicken and sour porridge and stays secluded in a room for 3 months after the birth without seeing any males. She abstains from sexual relations for up to 6 months. After children are born, mothers in rural areas cover their heads in public until the child's fontanelles close. Births of sons are celebrated more than births of daughters. Family planning and birth control services have small associated fees. With the onset of HIV/AIDS, men are offered free condoms, which are widely available, but they seem to be used extensively only in urban areas.

Death Rites: Swazis believe that death has supernatural causes. Neither organ donation nor autopsies are acceptable. Some traditionalists take the body to the *kraal* (an enclosure for cattle) to inform the ancestors that a person has died. A night vigil is held, and early in the morning the person is buried in a coffin with a straw mat and blanket.

Food Practices and Intolerances: In the rural areas, people eat primarily corn porridge, wild vegetables, pumpkins, peanuts, beans, cabbage, spinach, tomatoes, onions, chicken, eggs, milk, sour milk, avocados, and a little fruit. In rural areas, it is common to use the hands for eating, and people in urban areas use a spoon. At home, the older adults are served food first, and then the others are served according to their status; children are given the food that is left over. In the urban and semiurban areas, people are tending to eat more of a Western-style diet that comprises primarily fast food. School children are tending to eat more junk food, which often is sold close to the schools.

Infant Feeding Practices: Mothers often return to work soon after birth to supplement their families' incomes, but about 45% of them express their breast milk and feed it to the infant with a bottle for the first 3 months. Others use a combination of expressed milk and soft foods, which are introduced at 6 to 8 weeks, a practice that can slow the infant's growth. National policies support an intensive program that monitors and promotes growth in children and works to eliminate stunted growth.

Child Rearing Practices: Children sleep with their parents in the bed until the age of 4 years. Discipline is the responsibility of the oldest woman in the home. Child rearing practices are very strict, especially in rural areas. Children are expected to be quiet and obedient. Because mothers must supplement family incomes so soon after giving birth, alternate caregivers are sought out quickly.

National Childhood Immunizations: BCG at birth, DTP at 6,10, and 14 weeks and 18 months; OPV at birth, at 6, 10, and 14 weeks, at 18 months, and at 5 years; hep B at 6, 10, and 14 weeks; measles at 9 and 18 months; DT at 5 years; and TT CBAW ×5.

BIBLIOGRAPHY

Douglas P: Rehabilitation work in Swaziland, *Physiother Frontline* 2(6):17, 1996.

Moran R: Swazi safari, *Nurs Times* 88(40):54, 1992.

Upvall MJ: A Swazi nursing perspective on the role of indigenous healers, *J Cult Diversity* 2(1):16, 1995.

◆ SWEDEN (KINGDOM OF)

MAP PAGE (860)

Ulrike Kylberg

Location: This northern European country is located in eastern Scandinavia along the Baltic Sea. Sweden is a land of many lakes, and half of it is covered by forests. Its northern boundary extends into the Arctic Circle. The total land area is 449,964 km² (173,731 square miles). The country is divided into three regions: Götaland in the south, with large fields of corn, several industries, a strong economy, and major universities; Svealand in the central region, with its strong cultural roots, traditional, industries and mountains; and Norrland, an area of large forests, vast expanses, mountains, and Nordic tundra. Sweden has a high standard of living. The population is just less than 9 million.

Major Languages	Ethnic Groups	Major Religions
Swedish (official)	Swedish 90%	Evangelical
Samish (Lapps)	Lapp (Sami) 4%	Lutheran 90%
	Finnish 2%	Roman Catholic 4%
	Foreign born or	Other 6%
	first-generation immigrants	
	(Yugoslavian, Danish,	
	Norwegian, Greek,	
	Turkish) 4%	

Health Care Beliefs: Active role; health promotion important. The active involvement of Swedes in their health is apparent. Health promotion is important and organized by law for all inhabitants, but it primarily emphasizes prenatal and child care. People are expected to be responsible for their own health; however, many social services are available to assist them. Basic health care is provided for a small fee, and hospital care costs are based on patients' incomes. The focus of care is on health facilities rather than on the community and family settings.

Predominant Sick Care Practices: Biomedical. Biomedical treatment is offered by the national health care system and financed by income tax. Most companies offer health care services to their employees.

Ethnic/Specific or Endemic Diseases: The rates for osteoporosis are the highest in Europe among older men and women. Sjögren-Larsson syndrome is a frequently diagnosed syndrome among women in Sweden. Maternal and infant mortality rates are among the lowest in the world, which is the result of a targeted health promotion program for pregnant women and newborns.

Health Team Relationships: Receptionist nurses who are contacted by telephone are the first point of contact in the health care system. The doctor has an authoritarian role and is not questioned. Although patients are expected to say what they think, this is not encouraged by health professionals. Patients expect to help make decisions when planning medical treatment and nursing care.

Families' Role in Hospital Care: The staff meets all the patients' needs; however, the family can assist if they like. Flexible visiting hours are encouraged. Stipends are paid to individuals who provide care for a sick family member at home.

Dominance Patterns: Sweden has an egalitarian society; however, the women are usually responsible for household chores and purchasing and preparing food.

Eye Contact Practices: It is customary to maintain eye contact during conversations.

Touch Practices: Touching is uncommon, even in health care environments (other than during examinations).

Perceptions of Time: Northern Swedes are not as time conscious as southern Swedes from large cities. People are generally expected to be 15 to 30 minutes late. Swedes are present and future oriented and plan for important future events.

Pain Reactions: Inexpressive and expressive reactions to pain are both acceptable. When in pain, Swedes may contract muscles in the body or the face and verbally express their discomfort. Immediate pain relief is expected.

Birth Rites: Sweden has one of the lowest maternal mortality rates. Women can choose any position in which to give birth—even underwater. ABC-Clinics provide many choices for delivery, including births that include the participation of the father and siblings. For example, the father may cut the umbilical cord, after which the infant is placed on the mother's abdomen. The family is left alone for several hours. Rooming-in (keeping the infant and mother in the same room) is common.

Death Rites: Subdued or public expressions of grief are both acceptable. A dying person is not to be left alone and should have family members at the bedside. After death, bodies are placed in a coffin. Before the closure of the coffin in the mortuary, the family is allowed to say a final farewell.

Food Practices and Intolerances: Breakfast often consists of coffee or tea and a sandwich of cheese or ham, cereal, or porridge. A large meal is eaten at lunch or dinner, but fast food usually dominates lunch. Meat balls with potatoes and gravy are popular. Coffee breaks may include a sandwich at midmorning and sweets at midafternoon. Fish, meat, and bananas are common.

Infant Feeding Practices: Breast-feeding is preferred and encouraged and continues for about 1 year. Other foods are introduced at 4 or 5 months.

Child Rearing Practices: Children are raised in a permissive but safe environment. School starts at age 6. Nurses from government-sponsored day care centers supervise preschool children. Both parents are responsible for caring for children when they are not in school.

National Childhood Immunizations: BCG at 6 months; DTP at 3, 5, and 12 months; HIB at 3, 5, and 12 months; IPV at 3, 5, and 12 months and 6 years; MMR at 18 months and 12 years; and DT 10 years.

BIBLIOGRAPHY

Andrews MM, Boyle JS: *Transcultural concepts in nursing care,* ed 2, 1995, Philadelphia, Lippincott.

Gottlieb BH: Social support and the study of personal relationships, *J Soc Personal Relationships* 1(2):351–375 1985.

Green J: Death with dignity, *Nursing Times* 5–10(85), 1989.

Götherström C, Hamrin E, Gullberg M: Development of a tool for measuring the concept of good care among patients and staff in relation to Swedish legislation, *Int J Nurs Stud* 32(3):277, 1995.

Marklund B et al: Evaluation of the telephone advisory activity at Swedish primary health care centres, *Fam Pract* 7(3):184, 1990.

Sheehy B: Ideological exchange, *Nursing Times* 86(3):36, 1990.

◆ SWITZERLAND (SWISS CONFEDERATION)

MAP PAGE (860)
Location: Switzerland is a landlocked nation in central Europe, and the landscape includes the Alps, glaciers, lakes, and a large plateau where most people reside. France is to the west, Germany and Austria to the

east, Liechtenstein to the north, and Italy to the south and east. The capital is Bern. The rugged landscape does not support much agriculture. The climate is temperate but varies with the altitude, and strong Fohn winds can bring higher temperatures, avalanches, and red dust from the Sahara Desert. The total land area is 41,290 km^2 (15,938 square miles), approximately twice the size of New Jersey. The total population is 7,283,274. Switzerland has a stable market economy with a per capita gross domestic product (GDP) of $28,600, 20% higher than that of larger western European economies.

Major Languages	Ethnic Groups	Major Religions
German (official)	German 65%	Roman Catholic 46%
French (official)	French 18%	Protestant 40%
Italian (official)	Italian 10%	None, other 14%
Romansch	Romansch 1%	
	Other 6%	

Health Care Beliefs: Strong health promotion efforts.

Predominant Sick Care Practices: Biomedical. Good medical care is available throughout Switzerland.

Ethnic/Race Specific or Endemic Diseases: The Swiss are at risk for cardiovascular diseases and diabetes. Because of the terrain and winter temperatures, conditions such as altitude sickness, hypothermia, and sunburn are common. Endemic diseases include tick-borne fever and encephalitis, Lyme borreliosis, and human granulocytic ehrlichiosis. The Swiss are also at risk for goiter, Borna disease, echinococcosis, and in southern Switzerland imported leptospirosis (Weil's disease). The World Health Organization's (WHO) estimated prevalence rate for HIV/AIDS in adults ages 15 to 49 is 0.46%. The estimated number of children from birth to 15 years living with HIV/AIDS is less than 100. Approximately 150 deaths were attributed to AIDS in 1999. The number of newly diagnosed HIV infections is decreasing, particularly among those who use intravenous drugs and homosexual men. It is estimated that the total number of adults and children living with HIV/AIDS is 17,000.

Health Team Relationships: Each of the 26 cantons (states) has its own government, the 26 ministries of health have different laws regulating health care. Nurses fulfill primarily a technical role under the direction of the doctor, but clinical nurse specialists, nurse practitioners, and research nurses in major hospitals are more likely than doctors to perform procedures such as inserting peripheral intravenous catheters. Reform and academization of nursing education is currently in progress. Doctors and nurses are both extremely interested in pain management therapy.

Perceptions of Time: The Swiss are known for their punctuality.

Birth Rites: The birth rate is 10.12 births per 1000 people, and the infant mortality rate is 4.48 deaths per 1000 live births. Breast-feeding rates were recently reported to be 93.3% 1 day after birth, 62.5% at 3 months, 62.5% at 4 months, 51.1% at 6 months, 28.1% at a year. The median duration was 4.2 months. The duration of breast-feeding was shorter if the mother was employed and longer if the mother was originally from Africa, Asia, the Middle East, or Latin America. The total fertility rate is 1.47 children born per woman. Life expectancy at birth is 76.85 for men and 82.76 for women.

Food Practices and Intolerances: Swiss cuisine has German and French influences. Cheese is an important part of the diet; fondues of emmenthaler and gruyere cheese are a common dinner which has been adopted by other countries. The national dish for German Switzerland is *rosti,* or shredded and fried potatoes. Perch and trout from the many lakes are plentiful, and Swiss chocolate is known worldwide. Meals tend to be hearty, and filling soups are well liked.

National Childhood Immunizations: BCG for those at high risk only; DTP at 2, 4, 6, and 15 to 23 months and at 4 to 6 and 11 to 15 years; hep B at 11 to 15 years; HIB at 2, 4, 6, and 15 months; and MMR at 15 months and 5 to 6 years.

Other Characteristics: Switzerland is a transit country for and consumer of South American cocaine and Southwest Asian heroin.

BIBLIOGRAPHY

Bouvier P, Rougemont A: Breast-feeding in Geneva: prevalence, duration and determinants, *Soz Praventivmed* 43(3):116, 1998.
Clift JM: Nursing education in Austria, Germany, and Switzerland, *IMAGE: J Nurs Sch* 29(1):89, 1997.
Hulskers H, Niederer-Frei I: Nurse practitioners as counselors, *Pflege* 10(2):80, 1997.
Friedemann ML: Do nurse clinicians influence the working climate and quality of care? *Pflege* 10(3):132, 1997.
Panchaud C: Enhancing ethical thinking: the role of a national nurse' association, *Nurs Ethics* 2(3):243, 1995.
http://www.cia.gov/cia/publications/factbook/geos/sw.html

◆ SYRIA (SYRIAN ARAB REPUBLIC)

MAP PAGE (864)

Ismat Fayez Mikkey

Location: Syria is bordered on the north by Turkey, on the east by Iraq, on the south by Jordan, and on the west by Lebanon and the Mediterranean Sea. The Syrian Arab Republic has a total land area of 185,180 km^2 (71,498 square miles). The population is estimated to be 16.1 million. Approximately 40.5% is younger than 15 years of age, and 3% is older than 65.

Major Languages	Ethnic Groups	Major Religions
Arabic (official)	Arab 90%	Islam 90%
French	Kurdish, Armenian, other 10%	Christian 10%
English		

Syria is the only Arabian country that uses the Arabic language for university instruction in almost all sciences, including medicine and nursing. Tremendous efforts have been made in the past few years to translate textbooks into Arabic. Syrian society is composed of different cohesive groups characterized by their distinct linguistic and religious characteristics. These ethnic and religious groups tend to dwell in certain geographical regions and social classes. For instance, approximately 40% of Sunni Muslims are urban dwellers and of those, 80% live in the five largest cities in Syria. Alawis (Shia Muslims who believe in divine incarnation and the divinity of Ali) are poor and live in rural areas. Approximately 90% of the inhabitants of Jabal Al Arab are Druze, whereas Jews and Armenians are primarily urban traders. The cultural differences between groups extend beyond religious beliefs and rituals to differences in clothing, household architecture, etiquette, and agricultural practices. Kurds are believed to comprise 9% of the population, and most of them came from Turkey between 1924 and 1938. They speak their own language, Kirmanji. Numerous Armenians live in Syrian cities and towns. They speak their own language and are the largest unassimilated group, maintaining their own schools and newspapers. Other small ethnic groups live in Syria such as Turkomans, Circassians, and Assyrians.

Health Care Beliefs: Traditional and modern; passive role. Health care practices vary according to the nature of Syrian demography. The majority of citizens (80%), who live in the five major cities, are unlikely to consult indigenous healers or wear amulets as their first treatment option. They tend to consult health care professionals first, although they usually use more traditional therapies as a last resort when health care professionals cannot cure them. The use of drugs for other than therapeutic reasons is strictly forbidden. However, Syrians do smoke cigarettes, despite strong warnings by some Islamic scholars. Smoking is the most predominant unhealthy behavior among Syrians. Water-pipe smoking is a traditional and a widely practiced habit. Almost every home has one of these pipes, and streets are full of coffee shops for water-pipe smoking. Suicide is not a serious social problem in Syria as is true in all Arab nations. Islam forbids suicide, and strong family support helps prevent suicide attempts.

Predominant Sick Care Practices: Biomedical, indigenous and magical-religious. People from rural areas usually consult indigenous and other traditional healers such as those who use the Koran (the holy Islamic book) for healing. People with infertility problems generally seek medical advice from a doctor and a religious person *(shykh)* for amulets. *Shykhs* use traditional cures such as "closing the back" of a woman; a female healer rubs the women's pelvis with olive oil and places suction cups on her back. Some indigenous female healers also massage the abdomen around the ovaries and use vaginal herbal suppositories. The most prevalent practice is massaging children with warm olive oil. Traditional health practices are the domain of women, and some female healers are known in their communities for their skill in treating injuries and curing some disorders. In families, women assume responsibility for nutrition and treatment of illness. People's beliefs in the efficacy of traditional healers often prevent or postpone medical attention. The health system is based on primary health care that is delivered at three levels: village, district, and provisional. In 1988, 3.5% of recurrent government expenditures were for health and health services. In 1989, Syria had 10,114 doctors, 3,362 dentists, and 14,816 qualified nurses and midwives. Approximately 77% of doctors and 94% of dentists are employed in the private sector. In 1990, Syria had 41 general hospitals (8 of which were private), 152 specialized hospitals (136 of which were private), 391 rural health centers, and 151 urban health centers. The total number of beds was 13,164, 77% of which were in the public sector. Syria, which has a socialist government, provides free medical care to all citizens and imposes limits on charges by private hospitals.

Ethnic/Race Specific or Endemic Diseases: The use of vaccinations and other preventive measures in the 1980s significantly improved health conditions in Syria; the incidence of malaria and tuberculosis has decreased. However, gastrointestinal and parasitic diseases are endemic, particularly in rural areas. In the Damascus area, hepatitis E is endemic, and cutaneous leishmaniasis has been endemic in Aleppo for generations. Syrians are at risk for ascariasis (which often has the symptoms of biliary disease) and echinococcosis. In 1999, WHO reported 42 cases of malaria and 5447 cases of pulmonary tuberculosis. The World Health Organization's (WHO) estimated prevalence rate for HIV/AIDS in adults ages 15 to 49 years is 0.01%. WHO has no estimates for children.

Health Team Relationships: Doctors are dominant. They tend to discount nurses' knowledge and expertise; therefore patients seldom rely on nurses for health education. Nurses are considered subordinate to medical doctors; doctors issue the orders, and nurses follow them. This ideology is embedded in the social structure because the deans and educators in schools of nursing are doctors. Doctors' representation of nursing on national committees and councils continues to be the norm in some nursing programs. Nurse-doctor interactions are very limited and only occur during rounds (in the morning and evening) or when a nurse needs to call a doctor about a patient.

Families' Role in Hospital Care: Many close relatives accompany patients during the admission to the hospital to mitigate their uncertainties and worries and occasionally answer questions. Relatives tend to prepare nutritious food such as meat, vegetables, and rice for patients. Nurses rely on the patients' companions for basic nursing tasks such as assistance with bathing, eating, walking, and changing clothes. When visiting, food, chocolate, biscuits, or fruit are brought for the patient and family. Close relatives who stay most of the day show hospitality to visitors by serving them coffee, candy, or fruit. Visitors often do not comply with the visiting hours and policies set by health institutions, and hospitals use special security personnel to control visitors who could interfere with routine and emergency care. Visitors tend to come in groups during the day and though well intentioned, occasionally keep patients from getting enough rest and sleep.

Dominance Patterns: In a male-dominated society such as Syria, men are more valued than women, particularly because they carry on the family name and care for parents in their old age. The father is usually the head of the family and its breadwinner, whereas the mother plays the major role in raising children and maintaining the house. However, many educated women have jobs in health care, education, and private and public institutions. Grandmothers care for children whose mothers work outside the home. Older people in extended families are highly valued, so educated women may have difficulties obtaining health care for their children if they live in an extended-family household. Older women usually have more authority than the mother regarding decisions about the children's health and nutrition and health expenditures.

Eye Contact Practices: Body language is particularly important. A lowered gaze and shyness are the preferred behaviors for women during their interactions with men. In addition, it is inappropriate for children to make direct eye contact with their parents, grandparents, or older people. People of the same sex from the Middle East are likely to stand quite close to each other, but those of the opposite sex keep a wider distance.

Touch Practices: Arabs behave conservatively in public and keep their feelings private. Displays of affection between spouses (kissing, cuddling, hugging) are considered rude and extremely inappropriate in public areas. It is unacceptable for men and women to shake hands with strangers of the opposite sex. As a rule, health professionals treat patients who are the same sex unless too few professionals are available. Islam prohibits touching between males and females except during an emergency or when no competent health professional of the same sex is available.

Perceptions of Time: Schedules, deadlines, and punctuality are the American way. Arabs begin their meetings with social comments. Punctuality is not of great importance. Arabs serve many cups of tea or coffee and inquire about others' health and family before getting down to business. They tend to live more in the past and present and focus less on the future. Arabs do think ahead and have plans for the future but are reluctant to overwhelm themselves with thoughts of accomplishing the tasks. Financial and economic constraints and hardships are major barriers to planning for the future.

Pain Reactions: The cultural beliefs of Syrians play a major role in their expression of pain. They believe that their suffering will be counted on the Day of Judgment. They tend to attribute wellness and illness to God's will, so they often pray to cope with stressful experiences. Patients may not request a pain assessment or pain medication because they want to be considered "good" patients (i.e., patients who do not complain). Health care professionals do not expect patients to ask much of them. Men are particularly reluctant to mention their pain because it would be considered a weakness unless a health care professional asked about it. Men who endure pain and do not complain are considered more masculine, so it is more acceptable for women to mention pain and ask for analgesics. These behaviors are rooted in the roles of boys and girls that are established during the socialization process.

Birth Rites: When a woman gives birth to an infant, her relatives, friends, and neighbors visit to congratulate her and give her gifts, which are usually items for the infant. Most families believe that mothers should stay home for the first 40 days after delivery. During this time, she is cared for by her mother and sisters and occasionally by her husband's family. Circumcision is the norm for boys because it is part of the culture and considered necessary for cleanliness reasons. Most families prefer to circumcise their male infants during the first week of age, but others postpone it for many years. Despite discouragement from the medical community, most families still use *kuhl*, a charcoal-like powder, to dilate the pupils of female infants' eyes. Swaddling infants with a blanket and rope is still very common and used to strengthen the muscles, prevent scoliosis, and prevent movements that might frighten them during the night. Infants are usually kept in a crib close to their mother. During the postpartum period the mother is not allowed to perform religious rituals (e.g., pray, fast during Ramadan) or have sexual relations until completely free of postpartum discharge. The mother is encouraged to consume special drinks such as water with boiled cinnamon sticks and boiled *hilbah* seeds because it is believed this accelerates discharge and increases milk production. Depending on the financial status of the family, some shave the infant's head and estimate the weight of hair, calculating the price of an equivalent weight of gold or silver; the estimated amount of money is given to the needy. To thank God and welcome the infant, parents often slaughter a goat or lamb and invite all relatives and friends to have lunch at home.

Death Rites: Donation of human organs is allowed according to two specific Islamic rules: when "necessities overrule prohibition" and when there is a "choice of the lesser of the two evils if both cannot be avoided." In other words, organ donation that can save a life is more important than preserving the integrity of the body of the donor. Autopsy is permissible in Islam if it is conducted for the right purpose, such as to determine the cause of a suspicious death and for educational purposes. It is preferred to bury the dead body quickly in the same place (i.e., same country) where the person died, even if the death occurred far from the place of birth. Most people prefer burying the body at home. After death the body is washed and wrapped with white cloth and taken to the mosque for prayer. It then goes to the cemetery and is buried without a coffin in the ground. Relatives go back to the home and accept condolences for 3 days. Unsweetened coffee is traditionally served as a symbol of sadness for the deceased. Cremation is forbidden.

Food Practices and Intolerances: Pork and alcohol are strictly prohibited. Muslims fast during the month of Ramadan each year. They consume no food or drink and abstain from sexual intercourse between sunrise and sunset. People who are ill and older adults who cannot tolerate fasting do not have to. A popular dish is Middle Eastern shish kebabs, which are pieces of lamb or marinated chicken that are speared on a wooden stick and cooked over a charcoal fire with tomatoes and onions. Most food is eaten with a spoon and fork. Syrians are experts at making pastries, sweets, and desserts. Baklava, Turkish delights, *Qatayef,* and many other desserts and sweets are imported from Syria to other Arabian countries. They are eaten during the two major Islamic feasts: Eid al-Fiter and Eid Al-Adha. During these celebrations, people visit each other and bring sweets. Syrians have many other ethnic dishes. *Tabbouleh* is a Syrian salad of bulgur (wheat crumbles) mixed with flat-leaf parsley, fresh mint, green onion, diced tomato, lemon juice, olive oil, and salt. Eggplant dip *(baba ghannooj)* is baked, mashed eggplant blended with onion, garlic, lemon juice, oil, and salt. *Lahme bel ajin* is small balls of dough that are rolled out and filled with a mixture of finely chopped lamb, pine nuts, chopped onion, and green pepper, and served with *labani* (yogurt). *Hummus* is a dip or spread of finely mashed, cooked chickpeas that are mixed with tahini, olive oil, salt, parsley, garlic, and hot peppers.

Infant Feeding Practices: Breast-feeding is the norm. Working women, primarily those in urban cities, bottle-feed and then leave their infants with a close relative during the day. In rural areas, women usually follow the advice of health care professionals and breast-feed. Infants are introduced to solid food as young as 9 months. Infants are given starchy foods, primarily potatoes, at younger than 6 months. Anemia in young children is a serious problem due to the practice of giving them bread soaked in tea.

Child Rearing Practices: Children usually sleep in their parents' room up to 3 or 4 years. Because of housing and financial constraints, it may be impossible to separate young girls and boys, although it is preferable. Mothers are more responsible for discipline and tend to use less physical forms of punishment than fathers. Children tend to ask their mothers for assistance because the fathers are stricter. Older people in the extended family live in their older son's (or daughter's if they have no sons) home their entire lives—with respect and dignity. Older adults might assume some responsibility for disciplining their grandchildren even when the mother thinks that it interferes with her methods. Discipline of children is highly emphasized because unacceptable and inappropriate behaviors affect the reputation and honor of the family.

National Childhood Immunizations: BCG at birth; DTP at 3, 4, 5, and 18 months; OPV at birth and 3, 4, 5, and 18 months, school age-first class; hep B at birth and at 3 and 10 months; measles at 10 and 15 months; vitamin A at 9 months and after birth; DT at school age-first class; Td at sixth and ninth class; and TT CBAW.

BIBLIOGRAPHY

Al-Azmeh J et al: Hepatitis E in Damascus, Syria, *Infection* 27(3):221, 1999.

Al-Shakir HL: Public health and the health of the population of the Syrian Arab Republic, *Zdravookhr Ross Fed* 17(8):27, 1973.

Douba M, Mowakeh A, Wali A: Current status of cutaneous leishmaniasis in Aleppo, Syrian Arab Republic, *Bull WHO* 75(3):253, 1997.

Kamal I: Traditional birth attendant training: sharing experiences, *Int J Gynaecol Obstet* 38(suppl):55, 1992.

Sandouk F et al: Pancreatic-biliary ascariasis: experience of 300 cases, *Am J Gastroenterol* 92(12):2264, 1997.

http://www.arab.net/photos/arabicbread.html

◆ TAJIKISTAN (REPUBLIC OF)

MAP PAGE (861)

Location: This southeast central Asian country is more than 90% mountainous, and glaciers are the source of its rivers. Tajikistan is bordered by Kyrgyzstan to the northeast, China to the east, Afghanistan to the south and southwest, and Uzbekistan to the north and northwest. The total land area of the country is 143,100 km^2 (55,251 square miles), slightly smaller than Wisconsin. The capital is Dushanbe. Tajikistan has hot summers and mild winters, and the country is prone to earthquakes. The climate is semiarid to polar in the Pamir Mountains. The country became an independent state during the dissolution of the former Soviet Union and has been experiencing profound political and economic changes. Since 1991 the country has had three changes in government and a 5-year civil war. The total population is 6,578,681, and the gross domestic product (GDP) per capita is $1140.

Major Languages	Ethnic Groups	Major Religions
Tajik (official)	Tajik 65%	Sunni Muslim 80%
Russian (widely used in government and business)	Uzbek 25%	Shi'a Muslim 5%
	Russian 4%	Other, none 15%
	Other 6%	

Predominant Sick Care Practices: Traditional and biomedical when available. The medical infrastructure is significantly below Western standards. Medical equipment and medications are scarce, and many doctors have left the country because of the unsettled social and political climate. Those who have stayed often increase their meager incomes by expecting bonuses, or "presents," for providing medical treatment or care. Others have moved out of the health care sector to higher paying jobs in other areas. The republic inherited the Soviet system of health care in which doctors and other health care workers were poorly paid, and most were specialists. In 1994 the republic had 13,000 doctors, one for every 447 inhabitants—by far the worst ratio among the Central Asian republics. The number of other health care workers was 80.3 per 1000 inhabitants. The worst ratios were in rural areas. The government is slowly attempting to change the medical workforce and implement primary care strategies. However, after the several years of civil war that followed independence in 1991, economic and political pressures have made reform difficult. In the mid-1990s, more than 80% of Tajikistan's health care facilities were substandard, and most had no running water or central heating. Only one drug treatment program existed, in Dushanbe, and it had 20 to 30 beds. Acquiring medication was almost impossible for ordinary citizens and continues to be extremely difficult. A master plan has been developed for a complete reform of the health care system, and attempts to implement it are currently in progress. The plan calls for a shift to primary care, with family doctors rather than specialists forming the cornerstone of the system. Only 90 family doctors were trained in 2000, so an existing program is retraining massive numbers of current specialists and new family practitioners. Efforts are also being made to correct the uneven distribution of personnel so that rural citizens will have better health care access. Efforts are also being made to restore essential hospital services.

Ethnic/Race Specific or Endemic Diseases: According to the 1989 census the most common causes of death were infections, parasitic diseases, circulatory and respiratory disorders, tumors, and accidents. By the mid-1990s, serious health threats came from the water supply, which had pathogenic organisms and toxic chemicals from environmental pollution. Overall, the country has threats of significant disease outbreaks because of population shifts and the breakdown in immunizations. Hepatitis A and E (non-A and non-B) are hyperendemic. Endemic diseases include hepatitis B, resurgent tuberculosis, and falciparum malaria. Civil war, the mass return of refugees from Afghanistan, and the interruption of anti-malarial control measures are responsible for the large increase in malaria cases and the significant outbreak in 1995. In June 1997, the country had a major outbreak of typhoid fever in the Dushanbe area and in the south from polluted municipal water. The typhoid strain was resistant to multiple drugs and resulted in 95 deaths. The risk for cholera and other water-borne illnesses is high, mostly because of inadequate sanitation facilities. From 1993 to 1997 an epidemic of diphtheria occurred and was intense among unvaccinated and partially vaccinated populations. Population immunity as a whole was low, and the country had experienced breakdowns in disease surveillance and health care services. Shortages of qualified medical personnel, products, and resources, combined with increased migration further added to the problem. The number of cases began to decrease in 1995 because of routine immunizations, implementation of national immunization days, and use of a WHO-recommended system for patients and contacts. Tajikistan is hyperendemic for acute enteric diseases in children. *Shigella* infections accounted for 32.4% of the infections, enterovirus diarrhea 12.1%, and *Escherichia* infections 8.9%. Enterovirus diarrhea is 2.7 times more common in children in urban areas (15.9%) than those in rural areas. People are still at risk for contracting polio because eradication efforts were halted by armed conflicts. The country has had major epidemics of multidrug-resistant strains of salmonella and a high prevalence of iron-deficiency anemia in young women. The World Health Organization's (WHO) estimated prevalence rate for HIV/AIDS in adults ages 15 to 49 is 0.01%. The estimated number of children from birth to 15 years living with HIV/AIDS is less than 100. HIV testing is mandatory for blood donors, those at risk for HIV infection, and foreign residents. The excessive use of pesticides, which pollute the environment and enter water sources, is also a health hazard. In contrast to most areas of the world life, expectancy in Tajikistan decreased in the 1990s. Life expectancy at birth is 61.09 for men and 67.42 for women.

Health Team Relationships: Historically, nurses have not been allowed to perform to their full capacities. Although doctors are the head of the health care team, they often perform tasks more suitable for nurses.

Birth Rites: In 1988, women in Tajikistan were 1.6 times more likely to die during childbirth than women in other areas of the Soviet Union. By 1989, 40 of every 1000 infants did not survive until the age of 1 year. In many parts of southern Tajikistan the rate was more than 60 deaths per 1000. The birth rate is 33.23 births per 1000 people, and the infant mortality rate is unacceptably high—116.09 per 1000 live births. Factors contributing to infant mortality are family poverty; inadequate nutrition for nursing mothers, infants, and children; and a lack of safe drinking water. Environmental pollution is believed to be increasing the incidence of birth defects and maternal and child mortality. The total fertility rate is 4.29 children born per woman.

Infant Feeding Practices: Anemia prevention control programs have been established that include education, oral supplementation for high-risk groups, and fortification of wheat flour with iron and other micronutrients. The goal of this program, which is supported by the United Nations Children's Fund (UNICEF) and the International Nutrition Foundation, is to reduce iron-deficiency anemia in young children and females of child-bearing age.

Child Rearing Practices: According to studies from 1993 to 1995, most school children have diets with insufficient calories, protein, carbohydrates, and fats. The country has high morbidity rates (41.18%) associated with rotavirus gastroenteritis in children 14 years and younger; children ages 2 years and younger are at the greatest risk. Rotavirus is the cause of 25.8% of cases of gastroenteritis in children 14 years and younger and of 11% of cases in adults. Literacy rates were reported to be 99% for males and 97% for females in 1995, and 80.6% of boys and 71.7% of girls were enrolled in secondary school. It is quite possible that today's figures are lower because of socioeconomic conditions.

National Childhood Immunizations: BCG at birth; DTP at 2, 3, 4, and 16 months; OPV at birth and 2, 3, 4, and 12 months; measles at 9 months and 3 years; and Td at 5 to 6 and 15 to 16 years. The reported percentages of the target population vaccinated in 2000 were as follows: BCG, 99; first dose of DTP, 98; third dose of DTP, 97; MCV, 98; and Pol3, 97.

Other Characteristics: Tajikistan is a major transshipment zone for heroin and opiates from Afghanistan going to Russia and western Europe. The country also has limited illegal cultivation of cannabis, primarily for domestic consumption.

BIBLIOGRAPHY

Alidina S, Annett H: Going beyond triage in Tajikistan. Health reform in the former Soviet Union, *Healthcare Manag For* 13(4):45, 2000.

Aliev SP: Malaria in the republic of Tajikistan, *Med Parazitol (Mosk)* April-June(2):27, 2000.

Gleason-Gary R, Sharmanov T: Anemia prevention and control in four Central Asian republics and Kazakhstan, *J Nutr* 132(40):867, 2002.

Khairov Kh S: Nutritional status and physical development of schoolchildren in Dushanbe, Republic Of Tajikistan, *Vopr Pitan* 5:30, 1997.

Mermin JH et al: A massive epidemic of multidrug-resistant typhoid fever in Tajikistan associated with consumption of municipal water, *J Infect Dis* 179(6):1416, 1999.

Pitt S et al: War in Tajikistan and re-emergence of *Plasmodium falciparum*, *Lancet* 352(9136):1279, 1998.

Rafiev Kh K: The etiological structure of acute intestinal infections in children in the Republic Of Tajikistan, *Zh Mikrobiol Epidemiol Immunobiol* March-April (2): 42, 1999.

Rafiev Kh K: The spread of rotavirus gastroenteritis in the Republic of Tajikistan, *Zh Mikrobiol Epidemiol Immunobiol* May-June (3):26, 1999.

Reamy J, Gedik G: Health human resource reform in Tajikistan: part of a masterplan for change, *Cah Sociol Demogr Med* 41(3–4):327, 2001.

Usmanov I, Favorov MO, Chorba TL: Universal immunization: the diphtheria control strategy of choice in the Republic of Tajikistan, *J Infect Dis* 181(suppl 1):86, 2000.

http://www.cia.gov/cia/publications/factbook/geos/ti.html

http://lcweb2.loc.gov/cgi-bin/query/r?frd/cstudy:@field(DOCID=tj0046)

http://travel.state.gov/tajikistan.html

◆ TANZANIA (UNITED REPUBLIC OF)

MAP PAGE (863)

Gemma Burford (Consultants: Mohammed Yunus Rafiki and Lesikar Ole Ngila)

Location: The United Republic of Tanzania is located in eastern Africa, on the Indian Ocean, and incorporates the islands of Zanzibar, Pemba, and Mafia in addition to the mainland. The total land area is 945,090 km^2 (364,900 square miles). The climate is hot and humid on the coast, arid in the central area, and temperate in the northern highlands. The population is approximately 33 million.

Major Languages	Ethnic Groups	Major Religions
Swahili (official nd aprimary language)	Black African 99%	Christian 45%
English	Arab <1%	Muslim 35%
Indigenous (e.g., Maasai, Sukuma)	Indian, Pakistani <1%	Indigenous religions (Sikh, Hindu, and Bahá'i) 20%
Other minority languages (Punjabi, Arabic)	European <1%	

Tanzania has 120 separate ethnic groups, or tribes, representing five linguistic families; by far the largest family is Bantu (95%). Many tribes have become assimilated into the national culture, but others (particularly Maasai) have retained a distinct ethnic identity. Swahili is spoken by 99% of the population, and English is spoken in secondary education settings by approximately 6% of the population

Health Care Beliefs: Traditional; indigenous; passive role. It is difficult to generalize about health care beliefs because of the multiethnic nature of the country and variations in religion and education. In Swahili, health *(afya)* is associated with a physique that would be regarded in most industrialized countries as slightly overweight. Smooth, shiny skin is also an indicator of good health. Most ethnic groups have some traditional beliefs in social causes (e.g., witchcraft, sorcery, the "evil eye" [the belief a person can harm others by looking at them], possession, angry ancestral spirits) for at least some illnesses. These beliefs are more prominent in rural than in urban areas, are less common among those with a formal education, and are less prevalent among Christians and Muslims than followers of traditional religions. Mental illness is usually attributed to possession by demons or spirits and may be treated by private or public exorcism. Those with mental illness are stigmatized almost everywhere. Minor ailments such as coughs and diarrhea are usually thought to have natural causes or be "just the work of God." Some of the Bantu believe in the concept of *vital force,* a force that can be weakened by illnesses, wounds, disappointments, and suffering. Disease prevention involves observing dietary restrictions, using mosquito nets, and avoiding major climate changes when possible. Rural Maasai believe that all food should be consumed with plant preparations such as acacia-bark tea to strengthen the body and prevent disease. Some of these preparations have been shown to contain cholesterol-reducing substances. Injections are often considered superior to oral medication. Although no specific color symbolism is associated with medications, brightly colored capsules are considered more effective than white tablets, and antibiotics are overused.

Predominant Sick Care Practices: Traditional; magical-religious; biomedical where available. It is not unusual for an illness to be treated simultaneously or in succession by biomedical and traditional methods. The principal factors influencing health care decisions are practical ones such as cost and distance, although cultural factors and experience also play a role. The introduction of user fees for health and education in the 1980s during structural adjustment programs led to the near-collapse of government health facilities in some areas. As a result, traditional health services and the private clinic sector have expanded. Tanzania has a continuum of traditional health practitioners, ranging from herbalists who rely entirely on natural products to spiritualists practicing symbolic healing. A few specialize in bone setting or mental health practice. In cities, practitioners may dispense their own herbal tablets; in rural areas, they often provide amulets to be attached to children's wrists and bring blessings. Self-treatment for chronic illnesses is formalized among Maasai, who have holistic forest retreats involving song, dance, prayer, the use of plant-based medications, and the consumption of meat. Biomedical health services vary in distribution and quality. Although a few villages still have no formal health care facilities, most have at least one health post or dispensary staffed by a nurse or medical assistant. Tanzania has approximately 100 district-level hospitals and four regional hospitals. The doctor/ patient ratio is 1:26,000. The official attitude toward traditional health care is one of cautious acceptance, and the Ministry of Health licenses only herbalists who do not practice ritualism. Integration of traditional and biomedical approaches remains an ideal rather than a reality, with notable exceptions. The regional hospital in Tanga has allocated a whole floor to the Tanga AIDS Working Group, which has so far treated more than 2000 patients with HIV/AIDS using herbs prescribed by local healers. The herbs are claimed to alleviate opportunistic infections, improve appetite, and increase longevity.

Endemic Diseases: Chloroquine-resistant malaria is endemic throughout the country, although the risk varies with altitude and climate. Other common causes of morbidity and mortality are diarrhea, respiratory diseases, and parasitic infections. Forty-six percent of the population has no access to safe water, and typhoid and cholera are widespread. Trypanosomiasis is endemic in some areas. Bilharzia, onchocerciasis, tuberculosis, yellow fever, leprosy, and lymphatic filariasis also occur. The World Health Organization's (WHO) estimated prevalence rate for HIV/

AIDS in adults ages 15 to 49 years is 8.09%. The estimated number of children from birth to 15 years living with HIV/AIDS is 59,000. About 8% to 9% of the adult population is estimated to be living with HIV/AIDS.

Health Team Relationships: Within the health team, doctors (generally men) tend to be superior to nurses (who are almost always women), and some patients may prefer to see a doctor.

Families' Role in Hospital Care: Family members usually remain near the patient's bed side and provide assistance with hygiene, nutrition, and surveillance. If they consider a treatment to be ineffective, they may try to supplement it with herbal medications or ask for an early discharge, but usually the doctor's authority is respected.

Dominance Patterns: In almost every aspect of public life, men are dominant. Many people think that the sexes have different but complementary roles in society, and women wield considerable power in their own sphere, which includes treating minor ailments in children. Regardless, the men's public roles tend to be valued more than the women's private roles. Domestic violence is widespread, especially in areas where alcohol consumption is high. Because the family is emphasized more than the individual, language that reflects group ownership rather than individual ownership tends to be used. Age is also an important factor, especially in ethnic groups with a tradition of formal age-grades. Health professionals from the younger generation are often thought to lack wisdom or experience and may be ignored in favor of older relatives.

Eye Contact Practices: Eye contact is acceptable in almost all settings, although in some rural areas mothers of small children may be afraid of strangers "putting the evil eye" on their infants.

Touch Practices: The acceptability of touch depends on many factors, including ethnic group, gender, religion, relative ages of the people involved, and social setting. Even handshakes are unacceptable in certain circumstances (e.g., between a Muslim woman and an unrelated man). Health professionals should consult with the patient and family before beginning any health intervention that could be regarded as improper or disrespectful.

Perceptions of Time: In Swahili the system of time keeping is based on sunrise and sunset (which are considered 6 AM and 6 PM, respectively), not PM midday and midnight as it is in the West. Thus "hour 1" in the morning is 7 AM. In general, unplanned events and interactions play a greater role in daily life than schedules. If someone meets a friend or relative while on the way to another appointment, avoiding a conversation to avoid being late is considered rude. Plans for the future are almost always qualified by the phrase "God willing."

Pain Reactions: Many ethnic groups in Tanzania were warrior tribes fighting for land or other resources. The men of these societies were trained from early childhood to face pain without flinching. This attitude still persists, as reflected in the Swahili proverb "a man does not cry for nothing." Crying and screaming are acceptable for women in some cultures, but they are expected to be stoical in others.

Birth Rites: Pregnant women usually abstain from sexual intercourse and respect certain dietary taboos such as not eating eggs and fish heads (a practice of the Bantu). The Maasai believe that women should not be given rich food during the last 3 months of pregnancy because it makes the fetus grow too quickly and causes a difficult delivery. Nurse-midwives, traditional birth attendants, female relatives, or all of these assist at births. In some tribes the umbilical cord cannot be touched until it falls off, whereas in others it is smeared with cow dung or herbal preparations. The new mother may live with the infant at her own mother's house for several months after the birth. She also may stay at home and be assisted by older female relatives. She is usually given rich food such as chicken or mutton and confined indoors for 2 to 3 months to allow her to regain strength and protect the infant from illness and sorcery. In most areas, sons are preferred to daughters. Children are thought of in terms of wealth and as an investment for the future, so large families are preferred.

Death Rites: Family members are present at the death of a relative in almost all situations, and death rites depend on religious affiliation. Most people prefer to die at home rather than in a hospital and to be buried in their home territory. Rural funerals are often elaborate celebrations lasting up to 3 days, and all the deceased person's relatives and friends are expected to attend. Among Bantu peoples, the death of young adults may bring about accusations of witchcraft or sorcery. Autopsies and organ donations are not practiced.

Food Practices and Intolerances: Food is eaten with the fingers or a spoon. The main staple is *ugali,* a stiff corn porridge that is usually served with beans, meat or fish stew, or green leafy vegetables. Rice and plantains are also popular. Bananas, mangoes, and many other tropical fruits are commonly eaten. Modern food such as carbonated soft drinks, white bread, and doughnuts are becoming more popular, especially in towns. Very few pastoralists now subsist on milk, blood, and meat; their staple diet is usually boiled corn supplemented with milk, yogurt, and wild fruits, and meat is eaten on ceremonial occasions only. Fish, insects, and wild game are taboo for Maasai. In many areas, alcohol is only traditionally consumed by older adults, and it is rarely used in the predominantly Islamic coastal regions. Muslims follow dietary restrictions in accordance with their religion, namely not eating pork, and only eating meat that has been slaughtered in a certain way.

Infant Feeding Practices: Children may be breast-fed for as long as 3 to 4 years, but weaning with soft corn soup or millet porridge usually begins at 3 to 4 months. Crushed fruit and honey are often provided as well. In rural areas, mild plant-based medicines may be mixed with food to treat childhood illnesses.

Child Rearing Practices: During the preschool years, female relatives and neighbors help with child care. Child rearing is strict, and children are taught to work hard, respect elders, listen and obey without argument, and learn by rote. In Islamic societies, boys are circumcised as infants; those who practice indigenous religions often perform the procedure during puberty. Female genital mutilation is officially illegal but is still very common in the Arusha and Dodoma regions (with 81% and 68% of girls, respectively, being circumcised).

National Childhood Immunizations: BCG at birth; DPT at 6, 10, and 14 weeks; OPV at birth and 6, 10, and 14 weeks; measles at 9 months.

Other Characteristics: Swahili greeting rituals (e.g., asking for news of family members, discussing recent events in the person's life) occur before any other verbal interactions, even during professional consultations.

ACKNOWLEDGMENTS: The author would like to acknowledge the kind assistance of Gerard Bodeker, chairman of the Global Initiative for Traditional Systems of Health, University of Oxford, Oxford, England.

BIBLIOGRAPHY

Burford G, Rafiki MY, Ole Ngila L: The forest retreat of *orpul*: a holistic system of health care practised by the Maasai tribe of East Africa, *J Altern Complem Med* 7(5):547–551, 2001.

Burford G et al: Traditional medicine and HIV/AIDS in Africa: a report from the International Conference on Medicinal Plants, Traditional Medicine, and Local Communities in Africa, *J Altern Complem Med* 6(5):457–472, 2000.

Chhabra SC, Mahunnah RLA, Mshiu EN: Plants used in traditional medicine in eastern Tanzania, part I, *J Ethnopharmacol,* vols 21, 25, 28, 33, and 39.

Harjula R: *Mirau and his practice: a study of the ethnomedical repertoire of a Tanzanian herbalist,* London, 1980, Tri-Med Books.

Johns T et al: Saponins and phenolic content in plant dietary additives of a traditional subsistence community, the Batemi of Ngorongoro District, Tanzania, *J Ethnopharmacol* 66:1–10, 1999.

Johnsen N: The forest of medicines: Maasai medical practice and the anthropological representation of African therapy, *Folk* 38:53–82, 1996.

Juntunen A, Nikkonen M: Professional nursing care in Tanzania: a descriptive study of nursing care in Ilembula Lutheran Hospital in Tanzania, *J Adv Nurs* 24:536, 1996.

Karungula J: Measures to reduce the infant mortality rate in Tanzania, *Int J Nurs Stud* 29(2):113, 1992.

Kilimanjaro Christian Medical Center and College: http://www.kcmc.ac.tz

Ministry of Health: http://www.tanzania.go.tz/health.htm

Mshiu EN, Chhabra SC: Traditional healers and health care delivery in Tanzania, *Trop Doctor* 12:142–143, 1982.

UNAIDS: http://www.who.int/emc-hiv/fact_sheets/pdfs/Tanzania_EN.pdf

United Nations Children's Fund: Statistics—Tanzania, http://www.unicef.org/statis/
Country_1Page170.html
Wright J: Female genital mutilation: an overview, *J Adv Nurs* 24:251, 1996.

◆ THAILAND (KINGDOM OF)

MAP PAGE (867)

Markus Roselieb and Henry Wilde

Location: Thailand (formerly "Siam") is located in Southeast Asia. It borders Myanmar on the northwest, Laos on the northeast, Cambodia on the southeast, and Malaysia on the south. The total land area is 514,000 km^2 (198,456 square miles). The northwest is hilly to mountainous with some forests. The northeastern plains, the poorest part of the country, are arid, and the central plains are fertile. The south borders on two seas, the Gulf of Siam and the Andaman Sea. The population is almost 70 million, and its growth rate is about 1.1%, one of the lowest among developing countries. The literacy rate is 93% for males and 91% for females.

Major Languages	Ethnic Groups	Major Religions
Thai	Thai 75%	Buddhist 94%
Chinese	Chinese 14%	Islam 4%
English	Other 11%	Hindu, Christian 2%

Thai and different Chinese dialects (e.g., Toei Chiew, Mandarin, Cantonese) are spoken, and also English, Lao, Burmese, and Malay, although not as frequently. The vast majority of the population is Buddhist, but Muslims are predominant in the southern region. All religions have the patronage of the king.

Health Care Beliefs: Traditional and modern; active involvement. Thais and Chinese go to temples often for meditation, "merit making," or if they or a family member is ill. If children are frequently sick or otherwise "difficult," they are given to a monk, as a representative of Buddha, for a specified period of time or until the monk thinks it is no longer necessary. The Ministry of Public Health runs regular and well-publicized health promotion and illness prevention campaigns throughout the country.

Predominant Sick Care Practices: Biomedical, traditional and magical-religious. Thailand has a mix of modern medicine and traditional Thai, Chinese herbal, and magical practices such as using blessed amulets from holy monks that are believed to protect the wearers from bad luck and disease. However, if a serious illness strikes, the vast majority of people go to the nearest modern medical facility. The health care system is composed of a huge network of government district, provincial, and tertiary care centers that are crowded and have too little money. However, the country has an excellent private medical sector that is in many ways equal to that of most developed countries, although it is unaffordable for the majority of the Thai population. A new system that offers care to all registered inhabitants, whether they are rich or poor, for 30 Thai baht ($0.70 U.S. dollars) per clinic visit (including medications) was inaugurated during the last general election. It is now rapidly making the government health sector dysfunctional and will have to be revised in the near future.

Ethnic/Race Specific and Endemic Diseases: HIV, dengue fever, dengue hemorrhagic fever, all forms of viral hepatitis, Japanese B encephalitis, rabies, tuberculosis, melioidosis, leptospirosis, thalassemia, and lymphatic filariasis (in southern Thailand) are endemic in Thailand. Malaria and various other parasitic diseases are still present in the country, but their prevalence is decreasing. In addition to infectious diseases, liver cancer (mostly due to chronic hepatitis B), nasopharyngeal carcinoma, and other cancers, as well as the so-called "civilization diseases" are now becoming major problems. The World Health Organization's (WHO) estimated prevalence rate for HIV/AIDS in adults ages 15 to 49 is now under 2%. The estimated number of children from birth to 15 years living with HIV/AIDS is 13,900. The estimated HIV seropositivity rate in Thailand was 780,000 in 1997. Surprisingly, annual HIV serosurveillance has shown a decrease in the incidence of HIV infection, symptomatic HIV, and AIDS. This decrease has been particularly pronounced among commercial sex workers, pregnant women, and young military conscripts since 1997. The main reason for the improvement was likely a vigorous educational campaign that starts in grade school, as well as condom promotion. The life expectancy for men is 66 and for women is 72 years.

Health Team Relationships: Doctors have a high status in Thai society. Nurses are highly regarded as well and are usually very industrious and capable; they are often addressed by the same title as doctors *(Khun Moh)*. A significant difference exists between the health care facilities in the rural areas and large cities. The number of health care personnel in rural Thailand is still insufficient, although everybody works hard and team relationships are casual and very congenial. In Bangkok, health team relationships are more formal, and practitioners have clearly defined tasks. Licensing of foreign nurses, dentists, and doctors requires passing a qualifying examination. The examination is in Thai and fluency in spoken and written Thai is required.

Families' Role in Hospital Care: In rural government facilities, families may be in charge of the patient's hygiene and food. In cities such as Bangkok and in private hospitals, nurses take care of everything. Nevertheless, at least one family member remains with the patient at all times, and most private hospitals provide an extra bed in the patient's room for a family member or trusted servant.

Dominance Patterns: Officially, men are the heads of families, and sons are still considered more important than daughters. However, the women usually rule behind the scenes. They basically run the family and have their names on most property deeds.

Touch Practices: The head of the body is considered sacred, but it is acceptable to pat a child on the head. Reaching over a patient's body to pass something is considered impolite, and stepping over a patient who is lying on the floor also is considered very rude. Male doctors should not touch female patients without a nurse or another person present, preferably a female. The usual greeting is the *wai*—folding the hands in front of the upper chest and face. Shaking hands and other forms of social touching while talking are uncommon between Thais and foreigners but are acceptable. Pointing the feet at another person is unacceptable.

Perceptions of Time: The Thai are rather casual about punctuality and oriented to the present. Immediate gratification is preferred to delayed rewards. Past events are usually forgiven and forgotten quickly. The political enemies of today become the partners of tomorrow if it is beneficial.

Pain Reactions: Although Thais try not to express their pain too loudly, each person has an individual pain threshold.

Birth Rites: Thais believe that after childbirth, a new mother needs "fire." She is expected to sit near a fire, drink hot water and tea, and keep warm regardless of the ambient temperature because doing so keeps her healthy and gives her strength. These customs are now rapidly disappearing, particularly in the cities. A rest period of 1 month after birth is common, and oily food is avoided. In the north and northeast, it is believed that the wrists of infants must be bound with a string to prevent them from losing their soul. Other old traditional practices such as giving birth at home and burying the placenta are rapidly disappearing.

Death Rites: The dead are kept at home or in a temple from 3 days to many months depending on the financial and social background of the family. After this period is over, the bodies are be cremated. Many Chinese-Thai families still bury their dead. During the mourning period the monks have daily prayer sessions to which all can come to pay their respects. No religious or other customs prohibit organ donations or autopsies.

Food Practices and Intolerances: Rice is a staple. In the morning and late at night, rice gruel is the favorite food. Food is important and available everywhere at almost any time. Fish sauce, seafood, pork, and chicken are the main staples. Many Thais do not eat beef. The primary utensils used are spoons, forks, and chop sticks. Most Thais eat using a spoon in the right and a fork in the left hand, a practice that is acceptable even in the upper class. Many farmers still eat most food with their hands.

Infant Feeding Practices: During the first month, breast-feeding is common, but children are bottle-fed at young ages because their mothers have to return to work. In rural areas, cooked banana with mashed rice is a favorite substitute infant food, and introduced at a very young age in addition to breast-feeding.

Child Rearing Practices: Child rearing practices vary greatly between Bangkok and the rural areas. Although small, middle-class families are emerging in Bangkok, the vast majority still live with the extended family, and grandparents, especially grandmothers, play an important role in child rearing. Many families who work in towns leave their small children at their parents' rural homes and only see them during holidays. Seniority plays an important role in Thai daily life, and children are taught to be deferential to their elders. However, in general, children are given much space, and child rearing is fairly permissive.

National Childhood Immunizations: BCG at birth; DPT at 2, 4, 6, and 18 to 24 months and 4 to 6 years; OPV at 2, 4, 6 and 18 to 24 months and 4 to 6 years; HIB for newborns born to mothers infected with hepatitis B; MMR at 12 to 14 months and 4 to 6 years; hep B at birth and at 1 and 6 months; varicella at 12 to 18 months (not part of EPI). Optional vaccinations include Japanese encephalitis after age 1 and hep A and rabies preexposure after age 2 (not part of EPI).

Other Characteristics: Thai and Chinese patients tend to expect medication when consulting a doctor. If their symptoms are not better within 1 day, they often visit another doctor and ask for new medication. This practice is often a result of inadequate communication between doctors and patients. Thai doctors tend to prescribe too many medications, a practice that may be a result of patients' expectations and a traditional Chinese practice in which doctors did not charge for their professional services but did charge for medications. It is not uncommon, even in excellent hospitals, to be given a prescription for an antibiotic (usually the latest), one or two analgesics, a decongestant, a multivitamin, and a nighttime sedative to treat a common cold. Thailand is a relatively safe place to live, and women can still walk alone on the streets of big cities at night. Though burglaries and other crimes occur, they are much less common than they are in large American or European cities.

BIBLIOGRAPHY

Cassidy J: The unseen menace: Thailand, child health, HIV/AIDS, *Nurs Times* 92(8):50, 1996.

Chayovan N, Knodel J, Wongboonsin K: Infant feeding practices in Thailand: an update from the 1987 demographic and health survey, *Stud Fam Plann* 21(1):40, 1990.

Chow DC: AIDS in Thailand: a medical student's perspective, *J Comm Health* 19(6):417, 1994.

Dhamcharee V, Romyanan O, Ninlagarn T: Genetic counseling for thalassemia in Thailand: problems and solutions, *Southeast Asian J Top Med Public Health* 32(2): 413, 2001.

Fox PG, Komchum S: Primary health care in an unsettled area of northern Thailand, *Int Nurs Rev* 39(2):49, 1992.

Muecke MA: Worries and worriers in Thailand, *Health Care Women Int* 15(6):503, 1994.

Muecke MA, Srisuphan W: From women in white to scholarship: the new nurse leaders in Thailand, *J Transcultural Nurs* 1(2):21, 1990.

Stewart EC, Bennett MJ: American cultural patterns: a cross-cultural perspective, rev ed, Yarmouth, Me, 1991, Intercultural Press.

Triteeraprapab S et al: Lymphatic filariasis caused by *Brugia malayi* in an endemic area of Narathiwat Province, southern Thailand, *J Med Assoc Thailand* 84(suppl 1): 182, 2001.

van-Griensven F et al: Rapid assessment of sexual behavior, drug use, human immunodeficiency virus, and sexually transmitted diseases in northern Thai youth using audio-computer-assisted self-interviewing and noninvasive specimen collection, *Pediatrics* 108(1):13, 2001.

◆ TOGO (TOGOLESE REPUBLIC)

MAP PAGE (862)

Adama Dodji Gbadoé and Edoh Azankpé

Location: Located in West Africa on the Gulf of Guinea, Togo, with a total land area of 56,600 km^2 (21,848 square miles), is one of the smallest and poorest countries in Africa. It is bordered on the west by the Republic of Ghana, on the north by the Republic of Burkina Faso, and on the east by the Republic of Benin. The Atlantic ocean is to the south. Togo is divided in two zones by a long chain of mountains, and on both sides of the chain there are plains watered by two of the most important rivers of the country, Mono in the south and Oti in the north. The north has a tropical, humid climate, with only one rainy season from May to October and one dry and very hot season from November to April, characterized by the dry and dusty harmattan wind. The south is influenced by a subequatorial climate that has two dry seasons (from November to March and July to August) and two rainy seasons (from March to July and September to October). Overall, little rain falls, especially in the south, so forests are found only on mountains and adjacent to rivers. The plains are part savannah and part woodlands. Rich soils cover only 20% of the total area of the country. The capital is Lome. The southern part of the country is more populated than the northern region, and about 75% of the population lives in rural areas. The total population is 4,629,000. The gross domestic product (GDP) per capita is $340.

Major Languages	Ethnic Groups	Major Religions
French (official)	South: Adja/Ewe 44%	Christian 51%
Ewe and Mina (south)	Akposso/Akebou 4%	Animist 27%

Kotokoli-Tem and	Ana/Ife 3%	Muslim 11%
Kabye (north)	North: Kabye/Tem 30%	Other 11%
	Para-Gourma/Akan 14%	
	Foreign 5%	

Togolese people believe deeply in God and divinities, and traditional Togolese believe that there is a greatest god (God) who can be reached through small gods (divinities). These divinities are venerated in ceremonies, rituals, and prayers to ancestors. God is put first before the others. The gods the most adored are *Vaudou Sakpatè,* god of the earth, who expresses himself through smallpox, chicken pox, or measles; *Hèbiesso,* god of rain and justice, who expresses himself through thunderclaps and by killing thieves (e.g., striking them with lightning) whenever he is asked for justice; *Legba,* the protector god against enemies and bad spirits; *Mamiwata* (siren), the sea or ocean goddess who is the expression of wealth; and *Gnigblin,* the god of the forest and alliance, who is expressed by the rainbow. Togo has 40 local languages dominated by Ewe-Mina, Kotokoli-Tem, and Kabyè. Others include Tchokossi, Moba, Bassar, Ana, Akposso, Adja, and Fon. Other than French, only Ewe and Kabyè are acknowledged as national languages. English is studied as a second language, and is increasingly being used in social situations.

Health Care Beliefs: Traditional; passive role. People have an extreme fear of mental illness, and treatment is very different from than in occidental societies. The Togolese believe that mental illness is induced by another person or a spirit (vodou, or siren *Mami wata*), so people with mental problems are kept in the society. Families take charge of their family members and bring them to traditional healers or pastors for treatment. Ceremonies, amulets, scarifications, prayers, and potions of all sorts are methods of treatment. It is rare to confine these patients to an institution such as a psychiatric hospital, although it occasionally occurs in urban areas with more Westernized residents. Only one psychiatric hospital is available in Togo. Prevention and health education are carried out through programs. Priority is given to infectious and contagious disease programs such as those for HIV/AIDS, tuberculosis, leprosy, malaria, acute respiratory tract infections, and diarrheal diseases. Togo also has prevention programs for noninfectious diseases such as sickle cell disease, which affects 16% of the population, with 3% to 5% having homozygous or hemoglobin sickle cell disease. Most of these programs are sponsored by institutions such as the World Health Organization (WHO), the United Nations Children's Fund (UNICEF), USAID, the World Bank, and Care International. Although the people are interested in prevention, prevention efforts are adversely affected by traditional beliefs and lack of information because of the low literacy rate (45%). For example, 10% to 20% of the population thinks that malaria is caused by the sun, field work, or eating excessive amounts of cacahuets or palm oil. To prevent anemia, people treat themselves with beets or infusions of red herbs (because they are the color of blood), but they do not contain any of the iron, folic acid, or B_{12} vitamins that are normally recommended.

Predominant Sick Care Practices: Indigenous, magical-religious and biomedical where available. Togo is a poor country, so equipment in public hospitals is of poor quality. Togo has no health insurance system, and hospitals are overflowing with patients who could be treated in peripheral health units. With such an influx of patients, nursing performance in the hospitals is affected. People tend to go to hospitals rather than to health units because they believe that they can get better care, referrals from peripheral health units to hospitals is difficult, and the country does not have ambulances to transfer them because distances between facilities are long (17 km on average). A study by the International Center of Research in Childhood in Paris indicates that 31% of the population uses home remedies when they become ill. More than 25% resort to traditional medicine, primarily by consulting indigenous healers. Traditional medicine involving herbs was recently legalized by the national parliament. Togo also has a research team at the University of Lome that is studying the healing abilities of plants to bolster support for herbal medicine. Numerous Togolese also choose spiritual treatments, which are praying in churches or performing rituals for gods. For the most part, patients first consult a pastor, priest, traditional healer, or fetish priest before going to a modern health center. In most cases, spiritual treatments and medical treatments are combined, and the doctor is unaware of it. It is common for priests or prayer groups to be in hospitals during the day after a doctor has left and for traditional healers and fetish priests to be at hospitals at night.

Ethnic/Race Specific or Endemic Diseases: The ethnic groups in Togo are not very homogenous, so no diseases are specific to a particular ethnic group. Some diseases are specific to the northern part of the country such as onchocerciasis, which is endemic. Cerebrospinal meningococcal meningitis is endemic in the dry season (January to March). Schistosomiasis, cholera, goiter, malaria, and childhood illnesses such as mumps are endemic throughout the country. Because of the efficacy of childhood immunizations, pertussis, diphtheria, tetanus, and poliomyelitis are becoming rare. Goiter primarily affects the districts of Wawa, Koza, Doufelgou, Binah, and Amou. The National Service of Nutrition recommends consumption of iodized salt to compensate for iodine deficiencies in the water. Customs officers are even asked to seize all uniodized salt. Malaria is the disease that affects the country most and is the primary cause of mortality. It is endemic all year, with a recurrence at the end of rainy seasons. Each person in the country may have four to six attacks of malaria per year. *Plasmodium falciparum* is the most common species in 98% of cases, whereas *P. malariae* and *P. ovale* are diagnosed in 2% of cases. Severe malaria especially affects children ages 6 months to 6 years and pregnant women. Travelers and migrant workers who are not immune are also vulnerable. Approximately 2 weeks before coming to Togo, it is recommended that people have malaria chemoprophylaxis (chloroquine and paludrine). Common clinical features of severe malaria are hyperpyrexia, coma, convulsions, hypoglycemia, and anemia. Because of malaria's direct and indirect costs, it is considered a hindrance to the economic development of the country. (According to WHO data, malaria costs are approximately $12 billion per year in African endemic areas). Unfortunately, most people do not like using mosquito nets impregnated with repellent (because it makes them feel hot or like they are suffocating), which are considered by WHO to be the best and cheapest method of prevention. The World Health Organization's (WHO) estimated prevalence rate for HIV/AIDS in adults ages 15 to 49 years is 5.98%. The estimated number of children from birth to 15 years living with HIV/AIDS is 6300. Approximately 45% of males use condoms, and treatment of AIDS with antiretroviral drugs is less than 10% because of cost. The principal modes of transmission (>90%) are heterosexual and mother-to-child infections.

Health Team Relationships: Nurses have approximately 7 fewer years of school attendance and training than doctors, so they often feel inferior. Paradoxically, this creates good relationships within the medical staff. In the public health centers that receive many poor patients, relationships are fairly good between the medical staff and patients because the patients are not very demanding. However, in the private health centers, where everything costs money, demands for high-quality care occasionally lead to conflicts between patients and staff members.

Dominance Patterns: Socially and officially, children belong to the father; Togolese society is patriarchal. Children are the responsibility of their fathers, and only fathers get allowance money for children. Regardless, fathers are often absent from the home, so mothers (who are often un-employed if they live in urban areas) are the first educators of the children. When the father is absent for a long time or has died, his brothers or sisters assume an important role in the children's education, and they are obligated to support the widow and her children. In most ethnic groups the widow is automatically "given" (married) to a brother of her deceased husband so that she can have someone to support her and take respon-sibility for the education of her children. More than 80% of working women are in the agricultural sector, especially in rural areas. In urban areas, it is common to find women at many levels in public adminis-tration or private enterprise. Women are prominent in the trade sector. Togo is called the country of *nana Benz*—women who were part of the cloth trade in the West African subregion and became so rich that they were the first to own Mercedes Benz cars in West Africa. Today, a *nana Benz* is a rich woman.

Families' Role in Hospital Care: The health care system has too few nurses and "sick-nurses" and no effective health insurance. Families have an important role in the care of the patient. Once a patient is hospitalized, the family finds someone to remain with the person at the hospital. The support person's first objective is to provide the patient with food, but bathing, changing, washing clothes and bed sheets, and cleaning the room are other duties. In pediatric hospitals, mothers stay with their children in the same room and often in the same bed, and many patients are in the same ward. Parents are often asked to monitor intravenous fluids, food, and bathing of their children.

Eye Contact Practices: Whether a child is having a conversation or being reprimanded by an older person, it is considered improper and impolite to look directly into the eyes of an older adult.

Touch Practices: Traditionally, most widows and widowers do not shake hands with persons other than other widows and widowers. Children do not initiate a handshake when greeting an older adult because it is impolite. In some areas, men do not deliberately touch the wife of another man because it is regarded as adultery. If this occurs, the woman must be cleansed by rituals or she may become ill.

Perceptions of Time: People do not place much importance on punctuality, especially those who are less well educated. Lateness has become so common that people are not worried when they are not on time. It is common to hear people say that an event will start "on African time," meaning later than the scheduled time. This also has racial connotations and implies that all people other than Blacks do their best to be on time.

Pain Reactions: People react similarly when in pain. In public health centers, where care is less expensive, patients seem to be more stoical and talk very little about their pain to doctors because they do not want to annoy them. In private centers, patients are more demanding and may ask for morphine, which is not yet used in the hospitals. The pain of newborns is not considered. In general, the more someone is able to bear pain the more the person is appreciated and considered courageous. In some ethnic groups (e.g., Peuhls), stoicism is a proof of virility. Young people ready to be engaged are invited to flog one another; whoever expresses pain is considered weak and not eligible for marriage until the ritual can be completed with no outbursts.

Birth Rites: Pregnant women are treated with consideration because pregnancy is considered a sacred time for women and the society. All pray for an easy delivery. Traditionally, mothers prepare spiritually for future birth by asking divinities what to do to make the delivery easier. Some pregnant women wear amulets that protect the infant from witchcraft or will promote an easy birth. More than 50% of deliveries occur in the home attended by traditional "obstetricians" who have not actually received any education in obstetrics. Because health centers are far from homes, especially in rural areas, some nongovernmental organizations provide training for birth practitioners. Naming ceremonies are held for a single infant born with the head coming out first. On the eighth day after birth, family members, friends, and others are invited to the naming ceremony. An aunt (from the father's family) takes the infant out of the room seven times. On the seventh time, somebody throws water on the roof, and it drops on the infant, who is put on the ground temporarily. This ritual is performed after a prayer to the ancestors, and then a name is given to the infant. It may be chosen by the father or another member of the father's or mother's family. The name is chosen according to the infant's birth date or an event. Usually a second name (for Christians and Muslims) is chosen, even if the family members are not believers. After the ceremony, the infant can be taken outside at any time but must be well covered. Otherwise, it is believed that the infant should not be brought out for anything other than a medical visit or emergency. If any problems develop, the birth rites are postponed for 8 days. Twins are considered divines, expressing hope as well as fear; they also represent animals such as monkeys or buffalos according to geographical area. For the eighth-day birth ceremony of twins, the family organizes a very expensive and special event to integrate them into society. They are almost venerated. No member of the family of twins is allowed to eat or kill the animal the twins represent because legend says the twins will die. Special ceremonies also are performed for infants born legs first. They are given special names *(Agossou* or *Agossa* for boys and *Agossi* for girls). Every male infant is circumcised during the neonatal period or later. The birth rate is 37 per 1000. The mortality rate for children younger than 5 years is 146 per 1000, and 5.4 children are born per woman. The maternal mortality rate is 478 deaths per 100,000 live births. The life expectancy at birth is 55 years.

Death Rites: Death is always considered strange and abnormal. Every death is thought to be provoked spiritually by an enemy or angry gods, even if it is clinically proven to be caused by other factors. Instead of an autopsy, people consult an oracle or a necromancer in the belief that the spirit of the dead person will tell them who is responsible for the death or whether the person offended a god. Many rites and sacrifices are performed to calm down an angry god or allow the spirit of the deceased person to chase the murderer. At the burial, family members must be present, and most people travel many miles to help with the burial ceremonies of a parent, friend, or acquaintance. If a member of the family expected to be present does not come, the person is suspected. Older adults are not considered dead; they are thought to be in another world *(awlimé)*. Before burying someone, the cause of his death and the way a body is to be buried is prescribed by an oracle or a necromancer *(xoyoyo)*. Dead twins are symbolized by statuettes, and every member of the family, especially the parents, have to take care of them as if they are living beings (e.g., bathe and clothe them, serve them meals, put them to bed). The Togolese belief is that dead people can see and judge the acts of others, so no one wants to offend them. Organ donations and autopsies are not practiced because they are considered an offense to the dead person. Widowers and widows must put a piece of charcoal in their meal, or the late husband or wife is supposed to eat with them and kill them so that they can be together again. Likewise, to get rid of the deceased person's spirit, a widower or widow must use a special herb called *shame*. A widow has more restrictions than a widower. Although the widower only mourns for a few days, the widow has to spend numerous days and even months. They must shave their head, wear dark clothing, stay in their room at night, and wear a dark cloth rope around the waist.

Food Practices and Intolerances: The majority of people eat three times a day, eating the largest meal at lunch time (12 to 3 PM). Most poor people eat only once a day at noon. Meals do not adhere to scientific recommendations and are generally unbalanced. For example, the meal may only comprise a main course with no fruits or vegetables because they are expensive and considered a luxury. Vegetables and meat are always well cooked. Basic foods differ according to areas, but some foods are eaten all over the country. Pounded yam or cassava (*ayimolu,* the southern term or *watsé,* the northern term) is a meal made of rice and beans. Rice is consumed throughout the country. Rice was once a luxury food because it was imported and expensive, so people only cooked it only during festivities. Some meals such as *gari* (made out of cassava), *ademè, fétri* (vegetables), *akoumé* (which is made of corn) are especially popular in the south. Cereals such as sorghum or millet are eaten in the north. Some meals, such as beans combined with vegetable oil and *gari,* are very rich in protein and used in hospitals to rehabilitate malnourished children, although people consider this to be food for the poor. Mothers incorrectly think that pasta is a nutrient-rich food for their children. Most Togolese eat with their hands, although the use of spoons, forks, and knives was introduced during colonization. In rural areas, eating utensils are rarely used, although educated and financially comfortable families use them regularly. When in restaurants with foreigners, most Tongolese attempt to use utensils for convenience. Foods are usually cooked on a hearth using charcoal or firewood, even in urban areas. The use of cookers or electric stoves is considered a luxury.

Infant Feeding Practices: Until the last 10 years, because of occidental influences and advertising about cow's milk formulas, women, especially those with a Western education, substituted bottle-feeding for breast-feeding or reduced the duration of breast-feeding to 3 months at the most. Today, exclusive breast-feeding is practiced for about 6 months as recommended by WHO. From the seventh month to 2 years of age, cereal and solid foods are added to the breast-feeding. Many associations such as Groupe d'Action Pour l'Alimentation Infantile are working to promote breast-feeding and good infant nutrition, inviting hospitals to join the increasing group of Hôpitaux Amis de Bébés (Hospitals Friends of Babies). Nutritional diseases such as kwashiorkor and marasmas are common because of the poverty of the population, and lack of breast-feeding.

Children Rearing Practices: It is very rare for children to have their own room; children generally sleep with their parents. In some families, girls share a room with their mother, and boys do the same with their father to control the education of the children. Respect for adults, politeness, and obedience are the essential virtues taught to children. Children who call older adults by their names are considered to have bad manners. Children are not allowed to call their brothers or sisters by name; they call them *fofo, dada, fogan,* or *dagan,* meaning "grand-brother" or "grand-sister." About 47.7% of the population is 15 years of age or younger, and the literacy rate is 45%.

National Childhood Immunizations: BCG at birth; DTP at 6, 10, and 14 weeks; OPV at birth and 6, 10, and 14 weeks; measles at 9 months; vitamin A at birth to 59 months; and TT at 12 to 45 years. Childhood immunizations for tuberculosis, diphtheria, tetanus, pertussis, poliomyelitis, and measles are subsidized. Other vaccines may have a fee, such as those for infectious diseases such as influenza, pneumococcal infections, meningitis A and B, hepatitis A and B, typhoid fever, yellow fever, rubella, and mumps. According to 1998 statistics the percentages of fully immunized children from 12 to 23 months were as follows: BCG, 75.7%; DTP (three doses), 42%; poliomyelitis, (four doses), 46.6%; and measles 42.6%.

BIBLIOGRAPHY

Anipah K et al: *Enquête démographique et de santé, Togo,* 1998, Calverton, Md, Direction de la Statistique et Macro International Inc, 1999.

Assimadi K et al: Utilisation des structures de soins par les enfants de 0 à 5 ans au Togo: résultats d'une enquête épidémiologique menée dans un CHR (Atakpamé), *Bull Soc Path Ex* 87:251–252, 1994.

FNUAP/Direction Générale de la Statistique et de la Comptabilité Nationale: *La population Togolaise et les interventions du FNUAP au Togo,* p 62, Lomé, Togo, Décembre 2001.

Gbadoé AD et al: Priapism in sickle cell anemia in Togo: prevalence and knowledge of this complication, *Hemoglobin* 25:355–361, 2001.

Gbadoé AD: *L'utilisation des structures de soins par les enfants de 0 à 5 ans au Togo. Résultats de la première phase d'une enquête menée dans la région des Plateaux [Mémoire de DES de Pédiatrie],* p 74, Lomé, Togo, 1993, Université du Bénin.

Rivière C: *Union et procréation en Afrique: Rites de la vie chez les Evé du Togo,* p 223, Paris, L'harmattan, 1990.

United Nations Children's Fund: *The state of the word's children 2001,* New York, 2001, Oxford University Press.

◆ TONGA (KINGDOM OF)

MAP PAGE (856)

Munir A Khan, David Simmons, Patricia Jane Harry, and Isileli Fakakovi Vunileva

Location: Tonga (also called the "Friendly Islands") is an independent kingdom and a member of the Commonwealth of Nations; it is located in the western South Pacific northwest of New Zealand, and its western boundary is the eastern boundary of Fiji. The country consists of a cluster of approximately 180 small islands, with a total land area of 748 km² (289 square miles). The kingdom of Tonga is composed of four major island groups that extend from north to south: Niuas, Vava'u, Ha'apai, and Tongatapu. The largest island of Tonga is Tongatapu Island, on which is the capital, Nuku'alofa. Two thirds of the total population lives on Tongatapu. The islands are either of coral or volcanic origin. The islands were under British protection from 1900 until their independence on June 4, 1970. Tonga's estimated population in 2001 was 110,000. The geographical distribution of the population is very uneven, with 59% percent living in rural areas. Population density ranges from about 35 persons per square kilometer in the Niuas to more than 250 persons per square kilometer in Tongatapu. About 40% of the population is younger than 15 years and 6% is older than 60.

Major Languages	Ethnic Groups	Major Religions
Tongan (an Austronesian language)	Polynesian 98%	Christian
	European 2%	Free Wesleyan Church
English		

Tongan is a West Polynesian language and belongs to the Oceanic branch of Austronesian languages; it has minor local variations. Tongan and English are official languages, and both are used in schools. Almost all Tongans speak some English as their second language, so English-speaking visitors do not need a working knowledge of Tongan to communicate. Church ministers are very influential. The church has the power to influence politics and to raise large amounts of money. The Free Wesleyan Church has the most followers, followed by the (Methodist) Free Church of Tonga, the Church of England, Roman Catholic, Seventh Day Adventist, and Mormon. All commerce and recreation are prohibited on Sundays, the Christian day of rest, and much of the Tongan social life is structured around the church.

Health Care Beliefs: Traditional; indigenous; active role in health promotion. In spite of strong Christian beliefs, many Tongans still believe in the spirits, taboos, superstitions, medical charms, and Polynesian gods characteristic of the well-defined religious traditions that existed before the arrival of the missionaries. According to present-day folk beliefs in Tonga, the causes of some illnesses are a synthesis of previous religious folk ideas and Christian beliefs. It has been reported that the incidence of *te'ia*, a form of a culturally specific illness known as *avanga,* is increasing. *Te'ia* manifests as a range of particular symptoms and behaviors, and individuals who believe they have *te'ia* usually consult traditional healers. People with illnesses thought to be caused by spirits of the dead may see and identify the troublesome spirits or may consult a healer to do the same. Most healers pray to the Lord and ask for healing from God. They frequently suggest to patients that they should also pray for healing

Predominant Sick Care Practices: Biomedical; complementary; magical-religious. Tonga is a medically pluralist society, incorporating biomedical and traditional forms of health care. Complementary therapies such as herbal therapy, homeopathy, and acupuncture are considered alternatives to modern medicine. Tongans freely use traditional healing methods, herbal medications, and biomedicine without significantly changing their cultural identity. Their choices often are tempered by availability of treatment and past illness. Private health insurance is common in the middle and upper classes. Tongans have a high standard of health, comparable to that of more developed countries. This excellent health is primarily the result of primary health care programs, especially those for prenatal and children's health. Tongans have universal access to safe drinking water and treatment for common illnesses and injuries. A steady supply of medications is within 1 hour's travel time away (Demmke et al, 1996, p 51), and medication is free for Tongans. Like other developed nations, health promotion and illness prevention are emphasized. Medical services are best on Tongatapu, particularly Nuku'alofa, with its greater population density justifying the various medical specialists in Tonga's main clinical institution of Vaiola Hospital. Educational institutions, information availability, communication facilities, financial institutions, and entertainment are also more plentiful on the main island. Ha'apai and Vava'u also have hospitals. People with serious medical problems should be taken overseas for treatment.

Ethnic/Race Specific or Endemic Diseases: Tonga has few serious health risks. Fungal infections, heat exhaustion, heat stroke, watery and persistent diarrhea, dysentery, and fever are the common diseases. It is reported that the major causes of death per 100,000 people in 1993 were diseases of the circulatory system, 58.1; diseases of the nervous system, 51; senility, 27.6; diabetes mellitus, 17.3; and renal failure, 10.2. A pattern of high rates of obesity, diabetes, high blood pressure, and cardiovascular disease has emerged as Tongans have transitioned away from traditional diets. The annual admissions at Vaiola hospitals between 1971 and 1991 of patients with diabetes increased fourfold. A diabetes unit was established in 1994 to tackle the increased prevalence of diabetes and its complications. The Health and Weight Awareness Program was initiated in 1995 by the Tonga National Food and Nutrition Committee. Cancer is also a major cause of mortality, with large intestinal cancer among male and female Polynesians accounting for 39% and 29%, respectively, of all cancers. The World Health Organization (WHO) has not estimated prevalence rates for HIV/AIDS for adults or children in Tonga; it is rare. Less than 10 cases were reported in the last 10 years. Life expectancy is 72.2 years for women and 67.73 years for men.

Families' Role in Hospital Care: Families play a significant role in providing direct care for hospitalized family members. It is important to understand the role of each person in the family before communicating extensively with any one individual or groups of individuals. The members of the family and close relatives visit the patient during the stay in the hospital, bringing food and fruit. If permitted, at least one close relative stays with the patient 24 hours a day, frequently helping with personal tasks such as bathing. Members of the family cooperate fully with the doctors and nurses and have a voice in decisions about hospital procedures, including surgeries and referrals. Tongans prefer to care for older people at home.

Dominance Patterns: Although Tonga is a mixture of Western and Tongan cultures the country has retained much of its Polynesian culture. Tongans respect traditional authority and customs, and the lifestyle is conservative. Gender differences originate from *anga fakatonga* ("the Tongan way"). Usually, men head the family, and women typically play supportive roles. Women stay at home and do the indoor household work, whereas men do the outdoor work and have more freedom of movement away from the home. It is not customary for women to freely associate with men unless they are chaperoned, and women do not usually leave their homes alone. Gift giving is ubiquitous in Tonga. Tonga has a highly stratified and status-conscious society, and in any social interaction, cross-cutting hierarchies such as gender, kinship, and age determine the status of those involved. Low-status persons are expected to demonstrate respect and be unquestioningly obedient to those of high status. In families the higher status of sisters is reflected in their relationship with their brothers, which is characterized by *faka'apa'apa* (respect) and *faka'ehi'ehi'* (avoidance). The proper way to show respect in Tonga is by sitting on crossed legs and clasping the hands on the lap. When the royal car approaches, the proper procedure is to sit down in the grass at the road verges. Although caste is not as rigid and elaborate as it was before Europeans arrived, Tonga still has two clearly defined social classes: the nobles and the commoners. The royal family and the 33 hereditary nobles and their families are the highest ranking people in Tongan society. All other Tongans are commoners. Nobles cannot marry commoners unless they want to risk losing their royal titles. A commoner who marries a noble can never attain noble status.

Eye Contact Practices: Body language or direct eye contact is quite common between sexes and among social classes in Tonga. Raising the eyebrows is a way to say "yes" in answer to a question.

Touch Practices: Physical touching between men and women who do not know each other is unacceptable; some women may not even want to shake hands. Men usually greet each other verbally or by shaking hands. People who know each other extremely well embrace or kiss on both cheeks, which is also a sign of affection. Greetings during professional and formal interactions are limited to a handshake and verbal exchanges.

Perceptions of Time: Tongans are generally very punctual. Arriving late is often considered disrespectful.

Pain Reactions: Although some gender differences in pain reactions exist, both sexes tend to be stoical.

Birth Rites: Neither fathers nor any male members of the family are usually allowed to be present during childbirth, although close female relatives are usually present. In hospitals, mothers follow Western hospital procedures before and after a child is born. However, according to Tongan tradition, a messenger (usually the husband) is sent to retrieve a midwife when the delivery is imminent. It is believed that if the first person the messenger meets is female, the child will be a girl and vice versa. Members of the family play an active role as primary caregivers. For the first 10 days after childbirth, the mother's diet comprises exclusively yams and hot coconut milk *(veifua)*. Immediately after childbirth, the mother and child are painted with turmeric *(enga)* and oil, and the mother does not leave the house or bathe for 5 days. Each day for 2 or 3 months the mother and child are given a sponge bath and repainted with turmeric, which are thought to keep the mother and child warm and help the mother to produce plentiful milk quickly. The practice of burying the umbilical cord and of marking the burial spot is still the custom. Usually the cords are buried in mounds just outside the house, and often sweet-smelling flowers are planted over the spot. The *tope*, a long lock of hair worn by small boys over the temple is cut off at puberty; the boy's hair is cut in the style of an adult male. Male circumcision (modern procedure) and supercision (traditional procedure) are common in Tonga, and usually take place between 6 to 12 years. Boys are usually operated on in groups outdoors under a shady tree after they bathe in the sea. The boys sit naked on a rock, mat or tree root, and a razor is used as the cutting instrument. The spectators are adult male relatives. This is regarded as a sign of manhood, and any youth who refuses the procedure is forbidden to eat with other members of the household, cannot touch others' food, and is spurned by the girls. An uncircumcised person is called *kou* or *taetefe*. Tonga's birth rate is higher and its death rate is lower than the world average. According to the 1996 census, the birth rate was 27.8 per 1000 people, and the world average was 25 per

1000. The death rate was 5.9 per 1000, and the world average was 9.3 per 1000. The infant mortality rate was 37.9 deaths per 1000 live births. Women generally have three or more children, but population growth is limited because of migration to New Zealand, the United States, and Australia. One third of Tongans live overseas.

Death Rites: Death is considered an individual's physical departure from the family. The illnesses and even deaths of young children are frequently attributed to parental sins such as adultery or failure to behave properly to other family members. Burial is the preferred method. Relatives of equal or superior rank, such as *fae* (the mother, real or symbolic) or the *mehekitanga* (the aunt, real or symbolic), prepare the body of the deceased. The relatives of the deceased dig the grave and put the body in the grave. All the members of the family and community members gather to pay their last respects and bid farewell to the deceased. Funerals are considered very important and a major social event. When mourning for a relative or friend, Tongans dress in black and wear *ta'ovala*: distinctive pandanus mats tied around the waist with a cord of coconut sennit called a kafa. *Ta'ovala* are frequently worn by older people and by everyone when they enter a church, go to work, town, or a formal occasion, or whenever they might encounter someone of noble status. Every funeral has accompanying feasts and *kava* drinking. All who attend a funeral participate in the feast. When a member of the royal family dies, all Tongan people mourn for 6 months. During the 6 months of mourning, all Tongans are required to don *ta'ovala* and wear black.

Food Practices and Intolerances: The Tongan diet consists mostly of carbohydrates such as cassava *(Manihot esculenta),* yams *(Dioscorea alata),* taro *(Colocasia esculenta),* taro root, plantains *(Musa paradisiaca),* and breadfruit; coconut products; fresh fruit; pork; chicken; corned beef; fish; and imported food. Increasing quantities of fatty and refined foods, including imported foods, are now being consumed (e.g., bread, mutton flaps, imported chicken parts). Feasting is a national pastime based on centuries of believing that "big is beautiful." Educational programs have increased awareness of healthy food choices, and exercise and healthy eating are being encouraged. However, less healthy foods are often consumed because they are cheaper and more available.

Infant Feeding Practices: It is estimated that about 74% of mothers currently breast-feed their infants. However, a large proportion of mothers also give additional foods and drinks to their infants because they are not confident they have enough breast milk or that their infants are satiated. Bottle-feeding is also common. Boiled water, orange, or *lesi* (pawpaw) juice is usually given to infants within the first 2 months of life. Foods are introduced later than drinks; before the fourth month, mothers introduce foods, and papaw and bananas are the most common first foods. Older infants are also given different imported infant foods. In recent years the

National Food and Nutrition Committee (NFNC) and the Ministry of Health have established policies made public through the national media to encourage mothers to breast-feed their infants.

Child Rearing Practices: The extended family is the basic social unit in Tonga. Everyone is expected to contribute to the well-being of the extended family, which typically includes parents, siblings, grandparents, aunts, uncles, and cousins. Tongan extended families have no separate words for "brother," "sister," and "cousin." Aunts and uncles may also be referred to as "parents," and all older people may be called "grandparents" by the younger members. Parents have no real sense of possessing their children, and children are frequently shifted from one household to another. In the end, children are effectively reared by the entire family and may have several places to call home. Women have the most involvement in child rearing. Infants and young children sleep with their parents. Discipline is usually the father's duty. Most parents expect their children to be obedient and live according to their own culture. Education is free and compulsory for children from the ages of 6 to 14. The government operates most primary schools, whereas churches sponsor most secondary schools. At 99.6%, Tonga's literacy rate is among the highest in the Pacific.

National Childhood Immunizations: BCG at birth; DTP at 6 weeks and at 3 and 5 to 6 months; OPV at 6 weeks and at 3 and 5 to 6 months; hep B at birth, 6 weeks, and 5 to 6 months; measles at 9 months; DT at 15 months and 5 years; and yellow fever for individuals arriving from an infected area such as Africa or South America. The low rate of Tongan infant mortality is a result of government immunization and child health programs; 9 of 10 children are fully immunized before their first birthday.

Other Characteristics: The head of the body is *tapu* in Tongan culture, meaning individuals should never unexpectedly touch any part of another person's head. Traditionally, children do not touch the head of their father. Tongans are required by law to dress modestly. Men have fewer restrictions than women but are required to wear a shirt at all times in public. This rule does not apply to beaches, where men are permitted to go shirtless. Women cannot be topless at any time, and they usually cover their shoulders and chests completely and their legs at least to the knees. A Tongan woman who does not comply with the guidelines risks being considered disreputable. Men or women who wear short shorts in public are considered offensive. Visitors to Tonga are also requested to be respectful (e.g., to avoid wearing bikinis or short skirts in public). Cleanliness and presentable dress is a part of Tongan culture. Being clean and presentable indicates respect for yourself and others; conversely, being dirty is disrespectful. Respect is extremely important in Tongan culture, and respect for superiors is a principal basis of Tongan behaviors. Shame and embarrassment are taken very seriously and can lead to suicide, a fact that foreigners should heed. Gifts are given to new friends, especially if they are foreigners. Gifts are presented to kings and nobles by families after births, deaths, marriages, or university or high school graduations or in honor or memory of a family member.

BIBLIOGRAPHY

Cowling WE: Eclectic elements in Tongan folk belief and healing practice. In Herda P et al (eds): *Tongan culture and history,* 1990, Australian National University, Canberra.

Demmke A et al: *Tonga population profile: a guide for planners and policy-makers,* New Caledonia, 1996, South Pacific Commission Noumea.

Encyclopedia Britannica, 1997, Britannica Book of the Year, Chicago, Encyclopedia Britannica Inc.

Evans M et al: Globalization, diet, and health: an example from Tonga (nutritional evaluation), *Bull WHO* 79(9):856, 2001.

Fletcher M, Keeler N: *Tonga,* Hawthorn, Australia, 2001, Lonely Planet Publications.

Gifford EW: *Tongan society,* 1971, New York, Kraus Reprint Co. or use Gifford EW: Tongan society, Honolulu, Hawaii, 1929, Bernice P. Bishop Museum.

Halavatau V, Hughes R, Hughes MC: *1999 Tongatapu infant feeding survey,* SPC Technical Paper No 217, Noumea, New Caledonia, 2000, SPC.

Jozef V: *The Tongans,* Sydney, 1978, Pacific Publications.

Keller N, Swaney D: *Tonga,* Hawthorn, Australia, 1998, Lonely Planet Publications.

McGrath BB: Swimming from island to island: healing practice in Tonga, *Med Anthropol Quart* 13(4):483, 1999.

Morton H: Creating their own culture: diasporic Tongans, *The Contemporary Pacific* 10(1):1, 1998.

Sutton TD, Eide TJ, Jass JR: Trends in colorectal cancer incidence and histologic findings in Maori and Polynesian residents of New Zealand, *Cancer* 71(12):3839, 1993.

United Nations: *United Nations 2000 statistical yearbook,* New York, 2000, United Nations.

◆ TRINIDAD AND TOBAGO (REPUBLIC OF)

MAP PAGE (858)

Shirley Cooke

Location: Trinidad and Tobago are located in the Caribbean just off the Venezuelan coast. They are the southernmost pair of islands and are known as the "twin republic." Trinidad is the larger of the two and has the majority of the East Indian people. Trinidad has more of a city environment and many ethnicities, a faster pace, Indian-influenced food, more married people (partly because of Indian arranged marriages), and a stronger economic base. Tobago has more of a village atmosphere, is less developed, is slower paced, uses traditional locally grown foods, has fewer married people, and has a population that is primarily of African descent. The total land area is 5130 km^2 (1,981 square miles).

Major Languages	Ethnic Groups	Major Religions
English (official)	Black 43%	Roman Catholic 33%
Hindi	East Indian 40%	Hindu 25%
French	Mixed 14%	Anglican 15%
Spanish	White, Chinese, other 3%	Other Protestant 14%
		Muslim 6%
		Other or none 7%

Hindi is commonly spoken in cosmopolitan areas. Villages on Tobago comprise approximately 1000 people. The dominant language of the past was called *Patwa,* a colloquial form of French.

Health Care Beliefs: Traditional; passive role. People often believe illness is caused by evil spells that were put on them by others. Some also believe in *obeah,* or witchcraft, as a source of illness. One form of prevention involves the use of scents; perfume, incense, and scented oils are believed to chase the bad spirits away. Many people do not understand that unclean water and spoiled food can make them sick. It is common for patients to give an insufficient description of their symptoms to doctors.

Predominant Sick Care Practices: Combination of modern biomedicine and magical-religious. Baptist "healers" (who are not necessarily associated with an actual Baptist church) call on supernatural powers *(Simidemi)* to heal the sick. The patients are encouraged to fast for 2 days and nights, after which a ritual is performed involving burning incense. The patients enter into a trancelike state and begin to moan (hence the name "the moaning ritual"). Occasionally hexed patients are taken to a point where the sea meets a river. They are submerged to signify cleansing of their soul.

Ethnic/Race Specific or Endemic Diseases: Hypertension, adult-onset diabetes, and nutrition-related diseases are common. The World Health Organization's (WHO) estimated prevalence rate for HIV/AIDS in adults ages 15 to 49 is 1.05%. The estimated number of children from birth to 15 years living with HIV/AIDS is 180.

Health Team Relationships: Health care relationships are usually hierarchical and authoritarian. The doctor is like a god, and whatever the doctor says to do is expected to be done by nurse and patient without question. Doctors are considered to be in a different and higher class and are respected for their educational authority.

Families' Role in Hospital Care: Families are expected to help hospitalized relatives. They often must bring food because not enough food is available or it is of poor quality because of budget constraints. Physical care in the hospital is provided by a certified nurse's aide and the family. If a patient is in critical condition, the aid provides most of the care; in less critical situations the family provides items and assistance that are needed for activities of daily living.

Dominance Patterns: In the past, women were considered less important than men and often mistreated. It was not uncommon for men to beat their wives; the community expected and accepted it. It was thought that because men brought home the family money, it was their right to be abusive. With exposure to television and subsequently to other lifestyles, women are now less tolerant of abuse, and significant changes in women's independence have occurred during in the last 10 years. Women are no longer expected to marry, even if they become pregnant. People do not care if a woman gets pregnant when she is not married; no malice is directed toward her. Women who choose to marry are able to pick their spouses, and they are not pushed into marriage. Doctors and office workers such as bankers are considered to be in a higher class of people. They are visibly different in the community because of their dress, language, and walk.

Eye Contact Practices: Any direct eye contact maintained for too long is considered disrespectful. It is rude for young people to look older adults in the eye; children are expected to "know their place." Children also are not allowed to take part in adult conversations. If a guest comes into the home, children must leave to do other things; they are not allowed to stay in the room. At the age of 15 or so, children are gradually allowed to remain in the presence of adults.

Touch Practices: Touching is uncommon, regardless of gender or age. Waving is more acceptable than shaking hands, and people do not hug because it can have sexual connotations. It is considered masculine for men to shake hands. However, it is preferable for a man to lock his hand into a fist and hammer one hand into the other palm. Few displays of affection are seen, including toward children. Adults never kiss children on the lips, and they seldom even kiss them on the cheek.

Perceptions of Time: Time is irrelevant, regardless of the circumstances. The only situations in which time has importance are medical emergencies and school; children are punished if they are late to school and are usually beaten. For example, a person scheduled to arrive at 1:00 PM is expected to arrive around 2:30 PM. Similarly, a man who is supposed to work at a job for 8 hours and only works 6 usually gets full pay because he showed up. Because people often do not show up at all, it is acceptable to supervisors because those who do come to work are usually good workers; in addition, they realize that the heat and humidity make working difficult.

Pain Reactions: Pain is only expressed privately. When children are spanked, they are told not to cry. Adults seldom show pain in front of others and cry in private.

Birth Rites: During pregnancy, women do not eat gas-producing foods because they can cause "gripe" (colic) in the newborn. Stepping or walking over a pregnant person is a serious taboo. Births of sons and daughters are celebrated equally. Having a child is of great importance to a family, regardless of the child's gender. Women only take sponge baths for a week after birth. They do not wash their hair during this week and instead cover their head.

Death Rites: When a person is expected to die, much of the family is present; a person should never die alone. Incense is burned to ward off bad spirits. After death, everyone in the village is invited to the wake. They stay overnight and talk about the life of the person who died. When the body goes to the funeral home, incense continues to be burned, and the family bathes the body. The water is saved from the bath, brought to the home of the deceased, and poured on the floor in a corner where the person liked to spend time. Organ donations are not an option because people believe that those who die should leave the world with the organs they had from birth. Autopsies are seldom performed.

Food Practices and Intolerances: *Pelau* (rice) is the most common food. Rice, root provisions (e.g., sweet potato, *dashing* and *calaloo* [leaves of the dashing], yams, turnips), and land crabs are the staple foods. The favorite meal is land crab and *calaloo*. Most meals are placed on plates and in bowls, and spoons are the common eating utensils. Coconut is in most dishes, and bread and dumplings are also popular. Seasonal fruits are eaten, and drinks comprise locally made juices from fruits such as mango, grapefruit, pineapple, and pumpkin. The people carry out a traditional "thanks-giving" ritual several times a year on no specific dates. A large wooden tray is placed in the middle of the table. Meat without salt and rice are prepared and put on the tray with other foods, and all the people eat with their hands from the center tray. The origin of this tradition seems to be a mystery, but it is considered a special time for the family to gather.

Infant Feeding Practices: Breast-feeding is common, and many children are breast-fed until they are 5 years, although age 3 is the norm.

Child Rearing Practices: Parents are most responsible for rearing children, but many other people in the village are expected to help. If a child is disrespectful to a neighbor, the neighbor has the right to spank the child. Schools are allowed to spank children—the knuckles of the hand are rapped or the buttocks are spanked with paddles. It is not uncommon for some children to get broken knuckles from being beaten at school. A branch from the *tambern* tree is often used for school beatings, or "whoopings." Dirt under the nails, tardiness, not being prepared, and not wearing the proper uniform are all causes for beating. Children have home chores to do such as picking fruit, feeding chickens and goats, and milking goats. All the people in the village make sure that children do not misbehave; they may punish a child on the spot or notify the parents of a child's misdeeds. When parents are not present, older siblings are often put in charge.

National Childhood Immunizations: DTP at 3, 4 1/2, 6, and 18 months and 4 to 5 years; OPV at 3, 4 1/2, 6, and 18 months and 4 to 5 years; HIB at 3, 4 1/2, and 6 months; MMR at 12 to 15 months and 4 to 6 years; YFV at 12 to 15 months; and DT at 10 years.

Other Characteristics: Menstruation is considered secret, and no warnings are given to girls about their first menses. When it comes, the girl is usually frightened and embarrassed and asks an aunt or a sister about what is happening; she is referred to her mother. Her mother tells her that she must to be careful around boys and avoid them. Menstruating girls are considered dirty and are not supposed to prepare meals for men during this time because they might put spells on them.

BIBLIOGRAPHY

Adler MW, ed: Statistics from the World Health Organization and the Centers for Disease Control, *AIDS* 6(10):1229, 1992.

Andrews MM, Boyle JS: *Transcultural concepts in nursing care,* ed 2, Philadelphia, 1995, Lippincott.

Hezekiah J: Postcolonial nursing education in Trinidad and Tobago, *Adv Nurs Sci* 12(2):28, 1990.

McKee PL: A cultural exchange of values, *Act Adapt Aging* 19(2):17, 1994.

◆ TUNISIA (REPUBLIC OF)

MAP PAGE (862)

Afif Ben Salah

Location: Located in the Mediterranean basin between Algeria in the west and Libya in the southeast, Tunisia is part of North Africa. The size of the population is 9,673,300, and the total land area is 185,000 km^2 (71,410 square miles). Tunisia is divided into five main socioeconomic regions: northeast, northwest, center, southeast, and southwest. The climate is very different in the north above the Atlas chain of mountains (where it is cold) and the south (the continental area), which is characterized by desert and oasis. The central region and east coast are temperate. Tunisia has a relatively young population, and family planning programs have reduced the birth rate to 1.69% per year. An increase in life expectancy to 70.1 years for men and 74.1 years women in the last decade also has increased the size of the older adult age group. Tunisia is primarily an agricultural country, but the service sector has become more important because of increases in tourism, health services, and telecommunication.

Major Languages	Ethnic Groups	Major Religions
Arabic (official)	Arab-Berber 98%	Sunni Muslim 98%
French	European 1%	Christian 1%
	Jewish 1%	Jewish 1%

Arabic is typically used for administrative communication (in letters and for laws), but French is the language used in universities. More recently, English has taken on a more important role in education. In secondary schools and especially in the research sectors, English is required for international scientific communications. However, local Arabic is used in families. The Berber language is still used in some areas of southern Tunisia, where a few Berber tribes are still living in the hilly area of Tataouine in the south. Because of its geographical location and invasions throughout the centuries, the Tunisian population is a mixture of Berbers (the original ethnic group), Arabs, Turks, and Europeans. This genetic and sociocultural diversity is characteristic of the Tunisian population. Although Sunnite Islam is the major religion, Christianity and Judaism are also freely practiced and respected.

Health Care Beliefs: Traditional; passive role. Since achieving independence, five schools of medicine were built leading to strong promotion of modern medicine. However, traditional medicine is an important asset in the health care arena, particularly among people in rural areas and lower social classes. In this context of illiteracy or when the health care system cannot cure a person, the people may believe an illness has a supernatural origin and therefore needs a traditional treatment. It is also common for individuals to use herbs to treat illnesses or perform rituals to protect themselves against people with the "evil eye" (i.e., the ability to harm others by looking at them).

Predominant Sick Care Practices: Biomedical and magical-religious. Tunisia has a very decentralized health care system in which primary care constitutes the major component. Traditional medicine also continues to play a role, particularly in rural areas with less educated parents or when modern medicine cannot resolve an illness. Although health care accessibility is considered to be universal, it may take several consultations to properly diagnose visceral leishmaniasis, for example, because of a lack of continuity in care related to the high turnover of doctors, and inadequate access to health care in remote rural areas. A patient may have up to six consultations at different levels of the health care system (e.g., primary, emergency, private doctor) and receive symptom-related treatments such as aspirin, paracetamol, antibiotics, and iron. Parents who are not literate take their children to traditional healers and often receive a diagnosis of splenomegaly *(jilf)*. Splenomegaly is a common diagnosis in traditional culture, and healers prescribe herb recipes for treatment. When a diagnosis of splenomegaly is established by the healer, the community usually consults the pediatric medical specialist of the region who is known to be able to cure this disease. Therefore the path to treatment may involve simultaneous use of traditional and modern medical systems.

Ethnic/Race Specific or Endemic Diseases: Changes in the demographics of the country have resulted in epidemiological transitions that have influenced morbidity and mortality profiles. The country has experienced a shift from infectious diseases and malnutrition to cancer, atherosclerosis, diabetes, and accident-related deaths. However, infectious and emerging diseases are still serious health problems. For example, leishmaniasis (with 7509 cases in 1999), hepatitis (with 3317 cases in 2000), and tuberculosis (with 2000 cases in 2000) are the major causes of morbidity of all the compulsory notifiable diseases. The major causes of mortality are cardiovascular disease (23%), tumors (12%), accidents (9%), gastro-enteric disease (5%), infectious diseases (5%), hormonal diseases (4%), genitourinary tract diseases (3%), and unspecified causes (14.1%). Maternal mortality, although reduced to 20 deaths per 100,000 newborns, is still a public health problem in rural areas, where midwives, rather than doctors, continue to be consulted. Hemorrhage (27%), hypertension (19%), and infections (17.5%) remain the major causes of maternal mortality in Tunisia. The World Health Organization's (WHO) estimated prevalence rate for HIV/AIDS in adults ages 15 to 49 years is 0.04%. WHO has no estimates for children from birth to 15 years. As of 2000 the total number of HIV cases reached 1049 cases, 146 of whom were tourists seeking care or coming for holidays. Most of those infected (70.5%) were males 15 and older; 7.5% were infants. The route for transmission of HIV/AIDS in Tunisia has been primarily through heterosexual contact and intravenous drug use, not through homosexual contact.

Health Team Relationships: Doctors play the key role in case management of patients, particularly for specialized care such as surgery. However, in the primary health care setting, nurses are responsible for most of the preventive programs such as immunizations and water and food hygiene; therefore nurses tend to have more influence on the community. Practitioners must work together as a team, sharing roles and responsibilities according to their strengths. In addition, nurses must maintain a global focus on quality health care and patient satisfaction.

Families' Role in Hospital Care: In the Tunisian culture the family plays a key role in supporting its members when they are ill. Hospitalization is an important event because historically it was linked to serious conditions that generally led to death (e.g., patients with tuberculosis in the beginning of the century). Despite the evolution of the health care system and improvements in quality of care in hospitals and private clinics, the family continues to help care for hospitalized patients. They may decorate the room, bring in blankets, and feed the patients, especially women who are about to give birth. In private clinics, pregnant women usually are accompanied by their mothers for the entire stay. In the public hospitals, which have a limited number of beds, one family member usually visits the patient every day, brings food, and helps with personal and hygiene tasks.

Dominance Patterns: Historically, men have been more dominant in the Tunisian culture. However, since the independence of the country in

1956, conditions for women have improved and resulted in a better literacy level, liberal abortion laws, and effective integration of women into the workforce. Today, Tunisian women are very well represented in various professions, including medicine. The Tunisian government has a Ministry of Women's Affairs that influences social, cultural, and political life. Women play a key role in the family's health, particularly during pregnancies or childbirth or when children are ill.

Eye Contact Practices: Direct eye contact is avoided out of respect and obedience, particularly among rural people during interactions with parents or grandparents. This behavior is changing in urban and educated families, in which people use direct eye contact to be more convincing.

Touch Practices: Physical touching is part of Tunisian culture and denotes sympathy. During events such as religious feasts or marriages, women kiss each other when they first meet. Men may also kiss each other when greeting after a long separation. Men and women commonly shake hands. In the context of medical care, women consult male gynecologists, and breast palpations are just considered routine procedures in urban areas; however, those who live in rural areas may prefer to have female doctors for such intimate procedures.

Perceptions of Time: Time is not money, so punctuality is not a major issue. Delays of hours are not considered a problem, even when an appointment was made. People may not even make a phone call to apologize when they are late. With the increased use of mobile phones, it is possible that this behavior may change.

Pain Reactions: Pain reactions vary between those in urban and rural areas. In urban areas where communities have more medical amenities, pain is not tolerated. People in pain often consult doctors quickly, even when the pain is caused by factors such as stress or menstrual bleeding. In rural areas, people often react differently; they tend to be more tolerant of pain and ultimately consult a traditional healer or barber to perform scarification procedures to remove the pain.

Birth Rites: Birth is a desirable event in Tunisia, and both sexes are equally welcomed during the first pregnancy. After the first pregnancy, parents prefer that the next child be one of the opposite sex so that they can have boys and girl; they become particularly sad if they never have a son. When a child is born, the family meets and slaughters a lamb for a meal. Each person brings a present for the newborn such as new cloth or money. The infant mortality rate is 26.2 deaths per 1000 births.

Death Rites: Although a sad event, death is accepted in Tunisian society and believed to be God's will, which is a source of comfort for the family. Family members disseminate the news of a relative's death very quickly so that they can quickly congregate and console one another. Autopsies are performed when the cause of the death is suspicious (e.g., homicide, an unknown disease, sudden death of an apparently healthy person). Organ donations are encouraged by Tunisian law, and people are free to donate their organs after death, a preference they can write on their identification card.

Food Practices and Intolerances: Food habits vary from one region to the other in Tunisia, but generally couscous is the most famous dish in the country. Originally a traditional Berber food, couscous is made by most families at home with wheat. In the central region, it is often cooked with lamb and in the coastal region, with chicken or fish. Olive oil and fresh vegetables are also very popular among all social groups. Even though the country's calorie intake has not increased significantly during the last 20 years, the types of food they consume are beginning to change and signal a dietary transition. Consumption of sugar has increased significantly, as has consumption of meat and fat.

Infant Feeding Practices: Breast-feeding is the cornerstone of the Tunisian primary health care strategy for the prevention of diarrheal diseases and other infections. In 1996 the prevalence of breast-feeding was 93.8%, and the mean duration was 15 months. Furthermore, the mean for exclusive breast-feeding is 1.6 months. Early termination of breast-feeding is attributed to a new pregnancy (32.1%), insufficient milk production (31.7%), and illness of the child (9.9%). Subsequent pregnancies are a well-documented reason for cessation of breast-feeding in all developing countries and highlights inadequate contraceptive practices, which are important at the individual and community levels. Insufficient milk production is thought to shorten the period of amenorrhea associated with breast-feeding and is associated with stressful lifestyles—a biocultural phenomenon.

Child Rearing Practices: Child rearing practices vary depending on location. In urban areas, women usually work outside the home, and children from the age of 3 to 6 months are cared for in special facilities *(crêches),* which are either public or private. In rural areas, child rearing is the responsibility of women. Children are transported on their mother's backs, even when they go to work in the field. They also sleep close to their mothers. Discipline is usually the responsibility of both parents in urban areas but is mainly the responsibility of the father in rural and less wealthy communities. Grandparents also may play a key role in rearing children if both parents are employed outside the home or a large family lives in the same dwelling (a practice that is common in rural areas).

National Childhood Immunizations: BCG at birth and 6 years; DTP at 3, 4, 5, and 18 months; OPV at 3, 4, 5, and 18 months and 6, 12, and 18 years; hep B at 3, 4, and 9 months; measles at 15 months and 6 years; Td at 6, 12, and 18 years, CBAW. Since 1970, immunization campaigns have been in place for smallpox, tuberculosis, and poliomyelitis. In 1982, immunization schedules were organized according to WHO recommendations. In 2000, the coverage for vaccine-preventable diseases exceeded 90%: BCG, 94.6%; third dose of DTP, 96.8%; hepatitis, 94.4%; and measles, 95.8%. This program eradicated polyomyelitis and controlled measles in the country.

REFERENCES

American Academy of Pediatrics, Work Group on Breastfeeding: Breastfeeding and the use of human milk, *Pediatrics* 100:1035-1039, 1997.

Ben Salah A, Najah M, Marzouki M, Ducic S: The determinants of the duration of breastfeeding in semi-rural Tunisia, *EMR Health Serv J* 6:28-31, 1989.

Direction de soins de santé de base, Ministère de la santé publique: Rapport annuel, 2000.

Direction de soins de santé de base, Ministère de la santé publique: Enquête MICS2, 2000.

Duncan B, Ey J, Holberg CJ, Wright AL, Martinez FD, Taussig LM: Exclusive breastfeeding for at least 4 months protects against otitis media, *Pediatrics* 91(5):867-872, 1993.

Gendret D: Allaitement maternel et parsitoses intestinaux, *Archives Française de Pédiatie* 45:339-401, 1988.

Institut National de las statistique: Annuaire Statistique de la Tunisie, Décembre 2000.

Ministère de la santé publique: Enquête sur la morbidité et la mortalité hospitalère, 1996.

MSP, DSSB: *Enquête Tunisienne sur la santé de la mère et de l'enfant,* Tunis, 1992, Ministère de la santé publique: Office Nationale de la famille et de la population.

MSP, ONFP: Enquête Tunisienne sur la santé de la mère et de l'enfant, Tunis, 1996, Ministère de la santé publique: Office Nationale de la famille et de la population.

OMS/UNICEF: *L'allaitement maternel dans les années: initiative modiale,* Florence, Italie, 1990, Réunion coparraine par l'OMS/UNICEF.

Pisacana A, Graziano L, Mazzarella G, et al: Breastfeeding and urinary tract infections, *J Pediatr* 120(1):87-89, 1992.

Victoria CG: Evidence for protection by breastfeeding against infant deaths from infectious diseases is Brazil, *Lancet* 7:319-322, 1987.

◆ TURKEY (REPUBLIC OF)

MAP PAGE (860)

Nurgün Platin

Location: Turkey is a southeastern European country at the northeastern end of the Mediterranean Sea. The Black Sea is to the north, and the Aegean Sea is to the west. The total land area is 780,580 km^2 (301,382 square miles). Narrow coastal plain surrounds Anatolia, an inland plateau that becomes increasingly rugged as it progresses eastward. Although the coastal areas have milder climates, the inland Anatolian plateau experiences extremes, with hot summers and cold winters with limited rainfall.

Major Languages	Ethnic Groups	Major Religions
Turkish	Turkish 82%	Muslim 99%
Kurdish	Kurdish 18%	Other 1%
Arabic		

Health Care Beliefs: Passive role; acute sick care only. Health promotion is demonstrated but practiced very little. People accept treatment passively. Some may postpone elective medical treatment during the month of Ramadan or fasting.

Predominant Sick Care Practices: Biomedical; alternative; magical-religious. Biomedical treatment is valued, but the Turkish also consult various alternative medical and health care practitioners. Use of herbal teas, chiropractors, and folk medicine is fairly common. Particularly in rural areas, "the evil eye" (a curse from someone who looks at a child maliciously) is believed to cause childhood illnesses.

Ethnic/Race Specific or Endemic Diseases: Endemic diseases include chloroquine-sensitive malaria in the southeastern region, β-thalassemia on the Mediterranean coast and in the southeastern region, and goiter in the northern Black Sea area. Hepatitis A and tuberculosis are becoming more common. The World Health Organization's (WHO) estimated prevalence rate for HIV/AIDS is 0.01%. WHO has no estimates for children from birth to 15 years. By the end of 1999, 120 new HIV cases had been reported.

Health Team Relationships: Patients do not question doctors. Most doctors are men and have absolute authority; they are expected to use good judgment. Consent forms are generally not used, and information is not freely shared with patients. Information is often shared more freely with family members, and medical decisions are made in conjunction with families. Patients often address health professionals by title rather than name. Professional dialogue between doctors and nurses is weak. Almost all nurses are female, and they are not considered powerful by the health team. Women, especially those in rural areas, may prefer a nurse midwife or a female doctor for obstetrical and gynecological examinations, family planning treatments, or counseling.

Families' Role in Hospital Care: A family member usually stays with the patient day and night and is expected to help with personal and therapeutic care.

Dominance Patterns: Men generally make most major decisions, and they are traditionally accepted as the leader of the family. Women are passive and perceived as having a lower status in society, with variations between urban and rural areas. Rural women pass through four stages: young bride (ages 15 to 30) with low status; middle age (ages 30 to 45) with medium status; mature (ages 45 to 65) with highest status; and finally old (age 65 and older), when women are respected the most but are not powerful. Women are the quietly dominant decision makers in their homes, especially when health care decisions must be made. However, husbands are responsible for the official business such as filling out insurance forms for a hospital visit. Increasing numbers of women work outside the home. Parents expect to be cared for by their children in their old age.

Eye Contact Practices: Traditional groups consider sustained eye contact with authority figures to be impolite and disrespectful.

Touch Practices: Unlike in social settings, no physical contact occurs during greetings among health care professionals and patients. However, patting a patient on the back would be a sign of support. In social settings, kissing once on both cheeks and handshaking are customary for greetings.

Perceptions of Time: The Turkish have a relaxed attitude toward time. People are more oriented to the present and near future.

Pain Reactions: Tolerating pain and not verbalizing it are common. Pain is considered a part of life and not loudly discussed.

Birth Rites: Approximately 81% percent of births are attended by health personnel. Approximately 60% of infants in rural areas and 80% in urban areas are born in health institutions. A prone position on a flat surface and the kneeling position (which is used in some rural areas) are the most common delivery positions. Fathers are not present during deliveries, nor are relatives. Relatives and neighbors help with housework and infant care for 40 days after birth, during which the mother is considered to be vulnerable for infection.

Death Rites: The deceased are buried as soon as possible—the same day or the day after death. The time of the burial depends on the amount of paperwork involved or the arrival time of close relatives. For Muslim burials the body is wrapped in special pieces of cloth and buried without a coffin in the ground. A religious person *(imam)* recites a short prayer during the burial ceremony, and additional prayers are recited at home or the local mosque on the seventh, fortieth, and fifty-second days after the burial. Although this practice follows Islamic rituals, these gatherings for prayer provide a lot of support for the family. Live organ donations are becoming relatively common, but cadaver donations are uncommon because people prefer that the body be buried intact; for the same reason, autopsies are uncommon. Cremations are also not permitted.

Food Practices and Intolerances: People near the Black Sea coast consume a great deal of black cabbage. Pork is a forbidden food for Muslims. Fresh fruits and vegetables are favorites, and legumes, vegetables, and bread are food staples. Red meat and poultry are consumed throughout the country, whereas fish and seafood are primarily consumed in coastal areas and in big cities. Three meals per day are routine. Breakfast and dinner are the main meals in rural areas, and dinner is the main meal in urban areas. One month of fasting during Ramadan is practiced by all except for children and those who are sick. Tea is the most commonly consumed beverage.

Infant Feeding Practices: Approximately 95% of infants are breast-fed, but only about 14% of women exclusively breast-feed. Plain and fresh yogurt, fresh fruit juices, fruit purees, vegetable soup, and soups with grains are introduced at 3 months. Multivitamins are started at the end of the first month, especially for infants born in the winter. Breast-feeding usually continues for 12 months. Boys are breast-fed longer because of the belief that breast-feeding makes them stronger. According to studies, less educated mothers breast-feed longer than well-educated mothers. The use of commercial infant food is more common in urban areas.

Child Rearing Practices: In a traditional family, the father is the authority figure. The mother is the primary caregiver for children, but the paternal grandmother also has an important influence. Mother and child relationships are strong. Discipline is strict, and obedience and respect are valued. However, these attitudes are changing. Parents are more permissive with boys, whereas girls are taught to become productive, hard workers. Girls start helping with household chores when they begin school. Girls socialize with girls, and boys socialize with boys. Mothers are more protective of their sons than their daughters.

National Childhood Immunizations: BCG at 2 months and 6 to 7 years; measles at 9 months and 6 to 7 years; OPV at 1 to 2, 3, 4, and 16 to 18 months and 6 to 7 years; DTP at 2, 3, 4, and 16 to 18 months; DT at 6 to 7 and 11 years; TT at 6 to 7, 11, and 14 years; and hep B at 3, 4, and 9 months.

Other Characteristics: Families often believe in the "evil eye." Mothers may fasten an evil eye pin on a child's clothing over one shoulder for protection.

BIBLIOGRAPHY

Aksit B: *Rural health seeking, culture and the economy: changes in Turkish villages,* Cambridgeshire, England, 1993, Eothen Press.

Bedük T, Ozhan N: Inservice education in Turkey, *J Cont Educ Nurs* 25(2):86, 1994.

Dardick KR, Neumann HH: *Foreign travel and immunization guide,* ed 13, Oradell, NJ, 1990, Medical Economics Books.

Epidemiological fact sheets on HIV/AIDS and sexually transmitted infections, Turkey 2000 Update (revised), UNAIDS and the World Health Organization.

Hatipoglu S, Tatar K: The strengths and weaknesses of Turkish bone-setters, *World Health Forum* 16(2):203, 1995.

Pozanti MS, Bruder P: The Turkish healthcare system, *Hosp Topics* 73(2):28, 1995.

1998 Turkish demographic and health survey, Ankara, Turkey, 1999, Hacettepe University Institute of Population Studies and Macro International.

U.S. State Department: http://www.state.gov/www/backgroundnotes/turkey 9910bgn.html

The state of world's children 2001, United Nations Children's Fund.
WHO vaccines, immunizations, and biologicals, http://www-nt.who.int/vaccines/globalsummary/Immunization/ScheduleResult.cfm

◆ TURKMENISTAN

MAP PAGE (861)

Location: Once part of the Persian Empire, Turkmenistan became an independent republic with the dissolution of the Soviet Union in 1991. This earthquake-prone country is located in southwestern central Asia, with Kazakhstan to the north, Uzbekistan to the north and east, Iran to the south, Afghanistan to the southeast, and the Caspian Sea to the west. The terrain is flat to rolling sandy desert, with dunes rising to mountains in the south, and low mountains along the Iranian border. The great Garagum Desert occupies 80% of the country. The climate is subtropical desert. Turkmenistan has the fifth largest gas reserves in the world, oil reserves, and intensive agriculture in irrigated oases. The total land area is 488,100 km^2 (188,456 square miles), slightly larger than California. Ashgabat is the capital. The population is estimated to be 4,603,244, and the GDP per capita is $4300.

Major Languages	Ethnic Groups	Major Religions
Turkmen (official)	Turkmen 77%	Muslim (mostly Sunni) 89%
Russian	Uzbek 10%	Eastern Orthodox 9%
Uzbek	Russian 7%	Unknown 2%
English	Kazakh 2%	
Ethnic languages	Other 4%	

Turkmen is spoken by about 75% of the population. Russian was the official language before the 1992 constitution was established and is still often used in official communications. Many who are Muslim are said not to be active adherents.

Health Care Beliefs: Passive role; acute sick care only. Since it is currently difficult to receive adequate health care, particularly in rural areas, healers who use prayers and herbs are very common. In some areas, healers may provide the only care available.

Predominant Sick Care Practices: Traditional; biomedical where available. The Soviet free health care system is still in place, with its emphasis on specialist rather than primary care. In the early 1990s, supply shortages and poorly trained doctors led to inadequate levels of care, leading to the highest infant mortality rates and lowest life expectancy in central Asia. One study found that because 70% of the obstetricians and gynecologists of Dashhowuz Province lacked adequate surgical training, 50% of their patients died. In 1996, only 15% of maternity clinics had piped-in water. In 1999 the republic had 13,800 doctors (36.2 per 10,000 people), and the country had 40,600 other medical personnel (106.9 per 100,000). Today, medical care is far below Western European and North American standards. The country has private and public doctors and public hospitals, but modern technologies and medical supplies such as disposable needles, oral rehydration salts for children, vaccines, anesthetics, and antibiotics may be in short supply or unavailable. Sanitation is generally lacking. Health care is more available in urban areas than rural, but treatment is frequently primitive. The state still maintains control over the system. However, new statutory sickness benefit programs have been instituted and involve an employment-based strategy that restricts coverage to those who are formally employed. The programs are funded by employer and employee contributions. Ground water supplies have become considerably polluted because of excessive pesticide use, and pesticides have also contaminated the dust that blows across the region.

Ethnic/Race Specific or Endemic Diseases: The most common causes of death in the mid-1990s were cardiovascular diseases, cancer, respiratory diseases, and accidents. Poor diet, polluted drinking water, and industrial wastes and pesticides cause many health problems, especially in the areas near the Amu Darya and Aral Sea. Endemic diseases include malaria, tuberculosis, and poliomyelitis. The country recently had an outbreak of hepatitis E virus. The people (especially children and women of child-bearing age) are at risk for anemia, leishmaniasis, and cryptosporidiosis. Traffic accidents are a major source of injury for drivers, passengers, and pedestrians. The World Health Organization's (WHO) estimated prevalence rate for HIV/AIDS in adults ages 15 to 49 years is 0.01%. The estimated number of children from birth to 15 years living with HIV/AIDS is less than 100. Deaths from HIV are also estimated to be less than 100. Other sexually transmitted diseases such as syphilis, gonorrhea, and hepatitis B are increasing dramatically. AIDS is expected to follow.

Dominance Patterns: Turkmen society still recognizes a class structure based on a Marxist doctrine that divides people into intelligentsia, workers, and peasants. The Turkmen comprise the intelligentsia. Peasants, and the worker class are primarily made up of Russians. The intelligentsia is Western oriented and has control over many key positions in government, education, and industry. Most intelligentsia go to Russian schools, complete higher education in Russian, speak Russian by choice, and tend to live and work in urban areas. Turkmen are divided into territorial groups similar to tribes or clans (*khalk, il,* or *taipa* in Turkmen). In the past, tribes were differentiated by their dialects, carpet patterns, clothing, and headgear. Although Soviet policy diminished tribal consciousness, tribal identity still affects social relationships (e.g., in arranged marriages). In urban and rural settings the communities' elders retain the greatest power and are sources of wisdom and spirituality. Women have (although it is infrequent) become influential leaders in the system. Families still tend to be closely knit, and it is common for sons to remain with their parents after marriage. Turkmen refuse to put their relatives in homes for older adults. Although labor is divided into male and female tasks and women do not actively participate in politics, they have never worn veils or been kept in strict seclusion. Economic necessity has forced many women into the workforce, disrupting traditional Muslim values, and many have professional careers.

Birth Rites: The birth rate is 28.55 births per 1000 people. The infant mortality rate is 73.25 deaths per 1000 live births (the highest in the region) and is attributed to poor diet and health care by some and poor hygiene and lack of family planning by others. The maternal mortality rate is 55 per 100,000 live births, which is very high for the region. The total fertility rate is 3.58 children born per woman. Women in their child-bearing years and children seem to have the worst health and be the most susceptible to disease compared with others in the society. Life expectancy at birth is 57.43 for men and 64.76 years for women, reportedly the lowest in the region.

Child Rearing Practices: About 38% of the population is 14 years or younger. It is estimated that 99% of males and 97% of females older than 15 are literate; education is compulsory through the eighth grade. Much of the Soviet educational system is still in place.

National Childhood Immunizations: BCG at birth and 6 to 7 and 14 to 15 years; DTP at 2, 3, 4, and 18 months; OPV at birth and 2, 3, 4, 18, and 20 months and 6 to 7 years; measles at 9 months and 5 to 6 years; Td at 5 to 6 and 15 to 16 years. The reported percentages of the target population vaccinated are as follows: BCG, 99; first dose of DTP, 97; third dose of DTP, 97; MCV, 97; and Pol3, 98.

Other Characteristics: In Turkmen society, marriage is an important event and is often arranged by matchmakers *(sawcholar);* the ceremony includes a bride price *(kalong)* that may be excessive. Most couples freely consent to the arrangement, and divorce is relatively rare. Turkmenistan is a limited illegal cultivator of opium poppies, most of which is for domestic consumption; the country has a limited government eradication program. Turkmenistan is becoming more common as a transshipment point for illegal drugs from Southwest Asia to Russia and Western Europe and as a transshipment point for acetic anhydride for Afghanistan.

BIBLIOGRAPHY

Dixon J: A global perspective on statutory Social Security programs for the sick, *J Health Soc Pol* 13(3):17, 2001.

O'Hara SL et al: Exposure to airborne dust contaminated with pesticide in the Aral Sea region, *Lancet* 355(9204): 627, 2000.

Small I, van der Meer J, Upshur RE: Acting on an environmental health disaster: the case of the Aral Sea, *Environ Health Perspect* 109(6):547, 2001.

Strelkova MV et al: Mixed leishmanial infections in *Rhombomys opimus*: a key to the persistence of *Leishmania* major from one transmission season to the next, *Ann Trop Med Parasitol* 95(8):811, 2001.

http://lcweb2.loc.gov/cgi-bin/query/r?frd/cstudy:@field(DOCID+tm0007

http://www.odci.gov/cia/publications/factbook/geos/tx.html
http://travel.state.gov/turkmenistan.html

◆ TUVALU

MAP PAGE (856)

Location: Located just south of the equator, Tuvalu (formerly the Ellice Islands) is a chain of nine scattered, small islands about 560 km (350 miles) extending from north to south in the South Pacific. Kiribati is to the north, Fiji is to the south, and the Solomon Islands are to the west. Tuvalu is a constitutional monarchy with a parliamentary democracy. Most of the islands are low-lying, narrow coral atolls about 1.8 m (6 feet) above sea level with poor soil. The capital is Funafuti. The total land area is 26 km^2 (10 square miles), about a tenth the size of Washington, DC. The climate is tropical and moderated by trade winds, with the chief crops being fish and coconuts. The total population is 10,991, and the gross domestic product (GDP) per capita is $1480.

Major Languages	Ethnic Groups	Major Religions
Tuvaluan	Polynesian 96%	Church of Tuvalu
English	Other 4%	(Congregational) 97%
		Seventh-Day Adventist,
		Bahai, other 3%

Predominant Sick Care Practices: Traditional and biomedical where available. Through the United Nations Development Program (UNDP) and the Volunteer Specialist Scheme, the UNDP provides the Central Hospital in Funafuti with a fully qualified surgeon. The government is now helping to pay for this project.

Ethnic/Race Specific or Endemic Diseases: Endemic diseases include dengue fever, typhoid fever, and hepatitis A. The World Health Organization (WHO) has no estimated prevalence rates for HIV/AIDS for adults or children.

Dominance Patterns: Living standards are much better in Funafuti than they are on the outer islands. Women comprise about 78% of the subsistence farming workforce but only 37% of the cash employment market. Gender differences tend to be small in Tuvalu but are reflected in inequalities in professional employment, secondary school enrollment, and overseas training opportunities. Most public service jobs held by women are clerical or unskilled positions. Women outnumber men in small private businesses, and women's groups are actively promoting better living conditions on the islands, particularly in the areas of health and sanitation. Nongovernmental organizations are supporting programs that address gender concerns and promote outreach for women.

Birth Rites: The birth rate is 21.56 births per 1000 people, and the infant mortality rate is 22.65 deaths per 1000 live births. Life expectancy at birth is 64.52 for men and 68.88 years for women.

National Childhood Immunizations: BCG at birth and 6 years; DTP at 6, 10, and 14 weeks; OPV at birth and 6, 10, and 14 weeks; hep B at birth, 6 weeks, and 9 months; measles at 9 months; and TT for pregnant women. The reported percentages of target population vaccinated are as follows: BCG, 100; first dose of DTP, 80; third dose of DTP, 75; third dose of hep B, 78; Pol3, 80; and TT2plus, 65.

Other Characteristics: Tuvalu has no streams or rivers, and the groundwater is not potable. Water is collected in catchment systems with storage facilities; the Japanese government has built one desalination plant and plans to build another. The islands had three cyclones in 1997.

BIBLIOGRAPHY

http://www.odci.gov/cia/publications/factbook/geos/tv.html
http://www.undp.org.fj/tuv/tuvaluprog.htm

◆ UGANDA (REPUBLIC OF)

MAP PAGE (863)

Moses N. Katabarwa

Location: Uganda is in the eastern part of the African continent and has a total land area of 244,295 km^2 (94,322 square miles). Uganda has Kenya as its neighbor to the east, Tanzania to the south, Rwanda to the southwest, Democratic Republic of Congo to the west, and Sudan to the north. It is a landlocked country with many mountains, fertile valleys, forests, grasslands, lakes, and rivers. The river Nile, the longest in Africa, has it source in Uganda at Lake Victoria.

Major Languages	Ethnic Groups	Major Religions
English (official)	Baganda 17%	Roman Catholic 33%
Swahili	Karamojong 12%	Protestant 33%
Luganda	Basogo 8%	Islam 16%
Ateso	Iteso 8%	Indigenous beliefs 18%
Luo	Langi 6%	
	Rawanda 6%	
	Bagisu 5%	
	Acholi 4%	
	Lugbara 4%	
	Bunyoro 3%	
	Batobo 3%	
	European, Asian, Arab 1%	
	Other 23%	

Uganda has three major ethnic groups in the country—Bantu, Luo, and Nilo-Hamites—who collectively speak more than 32 languages with more than 50 dialects. English, although not a local language, is widely spoken especially in the urban areas. Swahili is spoken mainly in urban centers and by members of security organizations such as the army, police, and prisons.

Health Care Beliefs: Traditional and modern; active role. Prevention and health promotion are widely promoted by the government as its main strategies for disease control. For example, people in Uganda have been educated about how people contract sexually transmitted diseases, diseases endemic in the country, and especially incurable diseases such as AIDS. The use of condoms or abstinence for unmarried people and monogamy for those who are married are encouraged. This practice has helped improve the health of many Ugandans. Parents have also been encouraged to adopt family planning methods so that they can have the ideal number of children for their circumstances, although this tends to be disregarded in most rural areas. Mental illness is feared and has a negative impact on the families of those who are affected. In fact, potential suitors may not want to marry individuals from families with members who are mentally ill. The relatives of those who are mentally ill often do not want to see the affected family member, and some may even wish that the person were dead. Whether people wear amulets depends on where people are from. In some tribal communities, people wear amulets to protect themselves from harm or cure illness, especially illness "sent" by those who are envious. The society is in transition, but some people still wear amulets under their clothes because exposing them may solicit criticism. One traditional practice is making cuts on the body area that has pain, putting a small animal horn (from goats or antelopes) on the cut, and sucking blood through it. The horn is believed to have special powers to remove disease. Herbs also may be rubbed in the wound.

Predominant Sick Care Practices: Biomedical and magical-religious. Sick people generally seek out modern medical treatment in private clinics, government hospitals, or health units. However, the majority of people in rural areas seek treatment from traditional healers or obtain herbal medicine first. If they are not healed by traditional practitioners, they then consult biomedical health practitioners. Some people use herbal treatments and biomedicine concurrently and may also consult church leaders, witch doctors, or soothsayers.

Ethnic/Race Specific or Endemic Diseases: Human herpes virus-8 (which is believed to be the etiological agent of Kaposi's sarcoma) accounts for half of the reported cases of cancer in Uganda. In addition, AIDS-associated Burkitt's lymphoma is also endemic. Other endemic diseases include sleeping sickness (*Trypanosoma brucei gambiense* and *T. brucei rhodesiense*), onchocerciasis (in the Rukungiri district), lymphatic filariasis, nonfilarial elephantiasis (in Mt. Elgon), dracunculiasis, schistosomiasis, tuberculosis, *Shigella* infections, dengue fever, and endomyocardial fibrosis. The country has no risk for Rift Valley fever, West Nile virus, or meningococcal disease. Falciparum malaria affects the majority of the population, and people often buy modern medicine from private clinics or government health centers. Most who go to private clinics, especially in rural areas, and the poor in cities get less than the required dosage of malaria medicine because of limited resources. Therefore recurrent malaria is common and can cause death. Because of economic constraints, when many people in the same family are sick they share medications (even a single dose), so none of them receive enough. The government has attempted to control malaria by providing mosquito nets cheaply and spraying houses in areas where epidemics are common. Community members have also been educated about how to reduce mosquito breeding. The common cold is rampant, especially during the dry season. Although not a serious threat to adults, colds are a major cause of morbidity in infants. The minority Pygmies of western Uganda still live in the forests and have no exposure to modern health facilities. In most cases, they use local herbs to treat themselves. However, with government prohibitions on use of forests, most of these people have no land, are malnourished, and have no access to health care or resources. Vigorous and constant campaigns against HIV/AIDS have been launched by the government, president of the country, health departments, church leaders, and nongovernmental organizations. The World Health Organization's (WHO) estimated prevalence rate for HIV/AIDS is 8.3%. The estimated number of children from birth to 15 years with HIV/AIDS is 53,000. However, more recent country reports state that the number of people with the disease has been reduced from a high of 35% to 6% today, and rates are continuing to decrease.

Health Team Relationships: Nurses usually do a lot of work compared with doctors. However, they are both overworked (with 1 nurse per 7000 people and 1 doctor per 23,000 people). Generally, their professional working relationships are good. Patients' attitudes toward doctors and nurses are positive. However, medical work is mystifying, and visiting a clinic is still a traumatic experience for many people. Doctors are highly respected but also feared, which may explain why many people, but especially those from rural areas, prefer to visit clinics as a last resort.

Families' Role in Hospital Care: Family members stay with patients in the hospital and take complete care of their sick relatives. For example, they ensure that the relatives receive and take medicine from the hospital or a private pharmacy. They provide food and drinks, bathe the patient, wash clothes, and even notify medical personnel when the condition of the patient is questionable.

Dominance Patterns: Ugandan culture favors men. In times of illness, women cater to their male relatives. When married women are sick, their sisters or mothers have traditionally left their homes to take care of them. However, the culture is changing, especially in urban areas. Today, most husbands care for their sick wives.

Eye Contact Practices: Eye contact is used for communication. For example, a twinkle of the eye can be used to warn someone not to say anything when asked a question. If an adult or close relative twinkles an eye to a child, it may imply that the child should go away. Lovers and young people in particular use eye contact to convey loving messages, especially when they do not want other people to know about or suspect their love affair. Young people are not supposed to look directly into the eyes of an adult because it is rude. Eye contact between young women and men is discouraged, and women who make unrestrained eye contact with men are taken to be harlots. However, older women can look directly into the eyes of a mature man. It is as if at a certain age a woman (especially one who has mature and married daughters and sons) acquires the same status as a mature and responsible man. Her advice is sought and is taken seriously. She therefore has the confidence and cultural support to look directly into the eyes of a man without being ridiculed.

Touch Practices: Depending on a person's geographical area, physical touching may or may not be acceptable. For example, the Bakiga greeting involves embracing others regardless of sex or age but not if they are strangers. In other cultures, it is not culturally acceptable to touch others, especially members of the opposite sex or strangers.

Perception of Time: Punctuality is not an issue in Uganda's traditional cultural settings. People do not make appointments since people are generally allowed to visit others without telling them first. Two exceptions involve visits by many people, which require previous arrangements with the host, and appointments at hospitals or health units. Those who come first are served first. Even when a person makes an appointment to see a doctor at a certain time, the doctor will not see the patient at the agreed on time. However, procedures are gradually changing, and some people make appointments and adhere to their times.

Pain Reactions: Different people from different cultures react to pain differently. During childbirth, women from central Uganda are free to shout out and cry, whereas women in other areas may face the wrath of other women if they do so. Occasionally pain, especially from a medical procedure, is appreciated since people think a medical procedure that inflicts pain is more effective. Women and children enduring pain from the loss of a loved one normally express it by crying, whereas men are expected to be more reserved. On the whole, men rarely show that they are in pain. Culture dictates that men are supposed to be strong and brave so that they can protect the women, children, and older adults.

Birth Rites: During and after birth, various rituals are performed in some rural areas, whereas in others and in cities, generally nothing is done.

Mothers bathe immediately after giving birth and are given the best food that the family can afford. The traditional culture still favors and celebrates a son's birth more than a daughter's. In most homes with no sons, a man is allowed to marry another wife to have a son. This practice is gradually changing.

Death Rites: Death rites are observed, especially in the central and eastern parts of the country. People believe that someone must take the place of the person who died. When a woman dies and leaves behind young children, someone is appointed to take the place of the mother. When a man dies, a male relative is appointed to take care of the family. Appointed caretakers are highly respected by the people they care for. Death is feared and believed to be caused by someone. In traditional communities, every death is caused by someone. Hatred and family and community divisions may develop, and occasionally suspected families are attacked and ostracized. Those in strong Christian homes believe that God allows death and all people die at their predetermined time; therefore Christians do not believe that people could have caused a death. Family members may be present at the time of a relative's death depending on the nature of the death and whether the person was living with relatives or not. If a person has been at home and sick for some time, relatives are likely to be close. After learning of a family death, all close relatives and friends from near and far are informed either through radio announcements or messengers. All close relatives at the funeral participate in the burial arrangements in some way. Organ donations are uncommon, and very few people agree to autopsies because of fears and beliefs they have about the procedure; it is generally believed that removing body organs as part of an autopsy may cause bewitchment of the dead person's family members. Others do not approve of autopsy out of respect for the dead, a result of cultural beliefs about tampering with dead people.

Food Practices and Intolerances: In the past, certain foods were only eaten by certain sexes, although men were allowed to eat most foods. Banyankole women were not allowed to eat chicken, the tongue of any animal, or goat meat; if a woman ate a cow's tongue, she would become the main spokesperson for her family and leave the man in an inferior position. These practices are not common today. Uganda is an agricultural country with a variety of foods, and favorite foods vary among ethnic groups. People in the north prefer millet, *posho* (corn meal), meat, and beans at every meal. People from the western part of the country prefer to have a variety of *matooke* (bananas), meat, beans, millet, Irish potatoes, and milk. Those in the central part of the country are not impressed if a meal does not include *matooke*. People may use their hands or a fork, spoon, and knife; however, in rural areas, most people still use their hands while eating.

Infant Feeding Practices: Most mothers breast-feed their children, with the exception of a few employed and busy mothers who work far from their homes. These mothers bottle-feed during the day and breast-feed after office hours. Most mothers believe that as long as they are breast-feeding, they cannot become pregnant; breast-feeding is also used as a family planning method.

Child Rearing Practices: Child rearing may be permissive or strict depending on whether people live in a rural or an urban area. Whereas mothers in rural areas have a significant role in looking after their children, extended relatives such as grandparents or other relatives also take part in some way. They help feed the children and take care of them when their mothers are working. In rural areas, anyone looking after the children can discipline them when they do something wrong. In urban areas, child rearing is more complex because no extended family members are available. Parents hire maids to look after the children when they are not at home. In these situations, parents are responsible for most of the disciplining. The majority of parents, even in rural areas, do not sleep with their children in the same bed. They may sleep in the same room until the children can be alone in their rooms or huts or share accommodations with older siblings.

National Childhood Immunizations: BCG at birth or first contact; DTP at 6 weeks or first contact and at 10 and 14 weeks; OPV at birth and 6, 10, and 14 weeks; measles at 9 months or first contact; vitamin A at 9 months; and TT for pregnant women, CBAW 15 to 44 years. Childhood immunizations continue throughout the year. When coverage decreases, the government organizes immunization programs so that every eligible child is covered.

BIBLIOGRAPHY

Adler MW, ed: Statistics from the World Health Organization and the Centers for Disease Control, *AIDS* 6(10):1229, 1992.

Anderson SR et al: AIDS education in rural Uganda: a way forward, *Int J STD AIDS* 1(5):335, 1990.

Blair J: Health teaching in the context of culture: nursing in East Africa, *Kansas Nurse* 6(4):4, 1991.

Kater V: Health education in Jinja, Uganda, *IMAGE: J Nurs Sch* 28(2):161, 1996.

MacNeil JM: Use of culture care theory with Baganda women as AIDS caregivers, *J Transcultural Nurs* 7(2):14, 1996.

Sutton J: *AIDS in Uganda,* 1996, World Vision Childlife.

Wright J: Female genital mutilation: an overview, *J Adv Nurs* 24:251, 1996.

◆ UKRAINE

MAP PAGE (861)

Igor Y. Galaychuk

Location: Ukraine is located in southeastern Europe, and it shares borders with seven other countries, including Moldavia and Romania (on the southwest); Hungary, Slovakia, and Poland (on the west); Belarus (on the north); and Russia (on the east). To the south, Ukraine's borders are defined by the Black Sea and the Sea of Azov. The territory of the country extends 900 km from the north to the south and 1300 km from the east to the west. Ukraine has a total land area of 603,700 km^2 (233,100 square miles). After Russia, it is the second largest country on the European continent. The country has large areas with arable black soil, as well as the Carpathian and Crimean mountain chains. The population is about 48 million. Kyiv is the capital city and is located on the Dnieper River. Chernobyl, where the nuclear power plant disaster occurred in 1986, is located 100 km north of Kyiv. Ukraine regained its independence in 1991 with the dissolution of the former Soviet Union.

Major Languages	Ethnic Groups	Major Religions
Ukrainian	Ukrainian 73%	Orthodox 76%
Russian	Russian 22%	Ukrainian Catholic (Uniate) 14%
	Jewish 1%	Jewish 2%
	Other 4%	Baptist, Mennonite, Protestant, Muslim 8%

Health Care Beliefs: Traditional; modern; acute sick care. The population at large realizes that diseases can be prevented. However, smoking, alcohol abuse by young and middle-age people, hard manual labor in the rural areas, and stress connected with the economic crisis of the society are the background against which many mental and somatic diseases have emerged. Lately, so-called "healers" and extrasensory practitioners have expanded their practices, and patients who have not received proper qualified help in legal medical institutions consult these healers as a last resort. It is almost impossible to evaluate the effectiveness of their work because they do not gather any statistics.

Predominant Sick Care Practices: Biomedical; traditional. Ukraine has a state system of health promotion. The treatment and disease prevention service is established in hospitals that are divided into comprehensive (province, city, district) and specialized facilities, such as pediatric, communicable disease, oncology, endocrinology, ophthalmology, and maternity. Other facilities include out-patient clinics, polyclinic for adults and for children, women's clinics and maternity welfare centers, and village out-patient clinics. Doctors also provide health services in patient's homes. Ukraine has urgent care clinics as well. Doctors (e.g., therapists, cardiologists, general surgeons, traumatologists, pediatricians) go to the homes of sick people by ambulance or other vehicles, and provide medical help. If necessary, patients are admitted to a hospital. Sanatoriums and health resorts (e.g. general health resorts, children's sanatoriums) are popular for treatment. Another facility that is very popular is the balneological hospital—a resort where patients can be treated with mineral water, silt, salt, and other natural items. The origin of the word *balneology (balneotherapy)* is the Latin *balneum,* meaning "bathhouse" or "bathing." In Ukraine, natural resources are used extensively for treatment (e.g., mineral and spring waters for drinking and bathing, therapeutic mud and wax baths for skin, radon and oxygen baths, salt-mine air). Because of the current economic crisis, the financing of health promotion has been reduced dramatically, causing the closure of small hospitals in rural areas and a subsequent lack of care for these populations.

Ethnic Race/Specific or Endemic Diseases: The major illnesses affecting the population are cardiovascular diseases (e.g., high blood pressure, ischemia, cerebrovascular disease), infections and parasitosis, trauma, mental diseases, malignancies, and tuberculosis. Cardiovascular diseases are the major causes of mortality (with 847 deaths per 100,000 people in 1997) followed by malignant diseases (192 deaths), traumas (147), infectious diseases (22), tuberculosis (17), and mental disorders (6.6). Thyroid disease, caused by a lack of iodine in soil and water, is endemic in western Ukraine. The World Health Organization's (WHO) estimated prevalence rate for HIV/AIDS in adults ages 15 to 49 is 0.96%. The estimated number of children from birth to 15 years living with HIV/AIDS is 7500. The first cases of HIV infection were registered in 1987, but by 1995 infections were reaching epidemic proportions. According to WHO, the estimated number of adults and children living with HIV/AIDS at the end of 1999 was 240,000, of which 70,000 were women. In 1999, 570 AIDS cases were registered (441 male and 129 female). The total number of AIDS cases from 1988 to 1999 was 1277.

Health Team Relationships: Doctors are in a dominant position relative to nurses. Nurses generally carry out doctors' orders, and occasionally conflicts arise when nurses do not performed as expected. The relationships between the patient and the doctor and the patient and the nurse often involve "gifts" (bribes) from the patient.

Families' Role in Hospital Care: The majority of patients do not have medical insurance, and the state provides only a little medication. Patients have to buy the majority of their medications, bandages, and other supplies themselves in drug stores. Today, people can buy any type of medicine in drug stores, but they are very expensive and difficult on the family budget. The patients' relatives volunteer to look after them and prepare home-cooked meals. The meals in hospitals are served three times a day, but in most cases the food is low in calories and tasteless.

Dominance Patterns: According to the Constitution of Ukraine, men and women have equal rights. Women comprise approximately 75% of all the workers in the health system (e.g., hospital attendants, paramedics, nurses, doctors), and in 1999 and 2000 a woman was the Minister of Health.

Eye Contact Practices: Direct eye contact is acceptable.

Touch Practices: Ukrainians have no religious or sexual restrictions relating to touch during medical examinations.

Perceptions of Time: In general, punctuality depends on where people live and their social status. In urban areas, people try to be on time, whereas in rural areas the notion of time is often quite flexible.

Pain Reactions: People accept analgesics and usually try to relieve their pain. Narcotic analgesics for patients with cancer are paid for by the state fund.

Birth Rites: Most Ukrainian families have two children. Many hope that the first-born child will be a boy and the second will be a girl. No problems arise if this does not happen. In maternity hospitals, doctors and midwives assist women during childbirth, and it is not common for the fathers to be present at the time of delivery. After the delivery, mothers and infants are placed in different wards. During pregnancy and while breast-feeding, most mothers do not drink alcohol, smoke, or eat chocolate or citrus fruit. They avoid taking medications unless they are absolutely necessary.

Death Rites: The dominant religion in Ukraine is Christianity, and people accept the inevitability of death. If a person dies in a hospital, an autopsy is usually performed to identify the reason for death on a morphological level. If a person dies at home, family members are usually present. Ukraine has no hospice system. Death is followed by funerals with a priest, relatives, and neighbors. Ukraine has not yet legalized the sale of cadavers' organs.

Food Practices and Intolerances: In Ukraine the main meals are breakfast (until 9 AM), lunch (from 1 to 2 PM), and dinner (after 7 PM). Lunch usually consists of a first course (borscht, or soup), a second course (meat with potatoes) with a salad (of cabbage, tomatoes, or cucumbers), and a third course of tea or coffee and dessert. Traditionally the population eats a lot of bread, potatoes, and dairy products. Borscht with dumplings, *varenyky* (pirogy) with cottage cheese, and pork lard are all national Ukrainian dishes. Of the meat products, Ukrainians seem to prefer pork. Sugar is made from the sugar beets that are grown in large quantities in the country. Of the alcoholic drinks, *horilka* (40% vodka) is the most popular.

Infant Feeding Practices: Approximately 20% of mothers breast-feed during the first year. The majority of women begin bottle-feeding after several weeks or months of breast-feeding.

Child Rearing Practices: Children are reared by their families and in school. From early childhood, children are taught to be disciplined and obedient. From 1 to 6 years, children attend kindergarten, where they are cared for by teachers (from 8 or 9 AM to 5 or 6 PM). They are given food four times per day and have a nap after lunch. Teachers read books, tell fairy tales, organize games, and take children for outdoor walks. The number of kindergartens has drastically decreased because of the economic crisis.

National Childhood Immunizations: BCG at birth and at 7 and 14 years; DTP at 3 and 18 months; OPV at 3 and 18 months and 3, 6, and 14 years; measles at 12 months and 6 years; DT at 6 years; and Td at 11, 14, and18 years.

Other Characteristics: The country has developed machine-building, mining, metallurgical, and chemical industries, which are all connected with the country's environmental pollution problem. The pollution in 1 m^2 in industrial regions is 6.5 times higher than it is in the United States and 3.2 times higher than it is in other European countries. It is estimated that 21% of all diseases in Ukraine are caused by the polluted environment, and another 13% are directly attributed to polluted drinking water. The serious socioeconomic crisis of the last 8 to 10 years has affected the country's demographical situation. Since 1991, the population has not increased. Today the mortality rate exceeds the birth rate by more than 300,000 every year, and the average life expectancy has decreased from 70 to approximately 60 years.

BIBLIOGRAPHY

Ponomarenko VM, ed: *Health protection in Ukraine: the problems and perspectives,* Ternopil, "Ukrmedknyha", 1999.

Voronenko YV, Moskalenko VF, eds: *Social medicine and management of health protection*,Ternopil, "Ukrmedknyha", 2000.

Little RE et al: Outcomes of 17137 pregnancies in two urban areas of Ukraine, *Am J Public Health* 89:1832, 1999.

http://www.britannica.com/Ukraine

◆ UNITED ARAB EMIRATES

MAP PAGE (864)

Haider Al Attia (Consultant: Abdulbari Bener)

Location: Situated on the eastern side of the Arabian Peninsula, the country is primarily desert and rich in oil. Its boundaries are the Persian Gulf to the north, Gulf of Oman to the northeast, Oman to the east, Saudi Arabia to south and west, and a short frontier with Qatar to the northwest. The seven emirates are Ajman, Abu Dhabi, Dubai, Fujairah, Ras al-Khaimah, Sharjah, and Umm Al Qaiwain. The total land area is 82,880 km^2 (31,969 square miles). The emirate of Abu Dhabi comprises 85% of the total area, and the smallest emirate, Ajman, measures only about 100 square miles or 259 km^2. United Arab Emirates (UAE) has undergone rapid economic development since the discovery of oil and has become a center for commercial and financial activities in the region, especially Dubai Emirate.

Major Languages	Ethnic Groups	Major Religions
Arabic	Emirati 19%	Sunni Muslim 96%
Farsi (Persian)	Other Arab and	Other 4%
English	Iranian 23%	
Hindi	South Asian 43%	
Urdu	Westerners and	
	East Asians 7%	
	Other 8%	

The United Arab Emirates has had one of the highest population growth rates in the world during the past 26 years. Its vast economic development and increased demands for labor in all fields attract several thousands of expatriates and their families each year; it has one of the highest per capita incomes in the world. The population pyramid has a unique composition. It has a normal base for children and then broadens in the 20- to 50-year-old age group (a group comprising 42.8%, primarily men because of the influx of young expatriate male workers). The pyramid then gets narrower as the age exceeds 50 years; about 3% is older than 60. Compared with some other societies that have experienced rapid transformations because of oil wealth, the UAE has certain advantages relating to the geography of the country. The hinterland of desert, oases, wadis, and mountains and the sea, with its coast and remote islands, all provide opportunities for city dwellers to physically recapture the old way of life and reestablish contact with members of their family or tribe.

Health Care Beliefs: Traditional and modern; active and passive roles. The community is multicultural and multiethnic and has many different health beliefs. Individuals of higher status who can afford health care are more aware of health promotion and prevention programs, whereas by necessity the poor are more crisis oriented. The UAB has a ministerial Preventive Medicine Department at the Ministry of Health that is responsible for prevention programs. The programs include vaccinations, public health education (e.g., antismoking and anticancer campaigns). The ministry also runs school health programs and conducts surveys on various diseases such as diabetes mellitus and asthma. Early screening programs for children and adults, promotion of occupational health and safety, and promotion of a healthy lifestyle are gaining ground. Efforts should concentrate on health education for reducing mortality and morbidity of communicable and noncommunicable diseases. Early detection and efficient management of diseases should be stressed.

Predominant Sick Care Practices: Biomedical. Economic development has been accompanied by public health problems but also by an improvement in the health infrastructure and services since the establishment of the federation. The high quality and accessibility of health services are reflected by sharp decreases in infant mortality from 14.7% to 6.57% per 1000 live births in 1999. In addition, the high life expectancy at birth is close to the ages of Western and developed countries (74 years for men and 76 years for women). The Primary Health Care Clinics (PHC) is a package of comprehensive care offered to individuals, UAE citizens, expatriate workers, families, and the community. The Ministry of Health has made great efforts to develop the services of PHC to make them more equitable and accessible to all residents. The number of PHC centers increased from 45 clinics in 1977 to 105 health centers by the end of 1999. Health status and socioeconomic conditions of the population have markedly improved. Prosperity and modernization of the lifestyle in recent years has made many urban individuals more sensitive toward pain and disease. Their reactions to minor illnesses of loved ones, relatives, or members of their own tribe tend to be exaggerated and more expressive. Gravely morbid or terminal illnesses are fought relentlessly, and occasionally extraordinary measures are taken to prolong life merely to satisfy family or tribal members.

Ethnic/Race Specific or Endemic Diseases: Endemic diseases include hepatitis A and B, α- and β-thalassemia, cystic echinococcosis, and malaria (endemic or imported from Oman). People are at risk for brucellosis, Crimean Congo fever, and viral hemorrhagic fever. The incidence of cardiovascular disease is increasing fairly rapidly; in addition to accidents and cancer, cardiovascular disease is one of the major causes of death. Other noncommunicable diseases such as diabetes mellitus and congenital abnormalities have recently emerged as major causes of mortality. The World Health Organization (WHO) has no reported estimated prevalence rates in the UAE for HIV/AIDS for adults or children. However, the UAE has a comprehensive national HIV/AIDS plan in place that has screened 3 million people over the last 6 years. To reduce the spread of the disease, expatriates who are tested and found to be infected are deported to their home countries. A major decrease in rates of all infectious diseases in all age groups has evolved, especially among children, but non-communicable diseases have become the leading causes of morbidity and mortality; overall, the proportional mortality rates of the top five causes of death in 1998 clearly show this: cardiovascular disease (23.9%), motor vehicle crashes and injuries (16.8%), cancer (8.3%), congenital anomalies (5.1%), and respiratory diseases (2.7%). The prevalence of hypertension has increased to 14% in people 18 to 45 years and 42% in those older than 45. Diabetes mellitus seems to be highly prevalent in the adult Emirati population (15%). Because of these alarming data, great efforts have been directed toward the prevention and control of cardiovascular risk factors, hypertension, diabetes mellitus, and cancer. Hypertension, diabetes clinics, and nutrition clinics have become an essential part of the standard structure of PHC centers.

Health Team Relationships: Public hospitals have facilities for handling medical emergencies and accidents, as well as programs to handle disasters resulting in numerous casualties. Health services are available throughout the country, although their standards may vary. In large hospitals, the number of medical staff members seems adequate, but they have proportionally fewer health professionals than in Western countries. The inequitable geographical distribution of health care resources has long been recognized as a problem despite immense progress. Health care personnel, like many other professionals, tend to move to cities and large towns in numbers that exceed their need. Those who specialize in medicine, nursing, or one of many other health care professions have to be located to places with larger populations to ensure they have an adequate patient base. Nurses have recently begun migrating to Western countries because they offer better conditions overall.

Families' Role in Hospital Care: Family members or close friends stay with hospitalized patients and expect to participate in care or take on a vigilant, supervisory role.

Dominance Patterns: For all practical purposes the role of men within the society is frequently that of decision maker for all members of the family. The male head of the family is its provider, spokesman, and representative, although the women are often the primary decision makers. The man who heads the household upholds the Islamic norms of conduct for the outside world and embodies the social standing of the family within the community. If he is a true local, his children will never be considered anything less than full members of the local tribal society, even if their mother is foreign. The social standing of an individual man—and consequently of his entire family—depends first and foremost on the purity of his tribal Arab lineage. However, this does not mean that a man of pure tribal stock is invariably in a higher position than a wealthy man of uncertain tribal background. Social standing based on a man's wealth is determined by the level at which he can expected to arrange marriages for the members of his family. A woman has no position in the world outside the home, whereas her position within the family circle is a reflection of her personality and depends on the way she uses this confined environment to develop her abilities. Neither man nor woman has an identity other than in the context of the family to which they belong. In the Arab world, men marry their paternal uncle's daughter (i.e., cousin) so often that another name for a wife is "my uncle's daughter," even when couples are not related. In the UAE a cross-sectional population study showed that the frequency of consanguineous marriages in Al-Ain City, Abu Dhabi Emirate, and Dubai Emirate is very high and has increased (about 50.5%). Consanguinity is more common among women with educated husbands (with secondary or university educations) than among women with less educated husbands. Mothers, even educated ones, tend to stay at home, raise the children, and conform to the traditional role of women in an Islamic society. Regardless, changes have taken place in the last decade, and more and more women are developing careers. With better education, it is expected that cultural habits such as consanguineous marriages will decrease. They have not in the UAE, and arranged marriages are more common and there are few opportunities for members of the opposite sex to meet and socialize. When a husband and wife divorce or the husband dies, the sons are expected to support their mothers by providing a house and money if necessary or to take her into their own homes.

Eye Contact Practices: About 15% of adult women cover their faces with a veil. The majority of women do not cover their eyes; therefore direct eye contact is possible during conversations, although it must stay within the boundaries of modesty.

Touch Practices: Touch during professional examinations of patients has no gender restrictions. However, in general, female patients prefer female doctors and male patients often feel more comfortable with male doctors.

Perceptions of Time: People are fairly relaxed about punctuality.

Pain Reactions: Religious and socioeconomic issues and cultural background seem to have an important influence on how people react to pain. Individuals of *pathan* background (i.e., mountain people) seem to be more tolerant of pain than individuals in other communities. It has been observed that some Arabs tend to be more expressive than others as if they have a genetically determined pain threshold.

Birth Rites: Muslim parents usually read verses of the holy Koran to their infants. Immediate bathing after birth is discouraged if the baby is covered with vernix caseosa and is delayed for 12 to 24 hours.

Death Rites: The religious, socioeconomic, and cultural backgrounds of individuals also affect attitudes about death. Muslims who have a strong belief in Islamic teaching tend to be less emotionally expressive when in despair. They also consider death as not only the ultimate fate of each and every soul but also as an absolute surrender to Allah's will. Death is a test of the strength of their faith, so they should try to bear its pain with strength. Muslim doctors may recommend transfusions to save lives, and organ donations are permitted. Autopsies are uncommon because the deceased person must be buried intact, and cremations are not permitted. For Muslim burials the body is wrapped in special pieces of cloth and buried without a coffin in the ground immediately after death.

Food Practices and Intolerances: Pork, carrion, and blood are forbidden. The cuisine is similar to that of other Middle Eastern countries and consists of *falafel* (balls of chickpea paste that are deep fried and served in flat bread), *fuul* (fava beans, garlic, and honey paste), hummus (chickpeas with garlic and lemon), and *shawarma* (chicken or lamb served in flat bread). Food tends to be spicy. Alcohol is sold only in restaurants and bars of three-star hotels. Ramadan fasting is practiced by all except those who are sick or children.

Infant Feeding Practices: In infant-friendly hospitals such as those in the UAE, the importance of colostrum is well known and breast-feeding is highly encouraged within 30 minutes after delivery for healthy infants. A recent prospective cohort study of 221 infants described factors affecting initiation, patterns, and supplemental feeding in the UAE. None of the mothers opted not to breast-fed, but only 4% exclusively breast-fed during the first month (although 51% initiated breast-feeding on the first day of life). Factors associated with delaying initiation of breast-feeding after the first day of life included low birth weight, complicated delivery, ignorance about the advantages of colostrum, and young maternal age. Nonmilk supplements fed to babies included water, tea, juice, and *yansun* and *babunj* (local herbal drinks).

Child Rearing Practices: Child rearing in general is no longer as strict as it was. Although the UAE has a patriarchal society, boys and girls seem to do what they like. However, the attitudes and gestures of girls are more closely observed by other members of the family. Both parents seem to share the responsibility for disciplining their children, but the father has the upper hand.

National Childhood Immunizations: BCG at birth; DTP at 2, 4, 6, and 18 months; OPV at 2, 4, 6, and 18 months; hep B at birth and 1 and 9 months; HIB at 2, 4, 6, and 15 months; measles at 9 months; and MMR at 15 months. The steady decrease in childhood diseases is a positive indicator of the effectiveness of prevention and control strategies. Economic development has resulted in the spread of vaccination centers throughout the country, and health education has succeeded in attaining and sustaining a high coverage rate of more than 90%.

ACKNOWLEDGMENT: Abdulbari Bener was a consultant for infectious/noninfectious diseases.

BIBLIOGRAPHY

Al-Hosani H. Health for all in the United Arab Emirates, *Eastern Med Health J* 6:838–840, 2000.

Al-Mazroui MJ et al: Breastfeeding and supplemental feeding for neonates in Al-Ain, the United Arab Emirates, *J Trop Pediatr* 43:304–306, 1997.

Alwash R, Abbas A: Public health practice, the United Arab Emirates, *Public Health Med* 1:113–117, 1999.

Bener A et al: Consanguinity and associated socio-demographic factors in the United Arab Emirates, *Human Heredity* 46:256–264, 1996.

Bener A, Denic S, Al-Mazrouei M: Consanguinity and family history of cancer in children with leukemia and lymhomas, *Cancer* 92:1–6, 2001.

Bener A et al: The health services performance in United Arab Emirates, *Emirates Med J* 12:15–21, 1994.

Denic S, Bener A: Consanguinity decreases disk of breast cancer—cervical cancer unaffected, *Brit J Cancer* 85:1675–1679, 2001.

Heard-Bey F: From trucial states to United Arab Emirates: a society in transition, New York, 1984, Longman Group.

Preventive Medicine Department, Ministry of Health, United Arab Emirates: *Annual report 1998,* Abu Dhabi, United Arab Emirates, 1998.

World Health Organization (2001): *WHO vaccine-preventable diseases: monitoring system,* Geneva. Retrieved March 1, 2002, from http://www.who.int/vaccines/

◆ UNITED KINGDOM

MAP PAGE (860)

Angela Ellis

Location: The United Kingdom, which consists of England, Scotland, Wales, and Northern Ireland, is an island nation off the coast of France in the northern Atlantic Ocean. The total land area is 244,820 km² (94,525 square miles). It has about 60 million residents. The capital of the United Kingdom is London, the largest city in the country, with about 8 million people. Thanks to the moderating effects of the Gulf Stream, the United Kingdom enjoys a temperate climate despite its northern latitude.

Major Languages	Ethnic Groups	Major Religions
English	English 81%	Church of England
Welsh	Scottish 10%	Church of Wales
Scottish Gaelic	Irish, Welsh,	Church of Scotland
	Ulster 6%	Church of Ireland
	West Indian, Indian,	Roman Catholic,
	Pakistani, other 3%	Methodist,
		Congregational,
		Baptist, Jewish

English is the major language of the United Kingdom. Although Welsh and Scottish Gaelic are also officially recognized by the government, all adult Welsh or Scottish Gaelic speakers also know English. Some recent immigrants, many of whom come from former colonies of the United Kingdom, have yet to learn English.

Health Care Beliefs: Modern; increasingly active role in health prevention. Generally, Britons understand the need for prevention of disease through healthy living, but many fail to act on the knowledge. As in the United States and other affluent countries, the temptations of smoking, drinking, unhealthy eating, and physical inactivity can overwhelm people's will to maintain healthy lifestyles. Although Britons are coming to consider mental illness as less shameful, a certain stigma is still attached to diseases such as depression and schizophrenia, and people with these conditions often face discrimination from people who believe them to be potentially violent.

Predominant Sick Care Practices: Biomedical and complementary. Most Britons consult doctors when they are ill or injured. The National Health

Service provides medical care for all residents, but concerns about the quality and availability of treatment remain a main topic of debate in British politics. The last few decades have witnessed a growing interest in alternative forms of health care. According to a 1999 survey conducted for the British Broadcasting Corporation (BBC), 21% of respondents had relied on a form of alternative medicine in the past year, an increase from 10% 6 years ago. Popular choices include massage, aromatherapy, acupuncture, and herbal remedies. Perhaps a better term for this kind of treatment is *complementary medicine,* because although Britons have become more willing to consider new techniques, the majority also continues to rely simultaneously on more orthodox treatment options.

Ethnic/Race-Specific or Endemic Diseases: The leading killer of Britons is heart disease, and Scotland has the highest heart disease levels in the world. For every 100,000 deaths in the United Kingdom in 1999, 196.5 were from heart disease, whereas the deaths in Scotland alone were 241 per 100,000. Experts often attribute this dubious distinction to widespread smoking and poor eating habits among the Scots, but perhaps their susceptibility to heart attacks and strokes is a result of larger trend of northern poverty. In other words, Scots might often have cardiovascular disease not because they are Scots but because of the link between poverty and poor health. Furthermore, poor treatment by the National Health Service and long waits for its services aggravate the problem for all populations. Tooth decay also plagues the British, especially in the poorer north. Artificial fluoridation of drinking water has yet to become standard in the United Kingdom, and only 10% of Britons benefit from this method of strengthening teeth. The west Midlands has the highest levels of fluoridation in the nation, whereas Northern Ireland, parts of Scotland and Wales, the northwest of England, and inner London lag behind and have high levels of tooth decay. The efficacy of fluoridation in promoting British dental health is evidenced by statistics indicating that 5-year-olds in Birmingham in the west Midlands have three times less tooth decay and need three times fewer teeth extracted than their counterparts in Manchester in the northwest of England, where the water is not treated. Arguments that fluoride causes health problems such as Alzheimer's disease, Down syndrome, and cancer still carry weight among many Britons. Water companies, not the government, decide whether to fluoridate water, and many claim that their customers consider dental health to be a private concern. Previously rare communicable diseases have become a more significant problem in the United Kingdom. As the climate warms, British vacationers range farther afield, and immigrants from less developed countries enter the United Kingdom. British doctors have had to become more aware of illnesses such as malaria and tuberculosis. For example, in 2001 a particularly virulent strain of tuberculosis caused the worst outbreak in 2 decades at a school in Leicester. An area doctor had misdiagnosed the original carrier as having asthma, not tuberculosis. The vast majority of students at the school were of South

Asian ethnic origin; South Asia, in addition to sub-Saharan Africa, is a hotbed of the disease. However, health officials stress that the majority of people with tuberculosis in Britain are native to the United Kingdom, so the disease is not limited to immigrant populations. However, ethnic minorities in the United Kingdom, usually defined by the British Department of Health as coming from the Black Caribbean, Pakistan, Bangladesh, India, China, and Ireland, do face health problems specifically related to their minority status. Cardiovascular disease, diabetes, and obesity all affect members of immigrant groups at a higher rate than other Britons. Poverty is probably mostly to blame for ill health among ethnic minorities, but racism and lack of education about health also play a part. For example, on average, members of ethnic minority groups such as Bangladeshi men smoke more, which clearly is associated with the high rates of heart disease in this group. In addition, South Asian men develop oral cancer at a higher rate because of the cultural tradition of chewing tobacco and betel leaves. On a more positive note, other than the Irish, British ethnic minorities drink less alcohol than the average, and rates of tooth decay among minority children have decreased dramatically in recent years. The World Health Organization's (WHO) estimated prevalence rate for HIV/AIDS in adults ages 15 to 49 is 0.11%. The estimated number of children from birth to 15 years living with HIV/AIDS is 500. Of approximately 60 million Britons, slightly fewer than 50,000 are infected with HIV. The percentage of infections through heterosexual sex has increased, but it is probable that in some of those cases infection occurred abroad. The percentage of infections from intravenous drug use and homosexual sex has decreased.

Health Team Relationships: As part of an attempt to modernize the National Health Service (NHS), the United Kingdom's Department of Health recently implemented numerous new programs to break down traditional barriers between doctors, nurses, and other health care providers. For instance, to ameliorate the chronic shortage of doctors in the NHS system, nurses, who provide the vast majority of direct patient care, have received broader prescription powers within the last 3 years. Specially trained prescribing nurses can order drugs to treat minor injuries and ailments such as cuts and ear infections, medications that promote healthier living such as vitamins for pregnant women, and drugs that provide palliative care for chronic illnesses such as asthma and diabetes. Unfortunately, nurses, in addition to doctors, remain in short supply in the United Kingdom, partly because they receive low pay and insufficient recognition considering the highly trained, professional nature of their work. Furthermore, doctors often criticize changes that would allow other health care professionals to take on role responsibilities formerly reserved for doctors.

Families' Role in Hospital Care: Britons tend to consider health care as a service best provided by professionals. Families generally offer emotional support to hospitalized relatives but do not provide actual physical care. For example, despite widespread concern about the quality of hospital food, most patients in British hospitals still expect to eat food provided by the hospital rather than meals brought in by family members.

Dominance Patterns: Most Britons would agree that equality between men and women is desirable, but reality fails to achieve the ideal. Moreover, socioeconomic class distinctions are more fixed than they are in the United States. Nonetheless, younger generations are becoming less deferential toward their supposed social superiors, as the growing disinterest in and resentment of the royal family demonstrates.

Eye Contact Practices: In British culture, people do not avoid direct eye contact because of status or gender. Looking directly at a speaker indicates that the listener is paying attention, and not doing so suggests inattention. In large cities, many residents avoid eye contact with strangers in public as a way to maintain a sense of privacy in crowded surroundings but would not do so in a health care setting.

Touch Practices: As do the residents of many northern European countries, the British prefer to maintain an area of personal space. They also tend to reserve deliberate physical touching other than shaking hands for those they know well. British culture allows women and men and women and women to touch each other more freely than men and men. Younger generations are also more open to expressing physical affection. Most Britons allow health care providers to touch them as needed for diagnosis and treatment.

Perceptions of Time: The British place a high value on punctuality. Generally they strive to arrive at appointments on time and expect others to do the same.

Pain Reactions: The British tend to expect stoical toleration of physical and emotional pain. Outward displays of discomfort make others uncomfortable.

Birth Rites: The vast majority of British mothers deliver their children in hospitals under the care of doctors. During the last few years, some in the United Kingdom have expressed concern that 20% of British infants are delivered via cesarean section despite WHO's recommendation that cesareans should not constitute more than 10% to 15% of births. Numerous critics of the practice have suggested that perhaps British mothers have become "too posh to push," meaning that they prefer the convenience of a scheduled cesarean section to the pain and un-predictability of natural delivery. Still, at the same time, the country has experienced an increasing demand for midwives, so at least some pregnant women are hoping for less routine medical intervention in their deliveries. In mainstream British culture, Brits have no preference for boys or girls. At the very most, parents might hope for a boy if they already have a girl or a girl if they already have a boy. On the whole, British parents wish for healthy infants regardless of sex, and most have their wish granted because the United Kingdom's infant mortality rate of 5.7 per 1000 has decreased to an all-time low.

Death Rites: About three fourths of Britons now choose cremation over burial, partly because it is less expensive. A slight majority would also consider reusing of old graves to combat overcrowding in urban cemeteries. No widespread opposition to organ donation and autopsy exists in the United Kingdom. Still, not enough organs are donated to meet the needs of those who need them. Many British doctors argue for a system of presumed consent, which means people who do not want to donate their organs must deliberately opt out. Today, potential donors must register as such with the NHS and carry donor cards that identify them as willing donors. Even then, family members can block harvest after the potential donor's death.

Food Practices and Intolerances: Like people in many other first-world countries, the British enjoy the questionable privilege of being able to eat too much food with too many calories and too much fat, and obesity rates crept up throughout the 1990s. In England in 1994, 58% of men and 49% of women were obese, but by 1999, the rates were 63% and 54% respectively. At the same time, during the last 3 decades, Britons have cut their consumption of red meat and solid fats and increased their intake of poultry, fruits, and vegetables. Concern over developing Creutzfeldt-Jakob disease from eating tainted beef is partly but not entirely responsible for the decrease in beef consumption. Not surprisingly, those of higher educational and socioeconomic levels often eat more balanced diets than their less educated and poorer compatriots. Overall, Britons enjoy fried foods, such as the famous meal of fish and chips, and lesser known favorites such as deep-fried Mars candy bars. For the most part, Britons use forks, knives, and spoons for eating. Typically, if they are right handed, they put the knife in the right hand and the fork in the left and use both simultaneously. They also tend to mix foods on the plate and place a small portion of numerous items on the fork for a single bite.

Infant Feeding Practices: A slight but growing majority of British mothers try breast-feeding their infants at least once. Specifically, only 64% of mothers in England and Wales nursed their infants in 1990, but the percentage climbed to 68% in 1995 and to 70% in 2000. Scotland had a similar increase from 50% to 55% to 63%, whereas Northern Ireland's rate increased from 36% to 45% to 54%. Overall, older and better educated women from higher social classes are more inclined to breast-feed.

Child Rearing Practices: British child rearing practices are becoming more permissive. Although moderate corporal punishment of children by parents is legal in the United Kingdom, a growing number of parents have abandoned spanking as a form of punishment because studies suggest that it is not effective. Still, most parents defend the right of other parents to spank their own children if they choose. Most children sleep in their own beds from birth, and even infants often sleep in a different room than their parents. Ideally, at least among Britons who can afford it, children do not share bedrooms, and especially beds, with siblings of the opposite sex.

National Childhood Immunizations: BCG at 10 to 14 years; DTP at 2, 3, and 4 months and at 3 to 5 and 13 to 18 years; OPV at 2, 3, and 4 months and at 3 to 5 and 13 to 18 years; HIB at 2, 3, and 4 months; and MMR at 12 to 15 months and 3 to 5 years. The NHS strives for a 95% vaccination rate across the country and achieves it for most illnesses. However, a growing number of parents have expressed concern about the combined vaccination for measles, mumps, and rubella and the possibility that it may cause autism and bowel disease, and the immunization rate for these diseases has decreased to 88% (whereas rates for other childhood illnesses remain at 94% or 95%). Not surprisingly, outbreaks of measles, mumps, and rubella are now occurring more frequently.

BIBLIOGRAPHY

BBC News: news.bbc.co.uk
Department of Health: http://www.doh.gov.uk
Guardian Unlimited: www.guardian.co.uk
National Statistics: www.statistics.gov.uk
Royal College of Midwives: www.rcm.co.uk
Royal College of Nursing: http://www.rcn.co.uk
Royal Cosllege of Physicians: www.rcplondon.co.uk

◆ URUGUAY (ORIENTAL REPUBLIC OF)

MAP PAGE (859)

Hamlet Suarez

Location: Uruguay is situated in the Southern Cone of South America. It has borders with Brazil on the northeast, Argentina on the west and south, the River Plate to the south, and the Atlantic Ocean to the east. Its total land area is 176,215 km^2 (68,019 square miles).

Major Languages	Ethnic Groups	Major Religions
Spanish	White 88%	Catholic 66%
	Mestizo 8%	Protestant 2%
	Black 4%	Jewish 2%
		Unaffiliated, other 30%

Although Spanish is the official language, English, French, Italian, and Portuguese are taught in public secondary schools; the literacy rate is 97%. The country has 3,163,763 inhabitants, of which 89% live in urban areas and 11% live in rural areas. Montevideo, the capital city, has 1,344,839 people. Uruguay is a cosmopolitan society with successive European migration, primarily from Spain and Italy but also from small communities from England, Eastern Europe, and Germany. The per capita income is $6348 yearly.

Health Care Beliefs: Western; limited herbal therapy; active role. Most people go to a doctor or a hospital when they are ill. The use of alternative medicine such as homeopathy and herbs is only marginal. Some groups promote the use of herbs with medicinal properties for digestive or kidney function problems, and herbs are commonly used as therapies for obesity and asthma. Uruguay is a country created by European immigration and has no indigenous population, which explains the absence of witch doctors. Uruguay is one of the most secular countries in the Americas. The beliefs that relate health problems and their solutions to religious phenomena, which are more common in rural populations in Latin America, are not significant, although some semireligious practices used in Brazilian culture are found on the Uruguay-Brazil border. The National Health Prevention Programs, which have been in place since 1985, are responsible for increasing life expectancy by 2 years. Uruguay has many major initiatives for health promotion: *Promocion para la Salud de la Edad Adulta* (Promotion of Health for Adults), the Vascular Disease Prevention Program, the Hidatidosis Prevention Program, the Breast Cancer Prevention Program, the Mental Illness Prevention Program, *Programa Materno-Infantil* (the Mother-Infant Program, which includes the Pregnancy and Lactation Program), Health Care for Children and the Newborn, the HIV Prevention Program, and the *Comision Honoraria de Lucha Contra el Cancer* (the Honorary Commission for Policy Against Cancer). All of these programs focus on various approaches to disease prevention such as diet, exercise, and general lifestyle measures.

Predominant Sick Care Practices: Biomedical. Middle- and upper-class Uruguayans have private insurance, the most extensive health service in the country. Those in the lower classes are assisted by the public health system, which maintains a hospital network in the main cities and inland. Uruguay also has a form of extended health insurance coverage and the *Fondo Nacional de Recursos,* a national program for high-technology medicine, such as heart surgery and organ transplantation, that provides these procedures for the entire population as needed. Life expectancy is high for the region: 72.6 years. The infant mortality rate is 14.1%. Uruguay has one doctor for every 275 people. Uruguayans are at significant risk for developing cancer, especially lung and colon cancers; smoking and diet are contributing factors.

Ethnic/Race Specific or Endemic Diseases: Hidatidosis is the most characteristic endemic disease in the rural population. The disease is found in sheep and transmitted to humans through contact with dogs, which are fed raw animal organs on farms. Fortunately, the country's hidatidosis program was responsible for achieving a significant decrease in the number of yearly cases in the last decade. Flu is an endemic problem in winter, but the country has a free vaccination program for older adults. Dengue, malaria, and cholera have not colonized the country. Vaccination against hepatitis A and B is encouraged by the Public Health Ministry and is compulsory for high-risk populations such as health care professionals and workers. The major health problems in the population, in decreasing order of importance, are vascular disease (33.8%), cancer (22.6%), accidents (4.4%), infectious diseases (2.1%), and diabetes (2.1%). The World Health Organization's (WHO) estimated prevalence rate for HIV/AIDS in adults ages 15 to 49 is 0.33%. The estimated number of children from birth to 15 years living with HHIV/AIDS is less than 100. In 2001, Uruguay had 227 new cases of HIV/AIDS.

Health Team Relationships: Doctors have good working relationships with nurses but have always had the dominant position. Doctors are well respected in the country and have high standards. For example, ethical issues are addressed by a committee from the Association of Doctors *(Sindicato Medico de Uruguay)*. The professional role of the nurse has expanded in the last 20 years. Nurses are educated at a university and complete 5 years of course work at the University of the Republic School of Nursing. Plans for a doctoral nursing program were implemented 2 years ago.

Families' Role in Hospital Care: The family is extremely involved in health care in the public and private arenas of medicine. They actively participate in the care of hospitalized relatives and normally stay with them throughout the day and night to assist as needed. The practice of a family taking food to a hospitalized relative is more common in public hospitals. The poorest individuals are taken care of by the hospital; they have no hospital costs other than the cost of transportation for family members traveling from other parts of the country. Doctors tend to be protective of their patients. In cases of devastating illnesses such as cancer, doctors consult with families about prognosis and tend to avoid giving patients bad news so that they can remain hopeful.

Dominance Patterns: Although Uruguay has a Latin culture, male dominance is not very strong. Because most women work, decision making about finances and other issues involves men and women. Women actively participate in political activities, and Uruguay has a legislative commission that is currently considering the rights of female workers.

Eye Contact Practices: Direct eye contact is acceptable in social and medical environments alike.

Touch Practices: Because Uruguay has a Latin society, touch is an important way to express acceptance and friendship. A handshake during a formal greeting or kissing on the cheek when greeting families and friends is the norm.

Perceptions of Time: Punctuality is not a characteristic of Uruguayans, and arriving late to social events is common. For example, even weddings are expected to start at least 45 minutes later than their scheduled time. Time is more of an issue in the workplace, and people tend to be punctual for business appointments. Uruguayans focus heavily on past traditions.

Pain Reactions: Pain is expressed freely and usually elicits feelings of empathy and concern. In lower socioeconomic groups, controlling expressions of pain is valued for men. In general, men and women are very verbal about their pain. Love and support from family and friends are highly valued in painful situations.

Birth Rites: The health care system is heavily involved in pregnancy and childbirth. Uruguayans are equally happy when sons and daughters are born. The birth rates in Uruguay are low for Latin America, with an average of 2.5 children per family.

Death Rites: The family relationship is strong, and family members support each other when a loved one dies. Funerals are not particularly formal occasions, and people do not wear special clothes when attending. Women rarely wear black mourning clothes; this is only common among older women who emigrated from Spain or Italy. The funeral is carried out immediately after death, generally at funeral parlors, and lasts 18 to 24 hours. Family and friends express sympathy by sending flowers. Organ donations are encouraged.

Food Practices and Intolerances: Meat has a significant role in the Uruguayan diet, although during the last 30 years the consumption of vegetables and fruits has increased. The most typical food is *parrillada* (barbecue), which is roasted beef or lamb with sausages and *offal* (animal organs such as kidneys and certain glands) that are cooked on red-hot coals. The typical hot beverage is *mate,* an herbal infusion imported from Brazil and Paraguay that contains xanthine and is similar to tea and coffee. Uruguayans drink *mate* from a dry, empty pumpkin. Herbs and occasionally sugar are added through a hole in the top of the pumpkin. Hot water is added, and the individual drinks from a special silver tube called a *bombilla* (small pump).

Infant Feeding Practices: Breast-feeding is usual during the first month of life, and many women continue for 4 months. After the first month, foods are introduced gradually. The first food is usually mashed fruit, followed by mashed vegetables and then ground beef and chicken. Most mothers work outside of the home but still receive their salaries from the government during a 3-month leave after the birth. After 3 months, they must return to work on a part-time basis, and after 6 months they must return full time. Working mothers generally put their children in nurseries while they work or leave them with family members, often grandparents. Mothers with better paying positions may hire sitters to stay in their homes.

Child Rearing Practices: The Uruguayan society is quite permissive with children. Public education is secular, free, and compulsory at the primary and secondary levels. Children usually live with their parents for financial reasons until they marry or have a family. They become independent considerably later than do children in North America and Europe.

National Childhood Immunizations: BCG at birth and 5 years; DTP at 2, 4, 6, and 12 months and 5 years; OPV at 2, 4, 6, and 12 months; hep B for those at high risk only; HIB at 2, 4, 6, and 12 to 16 months; MMR at 1 and 5 years.

Other Characteristics: Agriculture is the main source of income for the country. Food, leather, and wool comprise more than 55% of Uruguayan exports. In the past 10 years, a forestation program began, including more than 200,000 hectares of plantations. Technological industries such as the software arena have been growing since 1990. Uruguay adopted a Democratic-Republican system in 1930. They have national elections every 5 years, during which the president and legislative powers are elected.

BIBLIOGRAPHY

Health in the Americas, 1998 edition, OPS No 569, vol 2, Washington, DC, 1998, Pan American Health Organization.

Medici A et al: *Diagnosis and perspectives of social security in Uruguay, health study,* Program of Technical Cooperation BID/704/OC/UR, 1994.

Miglionico A: *Analysis and tendencies of health in Uruguay,* Ministry of Public Health, Montevideo, Department of Statistics, 1999.

Ministry of Public Health, General Office of Health: *FIS, DELPHI Report, The health system in Uruguay, tendency and perspectives,* 1999.

United States Embassy: *Profile of Uruguay,* 1999. www.embassy.org/uruguay/

◆ UZBEKISTAN (REPUBLIC OF)

MAP PAGE (861)

Lori Rosenstein and Nodira Ochilova

Location: Formerly a part of the Soviet Union, Uzbekistan is located in central Asia between the Amu Darya and Syr Darya Rivers, Aral Sea, and the Tien Shan Mountains. It is bordered by Kazakhstan to the north and northwest, Kyrgyzstan and Tajikistan to the east and southeast, and Turkmenistan to the southwest. It includes the Karakalpakstan Autonomous Republic. The total land area is 447,400 km^2 (172,741 square miles). Two thirds is desert or semidesert.

Major Languages	Ethnic Groups	Major Religions
Uzbek	Uzbek 80%	Sunni Muslim 88%
Russian	Russian 6%	Eastern Orthodox 9%
Tajik	Tajik 5%	Other 3%
Other	Kazak 3%	
	Karakalpak, Tatar,	
	Korean, other 6%	

Beliefs: Traditional; acute sick care. Common colds, including ~~and~~ stomachaches, are generally believed to be caused by ~~ks~~, ice cream, and cold drafts (including those from fans and air conditioners). It is rare to see people chill water or other nonalcoholic beverages; most beverages are served at room temperature. Most ice cream stands are closed down during the winter season. During the hot summer season, many people do not roll down windows while using public transportation because they fear becoming ill. A cure for a cold and fever is considered to be a hot bowl of oily soup, and food is also used to cure stomach flu. Abrasions, cuts, and scrapes are often treated with vodka, which is used as an antiseptic. People who have a chest cold and cough may receive a vodka rub on the chest. Newborn infants wear a bracelet with a black and white eye-shaped bead, which is worn to protect the child from the "evil eye" (others who can harm people merely by looking at them). The term *girl* refers to virgins, and a *woman* is usually a married female who has had sexual intercourse. A girl who becomes a "woman" before marriage (i.e., has premarital sex) may have difficulty being married off by her father, a terrible situation for a woman. Young girls and women are discouraged from sitting on cement steps or curbs without a handkerchief or piece of paper because it is believed it can make her infertile. Attitudes toward hygiene and beliefs about the causes of illness are not always based on accurate information. For example, many families use only cold water and no soap to clean dirty dishes because they do not want to heat the water, and dish and laundry soap are expensive and strong. Some complain they can taste dish soap on clean dishes. In addition, after eliminating, people wash their hands with water but do not always use soap. These hygiene practices increase the risk of infection with bacteria and parasites.

Predominant Sick Care Practices: Biomedical; magical-religious. The health care system provides "first-aid" hospitals in every region. Some health care is provided for free, which is indicated on documents signed by patients; however, the government only allows the patient to receive free medical treatment for up to 5 days. The remaining expenses are paid by the patient. Occasionally a hospital stay can be very expensive. The hospitals tend to have Western medical equipment; however, some hospitals and clinics are very unsanitary. It is not uncommon to see cockroaches crawling on the floors and walls. Medications are widely available in the pharmacies and at the local markets, and people can buy what they need without a prescription, even drugs that are strong and have serious side effects. Western health professionals working in Uzbekistan have found very potent antibiotics that require prescriptions in the United States and most European countries being sold at pharmacies.

Ethnic/Race Specific or Endemic Diseases: Endemic diseases include leishmaniasis, hepatitis B and E, echinococcosis, and goiter. The Uzbek people are at risk for poliomyelitis, malaria, tuberculosis, and childhood anemia. The country had an epidemic of diphtheria from 1993 to 1996.

According to the Muslim religion, alcohol cannot be consumed, yet alcoholism is a significant health problem. Heavy alcohol consumption permeates Uzbek society. Many of the men also smoke cigarettes and chew tobacco. The diet consists of high amounts of starch, meat, fat, salt, and cottonseed oil. On the positive side, assorted fruits and vegetables are available seasonally. The World Health Organization's (WHO) estimated prevalence rate for HIV/AIDS in adults ages 15 to 49 is 0.01%. The estimated number of children from birth to 15 years living with HIV/AIDS is less than 100. By the end of 1998 a total of 36 cases had been reported, but Western scientists believe that AIDS is more prevalent than this. Most citizens refuse to believe that AIDS exists in Uzbekistan, although AIDS education is becoming more prevalent. For example, a television commercial about AIDS shows prostitutes approaching cars and getting in. Homosexuality is considered taboo, and the slang term *blue* is often used to refer to homosexuals. Those who even believe that homosexuality exists are often negative and even hostile about the topic, and most people only discuss homosexuality in private. When people speak about it, they are referring primarily to gay men.

Health Team Relationships: Doctors are highly respected by the population, although their salaries are very low. Only doctors diagnose and inform patients about their illness. Nurses assist the doctors with treating patients. The nurses speak with the families, give them information about health issues, and occasionally provide food for the patients.

Families' Role in Hospital Care: Families are responsible for preparing food for their hospitalized relatives. If a child needs surgery, the mother is allowed to stay overnight.

Dominance Patterns: The head of the family and the central decision maker in most Uzbek families is the father or patriarch. In social situations, men and women sit and eat in separate rooms.

Eye Contact and Touch Practices: It is acceptable to make direct eye contact with everyone. However, in some very traditional areas, women are not permitted to make eye contact with men or shake their hands. When younger men or women greet an older woman, they place their right hand on their heart, and the older woman pats them on the back. If a younger woman greets an older man, she may shake his hand if he offers his. If he does not, she shows respect by placing her right hand on her heart. Women greet each other by kissing two or three times on alternating cheeks.

Perceptions of Time: People in Uzbekistan often plan for the future, especially for the future of their children. In fact, they spend their lives preparing for their children's future. People are on time for doctor's appointments.

Pain Reactions: It is acceptable for women to express pain, as it is for men with severe injuries. However, people believe that men are strong, so it is relatively uncommon for a man to openly express his pain.

Birth Rites: Most women give birth in a hospital. Some very religious families prefer to give birth at home. The delivery practices are similar to Western ways, with women lying on their backs with their legs in stirrups. If a woman is in intense pain, she can request pain medication. It used to be customary for women to give birth with no family members in the room, but it is becoming more acceptable for women to have a family member present. The mother stays in the hospital for at least 3 days after birth but may stay 5 days if the delivery was abnormally difficult. In Western cultures, boys are circumcised shortly after birth, but Uzbek people circumcise boys at 5 years of age. Some traditional families arrange marriages within the family; for example, it is not uncommon for first cousins to marry. Recently, doctors have been educating families about the potential dangers in close familial marriages. However, children born with severe abnormalities may die; in rare cases, they are killed. Women may have at least 5 abortions in their lifetime. One 55-year-old woman known by the author has had twelve abortions. Until 5 years ago. abortions were performed without anesthetics, causing excruciating pain.

Death Rites: To preparing a body for burial, family members wash the body and dress it in new clothes. Only family members are allowed to see the body before the burial, and it is against customary laws to place anything inside the coffin. After 1 full day, a procession goes to the burial site; only men carry the coffin. Women and children are not permitted to be in the procession or at the burial site. The length of mourning depends on the age of the deceased. If the person was young, the family mourns and does not work for 40 days. If the relative was older, the family mourns for 1 year. People gather at the house of the deceased to pay their respects. They greet the mourning relatives, who stay outside the house crying and wailing, openly and loudly. Women dress in white and cover their heads with a white scarf. People who come to pay their respects enter the house, sit down, eat the national dish *(osh)*, and reminisce about the deceased. Men and women sit in separate rooms or areas.

Food Practices and Intolerances: Most people eat three meals a day. Breakfast consists mostly of nuts, fruit, bread, jam, rice pudding, or sweet cheese. Dinner is the largest meal of the day. The national dish, *osh,* consists of rice, meat, fat, and carrots cooked in heavy cottonseed oil. The flat, round bread that is served is considered very holy, and breaking the bread into pieces indicates a meal has begun. Pieces of bread are passed around to each person. If a guest is at the table, most of the bread is placed in front of the person as a sign of respect. It is unacceptable for the bread to be upside down or for a bottom part of the bread to be showing—this is considered very rude and an insult to the family and Allah.

Infant Feeding Practices: Breast-feeding is the most common way to feed an infant. Women know that it is healthier to feed an infant with the mother's breast milk than with formula, and it is cheaper as well.

Child Rearing Practices: Child rearing practices are gender specific. For example, boys are coddled and given a lot of freedom. If the youngest child is a boy, he is given the most physical affection from the mother. Young girls often do not get physical affection from their parents.

National Childhood Immunizations: BCG at birth and at 7 and 15 years; DTP at 2, 3, 4, and 16 months; OPV at birth and 2, 3, 4, and 16 months; measles at 9 and 16 months; mumps at 16 months; Td at 7, 16, 26, and 46 years. The reported percentages of target population vaccinated are as follows: BCG, 98; first dose of DTP, 97; third dose of DTP, 96; MCV, 99; and Pol3, 96.

BIBLIOGRAPHY

Beutels P et al: The disease burden of hepatitis B in Uzbekistan, *J Infection* 40(3):234, 2000.

Giebel HN, Suleymanova D, Evans GW: Anemia in young children of the Muynak District of Karakalpakistan, Uzbekistan: prevalence, type and correlates, *Am J Public Health* 88(5):805, 1998.

Niyazmatov BI et al: Diphtheria epidemic in the Republic of Uzbekistan, 1993–1996, *J Infect Dis* 181, Supplement 1: S104–109, 2000.

Semenza JC et al: Water distribution system and diarrheal disease transmission: a case study in Uzbekistan, *Am J Tropic Med Hyg* 59(6):941, 1998.

World Health Organization (June 2000): *Epidemiological fact sheets by country,* Geneva. Retrieved March 1, 2002, from http://www.unaids.org/hivaidsinfo/statistics/june00/fact_sheets/index.html

World Health Organization (2001): *WHO vaccine-preventable diseases: monitoring system,* Geneva. Retrieved March 1, 2002, from "http://www.who.int/vaccines/

◆ VANUATU (REPUBLIC OF)

MAP PAGE (856)

Location: Vanuatu (formerly the "New Hebrides") is a collection of about 80 islands in the southwestern Pacific Ocean. The total land area is 14,760 km² (1,571 square miles). Much of the land is covered with dense forests.

Major Languages	Ethnic Groups	Major Religions
English (official)	Indigenous	Christian 84%
French (official)	Melanesian 94%	Other 16%
Bislama/Bichelama	French 4%	
(pidgin; official)	Vietnamese, Chinese,	
	and Pacific	
	Islanders 2%	

Ethnic/Race Specific or Endemic Diseases: The World Health Organization (WHO) has no reported prevalence statistics for HIV/AIDS for Vanuatu.

National Childhood Immunizations: BCG at birth; DTP at 6, 10, and 14 weeks; OPV at 6, 10, and 14 weeks; hep B at birth and at 6 and 14 weeks; measles at 9 months; DT at primary school entry; and TT at first contact or very early during pregnancy, +4 weeks, +6 months or +1 year or next, +1 year or next pregnancy.

BIBLIOGRAPHY

World Health Organization. (2000, June). Epidemiological fact sheets by country, Geneva. Retrieved March 1, 2002, from
http://www.unaids.org/hivaidsinfo/statistics/june00/fact_sheets/index.html
World Health Organization. (2001). WHO vaccine-preventable diseases: monitoring system, Geneva. Retrieved March 1, 2002, from http://www.who.int/vaccines/

◆ VENEZUELA (REPUBLIC OF)

MAP PAGE (859)

Klaus Jaffe and Marino J. González

Location: Venezuela is located on the southern Caribbean coast of South America north of Brazil and east of Colombia. The climate is tropical but is influenced by changes in altitude from the coastline, to the plains and high plateaus, to the Andes Mountains. It is divided into 23 states. The total land area is 912,050 km^2 (352,144 square miles). The capital city is Caracas. Agriculture covers only about 5% of the country. The Orinoco River (2150 km) divides the country into the more densely inhabited north and the mostly uninhabited rain forests and savannas to the south that extend into the Amazon Basin north of Brazil.

Major Languages	Ethnic Groups	Major Religions
Spanish	Mestizo 67%	Roman Catholic 96%
Indigenous	White 21%	Protestant 2%
	Black 10%	Other, none 2%
	Amerindian 2%	

Spanish is the official language. Various indigenous languages are spoken in the remote interior. The population is estimated to be 23 million, and more men than women are younger than age 40; more women than men are older than 40. The 1999 literacy rate for individuals 15 years of age and older was 93.8%. In 2000 the per capita income (in purchasing power parity) was $6200, and 87.11% of the inhabitants lived in urban areas. Venezuela has African, Amerindian, Arab, and European (primarily Spanish, Portuguese, and Italian) influences. A heterogeneous and developing country, Venezuela has three distinct classes (rich, middle class, and poor). According to 1997 estimates, the distribution of classes was 1.5% rich; 31.3% middle class; and 67.2% poor.

Health Care Beliefs: Western and traditional; active and passive roles. The health services provided by the Ministry of Health and Social

Development (MSDS) place more emphasis on primary and secondary health care, whereas the social security system, which also attends nonsecured citizens, covers more specialized treatments, such as renal dialysis, transplantation, and antiretroviral drugs, among others. Health agents and public health monitors provide some community intervention. Those in the middle class are actively involved in health care, whereas those who are poor are more passive. Numbers of private health care providers are growing and providing service to most of the middle class and some of the lower economic classes. A large majority of Venezuelans (including Amerindians) believe in Western, or science-based, medicine. Only when science-based medicine does not work or official or private medical health care is too difficult or costly to obtain do people seek out alternative medicine. Alternative medicine is, for the most part, practiced by witches *(brujos)*. In addition to prayers, chants, and ceremonies, witches use herbs to cure their clients. Amulets and religious articles are used as protection against bad luck or bad influences from other people. Belief in astrology is widespread among all social classes.

Predominant Sick Care Practices: Biomedical and magical-religious. The Venezuelan health system can be divided according to its two major sources of financing and methods of delivery: public and private. The public system is financed through fiscal revenues and payroll taxes, and the private system is primarily financed through community and personal insurance plans. The public sector comprises national hospitals, social security institutions, and decentralized services (hospital and out-patient care services) at the state level. The major public institution is the MSDS, which accounted for 63% of the total public health expenditure in 2000. The public health expenditure per capita was $128 in 2000.

Ethnic/Race Specific or Endemic Diseases: Endemic diseases are dengue fever, hemorrhagic dengue fever, malaria (including chloroquine-resistant varieties), AIDS, cholera, tuberculosis, schistosomiasis, and measles. The population is at risk for transit accidents, malnutrition and dysentery, work-related problems, iatrogenic diseases, maternal and neonatal morbidity, and asthma and respiratory complaints. The World Health Organization's (WHO) estimated prevalence rate for HIV/AIDS in adults ages 15 to 49 is 0.49%. The estimated number of children from birth to 15 years living with HIV/AIDS is 580. The number of people infected with HIV is 62,000; and the total number of HIV deaths reported through December 1999 was 8047. The UNAIDS estimated morbidity rate was 2.4 cases per 1000 inhabitants. Life expectancy at birth in 2001 was estimated to be 70.29 years for men and 76.56 years for women.

Health Team Relationships: The term *doctor* is used indiscriminately as an expression of respect and affection. Nurses are addressed by the title *enfermera* or their first name. *Brujos* and *comadronas* are male or female healers who often serve rural populations and sections of suburban populations.

Families' Role in Hospital Care: The family is responsible for direct care, and family members may bring food or take turns staying with the patient 24 hours a day. It is common for the family to take part in decisions about procedures such as surgeries and referrals.

Dominance Patterns: The extended family can include godparents *(compadres),* who are occasionally chosen according to their social status in the community and as a form of recognition. Godparents are expected to help provide medical care for their godchildren if needed, although it is common for godparents and godchildren never to see each other after the baptism. The tradition of asking for the parents' blessing for marriage is weak in the younger generation but remains popular in many parts of Venezuela. When more than one last name is used, the mother's name follows the father's. Having the same last name gives families a sense of belonging.

Eye Contact Practices: Direct eye contact is common between sexes and social classes.

Touch Practices: Use of the body and touch during social contacts is the "tropical" way of relating. Two women greet each other by kissing on one cheek, as do men and women and men and men. The *abrazo* (embrace) is a common greeting among males. Handshaking occurs primarily with foreigners and on formal occasions. Touching while talking is common.

Perceptions of Time: Venezuelans are casual about punctuality and live in the present. The future is a very ambiguous and heterogeneous concept, and definitions of "early" and "late" are flexible. Arriving late can be a sign of a higher social standing. Immediate rewards for activity are preferred to delayed gratification.

Pain Reactions: Pain is expressed vocally through moans and groans, although men tend to be stoical. It is much more common for women to somaticize their problems.

Birth Rites: Fathers are not usually present during labor and delivery, although the presence of a family member is common. Male circumcisions are not routine. Girls may have their ears pierced soon after birth, frequently while they are still in the hospital. A rest period of 45 days after birth is typical for the mother, and fathers usually take some days off from work. Working parents continue to collect their salaries, and working mothers usually have flexible hours, including time off to breastfeed. The extended family may assume the role of primary caregiver when parents return to work. Tubal ligations in women after they have had two children (one boy and one girl) are common among those in the middle and upper class. This procedure is more difficult for those in the lower class to obtain. Childbirth is often by cesarean section. In 2000 the estimated birth rate was 22.52 births per 1000 people. The 1999 infant mortality rate was 19.1 deaths per 1000 live births.

Death Rites: Death rites are class dependent. The poor carry their dead to a cemetery, often in a cardboard casket. In small towns the funeral may involve the entire community, and many people join the family procession. Small businesses may be closed and activities suspended as a sign of sympathy and respect. Children often lead the procession by carrying a crown or cross of natural flowers. Male relatives such as brothers, sons, or grandsons are the pallbearers and are followed by close relatives and friends. Family and friends pray. Middle- and upper-class individuals are buried in wooden caskets. Family graves, in which several people may be buried, are becoming less and less common. Cremation is slowly becoming more popular but is not widely practiced. During a funeral service the body is surrounded by flowers, and only the head shows. Burial is usually the day after death. In the middle and upper classes the procession is done in cars. Cremation is becoming available in larger cities.

Food Practices and Intolerances: *Arepas* (corn bread) or bread with eggs, meat, cheese, and black beans are common for breakfast, although cereals and fruit are becoming popular as well. The main meal is eaten at noon and consists of rice, black beans, mashed bananas, pasta, and meat or fish. The consumption of vegetables and salads is increasing. The trend in middle-class families in which mothers and fathers work is to eat the noon meal at a self-service restaurant or in a luncheonette, although going back home is a popular choice because of the 2-hour lunch break allowed by most employers. Away from home, *arepa, empanada* (cornbread sandwich), or a sandwich is common. Supper is a light meal (of soup or leftovers from lunch) and is eaten in the evening, although it is not uncommon to eat a two- or three-course dinner.

Infant Feeding Practices: Breast-feeding is generally short term, and the attitude of the father can be the most significant factor in its duration. Filling formula made of a thickening agent (e.g., flour of manioc, corn, or rice) and water is often used, especially by poor families, to fill the stomach of a hungry infant or toddler. Slight obesity in infants or children is considered a sign of health.

Child Rearing Practices: Children are treated affectionately. Warm embraces by all family members are common. Grandmothers and friends play an active role in caregiving, especially in families in which the mother works outside the home. Middle- and upper-class children are enrolled in private or parochial schools. Lower class students receive a public school education. Young children are enrolled in a *crèche* (day care) or kindergarten. The normal school day is half a day (in the morning or afternoon). Children in the lowest socioeconomic class often work instead of going to school. Homeless children are a concern in large cities.

National Childhood Immunizations: BCG at birth; DTP at 2, 4, 6, and 18 months; OPV at 2, 4, and 6 months; hep B at birth and at 1 and

6 months; HIB at 2, 4, and 6 months; MMR at 1 year; and YFV younger than 6 months; anti-Sarampo.

BIBLIOGRAPHY

Biblioteca Nacional, Venezuela: http://www.bnv.bib.ve

Central Intelligence Agency: *The world factbook 2001* http://www.cia.gov/cia/publications/factbook/

González R, Marino J: Reformas del sistema de salud en Venezuela 1987–1999: balance y perspectivas. Santiago de Chile, *Serie Financiamiento del desarrollo,* No 111, 2001, CEPAL.

Oficina Central de Estadistica e Informatica: http://www.ocei.gov.ve

Pan American Health Organization: http://www.ops.org

Riutort M: El costo de erradicar la pobreza. In *UCAB-asociación civil para la promoción de estudios sociales,* vol 1, pp 15–26, Caracas, 1991, UCAB.

◆ VIETNAM (SOCIALIST REPUBLIC OF)

MAP PAGE (867)

Tinh Do Hoang

Location: Located on the Indochinese peninsula in southeastern Asia, Vietnam is long and narrow. The total land area is 329,560 km^2 (127,243 square miles). Most of the country is covered with mountains and plateaus, and the marshy Mekong River delta is in the south. The population density is high and concentrated along the coast and delta river ways. Vietnam is a poor country, with a per capita income of $1850.

Major Languages	Ethnic Groups	Major Religions
Vietnamese (official)	Vietnamese 87%	Buddhist 60%
French	Chinese 3%	Confucianist 13%
Chinese	Other 10%	Taoist 12%
English		Catholic 3%
Khmer		Other 12%

Ethnic minorities include the Muong, Thai, Meo, Khmer, Man, and Cham. Although the majority of the people are Buddhist, Vietnam also has Protestants, Cao Dai, Hoa Hao, and those with indigenous beliefs.

Health Care Beliefs: Traditional; acute sick care; passive and active roles. Vietnamese from different regions of the country have different beliefs about illness. Mountain people consider it to be a curse or punishment from the gods, whereas low-land rural communities and urbanites consider it to be a yin-yang imbalance or blocked *chi.* Herbs are considered important for staying healthy and can cause problems when mixed with Western medications that have similar pharmacological properties. Because of stigma against mental illness, emotional disturbances may be manifested somatically.

Predominant Sick Care Practices: Magical-religious, Eastern medicine and some biomedical. Self-medication and polypharmacy are customary methods for treating illness. Conventional treatments are only used when traditional methods have failed. Most Eastern medicine is classified as "cool," whereas most Western medicine is considered "hot." Water is classified as a "cold" substance, so it may be restricted when a person is sick (meaning they cannot drink it or take showers or baths). Illness is traditionally treated using self-care techniques and self-medication. Folk remedies include variations of acupuncture, massage, herbal remedies, and dermabrasive practices such as cupping, pinching, rubbing, and burning. Coin rubbing and cupping are used to draw illness out of the body. A heated coin or one smeared with oil is vigorously rubbed over the body, producing red welts, or cups with heated air *(moxibustion)* are placed on the body to suck out "bad winds" or unhealthy air currents. The resulting red marks are though to be evidence of the illnesses being brought to the surface of the body. The Vietnamese believe that the marks will only develop in people who are ill. It is important to take medicine that can restore the yin-yang and hot-cold balances.

Ethnic/Race Specific or Endemic Diseases: Vietnamese are at risk for the following diseases: choriocarcinoma, dysentery, tuberculosis, hepatitis, typhoid, dengue fever, Japanese encephalitis, cholera, and chloroquine-resistant malaria. After the Vietnam War, birth defects were caused by elevated levels of Agent Orange, a highly toxic herbicide. The World Health Organization's (WHO) estimated prevalence rate for HIV/AIDS in adults ages 15 to 49 is 0.24%. The estimated number of children from birth to 15 years living with HIV/AIDS is 2500.

Health Team Relationships: Young, recently educated doctors may be considered incompetent and asked the year they completed their training. Older health professionals with 20 years or more since their training are considered authority figures and experts. Patients are told little about their conditions, medications, or diagnostic procedures, so patients may know very little about their medical history. Educating patients and families is not a nurse's role either. Sparing a person's feelings is more important than telling the truth, so "yes" may actually mean "no." In traditional families the oldest male makes the health care decisions.

Families' Role in Hospital Care: The family essentially lives at the bedside of a hospitalized relative, sleeping on the patient's bed or on thin straw mats. Small wood stoves are used to cook. It is expected that food and help with hygiene tasks and personal comfort will be provided 24 hours a day by the family or a person hired by the family.

Dominance Patterns: The extended family is the basic family unit and consists of three or four generations living together. Decision making is influenced by the astrological and lunar calendar. Although women defer to men, women frequently control men, the home, the family's health care, and the economic power of the community. Children care for their aging parents until they die. People stand when speaking out of respect for others. Pointing a finger at someone is disrespectful.

Eye Contact Practices: Blinking means that a message has been received. Looking directly into another person's eyes while talking is considered disrespectful.

Touch Practices: A person's head is considered the center of the soul and is not touched by others. Only older adults are allowed to touch the heads of young children. Touching persons of the same sex is acceptable, and touching between women can be very affectionate. It is unaccept-able for a male to touch a female he does not know. The female breast is accepted dispassionately as an infant's food source; however, the lower torso is an extremely private area. The area between waist and knees is kept covered, even in private. Handshaking has gained wide acceptance with men but not women. A man does not extend his hand to a woman or a superior. Sisters and brothers do not touch or kiss each other.

Perceptions of Time: Time is thought to move in a recurring circle rather than in a linear direction.

Pain Reactions: Stoical reactions are the norm, and pain may be severe before a person requests relief. People may remain quiet or even smile when in pain.

Birth Rites: It is encouraged that families have no more than two children, and there are disincentives for having a third child. Some pregnant women avoid weddings and funerals and abstain from sexual intercourse because they believe they could harm themselves or the infant. The squatting position is preferred for delivery. Some type of "blooming" (such as the opening of closed flowers) may be used symbolically to help open the cervix during labor. The presence of a female friend may be desired during childbirth. Regardless of the temperature of the room or outdoors, women in labor drink only warm or hot water and keep warm by wearing socks and using blankets. Men, unmarried women, young girls, and husbands are usually not present during birth. In rural areas, delivery at home with a midwife is preferred. At birth the child is a year old. Hot coals may be placed under the mother's bed for about a month after delivery to make her skin firm and tight again and her body strong. Sitting over coals topped with herbs is believed to close the cervix, prevent cervical problems, and prevent gas and "bad fluids" from coming out later. To keep their yin-yang balanced, women following traditional Chinese practices do not bathe, drink juice or water, or wash their hair during the postpartum period. Some women believe they should not shower during the first month and must drink only liquor or wine that has been simmered with Chinese herbal medicine. This herbal concoction is believed to shrink the abdomen back to its previous size. Some women may not leave the house for 1 month after birth. On the last day of the month—before the mother is allowed to go outside again—she must bathe in the herb-liquor mixture and then squat over the coals again to be sure she is properly "dried"; if she is not, she may get arthritis when she is older. Circumcision is generally unknown. Newborns are not given compliments (i.e., are not called beautiful, healthy, or smart) for fear that they will be captured by evil spirits. Out-of-wedlock pregnancy is shameful and usually hidden from the family. The mother secretly aborts the fetus using Chinese herbs or conventional methods.

Death Rites: The Vietnamese prefer quality of life to quantity of life because they believe in reincarnation and expect to suffer less in the next life. The dying are helped to recall their past good deeds so that they can be in the proper mental state for their next life. Autopsies are permitted, and cremation is preferred. Death at home is preferred to death in a hospital. After death, the body is washed and wrapped in clean white sheets. The wife may prefer to do this task to ensure that it is done properly. In some areas a coin or jewels (in a wealthier family) or rice (in a poorer family) is put in the mouth of the deceased. The family believes that these items could help the soul during its encounters with gods and devils and help it be reincarnated rich in the next life. Relatives sew small pillows and place them under the neck, feet, and wrists of the deceased. The body is placed in a coffin, which is buried in the ground.

Food Practices and Intolerances: Vietnamese prefer using chop sticks. Their diet consists of rice, meat, seafood, fruit, and vegetables. Meals are eaten together, with all the foods in the center of the table; everyone shares. Lactose intolerance is not unusual in Vietnamese. Malnutrition affects approximately half the population of Vietnam.

Infant Feeding Practices: Almost all women breast-feed for the first 6 to 12 months. Children may use a bottle until they are 2 years old.

Child Rearing Practices: Methods for calculating the age of an infant may create a variance of as many as 2 years. Parents are relaxed about and enjoy the development of young children. The strict upbringing begins at age 6, when parents demand obedience and discourage independence. The oldest child, whether a boy or girl, is responsible for the younger siblings if the parents are dead, old, or ill.

National Childhood Immunizations: BCG at birth and 1 month; DTP at 2, 3, and 4 months; OPV at 2, 3, and 4 months; hep B at younger than 1 year ×3; measles at 9 to 11 months; TT for pregnant women in high-risk districts CBAW ×2.

Other Characteristics: Offensive behaviors include putting feet on furniture, photographing three people in a group, and voicing dissent. It is better to be silent than to disagree. Names are listed in order by family name, middle name, and given name, so the family is the primary source of a person's identity. Women retain their own names after marrying. Age, which is associated with wisdom and experience, is valued and respected. Education is more important than wealth. Vietnamese are polite and guarded. It is not common for them to share their feelings, even with family members. The American signal used to beckon someone else—moving the index finger with the palm of the hand up—is offensive because it is the Vietnamese motion used to call a dog.

BIBLIOGRAPHY

D'Avanzo CE: Barriers to health care for Vietnamese refugees, *J Prof Nurs* 8(4):245, 1992.

Fry A, Nguyen T: Culture and the self: implications for the perception of depression by Australian and Vietnamese nursing students, *J Adv Nurs* 23:1147, 1996.

Kristy SJ: Health issues in nursing in Vietnam, *Holist Nurs Practice* 9(2):83, 1995.

Laborde P (July 1996): *Vietnamese cultural profile,* University of Washington. Retrieved August 6, 2001, from http://healthlinks.washington.edu/clinical/ethnomed/vietnamesecp.html#traditional

Lawson LV: Culturally sensitive support for grieving parents, MCN, *Am J Matern Child Nurs* 15:76, 1990.

Marchione J, Stearne SJ: Ethnic power perspectives for nursing, *Nurs Health Care* 11(6):296, 1990.

Morrow M: Breastfeeding in Vietnam: poverty, tradition, and economic transition, *J Hum Lact* 12(2):97, 1996.

Poremba BA: After the storm: an American nurse visits Vietnam, *Nurs Health Care* 16(3):118, 1995.

Shanahan M, Brayshaw DL: Are nurses aware of the differing health care needs of Vietnamese patients? *J Adv Nurs* 22:456, 1995.

◆ YEMEN (REPUBLIC OF)

MAP PAGE (864)

Yahia Ahmed Raja'a

Location: The Republic of Yemen is located in the southern part of the Arabian Peninsula. It is bordered by the Kingdom of Saudi Arabia to the north, the Arabian Sea to the south, the Red Sea to the west, and the Sultanate of Oman to the east. Yemen has a total land area of about 550,000 km^2 (212,355 square miles) and is inhabited by 16.5 million people. Geographically, Yemen can be divided into five areas. The mountainous areas, which run parallel to the Red Sea and to the Gulf of Aden, have a highest peak of 3666 m above sea level. The coastal area extends along a strip that is approximately 2000 km long and 30 to 60 km wide. The plateau area runs parallel to and lies to the east and north of the mountainous highlands. Yemen also has a desert area (*Al-Ruba Al-Khali,* or "the empty quarter") and the Yemeni islands. Yemen has 112 islands scattered in its territorial waters. The largest and most important is Socotra Island, which is located in the Arabian Sea. It is the home of rare birds, as well as rare trees such as *Ormosia, Dracaena draco*, and *Pterocarpus draco* trees, from which gum and various medications and pigments are obtained. Kamaran Island, situated in the Red Sea, is another one of many other inhabited islands.

Major Languages	Ethnic Groups	Major Religions
Arabic	Arab 95%	Sunni and Shia Muslim 98%
	East Indian,	Other (Jewish, Christian,
	African 5%	Hindu) 2%

A minority of the population speaks the Mahri language, a Himyarite descendent language that was predominant more than 2000 years ago.

Health Care Beliefs: Both modern and traditional; acute sick care primarily. The vast majority of the population seeks modern medical care, especially for physical illnesses. Some people use herbs exclusively, whereas others combine herbs with modern medicine. It is not uncommon for people to have strong traditional beliefs about disease causation and treatment while simultaneously embracing modern medicine if they are not cured. Preventive care is valued, but financial constraints dictate that more crisis-oriented care is sought only after a person is extremely ill.

Predominant Sick Care Practices: Indigenous, magical-religious and biomedical if available. Practices such as *markh, essab, mysam*, and *hijama* are used to treat illness. *Markh* (neck, back, and abdomen massage) is used for headaches and backaches and to encourage pregnancy. Highly experienced persons (mostly women) practice *markh* combined with *essab* to treat infants with persistent diarrhea and vomiting. *Essab* is the practice of binding a child's abdomen with a piece of cloth to open blocked bowels. *Mysam,* placing a very hot metallic rod on a part of the body, is used to treat a wide range of conditions such as epilepsy, jaundice, or fear. The type of conditions determines where the rod is placed. *Hijamah* is sucking out blood (using a vacuumed animal horn or tin can) from puncture points in the back or joints and is usually done to promote health in older adults and to treat general fatigue. Many people attend holy Koran treatment sessions in the rapidly increasing numbers of treatment centers (with approximately 30 centers in Sana'a city alone, a city inhabited by 1 million people). These centers are mainly used to treat *muss,* a condition caused by a satanic soul's possession of the body. This soul orders people to commit sins and inhibits them from doing good deeds and achieving their ambitions; it also impairs many bodily functions. Another widely spread belief is that *fag'ah* (fear) affects many psychosomatic functions. For example, it can hemolyze blood and lead to jaundice. Mild *fag'ah* is managed by unexpected contact with a small piece of a hot coal, such as that on a lit cigarette, or with very cold water. It is thought that severe *fag'ah* must be treated with iron supplements (either in pharmaceutical preparations or home-extracted iron water).

Ethnic/Race Specific or Endemic Diseases: Diarrheal diseases, acute respiratory tract infections, and undernutrition in children younger than 5 are the most common health problems. Tropical diseases such as chloroquine-sensitive falciparum malaria, schistosomiasis (intestinal and urinary), and helminthiasis (especially the soil-transmitted form) are all highly endemic. Rates for HIV/AIDS are currently low. The World Health Organization's (WHO) estimated prevalence rate for HIV/AIDS in adults ages 15 to 49 is 0.01%. WHO has no estimates for children from birth to 15 years. Homosexuality is very rare, socially rejected, and punished by law.

Health Team Relationships: The doctor is usually the health team leader. Nurses, pharmacists, and laboratory technicians are subordinate to doctors, although the whole team is respected. Pharmacists are more likely to be considered businessmen than health professionals.

Families' Role in Hospital Care: A family member is expected to stay with and help care for hospitalized relatives. The family usually purchases drugs, brings food, assists with personal hygiene, and calls the medical staff when necessary.

Dominance Patterns: Males are dominant. Extended families are prevalent primarily in the rural areas, where 74.9% of the population resides. Most women (59%) are full-time housewives, but a considerable number, primarily in rural areas (24%), are actively engaged in cultivation activities and raising animal herds in addition to their household activities. The adult female illiteracy rate is 84.2%, and the median age of women at their first marriage is 16 years. At the dinner table the best foods are kept for the men, although women's nutritional status, as measured anthropometrically, is better than that of Yemeni males.

Eye Contact Practices: Direct eye contact is customary with everyone, including parents and authority figures. The given name is generally used during discussions. During professional meetings, the term *brother* precedes the first name.

Touch Practices: Physical touching is acceptable, but only between members of the same sex.

Perceptions of Time: Punctuality is not a very important value, and being 15 minutes late to a rendezvous is not even mentioned. People are generally present oriented, but the future is also of considerable concern.

Pain Reactions: People react to pain expressively, and complaining to friends is encouraged. Illnesses, such as psychiatric disorders, that involve cultural stigmas are mentioned only to close friends.

Birth Rites: A common saying is that *"Two marriages are easier than one birth."* The home is painted before the expected date of birth. If the delivery occurs at home, which is common (84%), more than half of them involve the assistance of the mother or a relative; or if they are absent, a trained birth attendant steps in. Only 22% of women have trained medical assistants during childbirth. Births to mothers younger than 20 years of age and first births are more likely to include help from health professionals. Medically assisted deliveries are more common among women living in urban areas, coastal regions, or plateau regions. When a newborn is a boy, three shrills are heard by the people waiting outside the delivery room. If only one shrill is heard, the newborn is a girl. Twenty-three percent of the infants born during the 1990s in the largest hospital in Yemen had low birth weight. A new razor blade is used to cut the umbilical cord in two thirds of the home deliveries. One quarter of the people use clean scissors, and only 5% use sterile medical instruments. The most common (58%) dressing used on the cord stump is a thread. Cauterization of the stump is involved in 15% of births, application of *kohl* in 8%, use of hot oil in 5%, use of cotton or sterile dressings in 4%, and 6% have no treatment. Mothers are expected to be still for several hours after delivery, and water and spicy foods are not allowed; only hot drinks are consumed. An entire hen is cooked for the new mother daily for 40 days, and friends and relatives visit her daily during this period. On day 40 a celebration is held, and the mother can resume sexual relations. Male children are usually circumcised on the seventh day after birth by the barber, who usually performs the operation at home. The occasion is celebrated by slaughtering one or two sheep, and neighbors and relatives are either invited for lunch or given the meat. Some female children (19.3%) are also circumcised. In the coastal area, 69% of all adolescent girls between 15 and 19 years of age have been circumcised, compared with 15% in the mountainous region and 5% in the plateau and desert regions. The median age of female circumcision is 8 days, and it is performed by birth attendants 68% of the time, grandmothers 19% of the time, and barbers and others 5% of the time. Razor blades are used for 75% of the procedures, although scissors and other instruments also may be used.

Death Rites: People consider death to be a sad fact of life. Yemenis believe in an afterlife. Close relatives are called to spend the last hours with a dying person, and the head of the person is directed toward Mecca. The dead body is washed and perfumed, wrapped in one continuous piece of hand-sewn white cloth, and buried in the ground without a coffin. The period between death and burial is only a few hours. Autopsies are uncommon, but organ donations are allowed, provided they are done for free. Mourning lasts from 3 to 10 days. The wife of a deceased husband dresses in black clothes and does not leave the husband's home for 4 months and 10 days. After this mourning period, she is free to marry again.

Food Practices and Intolerances: Yemenis commonly say that *"All foods call bread Sir."* Bread is available at every meal. Various other grains, oils, ghee, butter, other dairy products, and eggs are also consumed. Fish or the meat of hens, sheep, or cows is usually eaten once or twice per week. Foods are usually cooked fresh daily and served very hot with many spices; three meals per day is the norm. The family eats from the same dishes using the fingers of the right hand. Spoons are used when eating rice dishes, but forks and knives are not ordinarily used. Drinking tea at breakfast and dinner is common. Animals are slaughtered according to Islamic requirements; wine, blood, pork, donkeys, mules, canines, and birds with claws are forbidden.

Infant Feeding Practices: About 97% of Yemeni mothers breast-feed their children for long periods; the median duration is 17.8 months. Giving colostrum to a newborn is common (given by 91% of mothers) in Yemen, and about half of all infants begin breast-feeding within 1 hour of birth.

Child Rearing Practices: Attitudes towards child rearing are exemplified by the saying *"If your son becomes older, treat him as a brother."* Children younger than 5 years usually sleep with their parents, and older boys and girls sleep in separate rooms. Both parents (primarily the mother) participate in child rearing and discipline. During adolescence the mother predominantly takes care of the daughters and the father takes care of the sons.

National Childhood Immunizations: BCG at birth; DTP at 6, 10, and 14 weeks; OPV at birth and 6, 10, and 14 weeks; hep B at 6 and 10 weeks and 9 months; measles at 9 months; and TT at first contact, +1 month, +6 months, +1 year, +1 year.

Other Characteristics: Seven percent of currently married women are involved in polygamous marriages; 4% have one "co-wife" and 3% have two or three co-wives. Most of the men chew the soft leaves of the *khat* plant *(Katha edulis),* which is a stimulant. *Khat* is chewed and stored in the left side of the mouth under the cheek for approximately 3 hours per session. Friends usually attend *khat*-chewing sessions, and most of the houses in Yemen are prepared to receive the chewers. *Khat* sessions are held during every social event, at the end of the week, and occasionally daily. The practice of *khat* chewing is associated with many health problems: hypertension, duodenal ulcers, hemorrhoids, and mental disorders.

BIBLIOGRAPHY

Al-Hadrani AM: Khat induced hemorrhoidal diseases in Yemen, *Saudi Med J* 21:475, 2000.

Central Statistical Organization: *Results of the third round (July—September) of the family budget survey, 1998 (preliminary report),* 1999, Sana'a, Yemen, CSO.

Central Statistical Organization and Macro International Organization: *Yemen demographic and maternal and child health survey, 1997—1998,* Calverton, Md, CSO and MI.

Raja'a YA et al: *A decade study on birth outcomes in Al-Thawra hospital, Sana'a—Yemen,* The second Yemeni-Italian Medical Conference, Al-Mukalla, Yemen, 2001.

Raja'a YA et al: Khat chewing is a risk factor of duodenal ulcer, *Saudi Med J* 21:887, 2000.

◆ YUGOSLAVIA (THE FEDERAL REPUBLIC OF)

MAP PAGE (860)

Snezana Bosnjak and Draga Plecas

Location: The Federal Republic of Yugoslavia is located in southeastern Europe on the Balkan Peninsula. It borders Hungary on the north, and Croatia and Bosnia-Herzegovina on the west along the Adriatic Sea. Today, Yugoslavia consists of its former republics of Serbia and Montenegro. Serbia has two autonomous regions: Vojvodina/Kosovo and Metohija. Serbia contains the fertile Danube River plain, whereas Montenegro is very mountainous. The total land area is 102,173 km² (39,449 square miles) and the population is 10.6 million.

Major Languages	Ethnic Groups	Major Religions
Serbian	Serb 63%	Orthodox 65%
Albanian	Albanian 14%	Muslim 19%
Hungarian	Montenegrin 6%	Roman Catholic 4%
	Hungarian 9%	Protestant 1%
	Other 8%	Other 11%

Health Care Beliefs: Western; traditional; active and passive roles. People generally believe in biomedical care. With the exception of vaccination programs, preventive health care measures (including national programs) are insufficient and poorly implemented because of the insufficient health care budget. Programs for cancer prevention, early detection of cancer, and general public education about cancer are planned and organized by institutes of oncology, institutes of public health, medical faculties, and cancer societies in coordination with the health system or individually.

Predominant Sick Care Practices: Biomedical and traditional. All Yugoslavians are a part of a national health care system. Private practice exists as well. In Kosovo and Metohija the ethnic Albanian population has set up a parallel health care system. The resident population of the province occasionally uses the state and the parallel systems, although no official data exist on the latter.

Ethnic/Race Specific or Endemic Diseases: The five most commonly diagnosed diseases in 1996 were acute respiratory tract infections, hypertension, diseases of the skeleton and connective tissue, neurotic and personality disorders, and acute bronchitis. So-called "endemic nephropathy" (idiopathic tubulointerstitial nephropathy) is an endemic disease. The leading causes of death are circulatory diseases (accounting for more than 55% of deaths), malignancies (more than 16%), and respiratory diseases (approximately 4%). The World Health Organization's (WHO) estimated prevalence rate for HIV/AIDS in adults is 0.10%. WHO has no estimates for children from birth to 15 years. The Programme for AIDS Prevention and Control was established in 1995. In the past 3 or 4 years, the incidence of AIDS has been 5 to 9 cases per million people, and the AIDS mortality rate (AIDS deaths per million people) decreased from more 8 in 1995 to less than 4 in 2000. However, it is unclear whether all the cases of HIV/AIDS deaths were properly reported. (The last report from Kosovo and Metohija was in 1997, and it is unclear how the situation has changed since then.) Of the 860 AIDS cases that have been reported in the country, the most common modes of transmission were use of intravenous drugs (413 people), heterosexual contact (164), homosexual and bisexual contact (122), and mother-to-child transmission (7). No accurate HIV/AIDS statistics for the region of Kosovo and Metohija are available. Life expectancy is 72.2 years.

Health Team Relationships: Doctors have the leading role on the health team. Communication and cooperation with nurses is usually good, although they are subordinate to doctors. Generally, patients communicate more openly with nurses than with doctors. Recently, nurses have been making greater and more active contributions to the health team, especially those on multidisciplinary palliative care teams. Practitioners treating people with cancer, AIDS, and other chronic debilitating diseases are also beginning to include social workers, psychologists, and psychiatrists, as well as hospital chaplains, on their health care teams.

Families' Role in Hospital Care: Family and friends are important because they support hospitalized relatives. They visit patients very frequently and bring them food, sweets, and clothes. Mothers stay with hospitalized infants and young children when possible.

Dominance Patterns: Men are absolutely dominant in Kosovo and Metohija, as well as in other Muslim populations. In the rural populations of Serbia and Montenegro, men have the prominent role, and infant boys are more appreciated than infant girls. In urban or educated populations, differences in dominance patterns between men and women do not exist.

Eye Contact Practices: Direct eye contact is acceptable.

Touch Practices: Physical touching is acceptable, but in the Muslim population in Kosovo and Metohija, a medical service staffed by non-Muslim and non-Albanian practitioners is considered unacceptable.

Perceptions of Time: Yugoslavians are generally punctual, although traditionally timeliness has not been very important or appreciated. The people tend to focus on past traditions and be concerned about the present rather than the future.

Pain Reactions: It is common for Yugoslavians to accept and tolerate suffering. Individuals react to pain with a reasonable level of stoicism. Patients report pain reluctantly because they do not want to be considered weak or to be complainers. They also refuse to take pain medications, especially opioids, for chronic pain because of fears about addiction or because they believe that pain is necessary for salvation.

Birth Rites: Yugoslavia has a national program for prenatal health. The program includes pregnancy confirmations, laboratory tests, blood pressure and weight monitoring, obstetrical examinations, health behavior counseling, and ultrasounds. It is recommended that every pregnant woman visit a maternal care clinic at least four times during her pregnancy and 6 weeks after delivery. Antenatal classes that offer psychophysical preparation for childbirth are available. Nearly all deliveries are attended by a health care team that includes an obstetrician and a midwife. The proportion of hospital visits has consistently been in the high ninetieth percentiles, with the constant exception of Kosovo and Metohija (76.7% in 1990). Almost all births take place in one of the 74 maternity wards across the country, and some take place in one of the 12 out-patient maternity wards. Yugoslavia has 4.1 facilities providing basic essential obstetric care (EOC) per 500,000 people and 3.5 facilities providing basic and comprehensive EOC per 500,000 people. In Kosovo and Metohija, as well as in the rural populations of Serbia and Montenegro, the birth of a son is celebrated more than the birth of a daughter. In 2000 the birth rate per 1000 inhabitants was 11.8 (11.7 in Serbia and 14.03 in Montenegro). Birth rates are decreasing.

Death Rites: Yugoslavians generally focus on the quantity of life rather than its quality. The common belief is that the duty of a doctor is to postpone death. Human mortality is not a recognized concept, and dying is not considered as a normal process. Death is tragic. However, occasionally death provides relief from suffering and pain (e.g., for patients with cancer). Family members and close friends of a dying person are usually present. After the person dies, visits from all relatives, friends, and neighbors are expected. Family members and close friends of the deceased dress in black and are in mourning for at least 40 days after the death. No formal support system exists to help the family cope. Organ donations are acceptable although rare. Autopsies are performed if they are medically necessary but usually require a verbal consent from the family. In 2000 the death rate per 1000 inhabitants was 11.1 (11.29 in Serbia and 8.27 in Montenegro).

Food Practices and Intolerances: Diet varies according to region and religion. In the northern and central part of Serbia, the typical diet consists of milk and dairy products (e.g., soft cheese), vegetables, legumes, wheat- and corn-flour products, fruit, and meat (primarily pork, especially in Vojvodina). Fish is eaten occasionally. In the coastal part of Montenegro, the diet is Mediterranean. Those in the Kosovo province and other Muslim people eat mutton and beef (but no pork).

Infant Feeding Practices: Breast-feeding has never been completely abandoned. Breast-feeding is always the first choice. Bottle-feeding is used when a mother is not able to breast-feed and to supplement breast milk. The rate for exclusive breast-feeding up to 3 months of age is 10.6% and for complementary feeding until 6 to 9 months is 40.5%.

Child Rearing Practices: Child rearing practices are permissive but vary according to the educational level of the parents, location of the family, ethnicity, and religion. Children in Muslim communities in urban or rural settings must attend religious classes at local mosques during weekends.

National Childhood Immunizations: BCG at birth; DTP at 2, 3 1/2, and 5 months and 2 years; OPV at 2, 3 1/2, and 5 months and at 2 and 14 years; hep B at birth and 1 year; per at 4 years; MMR at 2 and 12 years; DT at 7 years; Td at 14 years; and TT at 18 years. Vaccination coverage rates are as follows: the BCG national coverage was 97.1% in 1997 and 98% in 2000, and in Kosovo and Metohija province it was 92.6%. The third dose of DTP national coverage was 94% in 1997 and 94.9% in 2000, and in Kosovo and Metohija province it was 89.3%. The third dose of OPV national coverage was 94% in 1997 and 98% in 2000, and in Kosovo and Metohija province it was 89.3%. The MMR national coverage was 91.9% in 1997 and 90.5% in 2000, and in Kosovo and Metohija province it was 84%.

BIBLIOGRAPHY

Benson ER: The legend of the Maiden of Kosovo and nursing in Serbia, *IMAGE J Nurs Sch* 23(1):57, 1991.

Sutton J: Why Bosnia lies bleeding, *World Vision Childlife* IX(2):6, 1996.

Monitoring progress towards the goals of the world summit for children, FRY 1996 Multiple Cluster Indicator Survey, Institute of Public Health of Serbia and Institute of Public Health of Montenegro, Belgrade 1997, United Nations Children's Fund.

Zdravstveno stanje stanovnistva Srbije 1986-1996, Institut za zastitu zdravlja Srbije dr Milan Jovanovic Batut, Beograd, 1998.

National report on follow-up to the World Summit for Children, 2001, The Government of FR Yugoslavia.

Savezni Zavod za Statistiku: Stanovnistvo i prirodno kretanje stanovnistva SR Jugoslavije u 20. I na pragu 21. veka, saopstenje 035, str 15, Beograd, 2002.

Savezni Zavod za Statistiku: Stanovnistvo, nacionalna pripadnost, podaci po naseljima i opstinama, Knjige popisa-knjiga 1, str 150, Beograd, 1993.

Savezni Zavod za Statistiku: Stanovnistvo, veroispovest, podaci po naseljima i opstinama. Knjige popisa-knjiga 2, str 142, Beograd, 1993.

Savezni Zavod za Statistiku: Stanovnistvo, nacionalna pripadnost, detaljna klasifikacija. Knjige popisa, knjiga 3, str 276, Beograd, 1993.

◆ ZAMBIA (REPUBLIC OF)

MAP PAGE (863)

Elizabeth N. Mataka

Location: Zambia, a landlocked south central African country, shares borders with Malawi to the east; Botswana, Zimbabwe, Namibia, Mozambique, and Angola to the south; and Zaire to the north. The total land area is 752,610 km^2 (290,583 square miles). Zambia is a highly urbanized country, and the majority of Zambians live in urban areas. Mobility is also very high; surveys have determined that 10% of Zambians have not lived in their present location for more than 5 years. More than 50% of the country's population is younger than 20 years of age. However, life expectancy at birth decreased from 54 years in the mid-1980s to 37 years in 1998.

Major Languages	Ethnic Groups	Major Religions
English	African 98%	Christian 50% to 75%
Local dialects	European,	Islam, Hindu 24% to 49%
	other 2%	Indigenous beliefs 1%

Zambia has a least 72 tribes. However, no strong ethnic feelings exist, as indicated by intertribal marriages and other associations. English is the official language, but most Zambians speak more than one local language.

Health Care Beliefs: Indigenous and modern; active and passive roles. Information on health issues, national campaigns, and promotions have helped most people understand the causes of various diseases. For example, vigorous anticholera campaigns, as well as antipolio drives have influenced people to seek immediate medical help to obtain immunizations against polio. People now understand that poisoning or witchcraft does not cause disease. However, certain mental conditions are associated with spirits (e.g., *mashawe*), and people resort to ancestral spirits for help with a cure.

Predominant Sick Care Practices: Traditional; magical-religious; bio-medical. The country has a comprehensive network of health institutions, hospitals, clinics, and health posts that are widely used. However, a parallel traditional health care service also exists. Zambia has thousands of traditional healers of different levels who use various practices and provide care to a large segment of the population. For chronic diseases such as infection with HIV/AIDS, people invariably consult traditional healers when they lose hope in conventional medicine. They may simultaneously consult and receive treatment from traditional healers and conventional medical doctors. Traditional healers have generally responded positively to education about cross-infections among their patients by modifying some of their practices; for example, they ask each patient to bring a new razor blade for any skin-piercing procedures. The country has also trained numerous traditional birth attendants, who provide care where health centers are not immediately accessible, a particular problem in rural areas. In five urban districts, syndrome management was integrated into maternal and child health service packages at the health-center level to improve pregnancy outcomes. Zambia has various levels of health care institutions. It has one university teaching hospital which is also a referral hospital, district hospitals, rural health centers, urban clinics, and church-run hospitals and health centers. These facilities are complemented by a wide range of privately owned surgery centers, clinics, and a growing number of private hospitals. All district, provincial, and central referral hospitals have blood transfusion facilities. All blood products used in these institutions are screened for HIV and syphilis, as well as hepatitis B (although not as thoroughly).

Ethnic/Race Specific or Endemic Diseases: Malaria, tuberculosis, HIV/AIDS-related diseases, and malnutrition are major health issues. Sporadic outbreaks of cholera, especially during the rainy season, are often quickly addressed and efficiently contained. The country has a very aggressive approach to the prevention of HIV/AIDS, and it has helped change perceptions about the disease. However, widespread denial exists within families. Traditional healers are thought to be very effective in treating conditions and symptoms such as epileptic seizures and mental illnesses and attempt to treat opportunistic infections in those with HIV/AIDS. Most Zambians use home remedies based on information passed from generation to generation or obtained from neighbors. Some of the home remedies are effective and have been trusted for years. Zambia is one of the sub-Saharan countries most affected by HIV/AIDS. The Ministry of Health reported that 20% of Zambians 15 years and older are infected with HIV. The World Health Organization's (WHO) estimated prevalence rate for HIV/AIDS in adults ages 15 to 49 is 19.95%. The estimated number of children from birth to 15 years living with HIV/AIDS is 40,000. The estimated number of adults and children who died of AIDS in 1999 was 99,000. The estimated number of children who have lost either their mother or both parents to AIDS since the beginning of the epidemic is 650,000. Countrywide surveys indicate that urban area rates are currently 27%, with 14.8% for rural areas. Infection rates have been improving among child-bearing women ages 15 to 19 years in four sites in Lusaka, which indicates a decrease in prevalence from 28% in 1993 to 15% in 1998.

Health Team Relationships: Doctors with various specialties are available in hospitals, although the country has a critical shortage of doctors and nurses. Clinics and rural health centers are primarily run by clinical officers and nurses. Patients prefer to be cared for by doctors but are willing to accept treatment by clinical officers and nurses on duty. The doctor/patient ratio is 1:16,130, and the nurse/patient ratio is 1:1571.

Families' Role in Hospital Care: The critical shortage of nursing staff makes care from family members essential. In addition, family members supplement patients' meals by bringing in food. Families also purchase medications from facilities outside the hospital as needed.

Dominance Patterns: Zambia, as in most of Africa, is a male-dominated country. However, the demand for gender equality is growing. The responsibilities of caring for those who are ill, orphans, and other vulnerable people fall on the shoulders of women.

Eye Contact Practices: It is generally accepted that lowering the eyes is a sign of respect to older adults and is the correct behavior when interacting with members of the opposite sex.

Touch Practices: Physical touching in public between members of the opposite sex is unacceptable. However, physical touching among friends of the same sex is acceptable and has no sexual connotations. Physical touching by children is not an issue.

Perceptions of Time: Punctuality is not important. Past traditions and ceremonies are practiced and celebrated. Tribe-specific ceremonies are becoming more important in the culture.

Pain Reactions: Pain and grief are openly expressed, and the community is very supportive of those in pain or who are grieving.

Birth Rites: It is estimated that more than 90% of child-bearing women use antenatal services. In urban centers, most births occur in hospitals and clinics. Some clinics in the compounds are specifically designated as maternity clinics and are run by qualified midwives. The country has also trained traditional birth attendants who serve primarily in rural areas; however, ordinary experienced women also assist in these areas. In traditional areas, some herbs are used to bathe the infant or are tied around the infant's neck or arm for protection against evil. The umbilical cord has tremendous significance; the infant is considered strong and mature after the umbilical stub withers and drops off, and most tribes do not name an infant until this happens. Furthermore, infant mortality in 1996 was 109 per 1000 live births, an increase from 90 per 1000 live births in 1990. HIV/AIDS and related infections and malaria are the leading cause of infant mortality.

Death Rites: Death is not readily accepted, so people blame others for the event. However, the HIV/AIDS epidemic has made death an everyday occurrence. This fact, combined with the harsh economy, has forced people to shorten their mourning period. Relatives, friends, and neighbors assemble at the funeral house until after the burial to give both physical and emotional support to the bereaved family.

Food Practices and Intolerances: *Nshima,* a thick cornmeal preparation, is a staple food for most Zambians; however, cassava and sorghum are used in some parts of the country. These dishes are eaten with a relish of some form and either meat, vegetables, or fish. Most people use their hands to eat.

Infant Feeding Practices: Working mothers are given a statutory 3 months of paid maternity leave. The clinics encourage breast-feeding for at least 6 months. Most working mothers use breast- and bottle-feeding for their infants. Infants' weight gain, immunizations, and general development are closely monitored by a countrywide comprehensive "younger-than-5 clinic" initiative.

Child Rearing Practices: Working mothers employ maids to supervise their infants while they work. Fortunately, numerous centers have been established to train these maids. It is not uncommon for young women, often relatives who have dropped out of school, to be called on to help out with an infant. Children mix freely and play with other children in nearby neighborhoods. Generally children are loved and protected by all in the neighborhood.

National Childhood Immunizations: BCG at birth or first contact; DTP at 6, 10, and 14 weeks and 18 months; OPV at birth and 6, 10, and 14 weeks; hep B at 6, 10, and 14 weeks; measles at 9 months; vitamin A every 6 months from 6 to 72 months; and TT CBAW ×5. This program also uses weight charts.

BIBLIOGRAPHY

Agha S: An evaluation of the effectiveness of a peer sexual health intervention among secondary school students in Zambia, *AIDS Education and Prevention: the official publication of the International Society for AIDS Education,* 14(4):269, 2002.

Kilpatrick S, Sarah J, Crabtree K, Kemp A, Geller S: Preventability of maternal deaths: comparison between Zambian and American referral hospitals, *Obstetrics and Gynecology,* 100(2):321, 2002.

Kwalombota M: The effect of pregnancy in HIV-infected women, *AIDS-Care,* 14(3):431, 2002.

Hjortsberg C, Mwikisa C: Cost of access to health services in Zambia, *Health policy and planning,* 17(1):71, 2002.

National 10-year human resources plan for public health, January 2001.

Situation analysis: Ministry of Health 1998.

◆ ZIMBABWE (REPUBLIC OF)

MAP PAGE (863)

Tafadzwa Steven Kasambira

Location: The Republic of Zimbabwe (known as "Rhodesia" during the decades of minority rule before its independence in 1980) is a landlocked country located in south central Africa. The total land area is more than 390,000 km² (156,000 square miles) of grassland and high plateau terrain, covering an area slightly larger than the state of Montana. Zimbabwe shares its borders with Zambia to the northwest, Botswana to the southwest, South Africa to the south, and Mozambique to the east and northwest. Nestled in the tropics, Zimbabwe enjoys a temperate climate with hot, rainy summers and warm, dry winters.

Major Languages	Ethnic Groups	Major Religions
Shona (major)	Shona 71%	Christianity 25%
English (official)	Ndebele 16%	Syncretic (part Christian,
Si'Ndebele	Mixed race ("colored"),	part indigenous) 50%
	Asians 1%	Traditional/indigenous
	White 1%	beliefs 25%
	Other indigenous	
	Africans 11%	

Health Care Beliefs: Indigenous; acute sick care; active or passive role. Diseases (*zvirwere* in Shona, or *izifo* in Si'Ndebele) are believed to be transmitted by *mamhepo*, air that is in a state of imbalance, containing a greater portion of bad elements than good. According to traditional medical thought, different manifestations of illness are explained by two types of this bad air. First, diseases that affect the body and cause minor problems such as coughing or headaches are believed to originate from bad air in the physical environment. Because of the natural source of the affliction, such diseases are considered fairly normal. An example is *nhova*, which is a sunken fontanel in infants. Although this condition is actually caused by dehydration, it is treated in traditional communities with *muti,* or African medicine. The second type of bad air is considered unnatural because grave health problems result from its influence. These diseases are considered unnatural—or caused by evil—because of the belief that God, in His infinite goodness, would not allow such ills to hurt humanity. It is believed also that those who are immoral or unhygienic, whether physically, spiritually, or socially, have lost the mediation with God that is provided by the ancestor's spirits and are subsequently more susceptible to bad airs and their consequences, such as sexually transmitted diseases (e.g., *runyoka,* or hepatitis B). Mental illness is still considered by most Zimbabweans to be an affliction that cannot be explained in regular medical terms. Most believe that the etiology is less organic than it is supernatural, whether it is possession by a spirit or the result of witchcraft and spells. The invading spirit can be good or evil; the good spirits are known as *vadzimu*, or family spirits, and are considered friendly. Evil spirits can be angry spirits, or *ngozi*, or may manifest as *mashara*, which are alien spirits. Mental illness is still an affliction that engenders shame should it affect a family member, so the help of a *nganga,* or traditional healer, is sought more often than not. These healers are believed to have the ability to identify the person who is responsible for the hex or to exorcise the alien spirit from the person with the mental illness.

Predominant Sick Care Practices: Traditional, magical-religious, biomedical primarily in urban settings. After independence was attained in Zimbabwe in 1980, the government undertook an almost complete restructuring of the health sector, providing free health care to all between 1980 and 1991 and building hundreds of hospitals and clinics in both urban and rural settings. The number of Zimbabweans with access to modern health care facilities increased from 14% before 1980, to 87% a decade later. Although the general health status of Zimbabweans was greatly improved by all of the measures taken, use of the many resources has been found to be less than ideal. Most Zimbabweans seek help from traditional healers before seeking allopathic remedies. However, those who live in urban areas tend to use Western medical services for their initial attempts at resolving illness. Traditional healers are primarily situated in rural settings, making them less accessible to urban populations. Their help is often sought by city dwellers when Western medications and treatments have failed to cure intractable diseases or when an affliction is thought to have a supernatural cause; in the latter situation, many individuals believe that Western medicine can do little if anything to alleviate symptoms.

Ethnic/Race Specific Endemic Diseases: Like many African countries, Zimbabwe struggles to cope with health problems that are primarily caused by a lack of public health resources rather than chronic diseases. Government spending on health decreased from $35 per capita per year in the 1980s to a mere $11 in 2000, primarily because of the extra burden that HIV/AIDS has placed on public health institutions. The infant mortality rate in 2000 was estimated to be 69 deaths per 1000 live births, a figure that has decreased substantially since independence in 1980. The primary causes of death in children younger than 5 years include respiratory tract infections and diarrhea, particularly in infants infected with HIV. Deaths are also caused, although to a lesser extent, from malnutrition, a comorbid condition that makes children susceptible to diarrhea and measles, among other conditions. Other communicable diseases such as schistosomiasis and intestinal parasites also affect many children. Significant health problems among adults include tuberculosis (often in combination with HIV), chloroquine-resistant malaria (in rural areas), and cholera (although it has been fairly controlled, despite two outbreaks in 1993 and 1998). The overriding and over-whelming disease that has devastated the health of Zimbabweans and has had an impact on the economic, social, and cultural landscape of the country is HIV infection. The majority of those infected were the most economically productive of all the country's citizens. The life expectancy of Zimbabweans at birth has decreased to 44 years from 66 in just a decade. It is estimated that 1.1 million Zimbabweans have died from HIV/AIDS since 1995, and almost 1 million children are orphans because of the scourge. The World Health Organization's (WHO) estimated prevalence rate for HIV/AIDS in adults ages 15 to 49 is 25.06%. The estimated number of children from birth to 15 years living with HIV/AIDS is 56,000.

Health Team Relationships: In Shona culture, the medical doctor is revered and respected. People believe that because doctors are so well educated, they are the only ones with the authority and the knowledge to treat illness. This attitude tends to negate the talents of nurses and trained community health care workers, who largely outnumber doctors and provide the bulk of general medical care for the populace. At large medical institutions and rural clinics alike, nurses are the first point of contact between the patient and the health care system. The roles they play vary according to the location of the institution and the number of doctors available. Community health workers, who are lay individuals trained in various skills, form an important part of the health care network in Zimbabwean rural society.

Families' Role in Hospital Care: The sick role is not a solitary one. When a person is admitted to a hospital, the extended family is informed immediately. A great mobilization usually occurs, with relatives phoning in or traveling from distant cities and rural areas to the hospital to provide comfort and help the immediate family. Those who have enough money donate funds to defray the costs of the hospital stay. It is not uncommon to see large numbers of family members, old and young, keeping watch at the bedside for hours on end. Once the patient is discharged from the hospital, relatives usually either take the person into their own homes during the convalescent period or stay at the person's home and provide assistance. Now more than ever, the role of families in hospital care has expanded beyond the expected. Today, essential drugs and even intravenous saline solutions and latex gloves are scarce. Many patients' families are told to purchase saline drips from an outside source, purchase expensive prescriptions, or bring in all the patients' meals; food and many other resources have become luxuries that hospitals can no longer afford to provide.

Dominance Patterns: Traditional Zimbabwean society is patriarchal in most aspects. The birth of a male child is often considered more of a blessing than that of a female child. If a woman bears only female children and her husband is very traditional, he may take a second wife to produce a son to continue the family name. Women are expected to marry and produce many children, all of whom belong to the husband and his family. Children take the father's surname and his *mutupo* (or "totem," the sacred family animal) and remain with the husband's family should his marriage fail. The man and his family are expected to pay *roora* or *lobola* (a "bride price") in the form of cattle (traditionally), money, or furniture to the family of the woman he wishes to marry. As people become more educated and embrace Western modes of living, the bride price has become more symbolic than binding, and women are not categorized in such rigid terms. However, these ideas remain part of the consciousness of Zimbabwean men and women alike, despite the practical cultural shifts of modern times. The dominance pattern does not change significantly during times of illness. Women are still expected to care for sick individuals at home and in the hospital. Men provide support to the ill individual and family but seldom take an active a role in caring for the patient.

Eye Contact Practices: Children avoid eye contact with authority figures as a sign of respect. A child who looks into the eyes of a parent directly, particularly when the child is being chastised, is an act of defiance and disrespect; the child is expected to look down. Eye contact is also avoided between people with inferiors and superiors (e.g., an employer and maids or gardeners, students and teachers). Medical practitioners may misinterpret this lack of eye contact. It may be interpreted as disinterest in the medical practitioners' discussion, when in actuality the patient is trying to be respectful and treat the doctor or nurse as an authority figure.

Touch Practices: Rules about physical contact in Zimbabwean culture are similar to those in most of the Western world. The notion of maintaining a personal space is not as prevalent as it is in Western culture, possibly because Zimbabweans grow up in an extended family in their community and are constantly surrounded by and sharing space with other people. Touching among relatives is acceptable but is not appropriate among those who are not related. Although women are free to hug one another in greeting, as are men, it is considered inappropriate for men and women to hug in public. Some exceptions to this societal rule exist, such as when a mother welcomes her son or husband home after a long absence. The usual mode of greeting between men and women and members of the same gender is a handshake.

Perceptions of Time: With the westernization of Zimbabwe has come the adoption of many Western attributes such as punctuality. Time is important in many situations but especially in business situations. However, a popular saying is that "there is no rush in Africa," which highlights the underlying nonchalance about the importance of timeliness. Often, people are expected to be late for engagements. This attitude can affect many interactions such as business interactions between friends and deadlines for payment; in fact, a friend would be reluctant to possibly offend another friend by reminding the person about an outstanding debt.

Pain Reactions: Men in Zimbabwe are expected to bear pain in silence with minimal expressions of sorrow, whereas women may react more overtly. When experiencing physical pain, such as the pain of childbirth, it is considered natural for a woman to verbally express her feelings. However, women are taught from birth, subtly and overtly, that pain leads to joy, therefore it behooves them to endure pain. For example, childbirth, which is obviously painful, results in a child, a happy occurrence. After a death in the family, especially when the deceased was a child or very close family members, these societal rules about pain are relaxed somewhat. It is not uncommon for men to express their emotional pain more openly, if only for a short time.

Birth Rites: Fertility is of paramount importance in Zimbabwean traditional culture, and women who are unable to bear children are often treated as social outcasts. A popular belief is that infertility is caused by witchcraft. The help of a *nganga* may be sought in these cases, for the sheer social stigma of not being able to bear a child can be overwhelming. Husbands may be allowed to divorce an infertile woman or simply take a second wife in the hopes of having a child. Pregnancy is cherished, and the family members become very excited about the upcoming birth. Social wealth is largely measured by a family's number of offspring. Prenatal care is provided by nurses to those who have access to medical facilities; traditional midwives, trained and untrained, are used in many areas that are underserved. Standard obstetric care is given to women who give birth at clinics and hospitals. Though uncommon, some women do give birth at home attended by traditional midwives. It is believed that a difficult labor is an indication of previous adultery; a woman must confess her indiscretions to ease the passage of the infant. It is rare for a husband to be present during the birth out of respect for the woman's privacy. News of the birth of a child spreads through the community quickly, and everyone rejoices. Certain rituals are followed after an infant is born. The umbilical cord has special significance so once it is has been cut, it is buried in the ground ceremoniously. Because traditional Zimbabweans believe that an infant is born pure, the infant is extremely vulnerable to evil and natural illnesses. As such, protection from these elements is provided with certain medications and observing taboos. An amulet may be tied around the infant's waist or wrist with a piece of string to ward off evil spirits. The child may also receive its first bath in a traditional herbal concoction with protective powers that has been obtained from a *nganga*. Infants are often kept away from strangers during the first few weeks after birth to protect the child from catching infections from people and to shield the infant from those who might have bad thoughts about the child or the family.

Death Rites: Death is not thought of as an event that is separate from the other aspects of life. When a person dies those who are left behind think about the cause of the death. It is believed by many that death has one of five causes, namely natural causes such as illness, supernatural causes such as *ngozi* (angry spirits), violence or accidents, behavioral indiscretions, and ill will of other people. News of the death of a family member is always met with shock and immediate despair. Relatives travel to the home of the deceased person within hours, and the home becomes a central place of mourning. The women, wearing wraps around their waists and head scarves, sit on the floor in a central room of the home, wailing and singing, taking turns preparing food in the kitchen, and comforting one other. The men sit on chairs in the same room or another, speaking among themselves. This ritual can go on for several days while burial arrangements are made by senior family members; few people get any sleep. The body is usually buried at the rural home of the deceased if the person was a man or at the home of her husband if the person was a woman. Children, who belong to the father, are buried at his home. The ceremony at the graveside is conducted by a priest for Christian families and in other families, traditional rituals are followed. The worldly possessions of the deceased must be distributed to the extended family, with almost all individuals receiving at least one of the items as a remembrance of the person who has passed away. Autopsies and organ donations are considered to be acceptable but unusual. Cutting open a corpse for any reason violates the body's resting state and is disrespect to the individual. Cremation also occurs, but relatives often feel guilty about the process because they are violating the sanctity of the body. The ashes of a cremated individual may even be placed in a coffin and buried in the ground.

Food Practices and Intolerances: The importance of food in Zimbabwean culture is revealed during special events such as funerals, birth celebrations, weddings, and even simple visits to an individual's house. The variety of foods traditionally consumed in Zimbabwe is fairly wide. Many people in urban areas grow their own vegetables in gardens behind the home, and subsistence farming is the norm in rural areas. A staple of the traditional Zimbabwe diet is *sadza*, a thick, malleable paste made from maize meal that has been cooked with water. When maize meal is scarce, individuals use bulrush millet, finger millet *(rapoko),* or sorghum meals as alternatives. *Sadza* may be consumed with fermented milk but is usually eaten with meat and leafy green vegetables such as *covo,* pumpkin leaves, *mbowa,* or *derere-munda*. A meal is not considered compete without meat, and the most popular types are beef and chicken. Many families in the rural areas raise goats and may eat them, especially during celebrations. Dried beans are an important part of the diets of certain individuals, as are bambara nuts when they are in season. Various types of fruit are grown domestically and found growing in the wild, such as guavas, mangoes, pawpaw, and avocados, in addition to more unique fruits such as *mazhanje* and baobab fruit. Little information on food intolerances is available. It has been shown that lactose intolerance is quite widespread, especially among children, although it is not often recognized. *Sadza* is usually eaten with the hands, whereas regular utensils (e.g., fork, knife, spoon) are used for most other foods.

Infant Feeding Practices: As in most developing countries, the majority of women in Zimbabwe breast-feed their infants. Knowledge about the enhanced nutritional value of breast milk is widespread, and the cost and lack of access to formula promotes breast-feeding. Shortly after birth, water is fed to infants in addition to milk, possibly with glucose. The families who can afford infant cereals may purchase them as well. The first supplemental food given to infants when they are a few months old is porridge made of corn meal. It may be given in a cup with a spoon, or if the child is very young, on the mother's fingertips. Certain items such as peanut butter *(dovi),* sugar, margarine, or oil may be added to the porridge to improve its palatability and nutritional value. Adult foods are generally introduced by approximately 9 months of age, though breast-feeding may continue while infants are receiving these solid foods. Some believe that traditional drinks such as *mahewu* are good for children because they increase the amount of blood, whereas foods such as groundnuts, boiled maize, and meat are often not provided because they are believed to be difficult to digest and able to cause diarrhea. Termination of breast-feeding occurs generally between 18 and 20 months of age. Weaning begins by giving the child sweet or adult foods or by putting bitter substances such as hot pepper on the nipples to deter the child from nursing. It is believed that breast milk becomes poisonous once a nursing mother becomes pregnant again, so breast-feeding ceases immediately as a result. If the child consumed the milk of a pregnant women, an emetic is provided by a traditional healer to cleanse the infant's gut. Wet nurses are a relatively foreign concept to Zimbabwean women, and women who cannot breast-feed usually give their infants formula instead.

Child Rearing Practices: In many ways, child rearing is the responsibility of the entire community, particularly in the rural areas, where the vast majority of the country's population resides. Discipline is meted out by adults who witness mischievous behavior, and parents are informed of the transgressions. The community as a whole takes joy in children's successes and bands together in times of trouble. Certain important traditions are taught to Zimbabwean children at an early age, such as respect for older adults, the importance of showing deference for those in authority, and how to act when people visit. The men and women in the community are models of conduct for children. Corporal punishment is considered essential and necessary. The disciplinarian is usually the father, but an uncle or older male relative takes on the role when the father if absent. Before its independence, Zimbabweans raised boys and girls very differently. The importance of schooling for boys was emphasized, and many girls were raised simply to be competent wives. However, since 1980, girls and boys have reaped the benefits of expanded opportunities for education, and schooling is considered essential for all children regardless of gender.

National Childhood Immunizations: BCG at birth; DTP at 3, 4, and 5 months; OPV at 3, 4, and 5 months; measles at 9 months; and hep B at 3, 4, and 9 months.

BIBLIOGRAPHY

Allain TJ et al: Diet and nutritional status in elderly Zimbabweans, *Age Ageing* 26:463–470, 1997.

Benhura MAN, Chitsaku IC: Seasonal variation in the food consumption patterns of the people of Mutambara District of Zimbabwe, *Central Afr J Med* 38(1), January 1992

Cosminsky S, Mhloyi M, Ewbank D: Child feeding practices in a rural area of Zimbabwe, *Soc Sci Med* 367:937–947, 1993.

Cubitt G, Joyce P: *This is Zimbabwe,* Harare, Zimbabwe, 1992, Baobab Books.

Folta JR, Deck ES: Rural Zimbabwean Shona women: illness concepts and behavior, *West J Nurs Res* 9(3): 301–316, 1987.

Kasambira T: Death of a nation: the AIDS crisis in Zimbabwe, *Pharos Alpha Omega Alpha Honor Medical Society* 63(1):12–15, 2000 Winter.

Mattson S: Maternal-child health in Zimbabwe, *Health Care Women Int* 19:231–242, 1998.

Mutambirwa J: Health problems in rural communities, Zimbabwe, *Soc Sci Med* 29(8):927–932, 1989.

Reynolds P: Zezuru turn of the screw: on children's exposure to evil, *Culture Med Psych* 14:313–337, 1990.

Sanders D, Davies R: The economy, the health sector and child health in Zimbabwe since independence, *Soc Sci Med* 27(7):723–731, 1988.

Shillington K: *History of Southern Africa,* England 1987, Longman Group UK Limited.

Winston CM and Patel V: Use of traditional and orthodox health services in urban Zimbabwe, *Int J Epidemiol* 24(5):1006–1012, 1995.

World Health Organization (June 2000): *Epidemiological fact sheet on HIV/AIDS: Zimbabwe.* Retrieved March 1, 2002, fromhttp://www.unaids.org/hivaidsinfo/statistics/june00/fact_sheets/index.html

World Health Organization (2001): *WHO vaccine-preventable diseases: monitoring system,* Geneva. Retrieved March 1, 2002, fromhttp://www.who.int/vaccines/

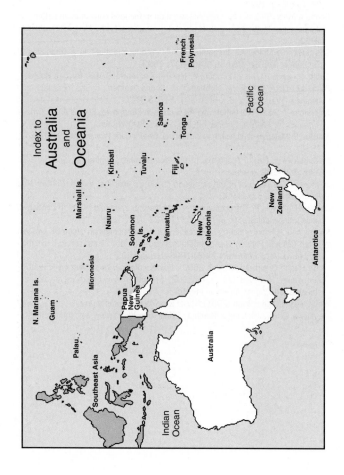

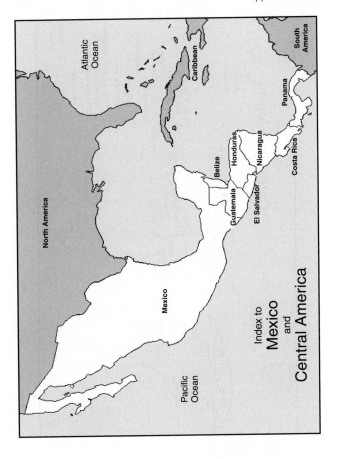

Index to
Mexico
and
Central America

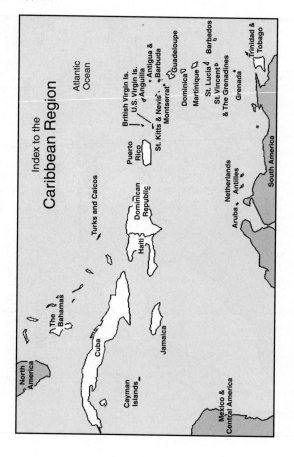

Index to the
Caribbean Region

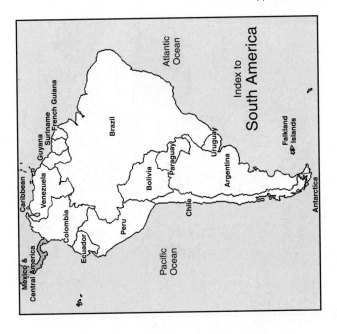

Index to
South America

Atlantic
Ocean

Brazil

Guyana
Suriname
French Guiana

Venezuela

Caribbean

Colombia

Ecuador

Peru

Bolivia

Paraguay

Uruguay

Argentina

Chile

Falkland
Islands

Antarctica

Pacific
Ocean

México &
Central America

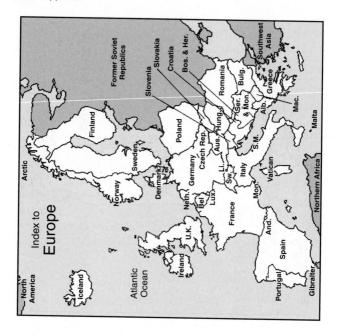

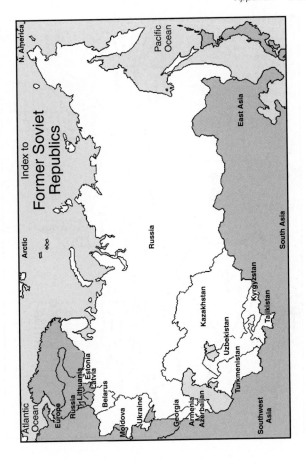

Index to
Former Soviet
Republics

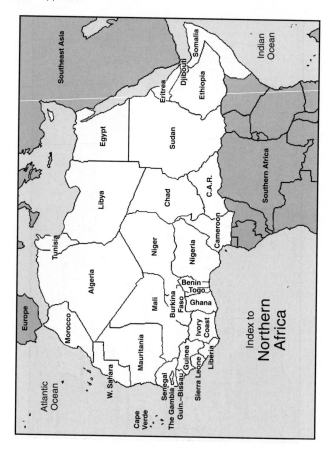

Index to Northern Africa

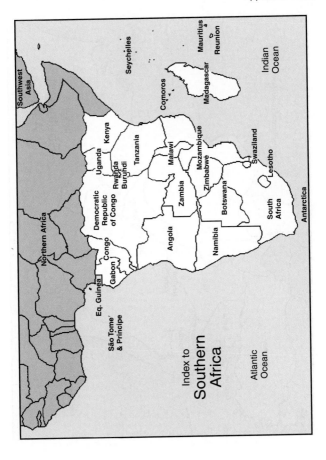

Index to
Southern
Africa

Southwest
Asia

Northern Africa

Seychelles

Comoros

Mauritius
Reunion

Madagascar

Indian
Ocean

Kenya

Uganda

Tanzania

Rwanda
Burundi

Malawi

Mozambique

Swaziland

Democratic
Republic
of Congo

Zambia

Zimbabwe

Lesotho

Congo

Angola

Botswana

South
Africa

Antarctica

Gabon

Eq. Guinea

Namibia

São Tomé
& Príncipe

Atlantic
Ocean

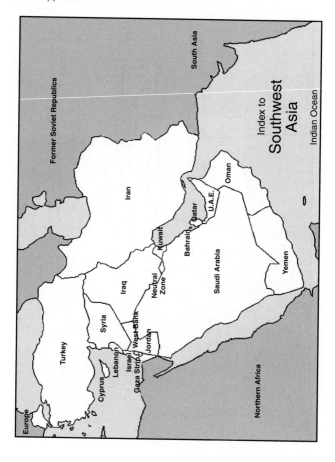

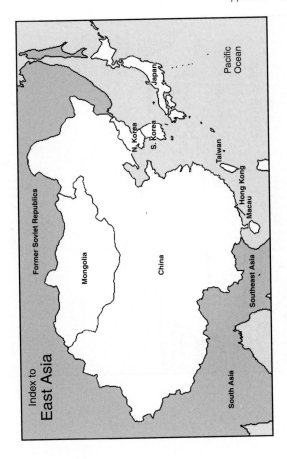

Index to
East Asia

Former Soviet Republics

Mongolia

China

N. Korea

S. Korea

Japan

Taiwan

Hong Kong

Macau

Pacific Ocean

Southeast Asia

South Asia

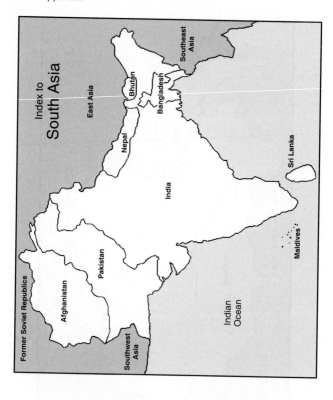

Index to
South Asia

Former Soviet Republics

East Asia

Southeast Asia

Bhutan

Bangladesh

Nepal

India

Sri Lanka

Pakistan

Maldives

Afghanistan

Southwest Asia

Indian Ocean

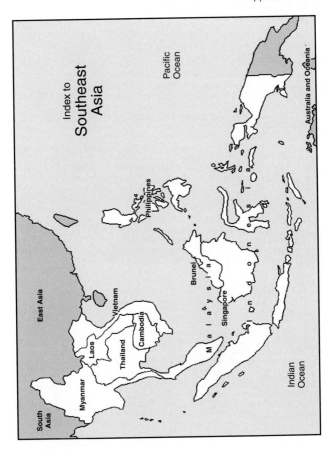

Index to Southeast Asia